Pain

Pain

Current Understanding, Emerging Therapies, and Novel Approaches to Drug Discovery

edited by

Chas Bountra
GlaxoSmithKline
Harlow, Essex, England

Rajesh Munglani
University of Cambridge and
Addenbrooke's Hospital
Cambridge, England

William K. Schmidt
Adolor Corporation
Exton, Pennsylvania

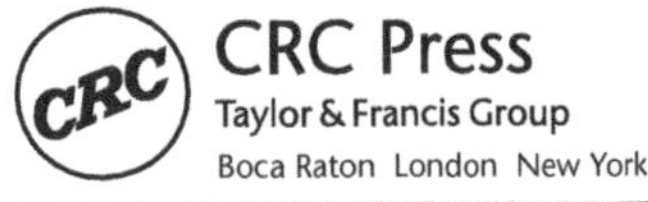

CRC Press
Taylor & Francis Group
Boca Raton London New York

CRC Press is an imprint of the
Taylor & Francis Group, an **informa** business

CRC Press
Taylor & Francis Group
6000 Broken Sound Parkway NW, Suite 300
Boca Raton, FL 33487-2742

First issued in paperback 2019

ISBN 13: 978-0-367-44673-4 (pbk)
ISBN 13: 978-0-8247-8865-0 (hbk)

Visit the Taylor & Francis Web site at
http://www.taylorandfrancis.com

and the CRC Press Web site at
http://www.crcpress.com

Preface

When we first drafted the outline of this book, we had a number of objectives and questions in mind:

1. What is the latest thinking in terms of pathological mechanisms (e.g., peripheral and central sensitization) underlying acute and chronic pain? Do these specific pathologies correlate with a particular symptom, irrespective of patient population? If so, will a novel molecule, which reverses or attenuates a particular symptom and thereby a particular mechanism, do so irrespective of patient population? What is the role of the immune system or peripheral nervous system in maintaining chronic pain? If we dampen or attenuate these peripheral changes, will they also reverse central pathological changes resulting in chronic pain?

2. Are technologies now available that we can apply both in preclinical animal disease models and in human volunteer models or patient groups? What nonpharmacological treatments are currently available, and how effective are they? How do we best classify pain in order to facilitate our understanding and development of novel pharmacological treatments (temporally—acute, chronic; disease association—cancer, diabetic neuropathy; etiology—nerve injury, tissue injury; site—headache, chronic back, visceral-abdominal, pelvic)? How do we best assess pain in clinical trials, e.g., evoked (mechanical, chemical, or thermal), postsurgical, hyperalgesic or allodynic, ongoing, or on movement? How do we demonstrate superiority over gold standards, without necessarily knowing how good gold standards are in specific patient populations (e.g., responder rate, ceiling of efficacy, dose-response, onset of action of tricyclic antidepressants or anticonvulsants in different types of neuropathic pain)? Are there imaging techniques (PET, fMRI, etc.) that can help with the diagnosis of specific pain states or serve as surrogate markers of efficacy in clinical trials of novel therapeutics? Of course, the challenge is made even greater by the demands in the pharmaceutical industry to demonstrate "superiority" or "differentiation" quickly and cheaply by doing proof-of-concept or proof-of-efficacy studies in small patient groups.

3. Why has it been so difficult to demonstrate proof-of-efficacy in humans with molecules targeting novel mechanisms? The classic example in the industry has been NK1 receptor antagonists. Pharmaceutical companies have worked with many of the world's pain experts at leading academic institutions to identify and evaluate such molecules in specific patient groups. They were unanimously unsuccessful in demonstrating a lack of efficacy. Why was this? Are animal

models not predictive of efficacy in the clinic? Could there be significant differences in target receptor affinity or function in rodents vs. humans, or differences in convergent pain pathways, or other factors that must be considered? Is it naive to assume that molecules targeting single molecular targets will have significant efficacy in patient groups where the presenting symptoms are a result of multiple pathologies? How can we better understand the complex heterogeneity of pain in the clinic and design predictive preclinical assays to facilitate prioritization of new chemical entities for clinical evaluation? How can we exploit novel target validation strategies? What is the role of genetics in this heterogeneity?

4. Many approaches are being pursued in this hungry quest for treating intractable pain. Many of these are reviewed in Part 4, ''New and Emerging Therapies.'' A key issue in using many novel targets is not simply demonstrating clinical efficacy in the right patient group but also showing that such targets/molecules have an adequate ''safety window'' or ''therapeutic index.'' It is, of course, a well-recognized possibility that many molecules are not able to achieve adequate therapeutic exposure in the appropriate compartment, prior to running into safety issues. Since patients generally prefer oral dosing regimes, once or twice a day, the result may be to expose the whole body compartment to a high concentration of a drug when all that is required is a lower therapeutic concentration in a specific region of the peripheral or central nervous system—a beautiful analogy likens this to pouring gas on the roof of a car and hoping that some of it reaches the tank. This dilemma has led to the quest for more tightly targeted formulations of drugs (e.g., topical, spinal) or other interventional techniques to control pain at its site of origin.

5. What analgesics are currently available or in development, and for what indications? How can we develop novel drug combinations? How do we ''hunt'' for new drugs, and from where are the next generation of pharmaceutical agents likely to emerge?

We have therefore deliberately structured this book in four broad sections devoted to basic aspects, clinical aspects, novel approaches to drug discovery, and new and emerging therapies.

The book offers a comprehensive review of many of the preceding aspects and challenges. It is designed to be a reference source for academic, clinical, and pharmaceutical researchers and to foster interaction among these various groups of professionals. We anticipate that it will appeal to both new and established researchers in this exciting and incredibly attractive field of research. We hope that such cross-functional/cross-disciplinary collaborations will result in major advances in our understanding of pain mechanisms and innovative approaches to drug discovery.

Some of the most pressing issues that remain for all of us to ponder include preclinical target validation, how we demonstrate proof of concept in humans, and how we develop combination treatments for pain (i.e., molecules with multiple activities or multiple molecules each with discrete molecular targets). For the latter, there are clear technical and regulatory challenges that extend beyond the scope of this book.

The book has taken longer to prepare than initially anticipated, due largely to the number of contributors and the breadth of the task. For that we apologize to the authors who submitted their chapters early in the process and offer in the Further Readings section recent references relevant to the respective chapters, which may guide the reader to additional thoughts and discovery.

There have doubtless been fantastic advances in pain therapeutics over the past few years. For example, gabapentin is providing significant therapeutic benefit for many neuropathic patient groups. Similarly, COX-2 inhibitors represent a major advance over existing NSAIDs for specific patient populations. We remain convinced that, with major advances in understanding the basic pathophysiology of pain and how it can be manipulated at the anatomical, physiological, immunological, pharmaceutical, and psychological levels, the most exciting discoveries remain before us.

We are all immensely optimistic that in the next decade we will continue to build on these advances, and hopefully deliver rationally designed, novel therapies to patients so that they may lead more manageable, less debilitating lives.

Chas Bountra
Rajesh Munglani
William K. Schmidt

Contents

Contributors

Sumihisa Aida, M.D., Ph.D. Department of Anesthesiology, Teikyo University School of Medicine, Tokyo, Japan

R. Arban, D.Pharm. Biology Department, Research Centre, GlaxoSmithKline S.p.A., Verona, Italy

Stephen P. Arneric, Ph.D. Department of Pharmacology, CNS Diseases Research, DuPont Pharmaceutical Company, Wilmington, Delaware, U.S.A.

Ralf Baron, M.D. Neurological Clinic, Christian-Albrechts University, Kiel, Germany

Allan I. Basbaum University of California, San Francisco, San Francisco, California, U.S.A.

Lino Becerra, Ph.D. Department of Radiology, Massachusetts General Hospital and Harvard Medical School, Boston, Massachusetts, U.S.A.

William G. Bensen, B.Sc., M.D., F.R.C.P.(C) St. Joseph's Hospital, McMaster University, Hamilton, Ontario, Canada

L. Bettelini Biology Department, Research Centre, GlaxoSmithKline S.p.A., Verona, Italy

Sharon Bingham SmithKline Beecham Pharmaceuticals, Harlow, Essex, England

Philip A. Bland-Ward Medicines Research Centre, GlaxoSmithKline, Stevenage, Hertfordshire, and Glaxo Institute of Applied Pharmacology, University of Cambridge, Cambridge, England

Sarah Booth, F.R.C.A., M.R.C.P. Palliative Care Service, Addenbrooke's Hospital, Cambridge, England

David Borsook, M.D., Ph.D. Departments of Radiology and Neurology, Massachusetts General Hospital and Harvard Medical School, Boston, Massachusetts, U.S.A.

Chas Bountra, Ph.D. GlaxoSmithKline, Harlow, Essex, England

S. Scott Bowersox, Ph.D. Director of Pharmacology, Elan Pharmaceuticals, Menlo Park, California, U.S.A.

David Bowsher, M.D., Ph.D., F.R.C.P.Ed., F.R.C.Path. Department of Research, Pain Research Institute, Liverpool, England

Kate J. Bradley School of Medical Sciences, University of Bristol, Bristol, England

Hans Breiter, M.D. Department of Psychiatry, Massachusetts General Hospital and Harvard Medical School, Boston, Massachusetts, U.S.A.

Lesley M. Bromley, M.B., B.S., F.R.C.A., M.H.M. Centre for Anaesthesia, University College London School of Medicine, London, England

Frank P. Bymaster, M.Sci. Neuroscience Research Division, Lilly Research Laboratories, Eli Lilly and Company, Indianapolis, Indiana, U.S.A.

David O. Calligaro, Ph.D. Neuroscience Research Division, Lilly Research Laboratories, Eli Lilly and Company, Indianapolis, Indiana, U.S.A.

C. Carignani, D. Pharm. Biology Department, Research Centre, GlaxoSmithKline S.p.A., Verona, Italy

Frank S. Caruso, Ph.D. Caruso Pharmaceutical Consultation Services, Cape May, New Jersey, U.S.A.

C. Patrick Case School of Medical Sciences, University of Bristol, Bristol, England

Fernando Cervero, M.D., Ph.D., D.Sc. Department of Physiology, University of Alcalá, Madrid, Spain

Kwen-Jen Chang, Ph.D. Ardent Pharmaceuticals, Inc., Durham, North Carolina, U.S.A.

Iain P. Chessell, Ph.D. Glaxo Institute of Applied Pharmacology, University of Cambridge, Cambridge, England

Boris A. Chizh, M.D., Ph.D. Grünenthal GmbH Research Centre, Aachen, Germany

R. W. Colburn, Ph.D. University of Cambridge, and Unit of Anaesthesia, Addenbrooke's Hospital, Cambridge, England

Alison Comite, M.S. Department of Anaesthesia, Massachusetts General Hospital and Harvard Medical School, Boston, Massachusetts, U.S.A.

Helen E. Connor, B.Pharm., Ph.D. Receptor Pharmacology Unit, Glaxo Wellcome R&D, Stevenage, Hertfordshire, England

M. Corsi, Ph.D. Neuropharmacology Department, Research Centre, GlaxoSmithKline S.p.A., Verona, Italy

G. Dal Forno, D.Biol. Biology Department, Research Centre, GlaxoSmithKline S.p.A., Verona, Italy

Gudarz Davar, M.D. Molecular Neurobiology of Pain Laboratory, Department of Anesthesia, Brigham and Women's Hospital, and Harvard Medical School, Boston, Massachusetts, U.S.A.

Philip Davey SmithKline Beecham Pharmaceuticals, Harlow, Essex, England

Diane L. DeHaven-Hudkins, Ph.D. Adolor Corporation, Malvern, Pennsylvania, U.S.A.

Neil W. DeLapp, Ph.D. Neuroscience Research Division, Lilly Research Laboratories, Eli Lilly and Company, Indianapolis, Indiana, U.S.A.

Alvaro M. Diaz, M.D., Ph.D. Departments of Physiology and Pharmacology, Universidad de Cantabria, Santander, Spain

R. Di Fabio, Ph.D. Medicinal Chemistry Department, Research Centre, GlaxoSmithKline S.p.A., Verona, Italy

Anthony H. Dickenson, Ph.D. Department of Pharmacology, University College London, London, England

Sudhir Diwan, M.D. Division of Pain Medicine, Department of Anesthesiology, New York Presbyterian Hospital, Cornell University, New York, New York, U.S.A.

Andy Dray, Ph.D. AstraZeneca R&D Montreal, Montreal, Quebec, Canada

Mary Eaton, Ph.D. The Miami Project to Cure Paralysis, University of Miami School of Medicine, Miami, Florida, U.S.A.

James C. Eisenach, M.D. Department of Anesthesiology, Wake Forest University School of Medicine, Winston-Salem, North Carolina, U.S.A.

Andreas G. Erdmann, F.R.C.A. University of Cambridge and Addenbrooke's Hospital, Cambridge, England

Wasyl Feniuk, Ph.D. Department of Pharmacology, Glaxo Institute of Applied Pharmacology, Cambridge, England

Mark J. Field, M.Sc. Department of Biology, Parke-Davis Neuroscience Research Centre, Cambridge University Forvie Site, Cambridge, England

Anders Fink-Jensen, Ph.D. Health Care Discovery, Novo Nordisk A/S, Måløv, Denmark

Elmar Friderichs Grünenthal GmbH, Aachen, Germany

Jeff Gelblum, M.D. Florida Neurological Associates, Mt. Sinai Medical Center, Miami, Florida, U.S.A.

Peter J. Goadsby, M.D., Ph.D., D.Sc., F.R.A.C.P., F.R.C.P. University Department of Clinical Neurology, Institute of Neurology, The National Hospital for Neurology and Neurosurgery, London, England

Ronald Goldblum, M.D. Elan Pharmaceuticals, San Diego, California, U.S.A.

Gil Gonzalez, M.D., Ph.D. Department of Radiology, Massachusetts General Hospital and Harvard Medical School, Boston, Massachusetts

M. Isabel Gonzalez, Ph.D. Neurodegeneration Research, Neurology CEDD, GlaxoSmithKline, Harlow, Essex, England

Sarah Greer, B.Sc., R.G.N. Rheumatology Research Unit, Addenbrooke's Hospital, Cambridge, England

C. Chan Gunn, M.D. Gunn Pain Clinic, Vancouver, British Columbia, Canada, and University of Washington School of Medicine, Seattle, Washington, U.S.A.

Brian L. Hazleman, M.A., M.B., F.R.C.P. Rheumatology Research Unit, Addenbrooke's Hospital, Cambridge, England

P. Max Headley, Ph.D. Department of Physiology, School of Medical Sciences, University of Bristol, Bristol, England

Gareth A. Hicks, Ph.D. GI Department, Neurology and GI Centre of Excellence for Drug Discovery, GlaxoSmithKline, Harlow, Essex, England

Raymond G. Hill, B.Pharm., Ph.D. Neuroscience Research Centre, Merck Sharp & Dohme, Harlow, Essex, England

Victor J. Hruby, Ph.D. Department of Chemistry, University of Arizona, Tucson, Arizona, U.S.A.

Michael Hudspith, F.R.C.A. University of Cambridge and Addenbrooke's Hospital, Cambridge, England

Patrick P. A. Humphrey, Ph.D., D.Sc. Pharmacology Department, Glaxo Institute of Applied Pharmacology, University of Cambridge, Cambridge, England

David J. Julius University of California, San Francisco, San Francisco, California, U.S.A.

Leslie L. Iversen, Ph.D. Department of Pharmacology, University of Oxford, Oxford, England

Wilfrid Jänig, Ph.D. Christian-Albrechts University, Kiel, Germany

Martin Koltzenburg, M.D. Institute of Child Health, University College London, London, England

Maria Koutantji, M.Sc., Ph.D. School of Health Policy and Practice, University of East Anglia, Norwich, England

Elizabeth A. Kowaluk, Ph.D. Pharmaceutical Discovery Department, Abbott Laboratories, Abbott Park, Illinois, U.S.A.

Jennifer M. A. Laird, B.Sc., Ph.D. Research Unit, University Hospital Principe de Asturias and University of Alcalá, Madrid, Spain

Patricia Lavand'homme, M.D. Service d'Anesthesie, Université Catholique de Louvain, Brussels, Belgium

Sally N. Lawson, B.Sc., Ph.D. Department of Physiology, School of Medical Sciences, University of Bristol, Bristol, England

Karen Lewis, B.Sc. Genetics Research, GlaxoSmithKline, Stevenage, Hertfordshire, England

Robert R. Luther, M.D. Elan Pharmaceuticals, Menlo Park, California, U.S.A.

Gordon Lyons, M.D., F.R.C.A. Obstetric Anaesthesia, St. James's University Hospital, Leeds, England

Halina Machelska, Ph.D. Department of Anesthesiology, Free University Berlin, Berlin, Germany

Jianren Mao, M.D., Ph.D. MGH Pain Center, Department of Anesthesia and Critical Care, Massachusetts General Hospital, and Harvard Medical School, Boston, Massachusetts, U.S.A.

Elizabeth A. Matthews, Ph.D. Department of Pharmacology, University College London, London, England

David J. Mayer, Ph.D.* Department of Anesthesiology, Medical College of Virginia, Richmond, Virginia, U.S.A.

Martha Mayo, Pharm.D. Elan Pharmaceuticals, Menlo Park, California, U.S.A.

Keith McCormack, Ph.D. Drug Research Group, McCormack Limited, Leighton Buzzard, Bedfordshire, England

Alexander J. B. McEwan, M.B., F.R.C.P.(C) Department of Oncology, Faculty of Medicine, University of Alberta, and Nuclear Medicine, Department of Oncologic Imaging, Cross Cancer Institute, Edmonton, Alberta, Canada

* Retired.

Andrew D. Medhurst SmithKline Beecham Pharmaceuticals, Harlow, Essex, England

Lorne M. Mendell, Ph.D. Department of Neurobiology and Behavior, State University of New York at Stony Brook, Stony Brook, New York, U.S.A.

Allan J. Miller, M.B., F.R.C.P., F.R.S.H., F.F.P.M. Napp Pharmaceuticals Ltd., Cambridge, England

Charles H. Mitch, Ph.D. Neuroscience Research Division, Lilly Research Laboratories, Eli Lilly and Company, Indianapolis, Indiana, U.S.A.

M. Mugnaini, Ph.D. Biology Department, Research Centre, GlaxoSmithKline S.p.A., Verona, Italy

Rajesh Munglani, M.B., B.S., D.A., D.C.H., F.R.C.A. University of Cambridge and Unit of Anaesthesia, Addenbrooke's Hospital, Cambridge, England

Alan Naylor, Ph.D. Neurology Centre of Excellence for Drug Discovery, GlaxoSmithKline, Harlow, Essex, England

Richard A. Newton School of Medical Sciences, University of Bristol, Bristol, England

Preben H. Olesen, Ph.D. Health Care Discovery, Novo Nordisk A/S, Maløv, Denmark

Andrew A. Parsons, Ph.D. SmithKline Beecham Pharmaceuticals, Harlow, Essex, England

Julie A. Payne Royal Albert Edward Infirmary, Lancashire, England

Shirley Pearce, M.Phil., Ph.D. School of Health Policy and Practice, University of East Anglia, Norwich, England

Martin N. Perkins, Ph.D. Pharmacology Department, AstraZeneca R&D Montreal, Montreal, Quebec, Canada

Roger G. Pertwee, M.A., D.Phil., D.Sc. Department of Biomedical Sciences, University of Aberdeen, Aberdeen, Scotland

Hugh O. Pettit, Ph.D. Ardent Pharmaceuticals, Inc., Durham, North Carolina, U.S.A.

Val Piercy SmithKline Beecham Pharmaceuticals, Harlow, Essex, England

Frank Porreca, Ph.D. Department of Pharmacology, University of Arizona Health Sciences Center, Tucson, Arizona, U.S.A.

G. C. Preston, M.A., D.Phil. Clinical Pharmacology Division, Glaxo Wellcome Research and Development, Greenford, Middlesex, England

Donald D. Price, Ph.D. Departments of Oral and Maxillofacial Surgery and Neuroscience, University of Florida, Gainesvillle, Florida, U.S.A.

M. Quartaroli, D.Pharm. Medical Department, Research Centre, GlaxoSmithKline S.p.A., Verona, Italy

Robert B. Raffa, Ph.D. Department of Pharmaceutical Sciences, Temple University School of Pharmacy, Philadelphia, Pennsylvania

E. Ratti, D.Biol. Psychiatry Centre of Excellence for Drug Discovery, Research Centre, GlaxoSmithKline S.p.A., Verona, Italy

Pravin Raval SmithKline Beecham Pharmaceuticals, Harlow, Essex, England

Andrew S. C. Rice, M.B., B.S., M.D., F.R.C.A. Department of Anaesthetics, Imperial College of Science, Technology, and Medicine, London, England

Jonathan Richardson, M.D., F.R.C.P., F.R.C.A. Anaesthetics and Pain Management Department, Bradford Royal Infirmary, Bradford, West Yorkshire, England

Wendye R. Robbins NeurogesX, Inc., San Carlos, and Stanford University, Stanford, California, U.S.A.

Howard Rosner, M.D. The Pain Center, Cedars-Sinai Medical Center, Los Angeles, California, U.S.A.

Anisa Sabrine, F.R.C.A. St. James's University Hospital, Leeds, England

Jacqueline Sagen, Ph.D. The Miami Project to Cure Paralysis, University of Miami School of Medicine, Miami, Florida, U.S.A.

Reijo Salonen Neurology and Psychiatry Therapeutic Development Group, Glaxo Wellcome, Inc., Research Triangle Park, North Carolina, U.S.A.

Christine Nai-Mei Sang, M.D., M.P.H. Clinical Trials Program, MGH Pain Center, Department of Anesthesia and Critical Care, Massachusetts General Hospital, and Harvard Medical School, Boston, Massachusetts

Gareth J. Sanger SmithKline Beecham Pharmaceuticals, Harlow, Essex, England

Philippe Sanseau, Ph.D. Genetics Research, GlaxoSmithKline, Stevenage, Hertfordshire, England

Margaret Saunders, M.B., M.R.C.P. Papworth Hospital, Cambridge, England

Per Sauerberg, Ph.D. Health Care Discovery, Novo Nordisk A/S, Måløv, Denmark

Marcus Schindler, Ph.D. Boehringer Ingelheim Pharma KG, Biberach, Germany

William K. Schmidt, Ph.D. Adolor Corporation, Exton, Pennsylvania, U.S.A.

Eileen M. Shalhoub, Ph.D. Johnson & Johnson Pharmaceutical Research and Development, Titusville, New Jersey, U.S.A.

Harlan E. Shannon, Ph.D. Neuroscience Research Division, Lilly Research Laboratories, Eli Lilly and Company, Indianapolis, Indiana, U.S.A.

Malcolm J. Sheardown, Ph.D. Health Care Discovery, Novo Nordisk A/S, Måløv, Denmark

Michael J. Sheehan, Ph.D. Receptor Pharmacology Unit, Glaxo Wellcome Research and Development, Stevenage, Hertfordshire, England

Koki Shimoji, M.D., Ph.D., F.R.C.A. Department of Anesthesiology, Niigata University School of Medicine, Niigata, Japan

Philip J. Siddall, M.B., B.S., Ph.D. Pain Management and Research Centre, University of Sydney and Royal North Shore Hospital, St. Leonards, New South Wales, Australia

Lakhbir Singh, Ph.D. Department of Biology, Parke-Davis Neuroscience Research Centre, Cambridge University Forvie Site, Cambridge, England

Judith A. Siuciak, Ph.D. CNS Discovery Research, Groton Laboratories, Pfizer Inc., Groton, Connecticut, U.S.A.

Kevin J. Smith, B.Sc., Ph.D. Napp Pharmaceuticals Ltd., Cambridge, England

Kathrin A. Stauffer, Ph.D. University of Cambridge and Addenbrooke's Hospital, Cambridge, England

Christoph Stein, M.D. Department of Anaesthesiology, Free University Berlin, Berlin, Germany

Abraham Sunshine, M.D. Analgesic Development Ltd. and NYU School of Medicine, New York, New York, U.S.A.

Michael D. B. Swedberg, Ph.D. Health Care Discovery, Novo Nordisk A/S, Måløv, Denmark

Y. Michael A. Tai, F.F.A.R.C.S.I., D.Obst., R.C.O.G. Anaesthetic Department, The Pain Clinic, Wexham Park Hospital, Slough, Berkshire, England

Simon Tate, B.Sc. Glaxo Wellcome Research and Development, Stevenage, Hertfordshire, England

Rolf-Detlef Treede, M.D. Institute of Physiology and Pathophysiology, Johannes Gutenberg University, Mainz, Germany

Derek J. Trezise Glaxo Wellcome Research and Development, Stevenage, Hertfordshire, England

D. G. Trist, Ph.D. Psychiatry Centre of Excellence for Drug Discovery, Research Centre, GlaxoSmithKline S.p.A., Verona, Italy

A. Ugolini, D.Pharm. Biology Department, Research Centre, GlaxoSmithKline S.p.A., Verona, Italy

John S. Ward, Ph.D. Neuroscience Research Division, Lilly Research Laboratories, Eli Lilly and Company, Indianapolis, Indiana, U.S.A.

Ursula Wesselmann, M.D., Ph.D. Department of Neurology, Johns Hopkins University School of Medicine, Baltimore, Maryland, U.S.A.

Daniel E. Womer, Ph.D. Neuroscience Research Division, Lilly Research Laboratories, Eli Lilly and Company, Indianapolis, Indiana, U.S.A.

Clifford J. Woolf, M.B., B.Ch., Ph.D., M.R.C.P. Neural Plasticity Research Group, Department of Anesthesia and Critical Care, Massachusetts General Hospital, and Harvard Medical School, Boston, Massachusetts, U.S.A.

Pain

1

Mechanism-Based Classifications of Pain and Analgesic Drug Discovery

Clifford J. Woolf and David Borsook
Massachusetts General Hospital and Harvard Medical School, Boston, Massachusetts, U.S.A.

Martin Koltzenburg
Institute of Child Health, University College London, London, England

I. INTRODUCTION

Two parallel processes characterize the contemporary pain field: first, enormous progress is being made in the discovery of the cellular and molecular mechanisms responsible for the pathogenesis of pain; second, there is a growing appreciation that multiple mechanisms contribute to common clinical pain syndromes. Both of these will have a considerable influence on novel analgesic development, the former in discovering novel molecular targets, and the latter in defining what therapeutic approaches are required for particular components of particular pain syndromes. The aim of this chapter is to show how a mechanism-based classification is likely to have profound implications; drugs may be developed that target distinct mechanisms, and clinicians may eventually be armed with more reliable and valid diagnostic tools for treatment and clinical investigation.

Current methods of classifying pain are unsatisfactory for several reasons: foremost is that pain syndromes are identified by parts of the body, duration, and causative agent, rather than the mechanism involved. Although the conventional anatomical-based classification of pain is clinicially useful for the differential diagnosis of the underlying cause, it tells us little about mechanisms, because the innervation of distinct anatomical regions is often analogous. Anatomical differences should be disregarded in favor of mechanisms that apply to either particular tissues (e.g., skin, muscle, joints, or viscera) or all parts of the body, rather than a particular part of the body. ''Acute'' and ''chronic'' also do not differentiate mechanistically. It is better to use the terms *transient* and *persistent* and define the particular mechanisms involved.

As far as causative agent is concerned, the same disease (e.g., herpes zoster) may produce pain by multiple mechanisms, and the reverse is also true, different causative agents may produce pain by similar mechanisms. Although disease-modifying treatment is always essential, where available, the disease and the generation of symptoms are not necessarily equivalent. For example, the virus that causes herpes zoster and the pain of acute zoster does not contribute directly to the pain of postherpetic neuralgia. Antiviral treatment has no place in the management of postherpetic neuralgia. The benign or malignant dichotomy has been used as a clinical guideline for the selection of treatment options for patients, but intrinsically has no mechanistic basis—the same pain-generating mechanisms may apply in both cases. The term cancer pain relates only to the disease from which the patient suffers, not the mechanism of any pain they may experience.

Great care is required for describing symptoms. Allodynia (pain evoked by a normally nonpainful stimulus) describes all situations in which pain thresholds are reduced. The phrase is commonly used clinically to describe pain evoked by lightly touching the skin that can either be caused by an Aβ low-threshold afferent input to a hypersensitivity state or by sensitized nociceptor central; therefore, it is not useful by itself to define the symptom responsible. The use of terms for pain hypersensitivity should be modified so that explicit reference is made to the particular mechanism involved. Symptoms are not equivalent to mechanisms and a symptom-based classification by itself is inadequate.

II. TOWARD A MECHANISM-BASED CLASSIFICATION OF PAIN

It is possible, we believe, to break pain down into a variety of syndromes and, then identify the mechanisms underlying each syndrome. Such an approach is likely to lead to specific phar-

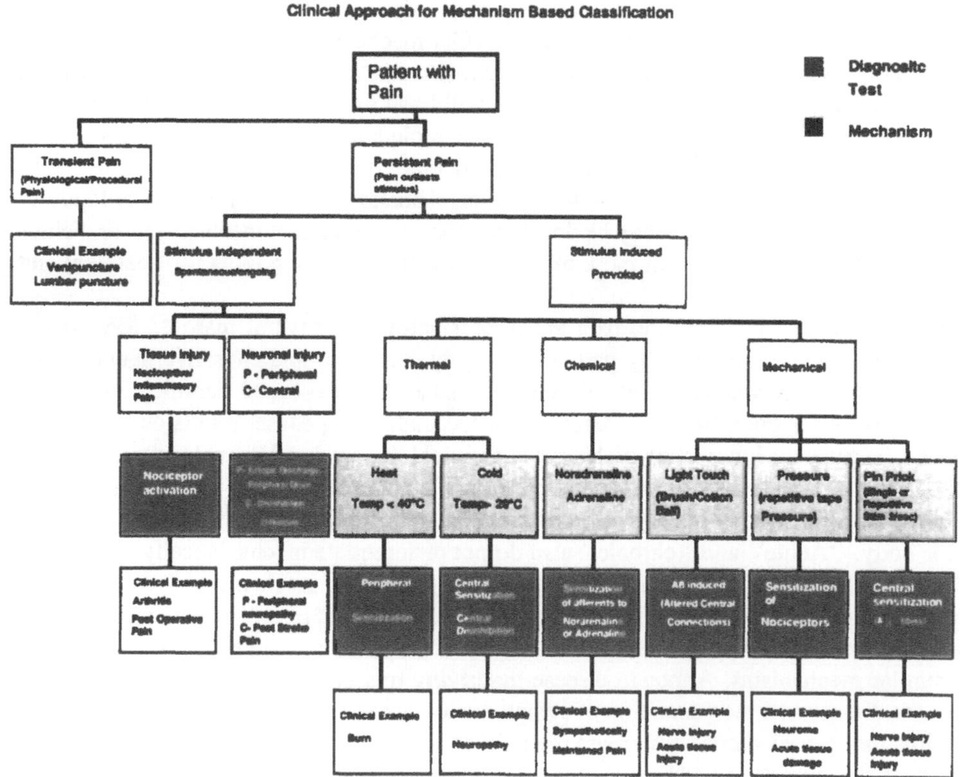

Figure 1 Clinical approach for mechanism-based classification

Table 1 Transient Stimulus-Induced Pains (Without Significant Tissue Alterations or Stimulus-Induced Pains Not Associated with Injury)

Activation of nociceptors (Aδ- and C-fibers)

macological intervention measures for each identified mechanims within the syndrome. An analogous example is the way cardiologists provide cocktails of drugs for their patients, which together combat the arrhythmia, contractility failure, and problems of coronary circulation that together constitute heart failure.

Advances in the pain area are, then, contingent on first determining the symptoms that constitute a syndrome and, then, finding mechanisms for each of these. For example, brush-evoked pain (a symptom), can be initiated by nerve injury and tissue injury, and there are several mechanisms involved in both. These different mechanisms may explain the differential susceptibility of individual patients to drugs but, in turn, certain commonalities, such as ongoing activity of nociceptors, whatever its initiating mechanism, will precipitate central changes in the excitability of the spinal cord that result in pain hypersensitivity.

It is clinically important to differentiate between two of the major components of pain: *stimulus independent* (ongoing) pain and *stimulus dependent* hyperalgesia (including what has previously been known as allodynia). Tables 1, 2, and 3 illustrate how different mechanisms contribute to different pains. A distinction is made between the pain that is generated in response to transient nondamaging stimuli (*transient pain,* see Table 1) that is an important component of the body's normal protective mechanisms and encountered clinically in many forms of procedural pains (venipuncture, lumbar puncture). These pains differ mechanistically from pain that presents clinically following tissue injury or injury to the peripheral or central nervous system (*persistent pain*; see Tables 2 and 3). A further dichotomy is made between *stimulus-independent pain* (spontaneous or ongoing pain; see Table 2) and *stimulus-induced pain* (provoked pain—hyperalgesia; see Table 3).

Table 2 Stimulus-Independent (Ongoing) Pains

Injury type/tissue	Location	Afferent involved	Possible mechanisms
Tissue injury	Region of tissue injury	Nociceptors (Aδ- and C-fibers)	Ongoing activity of nociceptors
Nerve injury	Projected to the region of the nerve injury	Nociceptors (Aδ- and C-fibers)	Ectopic ongoing discharge of nociceptors
CNS injury	"Projected"	None	Disinhibition, hyperactivity of central pain-signaling neurons

Note: Ongoing or ectopic activity in nociceptors will initiate central sensitization which must be considered, therefore, as part of the mechanism, and in turn, it will initiate stimulus-evoked pain. There is the theortical possibility that after tissue or nerve injury, nonnociceptive primary afferent fibers (-SAII-mechanoreceptors, sensitive cold receptors) that physiologically have ongoing activity can add to the magnitude of pain when central sensitization is present.

Table 3 Stimulus-Induced Pains: (Hyperalgesias—Defined as Increased Pain Sensation to a Simulus)

Type	Modality	Tissue	Location	Afferents involved[a]	Possible mechanisms
Thermal	Heat	Injury to skin (common) or cutaneous nerve (rare)	1° zone only	Nociceptors (C-fibers in hairy skin)	Sensitization of nociceptors
	Cold	Common after nerve injury, possible nil after skin injury	1° zone and 2° zone	Sensitive cold receptors	Central sensitization
		Common after nerve injury, possibly nil after skin injury	1° zone only?	Cold-sensitive nociceptors	Central disinhibition
Chemical	Chemical	Common after tissue injury	1° zone	Nociceptors	Sensitization of nociceptors
	Epinephrine Norepinephrine (SMP)	Nerve injury, tissue injury (probably rare)	1° zone (axotomized and non-axotomized fibers	Nociceptors: possibly Aβ-fibers, when central sensitization is present	Sensitization (expression of adrenoceptors?)
Mechanical	Light touch	Injury to skin or cutaneous nerve	1° and 2° zone	Aβ-fibers	Central sensitization initiated and maintained by nociceptor input
	Light touch	Injury to cutaneous nerve	1° and 2° zone	Aβ-fibers	Structural alterations of central connections
	Light touch	Trigeminal neuralgia	Trigger zone	Aβ LTM?	???
	Pinprick	Injury to skin or cutaneous nerve	1° and 2° zone	Aδ fibers	Central sensitization initiated, but not maintained by nociceptor input
	Blunt pressure	Tissue injury (S, M, J, V), nerve injury (S, M?)	1° zone	Nociceptors	Sensitization of nociceptors
Neuroma sign	Touch	Injured nerve	Trigger point/neuroma	Injured axons A and C	Mechanosensitivity of injured axons

SMP, sympathetically maintained pain; Aβ, Aδ LTM, light-touch mechanoreceptors.

III. PAIN CLASSIFICATION: ANIMAL AND HUMAN MODELS AND MOLECULAR TARGETS

Tables 1–3 illustrate some of the currently known mechanisms that operate to produce pain. Table 4 is an attempt to relate clinical pain syndromes with the mechanisms that are likely to operate together with the animal and human surrogate models that may be used to investigate the mechanisms. Considerable care must be exercised in extrapolating from animal models to clinical mechanisms, and the recent failures of NK1-antagonists in clinical pain trials in the face of impressive preclinical efficacy data are a warning sign. Animal models are only approximations. Ultimately, it is advisable to align preclinical, clinical, and human models with animal models to be certain of dissecting a particular mechanism. Table 5 identifies some of the molecular targets that have been identified as actually or potentially operating in the different mechanisms.

IV. IMPLICATIONS FOR DRUG DEVELOPMENT AND DIAGNOSIS

There are two important questions in clinical drug development: (1) Does the drug work? and (2) How commercially useful is it going to be? A mechanism-based classification is likely to be helpful in terms of setting targets for particular mechanisms and describing which patients are likely to benefit. The standard way of studying a population is to assemble the group on the basis of a classified disease-related symptom. The new classification suggests carrying out a study on a population with the same symptom (pathophysiological mechanism), but not necessarily the same disease. The standard method will indicate that a particular drug is efficacious for diabetic neuropathy, for example, but it may suggest nothing about postherpetic neuralgia. Testing a drug across a variety of etiologies may mean that development will continue because of the drug's generalized ability to treat that same symptom across different disease states. This type of approach has been used in other conditions, such as stroke prevention, in which the action of a compound has been used in groups of patients with various underlying risk factors. The modification of drug efficacy testing from treatment of individuals grouped in terms of disease to mechanism will require a novel approach to proof-of-concept analgesic drug evaluation in patients. A feature of this may well be the use of human surrogate models of particular pain mechanisms (see Table 4) as part of phase 1 tests, as well as much more targeted proof-of-concept testing in patients in phase 2 (see Table 5). Most clinical trials of novel drugs have been relatively unsophisticated in their evaluation of whether a particular mechanism has been modified. More sensitive outcome measures are required that are defined to provide information of targeted mechanisms.

V. CLINICAL IMPLICATIONS OF A MECHANISM-BASED PAIN CLASSIFICATION

Figure 1 illustrates how patients with pain could be analyzed from a pain–mechanism perspective. An individual patient may suffer from various pain problems, both stimulus-independent and stimulus-dependent, as a consequence of separate or overlapping mechanisms. These may manifest at different times during the natural history of the disease or simultaneously; hence, the importance of establishing operational criteria for identifying each definable mechanism. At present, such diagnostic tools are not available, and elucidating such tools represents the major challenge in the field. If drugs become available that act specifically on only a particular mecha-

Table 4 Different Pain Categories, Their Mechanisms, Animal and Human Models

Pain categories	Pain conditions	Pain mechanisms	Animal models	Human surrogate models
1. Transient stimulus-induced pains (nociceptive pain)	Procedural pain (injections/minor injuries)	Nociceptor activation	Thermosensitivity, mechanosensitivity, chemsensitivity	Cold pressor test Ischaemic pain Quantitative sensory testing
2. Tissue damage (inflammatory pain); spontaneous and provoked pain	Trauma/postoperative pain; arthritis/infection/migraine	Nociceptor activation; peripheral sensitization; central sensitization; phenotype switch	Chemical irritants Capsaicin, mustard oil, formalin Experimental inflammation Carageenan, UVB, Freund's adjuvant Cytokines/growth factors	Capsaicin Mustard oil Experimental burn
3. Injury: primary afferent (neuropathic pain); spontaneous and provoked pain	Peripheral nerve injury; diabetic neuropathy; toxic neuropathy; postherpetic neuralgia	Ectopic activity; phenotype switch; central sensitization; structural reorganization; disinhibition	Peripheral nerve section; partial nerve section; loose ligatures; experimental diabetes; toxic neuropathies	—
4. Injury: central neuron (neuropathic pain); spontaneous and provoked pain	Stroke; multiple sclerosis; spinal cord injury	Secondary ectopic activity; disinhibition; structural reorganization	Spinal cord injury; Ischemia; central disinhibition (i.e., strychnine/bicuculline)	—
5. Unknown mechanism	Tension-type headaches; fibromyalgia; irritable bowel syndrome	?Altered gain	?	—

Table 5 Potential Drug Targets for Different Pains and Clinical Proof-of-Concept Trials

Pain categories	Pain mechanisms	Potential drug and targets	Proof-of-concept
1. Transient stimulus-induced pains (nociceptive pain)	Nociceptor activation	VRs Na^+-TTXs MOR,nAChR	Minor surgical procedures
2. Tissue damage (inflammatory pain) spontaneous and provoked pain	Nocicetor activation Peripheral sensitization Central sensitization Phenotype switch	COX-2, EPR, 5-HTR, P_{2x}, BKR IL-β, TNR-α, TrkA, TrkB Na^+-TTX-R, ASIC, α_2, MOR, DOR, A_1, N-Ca^{2+}, NK1, nAChR NMDA-R, GluR5, mGluR, PKCγ	Dental postoperative pain Abdominal postoperative pain Thoracotomy Joint replacement, osteoarthritis Acute herpes zoster, migraine
3. Injury: primary afferent (neuropathic pain) spontaneous and provoked pain	Ectopic activity Phenotype switch Central sensitization Structural reorganization Disinhibition	Na^+–TTXr/TTXs α^2, NMDA-R, N-Ca^2, PKCγ NGF/GDNF Gaba, AEAs, gabapentin, lamotrigen, TCA, SNRIs	PHN, diabetic neuropathy Radiciular pain Disease vs. symptom (e.g., tactile allodynias)
4. Injury: Central neuron (neuropathic pain) spontaneous and provoked pain	Secondary ectopic activity Disinhibition Structural reorganization	GABA-R Na^+-TTXs AEAs TCA, SNRIs	Spinal cord injury/multiple sclerosis, central poststroke pain
5. Unknown mechanism	?Altered gain control	COX-2, NMDA-R, Na^+ channels	IBS/fibromyalgia

VR, vallinoid receptors; Na^+–TTXs, tetrodotoxin-sensitive sodium ion channels, MOR, μ-opiate receptors; nAChR, nicotinic acetylcholine receptor; COX-2, inducible cyclooxygenase inhibitors; EPR, Prostaglandin recepors; 5-HTR, serotonin receptors; P_{2x}, ligand-gated purino receptors/ion channels; BKR, bradykinin receptors; IL-β, interleukins; TNFα, tumor necrosis factor; TrkA, TrkB, high-affinity neurotrophin tyrosine kinase receptors; Na^+–TTX-R, tetrodotoxin-resistant sodium ion channels; ASIC, acid-sensitive ion channels; α_2, adrenergic receptors; DOR, delta opiate receptors; A_1 adenosine receptors; N-Ca^{2+}, voltage-gated calcium ion channels; NK1, neurokinin receptors; NMDA-R, *N*-methyl-D-aspartic acid receptors; GluR5, kainate receptors; mGluR, metabotropic glutamate receptors; PKCγ, protein kinase C; NGF/GDNF, nerve growth factor, glial derived neurotrophic factor; AEAs, antiepileptic agents; GABA-ergic compounds; TCA, tricyclic antidepressants; SNRIs, serotonin and norepinephrine reuptake inhibitors.

nism, they will be very useful as diagnostic aids as well as for therapy. In a patient it may be possible to dissect out how much of their pain is due to nociceptor activity, central sensitization, or a combination of these, and tailor the treatment accordingly.

VI. CONCLUSIONS

The opportunity exists for dramatic changes and indeed improvements in analgesic drug development. This requires, however, a major advance in the classification of pain from one based on anatomical area and disease, to one based on mechanism. It is the mechanism that needs to be the target for novel drugs, not particular disease states. The description of the mechanisms involved in pain needs to be intensified as well as progress made in identifying these mechanisms in individual patients. This will result in changes in the approach to the proof-of-concept testing in clinical drug development to one requiring more sophisticated tests in smaller groups of more homogeneous patients.

BIBLIOGRAPHY

Woolf CJ, Bennett GJ, Doherty M, Dubner R, Kidd B. Koltzenburg M, Lipton R, Loeser JD, Payne R. Torebjork E. Towards a mechanism-based classification of pain? Pain 1998; 77:227–229

Woolf CJ, Mannion RJ. Neuropathic pain: aetiology, symptoms, mechanisms, and management. Lancet 1999; 353:1959–1964.

Woolf CJ, Decosterd I. Implications of recent advances in the understanding of pain pathophysiology for the assessment of pain in patients. Pain 1999; 82(Suppl 6):S141–S147.

2
Sites of Analgesic Action

Michael Hudspith and Rajesh Munglani
University of Cambridge and Addenbrooke's Hospital, Cambridge, England

I. INTRODUCTION

The neurotransmitters, ion channels, receptors, and second-messenger systems of the neurons comprising pain transduction and perception represent potential targets for the manipulation of nociceptive information and, hence, the production of analgesia. To review the likely sites of action of current and future analgesics, it is necessary to briefly review the anatomy of the mammalian nociceptive system.

The diffusely ramifying unmyelinated terminals of Aδ- and C-fibers provide the initial transduction mechanism for mechanical, thermal, and chemical noxious insult. The resultant action potentials evoked in unmyelinated C-fibers and myelinated Aδ-fibers propagate to the spinal cord dorsal horn where they synapse with both spinal interneurons and projection neurons; however, it must also be appreciated that retrograde action potential transmission may evoke local "axon reflex"-mediated peripheral release of neuropeptides contributing to inflammation and peripheral sensitization following injury.

The axons of peripheral nociceptors, the cell bodies of which reside in the dorsal root (and trigeminal) ganglia, project to the spinal cord. C-fibers synapse primarily in laminae II, whereas Aδ-fibers synapse in both laminae I and V of the dorsal horn. Projection neurons form the spinothalamic, spinoreticular, and other ascending tracts that relay nociceptive information through thalamic nuclei to cortical centers of pain representation. Sensory discriminative components are relayed primarily by the lateral thalamic nuclei to somatosensory cortical areas SI and SII, whereas medial thalamic nuclei projecting to the anterior cingulate and prefrontal cortex mediate the affective–motivational components.

The pharmacology of cortical representation of pain is somewhat obscure, and it is at "subthalamic" levels that a clearer picture of the inhibitory mechanisms modulating afferent nociceptive input emerges. Thus, activation of areas such as the PAG, NRM, and locus caeruleus result in descending inhibition of afferent transmission at the level of the dorsal horn in addition to brain stem and thalamic inhibition of nociceptive traffic.

The potential pharmacological targets of analgesic action, from the peripheral nociceptor through the dorsal horn, toward higher centers will now be briefly reviewed.

II. PERIPHERAL NOCICEPTOR

Transduction of mechanical, thermal, and chemical stimuli into Aδ- and C-fiber action potentials occurs at the peripheral axon terminal of the primary afferent nociceptor, the cell body of which resides in the dorsal root ganglion (DRG). Peripheral nociceptor transduction is amplified following injury by the release of chemical mediators of inflammation, including ATP, bradykinin, prostanoids, histamine, (5-HT), adenosine, catecholamines, potassium and hydrogen ions (see Rang et al., 1994) with the development of peripheral sensitization (Dray, 1995) (Fig. 1). Furthermore, inflammation is associated with unmasking of "silent nociceptors" (Schmidt et al., 1995); thereby enhancing the number of functional nociceptors and amplifying pain transduction.

Mechanical and thermal transduction are mediated by mechanogated and thermally activated ion channels: the molecular structure and activation of mechanoreceptors are still poorly understood (Tanner et al., 1997); however, the recently cloned VR-1 vanniloid receptor is a likely candidate for thermal nociception. Although these provide theoretical targets of analgesic action, it is the modulation of nociceptor activation and attenuation of action potential generation that forms the basis of current peripheral analgesic action. Primary afferent nociceptors express a plethora of receptor types (see Rang et al., 1994). However, it must be appreciated that much of this data pertains to receptor types synthesized in the cell body in the DRG and the presence of mRNA encoding specific receptors, or the receptor protein itself within the DRG does not necessarily imply that the peripheral nociceptor terminal itself carries such receptors. For example, whereas both central and peripheral nociceptor terminals express NK-1 and B2 bradykinin receptor proteins, it remains uncertain whether ionotropic glutamate receptors (AMPA and NMDA), γ-aminobutyric acid (GABA) receptors, and glycine receptors, which are expressed on central nociceptor terminals (and play fundamental roles in modulating spinal pain transduction) are expressed on peripheral nociceptor endings (Coggleshall and Carlton, 1997). Moreover, nociceptor phenotype is determined by both local and axonally transported trophic factor availability and both inflammatory and neuropathic processes may alter receptor and ion channel expression from the naïve uninjured state (McMahon et al., 1997).

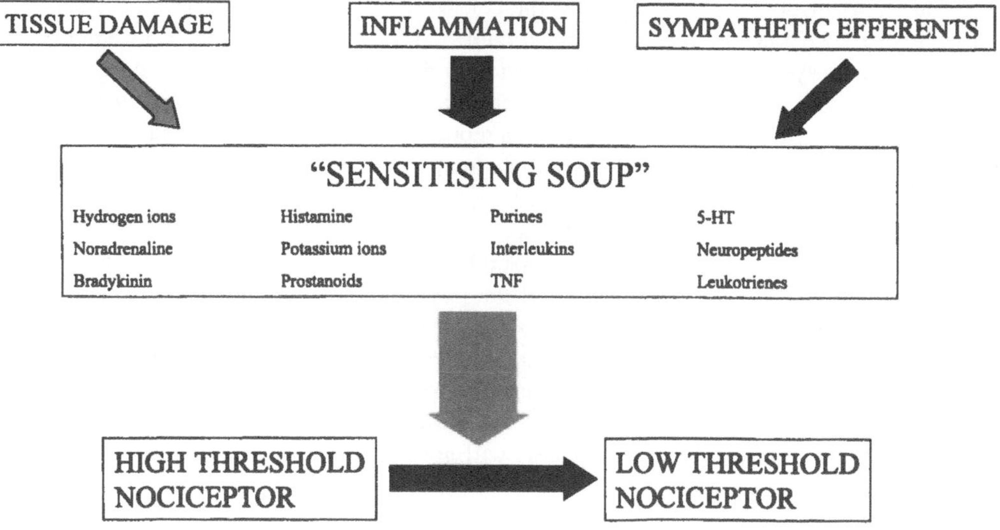

Figure 1 Factors leading to peripheral nociceptor sensitization.

The inflammatory mediators of peripheral sensitization (see Fig. 1) may activate the peripheral nociceptor either directly or indirectly by release of direct-acting agents from inflammatory cells and vascular endothelium. Modification of the synthesis or release of these mediators, or antagonism of their interaction with specific receptors, provide potential or realized analgesic targets.

A. NSAIDs

Many (although not all; see McCormack, 1994) of the analgesic actions of nonsteroidal anti-inflammatory drugs (NSAIDs) are attributed to inhibition of prostaglandin (PG) synthesis in the periphery (Vane, 1971) and the prevention of "peripheral sensitization" (Woolf and Chong, 1993). Nociceptors express receptors for both PGE_2 and PGI_2 prostaglandin products of arachidonic acid metabolism (Dray, 1995) which may be synthesized by both constitutive (COX-1) and inducible (COX-2) isoforms of the enzyme cyclooxygenase (COX) (Hla and Nielson, 1992; Feng et al., 1993). Inflammation-induced induction of COX-2 dictates that that NSAIDs that selectively target this isoform should have improved efficacy and side effect profiles when compared with established nonselective agents (Mitchell et al., 1993).

Although activation of PG receptors may directly potentiate nociceptor responses (Pitchford and Levine, 1991) their major action is to potentiate responses to inflammatory mediators. For example, as demonstrated in seminal studies by Ferreira (1972), experimental human pain induced by infusion of bradykinin or histamine is markedly enhanced by coadministration of prostaglandins. Although the inhibition of COX, demonstrable in vitro by NSAIDs (see McCormack, 1994) is a cornerstone of current analgesic therapy, many other chemical factors are central to nociceptor sensitization (Dray, 1995) and provide important potential analgesic targets.

B. Capsaicin

C- and Aδ-fibers express vanilloid receptor(s) to which capsaicin, the active ingredient of chili peppers, binds (see also Chaps. 10 and 41). The capsaicin receptor(s), a thermally activated ionotropic receptor involved in integration of nocigenic stimuli has been recently cloned (Caterina, 1997; Tominaga et al., 1998). Binding of vanilloids and receptor activation results in initial excitation of the nociceptor by Ca^{2+}-dependent entry, followed by subsequent functional desensitization and inhibition of excitatory amino acid and neuropeptide release (Wood and Docherty, 1997). As discussed in Chapters 10 and 41 in this volume, vanilloid ligands, therefore, provide potential mechanisms of nociceptor-specific blockade.

C. Opioids

In situ hybridization and immunohistochemical studies of opioid (OP) binding demonstrate the synthesis and expression of OP1 (δ), OP2 (κ), and OP3 (μ) receptors in the DRG (Maekawa et al., 1994; Ji et al., 1995); these receptors are transported peripherally by axonal transport, and a similar population of receptors exist on terminals of Aδ and C nociceptive fibers (Dado et al., 1993). In common with spinal and supraspinal opioid receptors, the binding of opioid agonists results in K^+-channel-mediated neuronal hyperpolarization, attenuation of Ca^{2+} entry through voltage-gated Ca^{2+} channels and reduced cAMP availability (Jordan and Devi, 1998), with resultant reduction in nociceptor activity.

As discussed by Dray (see Chap. 10), peripheral opioid-mediated antinociception is enhanced under conditions of inflammation where the axonal transport of opioid receptors from the DRG and peripheral expression of opioid receptors is increased (Hassan et al., 1995). Furthermore, opioid receptor binding and mRNA transcription has been demonstrated in peripheral immune cells (see Stein et al., 1997), indicating immunomodulatory roles for both endogenous and exogenous opioids in inflammatory pain in addition to analgesic actions at the peripheral nociceptor.

D. Future Directions

1. NGF–trkA Antagonists

Nerve growth factor (NGF) plays a key role in the etiology of inflammatory pain. NGF belongs to the family of neurotropic peptides including brain-derived neurotrophic factor (BDNF), neurotrophin 3 (NT3), NT4/5, and NT6, which specify the phenotypic development of central and peripheral neurons (McMahon et al., 1997). Neurotrophins interact with a low affinity P75 receptor, which may modulate the expression and function of specific high-affinity tyrosine kinase (trk) receptors for each individual neurotrophin. However, the biological effects of NGF are mediated by the trkA receptor.

The trkA receptor is expressed on small, unmyelinated nociceptive afferents coexpressing the peptide calcitonin gene-related peptide (CGRP) (Averill et al., 1995). A wide variety of tissues constitutively express NGF at low levels and such constitutive production of NGF may determine nociceptor phenotype in accordance with the "neurotrophic hypothesis." Inflammation (possibly by the cytokines interleukin [IL]-1β and tumor necrosis factor [TNF]) is associated with increased NGF expression and synthesis in peripheral tissues, suggesting that modulation of trkA receptor binding and activation has analgesic potential. Indeed, the rapid onset of hyperalgesia following experimental subcutaneous administration of NGF indicates a direct action of NGF mediating peripheral sensitization at the level of the nociceptor terminal (Lewin et al., 1994) and experimental local sequestration of NGF by trkA–IgG fusion molecules attenuates hyperalgesia following intraplantar carrageenan in the rat (McMahon et al., 1995).

2. Adenosine Antagonists

P2X Antagonists. The P2X3 receptor, an ATP-gated ion channel, selectively expressed by small-diameter nociceptive neurones, is implicated in peripheral sensitization (Burnstock, 1996). Further to the cloning of this receptor, the development of selective P2X3 antagonists may produce a novel class of peripherally active analgesic agents.

NK-1 Antagonists. The role of substance P in nociceptive processes has been suggested ever since the observation that SP peptide was concentrated in dorsal roots (see Chap. 40 and Munglani and Hill, 1999). Indeed NK_1 knockout mice show altered spinal windup and intensity coding of spinal reflexes, although baseline thresholds were unchanged. Furthermore similar responses have been seen in preprotachykinin (the precursor for substance P) knockout mice (De Felipe et al., 1998; Cao et al., 1998; Zimmer et al., 1998). With use of the nonpeptide antagonists of the NK_1 receptor, Longmore et al. (1996) have shown effectiveness in inflammatory hyperalgesia and hypersensitivity induced by experimental diabetes in animals, but not in humans (Reinhardt et al., 1998; Block et al., 1998).

III. AXON (± NEUROMA)

A. Local Anesthetics plus Anticonvulsants

Inactivation of voltage-gated Na^+ channels and reversible block of action potential conduction along the peripheral axons of Aδ- and C-fibers represent the major clinical applications of classic local anesthetic drugs, such as lignocaine and bupivacaine. The relative selectivity of bupivacaine and ropivacaine for nociceptive transmission primarily reflects pharmacokinetic aspects of penetration of myelinated and unmyelinated fibers in mixed nerves. However, sensory neurons express a structural and functional heterogeneity of voltage-gated Na^+ channels (Okuse et al., 1997), of which the tetrodotoxin insensitive (TTXi)-resistant channel is selectively expressed by small-diameter nociceptive neurons (Caffrey et al., 1992); Akopian et al., 1996).

B. Sodium Ion Channels*

Altered-gating characteristics of TTXi Na^+ channels contribute to nociceptor sensitization by inflammatory mediators (Gold et al., 1996) and spontaneous depolarization of neuromata and DRG neurons following nerve injury (Kral et al., 1999). The Na^+ channels are overexpressed in biopsies taken from painful neuromas (England et al., 1996) and also the slow, tetrodotoxin-resistant Na^+ current is the best target for a drug that will relieve pain, but have minimal side effects (Rizzo et al., 1996). This particular channel is overexpressed in inflammation on NGF-dependent unmyelinated nociceptive afferent fibers (Akopian et al., 1996; Friedel et al., 1997; Quasthoff et al., 1995). No compound that will block the TTX-resistant Na^+ sodium current in a selective way is yet available, but the channel has recently been cloned (Akopian et al., 1997). Currently, available agents are suboptimal. For example lignocaine does not select between Na^+ channels in neurons and those in other tissues, and in molar terms it is a rather weak blocker. It has a higher affinity for the TTX-sensitive current in myelinated fibers than for the TTX-resistant current in nociceptors (Scholz et al., 1998). When given intravenously, it is effective in the treatment of several neuropathic pain states, whereas efficacy against other pains is the subject of debate, with positive and negative studies being reported (Kral et al., 1999). The anticonvulsants phenytoin and carbamazepine also inhibit both TTX-resistant and TTX-sensitive currents in rat DRG cells (Rush and Elliot, 1997) and this may explain the clinical effectiveness of these agents in treating pain (McQuay et al., 1995). Mexiletene, and Lamotrigine, a more recently introduced Na^+ channel-blocking anticonvulsant are also proving useful in the treatment of neuropathic pain, and the recent demonstration that it reduces cold-induced pain in volunteer subjects may indicate a wider usefulness in treating other pains (Xie et al., 1995; Webb and Kamali, 1998). In addition, tricyclic antidepressants also may block neuronal Na^+ channels and this may account for some of the analgesic activity of this class of compound (Pancrazio et al., 1998).

IV. DORSAL HORN

Aδ and C-fiber nociceptors project to the superficial and deeper laminae of the dorsal horn where they synapse with both interneurons and projection neurons. Nociceptive afferent fibers corelease the excitatory amino acid transmitter glutamate with neurokinins (predominantly substance P), CGRP, and other peptide transmitters. At this locus, initial excitatory transmission is initiated by AMPA-receptor activation, Na^+ ion entry, and fast depolarization of postsynaptic neurons supplemented by K^+ channel inactivation through NK-1 receptor activation. Depolarization of sufficient duration and magnitude to remove Mg^{2+} block of the NMDA receptor channel results in Ca^{2+} entry, amplification of nociceptive transmission, and initiation of central sensitization at both pre- and postsynaptic sites (Woolf, 1996; Hudspith, 1998; Basbaum, 1999), which may be further supplemented by metabotropic glutamate receptor activation (Fisher et al., 1998).

* See also Hill and Munglani, 1999; and Trezise et al., this volume.

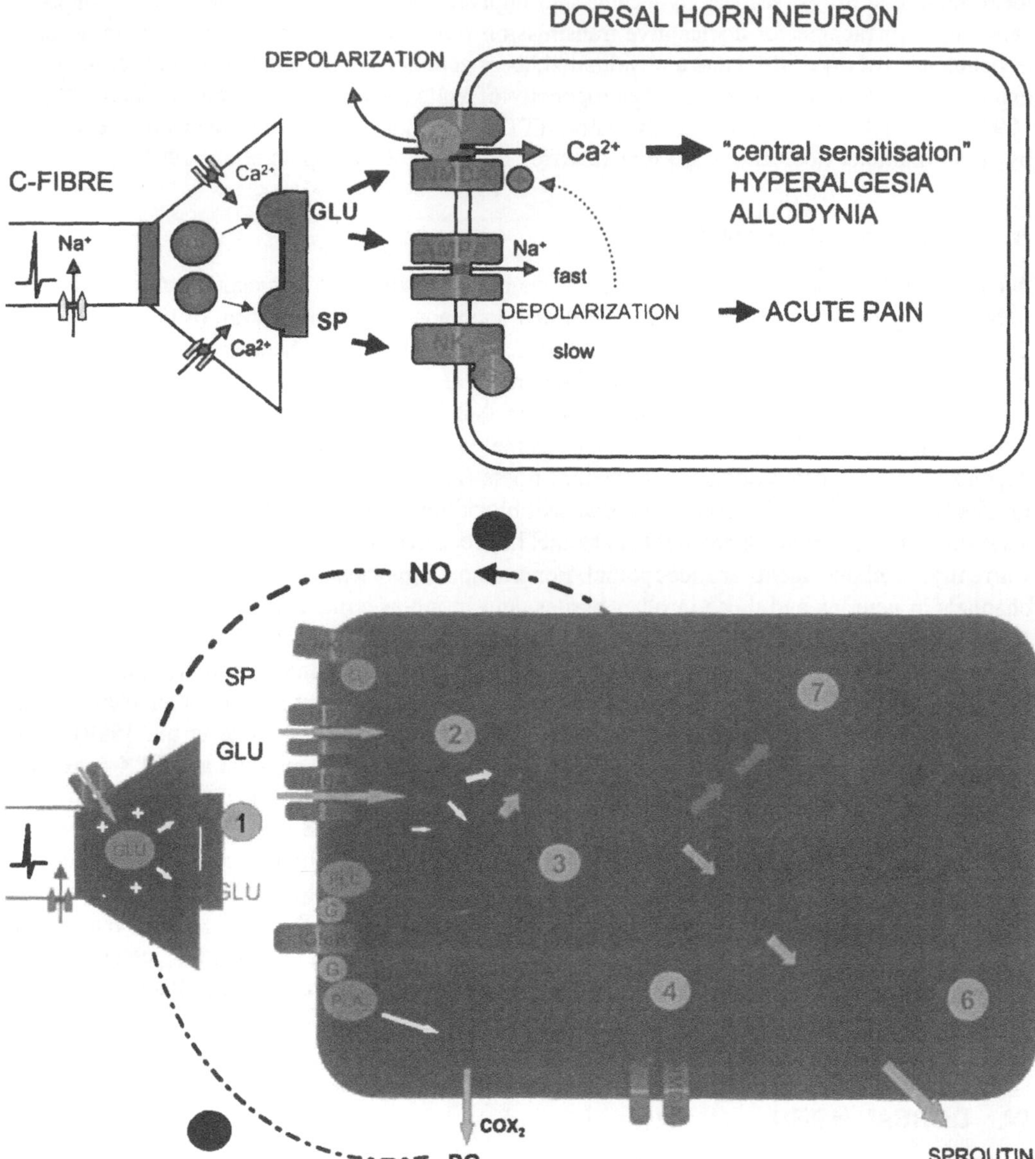

Figure 2 Mechanisms underlying central sensitization. The lower panel shows the development of long-term changes which may be present in chronic pain states.

Excitatory transmission within the dorsal horn is under complex inhibitory tone, mediated in part by GABA, glycine, catecholaminergic, and opioid systems (see Fields and Basbaum, 1994; Yaksh 1998). Critically, dorsal horn mechanisms of neural transmission exhibit remarkable plasticity as illustrated schematically in Figure 2 and readers are referred to specific chapters relating to neuropathic and inflammatory pain for further details.

The dorsal horn, therefore, provides a multiplicity of potential analgesic targets, few of which are currently exploited by analgesics in clinical use. Receptor classification and localization within the dorsal horn has recently been reviewed in a comprehensive manner (Coggleshall and Carlton 1997), and it is appropriate to consider briefly the role of certain of these as analgesic targets within the spinal cord dorsal horn.

A. Excitatory Targets

1. NMDA Receptors

The established role of the NMDA receptor in the initiation of central sensitization (Hudspith and Munglani, 1997) together with their anatomical localization to presynaptic (Liu et al., 1997) and postsynaptic (see Coggleshall and Carlton 1997) nociceptor synapses within the dorsal horn presents an attractive target and has generated a vast literature in multiple models of inflammatory and neuropathic pain. Current clinical applications (see Kohrs and Durieux, 1998) demonstrate analgesic efficacy of NMDA receptor blockade and the potential to exploit spinal subtype-specific NMDA receptors (Tolle et al., 1993) may limit psychotomimetic side effects. However, it must be appreciated that not all pain models are sensitive to NMDA receptor blockade (Zahn et al., 1998), and AMPA-receptor and metabotropic receptor mediated-mechanisms must be considered.

2. AMPA Receptors

GluR1 and GluR2/3 subunits of the AMPA receptor are concentrated in laminae I-II of the dorsal horn (Coggleshall and Carlton, 1997). Recent data suggests that, at least in acute or inflammatory pain models, for which NMDA receptor mechanisms are less significant, AMPA receptor blockade may be a useful analgesic target (Brennan, 1998; Zahn et al., 1998; Zahn and Brennan, 1998).

3. Neurokinin Receptors

Substance P and related neurokinins (NKs) are necessary for the perception of moderate to intense noxious stimuli and play a central role in neurogenic inflammation (Cao et al., 1998). NK-1 knockout animals exhibit a marked reduction in central sensitization following peripheral inflammatory stimuli, and neurokinin antagonists are analgesic in several experimental pain models. Targeting of neurokinin receptors with nonpeptide antagonists that may access dorsal horn receptor sites (Coggleshall and Carlton, 1997; Basbaum, 1999) may selectively block "pathological pain," while maintaining "physiological nociception."

4. Nitric Oxide Synthase

Calcium entry by NMDA receptor activation activates the neuronal isoform of nitric oxide synthase (*n*NOS) (Garthwaite et al., 1988; Bredt et al., 1990) localized within both primary afferent nociceptors in the dorsal root ganglia and neurons of the spinal cord dorsal horn (primarily laminae I-II and X) (Zhang et al., 1993). Nitric oxide, acting as a retrograde transmitter within the dorsal horn, thereby potentiating EAA and neurokinin release, contributes to central sensitization and plays a key role in nociceptive processing (Meller and Gebhart, 1993). Inhibition of NOS attenuates pain and hyperalgesia in several experimental pain models (e.g., Meller et al., 1992; Roche et al., 1996) and prevents or attenuates central sensitization. Selective inhibitors of *n*NOS may prove to be effective analgesics provided the cardiovascular consequences of endothelial NOS (*e*NOS) inhibition can be avoided (Handy and Moore, 1998).

5. Cyclooxygenase

Whereas NSAIDs are commonly considered peripherally acting analgesics, cyclooxygenase, notably the inducible isoform COX-2, plays a role in excitatory transmission within the CNS

(Kaufmann et al., 1996). Intrathecal administration of NSAIDs attenuate spinal cord neuropeptide release (Southall et al., 1998) and produce analgesia mediated by inhibition of dorsal horn prostaglandin synthesis (Malmberg and Yaksh, 1992, 1993). The analgesic effects of spinal NSAID administration are synergistic with those of spinal μ-opioid agonists and α_2-agonists (Malmberg and Yaksh, 1993), although mechanisms other than COX-1 or COX-2 inhibition have also been proposed (McCormack, 1994).

6. Cholecystokinin

The localization of cholecystokinin (CCK) immunoreactivity, together with that of its receptors CCK_A and CCK_B within the superficial dorsal horn of the spinal cord, mirrors that of endogenous opioids and their receptors (Coggleshall and Carlton, 1997). CCK receptors are localized on the central terminals of small nociceptive afferents (Coggleshall and Carlton, 1997) and CCK functions as an endogenous "antiopioid" system (Faris et al., 1983). Activation of CCK_B receptors may allosterically modulate opioid binding and promote the Ca^{2+}-mobilizing pathway of stimulatory opioid action. Furthermore, spinal administration of opioids results in release of endogenous CCK; this "antiopioid feedback" is attenuated in inflammatory pain, but up-regulated in neuropathic pain (De Araujo Lucas et al., 1998). Moreover, nerve injury is associated with up-regulation of spinal CCK immunoreactivity and receptor expression, which may partly underlie lack of opioid responsiveness in neuropathic pain.

CCK_B antagonists have antinociceptive actions at a spinal level, suppressing the development of pain behavior in rat models of nerve injury and potentiating the antiallodynic actions of opioids in experimental neuropathic pain (Xu et al., 1994; Nichols et al., 1996). Recent clinical data with the relatively weak nonspecific CCK antagonist proglumide indicates efficacy in human chronic pain (McLeane, 1998) and selective CCK_B antagonists are under development.

B. Inhibitory Targets

1. Opioid Receptors

Opioid administration remains the mainstay of clinical analgesia, and opioid efficacy reflects a combination of spinal, supplemented by supraspinal and peripheral actions.

Within the spinal cord, OP3 (μ), OP2 (κ), and OP1 (δ) opioid receptors are localized primarily within laminae I-II (and possibly deeper laminae) of the dorsal horn, although there is some discrepancy between ligand binding, immunohistochemical, and in situ hybridization data (Coggleshall and Carlton, 1997). Dorsal rhizotomy results in a variable loss (40–70%) of receptor expression within the superficial dorsal horn, indicating a predominant localization on presynaptic terminals of primary afferent nociceptors. In consequence, neuropathic pain following deafferentation may, to a greater or lesser degree, be opioid-resistant. Opioid receptors mediate spinal analgesia by presynaptic inhibition of nociceptive transmitter release from Aδ and C-fibers, together with attenuation of postsynaptic depolarization by inhibition of voltage-gated Ca^{2+} channels, activation of K^+ channels, and a reduction of cAMP (Jordan and Devi, 1998). Although the acute effects of opioid agonist–receptor interaction result in neuronal inhibition, opioids can paradoxically activate adenylate cyclase and potentiate synaptic Ca^{2+} signaling (Harrison et al., 1998). Stimulatory opioid effects with associated upregulation of NMDA receptor signaling are enhanced following nerve injury (Mao et al., 1995).

Leu- and met-enkephalin are found in high levels of the superficial dorsal horn, where they are endogenous ligands for the OP1 (δ) receptor and produce spinally mediated analgesia. Inhibitors of enkephalinase, such as RB120, are antinociceptive in animal models of nociceptive and inflammatory pain (Noble and Roques, 1997). Endogenous μ-ligands, such as endomorphin-

1 and endomorphin-2 (Zadina et al., 1997) are potent analgesics at dorsal horn targets (Chapman et al., 1997), although potentiation of their analgesic action through similar peptidase inhibitors has yet to be reported.

The orphan opioid receptor ORL1 and its endogenous ligand nociceptin have been recently described (see Darland and Grandy, 1998), and nociceptin has antihyperalgesic and antiallodynic effects (Hao et al., 1998) mediated by spinal ORL1 receptors identified in the dorsal horn. Although spinal ORL1 mechanisms mediate analgesia, ICV administration of nociceptin reverses opioid analgesia mediated by OP1, 2, and 3 receptors, indicating supraspinally mediated antalgesia that may limit the role of modulation of the ORL–nociceptin system as an analgesic target (see Darland and Grandy, 1998).

2. α_2-Receptors

Spinally administered α_2-agonists attenuate nocicieptive transmission within the dorsal horn and produce analgesia (Yaksh, 1985; Kamisaki et al., 1993). Binding sites for α_2-ligands are concentrated in laminae I-II of the dorsal horn although there is dispute over their relative pre- and postsynaptic distribution (Coggleshall and Carlton, 1997; Yaksh, 1998). Potentiation of endogenous release of norepinephrine from descending bulbospinal neurons (by inhibition of uptake-1 pathways) and consequent α_2-receptor activation, is likely to be the major mechanism of analgesic action of the "noradrenergic" tricyclic antidepressants such as amitriptyline.

Recent data indicates that (at least in neuropathic pain) α_2-mediated analgesia involves spinal muscarinic and cholinergic receptor activation with nitric oxide mechanisms (Pan et al., 1999) (Fig. 3), suggesting that α_2-receptors may be primarily located on spinal cholinergic interneurons. Spinal α_2-receptors (in conjunction with periaqueductal gray opioid receptors) mediate the analgesic actions of nitrous oxide (Guo et al., 1996). At least four subtypes of α_2-receptor have been identified that provide potential for the differentiation of spinally mediated analgesia, hypotension, and bradycardia (intermediolateral cell column) and supraspinal sedation (locus caeruleus) (see Kingery et al., 1997).

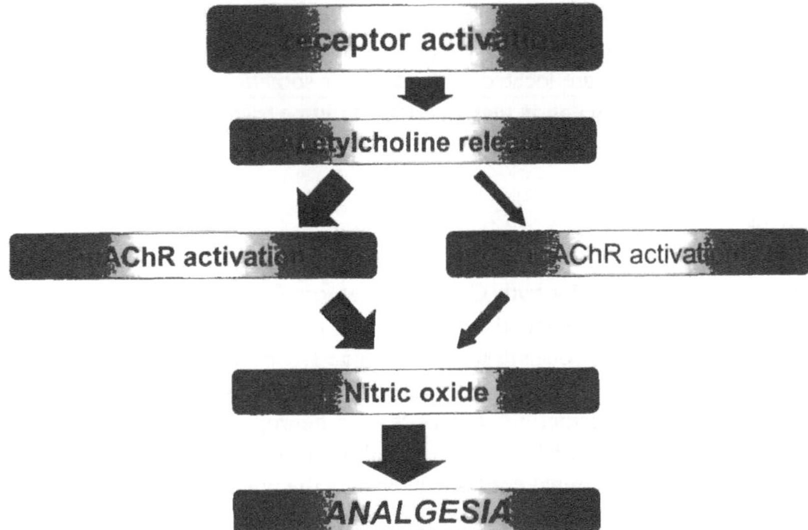

Figure 3 The mediation of muscarinic and nicotinic analgesic action may be in part through the release of nitric oxide.

3. Cholinergic Mechanisms

Acetylcholine release within the dorsal horn of the spinal cord from intrinsic interneurons or exogenous administration of cholinegic agonists produces both experimental antinociception and clinical analgesia (Yaksh et al., 1985; Hood et al., 1997). Cholinergic spinal analgesia involves primarily muscarinic (and to a lesser extent nicotinic) receptors mediating antinociception by nitric oxide synthesis and release. Spinal cholinergic mechanisms may play a key integrative role in both spinally mediated α_2-adrenergic and supraspinal opioid analgesia (see Pan et al., 1999 and references therein).

4. Adenosine

Nerve terminals releasing adenosine are concentrated within the superficial laminae of the dorsal horn where A_1 and A_2 adenosine receptors are situated on intrinsic spinal neurones (Geiger and Nagy, 1986; Choca et al., 1988). Intrathecal administration of adenosine agonists or potentiation of endogenous adenosine release results in antinociception in animal models of inflammatory and neuropathic pain (Delander and Keil, 1994; Poon and Sawynok, 1995; Poon and Sawynok, 1998; similar analgesia has been demonstrable in preclinical human studies (Rane et al., 1998). Endogenous adenosine release may partly mediate spinal opioid analgesia (Sawynok et al., 1989) and intrathecal coadministration of adenosine and morphine results in synergistic analgesic effects (Malmberg and Yaksh, 1993).

5. 5-HT Receptors

It is well established that release of serotonin (5-hydroxytryptamine; 5-HT) within the dorsal horn from serotonergic neurons plays an important role in descending modulatory analgesia (Stamford, 1995) and modulation of such pathways may contribute to the analgesic actions of antidepressant drugs with selective serotonin-reuptake inhibitor (SSRI) activity. However, intrathecal administration of 5-HT agonists has, in many studies, produced conflicting data dependent on experimental models and individual subtype specificity of the administered agent (see Stamford, 1995). This at least partly reflects the complexity of 5-HT receptor pharmacology, with at least seven cloned subtypes being identifiable, of which 5-HT_{1A}, 5-HT_3, and 5-HT_7 appear to predominate within the spinal cord (Coggleshall and Carlton, 1997). Within the superficial dorsal horn, many 5-HT receptors are located at dendritic or somatic, rather than "classic synaptic" loci, and serotonergic antinociception may involve "volume transmission" and multisynaptic mechanisms.

6. GABAergic Systems

γ-Aminobutyric acid (GABA) exerts a powerful inhibitory tone within the spinal cord dorsal horn (Game and Lodge, 1975) mediated by both GABA_A receptors (pre- and postsynaptic on primary afferents) and GABA_B receptors located principally on presynaptic sites (Hammond, 1997). GABAergic intrinsic neurons are concentrated in laminae I-II of the dorsal horn (Todd et al., 1996). Intrathecal administration of GABA_A agonists and GABA_B agonists produce antinociception in experimental models of acute, inflammatory, and neuropathic pain (Edwards et al., 1990; Smith et al., 1994). Modulation of GABAergic inhibition (together with inhibition of ectopic Na^+ channel activity) within the spinal cord dorsal horn is the predominant rationale for the use of various anticonvulsant drugs, such as sodium valproate (Boivie, 1994) and gabapentin (Wamil and Parris, 1997). Furthermore, enhancement of endogenous GABA release within the dorsal horn is still the most convincing mechanism of action of epidural spinal cord stimulation (Cui et al., 1996; Stiller et al., 1996; Yakhnitsa et al., 1999).

Although GABAergic inhibition may be up-regulated during peripheral inflammatory states (Castro–Lopes et al., 1992), GABAergic interneurons are vulnerable to excitotoxic or apoptotic death following nerve injury (Castro–Lopes et al., 1993; Ibuki et al., 1997; Azkue et al., 1998) resulting in "dark neuron" formation (Sugimoto et al., 1990) and a loss of inhibitory tone, contributing to hyperalgesia and allodynia.

7. Cannabinoids

The neuronal cannabinoid (CB1) receptor, cloned in 1990 (Matsuda et al., 1990), is a seven-transmembrane G_i protein-linked receptor that shares functional similarities with opioid mechanisms of action (Hirst et al., 1998). CB1 receptors are localized in the superficial dorsal horn (Herkenham et al., 1991) and intrathecal administration of CB1 agonists produce analgesia (Smith and Martin, 1992). Selective targeting of spinal CB1 receptors may provide an analgesic target without the supraspinally mediated psychotropic effects associated with systemic administration of cannabinoids.

8. Neuropeptide Y

In the central nervous system, neuropeptide Y-(NPY)-containing neurons and at least five distinct receptor subtypes are widely distributed throughout the brain and spinal cord (Hokfelt et al., 1998; Michel et al., 1998). The high density of NPY-positive interneurons in laminae I-II of the dorsal horn making synaptic contact with primary afferent neurons (Doyle and Maxwell, 1994) and their putative modulatory role in the spinal processing of nociceptive afferent input, indicates a likely role for NPY in spinal pain transduction (Cougnon et al., 1997).

NPY receptor activation has profound effects on neuronal excitability within the central nervous system (Colmers and Bleakman, 1994; Michel et al., 1998): such effects are clearly demonstrable at the level of the dorsal horn. Thus, NPY induces an outward (hyperpolarizing) current in small-diameter dorsal root ganglion neurons (Zhang et al., 1994) associated with a reduction in Ca^{2+} entry and transmitter release in vitro (Walker et al., 1988) and inhibits stimulus-evoked release of substance P within the dorsal horn in vivo (Duggan et al., 1991). Experimental intrathecal administration of NPY can produce analgesia to mechanical and thermal stimuli (Hua et al., 1991) and attenuate nociceptive spinal reflexes (Xu et al., 1994). However, the spectrum of receptor subtype(s) involved have not been definitively identified, and the net spinal effect may reflect a balance between Y_2-mediated analgesia and Y_1-mediated hyperalgesia (Hua et al., 1991; Xu et al., 1994; Cougnon et al., 1997). Paradoxically, the situation may be reversed at supraspinal sites where Y_1 receptor activation can produce analgesia (Broqua et al., 1996), although patterns of supraspinal analgesia or hyperalgesia appear test-specific (Mellado et al., 1996).

The dynamic changes in neuronal NPY expression, receptor number, and distribution following nerve injury or inflammation suggest that the role of this peptide transmitter system may be complex in chronic pain states and responses to acute administration of the peptide may not be predictive of longer-term administration.

V. SUPRASPINAL SITES

The neuroanatomy of ascending nociceptive pathways and descending inhibitory systems is beyond consideration within the scope of this volume (see, for example, Willis, 1985; Treede et al., 1999), and the neuropharmacology of the thalamocortical representation of pain is imprecisely understood. Nociceptive signaling and processing becomes increasingly complex as neurally encoded messages travel rostrally (Guilbaud et al., 1994); in consequence, only a very limited overview of supraspinal sites of analgesic action will be presented.

A. Modulation of Descending Inhibition

It is well established that there are powerful inhibitory (as well as facilitatory) influences on nociceptive transmission acting at many levels of the neuraxis (see Stamford, 1995). Descending inhibition may be activated by external factors such as stress (stress-induced analgesia) and noxious input (diffuse noxious inhibitory controls), or can be induced by peripheral or central nervous stimulation. There is also evidence for the ascending modulation of "higher" structures; stimulation in the periaqueductal gray matter can produce inhibition of the responses of neurons in the medial thalamus. Although it is possible that this inhibition may occur through the activation of descending pathways, it indicates that there are multiple interactions at many levels of the nervous system.

B. Brain Structures Involved in Descending Inhibition

Descending inhibitory influences arise from several supraspinal structures, including hypothalamus, periaqueductal gray matter (PAG), locus caeruleus, nucleus raphe magnus, and nucleus paragigantocellularis lateralis. Electrical stimulation or stereotactic administration of excitatory amino acids (EAA) into these regions produce antinociception or analgesia. It is essential to appreciate that although EAA mediate nociceptive responses at the dorsal horn (see Hudspith, 1997), their supraspinal effects include antinociception (Jensen and Yaksh, 1992; Jones, 1998) with consequent implications for systemic blockade of EAA receptor function.

The midbrain periaqueductal gray (PAG) plays a major role in descending inhibition (see Stamford, 1995; Siddall and Cousins, 1998). Stimulation in this region produces antinociception although the PAG does not project directly to the spinal cord. Descending fibers from the PAG project into several structures involved in descending inhibition: these include the nucleus raphe magnus (NRM) and the paragigantocellular nucleus (NRPG) situated lateral to the NRM. It has been demonstrated that analgesia obtained from the dorsal PAG is nonopioid in nature, whereas opioid analgesia is obtained from stimulation of the ventrolateral PAG (Bandler and Shipley, 1994).

Stimulation of the midline (NRM) or ventrolateral (NRPG) medulla results in antinociception. Fibers descend directly from these regions to the dorsal horn of the spinal cord, suggesting a role in descending inhibition and relaying information from the PAG. Tracts from these structures descend predominantly in the dorsolateral funiculus of the spinal cord and terminate in laminae I, II, and V. Furthermore, stimulation of the locus caeruleus, the main noradrenergic nucleus involved in nociception, results in inhibition of nociceptive-evoked dorsal horn activity (Stamford, 1995). This nucleus receives inputs from several brain structures and provides descending inputs to the spinal dorsal horn. These descending fibers travel ipsilaterally in the ventrolateral funiculus.

Terminations of descending pathways interact with several different neural elements in the dorsal horn. These include projection neurons that transmit information from spinal cord to the brain; local interneurons within the spinal cord and primary afferent terminals. Inhibition may occur presynaptically by modulation of transmitter release or postsynaptically by either producing an excitation of local inhibitory interneurons or a direct inhibitory action on second-order projection neurons. The pharmacology of spinal mechanisms of the major descending pathways have been considered in previous sections.

C. Neurosurgical Considerations

Many surgical and percutaneous procedures have been employed to disrupt specific tracts within the spinal cord cephalad to the first-order synapse within the dorsal horn: these include cordotomy, extraleminscal myelotomy, and commissural myelotomy (Tasker, 1994). The distribution of fibers associated with pain transmission within the anterolateral quadrant would suggest that section of these tracts using an anterolateral cordotomy should be a useful procedure in abolishing or relieving pain. This concept is based on the Cartesian or ''private line'' model of pain perception, and results are variable and often transient. Sometimes, excellent relief can be obtained in the short term, but long-term results are usually disappointing and complications include return of pain, motor weakness, and loss of bladder and bowel function. Similar limitations apply to stereotactic lesions of the thalamic nuclei and other supraspinal sites (see Tasker, 1994).

An alternative neurosurgical approach is the stereotactic implantation of electrodes to stimulate descending modulatory centers, such as PAG, NRM, or the ventroposterolateral (VPL) thalamic nuclei. Such invasive approaches have not been widely exploited and readers are referred elsewhere for further detail (Young and Rinaldi, 1994).

D. Selected Pharmacological Targets

1. Opioid and GABAergic Mechanisms

Opioid receptors, primarily μ (OP3) and κ (OP2), are synthesized and expressed in the PAG, NRM, and LC (Mansour et al., 1995) and may be tonically activated by endogenous peptide opioid ligands, including endomorphins 1 and 2, β-endorphin, and dynorphin. Although the mRNA and receptor protein for the orphan opioid receptor ORL1 has a similar distribution, its role in modulation of supraspinal analgesia or antalgesia is uncertain (Darland and Grandy, 1998). Supraspinal opioid analgesia is in part a result of increased (predominantly noradrenergic) descending control, enhancement of which is the primary analgesic mechanism of nitrous oxide (Guo et al., 1996). Supraspinal opioid receptors also mediate direct inhibition of nociceptive transmission at brain stem levels, indirect inhibition of brain stem projection neurons, ascending modulation, and corticothalamic inhibition (see Jensen, 1997 for further discussion).

Notably, opioid-mediated activation of descending pathways involves inhibition of GABAergic inhibitory interneurons evoking $GABA_A$ receptor-mediated inhibition of noradrenergic neurons; in consequence, supraspinal actions of $GABA_A$ agonists, such as midazolam, may produce antinociception and antagonize opioid analgesia (Luger et al., 1995). The role of supraspinal $GABA_B$ receptor mechanisms is less clear: stereotactic injection of the $GABA_B$ agonist baclofen into the NRM produces dose-dependent biphasic responses of analgesia and antalgesia (Hammond, 1997).

2. Serotonin

Serotonin (5-HT) has been long suggested as a major neurotransmitter candidate in descending controls; noxious stimuli are associated with an increased turnover of 5-HT in the NRM (Stamford, 1995), and serotonergic analgesia reflects a combination of medullary and spinal influences. Serotonin is contained within a high proportion of NRM cells, terminals of descending fibers in the dorsal horn contain 5-HT, and electrical stimulation of the NRM results in an increased release of 5-HT in the spinal cord. Agents that block the synthesis of 5-HT attenuate stimulation-produced analgesia, and application of some 5-HT agonists in the spinal cord results in inhibition of cells responsive to nociceptive stimuli.

3. Norepinephrine

Although there is ample evidence (see foregoing) for norepinephrine exerting analgesic actions through α_2-receptors at the level of the dorsal horn, there are no known noradrenergic neuronal cell bodies within the dorsal horn. The locus caeruleus (LC) is the major site of descending noradrenergic neurons and lesions of the LC markedly reduce spinal NA content (Ossipov et al., 1985). High concentrations of α_2-receptors are expressed in the LC, and intracerebroventricular administration of α_2-agonists can produce antinociception, perhaps by an opioid interneuronal circuit (Kingery et al., 1997). However, the more profound effect of LC α_2-receptor activation is EEG synchronization and sedation and the spinal α_2-receptor(s) is a more attractive analgesic target; recent data (Buerkle and Yaksh, 1998) indicates that sedation and analgesia may be differentially mediated.

4. Cannabinoids

In addition to the spinal actions of CB1 cannabinoid receptors, it has recently been reported that endogenous cannabinoid ligands (Di Marzo et al., 1998) mediate analgesia in the RVM involving brain stem circuitry and mechanisms analagous to that of supraspinal opioid analgesia (Meng et al., 1998). Brain stem respiratory centers do not express cannabinoid receptors, providing optimism that centrally acting cannabinoid analgesics may not produce respiratory depression.

VI. SUMMARY

Nociceptive signaling, transduction, and processing involve a highly complex set of neuronal pathways that potentially exhibit plasticity of processing at transducer, axonal, and synaptic loci. The nociceptive system is neither "hard-wired" nor wholly pharmacologically exclusive within the realm of currently available clinical analgesics. However, as is evident from this chapter, there exist a plethora of potential sites of analgesic action that may be exploited with the development of agents directed toward both peripheral and spinal targets. Within the peripheral and central nervous system, dynamic changes of neuronal phenotype in response to injury differ diametrically, dependent on the nature of the noxious stimuli. Such phenotypic changes, which many chapters in this volume describe, provide optimism for the reality of selective and effective analgesia tailored to specific pathologies.

REFERENCES

Akopian AN, Sivilotti L, Wood JN. A tetrodotoxin-resistant sodium channel expressed by sensory neurones. Nature 1996; 379:257–262.

Averill S, McMahon SB, Clary DO, Reichardt LF, Priestley JVP. Immunocytochemical localisation of trkA receptors in chemically identified subgroups of adult rat sensory neurones. Eur J Neurosci 1995; 7:1484–1494.

Azkue JJ, Zimmermann M, Hsieh T-F, Herdergen T. Peripheral nerve insult induced NMDA receptor-mediated delayed degeneration in spinal neurons. Eur J Neurosci 1998; 10:2204–2206.

Bandler R, Shipley MT. Columnar organisation of the midbrain periaqueductal gray. Trends Neurosci 1994; 17:379–389.

Basbaum AI. Spinal mechanisms of acute and persistent pain. Reg Anesth Pain Med 1999; 24:59–67.

Block G, Rue D, Panebianco D, Reines S. The substance P antagonist L-754,030 is ineffective in the treatment of postherpetic neuralgia. Am Acad Neurol, Annual Meeting, Minneapolis, April 1998.

Boivie J. Central pain. In: Wall PD, Melzack R, eds. Textbook of Pain. Edinburgh: Churchill Livingstone, 1994:871–902.

Bredt DS, Hwang PM, Snyder SH. Localisation of nitric oxide synthase indicating a neural role for nitric oxide. Nature 1990; 347:768–770.

Brennan TJ. AMPA/kainate receptor antagonists as novel analgesic agents [editorial]. Anesthesiology 1998; 89:1049–1050.

Broqua P, Wettstein JG, Rocher M–N, Gauthier–Martin B, Riviere PJM, Junien J–L, Dahl SG. Antinociceptive effects of neuropeptide Y and related peptides in mice. Brain 1996; 724:25–32.

Buerkle H, Yaksh TL. Pharmacological evidence for different alpha$_2$-adrenergic receptor sites mediating analgesia and sedation in the rat. Br J Anaesth 1998; 81:208–215.

Burnstock G. A unifying purinergic hypothesis for the initiation of pain. Lancet 1996; 347:1604–1605.

Caffrey JM, Eng DL, Black JA, Waxman SG, Kocsis JD. Three types of sodium channels in adult rat dorsal root ganglion neurons. Brain Res 1992; 592:283–297.

Cao YQ, Mantyh PW, Carlson EJ, Gillespie AM, Epstein CJH, Basbaum AI. Primary afferent tachykinins are required to experience moderate to intense pain. Nature 1998; 392:390–394.

Castro–Lopes JM, Tavaras I, Tolle TR, Coito A, Coimbra A. Increase in GABAergic cells and GABA levels in the spinal cord in unilateral inflammation in the hind limb in the rat. Eur J Neurosci 1992; 4:296–301.

Castro–Lopes JM, Tavares I, Coimbra A. GABA decreases in the spinal cord dorsal horn after peripheral neurectomy. Brain Res 1993; 620:287–291.

Caterina MJ, Schumacher MA, Tominaga M, Rosen TA, Levine JD, Julius D. The capsaicin receptors: a heat activated ion channel in the pain pathway. Nature 1997; 389:816–824.

Chapman V, Diaz A, Dickenson AH. Distinct inhibitory effects of spinal endomorphin-1 and endomorphin-2 on evoked dorsal horn responses in the rat. Br J Pharmacol 1997; 122:1537–1539.

Choca JI, Green RD, Proudfit HK. Adenosine A1 and A2 receptors of the substantia gelatinosa are located predominantly on intrinsic neurons: an autoradiographic study. J Pharmacol Exp Ther 1988; 247: 757–764.

Coggleshall RE, Carlton SM. Receptor localisation in the mammalian dorsal horn and primary afferent neurons. Brain Res Rev 1997; 24:28–66.

Colmers WF, Bleakman D. Effects of neuropeptide Y on the electrical properties of neurons. Trends Neurosci 1994; 17:373–379.

Cougnon N, Hudspith MJ, Munglani R. The therapeutic potential of neuropeptide Y in central nervous system disorders with special reference to pain and sympathetically maintained pain. Expert Opin Invest Drugs 1997; 6:759–769.

Cui J–G, Linderoth B, Meyerson BA. Effects of spinal cord stimulation on touch-evoked allodynia involve GABAergic mechanisms. Pain 1996; 66:287–295.

Dado RJ, Law P–Y, Loh HH, Elde R. Immunofluorescent identification of delta-opioid receptor on primary afferent nerve terminals. Neuroreport 1993; 5:341–344.

Darland T, Grandy DK. The orphanin FQ system: an emerging target in the management of pain? Br J Anaesth 1998; 81:29–37.

De Araujo Lucas G, Alster P, Brodin E, Wiesenfeld–Hallin Z. Differential release of cholecystokinin by morphine in rat spinal cord. Neurosci Lett 1998; 245:13–16.

De Felipe C, Herrero JF, O'Brien JA, Palmer JA, Doyle CA, Smith AJH, Laird JMA, Belmonte C, Cervero F, Hunt SP. Altered nociception, analgesia and aggression in mice lacking the receptor for substance P. Nature 1998; 329:394–397.

Delander GE, Keil GJ. Antinociception induced by intrathecal coadministration of selective adenosine receptor and selective opioid receptor agonists in mice. J Pharmacol Exp Ther 1994; 268:943–951.

Di Marzo V, Melck D, Bisogno T, De Petrocellis. Endocannabinoids: endogenous cannabinoid receptor ligands with neuromodulatory action. Trends Neurosci 1998; 521–528.

Doyle CA, Maxwell DJ. Light and electron-microscopic analysis of neuropeptide Y immunoreactive profiles in the cat spinal dorsal horn. Neuroscience 1994; 61:107–121.

Dray A. Inflammatory mediators of pain. Br J Anaesth 1995; 75:125–131.

Duggan AW, Hope PJ, Lang CW. Microinjection of neuropeptide Y into the superficial dorsal horn reduces stimulus evoked release of immunoreactive substance P in the anaesthetized cat. Neuroscience 1991; 44:733–740.

Edwards M, Serrao JM, Gent JP, Goodchild CS. On the mechanism by which midazolam causes spinally mediated analgesia. Anesthesiology 1990; 73:273–277.

England JD, Happel LT, Kline DG, Gamboni F, Thouron CL, Liu ZP, Levinson SR. Sodium channel accumulation in humans with painful neuromas. Neurology 1996; 47:272–276.

Faris PL, Komisaruk BR, Watkins LR, Mayer DJ. Evidence that the neuropeptide cholecystokinin is an antagonist of opiate analgesia. Science 1983; 219:310–312.

Feng L, Sun W, Xia Y, et al. Cloning two isoforms of rat cyclooxygenase: differential regulation of their expression. Arch Biochem Biophys 1993; 307:361–368.

Ferreira SH. Prostaglandins, aspirin-like drugs and analgesia. Nature 1972; 240:200–203.

Fields HL, Basbaum AI. Central nervous system mechanisms of pain modulation. In Melzack R, Wall PD, eds. Textbook of Pain. 3rd ed. Edinburgh: Churchill Livingstone, 1994:243–260.

Fisher K, Fundytus ME, Cahill CM, Coderre TJ. Intrathecal administration of the mGluR compound, (S)-4CPG, attenuates hyperalgesia. Pain 1998; 77:59–66.

Friedel RH, Schnurch H, Stubbusch J, Barde Y-A. Identification of genes differentially expressed by nerve growth factor- and neurotrophin-3-dependent sensory neurons. Proc Natl Acad Sci USA 1997; 94: 12670–12675.

Game CJA, Lodge D. The pharmacology of the inhibition of dorsal horn neurones by impulses in myelinated cutaneous afferents in the cat. Exp Brain Res 1975; 23:75–84.

Garthwaite J, Charles SL, Chess–Williams R. Endothelium-derived relaxing factor release on activation of NMDA receptors suggests role as intercellular messenger in the brain. Nature 1988; 336:385–388.

Geiger JD, Nagy JI. Distribution of adenosine deaminase activity in rat brain and spinal cord. J Neurosci 1986; 4:2303–2310.

Gold M, Reichling DB, Shuster MJ, Levine JD. Hyperalgesic agents increase a tetrodotoxin-resistant Na^+ current in nociceptors. Proc Nat Acad Sci USA 1996; 93:1108–1112.

Guilbaud G, Bernard JF, Besson JM. Brain areas involved in nociception and pain. In: Wall PD, Melzack R, eds. Textbook of pain. 3rd ed. Edinburgh: Churchill, 1994:113–128.

Guo T-Z, Poree L, Golden W, Stein J, Fujinaga M, Maze M. Antinociceptive response to nitrous oxide is mediated by supraspinal opiate and spinal a_2 adrenergic receptors in the rat. Anesthesiology 1996; 85:846–852.

Hammond DL. Inhibitory transmitters and nociception: role of GABA and glycine. In: Dickenson AH, Besson J-M, eds. Handbook of Experimental Pharmacology. The Pharmacology of Pain. Berlin: Springer-Verlag, 1997.

Handy RLC, Moore PK. Effects of selective inhibitors of neuronal nitric oxide synthase on carrageenan-induced mechanical and thermal hyperalgesia. Neuropharmacology 1998; 37:37–43.

Hao J–X, Xu IS, Wiesenfeld–Hallin Z, Xu X–J. Anti-hyperalgesic and anti-allodynic effects of intrathecal nocicieptin/orphanin FQ in rats after spinal cord injury, nerve injury and inflammation. Pain 1998; 76:385–393.

Harrison C, Smart, Lambert DG. Stimulatory effects of opioids. Br J Anaesth 1998; 81:20–28.

Hassan AHS, Ableitner A, Stein C, Herz A. Inflammation of the rat paw enhances axonal transport of opioid receptors in the sciatic nerve and increases their density in inflamed tissue. Neuroscience 1995; 55:185–195.

Herkenham M, Lynn AB, Johnson MR, Melvin LS, de Costa BR, Rice KC. Characterisation and localisation of cannabinoid receptors in rat brain. J Neurosci 1991; 11:563–583.

Hirst RA, Lambert DG, Notcutt WG. Pharmacology and potential therapeutic uses of cannabis. Br J Anaesth 1998; 81:77–84.

Hla T, Nielson K. Human cyclo-oxygenase-1 cDNA. Proc Nat Acad Sci USA 1992; 89:7389–98.

Hokfelt T, Broberger C, Zhang X, Diez M, Kopp J, Xu X–J, Landry M, Bao L, Schalling M, Koisinaho J, DeArmond SJ, Prusiner S, Gong J, Walsh JH. Neuropeptide Y: some viewpoints on a multifaceted peptide in the normal and diseased nervous system. Brain Res Rev 1998; 26:154–166.

Hood DD, Mallak KA, James RL, Tuttle R, Eisenach JC. Enhancement of analgesia from systemic opioid administration in humans by spinal cholinesterase inhibition. J Pharmacol Exp Ther 1997; 282:86–92.

Hua X, Boublik JH, Spicer MA, Rivier JE, Yaksh TL. The antinociceptive effect of spinally administered neuropeptide Y: systemic studies on structure–activity relationships. J Pharmacol Exp Ther 1991; 258:243–248.

Hudspith MJ. Glutamate: a role in normal brain function, anaesthesia, analgesia and CNS injury. Br J Anaesth 1997; 78:731–747.

Hudspith MJ, Munglani R. A role for presynaptic NMDA receptors in central sensitisation? Br J An 1998; 81:294–295.

Ibuki T, Hama AT, Wang XT, Pappas GD, Sagen J. Loss of GABA-immunoreactivity in the spinal dorsal horn of rats with peripheral nerve injury and promotion of recovery by adrenal medullary grafts. Neuroscience 1997; 76:845–858.

Jensen TS, Yaksh TL. The antinociceptive activity of excitatory amino acids in the rat brainstem: an anatomical and pharmacological analysis. Brain Res 1992; 569:255–267.

Jensen TS. Opioids in the brain: supraspinal mechanisms in pain control. Acta Anaesthesiol Scand 1997; 41:123–132.

Ji R–R, Zhang Q, Law P–Y, et al. Expression of μ-, δ-, and κ-opioid receptor-like immunoreactivity in rat dorsal root ganglia after carageenan-induced inflammation. J Neurosci 1995; 15:8156–8166.

Jones SL. Noxious heat-evoked fos-like immunoreactivity in the rat lumbar dorsal horn is inhibited by glutamate microinjections in the upper cervical spinal cord. Brain Res 1998; 788:337–340.

Jordan B, Devi LA. Molecular mechanisms of opioid receptor signal transduction. Br J Anaesth 1998; 81: 12–19.

Kamisaki Y, Hamada T, Maeda K, Ishimura M, Itoh T. Presynaptic a_2-adrenoceptors inhibit glutamate release from rat spinal cord synaptosomes. J Neurochem 1993; 60:522–526.

Kaufmann W, Worley PF, Pegg J, Bremer M, Isakson P. COX-2, a synaptically induced enzyme, is expressed by excitatory neurons at postsynaptic sites in rat cerebral cortex. Proc Nat Acad Sci USA 1996; 93:2317–2321.

Kingery WS, Davies MF, Maze M. Molecular mechanisms for the analgesic properties of alpha-2 adrenergic agonists. In: Borsook D, ed. Molecular Biology of Pain. Seattle: IASP, 1997:275–306.

Kohrs R, Durieux M. Ketamine: teaching and old drug new tricks. Anesth Analg 1998; 87:1186–1193.

Kral MG, Xiong Z, Study RE. Alteration of Na^+ currents in dorsal root ganglion neurons from rats with a painful neuropathy. Pain 1999; 81:15–24.

Lewin GR, Rueff A, Mendell LM. Peripheral and central mechanisms of NGF induced hyperalgesia. Eur J Neurosci 1994; 6:1903–1912.

Liu H, Mantyh PW, Basbaum AI. NMDA-receptor regulation of substance P release from primary afferent nociceptors. Nature 1997; 386:721–724.

Longmore J, Swain CJ, Hill RG. Neurokinin receptors. Drug News Perspect 1995; 8:5–23.

Luger TJ, Hayashi T, Weiss CG, Hill HF. The spinal potentiation effect and the supraspinal inhibitory effect of midazolam on opioid induced analgesia in rats. Eur J Pharmacol 1995; 275:153–162.

Maekawa K, Minami M, Yabuuchi K, et al. In situ hybridisation study of mu and kappa opioid receptor mRNAs in the rat spinal cord and dorsal root ganglia. Neurosci Lett 1994; 168:97–100.

Malmberg A, Yaksh T. Pharmacology of the spinal action of ketorolac, morphine, ST-91, U50488H, and L-PIA on the formalin test and an isobolographic analysis of the NSAID interaction. Anesthesiology 1993; 79:270–281.

Malmberg AB, Yaksh TL. Hyperalgesia mediated by spinal glutamate or substance P receptor blocked by spinal cyclooxygenase inhibition. Science 1992; 257:1276–1279.

Mansour A, Fox CA, Akil H, Watson SJ. Opioid receptor mRNA expression in the rat CNS: anatomical and functional considerations. Trends Neurosci 1995; 18:22–29.

Mao J, Price DD, Mayer DJ. Mechanisms of hyperalgesia and morphine tolerance: a current view of their possible interactions. Pain 1995; 62:259–274.

Matsuda LA, Lolait SJ, Brownstein MJ, Young AC, Bonner TI. Structure of a cannabinoid receptor and functional expression of the cloned cDNA. Nature 1990; 346:561–564.

McCormack K. Non-steroidal anti-inflammatory drugs and spinal nocicepetive processing. Pain 1994; 59: 9–43.

McLeane GJ. The cholecystokinin antagonist proglumide enhances the analgesic efficacy of morphine in humans with chronic benign pain. Anesth Analg 1998; 87:1117–1120.

McMahon SB, Bennett DLH, Priestley JV, Shelton D. The biological effects of endogenous NGF in adult sensory neurones revealed by a trkA–IgG fusion molecule. Nat Med 1995; 1:774–780.

McMahon SB, Bennett DLH, Michael GJ, Priestley JV. Neurotrophic factors and pain. In: Jensen TS, Turner JA, Wiesenfeld-Hallin Z, eds. Proceedings of the 8th World Congress on Pain. Seattle: IASP, 1997:353–379.

McQuay H, Carroll D, Jasdad AR, Wiffen P, Moore. Anticonvulsant drugs for management of pain: a systematic review. Br Med J 1995; 311:1047–1052.

Mellado ML, Gibert Rahola J, Chover AJ, Mico JA. Effect on nociception of intracerebroventricular administration of low doses of neuropeptide Y in mice. Life Sci 1996; 58:2409–14.

Meller ST, Gebhart GF. Nitric oxide (NO) and nociceptive processing in the spinal cord. Pain 1993; 52: 127–136.

Meller ST, Pechman PS, Gebhart GF, Maves TJ. Nitric oxide mediates the thermal hyperalgesia produced in a model of neuropathic pain in the rat. Neuroscience 1992; 50:7–10.

Meng ID, Manning BH, Martin MJ, Fields HL. An analgesia circuit activated by cannabinoids. Nature 1998; 395:381–383.

Michel MC, Beck–Sickinger A, Cox H, Doods HN, Herzog H, Larhammar D, Quirion R, Schwartz T, Westfall T. International Union of Pharmacology recommendations for the nomenclature of neuropeptide Y, peptide YY, and pancreatic polypeptide receptors. Pharmacol Rev 1998; 50:143–150.

Mitchell JA, Akarasereenont P, Thiemermann C, Flower RJ, Vane JR. Selectivity of nonsteroidal antiinflammatory drugs as inhibitors of constitutive and inducible cyclooxygenase. Proc Nat Acad Sci USA 1993; 90:11693–11697.

Munglani R, Hill R. New drugs including sympathetic block. In: Melzack R, Wall PD, eds. Textbook of Pain. 4th ed. Edinburgh: Churchill Livingstone, 1999.

Nichols ML, Bian D, Ossipov MH, Malan TP, Porreca F. Antiallodynic effects of a CCKB antagonist in rats with nerve ligation injury—role of endogenous enkephalins. Neurosci Lett 1996; 215:161–164.

Noble F, Roques BP. New research approach to the treatment of pain: the development of complete inhibitors of the enkephalin metabolism. In: Jensen TS, Turner JA, Wiesenfeld–Hallin Z, eds. Proceedings of the 8th World Congress on Pain. Seattle: IASP, 1997:759–782.

Okuse K, Akopian AN, Sivilotti L, Souslova VA, England S, Dolphin AC, Wood JN. Sensory neuron voltage-gated sodium channels and nociception. In: Borsook D, ed. Molecular Neurobiology of Pain. Seattle, IASP, 1997:239–257.

Ossipov MH, Chatterjee TK, Gebhart GF. Locus coeruleus lesions in the rat enhance the antinocicieptive potency of centrally administered clonidine but not morphine. Brain Res 1985; 41:320–330.

Pan H–L, Chen S–R, Eisenach JC. Intrathecal clonidine alleviates allodynia in neuropathic rats: interaction with spinal muscarinic and nicotinic receptors. Anesthesiology 1999; 90:509–514.

Pancrazio JJ, Kamatchi GL, Roscoe AK, Lynch C. Inhibition of neuronal Na^+ channels by antidepressant drugs? J Pharm Exp Ther 1998; 284:208–214.

Pitchford S, Levine JD. Prostaglandins sensitize nociceptors in cell culture. Neurosci Lett 1991; 132:105–108.

Poon A, Sawynok J. Antinociception by adenosine analogs and inhibitors of adenosine metabolism in an inflammatory thermal hyperalgesia model in the rat. Pain 1998; 74:234–245.

Poon A, Sawynok J. Antinociception by adenosine analogs and an adenosine kinase inhibitor: Dependence on formalin concentration. Eur J Pharmacol 1995; 286:177–184.

Quasthoff S, Grosskreutz J, Schroder JM, Schneider U, Grafe P. Calcium potentials and tetrodotoxin resistant sodium potentials in unmyelinated C fibres of biopsied human sural nerve. Neuroscience 1995; 69:955–965.

Rane K, Segersdal M, Goiny M, Sollevi A. Intrathecal adenosine administration (a phase 1 clinical safety study in healthy volunteers, with additional evaluation of its influence on sensory thresholds and experimental pain). Anesthesiology 1998; 89:1108–1115.

Rang HP, Bevan S, Dray A. Nociceptive peripheral neurons: cellular properties. In: Wall PD, Melzack R, eds. Textbook of Pain. 3rd ed. Edinburgh: Churchill Livingstone, 1994:57–78.

Reinhardt RR, Laub JB, Fricke J, Polis AB, Gertz BJ. Comparison of a neurokinin-1 antagonist, L-754,030, to placebo, acetaminophen and ibuprofen in the dental pain model. Am Soc Clin Pharm Ther, New Orleans, March 1998.

Rizzo MA, Kocsis JD, Waxman SG. Mechanisms of paresthesiae, dyesthesiae and hyperesthesiae: role of Na^+ channel heterogeneity. Eur Neurol 1996; 36:3–12.

Roche AK, Cook M, Wilcox GL, Kajander KC. A nitric oxide synthesis inhibitor (L-NAME) reduces licking behavior and Fos-labeling in the spinal cord of rats during formalin-induced inflammation. Pain 1996; 66:331–341.

Rush AM, Elliot JR. Phenytoin and carbamazepine: differential inhibition of sodium currents in small cells from adult rat dorsal root ganglia. Neurosci Lett 1997; 226:95–98.

Sawynok J, Sweeney MI, White TD. Adenosine release may mediate spinal analgesia by morphine. Trends Pharmacol Sci 1989; 10:186–189.

Schmidt R, Schmelz M, Forster C, et al. Novel class of responsive and unresponsive C nociceptors in human skin. J Neurosci 1995; 15:333–341.

Scholz A, Kuboyama N, Hempelmann G, Vogel W. Complex block of TTX-resistant Na^+ currents by lidocaine and bupivicaine reduce firing frequency in DRG neurons. J Neurophysiol 1998; 79:1746–1754.

Siddall PJ, Cousins MJ. Introduction to pain mechanisms. In: Cousins MJ, Bridenbaugh PO, eds. Neural Blockade. 3rd ed. Philadelphia: Lippincott–Raven, 1998:675–714.

Smith GD, Harrison SM, Birch PJ, Elliott PJ, Malcangio M, Bowery NG. Increased sensitivity to the antinociceptive activity of (+/−)-baclofen in an animal model of chronic neuropathic, but not chronic inflammatory hyperalgesia. Neuropharmacology 1994; 33:1103–1108.

Smith PB, Martin BR. Spinal mechanisms of delta-9 tetrahydrocannabinol-induced analgesia. Brain Res 1992; 578:8–12.

Southall MD, Michael RL, Vasko MR. Intrathecal NSAIDS attenuate inflammation-induced neuropeptide release from rat spinal cord slices. Pain 1998; 78:39–48.

Stamford JA. Descending control of pain. Br J Anaesth 1995; 75:217–227.

Stein C, Schafer M, Cabot PJ, Zhang Q, Zhou L, Carter L. Opioids and inflammation. In: Borsook D, ed. Molecular Neurobiology of Pain. Seattle: IASP, 1997:25–43.

Stiller C–O, Cui J–G, O'Connor W, Brodin E, Meyerson BA, Linderoth B. Release of gamma-amino butyric acid in the dorsal horn and suppression of tactile allodynia by spinal cord stimulation in mononeuropathic rats. Neurosurgery 1996; 367–375.

Sugimoto T, Bennett GJ, Kajander KC. Transsynaptic degeneration in the superficial dorsal horn after sciatic nerve injury: effects of a chronic constriction injury, transection, and strychnine. Pain 1990; 42:205–213.

Tanner KD, Gold MS, Reichling DB, Levine JD. Transduction and excitability in nociceptors: dynamic phenomena. In: Borsook D, ed. Molecular Neurobiology of Pain. Seattle: IASP, 1997:79–105.

Tasker RR. Stereotactic surgery. In: Wall PD, Melzack R, eds. Textbook of Pain. 3rd ed. Edinburgh: Churchill. 1994:1137–1158.

Todd AJ, Watt C, Spike RC, Sieghart W. Colocalization of GABA, glycine, and their receptors at synapses in the rat spinal cord. J Neurosci 1996; 16:974–982.

Tolle TR, Berthle A, Zieglgansberger W, Seeburg PH, Wisden W. The differential expression of 16 NMDA and non-NMDA receptor subunits in the rat spinal cord and periaqueductal gray. J Neurosci 1993; 13:5009–5028.

Tominaga M, Caterina MJ, Malmberg AB, et al. The cloned capsaicin receptor integrates multiple pain producing stimuli. Neuron 1998; 21:531–543.

Treede R–D, Kenshalo DR, Gracely RH, Jones AKP. The cortical representation of pain. Pain 1999; 79: 105–111.

Vane JR. Inhibition of prostaglandin synthesis as a mechanism of action for aspirin-like drugs. Nature 1971; 291:233–238.

Walker MW, Ewald DA, Perney TM, Miller RJ. Neuropeptide Y modulates neurotransmitter release and Ca^{2+} currents in rat sensory neurons. J Neurosci 1988; 8:2438–2446.

Wamil AW, Parris WCV. Consideration of the analgesic efficacy of gabapentin. Curr Rev Pain 1997; 1: 251–263.

Webb J, Kamali F. Analgesic effects of lamotrigine and phenytoin on cold induced pain: a cross over, placebo controlled study in healthy volunteers. Pain 1998; 76:357–363.

Willis WD. The Pain System. The Neural Basis of Nociceptive Transmission in the Mammalian Nervous System. Basel: Karger, 1985.

Wood JN, Docherty R. Chemical activators of sensory neurons. Annu Rev Physiol 1997; 59:457–482.

Woolf CJ. Windup and central sensitization are not equivalent. Pain 1996; 66:105–108.

Woolf CJ, Chong M. Pre-emptive analgesia-treating postoperative pain by preventing the establishment of central sensitization. Anaesth Analg 1993; 77:362–379.

Xie X, Lancaster B, Peakman T, Garthwaite J. Interaction of the antiepileptic drug lamotrigine with recombinant rat brain type IIA Na^+ channels. Pflugers Arch Eur J Physiol 1995; 430:437–446.

Xu X-J, Hao J-X, Hokfelt T, Wiesenfeld–Hallin Z. The effects of intrathecal neuropeptide Y on the spinal nociceptive flexor reflex in rats with intact sciatic nerves and after peripheral axotomy. Neuroscience 1994; 63:817–826.

Xu XJ, Hokfelt T, Hughes J, Wiesenfeld–Hallin Z. The CCK-B antagonist CI988 enhances the reflex-depressive effect of morphine in axotomized rats. Neuroreport 1994; 5:718–720.

Yakhnitsa V, Linderoth B, Meyerson BA. Spinal cord stimulation attenuates dorsal horn neuronal hyperexcitability in a rat model of mononeuropathy. Pain 1999; 79:223–233.

Yaksh TL, Dirksen R, Harty GJ. Antinociceptive effects of intrathecally injected cholinomimetic drugs in the rat and cat. Eur J Pharmacol 1985; 117:81–88.

Yaksh TL. Pharmacology of spinal adrenergic systems which modulate spinal nociceptive processing. Pharmacol Biochem Behav 1985; 22:845–858.

Yaksh TL. Physiologic and pharmacologic substrates of nociception and nerve injury. In: Cousins MJ, Bridenbaugh PO, eds. Neural Blockade. 3rd ed. Philadelphia: Lippincott–Raven, 1998:727–780.

Young RF, Rinaldi PC. Brain stimulation for relief of chronic pain. In: Wall PD, Melzack R, eds. Textbook of Pain. 3rd ed. Edinburgh: Churchill, 1994:1225–1233.

Zadina JE, Hackler L, Ge L–J, Kastin AJ. A potent and selective endogenous agonist for the μ-opiate receptor. Nature 1997; 386:499–502.

Zahn PK, Umali E, Brennan TJ. Intrathecal non-NMDA excitatory amino acid antagonists inhibit pain behaviors in a rat model of postoperative pain. Pain 1998; 74:213–223.

Zahn PK, Brennan TJ. Lack of effect of intrathecally administered *N*-methyl-D-aspartate receptor antagonists in a rat model for postoperative pain. Anesthesiology 1998; 88:143–156.

Zhang X, Bao L, Xu ZQ, Kopp J, Arvidsson U, Elde R, Hokfelt T. Localization of neuropeptide Y Y1 receptors in the rat nervous system with special reference to somatic receptors on small dorsal root ganglion neurons. Proc Nat Acad Sci USA 1994; 91:11738–11742.

Zhang X, Verge V, Wiesenfeldhallin Z, Ju G, Bredt D, Snyder SH, Hokfelt T. Nitric oxide synthase-like immunoreactivity in lumbar dorsal root ganglia and spinal cord of rat and monkey and effect of peripheral axotomy. J Comp Neurol 1993; 335:563–575.

Zimmer A, Zimmer AM, Baffi J, Usdin T, Reynolds K, Konig M, Palkovits M, Mezey E. Hypoalgesia in mice with a targeted deletion of the tachykinin I gene. Proc Natl Acad Sci USA 1998; 95:2630–2635.

3

From Acute to Chronic Pain
Peripheral and Central Mechanisms

Fernando Cervero
University of Alcalá, Madrid, Spain

Jennifer M. A. Laird
University Hospital Principe de Asturias and University of Alcalá, Madrid, Spain

I. INTRODUCTION

Perhaps the most significant advance in the field of pain research has been the realization that pain is not a single sensory experience and that the different forms of pain are mediated by different neurological mechanisms. Some years ago we proposed a conceptual framework and a series of models that addressed the mechanisms of both acute and chronic pain and the interrelation between different pain states (1). We argued that the neurophysiological mechanisms responsible for all of the various pain states are different and that normal (nociceptive) and abnormal (neuropathic) pain represent the endpoints of a sequence of possible changes that can occur in the nervous system. Normally, a steady state is maintained in which there is a close correlation between injury and pain. However, changes or oscillations induced by nociceptive input or by changes in the environment can result in variations in the quality and quantity of pain sensation produced by a particular noxious stimulus. Such changes would be temporary, unless there was further noxious input, as the system would always tend to restore the normal balance between injury and pain. However, long-lasting or very intense nociceptive input or the removal of a portion of the normal input would distort the nociceptive system to such an extent that the close correlation between injury and pain would be lost.

We considered three major stages or phases of pain and proposed that different neurophysiological mechanisms are involved, depending on the nature and time course of the originating stimulus. These three phases are (1) the processing of a brief noxious stimulus; (2) the consequences of prolonged noxious stimulation, leading to tissue damage and peripheral inflammation; and (3) the consequences of neurological damage, including peripheral neuropathies and central pain states (Fig. 1). However, it is important to point out that these phases are not exclusive, and that at any given time several of the neurophysiological mechanisms that underlie these pain states may coexist in the same individual.

II. PHASES OF PAIN

A. Phase 1 (Acute Nociceptive Pain)

The mechanisms subserving the processing of brief noxious stimuli (phase 1 pain) can be viewed as a fairly simple and direct route of transmission centrally toward the thalamus and cortex and

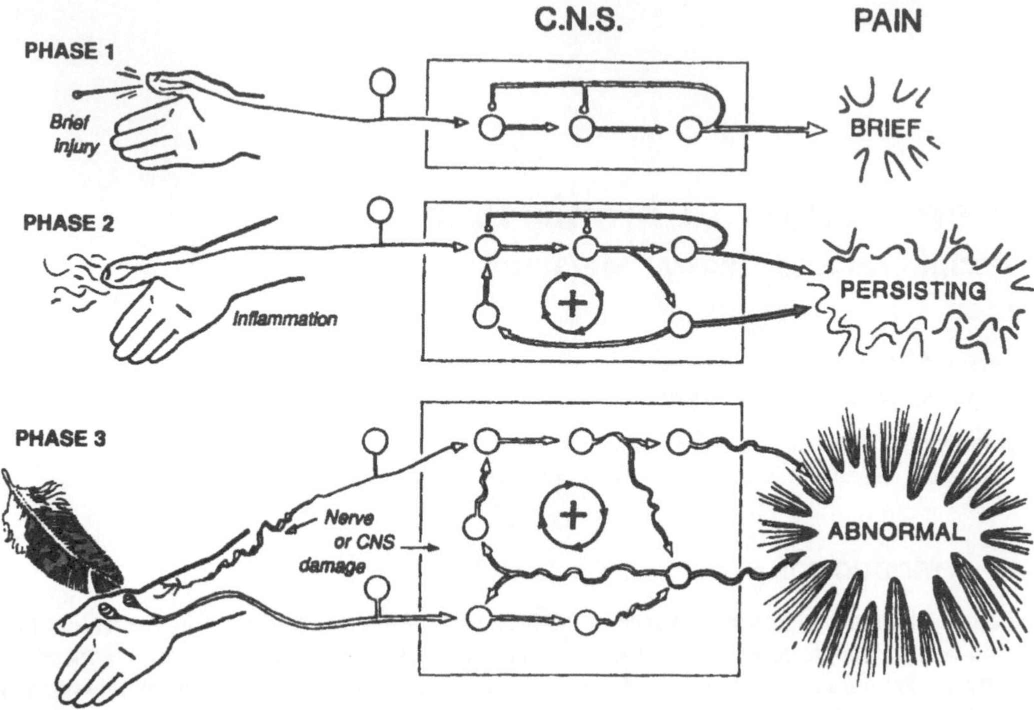

Figure 1 Three models of pain processing for the three phases of pain discussed in this chapter: For a detailed explanation see text. (From Ref. 1.)

thus the conscious perception of pain, with possibilities for modulation occurring at synaptic relays along the way (see phase 1 model in Fig. 1). The relative simplicity of this model reflects the experimental observation that, in humans undergoing phase 1 pain, there is a close correlation between the discharges in peripheral nociceptors and the subjective expression of pain. Phase 1 pain is the type that has been most studied experimentally, and on the basis of the large body of data from both humans and animals, it is reasonably easy to construct plausible and detailed neuronal circuits to explain the features of phase 1 pain. In our original proposal (1), we suggested that phase 1 pain can best be explained by models based on the specificity interpretation of pain mechanisms, that is, the existence within the peripheral and central nervous systems (CNS) of a series of neuronal elements concerned solely with the processing of these simple noxious events.

B. Phase 2 Pain (Inflammatory Pain)

The situation changes to what we have called phase 2 pain if a noxious stimulus is very intense, or prolonged, leading to tissue damage and inflammation. The pain state under these conditions is different from that in phase 1 pain, because the response properties of various components of the nociceptive system change. There is a greatly increased afferent inflow to the CNS from the injured area as a result of the increased activity and responsiveness of sensitized nociceptors. In addition, nociceptive neurons in the spinal cord modify their responsiveness in ways that are not merely an expression of the changes in their inputs from the periphery. These changes mean that the CNS has moved to a new, more excitable state as a result of the noxious input generated

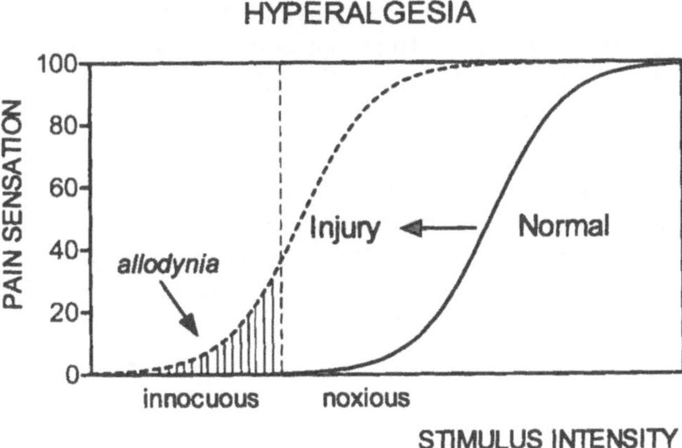

Figure 2 Diagram illustrating the changes in pain sensation induced by injury: The normal relation between stimulus intensity and the magnitude of pain sensation is represented by the curve at the right-hand side of the figure. Pain sensation is evoked only by stimulus intensities in the noxious range (the vertical dotted line indicates the pain threshold). Injury provokes hyperalgesia, defined as a leftward shift in the curve relating stimulus intensity to pain sensation. Under these conditions, innocuous stimuli evoke pain (allodynia), and stimulus intensities that normally evoke mild pain evoke more intense pain. (From Ref. 40.)

by tissue injury and inflammation. Phase 2 pain is characterized by its central drive, a drive that is triggered and maintained by peripheral inputs (see phase 2 model in Fig. 1).

In phase 2 pain, the subject experiences spontaneous pain, a change in the sensations evoked by stimulation of the injured area, and also of the undamaged areas surrounding the injury. This change in evoked sensation is known as hyperalgesia, defined as a leftward shift in the stimulus–response function describing the relation between stimuli and pain sensation (Fig. 2) (2). In this situation, normally innocuous stimuli, such as brushing and touch, are painful (allodynia), and normally mild painful stimuli; such as pinprick, are more painful (hyperalgesia) (3,4). Hyperalgesia in the area of injury is known as primary hyperalgesia, and in the areas of normal tissue surrounding the injury site, as secondary hyperalgesia.

C. Phase 3 Pain (Neuropathic Pain)

Phase 3 pains are abnormal pain states and are generally the consequence of damage to peripheral nerves or to the CNS itself. These are neuropathic pain states characterized by a lack of correlation between injury and pain. In clinical terms, phase 1 and 2 pains are symptoms of peripheral injury, whereas phase 3 pain is a symptom of neurological diseases that include lesions of peripheral nerves or damage to any portion of the somatosensory system within the CNS. Phase 3 pains are spontaneous, triggered by innocuous stimuli, or are exaggerated responses to minor noxious stimuli. These sensations are expressions of substantial alterations in the normal nociceptive system induced by peripheral or central damage (see phase 3 model in Fig. 1). The particular combination of mechanisms responsible for each one of the various phase 3 pain states is probably unique to the individual disease, or to a particular subgroups of patients. Phase 3-type syndromes are seen only in a few people. Even patients with seemingly identical damage to their nervous systems may or may not complain of pain. Thus, the development of phase 3 pain may involve genetic, cognitive, or emotional factors that have yet to be identified.

The loss of sensory function as a result of damage to the nervous system is conceptually easy to understand as the interruption of connections either within the CNS or between the CNS and the peripheral sensory receptors. However, the abnormal sensory symptoms that accompany many cases of neuronal damage require more explanation. Two groups of mechanisms probably account for these sensory symptoms: (1) pathological changes in the damaged neurones, and (2) reactive changes in response to nociceptive (damage-related) afferent input, and to the loss of portions of the normal afferent input. Whereas the pathological changes in damaged neurones are almost certainly unique to phase 3 pain, some of the reactive changes to nociceptive input may well be the expression of normal mechanisms also seen in phase 2-type pain. In phase 3 pain, the activation of these mechanisms may be abnormally prolonged or intense owing to the abnormal input from damaged neurons, or simply because the regenerative properties of neurons are very poor, healing never occurs.

III. ROLE OF PERIPHERAL MECHANISMS

An injury to the skin or to an internal organ evokes the initial discharge in the nociceptive afferents that innervate the damaged area and, as a consequence of the ensuing inflammatory process, sensitizes these nocpceptive endings (2). During the initial injury and for the duration of the repair process there will be increased nociceptive activity from the injured region. Sensitized nociceptors respond to peripheral stimuli with a lower threshold and an increased excitability; therefore, it is likely that the afferent discharges during the inflammatory process will be greater in magnitude and duration than the initial injury-related barrage.

These afferent barrages cause, in turn, central changes in excitability mediated by positive feedback loops between spinal and supraspinal neurons and by the enhanced synaptic actions of certain neurotransmitters, possibly involving an *N*-methyl-D-aspartate (NMDA) receptor mechanism (5–8). The central changes are maintained by the incoming discharges in sensitized nociceptors so that, in the absense of such discharges, the central alterations decline and the central system returns to normal sensory processing.

The afferent inflow to the CNS from a damaged and inflamed area increases dramatically as a result of the increased activity and responsiveness of sensitized nociceptors. In addition, nociceptive neurons in the spinal cord modify their responsiveness and increase their excitability (7,9–11). All of these changes indicate that the CNS has moved to a new, more excitable state as a result of the noxious input generated by tissue injury and inflammation. Only when this peripheral drive returns to normal will the central mechanism that amplifies and enhances the peripheral drive also return to normal processing.

Within the area of primary hyperalgesia, low-intensity mechanical stimuli and warmth evoke pain. It has long been known that an injury induces a process of nociceptor sensitization whereby the excitability of the nociceptors is increased and their thresholds lowered (12,13). Primary hyperalgesia can thus be explained in terms of nociceptor sensitization (2,14). However, the situation is quite different for secondary hyperalgesia. The alterations responsible for secondary hyperalgesia include two different components (see Fig. 2): (1) a change in the modality of the sensation evoked by low-threshold mechanoreceptors, from touch to pain, and (2) an increase in the magnitude of the pain sensations evoked by mechanically sensitive nociceptors (4,15). The first change results in touch-evoked pain (allodynia); that is, the perception of painful sensations following the activation of low-threshold mechanoreceptors. The second alteration produces hyperalgesia, an increased sensitivity to noxious stimuli. Both of these changes are mediated by alterations in the central processing of the sensory input and are induced by the arrival in the CNS of the afferent barrage that the originating injury evokes in peripheral nociceptors (4,16). Importantly, there is no thermal allodynia in areas of secondary hyperalgesia (4,17,18).

The sensitization of peripheral nociceptors is characterized by two main changes in their response properties. The first is the appearance of spontaneous activity that provides a continuous nociceptive afferent barrage that probably contributes to spontaneous pain. The second is a decrease in threshold to an extent that normally nonnoxious stimuli will activate the sensitized receptor. This drop in threshold is generally agreed to underlie primary hyperalgesia (2). A drop in threshold may also contribute to the development of continuous nociceptive input to the CNS and, thereby, spontaneous pain, depending on the site of injury. For example, the available evidence on the properties of visceral nociceptors indicates that a variety of noxious stimuli evoke not only an acute excitation of the nociceptors, but also cause prolonged sensitization of both the ''normal'' and the ''silent'' nociceptors (see Ref. 19 for review). In the sensitized state, visceral nociceptors respond to many of the innocuous stimuli that occur during the normal functioning of internal organs. As a consequence, after inflammation of an internal organ, the CNS will receive an increase barrage from peripheral nociceptors that is initially related to the extent of the acute injury, but for the duration of the inflammatory process initiated by the injury, will be dependent on the normal physiological activity of that organ until the peripheral

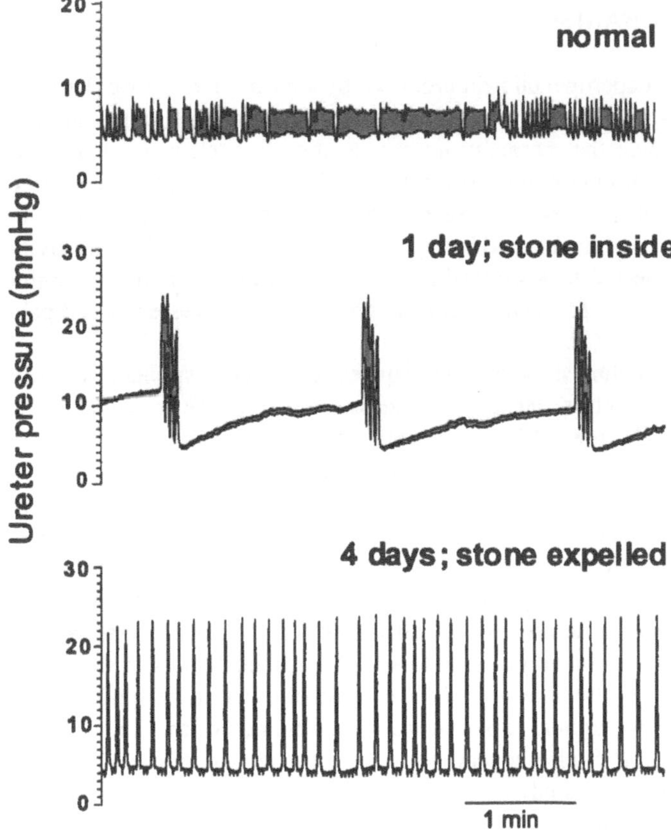

Figure 3 Effect of the presence of an experimental calculus on the motility of the rat ureter in vivo: Motility was measured by a fine catheter inserted into the lumen of the ureter, as changes in intraureteral pressure. The upper trace shows motility in a normal ureter. The middle trace shows abnormal ureter motility recorded 1 day after implantation of an artificial calculus. In these conditions, the ureter contractions reach pressures above the threshold of normal ureteric nociceptors and thus may contribute to the pain and hyperalgesia of ureteric calculosis. This abnormal motility also continues even after the natural explulsion of the calculus from the ureter (lower trace), suggesting that peripheral mechanisms may explain the frequently observed persistence of pain and hyperalgesia after calculus expulsion in patients with colic. (Data from Ref. 20.)

sensitization has completely resolved. Furthermore, an additional factor may be involved if the lesion alters the normal motility or secretion of the organ. Alterations in motility or secretion may evoke or increase activity in visceral nociceptors, even in those that were not directly affected or sensitized by the original lesion and, thereby, further contribute to the pain sensation.

We have recently observed that the induction of artificial ureteric calculosis in rats results in a very marked changed in the pattern of ureteric motility (Fig. 3). This is characterized by a large increase in the amplitude of contractions, such that they increase from a mean of near 5–10 mmHg, well below the nociceptive threshold in normal humans and animals of 20–25 mmHg, to values close to this level (20). In patients with ureteric calculosis, pain and hyperalgesia often last for some time after the elimination of the stone. Peripheral mechanisms may be responsible for this phenomenon, because we also found the same changes in ureteric motility in rats that spontaneously eliminated the artificial stone during the 1- to 8-day survival period between stone induction and recording (20).

IV. ROLE OF CENTRAL MECHANISMS

In normal human subjects, intense experimental pain produced by a burn injury, or by chemical stimulation of nociceptors with capsaicin, changes the responsiveness of an area of undamaged skin surrounding the injury site such that normally innocuous stimuli, such as brushing and touch, are painful (allodynia), and normally mild painful stimuli, such as pinprick, are more painful (hyperalgesia) (3,4). This phenomenon of "secondary hyperalgesia" is now known to be due to a central change, induced and maintained by input from nociceptors, such that activity in large myelinated afferents connected to low-threshold mechanoreceptors provokes painful sensations as well as tactile sensations (16), and input from nociceptors evokes enhanced pain sensations (15).

Psychophysical and animal studies show that the expressions of both spontaneous pain and of hyperalgesia are very dependent on ongoing afferent activity from the injury site. The elegant studies of LaMotte and colleagues (4,16) have shown that after the appearance of an area of secondary hyperalgesia around an intradermal capsaicin injection in normal human subjects, the secondary hyperalgesia disappears within seconds if the injection site is cooled with a piece of ice (a procedure known to block the ongoing activity in the nociceptors), and reappears if the ice is removed as the temperature returns to normal. Similarly, the duration of secondary hyperalgesia after a burn injury (21) or the application of mustard oil (22) is dependent on the afferent input from the site of injury. The presence of allodynia and hyperalgesia in patients with peripheral neuropathy, a phenomenon very similar to and perhaps identical with secondary hyperalgesia, can also be abolished by the injection of local anesthetic into a presumed source of nociceptive ectopic activity (23). In animal experiments, the magnitude of the changes seen in neurons at the first relay in the CNS also appears to be directly related to the amount of afferent input received. For example, in a study from this laboratory, the central changes in the excitability of trigeminal neurons in response to corneal injury were examined (24). In this study we were able to demonstrate a close correlation between the size of the nociceptive afferent barrage and the extent of the increase in excitability of the cells as measured by the increase in the size of their receptive fields.

Experiments in laboratory animals have provided evidence for the concept that noxious input to the CNS sets off a central process of enhancement of responsiveness that continues independently of peripheral afferent drive. Short periods of electrical stimulation at noxious intensity produce increases in excitability, with a time course similar to that of short-term potentiation (from a few seconds to tens of minutes) in single dorsal horn neurons (25,26), in

C-fiber–evoked potentials recorded in the superficial dorsal horn (27) and in spinal reflexes (6,28). Increases in excitability of dorsal horn C-fiber–evoked potentials, with a time course similar to that of long-term potentiation, have also recently been described (29). These increases in central excitability are also referred to as "central sensitization" (5,6).

States of central sensitization maintained for a period independently of further afferent input can be demonstrated experimentally, but it seems that the role of such a "self-sustaining" neurophysiological mechanism in the spontaneous pain and hyperalgesia produced by injury is relatively limited. On the one hand, in the normal situation, the nociceptive afferent barrage continues for as long as the injury takes to heal and, on the other hand, the available evidence from psychophysical and clinical studies shows that the expression of hyperalgesia and spontaneous pain is highly dependent on this continuing afferent input. Any central mechanism that is a candidate for an important role in the generation and maintenance of spontaneous pain and hyperalgesia should logically, therefore, also be strongly dependent on afferent input.

V. SOME NEUROTRANSMITTER SYSTEMS IMPLICATED IN PERSISTENT PAIN

The different pain states described by the three models in Figure 1 are due to changes in the neurophysiological mechanisms involved in the nociceptive pathway. However, it is clear that the neurochemistry of the nociceptive system changes with noxious input, and there is increasing evidence that the pharmacology of pain changes as one moves from phase 1 to phases 2 and 3, as different transmitter systems are recruited as part of the different mechanisms that underlie the different pain states. These pharmacological differences are already reflected in clinical practice, and they have important implications not just for the treatment of the different pain states, but also for the development of novel analgesic agents. Until recently, both industrial drug discovery programs and academic pain pharmacologists routinely used very simple animal models of pain that mostly represent phase 1 pain (e.g., tail-flick, hot-plate, and such). However, in recent years, there has been increased emphasis on the development of models of different pain states, and there is a growing body of literature showing that the pharmacology of several transmitter systems is different in the various pain states.

A. NMDA Receptors

Glutamate is a major transmitter in the spinal cord, and the *N*-methyl-D-aspartate (NMDA) glutamate receptor subtype has been proposed as having a particular role in mediating persistent pain and hyperalgesia in the spinal cord (30). Consistent with this view, NMDA receptor antagonists are not very effective in phase 1-type pain, but in behavioral tests in animals of phase 2-type pain, they reverse the hyperalgesia evoked by local inflammation of the hindlimb at doses that have no effect on the response to noxious stimulation of the contralateral, noninflamed limb (e.g., 31,32, and references therein).

In a recent study from our laboratory (33), we observed a differential effect of NMDA receptor antagonists on the reflex responses in anesthetized rats to acute noxious stimuli applied to normal somatic and visceral tissue. Although the responses to graded noxious distensions of the ureter were dose-dependently inhibited by the NMDa receptor ion channel blocker ketamine, the responses to graded pinch stimuli of one hindpaw were not affected. The results we obtained with ketamine were confirmed by results with the NMDA receptor glycine modulatory site antagonist, Mrz 2/576, which also had a differential effect (Fig. 4). This supports the conclusion

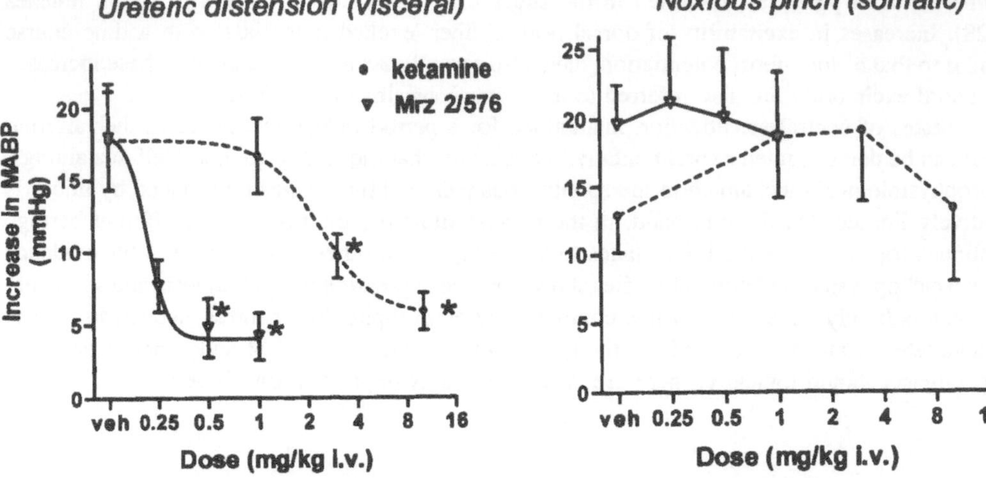

Figure 4 Effect of NMDA receptor antagonists on cardiovascular reflex responses to noxious stimuli applied to normal tissue in anesthetized rats: The left panel shows the dose-dependent inhibition of responses evoked by noxious distension of the ureter (80 mmHg, 30 s) by ketamine (closed circles) and by the Merz glycine site antagonist, Mrz 2/576 (open triangles). * indicates doses significantly different from vehicle. The right panel shows that these same compounds in the same animals had no effect on the responses to noxious pinch of the hindpaw (6 N, 30 s). (Data from Ref. 33.)

that the results are due to blockage of the NMDA receptor, because the two compounds have different structures and different mechanisms of action (33).

These data confirm the lack of participation of NMDA receptors in phase 1-type responses to noxious somatic stimulation, but suggests that they mediate the responses to acute noxious stimulation of viscera. We conclude that acute noxious stimulation of normal visceral tissue provokes intense responses that recruit neural mechanisms mediated by NMDA receptors, whereas in somatic pathways, these mechanisms are recruited only by an enhanced peripheral input, such as that produced after injury or inflammation. This suggests that acute visceral pain may be considered as a form of phase 2 pain.

NMDA receptor antagonists reduce some, but not all types of abnormal pain sensation in animal models of neuropathy (e.g., 34) and in case reports (e.g., 35), and in a small number of controlled trials in human pain patients (e.g., 36,37). However, the psychotomimetic and motor side effects of NMDA receptor blockade at present rule out widespread clinical use of these agents.

B. GABA and Presynaptic Inhibition

Most current models of hyperalgesic states have concentrated on postsynaptic events in the dorsal horn of the spinal cord and have considered either the properties of the network of second-order neurons or the functional properties of the neurotransmitters involved (7,38,39). This has overlooked a possible interaction between low-threshold mechanoreceptors and nociceptors occurring before their first synaptic relay, that is, by means of a presynaptic mechanism.

We have proposed a new model of allodynia based on a presynaptic interaction between the terminals of different types of primary afferents in the spinal cord (40). There is ample evidence for such a mechanism, as it forms the basis of the well-known process of presynaptic inhibition in the spinal cord, studied in great detail since the 1950s (for reviews see refs. 41,42). This mechanism generates depolarizations of primary afferents (PAD) and can evoke a form of antidromic spike activity in primary afferents known as dorsal root reflexes (DRRs) (41). Our model is based on such presynaptic interactions between low-threshold mechanoreceptors and nociceptors.

Our proposal is outlined in the following and illustrated indiagrammatic form in Figure 5. It has been described and discussed in detail in a recent review paper (40). Two situations are considered; normal and injured skin.

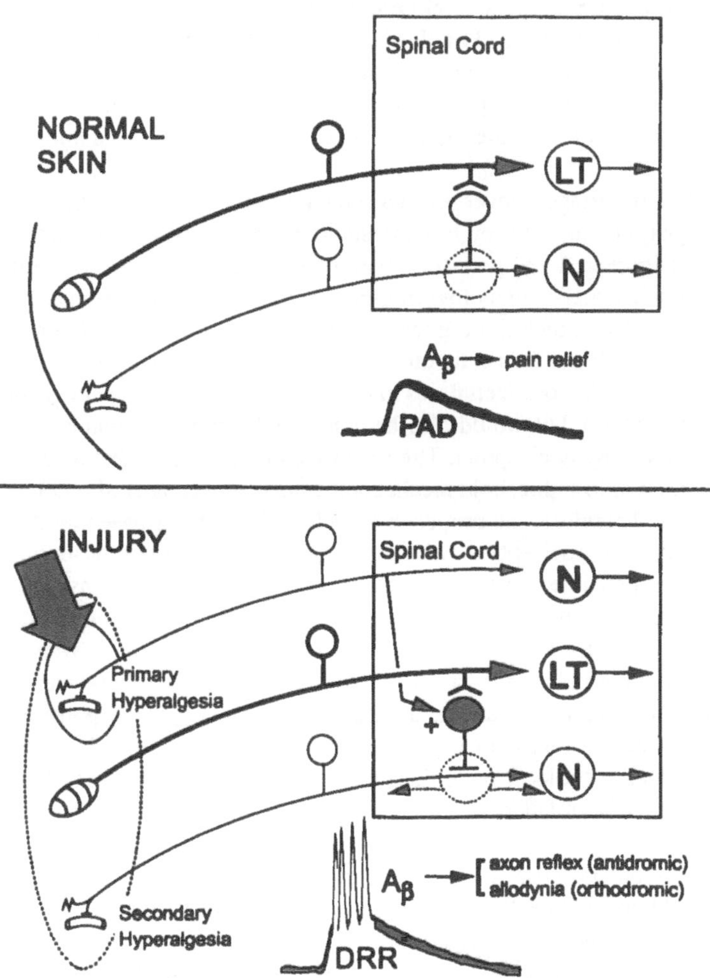

Figure 5 Diagrams illustrating the proposed model for the mechanisms of touch-evoked pain: (top) normal skin; (bottom) skin after an injury. Two types of afferent fiber are illustrated: large caliber connected to low-threshold mechanoreceptors and fine fibers connected to nociceptors (and showing an axon reflex arrangement). Key: LT, low-threshold cells; N, nociceptive cells; PAD, primary afferent depolarization; DRR, dorsal root reflex. In normal skin, stimulation of Aβ-afferents evokes PAD in C-fibers and pain inhibition; in hyperalgesic skin, the interneurons are sensitized (black neuron) by the nociceptive barrage and Aβ stimulation evoked antidromic DRRs (and flare) and orthodromic activation of the C-fiber terminals (and allodynia). (From Ref. 40.)

In normal skin, impulses in low-threshold mechanoreceptors activate second-order neurons, the discharges of which will lead to the perception of tactile sensations. Equally, activity in nociceptors will activate CNS systems that will eventually produce normal pain sensations. The central presynaptic link between these two kinds of afferent fiber contains at least one interneuron and results in PAD of the nociceptive afferents when low-threshold mechanoreceptors are stimulated. Thus, in normal conditions, activation of low-threshold mechanoreceptors with Aβ afferents evokes presynaptic inhibition of nociceptive afferents with C fibers and, therefore, produces a reduction in pain sensation. This mechanism was part of the original "gate control theory of pain" (43) and has been proposed to explain pain relief maneuvers such as "rubbing it better" or transcutaneous nerve stimulation (TENS).

Following an injury, the nociceptors in the area close to the lesion (primary hyperalgesia area) are activated and sensitized. This produces (1) a flare caused by the axon reflexes of the nociceptors at the site of injury; (2) an initial discharge in nociceptors induced by the injury; and (3) persistent activity in the sensitized nociceptors and thus a continuous afferent barrage in these fibers. Thus, the sensory result of an acute injury is persistent pain from the damaged site.

We proposed that this afferent barrage converges onto, among other sites, the spinal interneurons that mediate the presynaptic link between low-threshold mechanoreceptors and nociceptors. As a consequence of the increased and persistent barrage driving these neurons, their excitability is increased such that, when activated by low-threshold mechanoreceptors from areas surrounding the injury site, they produce much more intense PAD in the nociceptive afferents; which is capable of generating spike activity. This activation would be conducted antidromically in the form of DRRs and would thus evoke localized flares in the area of secondary hyperalgesia (by antidromic activation of nociceptors), but would also be conducted forward activating the second-order neurons normally driven by nociceptors. The sensory consequence of this mechanism is pain evoked by the activation of low-threshold mechanoreceptors from an area of secondary hyperalgesia, that is, allodynia. Therefore, the proposed model of allodynia is based on Aβ mechanoreceptors gaining access to the nociceptive channel by means of a presynaptic link.

The dorsal horn circuitry responsible for the production of PAD and DRRs involves γ-aminobutyric acid (GABA), for $GABA_A$ receptor antagonists, such as bicuculline inhibit PAD and DRRs (44–46). Several recent studies have shown that the spinal GABA energic system is up-regulated in animals with hyperalgesia as a result of inflammation of peripheral nerve injury (47–49). Increased spinal cord levels of glutamate decarboxylase (the enzyme responsible for GABA synthesis) mRNA are seen in rats with CFA-induced inflammation (50). Such increases in GABA synthesis and release could provide the substrate for an increase strength of PAD sufficient to result in the production of DRRs in hyperalgesic states produced by inflammation or nerve injury.

One of the consequences of our proposal is the prediction that, after a brief period of noxious stimulation, Aβ-afferent fibers could activate nociceptor-specific cells by means of Aβ-evoked DRRs on the C-fiber input of the neuron. In this respect, experiments from our laboratory indicate that Aβ excitation of nociceptor-specific cells from areas of cutaneous hyperalgesia evoked by capsaicin injection can be blocked by $GABA_A$ antagonists, suggesting a presynaptic link (Fig. 6).

It has also been shown that spinal cord reflexes in animals with a peripheral injury or an inflammatory process can express a frequency-dependent increase of their excitability (known as "windup") when Aβ-fibers are stimulated (51,52). We have also described that this kind of windup is dependent on $GABA_A$ receptors (53) demonstrating a presynaptic mechanism for this access of Aβ-fibers to a C-fiber-mediated function.

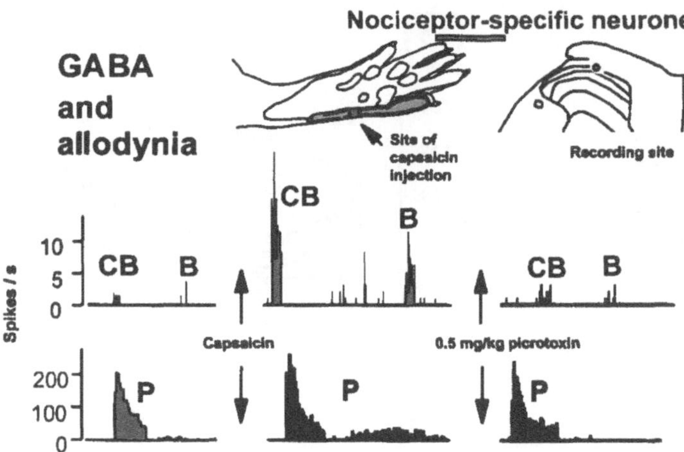

Figure 6 Effect of intradermal injection of capsaicin on the responses of a nociceptor-specific neuron recorded extracellularly in the dorsal horn of an anesthetized rat: The upper panel shows the receptive field of the neuron on the hindpaw of the rat (shaded area), and the location of the neuronal recording site in lamina I of the superficial dorsal horn. The lower panels show the responses of the neuron evoked by stroking the skin with a cotton bud (''CB''; 20 s), or a soft brush (''B''; 20 s) and to noxious pinch of the skin (''P''; 6 N, 20 s). These stimuli were applied under control conditions (left panel), after interdermal injection of capsaicin into the receptive field (center panel), and after administration of picrotoxin (0.5 mg/kg IV, right panel).

C. NK-1 Receptors and Substance P

Substance P has long been thought to be involved with nociceptive processing because it is expressed in small-diameter primary afferents, most of which are connected to peripheral nociceptors. However, the recent description of selective nonpeptide receptor antagonists for the neurokinin (NK)-1 tachykinin receptor, at which substance P is the highest affinity endogenous ligand (see Ref. 54, for review), has allowed direct investigation of the role of the NK-1 receptor in nociception. It seems that NK-1 receptors are not involved in phase 1 pain trasmission, because NK-1 receptor antagonists have no effect in simple behavioral analgesic tests in normal animals (tail-flick, paw pressure, etc.; e.g., 55). Similarly, NK-1 receptor antagonists do not affect the responses of dorsal horn neurons or spinal reflexes to brief noxious stimuli (e.g., 56–57). However, NK-1 receptors appear to have a role in the processing of phase 2 pain, because in electrophysiological experiments, NK-1 receptor antagonists inhibit the responses to more prolonged or intense stimulation (56,57), and also the enhanced responses of dorsal horn neurons provoked by joint inflammation (58) or the intradermal injection of capsaicin (59). Also, peripheral inflammation increases the expression of both NK-1 receptors and substance P in the spinal cord (60,61).

The published data on the effect of NK-1 receptor antagonists in phase 3 pain in animal models is somewhat contradictory. Thus, in some studies analgesic effects have been observed (62,63), in other studies, no effect on the responses of the animals was seen (64,65). However, after experimental nerve damage in mice that results in hyperalgesia, a substantial and maintained increase in NK-1 receptor expression in the spinal cord is observed (66).

The recent development of mutant mice strains with disruptions of the gene coding for the NK-1 receptor (67) or the gene coding for substance P and neurokinin A (preprotachyki-

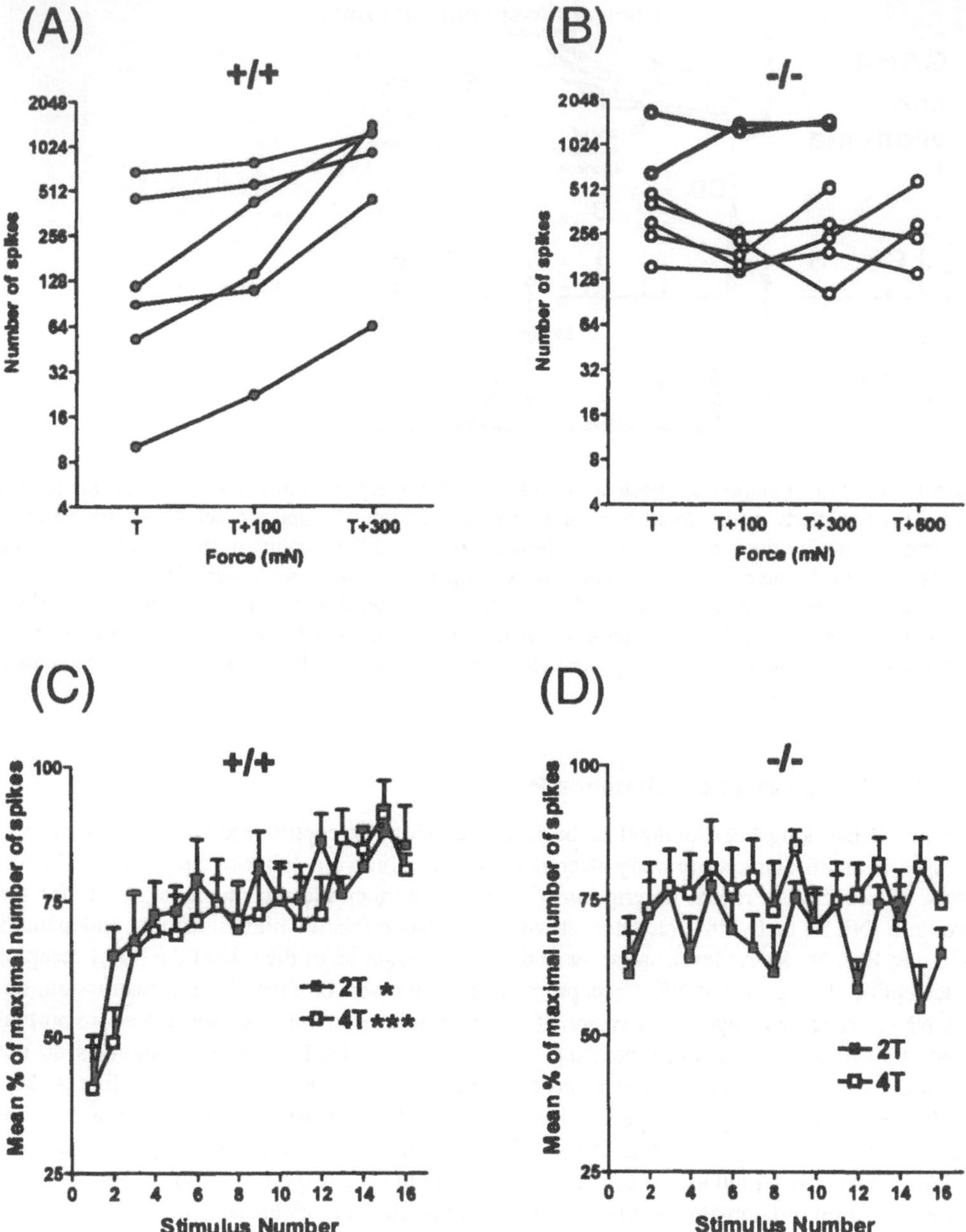

Figure 7 Nociceptive withdrawal reflex response following mechanical and electrical stimulation of the hind paw: (A and B) Responses to noxious mechanical stimulation at different intensities. Note the encoding of the responses in the NK1+/+ mice but not in those from the NK1−/− mice. (C and D). Electrical stimulation induced 'windup' in NK1+/+, but not in NK1−1− mice. (From Ref. 67.)

nin (A; pptA) (68,69) has provided an alternative method to investigate the role of substance P and NK-1 receptors in pain. In these mice, no differences were observed in tests of phase 1-type pain (hot plate, mechanical thresholds, or other) similar to the data obtained with NK-1 receptor antagonists, although the animals lacking substance P or its receptor did not encode the intensity of acute noxious stimuli (Fig. 7) (67). NK-1 receptor knockout mice also fail to show the characteristic amplification of nociceptive reflexes (windup), as shown in Figure 7 (67).

The NK-1 receptor has a greater role in phase 2 pain, judging by data obtained with NK-1 receptor antagonists (see foregoing). Similarly, the responses to inflammatory stimuli are also reduced in mice lacking substance P or the NK-1 receptor; for example, they show reduced responses in the formalin paw test (67,68), to intraplantar injection of capsaicin (68), and to acid injection into the colon (70).

The role of the NK-1 receptor and substance P in the development of hyperalgesia associated with inflammation is less clear. Freud's adjuvant injection into the hindpaw evokes inflammation and mechanical hyperalgesia in both NK-1 receptor and pptA knockout mice that is indistinguishable from normal (67,68). However, NK-1 receptor knockout mice show reduced plasma extravasation and lack of visceral hyperalgesia after instillation of acid in the colon (Fig. 8). This difference may be due to the difference in the nature of the stimulus; neurogenic (acid) versus nonneurogenic (Freud's adjuvant).

Models of phase 3 (neuropathic) pain have been tested only in the pptA knockout mice, where it was observed that partial ligation of the sciatic nerve produced equivalent signs of neuropathic pain in both wild-type and knockout mice (68).

In conclusion, the data from experiments using receptor antagonists and from experiments in mutant mice suggest that the role of substance P and the NK-1 receptor is particularly important in phase 2 pain, especially that with a neurogenic component.

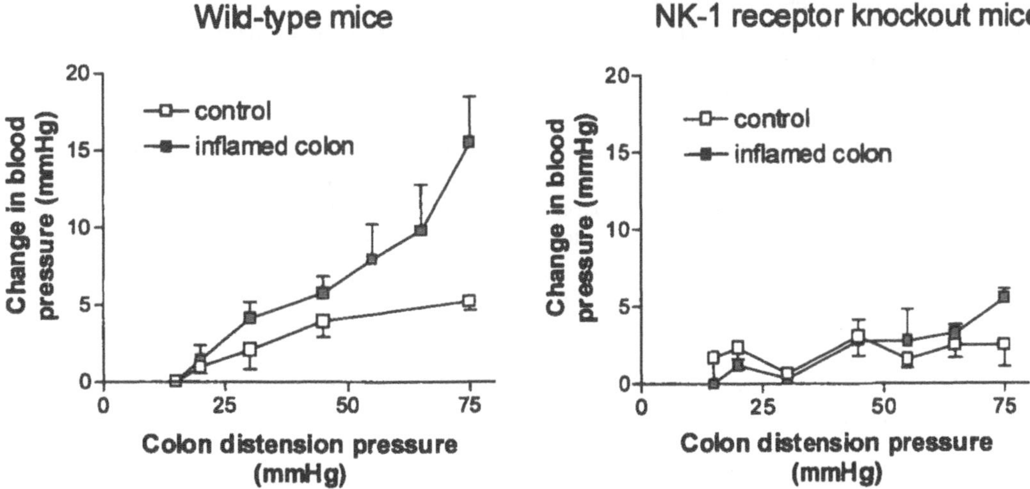

Figure 8 Cardiovascular reflex responses to graded distension of the colon in anesthetized mice, before and after inflammation of the mucosa produced by installation of acetic acid. In mice that express normal NK-1 receptors ("wild-type" mice), induction of colon inflammation results in greatly enhanced responses to colon distension, or visceral hyperalgesia. In contrast, in transgenic mice, in which the NK-1 receptor has been disrupted (knockout mice), a normal stimulus–response curve is obtained in control conditions, but there is no change in responsiveness after inflammation of the colon. These data suggest a specific role for substance P in visceral hyperalgesia. (Data from Ref. 70.)

REFERENCES

1. Cervero F, Laird JMA. One pain or many pains?: a new look at pain mechanisms. News Physiol Sci 1991; 6:268–273.
2. Treede R–D, Meyer RA, Raja SN, Campbell JN. Peripheral and central mechanisms of cutaneous hyperalgesia. Prog Neurobiol 1992;38:397–421.
3. Lewis T. Pain. New York: MacMillan, 1942.
4. LaMotte RH, Shain CN, Simone DA, Tsai E–FP. Neurogenic hyperalgesia: psychophysical studies of underlying mechanisms. J Neurophysiol 1991; 66:190–211.
5. Woolf CJ. Evidence for a central component of post-injury pain hypersensitivity. Nature 1983; 306: 686–688.
6. Woolf CJ, Thompson SWN. The induction and maintenance of central sensitization is dependent on *N*-methyl-D-aspartic acid receptor activation; implications for the treatment of post-injury pain hypersensitivity states. Pain 1991; 44:293–299.
7. Dubner R, Ruda MA. Activity-dependent neuronal plasticity following tissue injury and inflammation. Trends Neurosci 1992; 15:96–103.
8. Cervero F. Visceral pain: mechanisms of peripheral and central sensitization. Ann Med, 1995; 27: 235–239.
9. Woolf CJ, King AE. Subthreshold components of the cutaneous mechanoreceptive fields of dorsal horn neurons in the rat lumbar spinal cord. J Neurophysiol 1989; 62:907–916.
10. Cervero F, Laird JMA, Pozo MA. Selective changes of receptive field properties of spinal nociceptive neurones induced by visceral noxious stimulation in the cat. Pain 1992; 51:335–342.
11. Woolf CJ, Shortland P, Sivilotti LG. Sensitization of high mechanothreshold superficial dorsal horn and flexor motor neurones following chemosensitive primary afferent activation. Pain 1994; 58:141–155.
12. Burgess PR, Perl ER. Myelinated afferent fibres responding specifically to noxious stimulation of the skin. J Physiol (Lond) 1967; 190:541–562.
13. Bessou P, Perl ER. Responses of cutaneous sensory units with unmyelinated fibres to noxious stimuli. J Neurophysiol 1969; 32:1025–1043.
14. Meyer RA, Campbell JN. Myelinated nociceptive afferents account for the hyperalgesia that follows a burn to the hand. Science 1981; 213:1527–1529.
15. Cervero F, Meyer RA, Campbell JN. A psychophysical study of secondary hyperalgesia: evidence for increased pain to input from nociceptors. Pain 1994; 58:21–28.
16. Torebjörk HE, Lundberg LER, LaMotte RH. Central changes in processing of mechanoreceptive input in capsaicin-induced secondary hyperalgesia in humans. J Physiol (Lond) 1992; 448:765–780.
17. Raja SN, Campbell JN, Meyer RA. Evidence for different sensory mechanisms of primary and secondary hyperalgesia following heat injuryto glabrous skin. Brain 1984; 107:1179–1188.
18. Ali Z, Meyer RA, Campbell JN. Secondary hyperalgesia to mechanical but not heat stimuli following a capsaicin injection in hairy skin. Pain 1996; 68:401–411.
19. Cervero F. Sensory innervation of the viscera: peripheral basis of visceral pain. Physiol Rev, 1994; 74:95–138.
20. Laird JMA, Roza C, Cervero F. Effects of artificial calculosis on rat ureter motility: peripheral contribution to the pain of ureteric colic. Am J Physiol Regul Integr Comp Physiol 1997; 272:R1409–R1416.
21. Moiniche S, Dahl JB, Kehlet H. Time course of primary and secondary hyperalgesia after heat injury to the skin. Br J Anaesth 1993; 71:201–205.
22. Koltzenburg M, Lundberg LER, Torebjörk HE. Dynamic and static components of mechanical hypoeralgesia in human hairy skin. Pain 1'992; 51:207–219.
23. Gracely RH, Lynch SA, Bennett GJ. Painful neuropathy: altered central processing maintained dynamically by peripheral input. Pain 1992; 51:175–194.
24. Pozo MA, Cervero F. Neuronsin the rat spinal trigeminal complex drivben by corneal nociceptors: receptive-field properties and effects of noxious stimulation of the cornea. J Neurophysiol, 1993; 70: 2370–2378.

25. Cervero F, Schouenborg, J, Sjölund BH, Waddell PJ. Cutaneous inputs to dorsal horn neurones in adult rats treated at birth with capsaicin. Brain Res 1984; 301:47–57.
26. Cook AJ, Woolf CJ, Wall PD, McMahon SB. Dynamic receptive field plasticity in rat spinal cord dorsal horn following C-primary afferent input. Nature 1987; 325:151–153.
27. Schouenborg J. Functional and topographical properties of field potentials evoked in rat dorsal horn by cutaneous C-fibre stimulation. J Physiol (Lond) 1984; 356:169–192.
28. Wall PD, Woolf CF. Muscle but not cutaneous C-afferent input produces prolonged increases in the excitability of the flexion reflex in the rat. J Physiol (Lond) 1984; 356:443–458.
29. Liu X–G, Sandkühler J. Long-term potentiation of C-fiber-evoked potentials in the rat spinal corsal horn is prevented by spinal *N*-methyl-D-aspartic acid receptor blockage. Neurosci Lett 1995; 191: 43–46.
30. Dickenson AH. A cure for wind-up: NMDA receptor antagonists as potential analgesics. Trends Pharmacol Sci 1990; 11:307–309.
31. Ren K, Dubner R. NMDA receptor antagonists attenuate mechanical hyperalgesia in rats with unilateral inflammation of the hind-paw. Neurosci Lett 1993; 163:19–21.
32. Laird JMA, Mason GS, Webb J, Hill RG, Hargreaves RJ. Effects of a partial agonist and a full antagonist acting at the glycine site of the NMDA receptor on inflammation-induced mechanical hyperalgesia in rats. Br J Pharmacol 1996; 117:1487–1492.
33. Olivar T, Laird JMA. Differential effects of NMDA receptor blockade on nociceptive and visceral reflexes. Pain 1999; 79:67–73.
34. Tal M, Bennett GJ. Dextrorphan relieves neuropathic heat-evoked hyperalgesia in the rat. Neurosci Lett 1993; 151:107–110.
35. Kristensen JD, Svensson B, Gordh T. The NMDA-receptor antagonist CPP abolishes neurogenic ''wind-up pain'' after intrathecal administration in humans. Pain 1992; 51:249–253.
36. Felsby S, Nielsen J, Arendt–Nielsen L, Jensen TS. NMDA recepytor blockage in chronic neuropathic pain: a comparison of ketamine and magnesium chloride. Pain 1996; 64:283–291.
37. Max MB, Byas–Smith MG, Gracely R, Bennett GJ. Intravenous infusion of the NMDA antagonist ketamine in chronic post-traumatic pain with allodynia: a double-blind comparison with alfentanil and placebo. Clin Neuropharm 1995; 18:360–368.
38. Dougherty PM, Mittman S, Sorkin LS. Hyperalgesia and aminoacids: receptor selectivity based on stimulus intensity and a role for peptides. APS J 1994; 3:240–248.
39. Treede R–D, Mageri W. Modern concepts of pain and hyperalgesia: beyond the polymodal C-nociceptor. News Physiol Sci 1995;10:216–228.
40. Cervero F, Laird JMA. Mechanisms of touch-evoked pain (allodynia): a new model. Pain 1996; 68: 13–23.
41. Schmidt RF. Pre-synaptic inhibition in the vertebrate nervous system. Rev Physiol Biochem Pharmacol 1971; 63:21–101.
42. Rudomin P. Pre-synaptic inhibition of muscle spindle and tendon organ afferents in the mammalian spinal cord. Trends Neurosci 1990; 13:499–505.
43. Melzack R, Wall PD. Pain mechanisms: a new theory. Science 1965; 150:971–979.
44. Curtis DR, Lodge D. The depolarisation of feline ventral horn group la spinal afferent terminations by GABA. Exp Brain Res 1982; 46:215–233.
45. Evans RH, Long SK. Primary afferent depolarization in the rat spinal cord is mediated by pathways utilising NMDA and non-NMDA receptors. Neurosci Lett 1989; 100:231–236.
46. Rees H, Sluka KA, Westlund KN, Willis WD. The role of glutamate and GABA receptors in the generation of dorsal root reflexes by acute arthritis in the anaesthetised rat. J Physiol (Lond) 1995; 484:437–445.
47. Castro–Lopes JM, Tavares I, Tölle TR, Coito A, Coimbra A. Increase in GABAergic cells and GABA levels in the spinal cord in unilateral inflammation of the hindlimb in the rat. Eur J Neurosci 1992; 4:296–301.
48. Castro–Lopes JM, Tavares I, Tölle TR, Coimbra A. Carrageenan-induced inflammation of the hind foot provokes a rise of GABA-immunoreactive cells in the rat spinal cord that is prevented by peripheral neurectomy or neonatal capsaicin treatment. Pain 1994; 56:193–201.

49. Nahin RL, Hylden JLK. Peripheral inflammation is associated with increased glutamic acid decarboxylase immunoreactivity in the rat spinal cord. Neurosci Lett 1991; 128:226–230.
50. Castro–Lopes JM, Tölle TR, Pan BH, Zieglgänsberger W. Expression of GAD mRNA in spinal cord neurons of normal and monoarthritic rats. Mol Brain Res 1994; 26:169–176.
51. Thompson SWN, Dray A, Urban L. Injury-induced plasticity of spinal reflex activity: NK1 neurokinin receptor activation and enhanced A- and C-fiber mediated responses in the rat spinal cord in vitro. J Neurosci 1994; 14:3672–3687.
52. Thompson SWN, Dray A, McCarson KE, Krause JE, Urban L. Nerve growth factor induces mechanical allodynia associated with novel A fibre-evoked spinal reflex activity and enhanced neurokinin-1 receptor activation in the rat. Pain 1995; 62:219–231.
53. Weng H–R, laird JMA, Cervero F, Schouenborg J. GABA-A receptor blockade inhibits A beta fibre evoked wind-up in the arthritic rat. Neuroreport 1998; 9:1065–1069.
54. Maggi CA, Patacchini R, Rovero P, Giachetti A. Tachykinin receptors and tachykinin receptor antagonists. J Auton Nerv Syst 1993; 13:23–93.
55. Rupniak NMJ, Boyce S, Williams AR, et al. Antinociceptive activity of NK_1 receptor antagonists: non-specific effects of racemic RP67580. Br J Pharmacol 1993; 110:1607–1613.
56. De Koninck Y, Henry JL. Substance P-mediated slow excitatory postsynaptic potentials elicited in dorsal horn neurones in vivo by noxious stimulation. Proc Natl Acad Sci USA 1991; 88:11344–11348.
57. Laird JMA, Hargreaves RJ, Hill RG. Effect of RP 67580, a non-peptide $neurokinin_1$ receptor antagonist, on facilitation of a nociceptive spinal flexion reflex in the rat. Br J Pharmacol 1993; 109:713–718.
58. Neugebauer V, Schaible H–G, Weiretter F, Freudenberger U. The involvement of substance P and neurokinin-1 receptors in the responses ofrat dorsal horn neurones to noxious but not to innocuous mechanical stimuli applied to the knee joint. Brain Res 1994; 666:207–215.
59. Dougherty PM, Palecek J, Palecková V, Willis WD. Neurokinin 1 and 2 antagonists attenuate the responses and NK1 antagonists prevent the sensitization of primate spinothalamic tract neurons after intradermal capsaicin. J Neurophysiol 1994; 72:1464–1475.
60. Abbadie C, Brown JL, Mantyh PW, Basbaum AI. Spinal cord substance P receptor immunoreactivity increases in both inflammatory and nerve injury models of persistent pain. Neurosci 1996; 70:201–209.
61. Gary MG, Hargreaves KM. Enhanced release of immunoreactive CGRP and substance P from spinal dorsal horn slices occurs during carrageenan inflammation. Brain Res 1992; 582:139–142.
62. Corteix C, Lavarenne J, Eschalier A. RP-67580, a specific tachykinin NK1 receptor antagonist, relieves chronic hyperalgesia in diabetic rats. Eur J Pharmacol 1993; 241:267–270.
63. Field MJ, McCleary S, Boden PR, Suman–Chauhan N, Hughes J, Singh L. Involvement of the central tachykinin NK1 recept during maintenance of mechanical hypersensitivity induced by diabetes in the rat. J Pharmacol Exp Ther 1998; 285:1226–1232.
64. Malcangio M, Tomlinson DR. A pharmacologic analysis of mechanical hyperalgesia in streptozotocin/diabetic rats. Pain 1998; 76:151–157.
65. Yamamoto T, Yaksh TL. Effects of intrathecal capsaicin and an NK-1 antagonist, CP-96,345, on the thermal hyperalgesia observed following unilateral constriction of the sciatic nerve in the rat. Pain 1992; 51:329–334.
66. Malmberg AB, Basbaum AI. Partial sciatic nerve injury in the mouse as a model of neuropathic pain: behavioural and neuroanatomical correlates. Pain 1998; 76:215–222.
67. De Felipe C, Herrero JF, O'Brien JA, et al. Altered nociception, analgesia and aggression in mice lacking the receptor for substance P. Nature 1998; 392:394–397.
68. Cao YQ, Mantyh PW, Carlso EJ, Gillespie AM, Epstein CJH, Basbaum AJ. Primary afferent tachykinins are required to experience moderate to intense pain. Nature 1998; 392:390–394.
69. Zimmer A, Zimmer AM, Baffi J, et al. Hypoalgesia in mice with a targeted deletion of the tachykinin 1 gene. Proc Natl Acad Sci USA 1998; 95:2630–2635.
70. Laird JMA, Olivar T, Roza C, De Felipe C, Hunt SP, Cervero F. Deficits in visceral pain and hyperalgesia of mice with a disruption of the tachykinin NK1 receptor gene. Neuroscience 2000; 98:345–352.

4

Central and Peripheral Components of Neuropathic Pain

R. W. Colburn and Rajesh Munglani
University of Cambridge and Addenbrooke's Hospital, Cambridge, England

I. INTRODUCTION

The mechanisms by which a noxious or nociceptive stimulus is evoked, propagated, integrated, and finally perceived are extremely complex. At each of these functional steps there is a delicate balance betwen excitatory and inhibitory influences from local, remote, and global factors. In neuropathic conditions this process becomes profoundly more complicated owing to both the interruption of the normal "wiring" of the system and the dynamic compensatory responses that occur throughout the nervous system. Some of these changes, which encompass anatomical, immune, and endocrine responses, among many others, are gradually reversed in concert with "healing" of the nerve injury. Other changes are more permanent and persist despite resolution of the original neuropathic insult. This latter group is likely to correlate closely with, and may be in part responsible for, chronic neuropathic pain syndromes.

The first part of this chapter will review the various changes at sites along the neuroaxis that have been identified as contributing to the generation of neuropathic pain-like behaviors in animal models. The second part of the chapter will explore the evidence that neuroimmune responses and nonneuronal cell populations are intimately involved in how the body addresses and repairs a nerve injury and how they may contribute to neuronal sensitization. The development of novel local immunomodulatory agents capable of selectively titrating these neuroimmune responses may provide useful new tools to be used in conjunction with existing and emerging therapies for the prevention and treatment of neuropathic and inflammatory pain.

II. BASIC CONCEPTS

Neuropathic injury can result through vastly diverse mechanisms. It may take the form of a focal injury to a discrete nerve, as in acute mechanical trauma, or it may be a widespread, progressive, degenerative compromise within the nervous system as seen in diabetic neuropathy, amyotrophic lateral sclerosis (ALS), or multiple sclerosis (MS). Chemical (chemotherapy, toxins, heavy metals), viral (herpes zoster, HIV), genetic (hereditary polyneuropathies), vascular (diabetes, ischemia), mechanical (trauma, surgery), thermal (frostbite, burns), and autoimmune (MS, ALS) neuropathies are all well described clinically. However, the etiology of neuropathic

Table 1 Sites and Types of Injuries in Neuropathic Pain Models

Site/type	Ref.
Sciatic nerve	
Transection	121
Loose ligation (chromic)	122
Partial tight ligation (silk)	123
Cryoneurolysis	124–126
Photochemical	127, 128
Spinal nerve	
Transection	45, 129
Tight ligation (silk)	45, 129
Tight ligation (chromic)	Colburn, 1999 BNA abstr.
Cryoneurolysis	45
DRG	
Compression *Xing	130
Chemical	130–132
Dorsal root	
Transection	45
Loose ligation (chromic)	Hashizumi (Spine '99) 131, 132
Tight ligation (silk)	45
Cryoneurolysis	45
Spinal cord	
Chemical	133
Photochemical	134
Contusion	135

pain stemming from any of these injury sources is at best, only marginally understood. Basic scientific research into the causes and possible treatment of neuropathic pain has accelerated with the development of several animal models. The most common of these are the peripheral mononeuropathy models (Table 1 and Fig. 1; see also Chap. 27). The diferent types of lesions employed at various anatomical sites along peripheral nerves in these models give us clues to which injury characteristics are critical to the development of chronic neuropathic pain syndromes. Key elements associated with pain behaviors appear to be (1) the degree and duration of local neuritis evoked by the lesion; (2) the effect, either mechanical or chemical, directly on the neuronal cell body; (3) the integrity of the central neuronal process (dorsal root) to communicate electrical and axonally transported signals from the dorsal root ganglia (DRG) and periphery to the spinal cord; (4) the severity of axonal damage and resultant neuronal death, leading to sprouting and synaptic rewiring in the spinal cord; and (5) involvement of the sympathetic nervous system.

Studies using these animal models have also helped us more clearly characterize the behavioral modalities that constitute neuropathic pain syndromes. Hyperalgesia, a decreased threshold or increased response to a noxious stimulus, is closely tied to neuronal sensitization resulting from inflammatory processes. This sensitization occurs both directly at the nociceptor or injury site, as well as at the spinal dorsal horn level. Anti-inflammatory agents (steroids and cyclooxygenase inhibitors) are useful in reducing neuritis-induced hyperalgesia, whereas glutamate receptor antagonists show some benefit in mitigating the spinal sensitization component of hyperalgesia. Unfortunately, allodynia, the perception of a normally nonnoxious stimulus as painful, is the behavioral modality responsible for much of the debilitation caused by chronic neuropathic

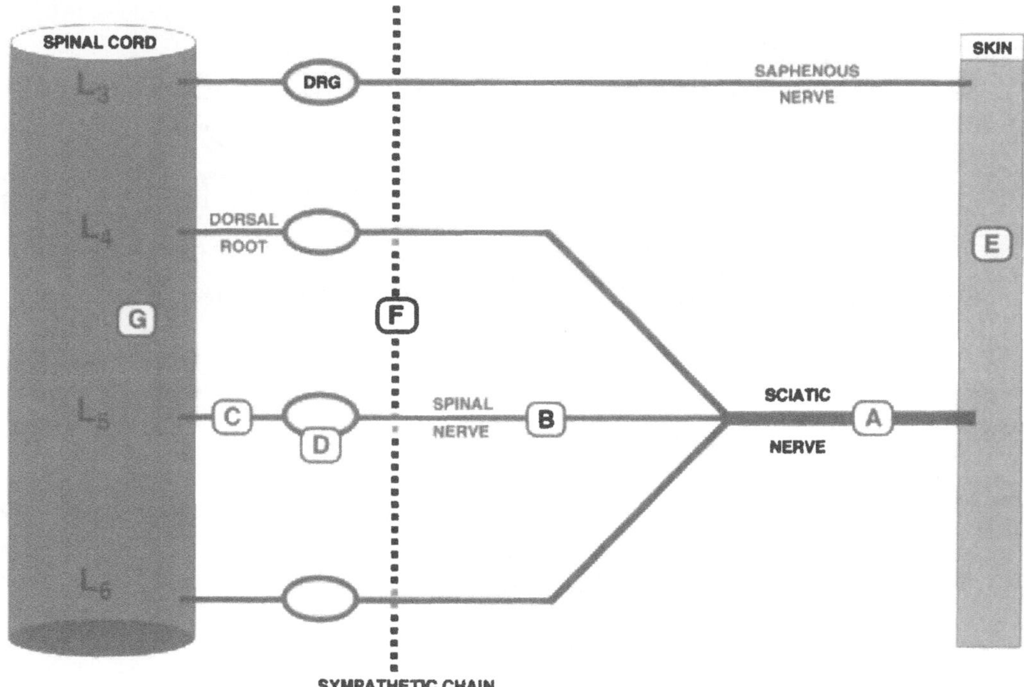

Figure 1 Nerve lesion sites, wiring diagram: Rat peripheral neuropathy models typically consist of (A) a partial lesion to the sciatic nerve or (B) a complete lesion to one (L5) or two (L5 and 6) of its constituent spinal nerves. The L4 spinal nerve is usually spared so as not to disrupt the motor function of the limb to a degree that evoked behaviors are comprised. Note that a complete lesion at A affects the spinal cord (G) from L4–6, whereas (B) the spinal nerve lesion provides a more discrete spinal disturbance. Other neuropathic pain models have been devised around injuries to (D) the DRG, (C) the dorsal root, or (G) the spinal cord itself (see Table 1). (F) The sympathetic nervous system responds to injuries of somatic nerves; therefore chemical, surgical, or immunosympathectomy is often performed to rule in/out its involvement in pain behaviors. (E) Nociceptors and nerves in the skin may respond to denervation by hyperreinnervation or collateral sprouting, respectively.

pain syndromes. Once established, mechanical allodynia is resistant to virtually all existing analgesic approaches. It appears to be centrally mediated, possibly through spinal synaptic rewiring and remapping. Prevention of these anatomical changes are a logical therapeutic intervention because there is little hope of selectively reversing them once they have occurred.

It has become obvious to many clinicians that the effective treatment of neuropathic pain requires an array of pharmacological tools (e.g., antidepressants, anticonvulsants, anti-inflammatory agents, and glutamate receptor antagonists) targeted at multiple sites along the neuroaxis. These sites correlate closely with those identified by basic researchers as sites important to the development and maintenance of neuropathic behaviors in animals (Fig. 2).

A. Possible Sites Responsible for the Generation of Neuropathic Pain

1. Peripheral Tissue

Denervated peripheral tissue (e.g., skin) does not sit passively and await reinnervation, but rather, it actively responds to the lack of electrical and chemical communication by inducing and direct-

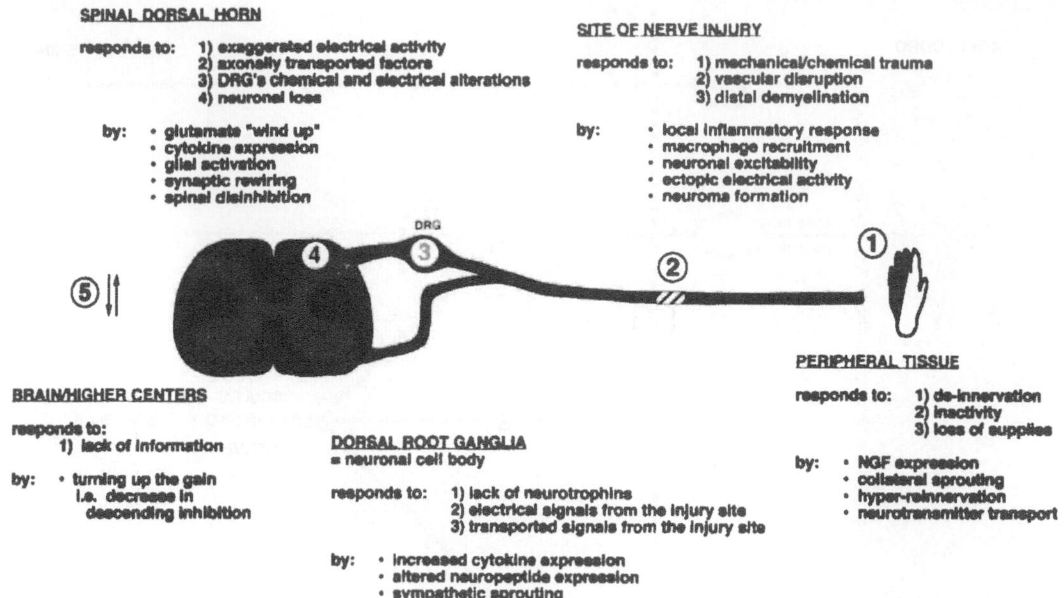

Figure 2 Possible sites for the generation of neuropathic pain.

ing the regenerative efforts of injured and collateral axons to regain appropriate connectivity with the CNS.

Target-derived neurotrophic factors, such as nerve growth factor (NGF), critical in directing the development of the nervous system, are expressed in abundance in the denervated tissue. This is likely an attempt to provide direction for the regenerating axons; however, uninjured neighboring or collateral nerve fibers also respond by sprouting into the denervated tissue and thereby expanding their receptive fields. For severe nerve injury this collateral innervation may be widespread enough to involve nerve fibers from an entirely different nerve thus representing multiple DRGs and spinal cord levels. Beyond its ability to induce neuronal sprouting, NGF is a direct mediator of hyperalgesia (1,2). Intact neurons respond to NGF by transporting activated NGF–Trk complexes to their DRGs, in turn, inducing a plethora of transcriptional activity. Some of the peptides or proteins that are induced include *N*-methyl-D-aspartate (NMDA) receptors, sodium channel proteins, cytokines, neuropeptides, and their receptors. These are all produced in the DRG and transported either centrally to the spinal cord or peripherally to the skin from the DRG following nerve injury (3–9). Therefore, even though a certain peripheral tissue is temporarily denervated it can very readily find ways to communicate with the CNS and, in turn, sensitize the spinal cord to incoming electrical signals. Reciprocally, some of these factors produced in the DRG are transported to the periphery where they sensitize local nociceptors. For example, elevated levels of the ionotropic glutamate receptor are found in nerves associated with inflammation (10). Their functional significance in neuropathic pain remains to be determined; however, their presence, coupled with a ready supply of glutamate in the skin or site of inflammation, would provide a simple direct mechanism for hyperalgesia. Similarly, the excitatory neuropeptide, substance P is elevated in the periphery following nerve injury (11,12). Neurokinin (NK) receptors capable of responding to substance P are located not only on neurons, but also on immune cells, such as macrophages and mast cells (13). These immune cells are particularly active at the nidus of the inflammation—the site of injury.

2. Site of Nerve Injury

The site of a nerve injury is perhaps the most obvious place to search for explanations of the processes involved in the generation of neuropathic pain. This is particularly true when the injury is caused by an acute focal lesion, as opposed to a chronic diffuse neuropathy. Local responses to nerve injury depend on the severity of the lesion and the extent to which inflammatory elements have been introduced or evoked. Clinical examples of inflammatory nerve injuries might include a penetrating wound causing trauma to a nerve, focal viral lesions such as those caused by herpes zoster (postherpetic neuralgia), repetitive stress injury (e.g., carpal tunnel syndrome), chemical "burns," or a herniated vertebral disk impinging on a spinal nerve root. Animal models have be developed that mimic some of these situations (see Table 1). The same inflammogens (e.g., bradykinin, histamine, and prostaglandins) active in acute tissue inflammation sensitize afferent fibers at the nerve injury site. Anti-inflammatory agents (e.g., NSAIDs and steroids) are effective at blocking hyperalgesia in this setting. However, if the nerve injury is severe enough to cause demyelination, a full inflammatory cascade ensues. Schwann cells and resident macrophages release tumor necrosis factor (TNF)-α which stimulates the production and release of interleukin (IL)-1β from resident macrophages. In turn, chemokines and cell adhesion molecules are produced that help recruit more inflammatory cells to the injured nerve to assist in the demyelination process (14). Recent evidence has shown that TNF-α microinjected into a nerve produces an inflammatory response, with variable demyelination, excessive neuronal firing, and pain-related behaviors (15–17). Similarly, functional TNF-α antagonists, such as TNF-binding protein, anti-TNF-α and MMP inhibitors, all are reported to block pain behaviors (18,19). Unfortunately, this area of study remains confusing because other studies show little effect of TNF-α injection or blockade on neuronal sensitization and neuropathic behaviors (Colburn RW, unpublished; DeLeo JA, personal communication, 1999).

Nerve injury may either accelerate or impede bidirectional axonal transport, depending on the severity of axonal damage. When impeded, anterogradely transported materials accumulate at the proximal axonal stump. Transported ion channel proteins that accumulate in this manner and are inserted into the axonal membrane at the stump. This density of ion channels creates a physiological basis for enhanced neuronal excitability and a foci for ectopic electrical activity (20). A similar source of ectopic signals is attributed to neuromas that form when axons of surviving neurons sprout chaotically (without appropriate neutropic support) in a misguided attempt to reinnervate their peripheral target tissue.

Severe focal nerve injuries affect all fiber types indiscriminately. Conversely, mild to moderate or chronic nerve insults may selectively deplete specific neuronal populations. Typically, the unmyelinated C fiber is the most vulnerable to neurotoxic or graded physical trauma. Depletion of a specific fiber type may result in errors in sensory processing, as modal fidelity may be jeopardized by reorganization of both the peripheral endings and the central terminals of the remaining neurons (21).

3. Neuronal Cell Body (e.g., Dorsal Root Ganglion)

Neurons located within the CNS retain very short central processes; for example, motor neurons and most cranial nerve neurons. However, for sensory neurons that send afferent fibers into the spinal dorsal horn, they are of the pseudo-unipolar type, with their cell bodies located in the DRG. The distance from remote transmembrane receptors in the spinal cord or periphery (e.g., in the foot) to the cell nucleus may be great (on the order of many centimeters). Because the neuronal cell body is the site where signals from all parts of the neuron converge, efficient axonal transport mechanisms are required to convey activated signaling complexes to the nucleus and, conversely, to send nuclear products either centrally to the spinal cord or to the periphery.

If this transport chain is disrupted, the nucleus responds by increasing or decreasing expression of neuropeptides and proteins, such as substance P, calcitonin gene-related peptide (CGRP), galanin, neuropeptide Y, growth factors, and cytokines (4,7,22–25). The specific impetus for these nuclear responses is unclear, but it is presumed to be linked to the abrupt withdrawal of constuitively transported neurotrophic factors or possibly lesion-induced factors (26).

The DRG may become a source for ectopic or spontaneous electrical signal generation following axonal injury. As mentioned earlier relative to spontaneous activity of neuromas, novel ion channel expression and accumulation of DRG neuronal membranes or the recruited firing of previously silent fibers could account for rogue signals emanating from the DRG (25,27). Another possible source of abnormal electrical signals is novel sympathosensory connections that form following nerve injury as adjacent sympathetic fibers sprout to form baskets around the cell bodies of DRG sensory neurons (28–31). The most extreme case of nuclear response to a nerve injury is the onset of apoptosis or programmed cell death (suicide). Whiteside et al. provide (32) an elegant triple-labeling technique to expose the postlesion time course of apoptosis in the DRG of neonatal rats following axotomy. However, they found no analogous neuronal apoptosis caused by axotomy in the DRG of adult animals.

4. Spinal Dorsal Horn

The spinal cord is the first major CNS site for the integration of sensory signals. Afferent fibers either terminate in the spinal dorsal horn or send projections to higher centers by the spinal dorsal columns. As reviewed in the foregoing, peripheral nerve injury, depending on its site and type, leads to neuronal loss and changes in gene expression of neuroactive factors that are transported centrally to the dorsal horn. Several chapters in this book provide excellent detailed reviews of dorsal horn physiology and pharmacology. Therefore, this section will mention only the two most obvious dorsal horn mechanisms for the generation and maintenance of neuropathic pain.

Glutamate Receptor (N-Methyl-D-Aspartate; NMDA)-Driven Sensitization of the Spinal Dorsal Horn. Glutamate is the primary excitatory neurotransmitter in the CNS and is released from presynaptic terminals of primary afferent neurons when they fire. On repetitive firing, synaptic glutamate levels rise as the capacity of reuptake transporters is exceeded. Elevations in glutamate and substance P release act synergistically to potentiate NMDA receptor-mediated postsynaptic excitation. Other endogenous agents, the expression of which change dramatically following peripheral nerve injury (e.g., neuropeptides, cytokines, or growth factors) also possess mechanisms for potentiating or mitigating glutamate transmission. Unfortunately, it is difficult to attribute the generation of pain behaviors to specific neuropeptide or cytokine changes, and it is likely that a several simultaneous cascades of events are responsible.

Neuronal Sprouting and Synaptic Rewiring. When an injured sensory neuron dies or sustains a lesion to its central axonal process (dorsal root), there is degeneration of the associated central axon and terminal connections. Associated spinal interneurons may also degenerate. The normal pattern of incoming electrical signals is replaced by either a barrage of signals, ectopic noise, or quiescence. These electrical changes, coupled with glial cell activation, provoke compensatory responses within the spinal dorsal horn, some of which may exacerbate the sensory malfunction. Degenerating or obsolete neuronal terminals are ''stripped'' by microglia, whereas astrocytes help guide uninjured primary neurons that are neurotropically coaxed to sprout into vacated sites. Sensory anomalies may result when this synaptic remapping represents a crossing of sensory modalities (e.g., pain vs. light pressure or touch). The exact contribution that glia and other nonneuronal cells make toward the generation or maintenance of pain behaviors is unclear; however, some of the possible mechanisms whereby this could occur are explored in the second part of this chapter.

B. Influences from Higher Centers

The influence that higher brain centers have in modulating pain perception is discussed in detail elsewhere in this book. To avoid redundancy, this section will merely state that descending spinal inhibition can have dramatic modulatory effects on spinal nociceptive processing and the ultimate central perception of a noxious stimulus. Emotional and psychological factors color our perception and response to acute pain; however, they are particularly prominent in neuropathic pain syndromes, in which the severity, duration, and inescapability of the pain can lead to chronic stress, depression, and numerous secondary maladies. The relation between the nervous system, the immune system, and psychological status is now a new area of study; however, recent interest in psychoneuroimmunology has been driven by its potential to help explain many of these mysterious interactions.

C. Summary

The nervous system attempts to balance its two primary, sometimes contradictory, missions: homeostasis and adaptability. Neuropathic insults severely tax these capabilities. In some pathological circumstances the CNS' best restorative efforts result in an outcome worse than being insensate; namely, chronic neuropathic pain. Efforts to decipher just where the repair efforts fail are hampered by the sheer complexity of the system. As we have seen (see Fig. 2) responses to a nerve injury occur at virtually every level of the neuroaxis and manifest as "permanent" anatomical changes, as well as transient or dynamic physiological adjustments. The CNS has the capability to dynamically respond to any perturbation: unfortunately, this includes most intended therapies. Therefore, the ideal approach to treating neuropathic pain syndromes would be to identify the key problems and to treat them, not in isolation, but simultaneously. Other chapters in this book attest to the progress that is being made to understand and design specific therapies for some of these maladaptive CNS responses. The remainder of this chapter will expose the significant role that nonneuronal cells play in the response to nerve injury, and how possible therapies might be generated from this knowledge.

III. NEUROIMMUNE RESPONSES

Central nervous system glial cells (e.g., microglia, astrocytes, and oligodendrocytes) were once thought of as merely a physical support system for neurons; however, recently, they have come to be appreciated as key neuromodulatory, neurotrophic, and neuroimmune elements in the CNS. Resident glial cells are in intimate physical and homeostatic contact with neurons (Figs. 3 and 4). There is, in fact, a rising tide of evidence to support the claim that astrocytes are full synaptic partners along with pre- and postsynaptic neurons (33). When a neuron is injured, adjacent glial cells are stimulated to mount a dramatic neuroimmunological response (34). This activation response includes glial cell hypertrophy, proliferation or migration, and the release of inflammatory cytokines and adhesion molecules. Following sciatic nerve lesions, we have seen spinal elevations of IL-1β, TNF-α, and IL-6 at times that coincide with the onset of glial responses and behaviors (35,36). Both microglia and astrocytes produce cytokines that sensitize spinal neurons; therefore, it is reasonable to suspect that glial cell activation may play a role in nocicep-

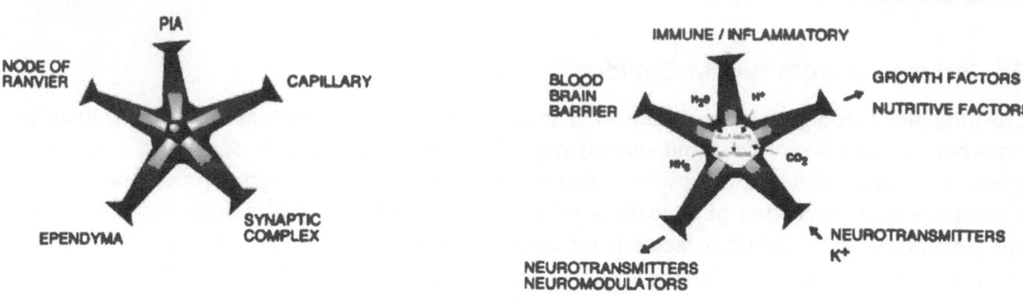

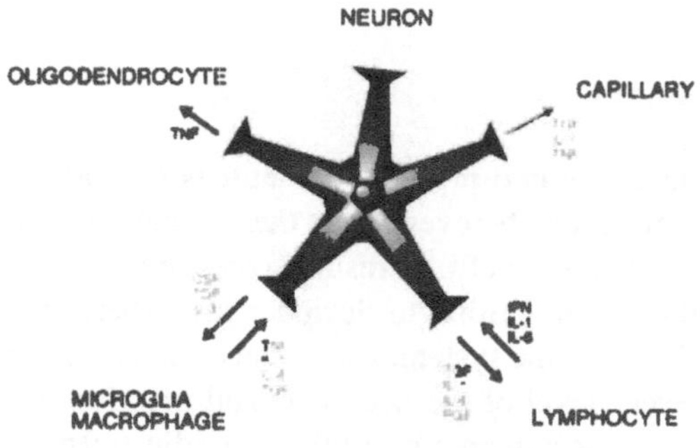

Figure 3 Possible astrocytic functions (see text for more details).

tive processing and may augment neuronal excitability in neuropathic pain states. Beyond neuromodulation, glia also provide neurotrophic support for regenerating neurons and play a critical role in synaptic remodeling that occurs spinally following neuronal loss (37,38). Thus, glia appear to be intimately involved in two primary correlates of chronic neuropathic pain; namely, spinal hypersensitization and synaptic remodeling.

A. Microglia

Microglia are the resident tissue macrophages of the CNS and, as such, are thought to be the first line of defense against injury or infection. Similar to all other monocytic cells they are originally derived from bone marrow. Having migrated into the CNS during development, their population turnover is very slow (e.g., years). They can, when needed, increase their numbers dramatically from relatively few cells to a virtual army of cells through proliferation and migration of resident microglia and recruitment of circulating monocytes. Their resting appearance is that of relatively quiescent cells with a distinct highly ramified "wispy" morphology; however, on activation they assume a more robust morphology, with short bold projections (Fig. 5) and express a variety of surface antigens and receptors such as major histocompatibility complex (MHC) I and II and CR3 (CD11b). Activated microglia undergo further functional

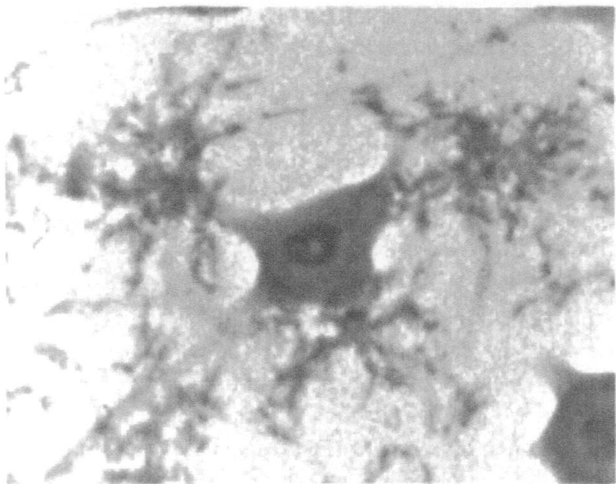

Figure 4 Photomicrograph of a neuron (NeuN-ir) surrounded by microglial (OX-42-ir) cells. Note that the microglia are nicely positioned for surveillance of the neural environment and are capable of rapidly responding to any perturbations through such tactics as migration, proliferation, release of cytotoxic mediators, and even differentiation into a phagocytotic macrophage if required.

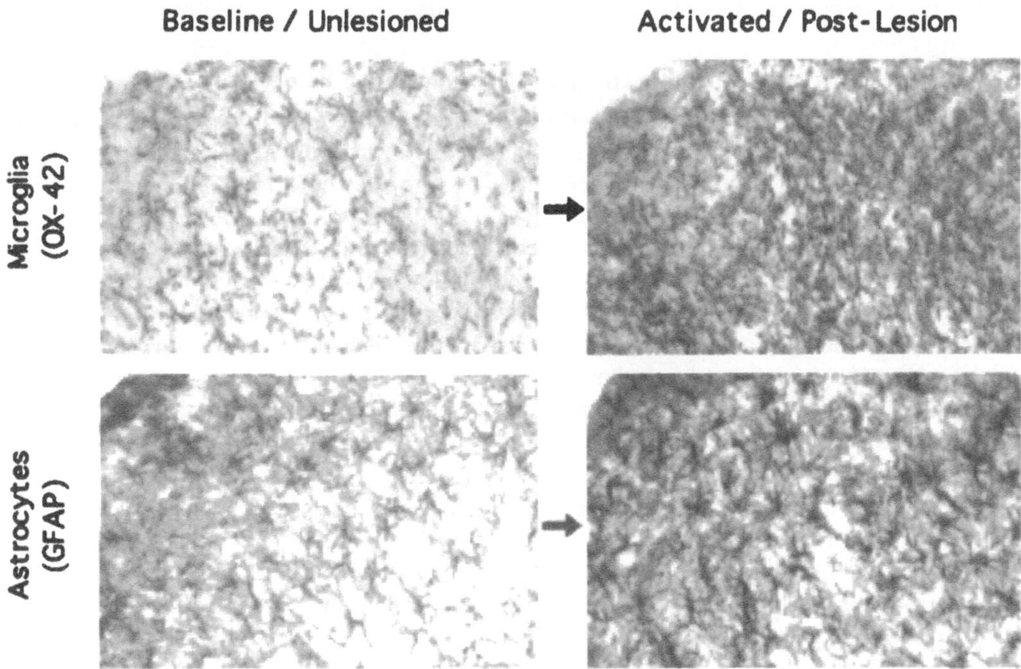

Figure 5 Photomicrographs of microglial and astrocytic staining in the L5 spinal dosal horn of a naive rat (left) and a L5 spinal nerve lesioned rat (right, 7 days postinjury, ipsilateral shown). Note the dramatic proliferation or migration of microglia and hypertrophy in astrocytes. There is also enhanced inflammatory cytokine (TNF-a, IL-1β, and IL-6) expression in these areas that appears to be primarily of neuronal and astrocytic origin. These changes occur gradually in the days following the lesion. It remains unclear whether these dramatic changes promote or protect against alterations in neuronal processing and pain behaviors.

changes, including the expression and release of cytotoxic or inflammatory mediators, including IL-1β, IL-6, TNF-α, proteases, and reactive oxygen intermediates, including nitric oxide (for reviews see Refs. 34,39).

1. Mechanisms of Microglial Activation

Microglia respond to a wide range of pathological stimuli including bacterial and viral infection, peripheral axotomy, neurotoxic insult, ischemia, autoimmune inflammation, and neurodegenerative disorders. Several molecules have been nominated as the primary trigger for microglial activation, and in particular, cytokines such as IL-1β and TNF-α, and the macrophage colony-stimulating factors (M–CSF, GM–CSF) appear to play key roles. The cellular source of these cytokines is not clear, although evidence points toward injured neurons and adjacent astrocytes as the likely producers (40–42). Other signals that may be capable of regulating microglial activation include neurotransmitters, such as epinephrine, adenosine, and substance P, which activate microglial adrenergic, purinergic, and neurokinin receptors, respectively. Chemokines, cell adhesion molecules, and factors from the complement cascade are also involved in the microglial response to neuronal injury. Microglial activation is not an all-or-none response, but rather, is carefully titrated to match the nature and severity of the injury. Microglia appear to be able to detect the difference between direct neurotoxic injury, as opposed to retrograde degeneration, and respond accordingly. This strengthens the hypothesis that injured neurons themselves are the source of the stimulatory signals, some of which may be transduced or relayed through local astrocytes (see Fig. 4). An example of this would be the production of M-CSF by astrocytes in response to alterations in synaptic glutamate levels or neuronally released IL-1β.

2. Ramifications of Microglial Activation for Neuropathic Pain

Microglia with their monocytic arsenal of cytotoxic tools have long been suspected as being the cells responsible for sensitizing neurons in the CNS under pathological conditions. Indeed microglia (or recruited macrophages differentiated as such) are key players in multiple sclerosis (MS), acquired immune deficiency syndrome (AIDS), Alzheimer's disease, amyotrophic lateral sclerosis (ALS), and other immune-related neurodegenerative diseases. However, their role in the neuroimmune response and pain behaviors that follow an acute neuropathic lesion has only recently drawn the attention of pain investigators. Initial observations showed a direct correlation betwen spinal microglial activation responses, inflammatory cytokine expression, and pain behaviors (43,44). More recent work, however, has identified several scenarios wherein robust neuropathic pain behaviors develop despite the apparent prevention or disruption of microglial activation responses. For example, selective L5 dorsal root transection results in robust mechanical allodynia akin to that seen following spinal nerve ligation; however, contrary to the latter, complete dorsal root transection produces no obvious microglial response when assessed at 1 week postlesion (45) (see Fig. 5). This result implies that (1) microglia respond to a signal transported centrally from the cell body (DRG) of the injured neuron and (2) that neither microglia nor incoming electrical signals (at the level of the lesion) are critical for the development of mechanical allodynia (Fig. 6). This latter conclusion must be qualified by two caveats. First, although microglia appeared quiescent at the time of sacrifice (7 days postlesion), it is possible that a very early, yet brief, microglial activation response occurred, setting a spinal neuroimmune cascade in motion. Although we have seen a very early generalized microglial "awakening" following peripheral inflammatory challenges (42), a vigorous focal (ipsilateral DH) microglial response is not observed for several days following spinal nerve lesions (Fig. 7). It is difficult to envision this type of profound focal response developing and then receding within several days. A second caveat is that microglial responses appear to be important in the synaptic strip-

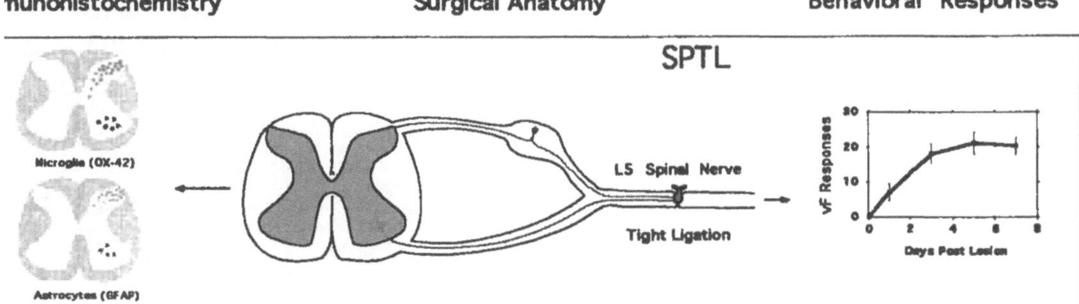

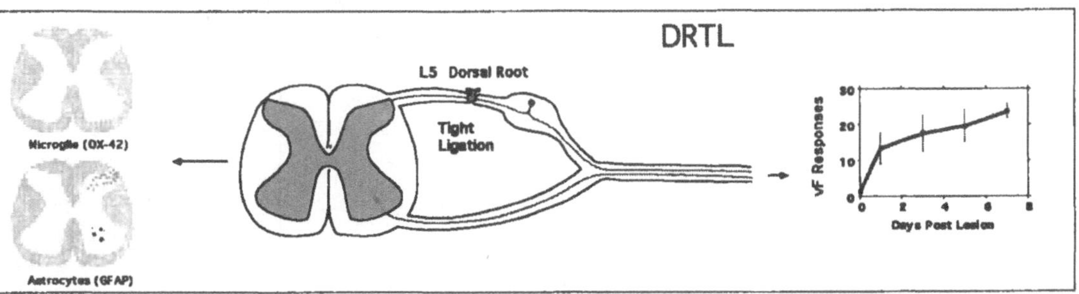

Figure 6 The site of a peripheral nerve injury has a dramatic bearing on the central neuroimmune response. Note the absence of a microglial response following a dorsal root lesion as compare with the robust microglia activation seen in response to a spinal nerve lesion. This finding implies that neuronal signals, mediated through the DRG and transported to the dorsal horn, are critical in stimulating microglia. Note also that the activation status of microglia has little association with mechanical allodynia, whereas astrocytes respond to neuronal injury regardless of site, and their activation reliably correlates with behaviors. Also noteworthy is the observation that, contrary to conventional wisdom, selective dorsal root lesion leads to mechanical allodynia, thus implying a central or collateral etiology. (From Ref. 45.)

ping and spinal reorganization that occurs following a nerve lesion which, in turn, may constitute the neuroanatomical basis for more chronic forms of neuropathic pain. The relatively short time course of these studies makes it difficult to assess this concept. Although the prevention of microglial activation responses is in its own right remarkable and may have relevance in deciphering microglial activation signals, this and similar studies (46) serve to shift suspicion onto astrocytes as the culprits that potentiate neuronal excitability.

B. Astrocytes

Astrocytes are the predominant cell type in the brain, outnumbering neurons by ten to one. They are located at virtually every interface between the CNS and the periphery, such that they may monitor, modulate, or respond to the entry of various factors (e.g., ions, metabolites, cytokines, drugs, infectious agents, or recruited cells; see Fig. 3). Their close physical presence next to neurons within the synaptic complex and at the nodes of Ranvier foretells their role in neurotransmission. Astrocytes are interconnected by gap junctions, such that ionic and metabolic coupling, both regionally and over distances, is possible. They possess a full complement of voltage- and ligand-gated channels, neuropeptide and neurotransmitter receptors, and second-messenger systems. Astrocytes perform a critical function in amino acid neurotransmission by taking up glutamate from the synaptic cleft and resupplying it to neurons as glutamine, which

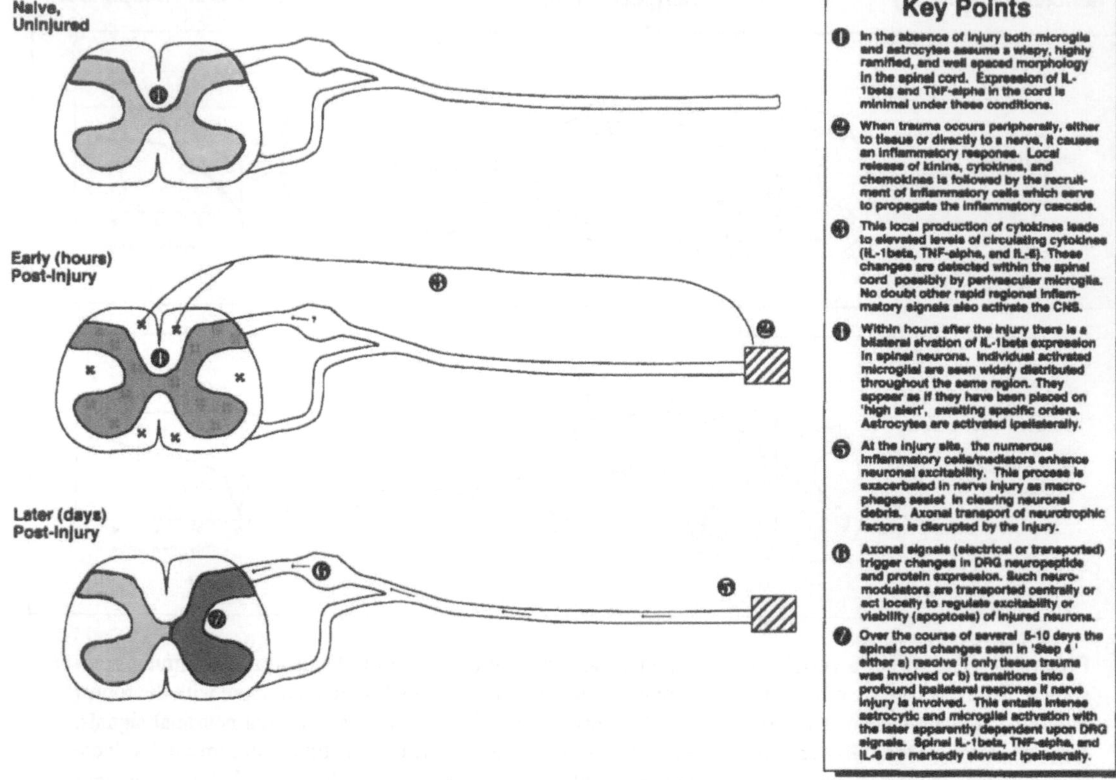

Figure 7 A schematic view of neuroimmune responses to tissue trauma or nerve injury.

is the precursor of both glutamate and γ-aminobutyic acid (GABA). This astrocytic glutamate-reuptake mechanism has been shown to be critical in the protection of neurons from glutamate excitotoxicity in pathological conditions, such as ischemia and trauma. Only recently has it come to be appreciated that astrocytes play a major role in neuroimmune responses. They produce, secrete, and respond to a large number of cytokines (such as IL-1β, TNF-α, IL-6, TGF-β, M-CSF), adhesion molecules, MHC antigens, complement, as well as prostaglandins and leukotrienes (for reviews see Refs. 33,46–49).

1. Mechanisms of Astrocytic Activation

By virtue of their close apposition to both neurons and the CNS vasculature, it is not surprising that astrocytes are among the first cells to respond to CNS injury. Their full repertoire of neurotransmitter and cytokine receptors keeps them closely informed on changes in the neuronal environment. On sensing a direct insult or even a remote disturbance, their prototypic response is to initiate a reactive gliosis, characterized by cellular hypertrophy and some degree of proliferation that appears to create a glial "scar." Expression of the intermediate filament, glial fibrillary acidic protein (GFAP), is enhanced within minutes of stimulation and has proved to be a clear marker for both resting and reactive astrocytes in the CNS (see Fig. 5). The vigorous astrocytic scar, rather than a simple impermeable barrier, actually subserves a neuroprotective role by capping and sheltering injured neurons from harmful or inappropriate stimulation. Astrocytes also provide neurotrophic support and guidance to facilitate regeneration in neurons.

2. Ramifications of Astrocytic Activation and Relevance to Neuropathic Pain

The intimate position of astrocytes at neuronal synapses and nodes of Ranvier provides them the opportunity to sense any electrical or chemical perturbation of neuronal activity. Astrocytic glutamate transporters are major regulators of synaptic glutamate concentration, thereby allowing astrocytes not only to continually sense neuronal activity, but also to modify neuronal activity by postsynaptic glutamate-mediated excitation and possibly "windup." Glutamate receptor antagonism diminishes both thermal hyperalgesia and astrocytic responses following sciatic chronic constriction injury (50). Neuronally released neuropeptides and cytokines bind receptors on astrocytes, which further alters astrocytic activation status. In turn, astrocytes express a full component of known neurotransmitters and cytokines, including specific microglial attractant and stimulatory factors (51,52). Ironically, retraction of astrocytic processes during the activation response may actually promote neuronal excitability by increasing interneuronal contact and by functionally reducing glutamate scavenging.

Astrocytic activation responses occur rapidly whenever there is nerve injury. It remains to be determined whether or not astrocytic activation plays a direct role in the generation of neuropathic pain behaviors. Unlike microglial activation responses, astroglial responses reliably coexist with and cannot be easily dissociated from pain behaviors (e.g., see Fig. 6). They are, however, not uniquely associated with such behaviors because astrocytic responses are also readily apparent following less severe nerve manipulations that do not lead to pain behaviors. Although activated astrocytes produce microglial-activating factors, as well as potentially hyperalgesic inflammatory cytokines, there is still a good deal of uncertainty over which glial cell type (microglia or astrocytes) first responds to nerve injury. As mentioned earlier (see Fig. 7), there is a generalized early microglia response (minutes to hours) possibly triggered by perivascular cells detecting circulating signals such as IL-1β. Astrocytes closely associated with the injured neurons respond within minutes, probably to fluctuations in synaptic glutamate or ion concentrations. The subsequent signaling between injured neurons and their glial partners helps determine which neurons survive and the degree to which regeneration and restoration of function is successful. Cytokines are key signaling molecules in these events.

C. Cytokines

1. Tumor Necrosis Factor-α

Tumor necrosis factor-α (TNF-α) is a major mediator of inflammatory and immune responses. Activated macrophages are the primary cellular source of TNF-α in the body; however, T cells, mast cells, microglia, and astrocytes can all be stimulated to release TNF-α. TNF-α's actions include enhancement of endothelial cell permeability, increased adhesion of circulating immune cells to endothelium, thereby fascilitating transendothelial migration of these cells, inducton of MHC molecules on a variety of cells types, as well as the induction of numerous cytokines (e.g., IL-1β, IL-6, and CSFs), including itself. TNF-α is produced primarily as a secreted protein that binds to either of two distinct transmembrane receptors (TNF-R1, 55 kDa, p55; and TNF-R2, 75 kDa, p75). The two receptors possess different cytoplasmic domains that utilize different intracellular-signaling pathways. Although activation of the TNF p55 receptor is intimately involved in inflammatory cytokine production and apoptosis, the p75 receptor is known to mediate cell proliferation and other cell survival characteristics. Intriguingly, many cells express both types of TNF receptor.

In the CNS, TNF-α is expressed by resident glial cells in response to various different stimuli, including exposure to ischemia, lipopolysaccharide (LPS), IL-1β, inteferon (IFN)-γ, and TNF-α itself. Astrocytes can respond to TNF-α stimulation by expressing GM–CSF and M–

CSF that further augments the migration of granulocytes and monocytes to the site. Both astrocytes and microglia are capable of responding to TNF-α by producing and releasing more TNF-α. This auto- or paracrine amplification of the inflammatory cascade continues with MHC and chemokine expression, leading to immune cell recruitment and potential oligodenrocyte or even neuronal cytotoxicity. One hypothesis for the mechanism of TNF-α neuronal cytotoxicity is that it can cause astrocytic depolarization, thereby disrupting voltage-dependent glutamate uptake, resulting in excitotoxic concentrations of synaptic glutamate. We have seen rapid expression of TNF-α in the spinal cord following a peripheral nerve injury (35). The distribution is bilateral in the dorsal horns, and double-labeling studies implicate astrocytes and neurons as the source in these types of mononeuropathy models. In more severe CNS inflammatory settings, such as experimental autoimmune encephalopathy (EAE), activated microglia and recruited macrophages also produce TNF-α.

The relevance of TNF-α to neuropathic pain lies in its ability (1) to directly excite neurons through an ill-defined mechanism; (2) to amplify local inflammatory cascades, resulting in the release of known neuron-sensitizing agents, such as prostaglandins, bradykinin, histamine, and NGF; and (3) to induce other cytokines such as IL-1β and IL-6, which also appear to have direct effects on neuronal function (Fig. 8). As mentioned earlier, a number of manipulations have been attempted to curtail these actions of TNF-α at the site of peripheral nerve injury. These will be discussed in more detail in the following anticytokine therapy section.

2. Interleukin-1β

Interleukin-1β is also a prominent molecule in the inflammatory cascade and immune responses (for reviews see Refs. 53–55). It is synthesized by peripheral immune cells as well as neurons, astrocytes, and microglia (56). Its actions are mediated primarily through specific membrane IL-1R receptors, and include triggering the release of IL-6, IL-8, and prostaglandins. IL-1β is a key modulator of fever and hyperalgesia associated with bacterial infection (e.g., LPS/endotoxin exposure) (57), as both responses are blocked by administration of an IL-1 receptor antagonist (IL-1ra). Spinal cord levels of IL-1β are elevated following peripheral LPS injection at times that coincide with hyperalgesia. Direct intradermal injection of IL-1β into the paw causes acute hyperalgesia (58–60), whereas intracerebroventricular or intraparenchymal injections in the brain can lead to either hyperalgesia or analgesia, depending on the site of application and the dose administered (61). Recent reports suggest IL-1β at femtomolar concentrations may be an endogenous inhibitory modulator of neuronal synaptic function; however, at higher (e.g., nano- to picomolar) concentrations the effect is reversed and neuronal sensitization results as per neuropathological scenarios.

In models of neuronal injury, such as cerebral ischemia, excitotoxicity, spinal contusion, and peripheral neuropathy, IL-1β is rapidly, albeit transiently, expressed in cells within the lesion site and occasionally in distant projections (62–64). Double immunohistochemical labeling has shown this expression is primarily astrocytic (65). We have observed neuronal IL-1β expression spinally in the dorsal horn ipsilateral to either spinal nerve lesion or intraplantar zymosan injection (42). This expression tends to correlate with both the severity of neuronal injury and the duration of pain behaviors. Attempts to mitigate or prevent pain behaviors by interceding in the physiological function of IL-1β have met some success; for example, IL-1ra or neutralizing antibodies to IL-1β have reversed acute hyperalgesia associated with systemic LPS or intraplatar IL-1β injection (57,66).

3. Interleukin-6

Interleukin-6 is another inflammatory cytokine mediating the acute-phase response and inflammation. It appears to be downstream from TNF-α and IL-1β in the classic inflammatory cascade;

Signals for Nerve Injury-Induced Glial Activation and Pain

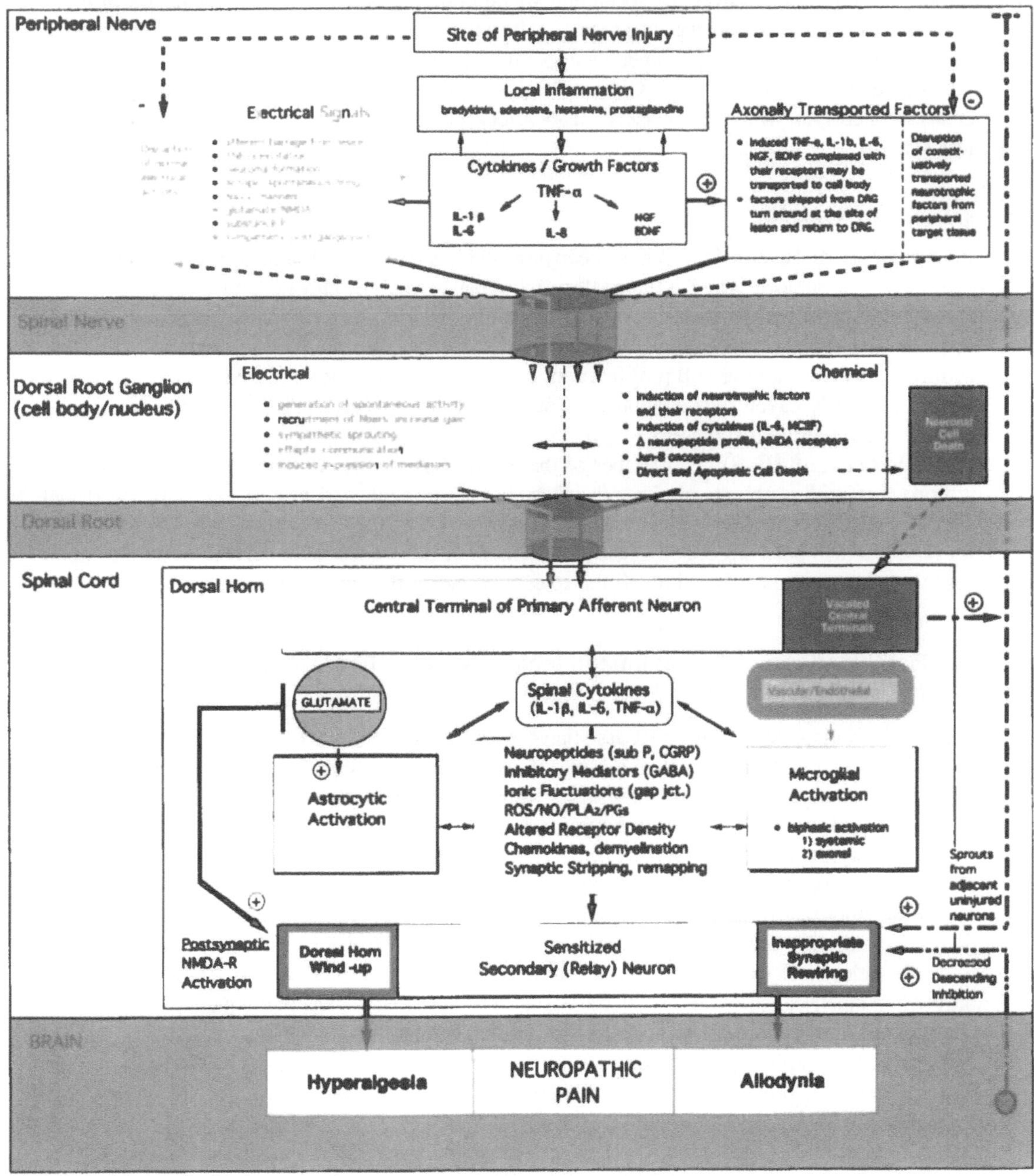

Figure 8 Overall view of the possible roles of glial responses in the generation of neuropathic pain.

however, there are also circumstances when it subserves an anti-inflammatory role (67). IL-6 exerts its activity through a high-affinity receptor complex that includes a specific IL-6R-binding protein, which then aligns with a 130-kDa signal-transducing glycoprotein (gp130) element that is shared with other ligands of the same family. IL-6 is synthesized in a wide variety of cells, including macrophages, endothelial cells, astrocytes, and microglia.

Following nerve injury, increases in IL-6 mRNA and protein are observed in neurons throughout the related DRG and ipsilateral spinal cord segments (26,40,68). This elevation in IL-6 may play a role in nociceptive processing because intrathecal (36) or intracerebroventricular (69) administration of IL-6 produced neuropathic pain behaviors in normal rats. IL-6 also exerts a stimulatory role on glial cells. Overexpression of IL-6 results in reactive astrocytes and increased microglia, while conversely, IL-6 knockout mice exhibit deficient glial activation (70,71).

4. Other Cytokines

Interleukin-4, IL-10, and TGF-β have been described as the anti-inflammatory cytokines. These cytokines are induced when inflammatory cytokine levels are elevated. In turn, they downregulate the expression of IL-1β and TNF-α, thereby serving as a feedback "braking" mechanism to limit the self-propagating inflammatory cascade. TGF-β in its various isoforms has additional effects on glial cell proliferation, migration, and chemokine production (72). These effects generally favor regeneration or wound healing; however, TGF-β is self-propagating through an autocrine mechanism.

Interleukin-8 (IL-8) is a member of the chemokine family. Chemokines, including IL-8, are proteins with a potent role in cell adhesion, recruitment, and migration. Both IL-1β and TNF-α (particularly together) can induce the expression of IL-8 and other chemokines. A role for IL-8 has also been suggested in the involvement of the sympathetic nervous system in nociceptive processing, possibly through the release of sympathomimetic amines (73).

D. Ramifications of Spinal Inflammatory Cytokine Expression for Neuropathic Pain

Peripheral trauma, particularly that associated with injury directly to a nerve, provokes a rapid and robust central (spinal) glial response and cytokine expression (see Fig. 8). This response appears to be biphasic with very rapid generalized (often bilateral) microglial activation and IL-1β expression occurring within hours, and then a focal (ipsilateral) microglial, astrocytic, and further cytokine expression (IL-1β, IL-6, and TNF-α) developing over several days postinjury. The mechanisms by which these responses are triggered are not well delineated. Because the initial microglial reaction and IL-1β expression are very rapid, they are not likely to be driven by axonally transported factors from the injury site. Indeed, studies by Molander help to dismiss electrical signals alone as the cause of microglial activation (74). They showed that only when electrical stimulation was increased to a level that caused nerve damage was subsequent microglial activation seen. These observations coupled with the finding that this "arousal" is rather global within the spinal cord (i.e., spread beyond the nerve terminals directly associated with injury) leads one to surmise that it is propagated by systemic factors, possibly circulating cytokines, such as IL-1β. Alternatively, peripheral monocytes may be recruited to the area of the spinal cord from the circulation. Once within the spinal parenchyma, they assume a microglial morphology, then migrate and proliferate. The later focal microglial response is likely directed by factors transported from the afferent fibers of the injured nerves because dorsal root rhizotomy eliminates much of the reaction. Astrocytic activation appears to be independent of transported factors and may be evoked by excessive neuronal firing or, conversely, neuronal quiescence. Latent focal expression of IL-1β, IL-6, and TNF-α appears to be primarily neuronal and astrocytic. It is not known whether the early global "arousal" is required for, permits, or potentiates the full local response. These glial and cytokine responses may directly or indirectly potentiate or propagate neuropathic syndromes much as they have been shown to do in other neurodegenerative diseases such as multiple sclerosis and Alzheimer's disease. There is good evidence that IL-1β is involved with TNF-α in the early global spinal response to peripheral trauma and associated hyperalgesic behaviors. TNF-α evokes neuronal excitation and pain behaviors when applied directly to a peripheral nerve. α-Melanocyte-stimulating hormone (α-MHS) inhibits the expression of both IL-1β and TNF-α, while at the same time, enhancing the anti-inflammatory cytokine, IL-10 (75). Studies are underway to assess the potential usefulness of α-MSH and a number of other anticytokine therapies in models of neuropathic pain (Colburn/Munglani IASP 1999 abstract).

E. Interventions to Control Neuroimmune Responses

To intervene in the neuroimmune responses to nerve injury one must consider whether the signals propagating these responses are systemic or local (see Fig. 7) and, if local, for example, at the spinal level or at the lesion site, are they restricted to specific immune cell populations?

1. Microglia or Macrophage-Directed Manipulations

Despite that the evidence linking macrophages or microglia with the development of pain behaviors following nerve injury is circumstantial, these cells are known to produce several cytotoxic and neuromodulatory factors that could readily sensitize exposed neurons. Similarly, these cells are crucial in promoting the inflammatory cascades that can lead to the further release of neuroactive substances, such as inflammatory cytokines, prostaglandins, nitric oxide, or other. There are two obvious sites at which to try to curtail a monocytic response: at the site of nerve injury and centrally. Although resident and invading macrophages are critical for myelin clearance and regeneration, it may be possible to modulate their response enough to reduce inflammation and neuronal sensitization without jeopardizing regeneration. Reducing neuronal firing in this way would diminish both ongoing electrical noise to the spinal cord and subsequent central compensatory responses. Focal perineural drug application of anti-inflammatory agents (steroids) (76,77), antiproliferative agents (colchicine) (78,79), local anesthetics (44,80), and anticytokine therapy (18,81–83) produce variable behavioral improvement depending on the nerve injury model employed.

Centrally, efforts to pharmacologically control microglial activation are hampered by a lack of certainty over the source of these activated microglia. Are they spinal parenchymal microglial that proliferate and migrate regionally in response to peripheral nerve lesion, or are many of these microglia recruited as monocytes from the circulation as in MS? To help answer this question, researchers have used experimental, global macrophage depletion through irradiation or selective phagocytotic ingestion of toxins (chlodronate) (84,85). These methods almost exclusively deplete circulating monocytes, as resting CNS microglia are not phagocytic and proliferate very slowly, thereby making them much less susceptible to these measures. As might be expected, circulating macrophage depletion dramatically reduces the inflammatory consequences of injury in situations where the blood–brain barrier is compromised and there is direct damage to the CNS because there is active leaking or recruitment of macrophages into the parenchyma. Similar effects are seen following administration of antichemokine and antiadhesion molecular therapy, as they too reduce the entry and consequences of recruited circulating inflammatory cells. Whether microglial activation at sites remote from the nerve lesion also triggers recruitment and invasion of monocytes is a fundamental question that has yet to be answered. A slightly more elegant approach to this question is the use of bone marrow chimeras in which peripheral monocytic stem cells are depleted and then replaced by those from a different strain (86). Any circulating cells that enter the CNS from the blood stream can then be easily detected by antibodies specific to the donor strain (DeLeo JA, personal communication).

2. Astrocyte-Directed Manipulations

Astrocytes are intimately involved in neuronal homeostasis and respond to a wide variety of perturbations. Therefore, it is extremely difficult to selectively inhibit or deplete astrocytes without jeopardizing neuronal function and viability. There are still relatively few studies directed toward this goal, particularly as relates to the role of astrocytes in neuropathic pain. Garrison et al. gave the NMDA antagonist, dizocilpine maleate (MK-801), to rats at the time of CCI lesion and observed reduced glial fibrillary acitic protein (GFAP)-labeled astrocyte activation as well as reduced thermal hyperalgesia (50). This supports the concept that synaptic glutamate plays a decisive role in astrocytic activation. A more extreme form of astrocytic inhibition is depletion. The metabolic gliatoxin, fluorocitrate, when applied centrally at low doses is purported to be selectively toxic for astrocytes (87,88). Meller et al. (89) administered fluorocitrate intrathecally to reversibly attenuate the persistent mechanical and thermal hyperalgesia produced by intraplantar injection of zymosan. Similarly, Watkins et al. (90) observed a reduction in formalin-induced hyperalgesia following intrathecal fluorocitrate. Another astrocyte-selective toxin is L-α-aminoadipate which, as an excitatory amino acid analogue, is thought to function by inhibiting glutamate transport (91,92). Intracerebral injection of α-aminoadipate depleted astrocytes in the region without causing obvious disruption to neurons or microglia (93); however, it has yet to be employed spinally in models of neuropathic pain.

The technical ability to manipulate genes has been coupled with the propensity for stimulated astrocytes to up-regulate expression of GFAP. An elegant method for selectively depleting activated astrocytes using this technology is described by Bush and Sofroniew (94,95). For this, the thymidine kinase gene of the herpes simple virus (HSV-TK) was linked to the GFAP promoter such that on stimulation (such as a stab wound to the brain) astrocytes would express thymidine kinase. Although not toxic on its own, this enzyme confers lethal sensitivity to subsequently administered ganciclovir by allowing its metabolism to toxic nucleotide analogues. This model allows the timing and location of astrocytic ablation to be regulated according to where and when the ganciclovir is administered; however, the toxicity is dependent on the degree of astrocytic proliferation. Several other transgenic mice have also been developed that link the GFAP promoter to a gene sequence coding for proteins such as IL-3, IL-6, TGF-β_1, TNF-α, and NGF. The result is an overexpression of the specific cytokine driven by conditions that stimulate astrocyte activation, such as a peripheral nerve injury. This affords researchers a tool to help deceipher which cytokines potentiate or, conversely, mitigate the development of neuropathic pain conditions.

3. Cytokine-Based Manipulations

Numerous potential cytokine-based therapies have been developed in an effort to limit the deleterious effects of inflammation following nerve injury or CNS damage. The obvious strategy has been to try to inhibit inflammatory cytokines, such as IL-1β and TNF-α. Mechanisms have been devised to interfere with these cytokines at numerous steps of their synthetic and functional pathways (96). For example, selective inhibition of TNF-α transcription is accomplished by CNI-1493, whereas inhibition of posttranslational modifications (97), particularly the cleaving pro- to active forms is accomplished by IL-1-converting enzyme (ICE) and TNF-α-converting enzyme (TACE) inhibitors (98). Cytokine binding proteins (e.g., TNF-bp) or soluble receptors (e.g., IL-1ra) act as functional cytokine antagonists by binding cytokines, thereby inhibiting their interaction with signal transducing cell membrane receptors. These agents have also been employed with some success in models of cerebral ischemia and experimental allergic encephalomyelitis.

Functional antagonism of inflammatory cytokines may also be accomplished by administering neutralizing antibodies targeted toward these cytokines or their receptors. Antibodies against TNF-α have been used to ameliorate acute hyperalgesic behaviors resulting from inflammogen injection. Ironically, repeated dosing of cytokine-related agents (e.g., IL-1ra or TNF-bp) can stimulate the production of autoantibodies that may negate or paradoxically reverse their beneficial effects in vivo. This concept can be used to advantage, however, by stimulating endogenous production of antibodies directed against inflammatory cytokines (99). The superantigenic Sant-1 molecule when linked with IL-6 subunits and administered as a vaccine stimulates the production of antibodies capable of neutralizing IL-6 (100). Whether this strategy can be employed effectively against neuropathic pain behaviors is currently under study (Arruda JL, personal communication).

An alternative strategy directed at reducing inflammatory cytokines is to enhance the availability of so-called anti-inflammatory cytokines, such as IL-10, IL-4, and TGF-β. These cytokines generally suppress the expression of IL-1β and TNF-α and are thought to endogenously regulate the duration and extent of the inflammatory cascade. Perineural IL-10 administration diminishes thermal hyperalgesia, inflammatory cell infiltration, and sciatic endoneurial TNF-α levels following CCI lesion (83). Similarly, systemic or intraplantar IL-10 administration reduced inflammatory responses and hyperalgesia associated with IL-1β or LPS injection (101,102). The effectiveness of IL-10 administration has been shown in stroke and spinal cord injury (103). A paradoxical reduction in the area of injury was observed following aggravation of the inflammatory response through the application of exogenous inflammatory cytokines in a spinal cord trauma model (64); perhaps advancing the inflammatory cascade expedites expression of more beneficial reparative cytokines (104). These examples are testament to the delicate fluctuations in concentrations and timing hat control cytokine interactions in vivo.

Recent reports of studies using cytokine and cytokine receptor knockout mice (71,105–112), cytokine overexpressing transgenic animals (113–117), and genetically engineered syngenic cell grafts (118) have provided insight into the roles of some of these cytokines. Many of these genetic models have yet to be specifically applied to deciphering the mechanisms of neuropathic pain; however, with great caution basic neuroimmune interactions can be extrapolated (119,120). On the other hand, we have also been confounded by some unexpected results that only serve to provide further evidence for the deeply complex nature of cytokine interactions.

F. Neuroimmune Responses: Summary

In summary, clinical chronic pain syndrome are based on a wide variety of nerve injury scenarios, most of which are much less specific than those performed experimentally in animals. To be able to identify the lesion, predict the course of sensory manifestations, and ultimately, intervene pharmacologically is the principal goal of pain researchers. We and others have confirmed the existence of a neuroimmune component to the central alterations that result in neuropathic pain behaviors. Future work needs to be directed at (1) more specific identification of the signals that independently activate microglia and astrocytes, (2) attempts to separate astrocytic activation responses from pain behaviors, (3) further identification and manipulation of the role of cytokines in spinal sensory processing, and (4) analysis of the crosstalk between classic neurotransmitters (substance P, glutamate, norepinephrine) and the neuroimmune response as manifest by neurons, astrocytes, microglia, and their cytokine products. Progress in these directions will provide not only new avenues for the treatment of chronic pain, but will also advance the understanding of deleterious neuroimmune interactions manifest in several neurodegenerative conditions.

IV. FINAL REMARKS

For centuries pain has been treated with aspirin and opioids. These two classes of drugs remain our primary therapy for acute pain, but typically they fail to provide relief from chronic neuropathic pain. Surgical interventions have been attempted with the intent of disconnecting the wiring to and from the offending body part. Unfortunately, central responses to peripheral injury reduce the usefulness of this approach since, as we have described in this chapter, all levels of the neuroaxis are involved in responding to nerve injury, and many of these responses involve relatively permanent anatomical changes. Ironically, many novel emerging therapies are both not selective enough (within the given system they are trying to modulate) and too focal (by virtue of modulating only one system). By targeting a single cytokine, peptide, ion channel, or neurotransmitter system, we fail to appreciate the immense interconnectivity and redundancy built into the nervous system. Frustratingly, neuropathic conditions appear to define a new homeostatic "setpoint" that singular therapies may favorably perturb briefly; however, they are readily compensated and overcome as the system regains the undesirable setpoint. Physicians often serendipitously create their own polypharmaceutical approach as they struggle with drug after drug to find a useful therapy for their patients with chronic pain. The hope is that ultimately, as our understanding of neuropathic pain mechanisms advancnes, it will be possible to define, on an individual-by-individual basis, which variables in the global pain algorithm need pharmacological attention and to tailor a multipronged therapeutic plan accordingly. Many of the subsequent chapters in this book describe novel therapies that we hope will lend new insight and an armamentarium toward fulfillment of this goal.

REFERENCES

1. Woolf CJ, Ma QP, Allchorne A, Poole S. Peripheral cell types contributing to the hyperalgesic action of nerve growth factor in inflammation. J Neurosci 1996; 16:2716–2723.
2. Lewin GR, Rueff A, Mendell LM. Peripheral and central mechanisms of NGF-induced hyperalgesia. Eur J Neurosci 1994; 6:1903–1912.
3. Ma W, Bisby MA. Increase of galanin mRNA in lumbar dorsal root ganglion neurons of adult rats after partial sciatic nerve ligation. Neurosci Lett 1999; 262:195–198.
4. Xian CJ, Zhou XF. Neuronal–glial differential expression of TGF-alpha and its receptor in the dorsal root ganglia in response to sciatic nerve lesion. Exp Neurol 1999; 157:317–326.
5. Donaldson LF, Harmar AJ, McQueen DS, Seckl JR. Increased expression of preprotachykinin, calcitonin gene-related peptide, but not vasoactive intestinal peptide messenger RNA in dorsal root ganglia during the development of adjuvant monoarthritis in the rat. Brain Res Mol Brain Res 1992; 16:143–149.
6. Lee SE, Shen H, Taglialatela G, Chung JM, Chung K. Expression of nerve growth factor in the dorsal root ganglion after periphral nerve injury. Brain Res 1998; 796:99–106.
7. Curtis R, Tonra JR, Stark JL, et al. Neuronal injury increases retrograde axonal transport of the neurotrophins to spinal sensory neurons and motor neurons via multiple receptor mechanisms. Mol Cell Neurosci 1998; 12:105–118.
8. Cho HJ, Kim JK, Park HC, Kim DS, Ha SO, Hong HS. Changes in brain-derived neurotrophic factor immunoreactivity in rat dorsal root ganglia, spinal cord, and gracile nuclei following cut or crush injuries. Exp Neurol 1998; 154:224–230.

9. Shen H, Chung JM, Chung K. Expression of neurotrophin mRNAs in the dorsal root ganglion after spinal nerve injury. Brain Res Mol Brain Res 1999; 64:186–192.
10. Carlton SM, Coggeshall RE. Inflammation-induced changes in peripheral glutamate receptor populations. Brain Res 1999; 820:63–70.
11. Donnerer J, Schuligoi R, Stein C, et al. Upregulation, release and axonal transport of substance P and calcitonin gene-related peptide in adjuvant inflammation and regulatory function of nerve growth factor. Regul Pept 1993; 46:150–154.
12. Carlton SM, Zhou S, Coggeshall RE. Localization and activation of substance P receptors in unmyelinated axons of rat glabrous skin. Brain Res 1996; 734:103–108.
13. Ahluwalia A, De Filipe C, O'Brien J, Hunt SP, Perretti M. Impaired IL-1beta-induced neutrophil accumulation in tachykinin NK1 receptor knockout mice. Br J Pharmacol 1998; 124:1013–1015.
14. Myers RR. 1994 ASRA Lecture. The pathogenesis of neuropathic pain. Reg Anesth 1995; 20:173–184.
15. Uncini A, Di MA, Di GG, et al. Effect of rhTNF-alpha injection into rat sciatic nerve. J Neuroimmunol 1999; 94:88–94.
16. Redford EJ, Hall SM, Smith KJ. Vascular changes and demyelination induced by the intraneural injection of tumour necrosis factor. Brain 1995; 869–878.
17. Wagner R, Myers RR. Schwann cells produce tumor necrosis factor alpha: expression in injured and non-injured nerves. Neuroscience 1996; 73:625–629.
18. Sommer C, Schmidt C, George A, Toyka KV. A metalloprotease-inhibitor reduces pain associated behavior in mice with experimental neuropathy. Neurosci Lett 1997; 237:45–48.
19. Sommer C, Schmidt C, George A. Hyperalgesia in experimental neuropathy is dependent on the TNF receptor 1. Exp Neurol 1998; 151:138–142.
20. Matzner O, Devor M. Hyperexcitability at sites of nerve injury depends on voltage-sensitive Na^+ channels. J Neurophysiol 1994; 72:349–359.
21. Nakamura S, Myers RR. Myelinated afferents sprout into lamina II of L3-5 dorsal horn following chronic constriction nerve injury in rats. Brain Res 1999; 818:285–290.
22. Bennett DL, Michael GJ, Ramachandran N, et al. A distinct subgroup of small DRG cells express GDNF receptor components and GDNF is protective for these neurons after nerve injury. J Neurosci 1998; 18:3059–3072.
23. Bradbury EJ, Burnstock G, McMahon SB. The expression of P2X3 purinoreceptors in sensory neurons: effects of axotomy and glial-derived neurotrophic factor. Mol Cell Neurosci 1998; 12:256–268.
24. Dib-Hajj SD, Black JA, Cummins TR, Kenney AM, Kocsis JD, Waxman SG. Rescue of alpha-SNS sodium channel expression in small dorsal root ganglion neurons after axotomy by nerve growth factor in vivo. J Neurophysiol 1998; 79:2668–2676.
25. Okuse K, Chaplan SR, McMahon SB, et al. Regulation of expression of the sensory neuron-specific sodium channel SNS in inflammatory and neuropathic pain. Mol Cell Neurosci 1997; 10:196–207.
26. Murphy PG, Borthwick LS, Johnston RS, Kuchel G, Richardson PM. Nature of the retrograde signal from injured nerves that induces interleukin-6 mRNA in neurons. J Neurosci 1999; 19:3791–3800.
27. Kral MG, Xiong Z, Study RE. Alteration of Na^+ currents in dorsal root ganglion neurons from rats with a painful neuropathy. Pain 1999; 81:15–24.
28. Kim HJ, Na HS, Sung B, Hong SK. Amount of sympathetic sprouting in the dorsal root ganglia is not correlated to the level of sympathetic dependence of neuropathic pain in a rat model. Neurosci Lett 1998; 245:21–24.
29. Lee BH, Yoon YW, Chung K, Chung JM. Comparison of sympathetic sprouting in sensory ganglia in three animal models of neuropathic pain. Exp Brain Res 1998; 120:432–438.
30. Thompson SW, Majithia AA. Leukemia inhibitory factor induces sympathetic sprouting in intact dorsal root ganglia in the adult rat in vivo. J Physiol (Lond) 1998; 506(pt 3):809–816.
31. Ramer MS, Bisby MA. Differences in sympathetic innervation of mouse DRG following proximal or distal nerve lesions. Exp Neurol 1998; 152:197–207.
32. Whiteside G, Doyle CA, Hunt SP. Differential time course of neuronal and glial apoptosis in neonatal rat dorsal root ganglia after sciatic nerve axotomy. Eur J Neurosci 1998; 10:3400–3408.

33. Araque A, Parpura V, Sanzgiri RP, Haydon PG. Tripartite synapses: glia, the unacknowledged partner. Trends Neurosci 1999; 22:208–215.
34. Perry VH, Gordon S. Microglia and macrophages. In: Keane RW, Hickey WF, eds. Immunology of the Nervous System. New York: Oxford University Press, 1997:155–172.
35. DeLeo JA, Colburn RW, Rickman AJ. Cytokine and growth factor immunohistochemical spinal profiles in two animal models of mononeuropathy. Brain Res 1997; 759:50–57.
36. DeLeo JA, Colburn RW, Nichols M, Malhotra A. Interleukin-6-mediated hyperalgesia/allodynia and increased spinal IL-6 expression in a rat mononeuropathy model. J Interferon Cytokine Res 1996; 16:695–700.
37. Kreutzberg GW, Graeber MB, Streit WJ. Neuron–glial relationship during regeneration of motorneurons. Metab Brain Dis 1989; 4:81–85.
38. Svensson M, Eriksson P, Persson JK, Molander C, Arvidsson J, Aldskogius H. The response of central glia to peripheral nerve injury. Brain Res Bull 1993; 30:499–506.
39. Raivich G, Bohatschek M, Kloss CUA, Werner A, Jones LL, Kreutzberg GW. Neuroglial activation repertoire in the injured brain: graded response, molecular mechanisms and cues to physiological function. Brain Res Rev 1999; 30:77–105.
40. Arruda JL, Colburn RW, Rickman AJ, Rutkowski MD, DeLeo JA. Increase of interleukin-6 mRNA in the spinal cord following peripheral nerve injury in the rat: potential role of IL-6 in neuropathic pain. Brain Res Mol Brain Res 1998; 62:228–235.
41. DeLeo JA, Colburn RW. Proinflammatory cytokines and glial cells: their role in neuropathic pain. In: Watkins LR, Maier SF, eds. Cytokines and Pain. Basel: Birkhauser, 1999:159–182.
42. Sweitzer SM, Colburn RW, Rutkowski M, DeLeo JA. Acute peripheral inflammation induces moderate glial activation and spinal IL-1beta expression that correlates with pain behavior in the rat. Brain Res 1999; 829:209–221.
43. Coyle DE. Partial peripheral nerve injury leads to activation of astroglia and microglia which parallels the development of allodynic behavior. Glia 1998; 23:75–83.
44. Colburn RW, DeLeo JA, Rickman AJ, Yeager MP, Kwon P, Hickey WF. Dissociation of microglial activation and neuropathic pain behaviors following peripheral nerve injury in the rat. J Neuroimmunol 1997; 79:163–175.
45. Colburn RW, Rickman AJ, DeLeo JA. The effect of site and type of nerve injury on spinal glial activation and neuropathic pain behavior. Exp Neurol 1999; 157:289–304.
46. Aldskogius H, Kozlova EN. Central neuron–glial and glial–glial interactions following axon injury. Prog Neurobiol 1998; 55:1–26.
47. Ridel JL, Malhotra SK, Privat A, Gage FH. Reactive astrocytes: cellular and molecular cues to biological function [published erratum appears in Trends Neurosci 1998 Feb; 21:80]. Trends Neurosci 1997; 20:570–577.
48. Vernadakis A. Glia–neuron intercommunications and synaptic plasticity. Prog Neurobiol 1996; 49: 185–214.
49. Norenberg MD. Astrocytes: normal aspects and response to CNS injury. In: Keane RW, Hickey WF, eds. Immunology of the Nervous System. New York: Oxford University Press, 1997:173–199.
50. Garrison CJ, Dougherty PM, Carlton SM. GFAP expression in lumbar spinal cord of naive and neuropathic rats treated with MK-801. Exp Neurol 1994; 129:237–243.
51. Oh JW, Schwiebert LM, Benveniste EN. Cytokine regulation of CC and CXC chemokine expression by human astrocytes. J Neurovirol 1999; 5:82–94.
52. Weiss JM, Berman JW. Astrocyte expression of monocyte chemoattractant protein-1 is differentially regulated by transforming growth factor beta. J Neuroimmunol 1998; 91:190–197.
53. Woiciechowsky C, Schoning B, Daberkow N, et al. Brain-IL-1beta induces local inflammation but systemic anti-inflammatory response through stimulation of both hypothalamic–pituitary–adrenal axis and sympathetic nervous system. Brain Res 1999; 816:563–571.
54. Rothwell NJ, Luheshi G, Toulmond S. Cytokines and their receptors in the central nervous system: physiology, pharmacology, and pathology. Pharmacol Ther 1996; 69:85–95.
55. Anforth HR, Bluthe RM, Bristow A, et al. Biological activity and brain actions of recombinant rat interleukin-1alpha and interleukin-1beta. Eur Cytokine Netw 1998; 9:279–288.

56. Benveniste EN. Cytokine actions in the central nervous system. Cytokine Growth Factor Rev 1998; 9:259–275.
57. Watkins LR, Maier SF, Goehler LE. Immune activation: the role of pro-inflammatory cytokines in inflammation, illness responses and pathological pain states. Pain 1995; 63:289–302.
58. Poole S, Bristow AF, Lorenzetti BB, Das RE, Smith TW, Ferreira SH. Peripheral analgesic activities of peptides related to alpha-melanocyte stimulating hormone and interleukin-1 beta 193–195. Br J Pharmacol 1992; 106:489–492.
59. Ferreira SH, Lorenzetti BB, Bristow AF, Poole S. Interleukin-1 beta as a potent hyperalgesic agent antagonized by a tripeptide analogue. Nature 1988; 334:698–700.
60. Safieh–Garabedian B, Poole S, Allchorne A, Winter J, Woolf CJ. Contribution of interleukin-1 beta to the inflammation-induced increase in nerve growth factor levels and inflammatory hyperalgesia. Br J Pharmacol 1995; 115:1265–1275.
61. Oka T, Aou S, Hori T. Intracerebroventricular injection of interleukin-1 beta induces hyperalgesia in rats. Brain Res 1993; 624:61–68.
62. Rothwell N, Allan S, Toulmond S. The role of interleukin 1 in acute neurodegeneration and stroke: pathophysiological and therapeutic implications. J Clin Invest 1997; 100:2648–2652.
63. Davies CA, Loddick SA, Toulmond S, Stroemer RP, Hunt J, Rothwell NJ. The progression and topographic distribution of interleukin-1beta expression after permanent middle cerebral artery occlusion in the rat. J Cereb Blood Flow Metab 1999; 19:87–98.
64. Klusman I, Schwab ME. Effects of pro-inflammatory cytokines in experimental spinal cord injury. Brain Res 1997; 762:173–184.
65. Pearson VL, Rothwell NJ, Toulmond S. Excitotoxic brain damage in the rat induces interleukin-1beta protein in microglia and astrocytes: correlation with the progression of cell death. Glia 1999; 25:311–323.
66. Safieh–Garabedian B, Kanaan SA, Haddad JJ, Jaoude PA, Jabbur SJ, Saade NE. Involvement of interleukin-1beta, nerve growth factor and prostaglandin E_2 in endotoxin-induced localized inflammatory hyperalgesia. Br J Pharmacol 1997; 121:1619–1626.
67. Gadient RA, Otten UH. Interleukin-6 (IL-6)—a molecule with both beneficial and destructive potentials. Prog Neurobiol 1997; 52:379–390.
68. Murphy PG, Ramer MS, Borthwick L, Gauldie J, Richardson PM, Bisby MA. Endogenous interleukin-6 contributes to hypersensitivity to cutaneous stimuli and changes in neuropeptides associated with chronic nerve constriction in mice. Eur J Neurosci 1999; 11:2243–2253.
69. Oka T, Oka K, Hosoi M, Hori T. Intracerebroventricular injection of interleukin-6 induces thermal hyperalgesia in rats. Brain Res 1995; 692:123–128.
70. Klein MA, Moller JC, Jones LL, Bluethmann H, Kreutzberg GW, Raivich G. Impaired neuroglial activation in interleukin-6 deficient mice. Glia 1997; 19:227–233.
71. Zhong J, Dietzel ID, Wahle P, Kopf M, Heumann R. Sensory impairments and delayed regeneration of sensory axons in interleukin-6-deficient mice. J Neurosci 1999; 19:4305–4313.
72. Flanders KC, Ren RF, Lippa CF. Transforming growth factor-betas in neurodegenerative disease. Prog Neurobiol 1998; 54:71–85.
73. Cunha FQ, Lorenzetti BB, Poole S, Ferreira SH. Interleukin-8 as a mediator of sympathetic pain. Br J Pharmacol 1991; 104:765–767.
74. Molander C, Hongpaisan J, Svensson M, Aldskogius H. Glial cell reactions in the spinal cord after sensory nerve stimulation are associated with axonal injury. Brain Res 1997; 747:122–129.
75. Lipton JM, Catania A. Anti-inflammatory actions of the neuroimmunomodulator alpha-MSH. Immunol Today 1997; 18:140–145.
76. Johansson A, Bennett GJ. Effect of local methylprednisolone on pain in a nerve injury model. A pilot study. Reg Anesth 1997; 22:59–65.
77. Clatworthy AL, Illich PA, Castro GA, Walters ET. Role of peri-axonal inflammation in the development of thermal hyperalgesia and guarding behavior in a rat model of neuropathic pain. Neurosci Lett 1995; 184:5–8.
78. Cougnon–Aptel N, Whiteside GT, Munglani R. Effect of colchicine on neuropeptide Y expression in rat dorsal root ganglia and spinal cord. Neurosci Lett 1999; 259:45–48.

79. Colburn RW, DeLeo JA. The effect of perineural colchicine on nerve injury-induced spinal glia activation and neuropathic pain behavior. Brain Res Bull 1999; 49:419–427.
80. Dougherty PM, Garrison CJ, Carlton SM. Differential influence of local anesthetic upon two models of experimentally induced peripheral mononeuropathy in the rat. Brain Res 1992; 570:109–115.
81. Sommer C, Marziniak M, Myers RR. The effect of thalidomide treatment on vascular pathology and hyperalgesia caused by chronic constriction injury of rat nerve. Pain 1998; 74:83–91.
82. Sorkin LS, Xiao WH, Wagner R, Myers RR. Tumour necrosis factor-alpha induces ectopic activity in nociceptive primary afferent fibres. Neuroscience 1997; 81:255–262.
83. Wagner R, Janjigian M, Myers RR. Anti-inflammatory interleukin-10 therapy in CCI neuropathy decreases thermal hyperalgesia, macrophage recruitment, and endoneurial TNF-alpha expression. Pain 1998; 74:35–42.
84. Popovich PG, Guan Z, Wei P, Huitinga I, van Rooijen N, Stokes BT. Depletion of hematogenous macrophages promotes partial hindlimb recovery and neuroanatomical repair after experimental spinal cord injury. Exp Neurol 1999; 158:351–365.
85. Koennecke LA, Zito MA, Proescholdt MG, van Rooijen N, Heyes MP. Depletion of systemic macrophages by liposome-encapsulated clodronate attenuates increases in brain quinolinic acid during CNS-localized and systemic immune activation. J Neurochem 1999; 73:770–779.
86. Hickey WF, Vass K, Lassmann H. Bone marrow-derived elements in the central nervous system: an immunohistochemical and ultrastructural survey of rat chimeras. J Neuropathol Exp Neurol 1992; 51:246–256.
87. Hassel B, Paulsen RE, Johnsen A, Fonnum F. Selective inhibition of glial cell metabolism in vivo by fluorocitrate. Brain Res 1992; 576:120–124.
88. Fonnum F, Johnsen A, Hassel B. Use of fluorocitrate and fluoroacetate in the study of brain metabolism. Glia 1997; 21:106–113.
89. Meller ST, Dykstra C, Grzybycki D, Murphy S, Gebhart CF. The possible role of glia in nociceptive processing and hyperalgesia in the spinal cord of the rat. Neuropharmacology 1994; 33:1471–1478.
90. Watkins LR, Martin D, Ulrich P, Tracey KJ, Maier SF. Evidence for the involvement of spinal cord glia in subcutaneous formalin induced hyperalgesia in the rat. Pain 1997; 71:225–235.
91. Tsai MJ, Chang YF, Schwarcz R, Brookes N. Characterization of L-alpha-aminoadipic acid transport in cultured rat astrocytes. Brain Res 1996; 741:166–173.
92. Bridges RJ, Hatalski CG, Shim SN, et al. Gliotoxic actions of excitatory amino acids. Neuropharmacology 1992; 31:899–907.
93. Khurgel M, Koo AC, Ivy GO. Selective ablation of astrocytes by intracerebral injections of alpha-aminoadipate. Glia 1996; 16:351–358.
94. Bush TG, Puvanachandra N, Horner CH, et al. Leukocyte infiltration, neuronal degeneration, and neurite outgrowth after ablation of scar-forming, reactive astrocytes in adult transgenic mice. Neuron 1999; 23:297–308.
95. Sofroniew MV, Bush TG, Blumauer N, Lawrence K, Mucke L, Johnson MH. Genetically-targeted and conditionally-regulated ablation of astroglial cells in the central, enteric and peripheral nervous systems in adult transgenic mice. Brain Res 1999; 835:91–95.
96. Poole S. Therapeutic applications of anti-cytokine strategies. Mol Psychiatry 1997; 2:137–138.
97. Cohen PS, Nakshatri H, Dennis J, et al. CNI-1493 inhibits monocyte/macrophage tumor necrosis factor by suppression of translation efficiency. Proc Natl Acad Sci USA 1996; 93:3967–3971.
98. Killer L, White J, Black R, Peschon J. Adamalysins. A family of metzincins including TNF-alpha converting enzyme (TACE). Ann NY Acad Sci 1999; 878:442–452.
99. Dalum I, Butler DM, Jensen MR, et al. Therapeutic antibodies elicited by immunization against TNF-alpha. Nat Biotechnol 1999; 17:666–669.
100. Ciapponi L, Maione D, Scoumanne A, et al. Induction of interleukin-6 (IL-6) autoantibodies through vaccination with an engineered IL-6 receptor antagonist [see comments]. Nat Biotechnol 1997; 15: 997–1001.
101. Kanaan SA, Poole S, Saade NE, Jabbur S, Safieh–Garabedian B. Interleukin-10 reduces the endotoxin-induced hyperalgesia in mice. J Neuroimmunol 1998; 86:142–150.

102. Poole S, Cunha FQ, Selkirk S, Lorenzetti BB, Ferreira SH. Cytokine-mediated inflammatory hyperalgesia limited by interleukin-10. Br J Pharmacol 1995; 115:684–688.
103. Spera PA, Ellison JA, Feuerstein GZ, Barone FC. IL-10 reduces rat brain injury following focal stroke. Neurosci Lett 1998; 251:189–192.
104. Streit WJ, Semple–Rowland SL, Hurley SD, Miller RC, Popovich PG, Stokes BT. Cytokine mRNA profiles in contused spinal cord and axotomized facial nucleus suggest a beneficial role for inflammation and gliosis. Exp Neurol 1998; 152:74–87.
105. Leon LR, Kozak W, Kluger MJ. Role of IL-10 in inflammation. Studies using cytokine knockout mice. Ann NY Acad Sci 1998; 856:69–75.
106. Marino MW, Dunn A, Grail D, et al. Characterization of tumor necrosis factor-deficient mice. Proc Natl Acad Sci USA 1997; 94:8093–8098.
107. Bruce AJ, Boling W, Kindy MS, et al. Altered neuronal and microglial responses to excitotoxic and ischemic brain injury in mice lacking TNF receptors. Nat Med 1996; 2:788–794.
108. Kulkarni AB, Karlsson S. Transforming growth factor-beta 1 knockout mice. A mutation in one cytokine gene causes a dramatic inflammatory disease. Am J Pathol 1993; 143:3–9.
109. Ramer MS, Murphy PG, Richardson PM, Bisby MA. Spinal nerve lesion-induced mechanoallodynia and adrenrgic sprouting in sensory ganglia are attenuated in interleukin-6 knockout mice. Pain 1998; 78:115–121.
110. Samoilova EB, Horton JL, Hilliard B, Liu TS, Chen Y. IL-6-deficient mice are resistant to experimental autoimmune encephalomyelitis: roles of IL-6 in the activation and differentiation of autoreactive T cells. J Immunol 1998; 161:6480–6486.
111. Bianchi M, Maggi R, Pimpinelli F, et al. Presence of a reduced opioid response in interleukin-6 knock out mice. Eur J Neurosci 1999; 11:1501–1507.
112. Xu XJ, Hao JX, Andell–Jonsson S, Poli V, Bartfai T, Wiesenfeld–Hallin Z. Nociceptive responses in interleukin-6-deficient mice to peripheral inflammation and peripheral nerve section. Cytokine 1997; 9:1028–1033.
113. Carrasco J, Hernandez J, Gonzalez B, Campbell IL, Hidalgo J. Localization of metallothionein-I and -III expression in the CNS of transgenic mice with astrocyte-targeted expression of interleukin 6. Exp Neurol 1998; 153:184–194.
114. Davis BM, Goodness TP, Soria A, Albers KM. Over-expression of NGF in skin causes formation of novel sympathetic projections to trkA-positive sensory neurons. Neuroreport 1998; 9:1103–1107.
115. Ramer MS, Kawaja MD, Henderson JT, Roder JC, Bisby MA. Glial overexpression of NGF enhances neuropathic pain and adrenergic sprouting into DRG following chronic sciatic constriction in mice. Neurosci Lett 1998; 251:53–56.
116. Stalder AK, Carson MJ, Pagenstecher A, et al. Late-onset chronic inflammatory encephalopathy in immune-competent and severe combined immune-deficient (SCID) mice with astrocyte-targeted expression of tumor necrosis factor. Am J Pathol 1998; 153:767–783.
117. Lundkvist J, Sundgren–Andersson AK, Tingsborg S, et al. Acute-phase responses in transgenic mice with CNS overexpression of IL- 1 receptor antagonist. Am J Physiol 1999; 276(3 pt 2):R644–R651.
118. Andreansky S, He B, van CJ, et al. Treatment of intracranial gliomas in immunocompetent mice using herpes simplex viruses that express murine interleukins. Gene Ther 1998; 5:121–130.
119. Woolf CJ, Mannion RJ, Neumann S. Null mutations lacking substance: elucidating pain mechanisms by genetic pharmacology [published erratum appears in Neuron 1998 Aug; 21:453]. Neuron 1998; 20:1063–1066.
120. Campbell IL. Structural and functional impact of the transgenic expression of cytokines in the CNS. Ann NY Acad Sci 1998; 840:83–96.
121. Devor M, Wall PD. Plasticity in the spinal cord sensory map following peripheral nerve injury in rats. J Neurosci 1981; 1:679–684.
122. Bennett GJ, Xie YK. A peripheral mononeuropathy in rat that produces disorders of pain sensation like those seen in man [see comments]. Pain 1988; 33:87–107.
123. Seltzer Z, Dubner R, Shir Y. A novel behavioral model of neuropathic pain disorders produced in rats by partial sciatic nerve injury. Pain 1990; 43:205–218.

124. Kerns JM, Braverman B, Mathew A, Lucchinetti C, Ivankovich AD. A comparison of cryoprobe and crush lesions in the rat sciatic nerve. Pain 1991; 47:31–39.
125. Kalichman MW, Myers RR. Behavioral and electrophysiological recovery following cryogenic nerve injury. Exp Neurol 1987; 96:692–702.
126. DeLeo JA, Coombs DW, Willenbring S, et al. Characterization of a neuropathic pain model: sciatic cryoneurolysis in the rat. Pain 1994; 56:9–16.
127. Gazelius B, Cui JG, Svensson M, Meyerson B, Linderoth B. Photochemically induced ischaemic lesion of the rat sciatic nerve. A novel method providing high incidence of mononeuropathy. Neuroreport 1996; 7:2619–2623.
128. Kupers R, Yu W, Persson JK, Xu XJ, Wiesenfeld–Hallin Z. Photochemically-induced ischemia of the rat sciatic nerve produces a dose-dependent and highly reproducible mechanical, heat and cold allodynia, and signs of spontaneous pain. Pain 1998; 76:45–59.
129. Kim SH, Chung JM. An experimental model for peripheral neuropathy produced by segmental spinal nerve ligation in the rat. Pain 1992; 50;355–363.
130. Kabuki S, Kikuchi S, Olmarker K, Myers RR. Acute effects of nucleus pulposus on blood flow and endoneurial fluid pressure in rat dorsal root ganglia. Spine 1998; 23:2517–2523.
131. Kawakami M, Weinstein JN, Chatani K, Spratt KF, Meller ST, Gebhart GF. Experimental lumbar radiculopathy. Behavioral and histologic changes in a model of radicular pain after spinal neve root irritation with chromic gut ligatures in the rat. Spine 1994; 19:1795–1802.
132. Kawakami M, Weinstein JN, Spratt KF, et al. Experimental lumbar radiculopathy. Immunohistochemical and quantitative demonstrations of pain induced by lumbar nerve root irritation of the rat. Spine 1994; 19:1780–1794.
133. Yezierski RP, Liu S, Ruenes GL, Kajander KJ, Brewer KL. Excitotoxic spinal cord injury: behavioral and morphological characteristics of a central pain model. Pain 1998; 75:141–155.
134. Hao JX, Xu XJ, Aldskogius H, Seiger A, Wiesenfeld–Hallin Z. Allodynia-like effects in rat after ischaemic spinal cord injury photochemically induced by laser irradiation. Pain 1991; 45:175–185.
135. Stokes BT, Reier PJ. Fetal grafts alter chronic behavioral outcome after contusion damage to the adult rat spinal cord. Exp Neurol 1992; 116:1–12.

5

A New Perspective on Signal Transduction in Neuropathic Pain

The Emerging Role of the G Protein βγ Dimer in Transducing and Modulating Opioid Signaling

Keith McCormack
McCormack Limited, Leighton Buzzard, Bedfordshire, England

I. PHENOTYPE EXPRESSION IN THE INJURED NERVE

A. Introduction

Neuronal injury evokes programs of survival or apoptosis that have a natural history of at least 500 million years. In this chapter, I present some elements of a hypothesis that emphasizes the absolute priority of these programs. If survival or regeneration is initiated, then it is essential that there is no distortion or interruption in signaling fidelity between the environment and cytoplasmic and nuclear processes of phenotype expression. It is now evident that many agents, notably the opioids, used to manage neuropathic pains, signal along pathways that converge with those of growth factors that regulate gene expression and promote survival. Through such convergence or "crosstalk," some analgesics may compromise processes of regeneration. Consequently, such intervention may be opposed by systems of indescribable complexity that have evolved to minimize such threats and maximize survival.

At clinical dosages, presynaptic actions of opioid agonists on transmitter release result from an opening of potassium channels or a closing of calcium channels, both of which lead to a reduction in Ca^{2+} influx into C-fiber terminals. Reduction of the voltage-sensitive calcium N current can be anticipated to result in diminished neurotransmitter release. However, following nerve injury, use of a drug to directly block voltage-sensitive calcium channels (VSCCs) may result in activation of fail-safe mechanisms that operate to oppose the blockade. Indeed, by contrast with normal neuronal function, it seems that nerve injury may be associated with, and characterized by, a limited tolerance of any exogenous modulation of synaptic transmission. That is, in the treatment of neuropathic pain, to what extent does the rightward shift in the opioid analgesic dose–response curve represent "antiopioid" effects that arise as a direct consequence of nerve injury? Such antiopioid effects would be distinct from the phenomenon of tolerance attributable, for example, to an uncoupling of transducer proteins (i.e., G proteins), with receptor desensitization and internalization.

B. Calcium Influx Is a Critical Determinant of Neuronal Phenotype

It is generally believed that some pathological events that subsequently lead to neuronal degeneration are triggered by "excess" levels of intracellular Ca^{2+} ($[Ca^{2+}]i$) (1–3). Theoretical considerations and indirect studies have suggested that nerve injury is associated with increases in $[Ca^{2+}]i$ to the millimolar level, several orders of magnitude above the range of calcium concentrations reached during normal physiological conditions within the intact uninjured neuron (4,5). Excess incoming calcium at various stages of neuronal injury, regeneration, and regrowth, are thought to trigger cytoskeletal depolymerization, beading, and degeneration of the axon or even the degeneration of the entire neuron (6,7).

However, more recently, Ziv and Spira (8) suggest that earlier analyses greatly underestimated neuronal $[Ca^{2+}]i$. Importantly, they found that despite an injury-induced elevation of $[Ca^{2+}]i$ well beyond the upper limits of physiological Ca^{2+} concentration, to levels higher than 1 mM, there were no apparent adverse effects on regenerative processes. These findings should be compared with the observations of Rehder et al. (9), who showed that Ca^{2+} influx below a critical level significantly retarded sealing of transected neurons. Paradoxically, these workers observed that a large increase in $[Ca^{2+}]i$ following entry through a lesion of the neuronal membrane and on depolarization, although hampering growth cone formation appeared to facilitate resealing. In summary, the results of these studies, together with those of other workers (10–12), suggest that Ca^{2+} influx must be controlled within optima that are compatible with the requirements for both survival and regrowth.

C. Modulation of Calcium Influx by Protein G $\beta\gamma$

Numerous reports indicate that the Go subclass of G proteins (GPs) mediates inhibitory coupling of opioid receptors to neuronal voltage-sensitive calcium channels (VSCCs), especially the N-type (13–20), and that such inhibition is likely mediated by direct interaction of the $G\beta\gamma$ subunit with the VSCC (21–24), following the ligand-stimulated functional dissociation of the heterotrimeric G protein. Naturally, these observations have been proposed as a molecular mechanism by which presynaptic G protein–complex receptors (GPCRs), such as those that bind morphine, for example, inhibit neurotransmission (21,25) (in addition to other mechanisms that include activation of an inwardly rectifying K^+ conductance).

D. Signal Integration by the VSCC

The recent report of protein kinase C (PKC)-dependent up-regulation of VSCC activity through antagonism of the $G\beta\gamma$ inhibitory action has been proposed as an additional mechanism for regulation and dynamic control of neurotransmitter release and synaptic efficacy (22). Although G protein-dependent inhibition occurs through binding of $G\beta\gamma$ to the VSCC, crosstalk resulting from the PKC-dependent phosphorylation of one of the $G\beta\gamma$-binding sites effectively *antagonizes* $G\beta\gamma$-induced inhibition. In some part, this antagonistic effect of PKC on $G\beta\gamma$-induced inhibition might explain why, in paradigms of neuropathic pain, the administration of cholecystokinin (CCK_B) receptor antagonists restores opioid sensitivity. (Stimulation of the CCK_B receptor with subsequent activation of the G protein, Gq, results in an increase in activity of phospholipase C [PLC] isoforms with resultant 1,2-diacylglycerol [DAG]-mediated activation of PKC).

By using enzymatically dissociated brain cells from newborn rats, Wang et al. (26) observed that KCl produced a significant increase in $[Ca^{2+}]i$ and that this increase could be prevented by administering antagonists of VSCCs. Although sulfated and desulfated forms of cholecystokinin octapeptide (CCK-8) did not affect the increase of $[Ca^{2+}]i$ following high K^+-induced membrane depolarization, they did reverse the suppression of high K^+-induced increase in $[Ca^{2+}]i$ by the μ agonist ohmefentanyl. Although the effects of CCK-8 on mobilization of intracellular Ca^{2+} as a result of inositol trisphosphate ($InsP_3$) formation, or after opioid-binding affinity (discussed later) cannot be discounted, the recent demonstration (27) that the antiopioid effects of CCK_B receptor stimulation are abolished by the PKC-specific inhibitor, calphostin, is in accord with this simple model. Moreover, elegant investigation of CCK_B receptor signal transduction mechanisms emphasize the dominant role occupied by DAG formation (and subsequent PKC activation and translocation) (28). In these studies it was demonstrated that whereas CCK_B receptor stimulation also results in rapid, but transient, elevations of $InsP_3$ (and subsequent intracellular Ca^{2+} mobilization), DAG levels demonstrate a more pronounced biphasic response. Interestingly, there is evidence to suggest that following stimulation by CCK-8, PKC activation inhibits $InsP_3$ formation and subsequent induction of cytosolic Ca^{2+} oscillations (29). Neuronal injury is associated with a very marked increase in the number of sensory neurons of all sizes expressing CCK_B receptor mRNA (30), together with a dramatic increase in the number of sensory neurons in dorsal root ganglia synthesizing CCK (31). Importantly, in the normal dorsal root ganglia in the rat, mRNA for the CCK_B receptor is present at very low levels. Thus, the injury-associated increase, described in the foregoing, suggests an increased sensitivity to CCK for many primary sensory neurons of different modalities (30). A crushing injury to sensory nerves either has no effect (32) or results in an increase (33) in levels of mRNA for isoforms of PLC that are activated by Gq. Taken together, these findings indicate an up-regulation of the pathway $CCK_B \rightarrow Gq \rightarrow PLC \rightarrow PKC$, which suggests an increase in PKC-mediated antagonism of $G\beta\gamma$-induced inhibition of VSCCs, in particular the N-type (22,25).

The following observations provide additional support for the foregoing suggestion:

1. In cultured dorsal root ganglion cells, activation of PKC partially reverses prior inhibition of VSCC current following G protein activation with the nonhydrolyzable GTP analogue, GTPγs (34,35) ($G\alpha \cdot GTP$ is the active moiety following subunit dissociation).

2. Inhibition of the Ca^{2+}–calmodulin-regulated protein phosphatase, calcineurin, greatly attenuates the pertussis toxin (PTX)-sensitive, G protein-coupled, receptor-induced inhibition of the N-type VSCC current in rat sympathetic neurons (36) (Gi/o are pertussis toxin (PTX)-sensitive G proteins). There is now considerable speculation that because PKC activation, in common with calcineurin inhibition, markedly attenuates GPCR-induced inhibition of the N-type channel activity, then PKC is likely the kinase that phosphorylates the calcineurin-regulated site and, consequently, PKC is indeed an important modulator of the N-type VSCC (36).

3. Immunophilins, protein receptors for immunosuppressant drugs, such as cyclosporine and tacrolimus (FK 506), are enriched far more in the brain than in the immune system. Indeed, levels within nervous tissue apparently exceed by manyfold those in immune tissues. Drug–immunophilin complexes bind to calcineurin, inhibiting its phosphatase activity and leading to immunosuppressant effects. It is noteworthy that facial nerve crush markedly augments expression of mRNA for the immunophilin, FKBP-12, with a time course paralleling changes in mRNA for the growth-associated protein, GAP-43 (37). Following sciatic nerve lesions, similar increases in FKBP-12 mRNA occur in lumbar motor neurons and dorsal root ganglia neuronal cells.

4. The expression of PKC isoforms is up-regulated following neuronal injury (38–41). A functional link between PKC and VSCCs in the spinal cord has been proposed (42), and protein kinases and calcineurin are suggested to be functionally linked by association with common anchoring proteins (43). High densities of immunophilins colocalize with calcineurin in neural tissue.

These changes are consistent with the notion that injury-induced increases in levels of the calcineurin inhibitor group of compounds, the immunophilins, accord with the antagonism by

PKC of Gβγ-mediated inhibition of VSCC activity. That is, activating PKC, similar to inhibiting calcineurin activity, greatly attenuates Gβγ-induced inhibition of N-type Ca^{2+} channels (36).

Taken together, all of these findings support the existence of the functional unit: VSCC/PKC/calcineurin/immunophilin. Finally, an increased expression of immunophilins augments depolarization-induced transmitter release from rat brain striatal synaptosomes. Synapsin I, a synaptic vesicle phosphoprotein, displays enhanced phosphorylation in the presence of immunophilin-stimulating drugs (e.g., FK 506) (44). It is worth emphasizing here that μ, δ, and κ opioid agonists attenuate the depolarization-induced phosphorylation of synapsin I (45) and that this action has reasonably been interpreted as representing a further mechanism whereby opioid receptor agonists inhibit neurotransmitter release (46).

E. Can Spontaneous Ectopic Discharges in Injured Nerves Antagonize Opioid-Mediated Analgesia?

Voltage-dependent inhibition of high–voltage-activated Ca^{2+} currents by Gβγ can be transiently relieved (an event synonymous with "facilitation" of current) by a depolarizing "prepulse" (for example, a pulse of depolarization applied immediately before the test pulse). However, until recently it remained to be established whether this phenomenon was merely an experimental artifact, or if it could be induced under physiological conditions by action potentials.

With use of patch-clamp methods, Womack and McCleskey (47) demonstrated that brief prepulses to very positive voltages increased (facilitated) the amplitude of current through Ca^{2+} channels during a subsequent test pulse in some, but not all, dorsal root ganglion sensory neurons. The amplitude of this facilitated current generally increased when the Ca^{2+} channels were inhibited by activation of the μ-opioid receptor. The facilitated current was blocked by the N-type VSCC blocker (within the picomolar range), ω-conotoxin GVIA. It was activated in the range of high-threshold Ca^{2+} channels, and was inactivated at relatively negative holding voltages. Thus, facilitated current passes through N-type Ca^{2+} channels, the same channels that are inhibited by opioids and control neurotransmitter release in sensory neurons. Although maximal facilitation occurred only at unphysiologically high membrane potentials (above +100 mV), some facilitation was seen after prepulses to voltages reached during action potentials. After return to the holding potential, facilitation persisted for hundreds of milliseconds, considerably longer than in other neurons. However, brief trains of pulses designed to mimic action potentials caused small facilitation (19% of maximal) in a fraction (8 of 24) of opioid-inhibited neurons. From these results, Womack and McCleskey concluded that prepulses to extremely positive voltages can cause partial recovery of Ca^{2+} channels inhibited by opioids; importantly, small, but detectable, facilitation was also seen after *physiological* stimulation in some dorsal root ganglion neurons. Thus, facilitation, largely considered a biophysical epiphenomenon because of the extreme voltages used to induce it, appears to be physiologically relevant during opioid inhibition of Ca^{2+} channels in dorsal root ganglion neurons.

More recently, Williams et al. (48), confirmed that physiological stimuli, such as action potentials, could promote facilitation of the N-type Ca^{2+} current. With dissociated cholinergic basal forebrain neurons of the guinea pig, they tested whether the inhibition of the N-type Ca^{2+} current by cholinergic agonists, carbachol or muscarine, could be relieved by using action potential-like depolarizations. As an example of their results, they observed that whereas application of muscarine caused a 70% reduction of the current, following a train of action potential-like depolarizations, this inhibition was only 22%. Most importantly, they concluded that their results also suggested that ". . . firing rates and patterns of discharge of neurons could influence their responsive to transmitters [i.e., agonists such as opioids at GPCRs] acting on N-type calcium channels."

Womack and McCleskey (47) further demonstrated that after inhibition of N-type VSCCs by activation of the μ-opioid receptor, facilitating depolarizations generally were more effective. Therefore, as they concluded, the facilitating prepulses diminish opioid inhibition of these channels. Such facilitation may be explained by the voltage-dependent release of G proteins (i.e., Gβγ) bound to the channel, with the facilitation decaying as Gβγ subunits rebind. By comparison with other neurons, facilitation (i.e., disinhibition of opioid block) persists so much longer in dorsal root ganglion neurons, and in some way this is due to a kind of "windup" during trains of action potentials (47).

Studies in patients with painful peripheral neuropathies have led to the hypothesis that ongoing discharge in primary afferent nociceptors has two harmful effects: it is a source of ongoing "spontaneous" pain, and it dynamically maintains a state of central hyperexcitability that underlies evoked-pain abnormalities such as hyperalgesia and allodynia. Temporary suppression of nociceptor discharge by a local anesthetic nerve block allows the central hyperexcitable state to normalize; hyperalgesia and allodynia are then absent or reduced, sometimes for many hours after the anesthetic block has dissipated. However, according to the hypothesis, the pain, hyperalgesia, and allodynia return because the resumption of nociceptor discharge rekindles the central hyperexcitable state. If the hypothesis is correct, then long-term suppression of spontaneous nociceptor discharge ought to be of therapeutic benefit. There is evidence that VSCCs, in particular the N-type, play a role in the genesis of spontaneous ectopic discharges and the abnormal pains that occur after nerve injury (49–51). However, to my knowledge, it has not previously been considered that continuous spontaneous ectopic discharges, although originating in some part from VSCCs within injured primary afferents, may also lessen the effectiveness of opioids to induce blockade of N-type VSCC. Although this additional formulation remains to be formally tested, it is worth reporting that clinicians have long noted that a local anesthetic nerve block can give a patient days or weeks of relief. This result is very difficult to understand in terms of the known duration of the pharmacological effect, and it is sometimes suspected to be a supernormal placebo effect, or presumptive evidence that the patient is neurotic or malingering. It is therefore of interest that rats with a chronic constriction injury likewise demonstrate prolonged relief (as measured by changes in the latencies of nocifensive withdrawal reflexes to painful stimulation) following application of a local anesthetic block. I speculate that temporary abolition of the spontaneous ectopic discharges, in addition to resulting in a diminution of dynamically maintained central hyperexcitability, may also produce an apparent increase in *endogenous* GPCR modulation of N-type VSCCs. Together these two mechanisms may nonlinearly augment (i.e., synergize) the effect of a local anesthetic nerve block on hyperalgesia and allodynia of neuronal injury.

II. OPIOIDS HAVE ACCESS TO NEURONAL PHENOTYPE BY Gβγ

A. Opioids and the Mitogen-Activated Protein Kinase Pathway

The ubiquitous mitogen-activated protein (MAP) kinases (MAPKs) constitute a family of serine/threonine kinases that are involved in the transduction of externally derived signals regulating cell growth, regeneration, division, and differentiation. On activation, MAP kinases translocate to the nucleus, where they phosphorylate and activate transcription factors for transcriptional regulation of several particular genes that are essential for the induction of survival (or apoptosis) and the subsequent regeneration process (52–54). Remarkably, it is becoming increasingly apparent that, similar to receptor protein tyrosine kinases (RTKs), many GPCRs are also involved in the regulation of cell growth and differentiation, and that many of these effects are mediated by the MAP kinase cascade. Indeed, there are a growing number of reports that opioid agonists are activators of the MAP kinase cascade (55–63).

The mechanisms by which GPCRs activate the MAP kinase-signaling cascade are poorly understood. Early investigations using transiently transfected COS-7 cells demonstrated that activation of receptors coupled to Gs, Gq, or Gi resulted in stimulation of the MAP kinase pathway (64). They further demonstrated that whereas β_1, β_2, γ_1, or γ_2 G protein subunits alone did not increase $p44^{MAPK}$ (44-kDa isoform of extracellular signal-regulated kinase; ERK) activity, the $\beta_1\gamma_2$ combination and, to a lesser extent, $\beta_1\gamma_1$ and $\beta_2\gamma_2$ did increase activity of $p44^{MAPK}$. Subsequently, using Chinese hamster ovary (CHO)-K1 cells, it was demonstrated that coexpression of Gβγ with the Ras guanine nucleotide exchange factor, son of sevenless (Sos)1, resulted in a synergistic increase in MAP kinase activation (65). Expression of either Gβγ or Sos alone resulted in a two- to threefold or a five-fold increase in MAP kinase activation, respectively, whereas coexpression of both Gβγ and Sos resulted in a 15- to 20-fold increase. These workers further demonstrated that as in COS-7 cells, the ability of Gβγ to synergize with Sos1 in CHO-K1 cells was dependent on activity of the pleckstrin homology (PH)-domain containing the enzyme phosphatidylinositol 3-kinase (PI-3K)γ. Ito and co-workers (66) in the same year also reported that in human embryonic kidney (HEK) 293 cells, overexpression of Gβγ induced the activation of Ras, c-Raf, and MAP kinase.

To activate a MAP kinase cascade, Gβγ subunits conditionally require the activity of a protein tyrosine kinase (PTK), for the PTK inhibitors genisten and herbimycin A attenuate Gβγ-stimulated MAP kinase activation in a dose-dependent manner. It seems that Gβγ uses the same pathway to stimulate MAP kinase as several tyrosine kinase-dependent cell-surface receptors that lack intrinsic tyrosine kinase activity. These cell-surface receptors appear to recruit Src (also known as $p^{60c\text{-}src}$ or c-Src) family of kinases (for review of Src kinases see Refs. 67, 68), such as Lck, Fyn, and c-Src. It has been proposed that association of Gβγ with an Src-like kinase initiates tyrosine phosphorylation of the Src homology 2/α-collagen-related adapter protein, Shc, which is then able to assemble a multiprotein complex for regulating activity of the low molecular weight G protein, p21 Ras (69). The tyrosine phosphorylation of Shc is accompanied by a simultaneous increase in complex formation between Shc and another adapter protein, Grb2 (65,70), which is constitutively associated with Sos1. These early events serve to recruit and translocate the p21–Ras guanine nucleotide exchange factor Sos1 to the cytoplasmic surface of the membrane. That is, translocated Sos1 activates p21-Ras by catalyzing GDP for GTP exchange (65). GTP-bound p21–Ras initiates activation of the MAP kinase cascade by activating the serine–threonine kinase, Raf-1, followed by the sequential phosphorylation and activation of MAPK kinase (MAPKK) which, in turn, mediates the activation of MAP kinase.

In summary, these observations, together with those of other workers (71,72) allow the conclusion that "free Gβγ" recruits PI-3Kγ to the plasma membrane, enhancing the activity of an Src-like kinase which, in turn, leads to the activation of the Shc–Grb2–Sos–Ras pathway, resulting in an increased MAP kinase activity (73). Alterations in the levels of expression of Gβγ will incluence the MAP kinase-mediated phosphorylation and activation of nuclear transcription factors that regulate nerve cell growth and regeneration. Depending on the cellular context, activated MAP kinases may mediate pleiotropic responses in the membrane, cytoplasm, nucleus, or cytoskeleton.

B. Opioids Are Coupled to Phospholipase A_2(PLA_2) by MAP Kinase (Is PLA_2 an Antiopioid Messenger?)

Fukuda et al. (55), using CHO cells, provided the first report of a functional coupling of μ-, δ-, and κ-opioid receptor subtypes with activation of both MAP kinase and PLA_2 (measured by an increase in release of arachidonate). Previously, this coupling had not been described for native opioid receptors in neuronal cells or opioid receptors expressed from cDNAs. Their results are entirely consistent with the view that full activation of cytosolic PLA_2 requires both phosphorylation by MAP kinase and an increased cytosolic Ca^{2+} concentration (74). Accordingly, they observed that staurosporine, which almost completely abolishes MAP kinase activity induced by activation of opioid receptors, strongly inhibits opioid receptor-mediated arachidonate release. Additionally, they showed that activation of the opioid receptor expressed in CHO cells leads to an increase in arachidonate release only in the presence of a calcium ionophore, confirming the requirement of elevation of intracellular Ca^{2+} for PLA_2 activation by opioid receptors. On the basis of these results, they speculate that PLA_2 activity within neurons is upregulated only when opioid receptors are activated coincidentally with a Gq/11-mediated increase in cytosolic levels of Ca^{2+} (e.g., following activation of the CCK_B receptor), or with an increase in opening probability of VSCCs, for example, as a direct result of depolarization-induced facilitation or disinhibition of $G\beta\gamma$-induced blockade.

Taken together, these data indicate a possible antiopioid action of PLA_2 that may be driven by the CCK_B receptor (Table 1). Interestingly, the inhibitory effects of glucocorticosteroids (75), ketamine (76–78), phenytoin (79), and imipramine (80) on PLA_2 activity, together with potentiation of impiramine binding to synaptosomal membranes by PLA_2 (81,82) may partly contribute to the reported efficacy of these drugs in managing neuropathic pains (see Table 1).

Table 1 PLA_2—an Anti-opioid Messenger of the CCK_B Receptor?

1. CCK-8 dose dependently increases cytosolic (c)PLA_2 activity in various cell lines stably expressing the Gq/11-coupled gastrin/CCK_B receptor (83–91).
2. Expression of μ-, δ-, or κ-opioid receptors in numerous cell lines (see text for refs.) allows agonist-mediated stimulation (i.e., phosphorylation) of MAP kinase, including $p42^{MAPK}$, $p44^{MAPK}$, and MEK. Interestingly, whereas chronic opioid administration in vivo results in activation of MAP kinases throughout the CNS (92–96), precipitated opioid withdrawal also results in brain region-specific activation of MAP kinase (97,98).
3. The opioid receptor-mediated stimulation of MAP kinases leads to an activation of cPLA_2 (following phosphorylation by MAP kinases) only in the presence of an increased cytosolic Ca^{2+} concentration (55,99). Consequently, it was recently proposed that in neuronal cells cPLA_2 is activated only when opioid receptors and coexisting Gq/11 Ca^{2+}-mobilizing (by IP_3) receptors, or VSCCs are activated coincidentally (99); cPLA_2 thus is a classic example of a "coincidence detector" (100).
4. Consistent with the foregoing observations, Gi/o-coupled (e.g., opioid) receptors activate cPLA_2 only when a Gq-coupled receptor is also activated (101,102).
5. Costimulation of a Gi/o-coupled receptor (e.g., opioid) and a Gq/11-coupled receptor (e.g., CCK) produce synergistic activation of MAP kinases (103) and cPLA_2 (104–106).
6. Following nerve injury there is a significant increase in CCK mRNA, CCK_B receptor mRNA (30,31), and induction of PLA_2 (107–112).
7. The PLA_2 products of phospholipid hydrolysis, such as fatty acids and lysophosphatides are potent inhibitors of high-affinity binding of opioids to neuronal membranes (106,113,114). It has been proposed that these in vitro effects of PLA_2 are of physiological significance (115).
8. Whereas prolonged morphine exposure may retard nerve regeneration and induce permanent neurological deficits (116,117), activity of PLA_2 appears critical for the induction and maintenance of nerve regeneration (118–123).
9. The inhibitory effects of glucocorticosteroids (75), ketamine (76–78), phenytoin (79), and imipramine (80), upon PLA_2 activity, together with potentiation of imipramine binding to synaptosomal membranes by PLA_2 (81,82) may partly contribute to the reported efficacy of these drugs in managing neuropathic pains.

III. A NEW MODEL OF NEUROPATHIC PAIN PROVIDES NEW INSIGHTS INTO Gβγ SIGNALING

A. Intrathecal PTX Produces Symptoms of Neuropathic Pain

Recently, Womer and colleagues at Lilly Research (124) conducted a series of elegant studies in which they investigated the effects of different doses of intrathecally (i.t.)-administered pertussis toxin (PTX) (0.01–0.5 μg/mouse) on the latency to withdrawal of the tail in water at various temperatures (35–55°C). An analysis of variance (ANOVA) with repeated measures demonstrated a significant difference ($p < 0.01$) between the PTX-treated groups and the vehicle-treated group at water temperatures of 40, 45, 50, and 55°C. During the course of tail-flick testing, Womer and colleagues observed that mice exhibited exaggerated tail-rattling after the tail was lightly touched, indicating the presence of mechanical allodynia. Using a nonnoxious stimulus (gauze), stroking of the tail [for further details of method see Ref. 124] elicited no positive responses out of 75 trials in the control mice. By contrast, in the PTX-treated mice there were 36 (48%) positive responses out of 75 trials. Following further characterization of the time course of the effects of a range of doses of PTX, Womer and co-workers (124) determined that the persistent thermal hyperalgesia and allodynia produced by PTX is similar to that produced by neuropathic pain models involving nerve ligation or section (125–127).

Although the mechanisms whereby PTX administration produces hyperalgesia and allodynia require further elucidation, Womer et al. (124) speculate that inactivation of Gi and Go by PTX leads to an inactivation of tonic and phasic inhibitory effector systems normally under the control of these G proteins. Inactivation of these regulatory systems would, they propose, lead to an apparent increase in activity of excitatory pathways. The result would be a windup of central pathways of nociceptive processing with exaggerated and aberrant responses to both innocuous and noxious stimulation. They conclude that the intrathecal administration of PTX causes hyperalgesia and allodynia that appears similar to the symptoms reported by patients suffering from neuropathic pain, and suggest that deficiencies in inhibitory systems, as compared with increases in excitatory systems, may play a role in the pathophysiology of at least some central or neuropathic pain states [see Ref. 124 for further details of clinical relevance].

B. The Enigma of Buprenorphine in a New Paradigm of Neuropathic Pain

The elegant characterization by Womer's group of the effects of PTX confirmed observations from earlier studies (128,129) that morphine-induced antinociception is blocked in a dose-dependent manner by PTX, resulting in complete blockade following a 0.3-μg dose of PTX. Other workers have similarly demonstrated that intrathecal PTX reduces the analgesic potency of etorphine and fentanyl (130), [D-Ala^2, D-Leu^5] enkephalin (DADLE), [D-Ala^2, *N*-Me-Phe^4, Gly^5-ol] enkephalin (DAMGO), and bremazocine (131) and that of the highly selective μ-agonist PL017 (132). Womer and co-workers (124) add that their observations with morphine are consistent with the fact that the analgesic signal transduced by morphine is mainly by PTX-sensitive inhibitory systems and that, clinically, morphine is relatively less effective in treating central and neuropathic pain states than in treating acute pain.

In the rat tail-flick test, buprenorphine-mediated antinociception was not affected by the prior administration of PTX, whereas in the same study, consistent with recent results (124), morphine antinociception was eliminated within the range of 0.1–30 mg kg^{-1} of morphine administered subcutaneously (SC) (128). In phase 2a of the formalin test in the adult rat, buprenorphine antinociception was modified by PTX only at the highest doses tested (more than 1 mg kg^{-1} SC), whereas with morphine, antinociception was significantly attenuated below 3 mg kg^{-1} of morphine SC. At high doses of morphine (10 and 20 mg kg^{-1} SC), the effects of PTX on morphine antinociception were progressively diminished (128). These novel data can be interpreted to imply that buprenorphine activates PTX-insensitive pathways in preference to PTX-sensitive pathways, the latter becoming progressively available only with increasing dose (133).

C. PTX-Insensitive Pathways and Gβγ

Using purified Gzα-subunits (i.e., the α-subunit of the PTX-insensitive Gz) obtained from a baculovirus infection of Sf9 cells, Fields and Casey (134) observed that once phosphorylated, Gzα has a greatly decreased ability to associate with Gβγ. Most importantly, these workers concluded that rapid phosphorylation of Gzα · GDP by activated PKC would not allow further recycling of Gzα. Support for this view was provided by Kozasa and Gilman (135), who examined nine Gα-subunits and observed that only the PTX-insensitive G proteins served as substrates for phosphorylation by various isoforms of PKC. Thus, they confirmed the earlier observations by Fields and Casey (134) that phosphorylated α-subunits of PTX-insensitive G proteins have reduced affinity for Gβγ by comparison with the unmodified Gα-subunits.

D. Gβγ and Neuronal Injury

Subsequently, it has been proposed by two independent groups (136,137) that this prevention of subunit reassociation could potentiate Gβγ-mediated signaling by creating a pool of free Gβγ that could continue to modulate effector activity. Support for a functional role of the selective phosphorylation by PKC of PTX-insensitive Gα-subunits follows the observation by Hinton et al. (138) that immunolocalization of PKC within the CNS corresponds closely with that of Gzα. Given the colocalization of opioid and CCK receptors throughout the CNS, then the CCK_B-mediated activation of PKC following neuronal injury in mediating the antiopioid effects of CCK paradoxically may also enhance analgesic signaling mediated by Gβγ along PTX-insensitive pathways. Fine tuning of this PKC-dependent Gβγ signal is suggested by the recent report (139) that phosphorylation in vitro of the $\beta_1\gamma_{12}$ dimer on the γ-subunit with PKC regulates its activity in an effector-specific fashion. These workers conclude that because the γ_{12}-subunit is highly expressed in all regions of the brain, and in most peripheral tissues, phosphorylation of Gβγ may be an important mechanism for ensuring signaling fidelity between receptor and a specific effector molecule.

IV. CONCLUDING REMARKS

A. Pharmacological Intervention Is no Match for an Evolutionary Need to Ensure Adequacy of Neurotransmission

Teleologically, even if survival is the ultimate goal (''survival'' may also necessitate apoptotic ''culling'' of functionally redundant neurons), then as part of this process, we can assume that pain has evolved as an important and necessary signal. However, when pain ceases to provide any obvious useful function, why are some chronic pains, especially those associated with neuronal dysfunction (i.e., neuropathic), frequently so difficult to eradicate? In this chapter, I propose that pharmacological intervention aimed at eliminating abnormal sensations, such as hyperalgesia or paresthesia arising as a direct result of nerve injury, activates adaptive processes that ensure adequacy of neurotransmission, regardless of whether such transmission ultimately evokes normal or abnormal sensations. Thus, even the most sophisticated novel pharmacological entities, when used to block the pain signal, represent substrates for evoking a repertoire of fail-safe mechanisms that have evolved throughout a history of challenge and response. Activation of these responses may explain why treatment of neuropathic pains, particularly with opioids, can be so frustrating.

If opioids represent substrates for evoking a repertoire of fail-safe mechanisms, then it is important to explore those signaling pathways along which clinically administered opioid agonists might impinge on programs of survival or apoptosis and subsequent expression of phenotype. It is becoming clear that the opioid-activated Gβγ-subunit enables opioid signaling to converge on pathways implicated in the regulation of neuronal growth and differentiation that are activated through growth factor-regulated receptor protein tyrosine kinases. Importantly, these new discoveries also bring an awareness of opportunities for further understanding the role of opioids in managing neuropathic pains. In a new model of neuropathic pain, buprenorphine-induced antinociception is apparently not modified by the intrathecal administration of PTX. This observation alone positions buprenorphine as a candidate for future studies designed to investigate how the Gβγ signal can be exploited in the management of neuropathic pain.

ACKNOWLEDGMENTS

The author gratefully acknowledges the expertise and advice of Helen Millins on methods of literature searching and retrieval. The author also thanks Professor Ilmar Jurna for advice and critical appraisal, and extends special gratitude to Professor Patrick D. Wall for providing the seeds of a notion that gave rise to the fail-safe theory.

REFERENCES

1. Kater SB, Mattson MP, Guthrie PB. Calcium-induced neuronal degeneration: a normal growth cone regulating signal gone awry? In: Khachaturian ZS, Cottmann CW, Pettegrew JW, eds. Calcium, Membranes, Aging and Alzheimer Disease. New York: New York Academy of Sciences, 1989; 568:252–261.
2. Mills LR, Kater SB. Neuron-specific and state-specific differences in calcium homeostasis regulate the generation and degeneration of neuronal architecture. Neuron 1990; 2:149–163.
3. Nicotera P, Bellomo G, Orrenius S. Calcium-mediated mechanisms in chemically induced cell death. Annu Rev Pharmacol Toxicol 1992; 32:449–470.
4. Mata M, Staple J, Fink DJ. Changes in intra-axonal calcium distribution following nerve crush. J Neurobiol 1986; 17:449–467.
5. Van Egeraat JM, Stasski R, Barach JP, Friedman RN, Wikswo JP Jr. The biomagnetic signature of a crushed axon: a comparison of theory and experiment. Biophys J 1993; 64:1299–1305.
6. Schlaepfer WW, Bunge RP. Effects of calcium ion concentration on the degeneration of amputated axons in tissue culture. J Cell Biol 1973; 59:456–470.
7. Schlaepfer WW, Lee C, Lee VMY, Zimmerman UJP. An immunoblot study of neurofilament degradation in situ and during calcium activated proteolysis. J Neurochem 1985; 44:402–509.
8. Ziv NE, Spira ME. Spatiotemporal distribution of Ca^{2+} following axotomy and throughout the recovery process of cultured *Aplysia* neurons. Eur J Neurosci 1993; 5:657–668.
9. Rehder V, Jensen JR, Kater SB. The initial stages of neural regeneration are dependent upon intracellular calcium levels. Neuroscience 1992; 51:565–574.
10. Gispen WH, Hamers FP. Calcium and neuronal dysfunction in peripheral nervous system. Ann NY Acad Sci 1994; 747:419–430.
11. LoPachin RM, Lehning EJ. Mechanism of calcium entry during axon injury and degeneration. Toxicol Appl Pharmacol 1997; 143:233–244.

12. Lu YM, Yin HZ, Chiang J, Weiss JH. Ca^{2+}-permeable AMPA/kainate and NMDA channels: high rate of Ca^{2+} influx underlies potent induction of injury. J Neurosci 1996; 16:5457–5465.
13. Bourinet E, Soong TW, Stea A, Snutch TP. Determinants of the G protein-dependent opioid modulation of neuronal calcium channels. Proc Natl Acad Sci USA 1996; 93:1486–1491.
14. Nah SY, Unteutsch A, Bunzow JR, Cook SP, Beacham DW, Grandy DK. μ and δ opioids but not κ opioid inhibit voltage-activated Ba^{2+} currents in neuronal F-11 cell. Brain Res 1997; 766:66–71.
15. Soldo BL, Moises HC. μ-Opioid receptor activation decreases N-type Ca^{2+} current in magnocellular neurons of the rat basal forebrain. Brain Res 1997; 758:118–126.
16. Suh HW, Song DK, Choi SR, Huh SO, Kim YH. Differential effects of ω-conotoxin GVIA, nimodipine, calmidazolium and KN-62 injected intrathecally on the antinociception induced by β-endorphin, morphine and (D-Ala[2], *N*-MePhe[4], Gly-ol[5])-enkephalin administered intracerebroventricularly in the mouse. J Pharmacol Exp Ther 1997; 282:961–966.
17. Wiley JW, Moises HC, Gross RA, MacDonald RL. Dynorphin A-mediated reduction in multiple calcium currents involves a Goα subtype G protein in rat primary afferent neurons. J Neurophysiol 1997; 77:1338–1348.
18. Kim CJ, Rhee JS, Akaike N. Modulation of high-voltage activated Ca^{2+} channels in the rat periaqueductal gray neurons by μ-type opioid agonist. J Neurophysiol 1997; 77:1418–1424.
19. Hall KE, Sima AA, Wiley JW. Opiate-mediated inhibition of calcium signaling is decreased in dorsal root ganglion neurons from the diabetic BB/W rat. J Clin Invest 1996; 97:1165–1172.
20. Hammond DL, Wang H, Naksahima N, Basbaum AI. Differential effects of intrathecally administered δ and μ opioid receptor agonists on formalin-evoked nociception and on the expression of Fos-like immunoreactivity in the spinal cord of the rat. J Pharmacol Exp Ther 1998; 284:378–387.
21. Qin N, Platano D, Olcese R, Stefani E, Birnbaumer L. Direct interaction of Gβγ with a C-terminal Gβγ-binding domain of the Ca^{2+} channel α_1 subunit is responsible for channel inhibition by G protein-coupled receptors. Proc Natl Acad Sci USA 1997; 94:8866–8871.
22. Zamponi GW, Bourinet E, Nelson D, Nargeot J, Snutch TP. Crosstalk between G proteins and protein kinase C mediated by the calcium channel α_1 subunit. Nature 1997; 385:442–446.
23. Chen Y, Penington NJ. QEHA27, a peptide that binds to G protein βγ subunits, reduces the inhibitory effect of 5-HT on the Ca^{2+} current of rat dorsal raphe neurons. Neurosci Lett 1997; 224:87–90.
24. DeWaard M, Liu H, Walker D, Scott VE, Gurnett CA, Campbell KP. Direct binding of G-protein βγ complex to voltage-dependent calcium channels. Nature 1997; 385:446–450.
25. Ikeda SR. Voltage-dependent modulation of N-type calcium channels by G protein βγ subunits. Nature 1996; 380:255–258.
26. Wang J, Ren M, Han J. Mobilization of calcium from intracellular stores as one of the mechanisms underlying the antiopioid effect of cholecystokinin octapeptide. Peptides 1992; 13:947–951.
27. Schafer M, Zhou L, Stein C. Cholecystokinin inhibits peripheral opioid analgesia in inflamed tissue. Neuroscience 1998; 82:603–611.
28. Seva C, Scemama JL, Pradayrol L, Sarfati PD, Vaysse N. Coupling of pancreatic gastrin/cholecystokinin-B (G/CCK_B) receptors to phospholipase C and protein kinase C in AR4-2J tumoral cells. Regul Pept 1994; 52:31–38.
29. Willems PH, Smeets RL, Bosch RR, Garner KM, Van Mackelenbergh MG, De Pont J. Protein kinase A activation inhibits receptor-evoked inositol trisphosphate formation and induction of cytosolic calcium oscillations by decreasing the affinity-state of the cholecystokinin receptor in pancreatic acinar cells. Cell Calcium 1995; 18:471–483.
30. Zhang X, Dagerlind A, Elde RP, Castel MN, Broberger C, Wiesenfeld–Hallin Z, Hökfelt T. Marked increase in cholecystokinin B receptor messenger RNA levels in rat dorsal root ganglia after peripheral axotomy. Neuroscience 1993; 57:227–233.
31. Xu XJ, Puke MJ, Verge VM, Wiesenfeld–Hallin Z, Hughes J, Hökfelt T. Up-regulation of cholecystokinin in primary sensory neurons is associated with morphine insensitivity in experimental neuropathic pain in the rat. Neurosci Lett 1993; 152:129–132.
32. Saika T, Kiyama H, Matsunaga T, Tohyama M. Differential regulation of phospholipase C isozymes in the rat facial nucleus following axotomy. Neuroscience 1994; 59:121–129.

33. Taylor GD, Fee JA, Silbert DF, Hofmann SL. PI-specific phospholipase C"α" from sheep seminal vesicles is a proteolytic fragment of PI-PLCδ. Biochem Biophys Res Commun 1992; 188:1176–1183.
34. Thomas G, Chung M, Cohen CJ. A dihydropyridine (Bay k 8644) that enhances calcium currents in guinea pig and calf myocardial cells. A new type of positive inotropic agent. Circ Res 1985; 56: 87–96.
35. Dolphin AC. Ca^{2+} channel currents in rat sensory neurons: interaction between guanine nucleotides, cyclic AMP and Ca^{2+} channel ligands. J Physiol (Lond) 1991; 432:23–43.
36. Zhu Y, Yakel JL. Calcineurin modulates G protein-mediated inhibition of N-type calcium channels in rat sympathetic neurons. J Neurophysiol 1997; 78:1161–1165.
37. Lyons WE, Steiner JP, Synder SH, Dawson TM. Neuronal regeneration enhances the expression of the immunophilin FKBP-12. J Neurosci 1995; 15:12985–12994.
38. Ekström PA, Bergstrand H, Edström A. Effects of protein kinase inhibitors on regeneration in vitro of adult frog sciatic sensory axons. J Neurosci Res 1992; 31:462–469.
39. Wiklund P, Ekström PA, Edbladh M, Tonge D, Edström A. Protein kinase C and mouse sciatic nerve regeneration. Brain Res 1996; 715:145–154.
40. Heacock AM, Agranoff BW. Protein kinase inhibitors block neurite outgrowth from explants of goldfish retina. Neurochem Res 1997; 22:1179–1185.
41. Roberts RE, McLean WG. Protein kinase C isozyme expression in sciatic nerves and spinal cords of experimentally diabetic rats. Brain Res 1997; 754:147–156.
42. Gandhi VC, Jones DJ. Protein kinase C modulates the release of (^{3}H)5-hydroxytryptamine in the spinal cord of the rat: the role of L-type voltage-dependent calcium channels. Neuropharmacology 1992; 31:1101–1109.
43. Coghlan VM, Perrino BA, Howard M, Langeberg LK, Hicks JB, Gallatin WM, Scott DJ. Association of protein kinase A and protein phosphatase 2B with a common anchoring protein. Science 1995; 267:108–111.
44. Steiner JP, Dawson TM, Fotuhi M, Synder SH. Immunophilin regulation of neurotransmitter release. Mol Med 1996; 2:325–333.
45. Nah SY, Saya D, Barg J, Vogel Z. Opiate receptor agonists regulate phosphorylation of synapsin I in cocultures of rat spinal cord and dorsal root ganglion. Proc Natl Acad Sci USA 1993; 90:4052–4056.
46. Matus–Leibovitch N, Ezra Macabee V, Saya D, Attali B, Avidor–Reiss T, Barg J, Vogel Z. Increased expression of synapsin I mRNA in defined areas of the rat central nervous system following chronic morphine treatment. Brain Res Mol Brain Res 1995; 34:221–230.
47. Womack MD, McCleskey EW. Interaction of opioids and membrane potential to modulate Ca^{2+} channels in rat dorsal root ganglion neurons. J Neurophysiol 1995; 73:1793–1798.
48. Williams S, Serafin M, Muhlethaler M, Bernheim L. Facilitation of the N-type calcium current is dependent on the frequency of action potential-like depolarizations in dissociated cholinergic basal forebrain neurons of the guinea pig. J Neurosci 1997; 17:1625–1632.
49. Xiao WH, Bennett GJ. Synthetic ω-conopeptides applied to the site of nerve injury suppress neuropathic pain in rats. J Pharmacol Exp Ther 1995; 274:666–672.
50. Chaplan SR, Pogrel JW, Yaksh TL. Role of voltage-dependent calcium channel subtypes in experimental tactile allodynia. J Pharmacol Exp Ther 1994; 269:1117–1123.
51. Sattler R, Tymianski M, Feyaz I, Hafner M, Tator CH. Voltage-sensitive calcium channels mediate calcium entry into cultured mammalian sympathetic neurons following neurite transection. Brain Res 1996; 719:239–246.
52. Egan SE, Weinberg RA. The pathway to signal achievement [News]. Nature 1993; 365:781–783.
53. Moodie SA, Willumsen BM, Weber MJ, Wolfman A. Complexes of Ras·GTP with Raf-1 and mitogen-activated protein kinase kinase. Science 1993; 260:1658–1661.
54. Wood KW, Sarnecki C, Roberts TM, Blenis J. Ras mediates nerve growth factor receptor modulation of three signal-transducing protein kinases: MAP kinase, Raf-1 and RSK. Cell 1992; 68:1041–1050.
55. Fukuda K, Kato S, Morikawa H, Shoda T, Mori K. Functional coupling of the δ-, μ-, and κ-opioid

receptors to mitogen-activated protein kinase and arachidonate release in Chinese hamster ovary cells. J Neurochem 1996; 67:1309–1316.
56. Li L–Y, Chang K–J. The stimulatory effect of opioids on mitogen-activated protein kinase in Chinese hamster ovary cells transfected to express μ-opioid receptors. Mol Pharmacol 1996; 50:599–602.
57. Berhow MT, Hiroi N, Nestler EJ. Regulations of ERK (extracellular signal regulated kinase), part of the neurotrophin signal transduction cascade, in the rat mesolimbic dopamine system by chronic exposure to morphine or cocaine. J Neurosci 1996; 16:4707–4715.
58. Chuang LF, Killam KF Jr, Chuang RY. Induction and activation of mitogen-activated protein kinases of human lymphocytes as one of the signaling pathways of the immunomodulatory effects of morphine sulfate. J Biol Chem 1997; 272:26815–26817.
59. Belcheva MM, Vogel Z, Ignatova E, Avidor–Reiss T, Zippel R, Levy R, Young EC, Barg J, Coscia CJ. Opioid modulation of extracellular signal-regulated protein kinase activity is *ras*-dependent and involves Gβγ subunits. J Neurochem 1998; 70:635–645.
60. Burt AR, Carr IC, Mullaney I, Anderson NG, Milligan G. Agonist activation of p42 and p44 mitogen-activated protein kinases following expression of the mouse δ opioid receptor in Rat-1 fibroblasts: effects of receptor expression levels and comparisons with G-protein activation. Biochem J 1996; 320:227–325.
61. Gutstein HB, Rubie EA, Mansour A, Akil H, Woodgett JR. Opioid effects on mitogen-activated protein kinase signaling cascades. Anesthesiology 1997; 87:1118–1126.
62. Lou LG, Zhang Z, Ma L, Pei G. Nociceptin/orphanin FQ activates mitogen-activated protein kinase in Chinese hamster ovary cells expressing opioid receptor-like receptor. J Neurochem 1998; 70: 1316–1322.
63. Fukuda K, Shoda T, Morikawa H, Kato S, Mori K. Activation of mitogen-activated protein kinase by the nociceptin receptor expressed in Chinese hamster ovary cells. FEBS Lett 1997; 412:209–294.
64. Faure M, Voyno Yasenetskaya T, Bourne HR. cAMP and βγ subunits of heterotrimeric G proteins stimulate the mitogen-activated protein kinase pathway in COS-7 cells. J Biol Chem 1994; 269: 7851–7854.
65. van Biesen T, Hawes BE, Luttrell DK, Krueger KM, Touhara K, Porfiri E, Sakaue M, Luttrell LM, Lefkowitz RJ. Receptor–tyrosine–kinase- and Gβγ-mediated MAP kinase activation by a common signalling pathway. Nature 1995; 376:781–784.
66. Ito A, Satoh T, Kaziro Y, Itoh H. G protein beta gamma subunit activates Ras, Raf, and MAP kinase in HEK293 cells. FEBS Lett 1995; 368:138–187.
67. Brown MT, Cooper JA. Regulation, substrates and functions of src. Biochim Biophys Acta 1996; 1287:121–149.
68. Rudd CE, Janssen O, Prasad KV, Raab M, da Silva S, Telfer JC, Yamamoto M. *src*-Related protein tyrosine kinases and their surface receptors. Biochim Biophys Acta 1993; 1155:239–266.
69. Luttrell LM, Hawes BE, van Biesen T, Luttrell DK, Lansing TJ, Lefkowitz DJ. Role of c-Src tyrosine kinase in G protein-coupled receptor- and Gβγ subunit-mediated activation of mitogen-activated protein kinases. J Biol Chem 1996; 271:19443–19450.
70. Sadoshima J, Izumo S. The heterotrimeric Gq protein-coupled angiotensin II receptor activates p21 ras via the tyrosine kinase-Shc-Grb2-Sos pathway in cardiac myocytes. EMBO J 1996; 15:775–787.
71. Sakanaka C, Ferby I, Waga I, Bito H, Shimizu T. On the mechanism of cytosolic phospholipase A_2 activation in CHO cells carrying somatostatin receptor: wortmannin-sensitive pathway to activate mitogen-activated protein kinase. Biochem Biophys Res Commun 1994; 205:18–23.
72. Rodriguez–Viciana P, Warne PH, Dhand R, Vanhaesebroeck B, Gout I, Fry MJ, Waterfield MD, Downward J. Phosphatidylinositol-3-OH kinase as a direct target of Ras. Nature 1994; 370:527–532.
73. Lopez–Ilasaca M, Crespo P, Pellici PG, Gutkind JS, Wetzker R. Linkage of G protein-coupled receptors to the MAPK signalling pathway through PI 3-kinase γ. Science 1997; 275:394–397.
74. Lin LL, Lin AY, Knopf JL. Cytosolic phospholipase A_2 is coupled to hormonally regulated release of arachidonic acid. Proc Natl Acad Sci USA 1992; 89:6147–6151.

75. Kitchen EA, Dawson W, Rainsford KD, Cawston T. Inflammation and possible modes of action of anti-inflammatory drugs. In: Rainsford KD, ed. Anti-Inflammatory and Anti-Rheumatic Drugs. Boca Raton, FL: CRC Press, 1985:21–87.
76. Denson DD, Worrell RT, Eaton DC. A possible role for phospholipase A_2 in the action of general anaesthetics. Am J Physiol 1996; 270:C636–C644.
77. Jain MK, Jahagirdar DV. Action of phospholipase A_2 on bilayers. Effects of inhibitors. Biochim Biophys Acta 1985; 814:319–326.
78. Bovill JG. Mechanisms of actions of anaesthetic drugs. Curr Opin Anaesthesiol 1997; 10:261–266.
79. Gupta C, Goldman AS. The arachidonic cascade is involved in the masculinizing action of testosterone on embryonic external genitalia in mice. Proc Natl Acad Sci USA 1986; 83:4346–4349.
80. Ishigooka J, Tanaka K, Suzuki Y, Katori M, Miura S. Selective inhibitory effects of chlorpromazine and imipramine on platelet aggregation. Int Pharmacopsychiatry 1980; 15:270–280.
81. Stockert M, Zieher LM, Medina JH. Interactions of phospholipids and free fatty acids with antidepressant recognition binding sites in rat brain. Adv Exp Med Biol 1992; 318:325–330.
82. Stockert M, Medina JH. Modulation of cerebral cortical (^{3}H)imipramine binding sites by phospholipase A_2: possible role of unsaturated free fatty acids. Neurosci Res Commun 1990; 6:89–94.
83. Ghrib F, Pyronnet S, Bastie MJ, Fagot–Revurat P, Pradayrol L, Vaysse N. Arachidonic–acid-selective cytosolic phospholipase A_2 is involved in gastrin-induced AR4-2J-cell proliferation. Int J Cancer 1998; 75:239–245.
84. Akagi K, Nagao T, Urushidani T. Calcium oscillations in single cultured Chinese hamster ovary cells stably transfected with a cloned human cholecystokinin CCK(B) receptor. Jpn J Pharmacol 1997; 75:33–42.
85. Yoshida H, Tsunoda Y, Owyang C. Cholecystokinin peptides stimulate pancreatic secretion by multiple signal transduction pathways. Am J Physiol 1997; 273:G735–G747.
86. Simonsson E, Karlsson S, Ahren B. Involvement of phospholipase A_2 and arachidonic acid in cholecystokinin-8-induced insulin secretion in rat islets. Regul Pept 1996; 65:101–107.
87. Tsunoda Y, Owyang C. High-affinity CCK receptors are coupled to phospholipase A_2 pathways to mediate pancreatic amylase secretion. Am J Physiol 1995; 269:G435–G444.
88. Tsunoda Y, Owyang C. The regulatory site of functional GTP binding protein coupled to the high affinity cholecystokin receptor and phospholipase A_2 pathway is on the Gβ subunit of Gq protein in pancreatic acini. Biochem Biophys Res Commun 1995; 211:648–655.
89. Tsunoda Y, Owyang C. A newly cloned phospholipase A_2-activating protein elicits Ca^{2+} oscillations and pancreatic amylase secretion via mediation of G protein β/phospholipase A_2/arachidonic acid cascades. Biochem Biophys Res Commun 1994; 203:1716–1724.
90. Tsunoda Y, Owyang C. Differential involvement of phospholipase A_2/arachidonic acid and phospholipase C/phosphoinositol pathways during cholecystokinin receptor activated Ca^{2+} oscillations in pancreatic acini. Biochem Biophys Res Commun 1993; 194:1194–1202.
91. Hidaka T, Naksno M, Shingu M, Sugiyama M, Inokuchi T, Ogura R. Stimulation of prostaglandin synthesis by cholecystokinin in primary culture cells of bovine gallbladder muscle. Prostaglandins Leukot Essent Fatty Acids 1989; 38:113–117.
92. Guitart X, Thompson MA, Mirante CK, Greenberg ME, Nestler EJ. Regulation of cyclic AMP response element-binding protein (CREB) phosphorylation by acute and chronic morphine in the rat locus coeruleus. J Neurochem 1992; 58:1168–1171.
93. Berhow MT, Russell DS, Terwilliger RZ, Beitner–Johnson D, Self SW, Lindsay RM, Nestler EJ. Influence of neurotrophic factors on morphine- and cocaine-induced biochemical changes in the mesolimbic dopamine system. Neuroscience 1995; 68:969–979.
94. Widnell KL, Self DW, Lane SB, Russell DS, Viadya VA, Miserendino MJD, Rubin CS, Duman RS, Nestler EJ. Regulation of CREB expression: in vivo evidence for a functional role in morphine action in the nucleus accumbens. J Pharmacol Exp Ther 1996; 276:306–315.
95. Nibuya M, Nestler EJ, Duman RS. Chronic antidepressant administration increases the expression of cAMP response element binding protein (CREB) in rat hippocampus. J Neurosci 1996; 16:2365–2372.
96. Ortiz J, Harris JW, Guitart X, Terwilliger RZ, Haycock JW, Nestler EJ. Extracellular signal-regu-

lated protein kinases (ERKs) and ERK kinase (MEK) in brain: regional distribution and regulation by chronic morphine. J Neurosci 1995; 16:1285–1297.
97. Schulz S, Höllt V. Opioid withdrawal activates MAP kinase in locus coeruleus in morphine-dependent rats in vivo. Eur J Neurosci 1998; 10:1196–1201.
98. Couceyro P, Douglass J. Precipitated morphine withdrawal stimulates multiple activator protein-1 signaling pathways in rat brain. Mol Pharmacol 1995; 47:29–39.
99. Lin LL, Wartmann M, Lin AY, Knopf JL, Seith A, Davis RJ. $cPLA_2$ is phosphorylated and activated by MAP kinase. Cell 1993; 72:269–278.
100. Bourne HR, Nicoll R. Molecular machines integrate coincident synaptic signals. Cell Neuron 1993; 72/10:65–75.
101. Shimegi S, Okajima F, Kondo Y. Permissive stimulation of Ca^{2+}-induced phospholipase A_2 by an adenosine receptor agonist in a pertussis toxin-sensitive manner in FRTL-5 thyroid cells: a new "cross-talk" mechanism in Ca^{2+} signalling. Biochem J 1994; 299:845–851.
102. Selbie LA, King NV, Dickenson JM, Hill SJ. Role of G-protein $\beta\gamma$ subunits in the augmentation of P2Y2 (P2U) receptor-stimulated responses by neuropeptide Y Y1 Gi/o-coupled receptors. Biochem J 1997; 328:153–158.
103. Dickenson JM, Blank JL, Hill SJ. Human adenosine A_1 receptor and P2Y2-purinoceptor-mediated activation of the mitogen-activated protein kinase cascade in transfected CHO cells. Br J Pharmacol 1998; 124:1491–1499.
104. Dickenson JM, Hill SJ. Synergistic interactions between human transfected adenosine A_1 receptors and endogenous cholecystokinin receptors in CHO cells. Eur J Pharmacol 1996; 302:141–151.
105. Dickenson JM, Hill SJ. Transfected adenosine A_1 receptor-mediated modulation of thrombin-stimulated phospholipase C and phospholipase A_2 activity in CHO cells. Eur J Pharmacol 1997; 321: 77–86.
106. Megson AC, Dickenson JM, Townsend–Nicholson A, Hill SJ. Synergy between the inositol phosphate responses to infected human adenosine A_1 receptors and constitutive P2-purinoceptors in CHO-K1 cells. Br J Pharmacol 1995; 115:1415–1424.
107. Scriabine A. Calcium channel antagonists as neuroprotective agents. In: Bär PR, Flint Beal M, eds. Neuroprotection in CNS Diseases. New York: Marcel Dekker, 1997:27–51.
108. Verity MA. Mechanisms of phospholipase A_2 activation and neuronal injury. Ann NY Acad Sci 1993; 679:110–120.
109. Walton M, Sirimanne E, Williams C, Gluckman PD, Keelan J, Mitchell MD, Dragunow M. Prostaglandin H synthase-2 and cytosolic phospholipase A_2 in the hypoxi-ischemic brain: role in neuronal death or survival? Brain Res Mol Brain Res 1997; 50:165–170.
110. Paul JA, Gregson NA. An immunohistochemical study of phospholipase A_2 in peripheral nerve during Wallerian degeneration. J Neuroimmunol 1992; 39:31–47.
111. Saal JS, Franson RC, Dobrow R, Saal JA, White AH, Goldthwaite N. High levels of inflammatory phospholipase A_2 in lumbar disc herniations. Spine 1990; 15:674–678.
112. Mitchell JA, Larkin S, Williams TJ. Cyclooxygenase-2: regulation and relevance in inflammation. Biochem Pharmacol 1995; 50:1535–1542.
113. Manjunath P, Sairam MP. Purification and biochemical characterization of three major acidic proteins (BSP-A1, BSP-A2 and BSP-A30) from bovine seminal plasma. Biochem J 1987; 241:685–692.
114. Makimura M, Ito Y, Murakoshi Y. Inhibitory mechanism of opioid binding to receptor by phospholipase A_2. Gen Pharmacol 1988; 19:707–712.
115. Lazar DF, Medzihradsky F. Differential inhibition of delta-opiate binding and low K_m GTPase stimulation by phospholipase A_2 treatment. Prog Clin Biol Res 1996; 328:113–116.
116. Sinatra RS, Ford DH. The effects of acute and chronic morphine treatment on the process of facial nerve regeneration. Brain Res 1979; 175:315–325.
117. Zagon IS, McLaughlin PJ. Morphine and brain growth retardation in the rat. Pharmacology 1977; 15:276–282.
118. Yawo H, Kuno M. How a nerve fiber repairs its cut end: involvement of phospholipase A. Science 1983; 222:1351–1353.

119. Nakamura S. Effects of manserin and fluoxetine on axonal regeneration of brain catecholamine neurons. Neuroreport 1991; 2:525–528.
120. Nakamura S. Involvement of phospholipase A_2 in axonal regeneration of brain noradrenergic neurones. Neuroreport 1993; 4:371–374.
121. Nakamura S. Effects of phospholipase A_2 inhibitors on the antidepressant-induced axonal regeneration of noradrenergic locus coeruleus neurons. Microsc Res Tech 1994; 29:204–210.
122. Edström A, Briggman M, Ekström PA. Phospholipase A_2 activity is required for regeneration of sensory axons in cultured adult sciatic nerves. J Neurosci Res 1996; 43:183–189.
123. Smalheiser NR, Dissanayake S, Kapil A. Rapid regulation of neurite outgrowth and retraction by phospholipase A_2-derived arachidonic acid and its metabolites. Brain Res 1996; 721:39–48.
124. Womer DE, De Lapp NW, Shannon HE. Intrathecal pertussis toxin produces hyperalgesia and allodynia in mice. Pain 1997; 70:223–228.
125. Wiesenfeld–Hallin Z. The effects of intrathecal morphine and naltrexone on autotomy in sciatic nerve sectioned rats. Pain 1984; 18:267–278.
126. Bennett GJ, Xie YK. A peripheral mononeuropathy in rat that produces disorders of pain sensation like those seen in man. Pain 1988; 33:87–107.
127. Kim SH, Chung JM. An experimental model for peripheral neuropathy produced by segmental spinal nerve ligation in the rat. Pain 1992; 50:355–363.
128. Wheeler–Aceto H, Cowan A. Buprenorphine and morphine cause antinociception by different transduction mechanisms. Eur J Pharmacol 1991; 195:411–413.
129. Wheeler–Aceto H, Cowan A. Effect of pertussis toxin (PTX) on the antinociceptive profile of buprenorphine (B) and morphine (M): evidence for differential regulation of pain transmission. In: Harris LS, ed. Problems of Drug Dependence 1991. Proceeding of the 53rd Annual Scientific Meeting, College on Problems of Drug Dependence, Research Monograph 119, NIDA, Rockville, MD, 1992:309.
130. Shah S, Duttaroy A, Davis T, Yoburn BC. Spinal and supraspinal effects of pertussis toxin on opioid analgesia. Pharmacol Biochem Behav 1994; 49:773–776.
131. Przewlocki R, Costa T, Lang J, Herz A. Pertussis toxin abolishes the antinociception mediated by opioid receptors in rat spinal cord. Eur J Pharmacol 1987; 144:91–95.
132. Wong CS, Su YF, Watkins WD, Chang KJ. Continuous intrathecal opioid treatment abolishes the regulatory effects of magnesium and guanine nucleotides on μ opioid receptor binding in rat spinal membranes. J Pharmacol Exp Ther 1992; 262:317–326.
133. McCormack K, Brune K, Budd K, Prather P. Experimental indices used to classify opioids as partial or full receptor agonists may have limited clinical utility [abstr 88]. In: 8th World Congress on Pain. Seattle: IASP Press, 1996:464.
134. Fields TA, Casey PJ. Phosphorylation of Gzα by protein kinase C blocks interaction with the beta gamma complex. J Biol Chem 1995; 270:23119–23125.
135. Kozasa T, Gilman AG. Protein kinase C phosphorylates G12α and inhibits its interaction with Gβγ. J Biol Chem 1996; 271:12562–12567.
136. Prather P, Brune K, Budd K, McCormack K. How far does functional promiscuity amongst receptor subtypes and G proteins explain diversity in clinical effects and interactions? [abstr 78] In: 8th World Congress on Pain. Seattle: IASP Press, 1996:460.
137. Fields TA, Casey PJ. Signalling functions and biochemical properties of pertussis toxin-resistant G proteins. Biochem J 1997; 321:561–571.
138. Hinton DR, Blanks JC, Fong HKW, Casey PJ, Hildebrandt E, Simons MI. Novel localization of a G protein, Gzα, in neurons of brain and retina. J Neurosci 1990; 10:2763–2770.
139. Yasuda H, Lindorfer MA, Myung C–S, Garrison JC. Phosphorylation of the G protein γ_{12} subunit regulates effector specificity. J Biol Chem 1998; 273:21958–21965.

6
Pain and the Somatosensory Cortex

Rolf-Detlef Treede
Johannes Gutenberg University, Mainz, Germany

I. INTRODUCTION

In their landmark paper on sensory disturbances from cerebral lesions, Head and Holmes (1) concluded from the lack of clear deficit in pain sensitivity with purely cortical lesions that the ''essential organ of the thalamus'' was the center of consciousness for those elements of sensation that evoke either pleasure or discomfort. In more modern terms, this would mean that the affective component of pain is felt in the medial and intralaminar thalamus (2) and that there is no cortical representation of pain. This view was contradicted by several reports that demonstrated sensory deficits for pain following small cortical lesions or resections (3–6).

Nevertheless, this issue remained dormant until 1991, when the first studies were published that used positron emission tomography (PET) to investigate cortical activation by painful heat stimuli (7,8). Both studies demonstrated a significant increase in blood flow in the anterior cingulate gyrus, a neocortical part of the limbic system. The studies disagreed on whether or not the somatosensory cortex was also activated. Since then, many additional PET studies on the cortical representation of pain have been published (for a recent review see Ref. 9).

Earlier evoked potential studies in humans using electrical stimulation of the tooth pulp (10) or laser radiant heat stimulation of the hairy skin (11) had also suggested cortical activation by painful stimuli. Although there was evidence for generation of some evoked potential components in the secondary somatosensory cortex (10,12,13), a thalamic generator was upheld particularly for the large vertex potential with its maximum amplitude in the midline (14). Only more recently, evidence has accumulated that the vertex potential may partly derive from the anterior cingulate gyrus (15–18).

These multiple converging lines of evidence for involvement of the anterior cingulate gyrus in pain sensation are of particular significance, because this cortical area is part of the so-called medial pain system. The medial pain system is named for the medial and intralaminar thalamic nuclei through which it projects (Fig. 1). It is thought to be responsible for the affective–motivational component of pain (2), and this system is the one that was suggested to end in the ''essential organ of the thalamus'' (1).

The primary and secondary somatosensory cortex (SI and SII) are part of the lateral pain system that projects through specific lateral thalamic nuclei (see Fig. 1). In both SI and SII, nociceptive neurons have been identified with single-cell recordings (reviewed in Ref. 19). In addition, part of the anterodorsal insula, next to the visceral and gustatory areas, may contain a specific nociceptive area (20). The insula takes up an intermediate position, for it receives its

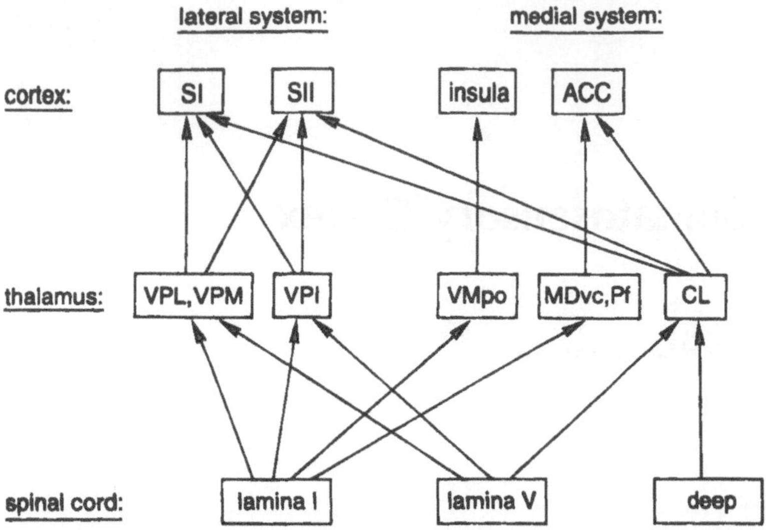

Figure 1 Distribution of information on painful stimuli from the spinal cord to various cortical areas: Main spinothalamic and thalamocortical projections were summarized and simplified from several reports on the central nociceptive pathways in the monkey (20,111,115,116). Corticocortical connections are not shown. ACC, anterior cingulate cortex; CL, centrolateral nucleus; MDvc, ventrocaudal part of medial dorsal nucleus; Pf, parafascicular nucleus; SI, primary somatosensory cortex; SII, secondary somatosensory cortex; VMpo, posterior part of ventromedial nucleus; VPI, ventral posterior inferior nucleus; VPL, ventral posterior lateral nucleus; VPM, ventral posterior medial nucleus. (From Ref. 117.)

major input from the lateral system, but itself, projects to the limbic system. Thus, the division into lateral and medial pain systems is somewhat artificial, but it still provides a useful framework to discuss the functional role of the cortical projection targets of the nociceptive system (21).

The lateral pain system is thought to subserve sensory–discriminative aspects of pain sensation (2), such as stimulus localization, and intensity discrimination. Historically, these capacities have been ascribed to the lemniscal system, which is likely coactivated by most cutaneous stimuli and also projects by lateral thalamic nuclei to the primary somatosensory cortex. The aim of this chapter is to summarize the evidence that the discriminative functions of pain sensation are mediated by its own central apparatus that is independent of the lemniscal system. The possible functions of the anterior cingulate gyrus have recently been discussed elsewhere (22,23).

II. SPATIAL DISCRIMINATION

A. Psychophysical Observations

Traditionally, pain was considered to be poorly localized. If tactile discrimination at the lips and fingertips (the tactile fovea) is compared with the mislocalization of visceral pain (see also later discussion), this impression is obvious. Cutaneous pain, however, is localized much more precisely. Using painfully hot thermodes, for example, the mean distance between stimulus site and perceived site (indicated by pointing) was 17 mm on the foot and 10 mm on the palm or dorsum of the hand (24–26). A contribution from tactile afferents was excluded by a compression nerve block that inhibits conduction in Aβ-fiber mechanoreceptors (24,26). Likewise, the site on the hand that had been stimulated with radiant heat could be pointed out with a mean error of 14 mm (27). The accuracy of pointing to the stimulated spot depends not only on sensory, but also on motor performance. To determine the sensory limits of heat pain localization on the dorsum of the hand, we used a two-alternative forced choice paradigm (28). The average threshold for 75% correct identification, which one of two sites had been stimulated by laser radiant heat, was 8.8 mm. In the same skin area, the threshold for 75% correct detection of a light touch stimulus was 8.6 mm. Both values were clearly worse than those for touching the lips or finger tips, but outside the tactile fovea, pain was located equally as well as touch.

B. Somatotopic Representation in the Nociceptive System

The psychophysical findings just mentioned suggest that selective activation of nociceptive afferents in humans encodes sufficient spatial information to account for our capacity to know where it hurts. A precise spatial coding in the central nociceptive system is necessary to provide the neural basis for this capacity. Tracing studies in the rat have shown that the terminal fields of different peripheral nerves have predictable and nonoverlapping positions in the dorsal horn of the spinal cord (29,30). In this way, a faithful somatotopic map of the skin surface with contiguous peripheral fields is represented centrally by contiguous terminal fields in the dorsal horn. The somatotopic maps of nociceptive C-fiber afferent terminals in lamina II and mechanoreceptive Aβ-fiber afferent terminals in laminae III and IV are similar. The receptive field properties of some dorsal horn neurons deviate from this pattern, probably because of interneuronal connections. Nevertheless, spatial information is largely preserved in the first synaptic relay of the nociceptive pathways.

The spinothalamic tract in humans terminates in the lateral thalamic nuclei, including the principal sensory nucleus (also a projection target of the medial lemniscus), and in medially located nuclei including the intralaminar nucleus centralis lateralis (31). This termination pattern is similar to that in the monkey, in spite of differences in nomenclature (e.g., ventrocaudal in humans corresponds to ventroposterior in monkey). Within the lateral thalamus, different regions of the body are represented in parasagittal planes or lamellae. From medial to lateral, these lamellae contain neurons with receptive fields in the face, thumb, fingers, arm, and leg. This mediolateral somatotopy has been identified with tactile stimuli. Nociceptive cells in the human lateral thalamus appear to be mostly located in its posterior inferior parts. Because the segregation relative to modality is perpendicular to the somatotopy, it is likely that the nociceptive neurons are arranged in the same mediolateral somatotopic sequence.

The human lateral thalamic nuclei that receive spinothalamic input project to the postcentral parietal cortex (including SI), inferior parietal lobule (including parietal operculum and SII), anterior insula, posterior insula, and superior temporal gyrus (31). Although no detailed mapping of the somatotopy in SI has been performed with noxious stimuli, several lines of evidence indicate that it is no different from the one outlined with tactile stimuli (the well-known sensory homunculus, where the leg is represented most medially near the interhemispheric fissure and the face most laterally toward the Sylvian fissure). In both monkey and rat, nociceptive neurons with receptive fields in the hindlimb were found more medially than those with receptive fields in the forelimb (32,33). An estimation of hand and foot representation in the human SI derived from a dipole source analysis of heat-evoked potentials is shown in Fig. 2. Likewise, in those PET studies that showed activation of SI, increased blood flow following hand stimulation was found approximately within the hand area of the sensory homunculus (8,34–36). The receptive fields of nociceptive neurons in monkey SI tend to be smaller than in the spinal cord and thalamus, possibly owing to lateral inhibition, and some receptive fields are small enough to explain

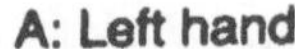

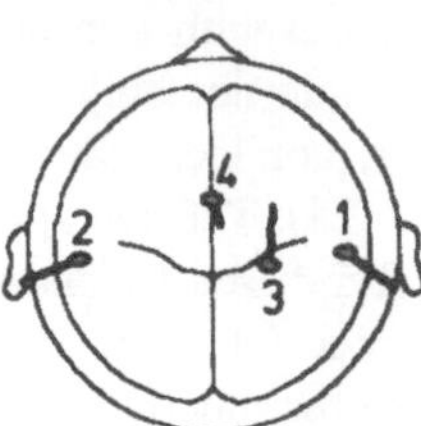

B: Right hand

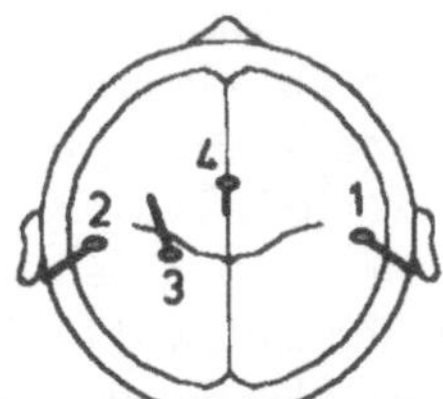

C: Left foot

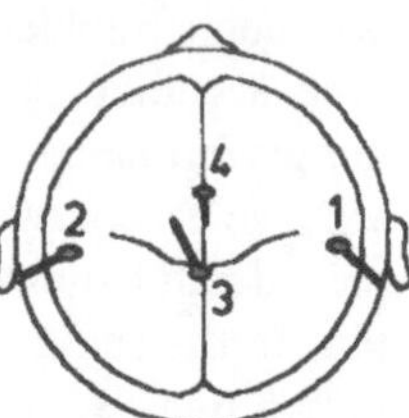

Figure 2 Somatotopy of heat pain representation in the primary somatosensory cortex: Pain-related evoked cerebral potentials were measured in 24 healthy subjects (13) and the grand mean averages across subjects were submitted to a dipole source analysis. Bilaterally symmetrical sources (1 and 2) in the secondary somatosensory cortex alone were insufficient to explain the scalp topography of the evoked potential and had to be supplemented by a source in the primary somatosensory cortex (3) and another source in the midline (4), possibly representing the anterior cingulate gyrus. Comparison of data from stimulation of (A) the left hand, (B) right hand, and (C) the left foot demonstrated shifts in the location of source 3 that were consistent with their generation in the primary somatosensory cortex. (Modified from Ref. 15.)

the psychophysical capacity to localize painful stimuli (33,37). Thus, all existing evidence favors the view that SI is involved in stimulus localization for the nociceptive system as well as for the tactile system.

The central representation of how our body looks (body image), however, does not reside in SI, as shown by observations on phantom limb phenomena and cortical reorganization (38). In monkeys as well as in humans, digit amputations result in reorganization of the cortical map in such a way that the deafferented cortex (representation area of the amputated finger) moves its receptive fields to neighboring fingers (39,40). With large denervations, this cortical reorganization can be extensive, suggesting participation of subcortical mechanisms (41). This type of cortical plasticity can be induced within minutes by nerve blocks (42). If the body image resides in SI, these plastic changes would imply that the brain "forgets" that the amputated body part had ever existed (i.e., the reorganization might be an adaptive process that protects the amputee from phantom limb pain). The opposite, however, seems to be true: patients with phantom limb pain revealed particularly pronounced cortical reorganization (43).

These observations are consistent with the concept that SI is a relatively "low" somatosensory center (analogous to V1 in the visual system), and that the body image resides in one of its projection targets, such as the posterior parietal cortex (44,45). In this framework, receptive field reorganization in SI would be inadequate and would lead to sensations projected into the nonexisting body part when adjacent areas are stimulated (46). A few studies have investigated, in which the body site projected sensations were felt when neurons that had developed new receptive fields were activated. One upper-limb amputee (without phantom pain), who had to undergo surgery for a brain tumor, experienced phantom sensations after intraoperative stimulation of the deafferented cortical hand area (47). In a few patients, a large representation of the stump of the amputated limb was found during stereotactic procedures in the thalamus; microstimulation of thalamic neurons responsive to tactile stimuli in the stump evoked sensations in the phantom limb (48).

C. Clinical Relevance

Although textbook knowledge states that pain is poorly localized, practicing clinicians implicitly assume that this is false. Asking the patient whether he or she is suffering from pain is part of regular history taking. The location of the painful body part plays a major role in guiding further diagnostic procedures [trivial example: if a finger hurts, examine the finger for signs of inflammation]. Correct localization of pain is so common in clinical practice that we have derived special terms for cases of mislocalization: projected pain and referred pain. Referral of pain describes the situation, where pain is felt in a different body part than the one that is stimulated, whereas projected pain refers to the situation where parts of the somatosensory pathways are directly activated.

Projected pain reflects the fact that all sensations are perceived in the brain and are projected into the receptive fields of the cortical areas activated (e.g., part of the visual field for a visual stimulus, or part of the body surface for touch or pain). If the neural activity is generated by a stimulus in that field, the projection is adequate. If the activity is generated at a more proximal site along the sensory pathways, a projected sensation is generated (e.g., in the little finger, if the ulnar nerve is stimulated in the course of a clinical neurophysiological examination; or tinnitus if the central auditory pathway generates spontaneous activity). On this background, phantom limb pain is just an extreme example of a normal physiological process, and the absence of phantom sensations after recovery from amputation is an active accomplishment of the CNS. However, the factors determining that one patient develops phantom limb pain, whereas another patient does not, still remain largely unknown. The somatotopic reorganization after amputations, discussed above has been demonstrated only for tactile receptive fields and not for nociceptive receptive fields. This reorganization would explain the occurrence of referred sensations (e.g., stimulation of the face is also felt in the phantom), rather than the actual sensation of a phantom limb (49). Empirically, however, there is only a weak correlation of the extent of reorganization with the occurrence of referred sensations, but a strong correlation with phantom limb pain (43,50).

Referred pain from the viscera is another example of erroneous projection of pain (51). The neural basis of referred visceral pain is a convergence of afferent pathways from skin and viscera (convergence–projection theory). There is only little evidence that two branches of the same primary afferent could innervate skin and viscera, but viscerosomatic convergence is the rule, rather than an exception, in the spinal cord (52). Central convergence within the spinal cord dorsal horn, therefore, is thought to provide the basis for referred pain. A second center with viscerosomatic convergence is the lateral thalamus (53), and some authors have proposed thalamic mechanisms for referred pain (54). In any event, projection of pain sensation is part of the mechanism of referred pain, but this projection occurs inappropriately into the cutaneous, instead of the visceral receptive field.

III. INTENSITY DISCRIMINATION

A. Psychophysical Observations

Pain is not an all-or-none phenomenon. For example, temperature changes as small as 0.3°C are detected when delivered on a painful baseline of 47°C (55). Psychophysical studies using cross-modality matching have shown that humans can accurately scale both the intensity and the unpleasantness of experimental pain at a ratio scale level (56,57). Quantitative assessment of pain can also be given by patients, using either visual analog scales (58), or verbal descriptor scales, such as the McGill Pain Questionnaire (59). Figure 3 shows a graph plotting a quantitative evaluation of McGill Pain Questionnaire data from several experimental and clinical studies for the two dimensions intensity and unpleasantness (60). Each point represents one group of subjects or patients. All entries lie below the main diagonal, suggesting that unpleasantness is partly correlated to intensity. For the same perceived intensity, however, the perceived unpleasantness

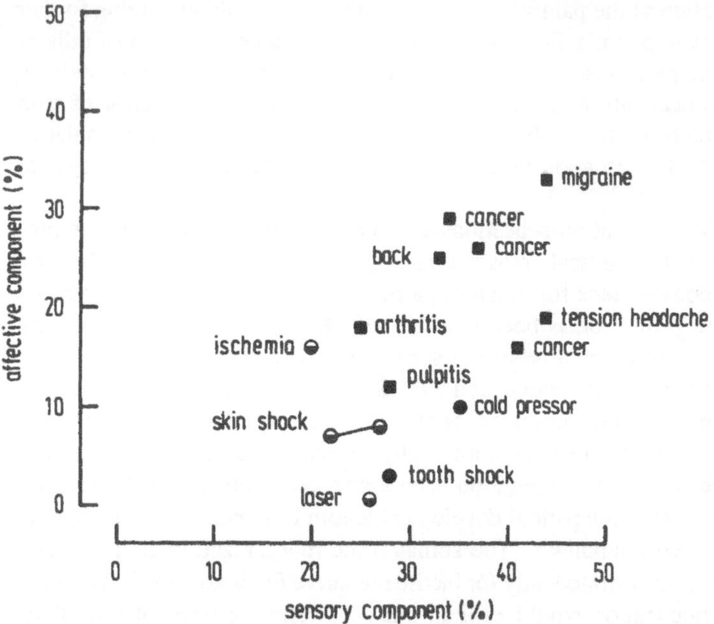

Figure 3 Sensory and affective components of experimental and clinical pain: Each point in this graph represents the mean value of one study that used the McGill Pain Questionnaire (squares, patient groups; circles, experimental studies; semifilled circles, data from authors' laboratory). The pain rating index (PRI) values for sensory and affective words were plotted as percentages of the maximum possible values. The two values for skin shock show the analgesic effect of heterotopic noxious conditioning stimuli. Note that only the experimental pain of ischemic muscle work reaches a similar affective rating as the clinical pain states. (Data from Ref. 60.)

may vary considerably (compare tooth shock and pulpitis). In general, clinically relevant pain and pain of longer duration tend to be associated with a higher affective component than brief experimental stimuli. Some experimental manipulations, such as warning signals, can influence the affective component selectively (61). Frequently, however, changes in perceived unpleasantness of the stimulus are, at least partially, a consequence of alterations in the perceived intensity of the stimulus (62,63). Opioids (64) and even surgical interruptions of the subcortical input to the anterior cingulate and frontal cortex (65,66) influence both perceived intensity and unpleasantness of experimental pain.

B. Intensity Coding in the Nociceptive System

The capacity to discriminate different perceived intensities of potentially or actually tissue-damaging stimuli depends on an accurate encoding of stimulus intensity in primary nociceptive afferents. Encoding of heat stimulus intensity has been demonstrated for polymodal C-fiber nociceptors (67–69), as well as polymodal A-fiber nociceptors (70,71), whereas nonnociceptive warm fibers reach saturation, or even decrease their response, when stimulus intensity reaches noxious levels (67). For mechanical stimuli, a correlation with noxious stimulus intensity was found in the discharges of C-fiber and A-fiber nociceptors, but not low-threshold mechanoreceptors (72–74). Nociceptive primary afferents also encode the intensity of noxious chemical stimuli such as bradykinin (75) or acids (76). Increasing the stimulus intensity results in not only increasing action potential rates, but also leads to recruitment of insensitive nociceptors or silent afferents (77–80). Also, in the CNS, one of the criteria to identify nociceptive neurons is intensity coding in the noxious range (81). This criterion is fulfilled by nociceptive neurons in the spinal cord dorsal horn and in the thalamus (82).

Intensity coding has also been demonstrated for nociceptive neurons in SI and to a certain extent also in SII (19,33). Heat-evoked responses in nociceptive SI neurons of awake monkeys are significantly correlated with the monkey's detection speed for the same stimuli (83). The heat responses of neurons in SI reflect the heat sensitivity of primary nociceptive afferents, as well as the changes in their heat sensitivity owing to peripheral sensitization (84). Responsiveness of rat nociceptive SI neurons is enhanced following skin inflammation (85) or nerve lesions (86). Spinal intrathecal morphine reduces the heat-evoked potential from rat SI in a dose-dependent manner, by reducing its spinothalamic input, without affecting the tactile responses in SI (87). Thus, intensity coding is preserved up to the cortical projection targets of the lateral pain system.

Intensity coding has also been observed in structures that belong to the medial pain system. Neurons in the medullary reticular formation of rats (88) and in medial thalamic nuclei of primates encode the intensity of noxious heat stimuli (89), and neurons in rabbit anterior cingulate cortex encode the intensity of noxious mechanical stimuli (90). Thus, intensity coding is a poor criterion to identify neurons involved in sensory-discriminative aspects of pain, because the affective–motivational component of pain also depends on stimulus intensity.

C. Targets for Analgesic Actions

Intensity coding in the nociceptive system also provides the basis for analgesic efficacy and potency of drugs. In most animal studies, analgesic effects are deduced from changes in withdrawal reflexes. Because reflexes and pain may become uncoupled (e.g., by muscle relaxants) and reflex pathways and centrally projecting pathways begin to separate in the dorsal horn (91), a method to measure the nociceptive input to SI would be valuable (e.g., by measuring evoked potentials) (87).

In humans, many analgesic drugs have been assessed with evoked potential measures, including acetylsalicylic acid, acetaminophen (paracetamol), and ibuprofen (92–94); nitrous oxide (95,96); systemic (97,98) and epidural opioids (99); and antidepressants (100,101) as well as ketamine (102). Some of the measured effects may represent projections of reduced neuronal discharges in peripheral nerves, spinal cord, or the thalamus, rather than showing genuine effects on cortical neurons. Moreover, nonspecific effects by sedation need to be differentiated from specific analgesic effects (101,103). The evoked potential components studied in humans are late components, which are most likely generated outside of the somatosensory cortex by widespread cortical sources.

Thus, there is little evidence that analgesic drugs act specifically on the cortical areas of the lateral pain system (SI, SII, and anterior insula). The anterior cingulate cortex, however, a projection target of the medial pain system, may be one of the sites of action of opioids. The anterior cingulate cortex is one of the generators of the late-evoked potentials (15–18) that are reduced by opioids (97,98). Within the brain, it has one of the highest densities of opioid receptors (104–106), and PET studies have shown metabolic activation in this area by fentanyl (107,108). These findings suggest that opioid effects on the lateral pain system are mostly subcortical, but in the medial pain system, the cortex itself may be a target of analgesic action.

Several transmitter systems potentially modulate the processing of nociceptive information in the CNS: excitatory amino acids (e.g., glutamate); inhibitory amino acids (e.g., GABA); monoamines (norepinephrine, serotonin, and dopamine); acetylcholine, adenosine, histamine, and several peptides (opioids, CCK, and others). Relatively little, however, is known concerning the neurotransmitters and receptors utilized by nociceptive neurons or the modulatory inputs to these neurons at the cortical level (21). The introduction of PET-imaging techniques may provide new tools for directly measuring antinociceptive actions in the brain under normal and pathological conditions (109).

IV. CONCLUSIONS

Anatomical tracing studies in animals, single-unit recordings in animals, evoked potential studies in humans, metabolic and perfusion-imaging studies in humans, as well as observations on the sensory consequences of cortical lesions in patients, all suggest that the nociceptive system has cortical projection targets. According to the traditional separation, the lateral pain system projects to SI, SII, and the anterior insula, whereas the medial pain system projects to the anterior cingulate cortex, in addition to subcortical projection targets. The lateral pain system has been associated with the sensory–discriminative component of pain, and the medial system with the affective–motivational component. These two components, both of which are represented in parts of the cerebral cortex, are reflected in the definition of *pain* according to the International Association for the Study of Pain:

> Pain is an unpleasant sensory and emotional experience associated with actual or potential tissue damage or described in terms of such damage (110).

As outlined in the foregoing, multiple lines of evidence indicate that SI participates in the coding of the sensory–discriminative aspects of pain, particularly in spatial and intensity discrimination. The clinical relevance of this pain component is reflected in that most analgesics reduce the sensory as well as the affective component of pain. The roles of SII and the anterior insula for pain perception are much less clear. SII receives nociceptive input at least partly through direct thalamocortical projections, rather than indirectly from SI (111). Lesions in SII tend to lead to loss of pain sensitivity (112), but these lesions often involve both SII in the parietal operculum and parts of the insula. Only few recordings of single neurons have been performed in SII and its vicinity, showing relatively poor spatial and intensity coding (113,114). No detailed information is available on neuronal properties of nociceptive neurons in the anterior insula.

In summary, the known cellular properties of the nociceptive system (from primary afferents to the primary somatosensory cortex) can account for the sensory–discriminative capacity of pain perception. Similar to the visual system, in which, for example, color and shape are processed in parallel by different cortical circuits, it appears that there is a parallel processing of sensory, affective, and other dimensions of pain by different parts of the nociceptive system.

ACKNOWLEDGMENTS

My colleague Dr. Gerd Böhmer deserves special thanks for critical reading of this manuscript.

REFERENCES

1. Head H, Holmes G. Sensory disturbances from cerebral lesions. Brain 1911; 34:102–254.
2. Melzack R, Casey KL. Sensory, motivational, and central control determinants of pain. A new conceptual model. In: Kenshalo DR, ed. The Skin Senses. Springfield, Illinois: Charles C Thomas 1968:423–443.

3. Echols DH, Colclough JA. Abolition of painful phantom foot by resection of the sensory cortex. JAMA 1947; 134:1476–1477.
4. Marshall J. Sensory disturbances in cortical wounds with special reference to pain. J Neurol Neurosurg Psychiatry 1951; 14:187–204.
5. Lende RA, Kirsch WM, Druckman R. Relief of facial pain after combined removal of precentral and postcentral cortex. J Neurosurg 1971; 34:537–543.
6. Greenspan JD, Winfield JA. Reversible pain and tactile deficits associated with a cerebral tumor compressing the posterior insula and parietal operculum. Pain 1992; 50:29–39.
7. Jones AKP, Brown WD, Friston KJ, Qi LY, Frackowiak RSJ. Cortical and subcortical localization of response to pain in man using positron emission tomography. Proc R Soc Lond B 1991; 244:39–44.
8. Talbot JD, Marrett S, Evans AC, Meyer E, Bushnell MC, Duncan GH. Multiple representations of pain in human cerebral cortex. Science 1991; 251:1355–1358.
9. Casey KL, Minoshima S. Can pain be imaged? In: Jensen TS, Turner JA, Wiesenfeld–Hallin Z, eds. Proceedings of the 8th World Congress on Pain, Progress in Pain Research and Management Seattle: IASP Press, 1997:855–866.
10. Chatrian GE, Canfield RC, Knauss TA, Lettich E. Cerebral responses to electrical tooth pulp stimulation in man. Neurology 1975; 25:745–757.
11. Carmon A, Mor J, Goldberg J. Evoked cerebral responses to noxious thermal stimuli in humans. Exp Brain Res 1976; 25:103–107.
12. Hari R, Kaukoranta E, Reinikainen K, Huopaniemi T, Mauno J. Neuromagnetic localization of cortical activity evoked by painful dental stimulation in man. Neurosci Lett 1983; 42:77–82.
13. Treede R–D, Kief S, Hölzer T, Bromm B. Late somatosensory evoked cerebral potentials in response to cutaneous heat stimuli. Electroenceph Clin Neurophysiol 1988; 70:429–441.
14. Kakigi R, Shibasaki H, Ikeda A. Pain-related somatosensory evoked potentials following CO_2 laser stimulation in man. Electroenceph Clin Neurophysiol 1989; 74:139–146.
15. Tarkka IM, Treede R–D. Equivalent electrical source analysis of pain-related somatosensory evoked potentials elicited by a CO_2 laser. J Clin Neurophysiol 1993; 10:513–519.
16. Bromm B, Chen ACN. Brain electrical source analysis of laser evoked potentials in response to painful trigeminal nerve stimulation. Electroencephalogr Clin Neurophysiol 1995; 95:14–26.
17. Valeriani M, Rambaud L, Mauguière F. Scalp topography and dipolar source modelling of potentials evoked by CO_2 laser stimulation of the hand. Electroencephalogr Clin Neurophysiol 1996; 100: 343–353.
18. Lenz FA, Rios M, Zirh A, Chau D, Krauss G, Lesser RP. Painful stimuli evoke potentials recorded over the human anterior cingulate gyrus. J Neurophysiol 1998; 79:2231–2234.
19. Kenshalo DR, Douglass DK. The role of the cerebral cortex in the experience of pain. In: Bromm B, Desmedt JE, eds. Pain and the Brain: From Nociception to Cognition. New York: Raven Press, 1995:21–34.
20. Craig AD. An ascending general homeostatic afferent pathway originating in lamina I. Prog Brain Res 1996; 107:225–242.
21. Craig AD, Dostrovsky JO. Processing of nociceptive information at supraspinal levels. In: Yaksh TL, ed. Anesthesia: Biologic Foundations. Philadelphia: Lippincott–Raven 1997:625–642.
22. Devinsky O, Morrell MJ, Vogt BA. Contributions of anterior cingulate cortex to behaviour. Brain 1995; 118:279–306.
23. Vogt BA, Derbyshire S, Jones AKP. Pain processing in four regions of human cingulate cortex localized with co-registered PET and MR imaging. Eur J Neurosci 1996; 8:1461–1473.
24. Jorum E, Lundberg LER, Torebjörk HE. Peripheral projections of nociceptive unmyelinated axons in the human peroneal nerve. J Physiol 1989; 416:291–301.
25. Ochoa J, Torebjörk HE. Sensations evoked by intraneural microstimulation of C nociceptor fibers in human skin nerves. J Physiol 1989; 415:583–599.
26. Koltzenburg M, Handwerker HO, Torebjörk HE. The ability of humans to localise noxious stimuli. Neurosci Lett 1993; 150:219–222.
27. Moore CEG, Schady W. Cutaneous localisation of laser induced pain in humans. Neurosci Lett 1995; 193:208–210.

28. Schlereth T, Magerl W, Treede R-D. Spatial discrimination thresholds for pain and touch in human hairy skin. Pain 2001; 92:187–194.
29. Swett JE, Woolf CJ. The somatotopic organization of primary afferent terminals in the superficial laminae of the dorsal horn of the rat spinal cord. J Comp Neurol 1985; 231:66–77.
30. Woolf CJ, Fitzgerald M. Somatotopic organization of cutaneous afferent terminals and dorsal horn neuronal receptive fields in the superficial and deep laminae of the rat lumbar spinal cord. J Comp Neurol 1986; 251:517–531.
31. Lenz FA, Dougherty PM. Pain processing in the human thalamus. In: Steriade M, Jones EG, McCormick DA, eds. Thalamus. Experimental/Clinical Aspects. Vol 2. Oxford: Elsevier, 1997:617–651.
32. Lamour Y, Guilbaud G, Willer JC. Rat somatosensory (SmI) cortex: II. Laminar and columnar organization of noxious and non-noxious inputs. Exp Brain Res 1983; 49:46–54.
33. Kenshalo DR, Willis WD. The role of the cerebral cortex in pain sensation. In: Peters A, ed. Cerebral Cortex. Vol 9. New York: Plenum Press, 1991:153–212.
34. Casey KL, Minoshima S, Berger KL, Koeppe RA, Morrow TJ, Frey KA. Positron emission tomographic analysis of cerebral structures activated specifically by repetitive noxious heat stimuli. J Neurophysiol 1994; 71:802–807.
35. Craig AD, Reiman EM, Evans A, Bushnell MC. Functional imaging of an illusion of pain. Nature 1996; 384:258–260.
36. Derbyshire SWG, Jones AKP, Gyulai F, Clark S, Townsend D, Firestone LL. Pain processing during three levels of noxious stimulation produces differential patterns of central activity. Pain 1997; 73: 431–445.
37. Biedenbach MA, Van Hassel HJ, Brown AC. Tooth pulp-driven neurons in somatosensory cortex of primates: role in pain mechanisms including a review of the literature. Pain 1979; 7:31–50.
38. Melzack R, Israel R, Lacroix R, Schultz G. Phantom limbs in people with congenital limb deficiency or amputation in early childhood. Brain 1997; 120:1603–1620.
39. Merzenich MM, Nelson RJ, Stryker MP, Cynader MS, Schoppmann A, Zook JM. Somatosensory cortical map changes following digit amputation in adult monkeys. J Comp Neurol 1984; 224:591–605.
40. Weiss T, Miltner WHR, Dillmann J, Meissner W, Huonker R, Nowak H. Reorganization of the somatosensory cortex after amputation of the index finger. Neuroreport 1998; 9:213–216.
41. Pons TP, Garraghty PE, Ommaya AK, Kaas JH, Taub E, Mishkin M. Massive cortical reorganization after sensory deafferentation in adult macaques. Science 1991; 252:1857–1860.
42. Birbaumer N, Lutzenberger W, Montoya P, Larbig W, Unertl K, Töpfner S, Grodd W, Taub E, Flor H. Effects of regional anesthesia on phantom limb pain are mirrored in changes in cortical reorganization. J Neurosci 1997; 17:5503–5508.
43. Flor H, Elbert T, Knecht S, Wienbruch C, Pantev C, Birbaumer N, Larbig W, Taub E. Phantom-limb pain as a perceptual correlate of cortical reorganization following arm amputation. Nature 1995; 375:482–484.
44. Stein JF. Representation of egocentric space in the posterior parietal cortex. QJ Exp Physiol 1989; 74:583–606.
45. Steinmetz MA. Contributions of posterior parietal cortex to cognitive functions in primates. Psychobiology 1998; 26:109–118.
46. Yang TT, Gallen CC, Ramachandran VS, Cobb S, Schwartz BJ, Bloom FE. Noninvasive detection of cerebral plasticity in adult human somatosensory cortex. Neuroreport 1994; 5:701–704.
47. Ojemann JG, Silbergeld DL. Cortical stimulation mapping of phantom limb rolandic cortex—case report. J Neurosurg 1995; 82:641–644.
48. Davis KD, Kiss ZHT, Luo L, Tasker RR, Lozano AM, Dostrovsky JO. Phantom sensations generated by thalamic microstimulation. Nature 1998; 391:385–387.
49. Ramachandran VS. Behavioral and magnetoencephalographic correlates of plasticity in the adult human brain. Proc Natl Acad Sci USA 1993; 90:10413–10420.
50. Knecht S. Reorganizational and perceptional changes after amputation. Brain 1996; 119:1213–1219.
51. Head H. On the disturbances of sensation with especial reference to the pain of visceral disease. Brain 1893; 16:1–133.

52. Ness TJ, Gebhart GF. Visceral pain: a review of experimental studies. Pain 1990; 41:167–234.
53. Al-Chaer ED, Lawand NB, Westlund KN, Willis WD. Visceral nociceptive input into the ventral posterolateral nucleus of the thalamus: a new function for the dorsal column pathway. J Neurophysiol 1996; 76:2661–2674.
54. Apkarian AV, Brüggemann J, Shi T, Airapetian LR. A thalamic model for true and referred visceral pain. In: Gebhart GF, ed. Progress in Pain Research and Management. Vol 5. Visceral Pain. Seattle: IASP Press, 1995:217–259.
55. Bushnell MC, Taylor MB, Duncan GH, Dubner R. Discrimination of innocuous and noxious thermal stimuli applied to the face in human and monkey. Somatosens Res 1983; 1:119–129.
56. Gracely RH, McGrath P, Dubner R. Ratio scales of sensory and affective verbal pain descriptors. Pain 1978; 5:5–18.
57. Price DD, McGrath PA, Rafii A, Buckingham B. The validation of visual analogue scales as ratio scale measures for chronic and experimental pain. Pain 1983; 17:45–56.
58. Collins SL, Moore RA, McQuay HJ. The visual analogue pain intensity scale: what is moderate pain in millimetres? Pain 1997; 72:95–97.
59. Melzack R. The McGill Pain Questionnaire: major properties and scoring methods. Pain 1975; 1: 277–299.
60. Chen ACN, Treede R–D. The McGill Pain Questionnaire in the assessment of phasic and tonic experimental pain: behavioral evaluation of the "pain inhibiting pain" effect. Pain 1985; 22:67–69.
61. Price DD, Barrell JJ, Gracely RH. A psychophysical analysis of experiential factors that selectively influence the affective dimension of pain. Pain 1980; 8:137–149.
62. Miron D, Duncan GH, Bushnell MC. Effects of attention on the intensity and unpleasantness of thermal pain. Pain 1989; 39:345–352.
63. Rainville P, Feine JS, Bushnell MC, Duncan GH. A psychophysical comparison of sensory and affective responses to four modalities of experimental pain. Somatosens Motor Res 1992; 9:265–277.
64. Price DD, von der Gruen A, Miller J, Rafii A, Price C. A psychophysical analysis of morphine analgesia. Pain 1985; 22:261–269.
65. Davis KD, Hutchison WD, Lozano AM, Dostrovsky JO. Altered pain and temperature perception following cingulotomy and capsulotomy in a patient with schizoaffective disorder. Pain 1994; 59: 189–199.
66. Talbot JD, Villemure JG, Bushnell MC, Duncan GH. Evaluation of pain perception after anterior capsulotomy: a case report. Somatosens Motor Res 1995; 12:115–126.
67. LaMotte RH, Campbell JN. Comparison of responses of warm and nociceptive C-fiber afferents in monkey with human judgments of thermal pain. J Neurophysiol 1978; 41:509–528.
68. Gybels J, Handwerker HO, van Hees J. A comparison between the discharges of human nociceptive nerve fibres and the subject's ratings of his sensations. J Physiol 1979; 292:193–206.
69. Robinson CJ, Torebjörk HE, LaMotte RH. Psychophysical detection and pain ratings of incremental thermal stimuli: a comparison with nociceptor responses in humans. Brain Res 1983; 274:87–106.
70. Adriaensen H, Gybels J, Handwerker HO, van Hees J. Response properties of thin myelinated (A-δ) fibers in human skin nerves. J Neurophysiol 1983; 49:111–122.
71. Treede R–D, Meyer RA, Campbell JN. Myelinated mechanically insensitive afferents from monkey hairy skin: heat response properties. J Neurophysiol 1998; 80:1082–1093.
72. Campbell JN, Meyer RA, LaMotte RH. Sensitization of myelinated nociceptive afferents that innervate monkey hand. J Neurophysiol 1979; 42:1669–1679.
73. Handwerker HO, Anton F, Reeh PW. Discharge patterns of afferent cutaneous nerve fibers from the rat's tail during prolonged noxious mechanical stimulation. Exp Brain Res 1987; 65:493–504.
74. Garell PC, McGillis SLB, Greenspan JD. Mechanical response properties of nociceptors innervating feline hairy skin. J Neurophysiol 1996; 75:1177–1189.
75. Lang E, Novak A, Reeh PW, Handwerker HO. Chemosensitivity of fine afferents from rat skin in vitro. J Neurophysiol 1990; 63:887–901.
76. Steen KH, Reeh PW, Anton F, Handwerker HO. Protons selectively induce lasting excitation and

sensitization to mechanical stimulation of nociceptors in rat skin, in vitro. J Neurosci 1992; 12:86–95.

77. Schaible H–G, Schmidt RF. Time course of mechanosensitivity changes in articular afferents during a developing experimental arthritis. J Neurophysiol 1988; 60:2180–2195.
78. Meyer RA, Davis KD, Cohen RH, Treede R–D, Campbell JN. Mechanically insensitive afferents (MIAs) in cutaneous nerves of monkey. Brain Res 1991; 561:252–261.
79. Michaelis M, Häbler HJ, Jänig W. Silent afferents: a separate class of primary afferents? Clin Exp Pharmacol Physiol 1996; 23:99–105.
80. Schmelz M, Schmidt R, Ringkamp M, Forster C, Handwerker HO, Torebjörk HE. Limitation of sensitization to injured parts of receptive fields in human skin C-nociceptors. Exp Brain Res 1996; 109:141–147.
81. Dubner R, Price DD, Beitel RE, Hu JW. Peripheral neural correlates of behavior in monkey and human related to sensory–discriminative aspects of pain. In: Anderson DJ, Matthews B, eds. Pain in the Trigeminal Region. Amsterdam: Elsevier/North Holland; 1977:57–66.
82. Willis WD. The Pain System. Basel: Karger, 1985.
83. Kenshalo DR, Chudler EH, Anton F, Dubner R. SI nociceptive neurons participate in the encoding process by which monkeys perceive the intensity of noxious thermal stimulation. Brain Res 1988; 454:378–382.
84. Kenshalo DR, Isensee O. Responses of primate SI cortical neurons to noxious stimuli. J Neurophysiol 1983; 50:1479–1496.
85. Vin–Christian K, Benoist JM, Gautron M, Levante A, Guilbaud G. Further evidence for the involvement of SmI cortical neurons in nociception: modification of their responsiveness over the early stage of a carrageenin-induced inflammation in the rat. Somatosens Motor Res 1992; 9:245–261.
86. Guilbaud G, Benoist JM, Gautron M, Willer JC. Primary somatosensory cortex in rats with pain-related behaviours due to a peripheral mononeuropathy after moderate ligation of one sciatic nerve: neuronal responsivity to somatic stimulation. Exp Brain Res 1992; 92:227–245.
87. Kalliomäki J, Luo X–L, Yu Y–B, Schouenborg J. Intrathecally applied morphine inhibits nociceptive C fiber input to the primary somatosensory cortex (SI) of the rat. Pain 1998; 77:323–329.
88. Villanueva L, Bouhassira D, Le Bars D. The medullary subnucleus reticularis dorsalis (SRD) as a key link in both the transmission and modulation of pain signals. Pain 1996; 67:231–240.
89. Bushnell MC, Duncan GH. Sensory and affective aspects of pain perception: is medial thalamus restricted to emotional issues? Exp Brain Res 1989; 78:415–418.
90. Sikes RW, Vogt BA. Nociceptive neurons in area 24 of rabbit cingulate cortex. J Neurophysiol 1992; 68:1720–1732.
91. Jasmin L, Carstens E, Basbaum AI. Interneurons presynaptic to rat tail-flick motoneurons as mapped by transneuronal transport of pseudorabies virus: few have long ascending collaterals. Neuroscience 1997; 76:859–876.
92. Chen ACN, Chapman CR. Aspirin analgesia evaluated by event-related potentials in man: possible central action in brain. Exp Brain Res 1980; 39:359–364.
93. Bromm B, Forth W, Richter E, Scharein E. Effects of acetaminophen and antipyrine on non-inflammatory pain and EEG activity. Pain 1992; 50:213–221.
94. Kobal G, Hummel C, Gruber M, Geisslinger G, Hummel T. Dose-related effects of ibuprofen on pain-related potentials. Br J Clin Pharmacol 1994; 37: 445–452.
95. Chapman CR, Colpitts YM, Benedetti C, Butler S. Event-related potential correlates of analgesia; comparison of fentanyl, acupuncture, and nitrous oxide. Pain 1982; 14:327–337.
96. Kochs E, Treede R–D, Schulte am Esch J, Bromm B. Modulation of pain-related somatosensory evoked potentials by general anesthesia. Anesth Analg 1990; 71:225–230.
97. Bromm B, Meier W, Scharein E. Antagonism between tilidine and naloxone on cerebral potentials and pain ratings in man. Eur J Pharmacol 1983; 87:431–439.
98. Hill H, Walter MH, Saeger L, Sargur M, Sizemore W, Chapman CR. Dose effects of alfentanil in human analgesia. Clin Pharmacol Ther 1986; 40:178–186.
99. Arendt–Nielsen L, Anker–Moller E, Bjerring P, Spangsberg N. Hypoalgesia following intrathecal morphine: a segmental dependent effect. Acta Anaesthesiol Scand 1991; 35:402–406.

100. Bromm B, Meier W, Scharein E. Imipramine reduces experimental pain. Pain 1986; 25:245–257.
101. Hummel T, Hummel C, Friedel I, Pauli E, Kobal G. A comparison of the antinociceptive effects of imipramine, tramadol and anpirtoline. Br J Clin Pharmacol 1994; 37:325–333.
102. Kochs E, Scharein E, Möllenberg O, Bromm B, Schulte am Esch J. Analgesic efficacy of low-dose ketamine: somatosensory-evoked responses in relation to subjective pain ratings. Anesthesiology 1996; 85:304–314.
103. Scharein E, Bromm B. The intracutaneous pain model in the assessment of analgesic efficacy. Pain Rev 1998; 5:216–246.
104. Pfeiffer A, Pasi A, Mehraein P, Herz A. Opiate receptor binding sites in human brain. Brain Res 1982; 248:87–96.
105. Jones AKP, Qi LY, Fujirawa T, Luthra SK, Ashburner J, Bloomfield P, Cunningham VJ, Itoh M, Fukuda H, Jones T. In vivo distribution of opioid receptors in man in relation to the cortical projections of the medial and lateral pain systems measured with positron emission tomography. Neurosci Lett 1991; 126:25–28.
106. Vogt BA, Watanabe H, Grootoonk S, Jones AKP. Topography of diprenorphine binding in human cingulate gyrus and adjacent cortex derived from coregistered PET and MR images. Hum Brain Mapping 1995; 3:1–12.
107. Firestone LL, Gyulai F, Mintun M, Adler LJ, Urso K, Winter PM. Human brain activity response to fentanyl imaged by positron emission tomography. Anesth Analg 1996; 82:1247–1251.
108. Adler LJ, Gyulai FE, Diehl DJ, Mintun MA, Winter PM, Firestone LL. Regional brain activity changes associated with fentanyl analgesia elucidated by positron emission tomography. Anesth Analg 1997; 84:120–126.
109. Jensen TS. Opioids in the brain: supraspinal mechanisms in pain control. Acta Anaesthesiol Scand 1997; 41:123–132.
110. Merskey H, Albe–Fessard D, Bonica JJ, Carmon A, Dubner R, Kerr FWL, Lindblom U, Mumford JM, Nathan PW, Noordenbos W, Pagni CA, Renaer MJ, Sternbach RA, Sunderland S. Pain terms: a list with definitions and notes on usage. Recommended by the IASP subcommittee on taxonomy. Pain 1979; 6:249–252.
111. Apkarian AV, Shi T. Squirrel monkey lateral thalamus. I. Somatic nociresponsive neurons and their relation to spinothalamic terminals. J Neurosci 1994; 14:6779–6795.
112. Biemond A. The conduction of pain above the level of the thalamus opticus Arch Neurol Psychiatry 1956; 75:231–244.
113. Robinson CJ, Burton H. Somatic submodality distribution within the second somatosensory (SII), 7b, retroinsular, postauditory, and granular insular cortical areas of *M. fascicularis*. J Comp Neurol 1980; 192:93–108.
114. Dong WK, Salonen LD, Kawakami Y, Shiwaku T, Kaukoranta EM, Martin RF. Nociceptive responses of trigeminal neurons in SII-7b cortex of awake monkeys. Brain Res 1989; 484:314–324.
115. Vogt BA, Rosene DL, Pandya DN. Thalamic and cortical afferents differentiate anterior from posterior cingulate cortex in the monkey. Science 1979; 204:205–207.
116. Albe–Fessard D, Berkley KJ, Kruger L, Ralston HJ, Willis WD. Diencephalic mechanisms of pain sensation. Brain Res Rev 1985; 9:217–296.
117. Treede R–D, Kenshalo DR, Gracely RH, Jones AKP. The cortical representation of pain. Pain 1999; 79:105–111.

7

Descending Pathways in Spinal Cord Stimulation and Pain Control

Sumihisa Aida
Teikyo University School of Medicine, Tokyo, Japan

Koki Shimoji
Niigata University School of Medicine, Niigata, Japan

I. INTRODUCTION

Certain somatic stimuli, such as electrical stimulation, can produce analgesia. Therapeutic electrical stimulation has a long history. As early as 46 AD, during the period of the ancient Romans, shock from electric rays were used for pain relief in patients with gout and headache (1). Several forms of therapeutic stimulation, including acupuncture, acupressure, transcutaneous electrical nerve stimulation (TENS), and spinal cord stimulation (SCS) have been widely applied to the treatment of intractable pain. Beginning in the 1960s, Shealy (2) and co-workers (3) showed that electrodes implanted on the dorsal surface of the cord could produce an analgesic effect. Their results were partly explained by gate control theory proposed by Melzack and Wall in 1965 (4). Although the details of the mechanism underlying therapeutic stimulation still remains unclear, recent studies of diffuse noxious inhibitory controls (DNIC) (5,6) and the descending inhibitory system (7) have begun to elucidate the process in greater detail.

The clinical use of SCS for analgesia has had variable success. The SCS methods pioneered by Shealy (2,3) required that an electrode be situated close to the dorsal spinal cord. However, this requires spinal cord surgery, and can occasionally cause serious complications, such as leakage of cerebrospinal fluid (CSF), infection, compression of the spinal cord and root, or spinal cord injury (8). Shimoji et al. demonstrated (9,10) that fine-catheter electrodes implanted into the epidural space could be used to stimulate the spinal cord and to record spinal cord potentials (SCPs) (11,12). Their method was based on the techniques developed for continuous epidural blocks. Because placement of fine epidural electrodes produces minimal side effects, these techniques have became widely used both for SCS analgesia and for making detailed recordings of spinal cord function. These techniques have been used on human subjects in our own institute and in other laboratories.

II. PAIN ALLEVIATING SYSTEM IN THE SPINAL CORD AND SPINAL CORD STIMULATION

A. Classic Theories

1. High-Frequency Stimulation

Conduction blocks can be induced by high-frequency train–pulse stimulation of nerve fibers (13). Nociceptive inputs are blocked by the high-frequency stimulation applied to the dorsal column and spinal roots. With stronger stimulation, however, such treatment can cause numbness or an uncomfortable sensation (13,14).

2. Gate Control Theory

Stimulation of the large Aβ-primary afferent fibers may inhibit nociceptive secondary neurons. These secondary neurons receive inputs from primary afferent Aδ- or C-fibers and project to the thalamus through the spinothalamic tract. Their inhibition is caused by the generation of inhibitory postsynaptic potentials (IPSPs) in the substantia gelatinosa (SG) interneurons. This model is called gate control theory (4). This was the first theory to propose that the central nervous system (CNS) controls nociception. This theory may explain why some patients feel a decrease in pain intensity when skin near the pain region is rubbed with a hand. Gate control theory has been debated by many investigators (5,6,8–10,13–15).

B. Segmental Inhibition

1. Primary Afferent Depolarization in Response to Segmental Peripheral Nerve Stimulation

Typical segmental SCPs, consisting of the initial positive spike (P_1 wave) and the following negative (N_1 wave), and slow positive (P_2 wave) potentials, can be observed in the cervical and lumbosacral enlargements evoked by the spinal cord, the nearby nerve root, or the peripheral nerve stimulation. The P_1 wave is thought to consist of compound action potentials propagating through the roots. The N_1 wave is thought to be caused by synchronized activities (postsynaptic spikes; EPSPs, and IPSPs) of secondary neurons or interneurons. The P_2 wave is thought to reflect primary afferent depolarization (PAD), the same origin as the dorsal cord positive potential or the dorsal root potential (DRP_v by Lloyd's terminology; 16).

PAD inhibits dorsal horn neuronal activities in studies using a micropipette-recording method in animals (17–20). Judging from the similarities of the time courses of the inhibition of unit activities of the dorsal horn and the slow positive potentials (15,18), it has been suggested that the slow positive potentials (P_2 in the segmental or slow P in the descending SCPs) are manifestations of PAD (21) (Fig. 1).

2. Antidromic Stimulation of the Dorsal Column

Waveforms of N and P waves in SCPs evoked by descending volleys (descending SCPs) are similar to those of the N_1 and P_2 waves of the segmental SCPs, respectively. Occasionally, a very slow negative wave with low voltage (N_2) follows the P_2 or P wave. The N and P waves in "descending SCPs" are thought to be produced by the antidromic volleys of the dorsal column, but not by lateral or ventral column volleys (22). Detailed waveform characteristics have been described elsewhere (22–30).

On the other hand, waveforms can be significantly altered by other types of stimulation. When conditioning stimulation is applied to the dorsal column at the cervical enlargement, and test stimulation is applied to the segmental nerve, recordings at the lumbosacral enlargement show an occlusion or reduction in the N_1 wave and a biphasic effect on P_2 wave (occlusion with short interval within 20 ms and facilitation beyond 20 ms) was observed (30) (Fig. 2). When both the conditioning and testing shocks were given antidromically to the dorsal column, occlusion or inhibition of slow N and P waves in the descending SCP also occurred (30). These phenomena—the occlusion or inhibition of N_1/N and P waves, and the facilitation of P_2 wave—are thought to be responsible for the segmental inhibition of sensory transmission (probably

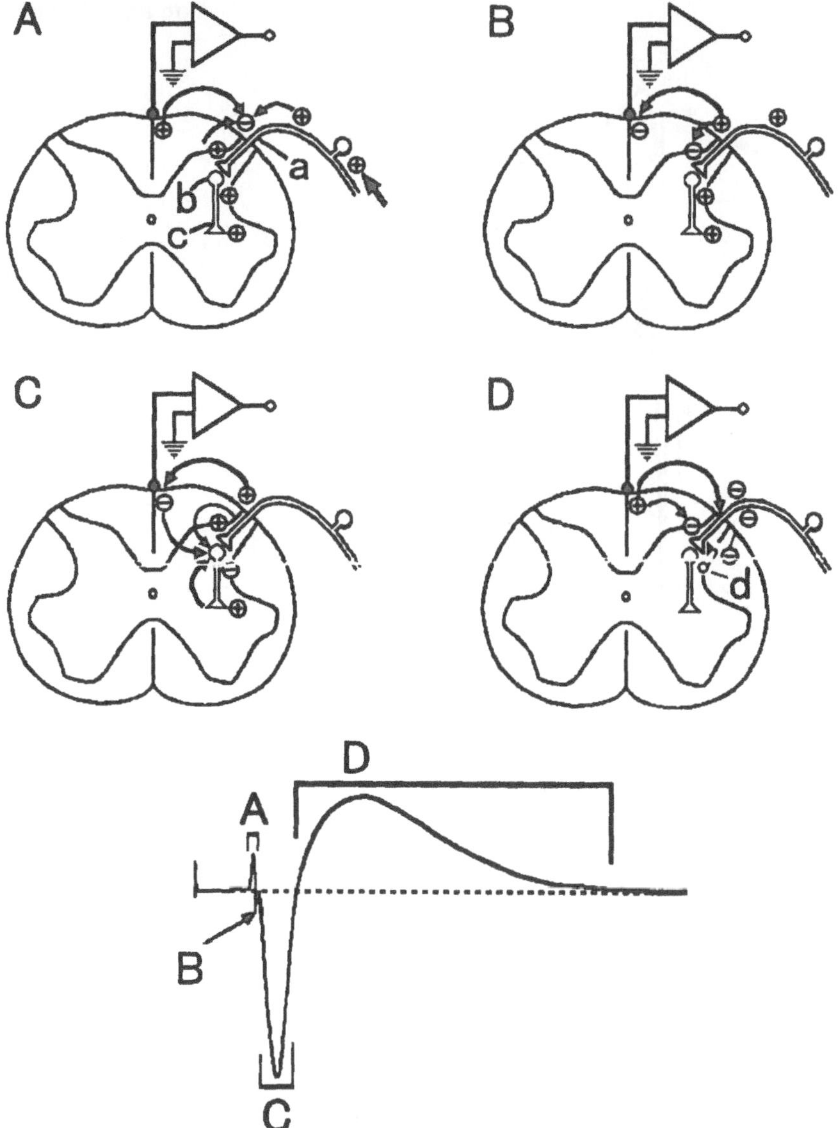

Figure 1 Schematic presentation of the mechanisms by which the components of the spinal cord potential (SCP) are generated: The initial positive spike represents the action potential occurring through the roots into the spinal cord. This action potential reaches a node of Ranvier where it creates a positive capacitative current, which is conducted down the axon and creates (A) a positive spike. The capacitative current depolarizes the cell membrane at the next node to threshold, initiating an influx of Na^+, and resulting in a negative charge in the extracellular space and the production of an action potential. This event is recorded (B) as the negative component of the triphasic spike. The negative charge causes a K^+ efflux from the axon into the extracellular space, recorded as the second positive component of the triphasic spike. (C) The slow sharp negative wave of spinal cord potential reflects changes in the extracellular environment produced by activity of dorsal horn interneurons. When the interneurons are synaptically activated, a positive ionic current leaves the extracellular space at the synapses (sinks) and reappears along the ventrally projecting axons of the cells (sources). (D) The slow positive wave of the cord dorsum potential is the result of primary afferent depolarization (PAD). A positive ionic current leaves the extracellular space at excited axoaxonal synapses (sinks) and reappears along the primary afferents (sources). Thus, the dorsal spinal cord becomes positively charged a, primary afferent; b, soma and dendrites of interneuron; c, axon of interneuron; d, interneuron making axoaxonal synapse. (From Ref. 21.)

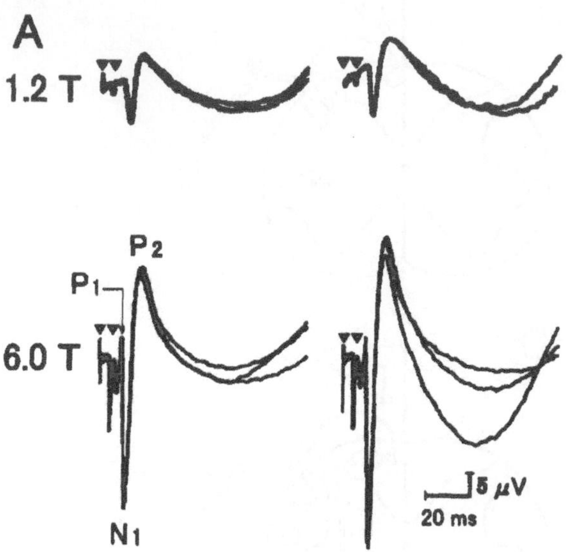

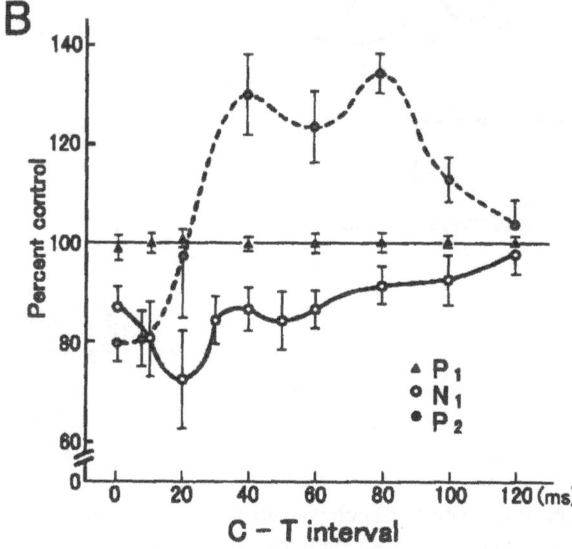

Figure 2 Effects of conditioning stimulation on spinal cord potentials (SCPs): Conditioning stimulation was applied to the cervical enlargement from the posterior epidural space of a human subject. (A) Individual recordings of the interaction of two SCPs produced with an interval between the segmental and descending volleys (left) or with a summation of the volleys (right). The two interval deflections are stimulus artifacts of the segmental and descending volleys, respectively. Note that degree of occlusion or inhibition is greater at six times threshold (6.0 T) than at near threshold (1.2 T). (B) Changes in the sizes of the N_1 and P_2 waves as a function of the interval between the conditioning stimulus and the testing stimulus. Note that the N_1 wave is inhibited by the descending conditioning volley up to 120 ms, and the P_2 wave is initially inhibited and thereafter facilitated. Stimuli were delivered at 6.0 T. Values are expressed as means and SE. P_1, the initially positive spike; N_1, slow (sharp) negative wave; P_2, slow positive wave. (From Ref. 30)

including pain transmission) in the human spinal cord by antidromic stimulation of the dorsal column.

3. Segmental Effects of Dorsal Column Stimulation on Substance Gelatinosa Neurons

Baba et al. (31) noted three types of IPSPs generated in SG neurons in slice preparations of rat spinal cord following dorsal column stimulation: glycinergic interneurons with fast IPSPs; GABAergic interneurons with slow IPSPs; and interneurons that were insensitive to strychnine and bicuculline and had long-lasting slow IPSPs. Excitatory postsynaptic potentials (EPSPs) evoked by dorsal root stimulation are suppressed by repeated stimulation of the dorsal column. This response may be mediated by Aδ-, but not C-fibers. This observation in rat spinal cord slices might partly explain the segmental analgesic mechanism of SCS, showing the close relation between dorsal column or dorsal root stimulation and inhibition by SG interneurons of sensory inputs to the pain-transmission cells in the spinal cord.

C. Feedback Inhibition

1. Is There a Feedback?

Supraspinal structures have been known to modify pain perception and spinal afferent neuronal activity. In 1969, Reynolds (7) first documented stimulation-produced analgesia (SPA), demonstrating strong analgesia without behavioral change (specific nociceptive blockade), produced by weak stimulation of the periaqueductal gray matter (PAG) in rats. SPA by stimulation of PAG and periventricular gray matter has also been confirmed in humans by Richardson and Akil (32,33) as well as Hosobuchi et al. (34). Thereafter, the rostral ventromedial medulla (RVM) including the nucleus raphe magnus (NRM), the nucleus reticularis gigantocellularis (NRGC), and the nucleus reticularis paragigantocellularis (NRPG) were also demonstrated to be crucial sites for SPA (35). A more rostral structure, the anterior pretectal nucleus (APtN), has also been suggested to produce SPA by Roberts and Rees (36).

Hughes et al. (37) identified two brain peptides that act as endogenous opioids: methionine-enkephalin and leucine-enkephalin. Kuranishi et al. (37) as well as Yaksh and Rudy (39) have suggested that the foregoing nuclei are the sites of analgesic action of opioids. On the other hand, most SPAs have been inhibited by an opioid antagonist, naloxone (40). Thus, the close relation between the SPA and action of opioids has been demonstrated. Basbaum et al. (41–43) found that the fibers originating in the PAG projected to dorsal horn neurons through the dorsolateral funiculus, after relay at RVM, by confirming the reversal of morphine analgesia and SPA by the transection of this pathway, the so-called descending inhibitory system (Fig. 3).

In addition, several hypotheses concerning central sensory control by peripheral stimulation have been proposed. These hypotheses suggest that supraspinal feedback is involved in SPA. For example, activation of PAD by segmental and heterosegmental stimulation was shown in cats (44,45), and DNIC was shown in rats (5,6). Similar mechanisms may be activated in acupuncture analgesia (46) and stress-induced analgesia (47).

2. Primary Afferent Depolarization Generated by Supraspinal or Heterosegmental Stimulation

As described in the foregoing, the slow positive potentials (the P_2 wave in the segmental SCP and the P wave in the descending SCP) are now thought to be manifestations of PAD. There

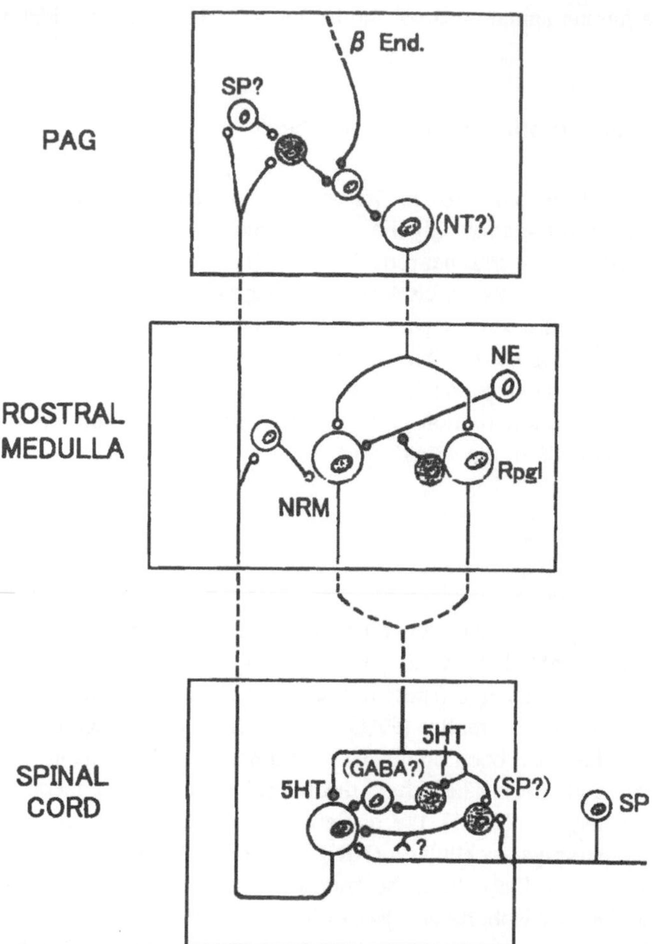

Figure 3 The descending inhibitory system: The proposed midbrain (PAG), medullary, and spinal circuitry related to the control of spinal nociceptive neurons. Unfilled "boutons" indicate release of an excitatory transmitter, filled "boutons" indicate an inhibitory input. In the PAG, the output neuron is depicted as an excitatory neurotensinergic (NT) neuron that activates cells of the nucleus raphe magnus (NRM) and of the lateral Rpg1 of the rostral medulla. An endogenous opioid peptide neuron (stippled) in the PAG is presumed to inhibit an inhibitory interneuron that, in turn, controls the PAG output neuron. Input to the opioid interneuron may derive from ascending nociceptive pathways, by a local substance P-containing (SP) neuron. Inputs from β-endorphin cells of the hypothalamus may also contribute to the opioid link in the PAG. It is not known whether all of the endorphin subtypes act in a similar fashon in the PAG. (From Ref. 35.)

have been several lines of evidence showing that stimulation of certain areas of the brain stem (48) or even the cortex (49) produces a dorsal root potential (DRP), which may also be a reflection of PAD. Following segmental and heterosegmental stimulations of the dorsal root, Besson and Rivot found that convergent neurons (or wide dynamic range [WDR] neurons) in the dorsal horn first increase their firing and then show a DRP (Fig. 4) (44,45). From these facts, WDR neuron activity is strongly suggested to be related to PAD, which is generated not only by

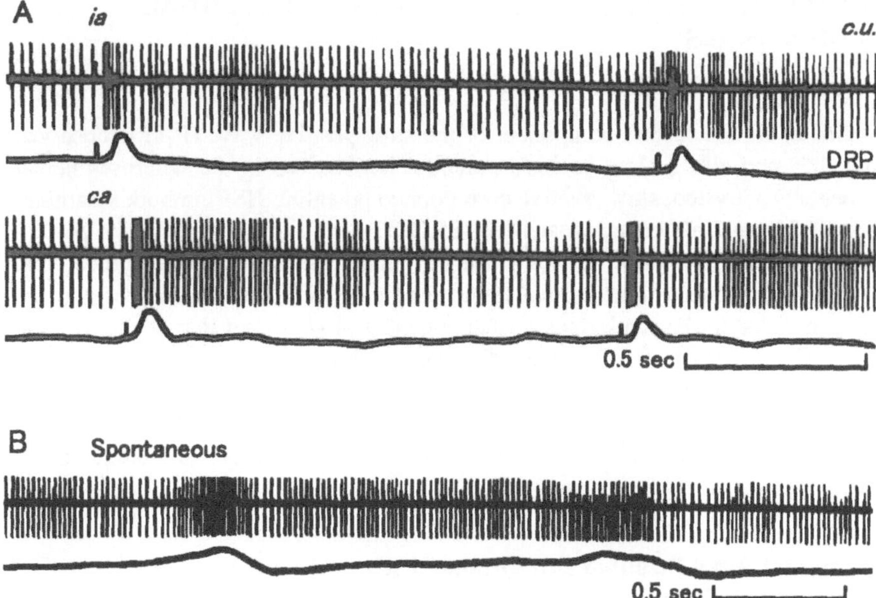

Figure 4 Convergent unit (wide dynamic range neuron) and dorsal root potentials (DRPs): (A) Recordings of a single WDR neuron in the cat. Convergent unit (c.u.) showing a high rate of spontaneous firing. The frequency is increased by heterotropic stimulation at the ipsilateral anterior limb (ia) or the contralateral anterior limb (ca). This increase precedes the occurrence of DRPs. (B) Same cell; spontaneous variations in firing rate accompanied by simultaneous fluctuations in polarization of the dorsal root. (From Ref. 45.)

primary afferent inputs, but also by feedback mechanisms through supraspinal structures, thus controlling the nociceptive inputs of these structures.

3. Diffuse Noxious Inhibitory Controls

Le Bars et al. (5,6) advocated DNIC, based on the following facts: (1) activity of spinal wide dynamic range (WDR) neurons (or convergent neurons) is powerfully inhibited by diffuse noxious stimuli applied to various parts of the body; and (2) the effect of DNIC was not demonstrated in the spinal animal. Because DNIC was demonstrated to remain even after PAG and NRGC lesions, it has been considered to be an mechanism independent from the SPA or conventional descending inhibitory system (50). However, an indirect relation between DNIC and the descending inhibitory system may exist, as naloxone occasionally induces partial attenuation of DNIC, and morphine antagonizes DNIC, but not after PAG lesioning (50). Thus DNIC is thought to play a role in some folk remedies, such as counterirritation and hyperstimulation analgesia.

4. Acupuncture Analgesia and Stress-Induced Analgesia

Both acupuncture analgesia and stress-induced analgesia are thought to be associated with certain supraspinal feedback loops. Analgesic mechanisms of acupuncture appear to be closely related to the descending inhibitory system, because both analgesic effects are depressed by naloxone or serotoninergic or adrenergic antagonists (51,52). Stress-induced analgesia is inhibited by adrenal glucocorticoids, suggesting another descending route, the hypothalamic–pituitary–adrenal pathway (53,54).

III. DEMONSTRATION OF FEEDBACK BY SPINAL CORD POTENTIAL IN MAN AND ANIMALS

A. The P_2s Wave and Its Feedback Center

During strong stimulation, the second component of the slow positive wave (P_2s) is observed in the segmental SCP and also a slow positive potential is observed in the heterosegmental SCP (heterosegmentally activated, slow positive cord dorsum potential; HSP) in both ketamine-anesthetized rats (26,28) and in awake humans (23–25,29).

Central latencies to the peaks of the P_2s wave in humans are 29–33 ms at the cervical enlargement and 42–48 ms at the lumbosacral enlargement. Thus, the central latency to the peak of P_2s wave recorded at the lumbosacral enlargement is slower than that at the cervical enlargement, as expected (24,26). The P_2s wave disappears after barbiturate administration or during sleep (26,27). P_2s is observed in ketamine-anesthetized animals and abolished by spinal transection at a high spinal level (26). Therefore, the feedback center must be situated in a supraspinal structure (Fig. 5). These characteristics of the P_2s wave suggest that there are polysynaptic feedback loops in supraspinal structures.

B. Heterosegmental Slow Positive Potentials (HSP_1 and HSP_2) and Their Feedback Center

More details of the slow positive spinal cord potentials evoked by segmental and heterosegmental stimuli have been documented in awake human subjects (Fig. 6). HSPs have been clearly demonstrated in the spinal cord of rats anesthetized with ketamine, but not with barbiturates, in response to forepaw or hindpaw stimulation. However, HSPs are not observed, even after strong stimulation of the median nerve at the wrist or posterior tibial nerve at the popliteal space, in wakeful human subjects (23). When more rostral peripheral nerves, such as the brachial plexus (Erb's point) or the cauda equina, are stimulated at the L1–5 levels, HSPs can be produced (29). The difficulty in producing a clear configuration of HSP in humans may be due to (1) spinal dispersion owing to the long distance between stimulus site and the supraspinal feedback center, or (2) an insufficiency of incoming afferent volleys (29). By contrast, the short distance between the fore- or hindpaw and the supraspinal nucleus might make it possible to produce the HSP waveform in the rat (26,28). In the human lumbosacral enlargement, two HSPs (HSP_1 and HSP_2) can be generated by strong heterosegmental stimulation at Erb's point (29). Furthermore, another slow wave, the late positive potential (late P), was also noted in the segmental SCP in 44.4% of subjects (29). HSPs as well as P_2s waves with slow latencies and long durations are suggested to be PAD generated by feedback signals by supraspinal structures.

Two HSPs, HSP_1 and HSP_2, are observed in awake humans, whereas only one HSP is observed in ketamine-anesthetized rats. As the spinal cord of humans is long compared with that of rats, perhaps the HSPs separate into two peaks in humans. Alternatively, anesthetics may interfere with the appearance of these slow, positive waves in the rat spinal cord. Thus, there may be multiple supraspinal feedback nuclei or reverberating circuits between the spinal cord and supraspinal structures for producing HSPs when SCS or peripheral nerve stimulation is applied.

C. Localization of the Feedback Centers for Heterosegmental Slow Positive Potentials

As suggested by disappearance of HSPs following spinal transection or anesthetic administration and by the difference in the latencies of the HSPs, there might be several feedback centers with

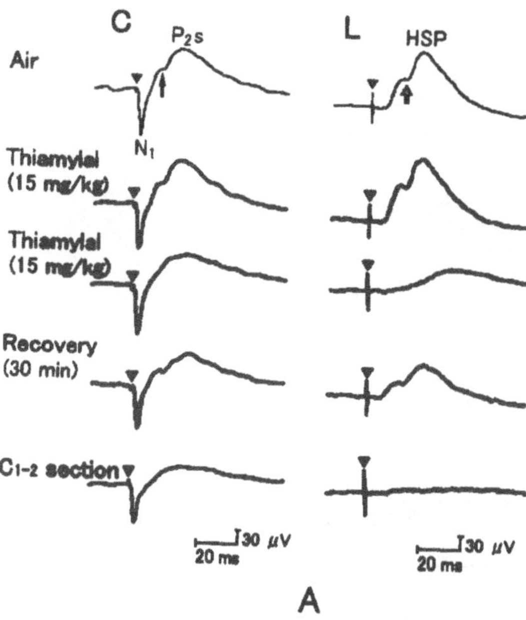

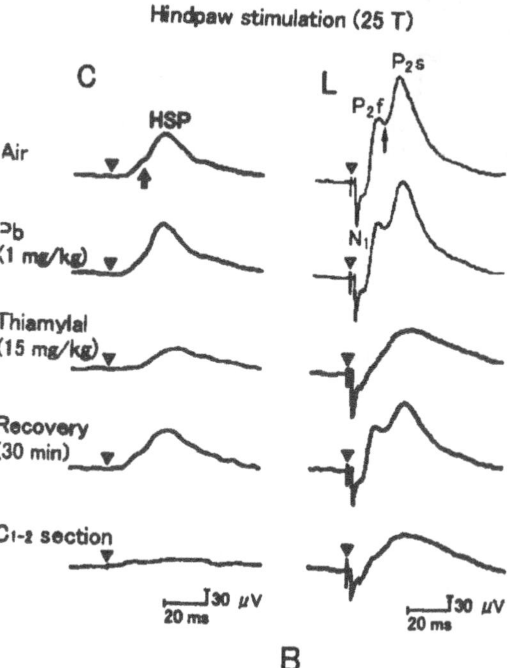

Figure 5 Heterosegmental slow, positive potentials (HSPs) in the rat: Following stimulation (A) of the forepaw or (B) hindpaw, HSPs and segmental P_2s potentials were recorded. Large and small arrows show the negative dips in HSP and the P_2, respectively. Reverse triangles identify stimulus artifacts. Note that both HSPs and P_2s are highly vulnerable to thiamylal and spinal cord transection (C1-2). L, recordings from the lumbosacral enlargement; C, recordings from the cervical enlargement; Pb, pancuronium bromide. (From Ref. 26.)

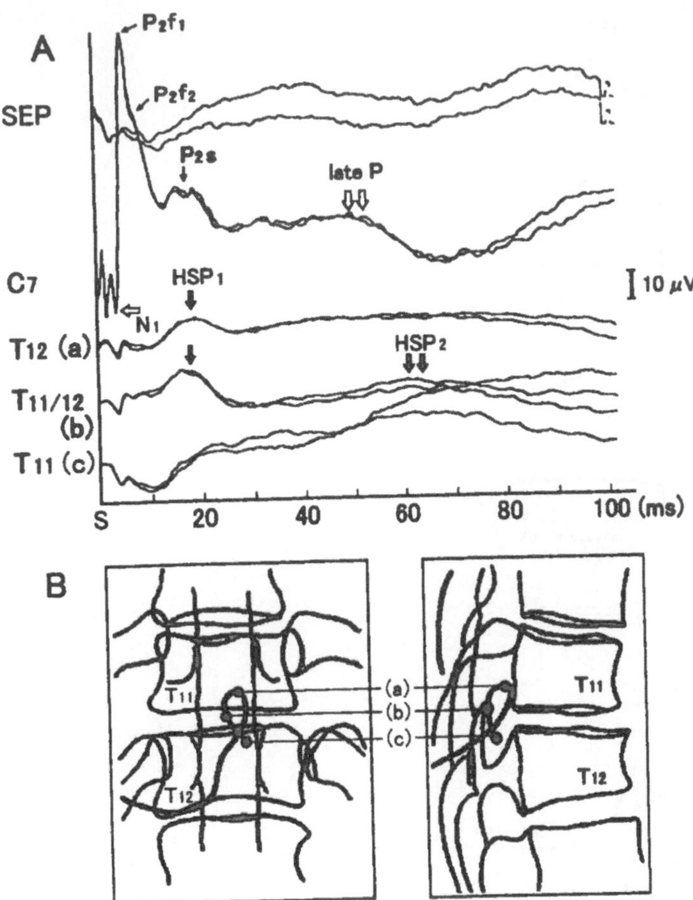

Figure 6 Slow, positive spinal cord potentials (SCPs) in humans: Erb's point was stimulated at ten times threshold, and potentials were recorded from the cervical enlargement (C7), lumbosacral enlargements (T11, T11–12, and T12 segments) and the scalp (C3) (SEP, somatosensory evoked potential). (A) Several slow positive waves are produced in the spinal cord: P_2f_2, P_2s, late P, HSP_1, and HSP_2. (B) Pencil tracing of the electrode positions. The epidural catheter electrode had three lead wires with the respective contact points 15 mm apart, and could record SCP at three points, a, b, and c. (From Ref. 29.)

polysynaptic pathways or reverberating circuits in the brain (26). We performed experiments to localize the feedback centers in rats during ketamine anesthesia (Fig. 7). After transection between the pons and medulla, the amplitude of the HSP did not change. Transection at the middle of the medulla oblongata caused a partial reduction of HSP amplitude. Total disappearance of the HSP was demonstrated by transection between the caudal end of medulla and the spinal cord. From these results, it appears that the main feedback center for HSPs may be located diffusely in the medulla (28).

D. Pathway of Heterosegmental Slow Positive Potential and Inhibition of Wide Dynamic Range Neurons

In humans, HSP was detected only when the epidural electrode was situated within approximately 5 mm from the midline of the human spinal cord in the posterior epidural space (see

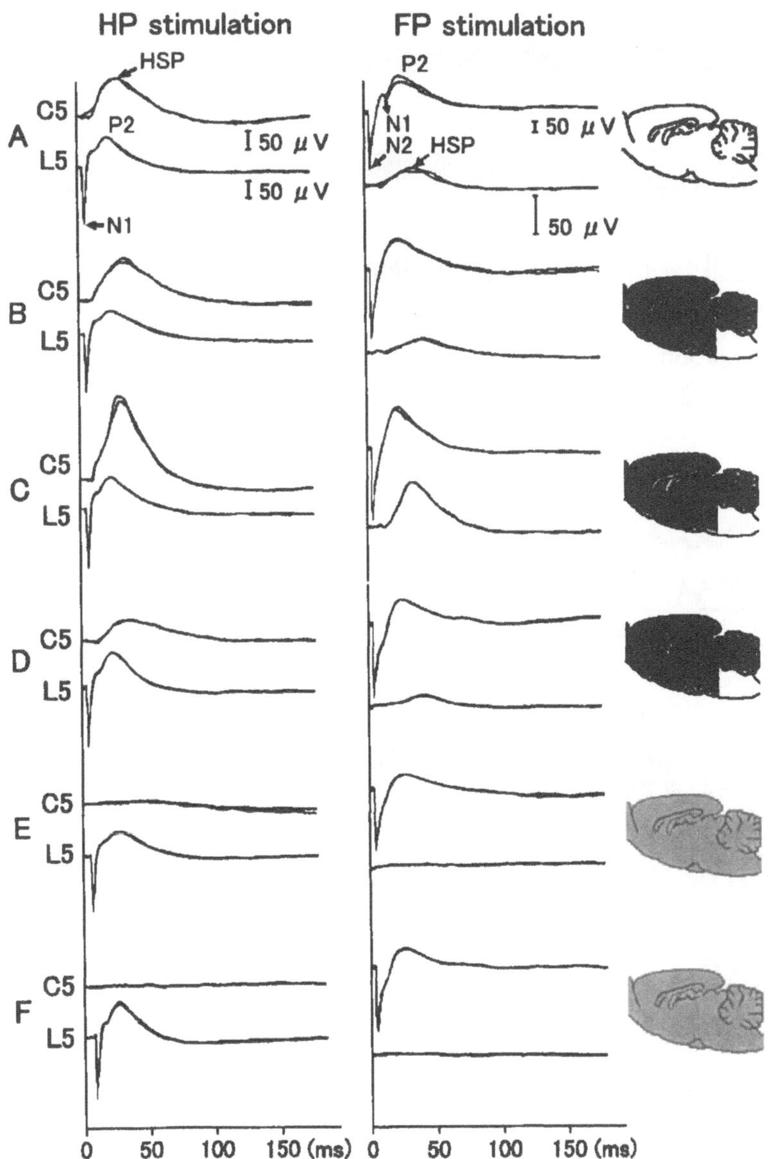

Figure 7 Changes in HSP induced by brain lesions and by ketamine in the rat: (A) Before brain lesion during ketamine anesthesia. HP, hindpaw; FP, forepaw. Upper sweep, recorded at the C5 level; lower sweep, recorded at the L5 level. (B) Transection between the pons and medulla under ketamine anesthesia. (C) Transection between the pons and medulla 30 min after stopping ketamine infusion. (D) Transection at the middle of the medulla under ketamine anesthesia. (E) Transection between the medulla and spinal cord under ketamine anesthesia. (F) Transection between the medulla and spinal cord 30 min after stopping ketamine infusion. Reduction or total disappearance of HSP are noted in D, E, and F. Cessation of anesthesia augmented HSP in C, whereas HSP no longer appears in F. (From Ref. 28.)

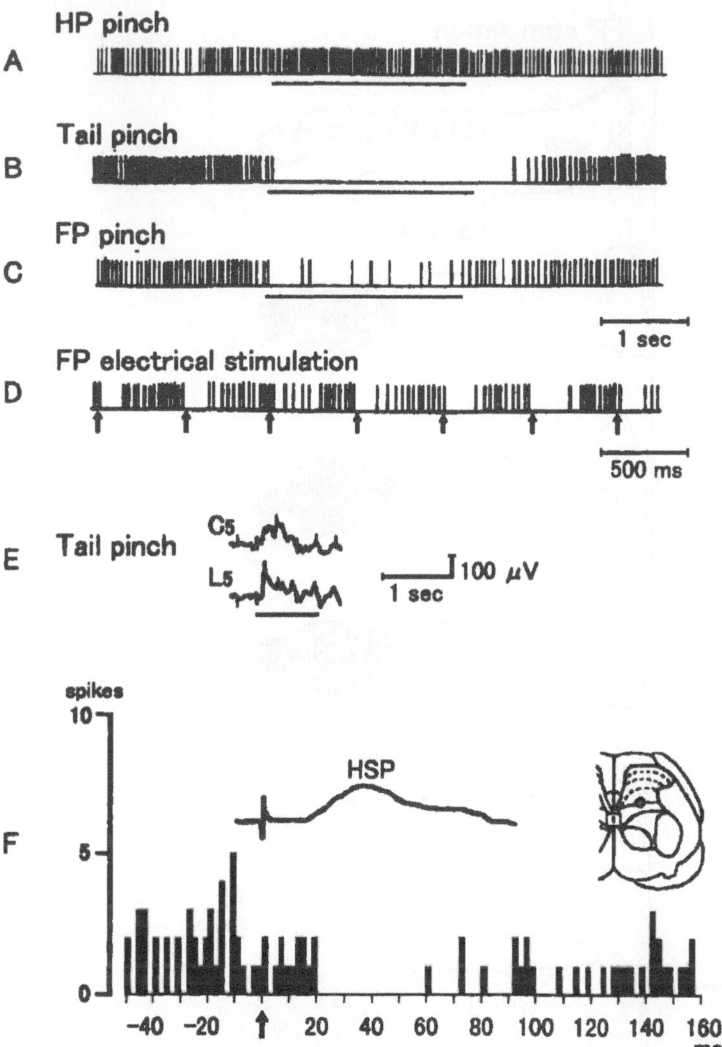

Figure 8 Relation between HSP and firing of wide dynamic range (WDR) neurons in the rat: (A–D) Polygraphic records of square wave pulses at the lumbosacral enlargement. Pulses were triggered by a discriminator and indicate WDR neuron spikes. Horizontal lines under the traces indicate the time periods of stimulation. Arrows in D denote the time of electrical stimuli. (E) Polygraphic traces of cord dorsum potentials recorded from C5 and L5 levels in response to tail pinch. The spike-like potentials overlapping the traces are ECG artifacts. (F) The HSP and peristimulus time histogram of the WDR neuron firing, in response to forepaw (FP) electrical stimulation, displayed on the same time scale. The spike artifact on the HSP trace and the arrow under the histogram represent the time of electrical stimulation. Location of the WDR neuron is illustrated on the right. (From Ref. 26.)

Fig. 6A). Therefore, the HSP might be relatively small and localized in the dorsal cord (29). P waves are also recorded most dominantly from the dorsal cord (22,29). These facts suggest that the HSP and the P_2 wave are manifestations of PAD and are produced by interneurons in the dorsal horn. On the other hand, transection of the ipsilateral or contralateral ventral portions of the spinal cord caused complete or partial loss of HSP, respectively (28). This finding may indicate that the descending pathway of the HSP is included in the ventral portion of the spinal cord.

SCS may facilitate PAD (44,45) and suppress dorsal horn pain transmission cells through SG neurons (31). On the other hand, PAD has been produced by stimulation of not only the dorsal column but also the cerebral cortex (44,45,49), brain stem (48,55), and cerebellum (48). These observations suggest that there is a descending inhibition on spinal sensory (including pain) transmissions from supraspinal structures. Increases in WDR neuron activities in the rat lumbosacral enlargement in response to hindpaw touch and pinch as well as to graded electrical hindpaw stimuli have been suppressed by heterosegmental stimuli such as tail or forepaw pinch and electrical shock to the forepaw (26). Pinch stimulation also evoked slow cord dorsum positive waves at both cervical and lumbar spinal cord levels. The time courses of both the HSP and inhibition of WDR neuron activity are similar, suggesting that the HSP reflects heterosegmentally activated PAD caused by feedback from the brain stem to the dorsal spinal cord (Fig. 8) (23). This finding suggests that HSP is a reflection of PAD generated by a feedback signal through the brain stem, not only by the heterosegmental peripheral nerve, but also by heterosegmental dorsal column stimulations that inhibit sensory as well as pain transmission cells.

IV. PAIN RELIEF BY SPINAL CORD STIMULATION AND DESCENDING INHIBITION

Nociception inhibitory fibers from the PAG project to the spinal dorsal horn by relays in the rostral ventromedial medulla (RVM), including NRM, NRGC, and NRPG, with descending axons in the dorsolateral funiculus (DLF) (41,42,54). The concept of the "descending inhibitory system" (7) and features of the descending activities for producing slow, positive SCPs (P_2s and HSP) are thought to be overlapping in part. It is noteworthy that this descending inhibitory system is believed to produce analgesia by inhibition of dorsal horn pain neurons through the medulla and the dorsolateral pathway of the spinal cord (41–43), whereas HSP is probably an activity of the descending inhibitory system on general sensory inputs, manifesting itself as a slow positive potential.

Furthermore, stimulation of a more rostral structure, the anterior pretectal nucleus (APtN), also produces SPA, and this nucleus has also been suggested to be one of the feedback centers for SCS analgesia (36). The feedback center for the HSP of the rat spinal cord appears to be located at the medulla, including the NRM, NRGC, and NRPG, in brain transection experiments (28). The SCS used by Shimoji et al. (9,10) was at low frequency (0.5–5.0/s), whereas those by other groups were at high frequency (50–100/s). Although very slow HSP (HSP_2) is found in the human spinal cord (29), its origin remains to be studied (Fig. 9). It is conceivable that HSP_2 or segmental late P (see Fig. 6) of human SCP is related to the feedback potentials by a more rostral center such as APtN. Further studies should be carried out to localize the feedback nuclei producing these slow, positive potentials of the SCP, and to determine the relation between these slow potentials and SCS analgesia.

IV. CONCLUSION

Thus, the underlying mechanism in SCS analgesia appears to be the inhibition of pain-transmitting neurons of the spinal cord by activation of segmental and descending inhibitions. The evidence supporting this mechanism is (1) the inhibition of pain-transmission neurons by antidromic or orthodromic activation of the dorsal column, which results in facilitation of PAD or postsyn-

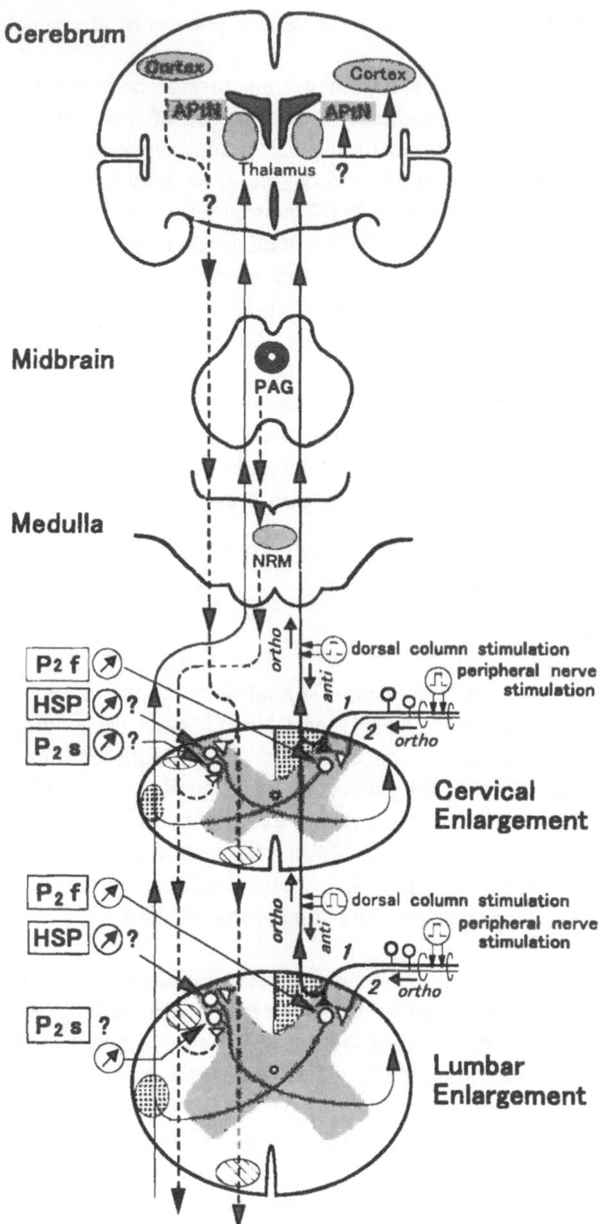

Figure 9 Model of the feedback centers producing slow, positive waves: Solid lines show ascending pathways, and broken lines show descending pathways. APtN, anterior pretectal nucleus; PAG, periaqueductal gray matter; NRM, nucleus raphe magnum; Ortho, orthodromic stimuli; Anti, antidromic stimuli; Empty buttons, excitatory synapses; filled buttons, inhibitory synapses. 1, Aα and Aβ fibers; 2, Aδ and C fibers. Refer to Fig. 6 for HSP, P_2f and P_2s.

aptic inhibition at the segmental level, viewed from the segmental SCPs and activities of SG neurons; (2) facilitation of descending inhibitory mechanisms through dorsal column system by feedback nuclei situated mostly in the medulla oblongata; this may generate PAD, seen as HSPs and P_2s waves in heterosegmental and segmental SCPs, respectively.

Other mechanisms for the inhibition of nociception, such as diffuse noxious inhibitory controls (5,6) or stress-induced analgesia (47), have been proposed. SCS analgesia may be fundamentally different from these two mechanisms, because therapeutic SCS induces neither pain nor stress. Indeed, patients receiving therapeutic SCS usually experience a pleasant feeling, rather than stress or pain (23,29). Thus, SCS analgesia by heterosegmental stimulation at low frequency is probably produced by activation of the descending inhibitory system. Future experimental work will further elucidate the details of the mechanisms of SCS analgesia, and we hope, lead to advances in its clinical application.

REFERENCES

1. Kane K, Taub A. A history of local electrical analgesia. Pain 1975; 1:125–138.
2. Shealy CN. Electrical inhibition of pain by stimulation of the dorsal columns: preliminary clinical report. Anesth Analg 1967; 46:489–491.
3. Shealy CN, Mortimer JT, Hagtors NR. Dorsal column electro-analgesia. J Neurosurg 1970; 32:560–564.
4. Melzack R, Wall PD. Pain mechanism: a new theory. Science 1965; 150:971–979.
5. Le Bars D, Dickenson AH, Besson JM. Diffuse noxious inhibitory controls (DINC). I. Effects on dorsal horn convergent neurones in the rat. Pain 1979; 6:283–304.
6. Le Bars D, Dickenson AH, Besson JM. Diffuse noxious inhibitory controls (DINC). II. Lack of effect on non-convergent neurones. Supraspinal involvement and theoretical implications. Pain 1979; 6:305–327.
7. Reynolds DV. Surgery in the rat during electrical analgesia induced by focal stimulation. Science 1969; 164:444–445.
8. Simpson BA. Spinal cord stimulation. Pain Rev 1994; 1:199–230.
9. Shimoji K, Higashi H, Kano T, Asai S, Morioka T. Electrical management of intractable pain. Jpn J Anesthesiol 1971; 20:444–447.
10. Shimoji K, Kitamura H, Ikezono E, Shimizu H, Okamoto K, Iwakura Y. Spinal hypalgesia and analgesia by low-frequency electrical stimulation in the epidural space. Anesthesiology 1974; 41: 91–94.
11. Shimoji K, Higashi H, Kano T. Epidural recording of spinal electrogram in man. Electroencephalogr Clin Neurophysiol 1971; 30:236–239.
12. Shimoji K, Kano T, Higashi H, Morioka T, Henschel MO. Evoked spinal electrograms recorded from epidural space in man. J Appl Physiol 1972; 33:468–471.
13. Campbell JN, Taub A. Local analgesia from percutaneous electrical stimulation. A peripheral mechanism. Arch Neurol 1973; 28:347–350.
14. Lindblom U, Meyerson BA. Influence on touch, vibration and cutaneous pain of dorsal column stimulation in man. Pain 1975; 1:257–270.
15. Besson JM, Rivot JP. Spinal interneurones involved in presynaptic controls of supraspinal origin. J Physiol 1973; 230:235–254.
16. Lloyd DPC. Electrons in dorsal nerve roots. Cold Spring Harbor Symp Quant Biol 1952; 17:203–219.
17. Eccles JC, Kostyuk PG, Schmidt RF. Central pathways responsible for depolarization of primary afferent fibres. J Physiol 1962; 161:62–93.
18. Eccles JC, Malcolm JL. Dorsal root potentials of the spinal cord. J Neurophysiol 1946; 9:139–160.
19. Wall PD. Excitatory changes in afferent fibre termination and their relation to slow potentials. J Physiol 1958; 142:1–21.

20. Frank K, Fuortes MGF. Presynaptic and postsynaptic inhibition of monosynaptic reflex. Fed Proc 1957; 16:39–40.
21. Shimoji K. Origins and properties of spinal cord evoked potentials. In: Dimitrijevic MR, ed. Atlas of Human Spinal Cord Evoked Potentials. Newton, MA: Butterworth–Heinemann, 1995: 1–25.
22. Tomita M, Shimoji K, Denda S, Tobita T, Uchiyama S, Baba H. Spinal tracts producing slow components of spinal cord potentials evoked by descending volleys in man. Electroencephalogr Clin Neurophysiol 1996; 100:68–73.
23. Shimoji K, Matsuki M, Ito Y, Masuko K, Maruyama M, Iwane T, Aida S. Interactions of human cord dorsum potential. J Appl Physiol 1976; 40:79–84.
24. Shimoji K, Matsuki M, Shimizu H. Wave-form characteristics and spatial distribution of evoked spinal electrogram in man. J Neurosurg 1977; 46:304–313.
25. Shimizu H, Shimoji K, Maruyama Y, Sato Y, Kuribayashi H. Interaction between human evoked electrograms elicited by segmental and descending volleys. Experientia 1979; 35:1199–1200.
26. Shimoji K, Sato Y, Denda S, Takada T, Fukuda S, Hokari T. Slow positive dorsal cord potentials activated by heterosegmental stimuli. Electroencephalogr Clin Neurophysiol 1992; 85:72–80.
27. Shimoji K, Ito Y, Ohama K, Sawa T, Ikezono E. Presynaptic inhibition in man during anesthesia and sleep. Anesthesiology 1975; 43:388–391.
28. Denda S, Shimoji K, Tomita M, Baba H, Yamakura T, Masaki H, Endoh H, Fukuda S. Central nuclei and spinal pathways in feedback inhibitory spinal cord potentials in ketamine-anaesthetized rats. Br J Anaesth 1996; 76:258–265.
29. Shimoji K, Tomita M, Tobita T, Baba H, Takada T, Fukuda S, Aida S, Fujiwara N. Erb's point stimulation produces slow positive potentials in the human lumbar spinal cord. J Clin Neurophysiol 1994; 11:365–374.
30. Shimizu H, Shimoji K, Maruyama Y, Matsuki M, Kuribayashi H, Fujioka H. Human spinal cord potentials produced in lumbosacral enlargement by descending volleys. J Neurophysiol 1982; 48: 1108–1120.
31. Baba H, Yoshimura M, Nishi S, Shimoji K. Synaptic responses of substantia gelatinosa neurones to dorsal column stimulation in rat spinal cord in vitro. J Physiol 1994; 478:87–99.
32. Richardson DE, Akil H. Pain reduction by electrical brain stimulation in man. Part 1: acute administration in periaqueductal and periventricular sites. J Neurosurg 1977; 47:178–183.
33. Richardson DE, Akil H. Pain reduction by electrical brain stimulation in man. Part 2: chronic self-administration in the periventricular gray matter. J Neurosurg 1977; 47:184–194.
34. Hosobuchi Y, Adams JE, Linchitz R. Pain relief by electrical stimulation of the central gray matter in humans and its reversal by naloxone. Science 1977; 197:183–186.
35. Basbaum AI, Fields HL. Endogenous pain control systems: brainstem spinal pathways and endorphin circuitry. Annu Rev Neurosci 1984; 7:309–338.
36. Roberts MHT, Rees H. Physiological basis of spinal cord stimulation. Pain Rev 1994; 1:184–193.
37. Hughes J, Smith TW, Kosterlitz HW, Fothergill LA, Mogan BA, Morris HR. Identification of two related pentapeptides from the brain with potent opiate agonist activity. Nature 1975; 258:577–579.
38. Kuranishi Y, Satoh M, Harada Y, Akaike A, Shibata T, Takagi H. Analgesic action of intrathecal and intracerebral β-endorphin in rats: comparison with morphine. Eur J Pharmacol 1980; 67:143–146.
39. Yaksh TL, Rudy TA. Narcotic analgesics: CNS sites and mechanism of action as revealed by intracerebral injection techniques. Pain 1978; 4:299–359.
40. Akil H, Liebeskind JC. Antagonism of stimulation-produced analgesia by naloxone, a narcotic antagonist. Science 1976; 191:961–962.
41. Basbaum AI, Marley NJE, O'Keefe J, Clanton CH. Reversal of morphine and stimulus-induced analgesia by subtotal spinal cord lesions. Pain 1977; 3:43–56.
42. Basbaum AI, Clanton CH, Fields HL. Three bulbospinal pathways from the rostral medulla of the cat: an autoradiographic study of pain modulating systems. J Comp Neurol 1978; 178:209–224.
43. Basbaum AI, Fields HL. The origin of descending pathways in the dorsolateral funiculus of the spinal cord of the cat and rat: pain modulation. J Comp Neurol 1979; 187:513–532.

44. Besson JM, Rivot JP. Heterosegmental, heterosensory and cortical inhibitory effects on dorsal interneurones in the cat's spinal cord. Electroencephalogr Clin Neurophysiol 1972; 33:195–206.
45. Besson JM, Rivot JP. Spinal interneurones involved in presynaptic controls of supraspinal origin. J Physiol 1973; 230:235–254.
46. Hsu DT. Acupuncture. A review. Reg Anesth 1996; 21:361–370.
47. Tricklebank MD, Curzon G. Stress-Induced Analgesia. Chichester: John Wiley & Sons, 1984.
48. Carpenter D, Engberg I, Lumberg A. Primary afferent depolarization evoked from the brain stem and the cerebellum. Arch Ital Biol 1966; 104:73–85.
49. Anderson P, Eccles JC, Sears TA. Presynaptic inhibitory action of cerebral cortex on the spinal cord. Nature 1962; 194:740–741.
50. Bouhassira D, Bing Z, Bars DL. Studies of brain structures involved in diffuse noxious inhibitory controls in the rat: the rostral ventromedial medulla. J Physiol 1993; 463:667–687.
51. Mayer DJ, Price DD, Rafii A. Antagonism of acupuncture analgesia in man by the narcotic antagonist naloxone. Brain Res 1977; 121:368–372.
52. Shen E, Tsai TT, Lan C. Supraspinal participation in the inhibitory effect of acupuncture on viscerosomatic reflex discharges. Clin Med J 1975; 1:431–440.
53. Lewis JW, Cannon JY, Liebeskind JC. Opioid and nonopioid mechanisms of stress analgesia. Science 1980; 208:623–625.
54. Takahashi M, Sugimachi K, Kaneto H. Role of adrenal glucocorticoids in the blockade of the development of analgesic tolerance to morphine by footshock stress exposure in mice. Jpn J Pharmacol 1991; 56:121–126.
55. Martin RF, Haber LH, Willis WD. Primary afferent depolarization of identified cutaneous fibers following stimulation in medial brain stem. J Neurophysiol 1979; 42:779–790.
56. Yaksh T, Hammond DL, Tyce GM. Functional aspects of bulbospinal monoaminergic projections in modulating processing of somatosensory information. Fed Proc 1981; 40:2786–2794.

8

Local Neuroimmune Interactions in Visceral Hyperalgesia

Bradykinin, Neurotrophins, and Cannabinoids

Andrew S. C. Rice
Imperial College of Science, Technology and Medicine, London, England

I. INTRODUCTION

The physiology of visceral nociception has traditionally been elucidated by the examination of responses to ephemeral stimuli, such as the rapid distension of a viscus. However, it is now appreciated that such physiological studies are of only limited relevance to clinical pain, a situation in which the adaptive responses of a dynamic nervous system profoundly influence the processing of sensory traffic, clinically manifested by the appearance of allodynia and hyperalgesia (1). The effects of tissue injury and the subsequent inflammatory response are critical in determining the functional status of the sensory nervous system so that pain continues to be perceived long after a transient noxious stimulus has ceased. Therefore, the pathophysiology of visceral pain must be reexamined in models that incorporate a significant tissue injury and inflammatory components, so that the findings might be clinically relevant.

This chapter will focus on experiments that sought to elucidate the complex local neuroimmune interactions that underlie the hyperalgesia which accompanies visceral inflammation. For this, we have used an established model of visceral inflammation first described by McMahon and Abel (2) (a chemical cystitis induced by intravesical instillation of turpentine). Several features of this model have been described that enhance its credibility as a model of persistent visceral pain:

1. Viscerovisceral hyperreflexia (VVH) (2) (Fig. 1): Inflammation is accompanied by an enhancement of the spinal reflexes that control micturition, as measured by means of serial cystometrograms. Although this increase in bladder motility mirrors associated features of cystitis, such as frequency of micturition, rather than pain, it is a very consistent and reproducible feature of the model and has tended to be a "gold standard."

2. Sensitization of primary afferent neurons (3,4): Direct extracellular recording of primary afferent neurons innervating the urinary bladder has revealed that inflammation is associated with an increased excitability state of such neurons. Additionally, the existence of a population of primary afferent neurons innervating the urinary bladder that are not normally activated by physiological stimuli has been reported; once the bladder is inflamed the threshold of such neurons falls to within the physiological range (5,6). The net effect of this recruitment of "silent nociceptors" is to increase the overall barrage of sensory information reaching the spinal cord.

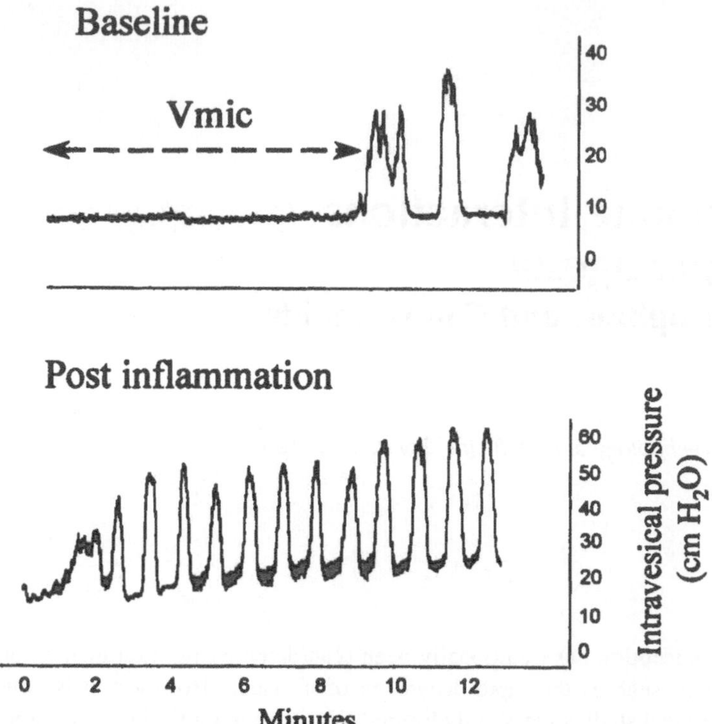

Figure 1 Examples of serial cystometrograms (CMG), obtained from an anesthetized female Wistar rat, by continuous measurement of intravesical pressure (*y* axis) during infusion of saline (0.05 mL/min to 0.7 mL): (Upper trace), a typical baseline CMG: Note the onset of regular rhythmic increases in intravesical pressure, typically at an intravesical volume of 0.4–0.5 mL, representing micturition contractions. The intravesical volume at which this event occurs is the micturition threshold (Vmic). (Lower trace), taken from the same animal, was recorded after intravesical application of 50% turpentine for 1 h. The fall in V_{mic} indicates a viscerovisceral hyperreflexia.

3. Dorsal horn neuronal sensitization (3): In an effort to ascertain the contribution of central sensitization to visceral hyperalgesia, the excitability of dorsal horn neurons innervating the urinary bladder has been enhanced following turpentine administration. Such spinal events following bladder inflammation are mediated by glutaminergic and nitric oxide-dependent systems (7,8).

4. Viscerosomatic hyperalgesia (VSH) (Fig. 2): A classic clinical characteristic of pain following visceral injury is that the sufferer often perceives it as arising from a (sometimes distant) somatic structure. Although the precise mechanism of this "referred" pain is unknown, the most widely accepted explanations rely on a convergence of somatic and visceral neuronal traffic at a spinal level (9). Recently, we have shown that experimental inflammation of the urinary bladder is associated with the development of a referred somatic hyperalgesia to both mechanical and thermal stimuli in a somatotopically appropriate area, the hindpaw (10,11).

5. Early-immediate gene expression: The protein product of the early-immediate gene c-*fos* is expressed in appropriate regions of the spinal cord following instillation of irritant chemicals into urinary bladder (12–14). Although the exact significance of this phenomenon is unknown, it does indicate that spinal nociceptive systems have been activated by this noxious insult. The prevention of stimulus-induced Fos expression is a useful tool in the identification of novel analgesic molecules (15).

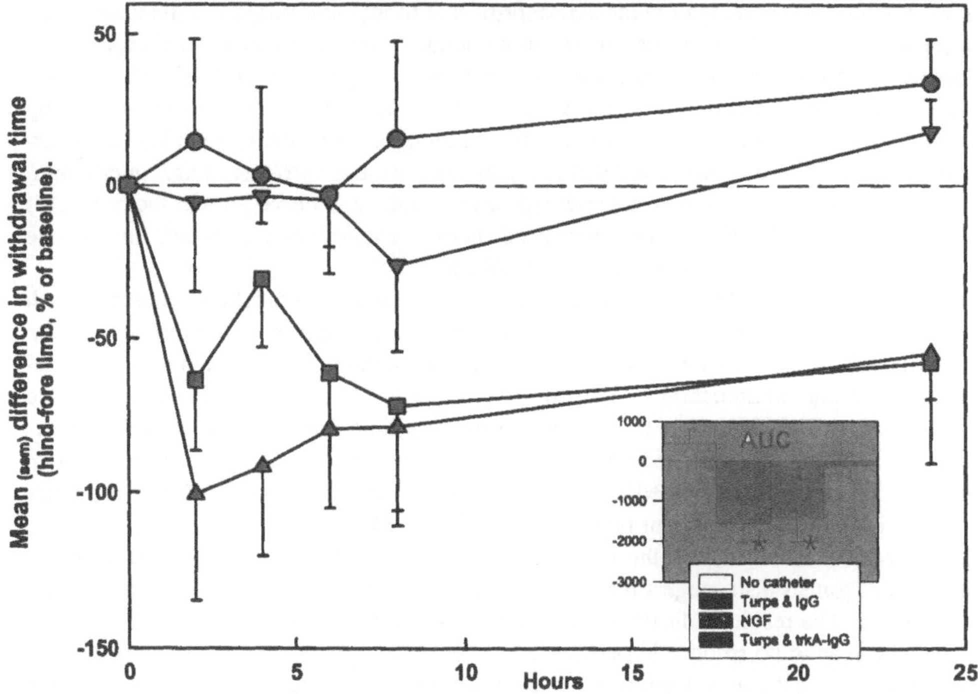

Figure 2 Referred hyperalgesia following urinary bladder inflammation is NGF-dependent: The main graph represents the relative change in limb withdrawal time (expressed as a difference in contemporaneously measured fore- and hindlimb withdrawal times) from a radiant heat stimulus, in the 24 h following inflammation of the urinary bladder. Thus, a negative deflection on the *y* axis represents a relative hyperalgesia of the hindlimb. The insert graph shows the mean area under the curve (AUC) for all treatment groups, this provides a single measure for each group, on which statistical analysis was performed (*p < 0.05 (Student's *t* test) versus control group). In the control group (no bladder catheterization, ●) there is no significant change from baseline values. However, when the bladder is inflamed with turpentine (50%, 1 h, ▲) there is a significant change indicating relative hyperalgesia of the hindlimb, which persists for at least 24 h after the instillation of turpentine. This referred hyperalgesia is replicated by intravesical instillation of human recombinant NGF (10 μg, ■) in place of turpentine. Furthermore, if turpentine instillation (50%, 1 h, ▼) is accompanied by systemic administration of an NGF sequestering molecule (trkA–IgG, 1 mg/kg IV) then the referred hyperalgesia associated with turpentine is prevented. $n = 6$ for all groups. NGF and trKA–IgG were gifts of Genentech.

With this model, we have investigated the local inflammation-driven events responsible for visceral hyperalgesia. Although a wide range of molecules are involved in this process, we have concentrated on three key groups of molecules: bradykinin, nerve growth factor (NGF), and cannabinoids.

II. BRADYKININ

The potent algogenic actions of the locally cleaved autacoid bradykinin have been appreciated for sometime. Nevertheless, the recent elucidation of bradykinin receptor subtypes has led to renewed interest in this compound, particularly from the standpoint of the development of novel analgesics. A considerable body of evidence confirms that bradykinin directly activates primary afferent nociceptors (16–19). However, bradykinin not only directly stimulates nociceptors, but is also implicated in the sensitization process and thus primary hyperalgesia (19,20). This sensitization is probably not a direct effect of bradykinin itself on nociceptive neurons, for during inflammation a complex synergy exists between bradykinin, its metabolites, and other prohyperalgesic molecules, such as neuropeptides (e.g., substance P) and cytokines (e.g., interleukin-1β[IL-1β] and tumor necrosis factor-α [TNF-α]), prostanoids, and nerve growth factor (NGF) (17–19,21–23). Unlike NGF, bradykinin-induced thermal hyperalgesia does not involve the participation of the sympathetic nervous system (24,25).

It is now understood that there are at least two subtypes of bradykinin receptor, both members of the G protein superfamily (26): The B_2 receptor is constitutively present, whereas the physiologically low expression of the B_1 receptor is considerably up-regulated by a cytokine-driven process during inflammation (17,19,26). Bradykinin itself is a preferential agonist at the B_2 receptor, whereas the kinase I metabolite des-Arg^9-bradykinin appears to be the most important endogenous ligand at the B_1 receptor. Further evidence for the role of the B_1 receptor in inflammatory hyperalgesia is provided by the finding that des-Arg^9-bradykinin is found in greater concentration in inflamed tissue than bradykinin itself (27,28).

Experiments that investigated the antihyperalgesic potential of bradykinin B_1 and B_2 receptor-selective antagonists also suggest that the two receptors have disparate roles in nociception and hyperalgesia. The results indicate that B_2 receptor antagonists attenuate acute nociceptive events (and continue to do so once hyperalgesia has developed), whereas antagonist activity at the B_1 receptor inhibits the sensitization associated with hyperalgesia, probably by an interaction with other hyperalgesia mediators (20,29). Although the B_2-mediated stimulatory effects can be attributed to a direct activation of receptors localized on primary afferent nociceptive neurons, the B_1-mediated sensitizing effects are more complex. Because it has not yet been possible to identify B_1 receptors located on sensory neurons, even in the presence of inflammatory mediators, it is probable that the prohyperalgesic effects of B_1 receptor activation are mediated by mechanisms other than a direct effect on nociceptors (22). The complexity of the relation between bradykinin-mediated events and hyperalgesia has been further underlined by studies using genetically modified animals in which the gene encoding the B_2 receptor has been disrupted (30). The B_2 receptors appears to be important in initiating hyperalgesia in some inflammatory models (e.g., carrageenan), but not others (e.g., formalin or Freund's adjuvant) for which B_1 effects are more important.

In the light of these observations, we examined the effects of competitive antagonists at the B_1 and B_2 receptors in the model of vesical inflammation (29). Neither the B_1 antagonist (des-Arg^9[Leu^8]-bradykinin) nor the B_2 antagonist icatibant acetate (HOE 140) had any significant effect on the normal micturition reflex in the absence of inflammation. However, if the antagonists were administered at the onset of inflammation then only HOE 140 prevented the inflammation-associated decline in micturition threshold in the dose range of 1–7.5 mg/kg. The B_1 antagonist was without such an effect in the same dose range. This phenomenon was maintained in the early stages of the inflammatory process. However, when the antihyperalgesic effect of these compounds was reexamined when the inflammatory hyperalgesia was well established, then both compounds were able to reverse the inflammation-associated decline in micturition threshold. Interestingly, neither bradykinin receptor antagonist influenced a measure of the inflammatory response (plasma protein extravasation), so that it would appear that bradykinin participates in the process of hyperalgesia, while not influencing the inflammatory process per se. The obvious implication of these findings is that B_2 antagonists will have some potential as acute antinociceptive agents, whereas both B_1 and B_2 effects are important for the analgesia in more persistent and chronic inflammatory states.

Therefore, there is logic in developing antagonists at both bradykinin receptor subtypes as potential analgesics. However most of the bradykinin receptor antagonists currently under investigation (e.g., HOE 140 or des-Arg^9[Leu^8]-bradykinin) are peptide analogues of bradykinin and consequently have a relatively limited duration of action. It is expected that nonpeptide antagonists with a more clinically relevant duration of action will become available for experimental use in the near future. Notwithstanding this, the complexity of the relative contributions of B_1 and B_2 receptor effects remain poorly understood and requires further clarification.

III. NERVE GROWTH FACTOR

In the fetus and neonate the target-derived neurotrophin nerve growth factor (NGF) is vital for the survival and phenotypic development of small-diameter afferent and sympathetic efferent neurons (31). However, in the developed animal NGF assumes a different role; it is no longer necessary for the survival of sensory neurons, but it is capable of sensitizing nociceptors under inflammatory conditions. Following tissue injury, NGF is released by various connective tissue and inflammatory cells in response to inflammatory cytokines (e.g., IL-1β and TNF-α) (31–33).

There are two receptor types that bind neurotrophins (34): the high-affinity tyrosine kinase (trk) clan of receptors are specific for each member of the neurotrophin family, with the trkA receptor mediating the physiological functions of NGF. The low-affinity p75 receptor binds all neurotrophins and plays a limited role in modulating the physiological functions of trks. In particular, trk selectivity for the various neurotrophins may be modulated by the p75 receptor.

Several lines of evidence suggest that NGF is pivotal to the development of inflammatory hyperalgesia (see Ref. 34 for a comprehensive overview):

1. Endogenous NGF protein and its mRNA are expressed in acutely inflamed tissue taken from experimental animals (35,36) and patients (37). Increased NGF expression has also been found in biopsy material taken from patients suffering from interstitial cystitis, suggesting a similar role for NGF in persistent visceral pain (38).
2. Primary afferent nociceptors express the trkA receptor. This is of particular relevance to the viscera, because the proportion of neurons expressing trkA is higher in the visceral (~90%), as opposed to the somatic domain (~40%) (34,39).
3. Electrophysiological experiments demonstrate that administration of exogenous NGF directly sensitizes visceral primary afferent nociceptors and participates in the recruitment of "silent" nociceptors (9,40).
4. Administration of exogenous NGF evokes hyperalgesic responses similar to those observed in inflammatory pain models (41–43). Administration of NGF also evokes persistent pain and a biphasic hyperalgesia in human volunteers (41,44). Of particular relevance to the visceral domain is the finding that intravesical administration of exogenous NGF precisely replicates the viscerovisceral hyperreflexia observed following turpentine administration (42).
5. Intravesical administration of exogenous NGF provokes expression of the protein product of the early-immediate gene c-*fos* and its protein product in the spinal cord (14).
6. Sequestration of NGF is associated with hypoalgesia in normal animals (45) and attenuates viscerovisceral hyperreflexia observed following turpentine treatment of the urinary bladder (42).
7. By using an NGF-sequestering molecule, we have demonstrated the vital role of endogenous NGF in the development of referred hyperalgesia. We have also shown

that intravesical application of exogenous NGF replicates the referred hyperalgesia observed in inflammatory models (see Fig. 2) (11).

8. Nociceptive neurons fail to develop in genetically modified animals that have had the NGF-encoding gene disrupted. These animals also exhibit elevated thresholds to noxious stimuli (46). Similarly, animals that overexpress the NGF-encoding gene are hypersensitive to sensory stimuli (47).

How are the prohyperalgesic actions of NGF mediated at a local level (Fig. 3)? Direct sensitization of primary afferent nociceptors by the trkA receptor is probably the major event underlying NGF-evoked hyperalgesia (34,40). In dorsal root ganglion cells the concentration of various nociceptive neurotransmitters, including the neuropeptides substance P and calcitonin

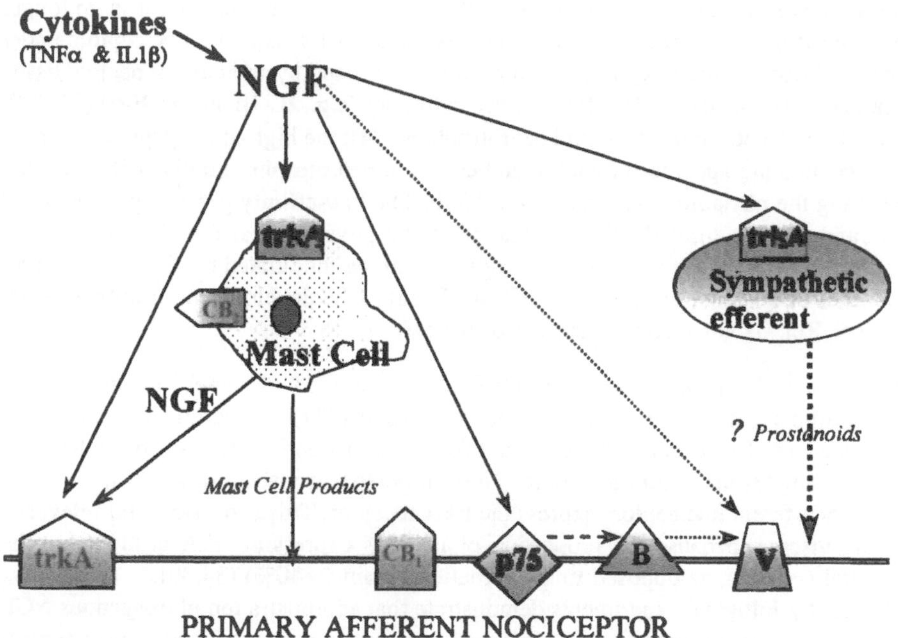

Figure 3 Peripheral mechanisms of nerve growth factor (NGF)-induced hyperalgesia. Following a cytokine-driven release of NGF from connective tissue and other cell types, there are several pathways by which NGF can alter nociceptor sensitivity.

1. NGF directly interacts with trkA receptors expressed on primary afferent nociceptors.
2. The effects of NGF are amplified by agonist activity at mast cell trkA receptors provoking further release of NGF.
3. Degranulation of mast cells also results in release of other prohyperalgesic mediators (e.g., histamine and serotonin) which are capable of directly sensitizing nociceptors.
4. NGF regulates the responsiveness of nociceptors to bradykinin (B, bradykinin receptor).
5. NGF-induced hyperalgesia requires the functional presence of sympathetic efferent neurons. This effect possibly involves prostanoids, released from sympathetic neurons, interacting with nociceptors.
6. NGF regulates the responsiveness of primary afferent neurons to capsaicin and protons, possibly by a mechanism involving the vanniloid receptor (VR_1).

gene-related peptide (CGRP), are increased by NGF (48). However, additional NGF-driven events enhance and amplify the actions of NGF in promoting the development of inflammatory hyperalgesia:

1. Mast cells amplify the NGF signal (34,49). The activity of mast cells is required for the prohyperalgesic effects of NGF, because the response to NGF is attenuated in animals prophylactically treated with a mast cell degranulating compound (41,50). Mast cells express trkA receptors and NGF-induced degranulation of mast cells provokes release of other mediators (e.g., histamine and serotonin) which, in turn, directly sensitize primary afferent nociceptors (51–53). In addition, the mast cell is capable of further NGF synthesis and release (53,54). Furthermore, mast cells play a role in the clinical scenario of visceral hyperalgesia (55–58).
2. NGF-induced hyperalgesia requires the functional presence of sympathetic efferent neurons (59). Moreover, it has been hypothesized that prostaglandins produced by such neurons in response to NGF stimulation participate by directly sensitizing nociceptors (59).
3. NGF up-regulates the responsiveness of nociceptors to the potent algogens bradykinin (21,60,61), capsaicin, and protons (62,63).

So far, there has been limited success in developing conventional pharmacological competitive antagonists for NGF at the trkA receptor. However, alternative strategies have been somewhat rewarding: One approach has been to attempt to sequester NGF so that little is available for binding to trkA. A novel molecule manufactured by dimerization of the extracellular domains of two trkA receptors and fusion to an IgG molecule (64) has been successful in animal experiments (42,45). NGF antibodies have also been employed to a similar end (33). Another approach is to attenuate the intracellular consequences of the NGF–trkA interaction (65).

Thus, NGF occupies a pivotal position in the induction of visceral hyperalgesia, and manipulation of this finding may result in the production of a novel class of analgesics for inflammatory pain.

IV. CANNABINOIDS

Although cannabis has been suspected of possessing analgesic qualities for some time, there is, as yet, little sound clinical evidence to support its widespread therapeutic use (66,67). Rational clinical and political concerns over side effects have curtailed legal clinical investigation of cannabis as an analgesic (66). As herbal cannabis contains at least 60 compounds that interact in various ways with cannabinoid (CB) receptors, it has been recommended that one direction for future research should be aimed at identifying the precise mechanism of cannabis-induced analgesia (66). To this end, the discovery of endogenous ligands and two distinct forms of cannabinoid receptor and their subsequent cloning were major advances (68–74).

Several endocannabinoids have been identified, all of which are structurally related to arachidonic acid. The best characterized endogenous ligand is the brain constituent anandamide (ANA) (75,76). A second endogenous CB ligand, 2-arachidonyl glycerol, has more recently been located within the CNS and peripheral tissues (77), and a third, palmitoylethanolamide (PEA), has been identified in inflamed nonneural tissue (49). However, the extent to which the biological effects of PEA are CB receptor mediated is still controversial and unclear.

The CB_1 receptor is constitutively expressed predominantly within the brain and spinal cord and a large body of evidence points to analgesic effects of cannabinoids at these levels (78–82). However, there is also evidence of a peripheral inflammation-associated site of action, exploitation of which might provide an avenue for divorcing the analgesic effects of cannabinoids from their CNS-mediated side effects (83,84). Further support for such a peripheral site of action is provided by the discovery that CB_2 receptor expression appears to be restricted to cells of immune origin, and of particular relevance to persistent visceral pain is its location on mast cells (49,68,69,72,85,86).

Given the central role of NGF in the generation of visceral hyperalgesia, it is germane to the development of novel analgesics to examine methods of antagonizing its effects. One approach is to investigate ligand trap sequestration molecules, as described in the foregoing, another is to examine potential avenues of "physiological antagonism." One group of candidates for such a role are the endogenous cannabinoids, and there is evidence implicating both CB_1 and CB_2 receptor subtypes in this process.

We have studied the expression of the CB_1 receptor in spinal cord using immunohistochemical double-labeling techniques and found that CB_1 expression colocalizes in the same regions of the dorsal horn as the central terminals of the NGF-dependent peptidergic class of primary afferent nociceptors (unpublished data). [Primary afferent nociceptive neurons can be classified into two broad groups on the basis of their peptide (or purine) content: neurotrophin-dependency, and spinal terminations (87)]. A further finding that cannabinoids attenuate capsaicin-evoked neurotransmitter release from peptidergic primary afferent neurons lends further support to the concept of a close relation between cannabinoids and the NGF-dependent class of primary afferent nociceptor (83). In the primary afferent neurons, the gene encoding the CB_1 receptor has been identified in dorsal root ganglion cells that are NGF, but not neurotrophin 3 (NT-3), dependent (88). Furthermore, CB_1 mRNA is found in dorsal root ganglion cells, and the data suggest that a proportion of this expression occurs on the peptidergic class of cell (89). CB_1 receptors also undergo axonal transport in peripheral nerves (90), and there is some evidence to support a role for CB receptors in tissues of the urogenital tract (91).

Both CB_2 and trkA receptors have been identified on mast cells (53,86), which are known to be of importance in the pathophysiology of chronic visceral hyperalgesia (56–58,92). Mast cells not only express the trkA receptor, but also amplify the NGF signal during inflammation (54). What are the biological controls on this process? Certainly, there is mounting evidence that the endocannabinoid PEA attenuates this amplification of NGF effects by participating in the process of "autacoid local inflammation antagonism" (ALIA) (49,86,93): PEA accumulates in inflamed tissue, binds to mast cell CB_2 receptors, prevents mast cell degranulation, and suppresses inflammatory hyperalgesia and edema (86,93). Other inflammatory cells may also be involved in the process of ALIA, for example, leukocytes both biosynthesize and take up and degrade both ANA and PEA (94).

In the model of visceral hyperalgesia described earlier, we have demonstrated that both ANA and PEA reverse the inflammation-related signs of an established turpentine-induced VVH in a dose-related fashion (95) (Fig. 4). At the effective doses neither PEA, nor ANA has an adverse effect on micturition reflexes in the absence of inflammation (96). Additional unpublished data support the concept of such an antihyperalgesic effect, in that cannabinoids prevent the expression of Fos protein in spinal cord following bladder inflammation with turpentine. When "preemptive " effects were examined, only ANA was effective in preventing VVH when administered at the start of inflammation (96). One implication of this finding is that the requisite mechanisms for ANA-induced analgesia are constitutively present, whereas the inflammatory process must be established before PEA becomes effective. This would concur with the hypothesis that PEA exerts its effects through CB_2 receptors located on immune cells that migrate into areas of inflammation, such as mast cells. This evidence of ANA- and PEA-induced analgesia is supported by evidence from the somatic domain that revealed that these compounds both attenuated the behavioral response to subcutaneous formalin injection (95). Others have shown

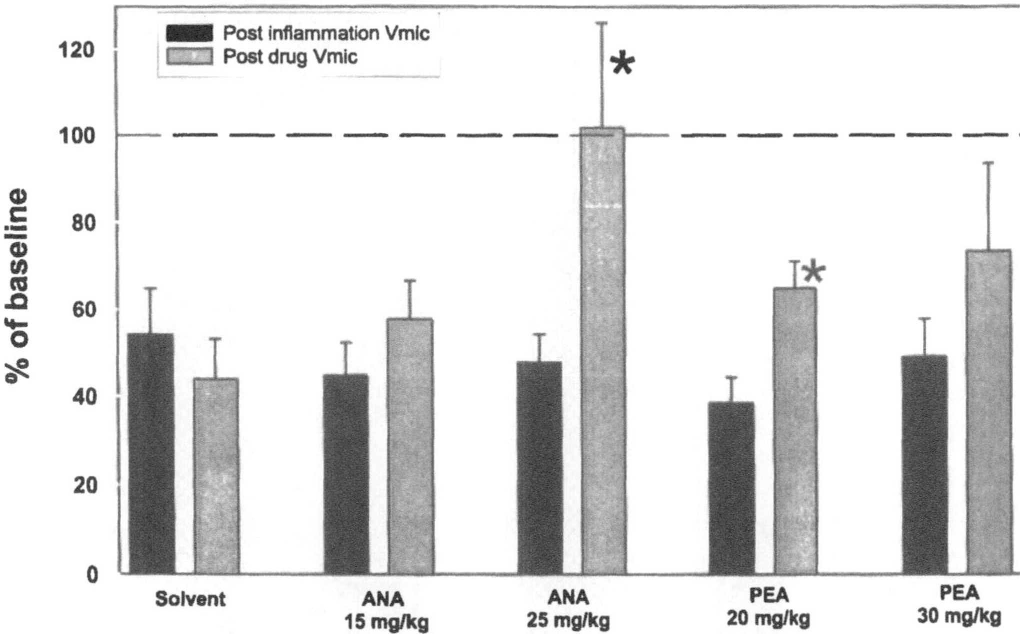

Figure 4 Endocannabinoids reverse the viscerovisceral hyperreflexia associated with inflammation of the urinary bladder: The filled bars demonstrate the decline (normalized as percentage of baseline values) in the micturition threshold (V_{mic}) following intravesical treatment with 50% turpentine. There is an inflammation-associated 40–50% decline in V_{mic} associated with turpentine application in all groups. However, this decline in V_{mic} is reversed by subsequent treatment with either anandamide (ANA, 25 mg/kg i.a.) or palmitoylethanolamide (PEA, 20–30 mg/kg i.a.) in a dose-dependent fashion. * $p < 0.05$ vs. post inflammation V_{mic} (ANOVA).

similar effects for ANA, PEA, and synthetic cannabinoids in the formalin model (84), in models of inflammatory arthritis (97), neuropathic pain (98), and of afferent-induced hyperexcitability of dorsal horn neurons (81,82).

There is also direct evidence of cannabinoid involvement in the attenuation of NGF-induced hyperalgesia in the visceral domain: both ANA and PEA dose-dependently prevent the VVH associated with NGF treatment of the urinary bladder (99,100) (Fig. 5). The effects of ANA are reversed by SR141716A and partially by SR144528 implying that its effects may be mediated by both CB_1 and CB_2 receptors (100). The antihyperalgesic effect of PEA is reversed only by SR144528, confirming a CB_2-mediated effect. In support of this, we have obtained preliminary evidence that the appearance of Fos protein in the dorsal horn following NGF treatment of bladder is attenuated by cannabinoids (unpublished data).

The question of whether ANA and PEA analgesia is mediated by CB_1 or CB_2 receptors, is currently being clarified. ANA binds to the CB_1 receptor, displaces the radiolabeled receptor probe HU 210 and stimulates receptor-mediated signal transduction (75,101), ANA also binds to CB_2 receptors (86,102). One study did demonstrate that ANA inhibited adenylate cyclase activity by CB_2 receptors (102), but other evidence suggests that ANA is not a CB_2 agonist, nor does it induce down-regulatory activity on mast cell function (86,103). However, ANA attenuation of NGF-induced visceral hyperalgesia is prevented by both CB_1 and CB_2 receptor antagonist administration (100). In an inflammatory arthritis model, the analgesic effects of ANA were not reversed by high-dose SR141716A, implying a possible action mediated at other,

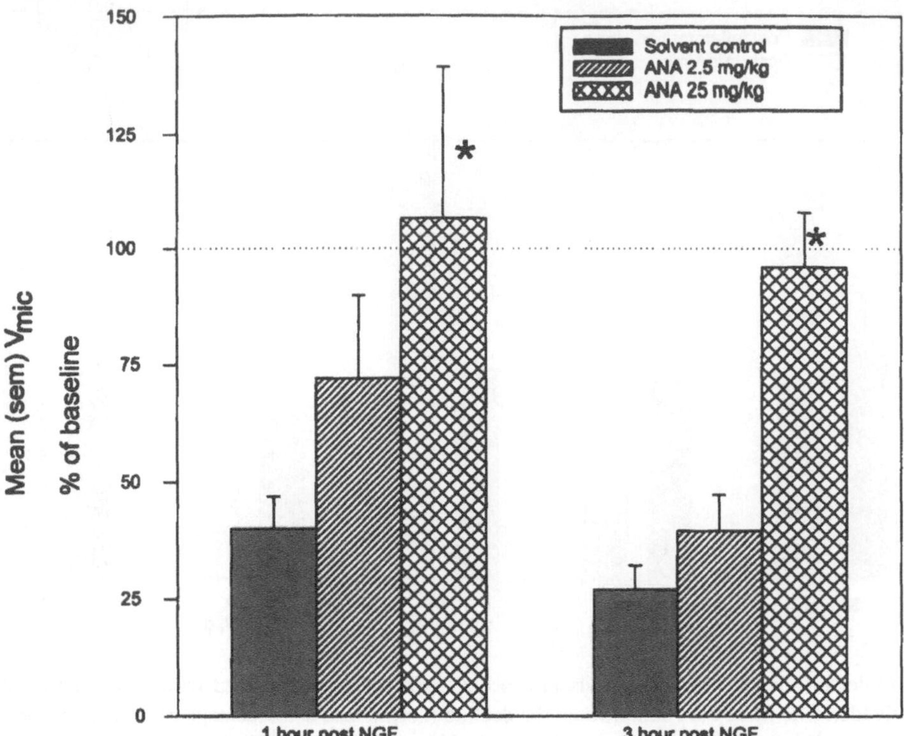

Figure 5 Anandamide (ANA) prevents NGF-induced viscerovisceral hyperreflexia: Intravesical instillation of NGF (10 μg) is associated with a decline in micturition threshold (V_{mic}) compared with baseline values. This effect is prevented by systemic administration of ANA at a dose of 25 mg/kg i.a., but not 2.5 mg/kg i.a. This is maintained for at least 3 h following the end of the NGF treatment, a period much longer than the duration of pharmacological activity of ANA. $^*p < 0.05$ vs. control V_{mic} (ANOVA).

as yet undiscovered, CB receptors (97). Another possibility is of nonreceptor-mediated effects, a phenomenon not altogether inconceivable for such a highly lipophilic molecule.

The analgesic actions of PEA appear to be mediated by CB_2 receptors, because PEA-induced analgesia and attenuation of NGF-induced visceral hyperalgesia is reversed by SR144528, but not by SR141716A (84,100). However, the location of these receptors is debated. Mast cells express the CB_2-encoding gene and functional CB_2 protein (86). PEA binds to CB_2 receptors located on mast cells, displaces a CB probe and down-modulates mast cell function (86). However, PEA only weakly displaces the same probe from CB_2 transfected cells (104). Notwithstanding this latter finding, PEA did not activate receptor-mediated signal transduction in Chinese hamster ovary (CHO) cells expressing only the CB_1 receptor (101). Furthermore, studies using CHO cells transfected with the cDNA encoding either the CB_1 or CB_2 receptor gene and similarly examining forskolin-stimulated cAMP production, have demonstrated an IC_{50} for PEA of 239 nM in CB_1-transfected cells, whereas this value was 1.94 nM in CB_2-transfected cells, thereby both confirming the selectivity and activity of PEA at the CB_2 receptor (105). Piomelli's group (84) have confirmed that the analgesic effect of co-administration of ANA and PEA is synergistic, thus lending further support to the concept that they act through different receptor systems.

Do cannabinoids physiologically attenuate inflammatory hyperalgesia? There are no direct data pertaining to the viscera, but in mice, using intrathecal administration of the CB_1 antagonist

SR141716A, Hargreaves and colleagues have demonstrated an antagonist-induced elevation of "hot plate" latencies, implying that endogenous CB_1 agonists topically regulate the threshold for noxious heat (106). Similarly, others have demonstrated an enhancement of various phases of the behavioral response to subcutaneous formalin injection in mice using both CB_1 and CB_2 antagonists (84). However, we have been unable to reproduce these findings in the rat (107), and the early results from CB_1 knockout mice would not tend to support the existence of an endogenous cannabinoid analgesic tone, in that a greater degree of hyperalgesia, following an inflammatory insult, is generally not observed in comparison with wild-type controls (108,109).

Although cannabinoid-induced analgesia has been suspected from anecdotal clinical reports, until the results of randomized controlled studies it has to be concluded that there is still no firm evidence of such an effect in humans (66,67). However, the recent exciting developments in elucidating the physiology of endogenous cannabinoid systems and their role in regulating the NGF-mediated component of visceral hyperalgesia, in particular the identification of the receptors and endogenous ligands, augers well. Furthermore, the recent announcement of a genetically modified mouse in which the gene encoding the CB_1 receptor has been disrupted (108,109), together with the almost inevitable appearance of highly selective CB_1 and CB_2 agonists, indicates that far more will soon be known about these systems.

ACKNOWLEDGMENTS

Supported by the Association of Anaesthetists of Great Britain and Ireland; Joint Standing Research Committee St. Mary's Hospital; and Academic Foundation of the Royal College of Anaesthetists.

REFERENCES

1. Coderre TJ, Katz J, Vaccarino A, Melzack R. Contribution of central neuroplasticity to pathological pain: review of clinical and experimental evidence. Pain 1993; 52:259–285.
2. McMahon SB, Abel C. A model for the study of visceral pain states: chronic inflammation of the chronic decerebrate rat urinary bladder by irritant chemicals. Pain 1987; 28:109–127.
3. McMahon SB. Neuronal and behavioural consequences of chemical inflammation of rat urinary bladder. Agents Actions 1988; 25:231–233.
4. McMahon SB, Koltzenburg M. Mayer EA, Raybould H, eds. Changes in the afferent innervation of the inflamed urinary bladder. In: Basic and Clinical Aspects of Chronic Abdominal Pain. Amsterdam: Elsevier, 1993:155–172.
5. Habler HJ, Janig W, Koltzenburg M. A novel type of unmyelinated chemosensitive nociceptor in the acutely inflamed urinary bladder. Agents Actions 1988; 25:219–221.
6. McMahon SB, Koltzenburg M, Fields HL, Liebeskind JC, eds. Silent afferents and visceral pain. In: Pharmacological Approaches to the Treatment of Chronic Pain: New Concepts and Critical Issues. Seattle: IASP Press, 1994:11–30.
7. Rice ASC, McMahon SB. Pre-emptive intrathecal administration of an NMDA receptor antagonist (AP-5) prevents hyper-reflexia in a model of persistent visceral pain. Pain 1994; 57:335–340.
8. Rice ASC. Topical spinal administration of a nitric oxide synthase inhibitor prevents the hyper-reflexia associated with a rat model of persistent visceral pain. Neurosci Lett 1995; 187:111–114.
9. McMahon SB, Dmitrieva N, Koltzenburg M. Visceral pain. Br J Anaesth 1995; 75:132–144.
10. Scott HCF, Jaggar SI, Rice ASC. Mechanical hyperalgesia is referred to the hind limb following inflammation of the urinary bladder in the rat. J Physiol (Lond) 1998; 507:18.
11. Jaggar SI, Scott HCF, Rice ASC. Inflammation of the rat urinary bladder is associated with a referred hyperalgesia which is nerve growth factor dependant. Br J Anaesth 1999; 83:442–448.

12. Birder LA, de Groat WC. Increased c-*fos* expression in spinal neurones after irritation of the lower urinary tract in the rat. J Neurosci 1992; 12:4878–4883.
13. Cruz F, Avelino A, Lima D, Coimbra A. Activation of the c-*fos* proto-oncogene in the spinal cord following noxious stimulation of the urinary bladder. Somatosens Mot Res 1994; 11:319–325.
14. Dmitrieva N, Iqbal R, Shelton D, McMahon SB. c-*fos* Induction in a rat model of cystitis: role of NGF. Soc Neurosci Abstr 1996; 22:301.6.
15. Chapman V, Besson JM. Dickenson AH, Besson JM, eds. Pharmacological studies of nociceptive systems using the c-*fos* immunohistochemical technique: an indicator of noxiously activated spinal neurones. In: The Pharmacology of Pain. Berlin: Springer; 1997:235–280.
16. Lang E, Novak A, Reeh PW, Handwerker H. Chemosensitivity of fine afferents from rat skin in vitro. J Neurophysiol 1990; 63:887–901.
17. Dray A. Tasting the inflammatory soup: the role of peripheral neurones. Pain Rev 1994; 1:153–171.
18. Dray A. Inflammatory mediators of pain. Br J Anaesth 1995; 75:125–131.
19. Dray A, Perkins MN. Bradykinin and inflammatory pain. Trends Neurosci 1993; 16:99–104.
20. Perkins MN, Campbell E, Dray A. Antinociceptive effects of the bradykinin B_1 and B_2 receptor antagonists des-Arg^9, [Leu^8]-BK and HOE 140, in two models of persistent hyperalgesia in the rat. Pain 1993; 53:191–197.
21. Rueff A, Dawson AJLR, Mendell LM. Characteristics of nerve growth factor induced hyperalgesia in adult rats: dependence on enhanced bradykinin-1 receptor activity but not neurokinin-1 receptor activation. Pain 1996; 66:359–372.
22. Davis CL, Naeem S, Phagoo SB, Campbell EA, Urban L, Burgess GM. B_1 bradykinin receptors and sensory neurones. Br J Pharmacol 1996; 118:1469–1476.
23. Stucky CL, Thayer SA, Seybold VS. Prostaglandin E_2 increases the proportion of neonatal rat dorsal root ganglion cells that respond to bradykinin. Neuroscience 1996; 74:1111–1123.
24. Koltzenburg M, Kress M, Reeh PW. The nociceptor sensitization by bradykinin does not depend on sympathetic neurons. Neuroscience 1992; 46:465–473.
25. Meyer RA, Davis KD, Raja SN, Campbell JN. Sympathectomy does not abolish bradykinin induced cutaneous hyperalgesia in man. Pain 1992; 51:323–327.
26. Hall JM. Bradykinin receptors: pharmacological properties and biological roles. Pharmacol Ther 1992; 56:131–190.
27. Burch RM, De Haas C. A bradykinin antagonist inhibits carageenin oedema in the rat. Naunyn Schmiedebergs Arch Pharmacol 1988; 342:189–193.
28. Dray A. Dickenson AH, Besson JM, eds. Peripheral mediators of pain. In: The Pharmacology of Pain. Berlin: Springer-Verlag, 1997:21–41.
29. Jaggar SI, Habib S, Rice ASC. The modulatory effects of bradykinin B_1 and B_2 antagonists upon viscero-visceral hyper-reflexia in a rat model of visceral hyperalgesia. Pain 1998; 75:169–176.
30. Rupniak NM, Boyce S, Webb JK, Williams AR, Carlson EJ, Hill RG, Borkowski JA, Hess JF. Effects of the bradykinin B_1 receptor antagonist des-Arg^9[Leu^8] bradykinin and genetic disruption of the B_2 receptor on nociception in rats and mice. Pain 1997; 71:89–97.
31. Lewin GR, Mendell LM. Nerve growth factor and nociception. Trends Neurosci 1993; 16:353–359.
32. Safieh Garabedian B, Poole S, Allchorne A, Winter J, Woolf CJ. Contribution of interleukin-1 beta to the inflammation-induced increase in nerve growth factor levels and inflammatory hyperalgesia. Br J Pharmacol 1995; 115:1265–1275.
33. Woolf CJ, Safieh Garabedian B, Ma QP, Crilly P, Winter J. Nerve growth factor contributes to the generation of inflammatory sensory hypersensitivity. Neuroscience 1994; 62:327–331.
34. McMahon SB, Bennett DLH, Dickenson AH, Besson JM, eds. Growth factors and pain. In: The Pharmacology of Pain. Berlin: Springer; 1997:135–157.
35. Andreev NY, Bennett DLH, Priestley JV, et al. NGF mRNA is increased by experimental inflammation of adult rat urinary bladder [abstr]. Soc Neurosci Abstr 1994; 20:108.18.
36. Oddiah D, Anand P, McMahon SB, et al. Rapid increase of NGF, BDNF and NT-3 mRNAs in inflamed bladder. Neuroreport 1998; 9:1455–1488.
37. Aloe L, Tuveri M, Cacassi U, Levi–Montalcini R. Nerve growth factor in the synovial fluid of patients with chronic arthritis. Arthritis Rheum 1992; 35:351–355.

38. Lowe EM, Anand P, Terenghi G, Williams–Chestnut RE, Sinicropi DV, Osborne JL. Increased nerve growth factor levels in the urinary bladder of women with idiopathic sensory urgency and interstitial cystitis. Br J Urol 1997; 79:572–577.
39. McMahon SB, Armanini MP, Ling LH, Phillips HS. Expression and coexpression of trk receptors in subpopulations of adult primary sensory neurons projecting to identified peripheral targets. Neuron 1994; 12:1161–1171.
40. Dmitrieva N, McMahon SB. Sensitisation of visceral afferents by nerve growth factor in the adult rat. Pain 1996; 66:87–97.
41. Lewin GR, Rueff A, Mendell LM. Peripheral and central mechanisms of NGF-induced hyperalgesia. Eur J Neurosci 1994; 6:1903–1912.
42. Dmitrieva N, Shelton D, Rice ASC, McMahon SB. The role of nerve growth factor in a model of visceral inflammation. Neuroscience 1997; 78:449–459.
43. Lewin GR, Ritter AM, Mendell LM. Nerve growth factor induced hyperalgesia in the neonatal and adult rat. J Neurosci 1993; 13:2136–2148.
44. Petty BG, et al. The effect of systemically administered recombinant human nerve growth factor in healthy human subjects. Ann Neurol 1994; 36:244–246.
45. McMahon SB, Bennett DLH, Priestley JV, Shelton D. The biological effects of endogenous NGF on adult sensory neurones revealed by a trkA–IgG fusion molecule. Nat Med 1995; 1:774–780.
46. Crowley C, Spencer SD, Nishimura MC et al. Mice lacking nerve growth factor display perinatal loss of sensory and sympathetic neurons yet develop basal forebrain cholinergic neurons. Cell 1994; 76:1001–1011.
47. Davis BM, Lewin GR, Mendell LM, Jones ME, Albers KM. Altered expression of nerve growth factor in the skin of transgenic mice leads to changes in response to mechanical stimuli. Neuroscience 1993; 56:789–792.
48. Donnerer J, Schuligoi R, Stein C. Increased content and transport of substance P and calcitonin gene-related peptide in sensory nerves innervating inflamed tissue: evidence for a regulatory function of nerve growth factor in vivo. Neuroscience 1992; 49:693–698.
49. Levi–Montalcini R, Skaper SD, Dal Toso R, Petrelli L, Leon A. Nerve growth factor: from neurotrophin to neurokine. Trends Neurosci 1996; 19:514–520.
50. Woolf CJ, Ma QP, Allchorne A, Poole S. Peripheral cell types contributing to the hyperalgesic action of nerve growth factor in inflammation. J Neurosci 1996; 16:2716–2723.
51. Horigome K, Pryor JC, Bullock ED, Johnson EM Jr. Mediator release from mast cells by nerve growth factor. Neurotrophin specificity and receptor mediation. J Biol Chem 1993; 268:14881–14887.
52. Tal M, Liberman R. Local injection of nerve growth factor (NGF) triggers degranulation of mast cells in rat paw. Neurosci Lett 1997; 221:129–132.
53. Nilsson G, Forsberg Nilsson K, Xiang Z, Hallbook F, Nilsson K, Metcalfe DD. Human mast cells express functional trkA and are a source of nerve growth factor. Eur J Immunol 1997; 27:2295–2301.
54. Leon A, Buriani A, Dal Toso R, Fabris M, Romanello S, Aloe L, Levi–Montalcini R. Mast cells synthesize, store, and release nerve growth factor. Proc Natl Acad Sci USA 1994; 91:3739–3743.
55. Lynes WL, Flynn SD, Shortliffe LD, Lemmers M, Zipser R, Roberts LJ, Stamey TA. Mast cell involvement in interstitial cystitis. J Urol 1987; 138:746–752.
56. Sant GR, Theoharides TC. The role of the mast cell in interstitial cystitis. Urol Clin North Am 1994; 21:41–53.
57. Boucher W, el Mansoury M, Pang X, Sant GR, Theoharides TC. Elevated mast cell tryptase in the urine of patients with interstitial cystitis. Br J Urol 1995; 76:94–100.
58. Theoharides TC, Sant GR, el Mansoury M, Letourneau R, Ucci AA Jr, Meares EM Jr. Activation of bladder mast cells in interstitial cystitis: a light and electron microscopic study. J Urol 1995; 153:629–636.
59. Andreev NY, Dmitrieva N, Koltzenburg M, McMahon SB. Peripheral administration of nerve growth factor in the adult rat produces a thermal hyperalgesia that requires the presence of sympathetic post-ganglionic neurones. Pain 1995; 63:109–115.

60. Petersen M, Segond von Banchet G, Heppelmann B, Koltzenburg M. Nerve growth factor regulates the expression of bradykinin binding sites on adult sensory neurons via the neurotrophin receptor p75. Neuroscience 1998; 83:161–168.
61. Bennett DLH, Koltzenburg M, Priestley JV, Shelton D, McMahon SB. Endogenous nerve growth factor regulates the sensitivity of nociceptors in the adult rat. Eur J Neurosci 1998; 10:1282–1291.
62. Bevan S, Winter J. Nerve growth factor (NGF) differentially regulates the chemosensitivity of adult rat cultured sensory neurons. J Neurosci 1995; 15:4918–4926.
63. Winter J, Forbes CA, Sternberg J, Lindsay RM. Nerve growth factor (NGF) regulates adult rat cultured dorsal root ganglion neuron responses to the excitotoxin capsaicin. Neuron 1988; 1:973–981.
64. Shelton D, Sutherland J, Gripp J, Camerato MP, Armanini MP, Phillips HS, Carroll K, Spencer SD, Levinson AD. Human trks: molecular cloning, tissue distribution and expression of extracellular domain adhesins. J Neurosci 1995; 15:477–491.
65. Berg MM, Sternberg DW, Parada LF, Chao MV. K-252a inhibits nerve growth factor-induced *trk* proto-oncogene phosphorylation and kinase activity. J Biol Chem 1992; 267:13–16.
66. Ashton CH. Morgan DR, eds. Therapeutic Uses of Cannabis. Amsterdam: British Medical Association/Harwood, 1997.
67. Lachmann PJ, Edwards JG, Pertwee RG, et al. The use of Cannabis and Its Derivatives for Medical and Recreational Purposes. London. The Royal Society/The Academy of Medical Sciences, 1998; June.
68. Munro S, Thomas KL, Abu Shaar M, Molecular characterization of a peripheral receptor for cannabinoids. Nature 1993; 365:61–65.
69. Galiegue S, Mary S, Marchand J, Dussossoy D, Carriere D, Carayon P, Bouaboula M, Shire D, Le Fur G, Casellas P. Expression of central and peripheral cannabinoid receptors in human immune tissues and leukocyte subpopulations. Eur J Biochem 1995; 232:54–61.
70. Howlett AC. Pharmacology of cannabinoid receptors. Annu Rev Pharmacol Toxicol 1995; 35:607–634.
71. Pertwee RG. Pharmacology of cannabinoid CB_1 and CB_2 receptors. Pharmacol Ther 1997; 74:129–180.
72. Abood ME, Martin BR. Molecular neurobiology of the cannabinoid receptor. Int Rev Neurobiol 1996; 39:197–221.
73. Hohmann AG, Herkenham M. Localization of central cannabinoid CB_1 receptor messenger RNA in neuronal subpopulations of rat dorsal root ganglia: a double-label in situ hybridization study. Neuroscience 1999; 90:923–931.
74. Devane WA, Dysarz FA 3d, Johnson MR, Melvin LS, Howlett AC. Determination and characterization of a cannabinoid receptor in rat brain. Mol Pharmacol 1988; 34:605–613.
75. Devane W, Hanus L, Breuer A, Pertwee RG, Stevenson LA, Griffin G, Gibson D, Mandelbaum A, Etinger A, Mechoulam R. Isolation and structure of a brain constituent that binds to the cannabinoid receptor. Science 1992; 258:1946–1949.
76. Mechoulam R, Ben Shabat S, Hanus L, Fride E, Vogel Z, Bayewitch M, Sulcova AE. Endogenous cannabinoid ligands—chemical and biological studies. J Lipid Mediat Cell Signal 1996; 14:45–49.
77. Stella N, Schweitzer P, Piomelli D. A second endogenous cannabinoid that modulates long-term potentiation. Nature 1997; 388:773–778.
78. Meng ID, Manning BH, Martin WJ, Fields HL. An analgesic circuit activated by cannabinoids. Nature 1998; 395:381–383.
79. Tsou K, Lowitz KA, Hohmann AG, Martin WJ, Hathaway CB, Bereiter DA, Walker JM. Suppression of noxious stimulus-evoked expression of FOS protein-like immunoreactivity in rat spinal cord by a selective cannabinoid agonist. Neuroscience 1996; 70:791–798.
80. Richardson JD, Aanonsen L, Hargreaves KM. Antihyperalgesic effects of spinal cannabinoids. Eur J Pharmacol 1998; 345:145–153.
81. Hohmann AG, Martin WJ, Tsou K, Walker JM. Inhibition of noxious stimulus-evoked activity of spinal cord dorsal horn neurons by the cannabinoid WIN 55,212-2. Life Sci 1995; 56:2111–2118.

82. Chapman V. The cannabinoid CB_1 receptor antagonist, SR141716A, selectively facilitates nociceptive responses of dorsal horn neurones in the rat. Br J Pharmacol 1999; 127:1765–1767.
83. Richardson JD, Kilo S, Hargreaves KM. Cannabinoids reduce hyperalgesia and inflammation via interaction with peripheral CB_1 receptors. Pain 1998; 75:111–119.
84. Calignano A, La Rana G, Giuffrida A, Piomelli D. Control of pain initiation by endogenous cannabinoids. Nature 1998; 394:277–281.
85. Lynn AB, Herkenham M. Localization of cannabinoid receptors and nonsaturable high-density cannabinoid binding sites in peripheral tissues of the rat: implications for receptor-mediated immune modulation by cannabinoids. J Pharmacol Exp Ther 1994; 268:1612–1623.
86. Facci L, Dal Toso R, Romanello S, Buriani A, Skaper SD, Leon A. Mast cells express a peripheral cannabinoid receptor with differential sensitivity to anandamide and palmitoylethanolamide. Proc Natl Acad Sci USA 1995; 92:3376–3380.
87. Snider WD, McMahan SB. Tackling pain at the source: new ideas about nociceptors. Neuron 1998; 20:629–632.
88. Friedel RH, Schnurch H, Stubbusch J, Barde Y. Identification of genes differentially expressed by nerve growth factor and neurotrophin-3 dependent sensory neurons. Proc Natl Acad Sci USA 1997; 94:12670–12675.
89. Hohmann AG, Herkenham M. Localization of central cannabinoid CB_1 receptor messenger RNA in neuronal subpopulations of rat dorsal root ganglia: a double-label in situ hybridization study. Neuroscience 1999; 90:923–931.
90. Hohmann AG, Herkenham M. Cannabinoid receptors undergo axonal flow in sensory nerves. Neuroscience 1999; 92:1171–1175.
91. Pertwee RG, Fernando SR. Evidence for the presence of cannabinoid CB_1 receptors in mouse urinary bladder. Br J Pharmacol 1996; 118:2053–2058.
92. Ratliff TL, Klutke CG, Hofmeister M, He F, Russell JH, Becich MJ. Role of the immune response in interstitial cystitis. Clin Immunol Immunopathol 1995; 74:209–216.
93. Mazzari S, Canella R, Petrelli L, Marcolongo G, Leon A. *N*-(2-Hydroxyethyl)hexadecanamide is orally active in reducing edema formation and inflammatory hyperalgesia by down-regulating mast cell activation. Eur J Pharmacol 1996; 300:227–236.
94. Bisogno T, Maurelli S, Melck D, De Petrocellis L, Di Marzo V. Biosynthesis, uptake, and degradation of anandamide and palmitoylethanolamide in leukocytes. J Biol Chem 1997; 272:3315–3323.
95. Jaggar SI, Hasnie FS, Sellaturay S, Rice ASC. The anti-hyperalgesic actions of the cannabinoid anandamide and the putative CB_2 agonist palmitoylethanolamide investigated in models of visceral and somatic inflammatory pain. Pain 1998; 76:189–199.
96. Jaggar SI, Sellaturay S, Rice ASC. The endogenous cannabinoid anandamide, but not the CB_2 ligand palmitoylethanolamide, prevents the viscero-visceral hyper-reflexia associated with inflammation of the rat urinary bladder. Neurosci Lett 1998; 253:123–126.
97. Smith FL, Fujimore K, Lowe J, Welch SP. Characterisation of delta^9 tetrahydrocannabinol and anandamide antinociception in nonarthritic and arthritic rats. Pharmacol Biochem Behav 1998; 60: 183–191.
98. Herzberg U, Eliav E, Bennett GJ, Kopin IJ. The analgesic effects of *R*(+)-WIN55,212-2 mesylate, a high affinity cannabinoid agonist, in a rat model of neuropathic pain. Neurosci Lett 1997; 221: 157–160
99. Farquhar–Smith WP, Jaggar SI, Rice ASC. The endogenous cannabinoid anandamide attenuates nerve growth factor induced hyper-reflexia in a model of visceral hyperalgesia. 9th World Congress of Pain Abstracts, 1999:524.
100. Farquhar–Smith WP, Jaggar SI, Rice ASC. Cannabinoids attenuate NGF-induced viscero-visceral hyper-reflexia (VVH) via CB_1 and CB_2 receptors. Soc Neurosci Abstr 1999; 25:924.
101. Felder CC, Briley EM, Axelrod J, Simpson JT, Mackie K, Devane WA. Anandamide, an endogenous cannabimimetic eicosanoid, binds to the cloned human cannabinoid receptor and stimulates receptor-mediated signal transduction. Proc Natl Acad Sci USA 1993; 90:7656–7660.
102. Felder CC, Joyce KE, Briley EM, Mansouri J, Mackie K, Blond O, Lai Y, Ma AL, Mitchell RL.

Comparison of the pharmacology and signal transduction of the human cannabinoid CB_1 and CB_2 receptors. Mol Pharmacol 1995; 48:443–450.

103. Bayewitch M, Avidor Reiss T, Levy R, Barg J, Mechoulam R, Vogel Z. The peripheral cannabinoid receptor: adenylate cyclase inhibition and G protein coupling. FEBS Lett 1995; 375:143–147.
104. Showalter LA, Compton DR, Martin BR, Abood ME. Evaluation of binding in a transfected cell line expressing a peripheral cannabinoid receptor (CB_2): identification of cannabinoid receptor subtype selective ligands. J Pharmacol Exp Ther 1996; 278:989–999.
105. Ross RA, Templeton F, Green A, Pertwee RG. L759633, L759656 and palmitoylethanolamide: are they CB_2 selective agonists? 1998 Symposium on the Cannabinoids, Burlington, VT:International Cannabinoid Research Society 1998:83.
106. Richardson JD, Aanonsen L, Hargreaves KM. SR141716A, a cannabinoid receptor antagonist, produces hyperalgesia in untreated mice. Eur J Pharmacol 1997; 319:R3–4.
107. Beaulieu P, Punwar S, Farquhar-Smith WP, Rice ASC. Effects of cannabinoid receptor antagonists on the formalin test in rats. 9th World Congr Pain Abstr 1999:523.
108. Ledent C, Valverde O, Cossu G, Petitet F, Aubert JF, Beslot F, Bohme GA, Imperato A, Pedrazzini T, Roques BP, Vassart G, Fratta W, Parmentier M. Unresponsiveness to cannabinoids and reduced addictive effects of opiates in CB_1 receptor knockout mice. Science 1999; 283:401–404.
109. Zimmer A, Zimmer AM, Hohmann AG, Herkenham M, Bonner TI. Increased mortality, hypoactivity, and hypoalgesia in cannabinoid CB_1 receptor knockout mice. Proc Natl Acad Sci USA 1999; 96:5780–5785.

9

Pain Processing in the Periphery

Development of Analgesics

Andy Dray
AstraZeneca R&D Montreal, Montreal, Quebec, Canada

I. INTRODUCTION

All tissues, with the exception of the neuropil, of the central nervous system (CNS) are innervated by fine afferent C- and Aδ fibers. Under physiological circumstances many, but not all, of these sensory fibers act as nociceptors by responding to a range of noxious chemicals, to cold, to intense heat, and to pressure stimuli. Afferent fiber activity and the intensity of pain are directly related to the stimulus, but during a variety of pathological conditions, such as inflammation and nerve injury, this relation is lost. Pain signaling may become enhanced or spontaneous, poorly related to the stimulus and, therefore, no longer reliable or necessary as a physiological warning mechanism.

The chemical environment around receptive regions of the sensory neuron is the major factor that determines the ways in which nociception and pain processing are changed. Chemically receptive regions may be changed or new ones expressed by pathophysiological processes such as nerve injury or inflammation. The chemical products of inflammation and tissue damage induce *hyperalgesia* (an exaggerated response to a noxious stimulus) and *allodynia* (pain induced by stimuli that are normally innocuous). Activation and sensitization of peripheral nociceptors by a variety of chemical mediators partially accounts for this (1–3). But persistent alteration (''windup'' and central sensitization) of the central processing of sensory signals also occurs as a result of prolonged nociceptor activation. This allows signals from normally innocuous stimuli, such as gentle touch or stroking (mediated by large Aβ-fibers), to be abnormally processed and thus perceived as pain (4–6). In addition, peripheral nerve injuries induce spontaneous and abnormal electrical activity from the neuroma formed at the nerve lesion site, while ectopic activity is generated from undamaged sensory ganglion neurons, which may be remote from the injured site (6,7). These sites are also sensitive to exogenous chemicals and may be targeted for therapeutic intervention. More recently, postinjury-induced plasticity in postganglionic sympathetic fibers and the expression of adrenergic receptors have also been shown to influence afferent fiber excitability (8–9). Such activity also contributes to the spontaneous pain and abnormal sensitivity to innocuous stimuli that occur in painful neuropathies.

A variety of mechanisms account for the changes in peripheral and central pain processing. These range from changes in expression of sensory nerve neurochemistry, induced by changes in gene regulation, as well as abnormal, postinjury, sprouting and reorganization of afferent and sympathetic fibers. It is likely that most of these changes of cellular phenotype occur through a multitude of chemical interactions designed to rebalance excitability and begin the processes of tissue repair and regeneration. Simultaneously, these changes offer a variety of new targets on which to base strategies for effective chronic pain therapy (2,10,11); ideally encompassing aspects of symptomatic pain relief and tissue regeneration. These strategies are now being aggressively explored to offer safer and more effective alternatives to conventional analgesics.

II. WHY IS PERIPHERAL ANALGESIA DESIRABLE?

Analgesia may be approached simply and effectively by blocking afferent fibers and the initiation of pain signaling. This will also attenuate the peripheral input essential for the initiation and maintenance of central hyperexcitability. Ideally, exaggerated or abnormal nociception (hyperalgesia and allodynia) would be prevented and physiological nociception restored without the occurrence of sensory abnormalities. Other advantages of a peripheral analgesic over centrally mediated analgesic would be the absence of potential central side effects. New initiatives for peripheral analgesia have focused (1) on inhibiting the formation or preventing the actions of pathological chemical factors (e.g., inflammatory mediators) that are important for pain generation and (2) on ways, e.g. (ion channel blockers) to inhibit abnormal sensory nerve excitability associated with pathological pain. Several new approaches are in progress and some of these have been summarized in Table 1. This chapter will focus on only two of these targets, peripherally opioid receptors and vanilloid receptors.

III. PERIPHERAL OPIOIDS

Opioids inhibit nociception by attenuating transmission in the spinal cord (12) by acting on μ (MOR), δ (DOR), and κ (KOR) subtypes of receptors specifically located in the superficial dorsal horn as well as on central terminals of primary afferent fibers (13–15). Several studies have shown that opioid receptors are also expressed in the periphery. Thus, all three opioid receptor subtypes are made in primary sensory neurons (16) and can be visualized in fine cutaneous nerves (17–19). Although these receptors appear to be more abundant on small sensory neurons, they have also been reported to occur in larger fibers (20).

The occurrence of opioid receptors on periphery fibers has highlighted the possibility that they are present to modulate the excitability of sensory neurons and, thereby, may induce a local analgesia. However, their function, under physiological and pathophysiological conditions, requires further clarification. Under normal physiological conditions, where access to receptors may be denied by physical barriers, exogenously administered opioids may have little effect on nerve excitability and have little or no analgesic efficacy (21–24). However, if neural barriers are avoided (25,26) or receptors are exposed by mechanical nerve injury (27), disruption of the perineurial barriers by osmotic stress or by inflammatory mediators (18,28), then access of endogenous as well as exogenous opioids to receptors is facilitated with consequent functional changes in nerve activity.

Interestingly, opioid receptor expression in peripheral nerves and sensitivity to receptor-selective ligands is differentially modulated by pathology. There is an increased expression of MOR (16) during inflammation as well as a concomitant up-regulation of opioid peptide production and release from immune cells that become concentrated in the inflamed regions, often in close apposition to peripheral afferent nerve endings (29). Under these circumstances, there is

Table 1 Summary of Peripheral Pain Mechanisms and Potential Targets for New Analgesics

Peripheral mechanism	Peripheral target	Type of drug
Nociceptor activation	Sodium channels	TTX-s channel blocker
Ectopic activity (neuroma, DRG)		TTX-r (SNS, NaN) channel blocker
Nociceptor sensitization	Calcium channels	N-channel blocker
		L-channel blocker
	ASICs	Channel blocker
	P 2 × 3 receptor	Receptor antagonist
	VR1 receptor	Receptor agonist or antagonist?
	Opioid receptors	MOR, DOR, or KOR agonists
	Cannabinoid receptors	CBI and CB2 agonists
	Nicotinic receptors	Receptor agonist
	Adrenergic receptors	α_2-agonist
		α_1-antagonist
Nociceptor sensitization	Prostanoid receptors	EP, antagonist
	Prostanoid production	COX I/II inhibitors
	Serotonin receptors	5-HT_1D agonist
		5-HT_2 antagonist
	Kinin receptors	B1 antagonist
		B2 antagonists
	Glutamate receptors	NMDA antagonists
	NGF	Trk A receptor antagonist
	Cytokines	IL-1β receptor antagonist
		ICE inhibitor
	PKCγ	TNF-α receptor antagonist
		Kinase isotype inhibitor

TTX-s, tetrodotoxin-sensitive ion channel; TTX-r, tetrodotoxin-resistant ion channel; ASIC, acid-sensing ion channel; VR, vanilloid receptor; MOR, μ-opioid receptor; DOR, δ-opioid receptor; KOR, κ-opioid receptor; NGF, nerve growth factor; PKCγ, protein kinase C; ICE, interleukin-converting enzyme.

compelling data for analgesic effects of opioids (30) where μ, δ, and κ selective opioid ligands produce analgesia and anti-inflammatory activity by depressing afferent nerve excitability and the release of proinflammatory neurogenic factors, such as substance P. Such data suggest that endogenously released opioids have an important regulatory function to modulate sensory nerve excitability as well as the release of sensory chemotactic and trophic factors. Interestingly, inflammation in the viscera has been associated with striking overexpression of KOR rather than MORs (31), with KOR-selective rather than MOR-selective ligands producing analgesia to painful colorectal distention.

In keeping with the presence of receptors, MOR-selective ligands reduce the algesic effects and hyperresponsiveness produced by peripherally administered chemical excitants and irritants, including glutamate (17); prostaglandin-E_2 (PGE_2) (32), formalin (33), or capsaicin (34), and hyperexcitability of the primary afferent nerves produced by ultraviolet irradiation of the skin (35). These data are supported by studies in primates (34) as well as in humans (36–38). Thus, local subcutaneous (SC) administrations of low concentrations of MOR (DAMGO, fentanyl) and KOR (U-50488) agonists in the tail of the rhesus monkey reduce thermal allodynia induced by capsaicin sensitization (34). These effects were attenuated by the MOR antagonist quadazocine and quaternary naltrexone and by the κ-receptor antagonist norbinaltorphimine, respectively, when administered locally, but not systemically at the same dose.

Overall, data for the involvement of DORs in the modulation of afferent nerve excitability

Table 2 The MOR Tetrapeptide BCH-2687(−*H*-Tyr-D-Arg-Phe-Phe-NH_2) bishydrochloride salt is Highly Selective Toward Human MOR (nM)

	Receptor selectivity			*Analgesia*: *Mouse* (ED_{50}, μmol/kg SC)			
	hMOR/EC_{50}	μ/δ	μ/κ	Formalin	PBQ	Tail-flick	Hot plate
BCH-2687	0.68	2841	436	0.3	1.0	43	>170
Morphine	0.8	176	153	6.4	0.5	2.0	2.5

A mainly peripheral site of analgesic action is suggested by its higher efficacy in the formalin and phenyl quinone abdominal constriction (PBQ) assays, rather than tail-flick and hot plate assays which are indicative of central sites of action.

and the production of peripheral analgesia are less compelling because selective ligands for this receptor (e.g., DPDPE) were ineffective in several circumstances when administered locally (17,32,35). It is significant, however, that a highly selective DOR agonist, such as SNC80 produced analgesia in primates after systemic administration suggestive of a predominantly central site of action (39). This effect was attenuated by the DOR antagonist, naltridole, but not by the MOR antagonist quadazocine.

These findings have stimulated and underpinned the development of receptor-selective opioids for application as peripheral analgesics. Peripherally mediated analgesia would reduce typical central opioid side effects, including sedation, respiratory depression, dysphoria and dependence, and urinary retention. Further development of this concept has been provided by the development of the MOR-selective tetrapeptide BCH-2687 (Table 2), which has been suggested to induce a peripherally localized analgesia based on the differential potency in tests predictive of a peripheral (abdominal constriction), rather than a central, site of action. On the other hand, κ- rather than μ- or δ-selective opioid ligands were efficacious in suppressing activity in a number of visceral pain models (31,40,41). In particular, asimadoline (EMD-61753; Fig. 1), a peripherally selective κ agonist (42), has been projected as having therapeutic efficacy in visceral pain, as it attenuated painful colorectal distention in rats (31). Its effects, as well as

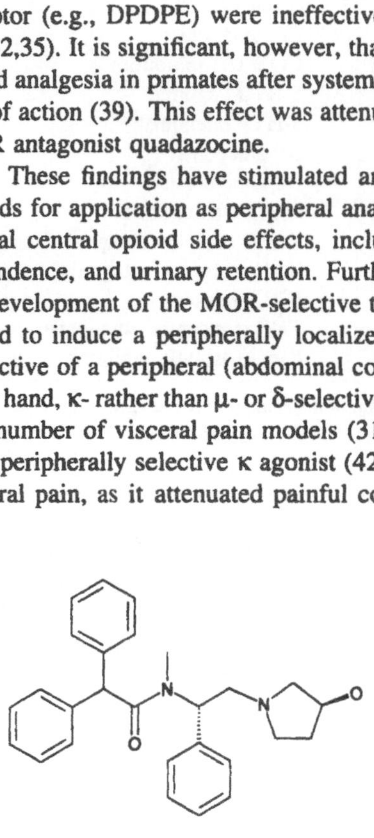

Receptor binding (RVD)	Formalin	MAC
IC_{50} = 54nM	3-10 mg kg p.o.	8.4 mg kg p.o.

Figure 1 In vitro and in vivo data showing asimiadoline (EMD-61753) activity in KOR assay in the rat vas deferens (RVD) and antinociceptive activity in the rat formalin and mouse abdominal constriction assay (MAC).

that of other KOR ligands, were naloxone-reversible but were not antagonized by KOR antagonists, such as norbinaltorphimine, indicating possible differences in peripheral and central KOR. Earlier studies with fedotozine, characterized as a peripheral κ agonist, with efficacy in the colorectal distention model (40) and in functional dyspepsia (43), reported efficacy in the gastric discomfort associated with irritable bowel syndrome (44).

A. Capsaicin and Resiniferatoxin

Capsaicin is a naturally occurring vanilloid (Fig. 2) that selectively *activates*, and at higher doses selectively *inactivates*, and ultimately damages, several types of fine sensory C and Aδ-fibers (45–47). Thus, application of capsaicin to skin or mucous membranes produces a burning pain, hyperalgesia, and allodynia, but after repeated administrations the initial pain is attenuated and conduction in nociceptors is blocked, leading to analgesia without any other sensory nerve deficit. These properties of capsaicin have been exploited to treat many painful conditions such as cluster headache and neuropathic pain, that are resistant to conventional analgesics (see Table 2) (48,49). Based on these and other findings the molecular mechanism of action of capsaicin has been vigorously persued to develop other vanilloids as novel peripheral treatments for chronic pain.

B. Therapeutic Efficacy of Capsaicin and Other Vanilloids

In humans intradermal injection or repeated topical application of capsaicin to the skin produces an initial concentration-dependent burning sensation and a flare response. The immediate area of capsaicin administration becomes insensitive to mechanical or thermal stimulation for several

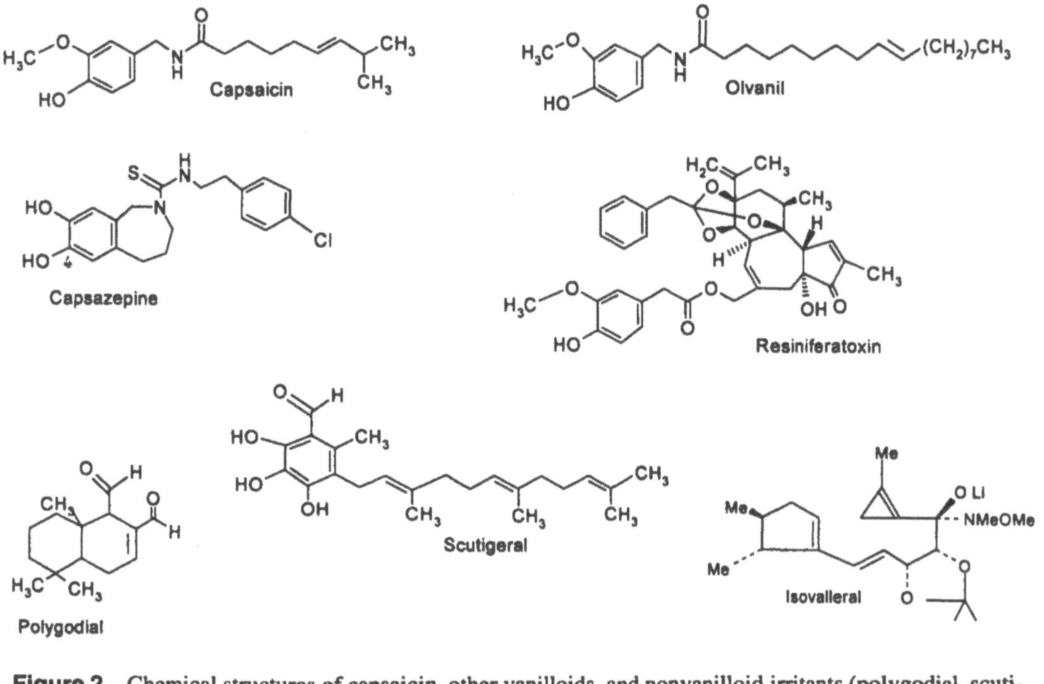

Figure 2 Chemical structures of capsaicin, other vanilloids, and nonvanilloid irritants (polygodial, scutigeral, isovalleral) that act on "vanilloid receptors."

Table 3 Clinical Tests in Which Topical or Locally Administered Capsaicin, Resiniferatoxin, or Other Vanilloids Improved Pain Scores

Capsaicin	Resiniferatoxin	Vanilloids
Pruritus		
Psoriasis		
Skin allergy		
Postherpetic neuralgia		
Diabetic neuropathy		
Rhinopathy		
Postmastectomy pain		
Stump pain		
Reflex sympathetic dystrophy		
Trigeminal neuralgia		
Oral mucositis		
Osteoarthritis		
Rheumatoid arthritis		
Cluster headache		
Fibromyalgia		
Urinary bladder hyperreflexia	Bladder hyperreflexia	
Cystitis pain	Cystitis pain	
Experimental burn pain		NE-21610

Source: Refs. 49, 62, 63, 69, 108.

hours, but within the area of the flare, a primary hyperalgesia develops, with increased pain to mechanical and thermal stimuli. Beyond the flare, an area of secondary (mechanical) allodynia develops (50–52) and is thought to be due to a central sensitization mechanism resulting from the capsaicin-induced C-fiber afferent barrage (53,54). Repeated topical administrations produces analgesia (50,55) and loss of flare responses to a variety stimuli only after several days or weeks of treatment (56,57).

Overall, analgesia produced by topical capsaicin appears variable and dependent on the amount of capsaicin that penetrates the skin (58–61) so that the frequency of capsaicin administration, as well as the choice of vehicle or formulation, are important. In addition instillation of capsaicin or another vanilloid, resiniferatoxin into the urinary bladder has been used to treat bladder hyperreflexia and bladder pain after spinal cord injury or cystitis, respectively (62,63), whereas topical capsaicin can also prevent itching in chronic pruritus (Table 3 for references).

Several improved vanilloid analogues have been developed that have also induced analgesia with a minimum of initial irritability, which often limits the therapeutic acceptability of capsaicin (see Fig. 2). These compounds include NE-19550 (olvanil), NE-21610 (nuvanil) (64–66), and nonivamide acetate (67,68). In humans, NE-21610 was much less excitatory than capsaicin and was effective in inhibiting burn-induced hyperalgesia and allodynia (69).

C. Mechanisms of Action of Capsaicin and Evidence for Receptors

Capsaicin induces concentration-dependent activation of fine afferent fibers and small sensory neurons, although effects on larger cells have also been acknowledged (70–72). Activation is due to membrane depolarization and an increase in membrane permeability to cations (73).

The analgesic, anti-inflammatory, and antipruritic effects of capsaicin are due to a block of nerve conduction in subsets of fine afferents, with a subsequent loss of responsiveness to sensory stimuli and spontaneous activity in these fibers (74,75). A combination of calcium-independent, calcium-coupled, and osmotically induced inactivation largely accounts for these neurogenic effects (47,76,77). Sensory fiber inactivation also induces a reversible inhibition of sensory neurotransmitter (neuropeptides, glutamate) release in the spinal cord and in the periphery (78,79). However the concentrations of sensory neurochemicals is not significantly affected, suggesting that loss of sensory transmission is not due to exhaustion of sensory neurochemicals and thus cannot be the major reason for capsaicin's therapeutic effects. These reversible effects should be distinguished from the irreversible neurotoxicity and neurochemical depletions that capsaicin can induce at high concentrations with repeated systemic doses (47,80).

D. Vanilloid Receptors

It is now clear that the actions of capsaicin and vanilloid analogues that account for the sensory effects and probably the therapeutic effects are mediated through specific membrane receptors on sensory fibers. The presence of such receptors was originally supported by structure–activity studies with vanilloid analogues (81–84) complemented by the use of resiniferatoxin (RTX) (see Fig. 2), obtained from the latex of ***Euphorbia resinifera***. [^{3}H]RTX showed specific, saturable, capsaicin-displaceable binding (85) localized to small sensory, but not sympathetic neurons, as well as binding to regions of the spinal dorsal horn and to various central sensory nuclei in the brain stem (e.g., nucleus of the solitary tract, area postrema, or trigeminal nucleus) (85,86). This highly potent irritant also activated small sensory neurons in a manner identical to that of capsaicin (46,87). Detailed analysis of RTX binding indicated that the receptor might exist as a multimeric complex of 270-kDa protein subunits, showing positive cooperativity, indicative of two interactive binding sites (85).

Further evidence for vanilloid receptors has come from studies using capsazepine (see Fig. 2) which reversibly and competitively inhibits the excitatory effects of capsaicin (47,88) as well as the secondary release of neuropeptides from sensory neurons (89,90). These studies also indicated differences in vanilloid receptors and possible receptor heterogeneity in different tissues. Thus, capsazepine was equipotent in displacing RTX binding from dorsal root ganglia and from the spinal cord and in blocking vanilloid-evoked sensory neuropeptide release, but much less potent in displacing RTX from airway binding (85,90). Indeed, there may be different receptors within populations of sensory neurons because capsaicin evoked at least two types of membrane activation in sensory neurons (91,92), while capsazepine attenuated only a proportion (early component) of the response to capsaicin, and *protected* this component from undergoing desensitization following prolonged exposure to capsaicin (93).

The likelihood of receptor heterogeneity has prompted the classification of vanilloid receptors into C- and R-receptor subtypes based on the relative differences in potency of capsaicin and RTX in stimulating calcium accumulation (C-type) or the binding of [^{3}H]RTX (R-type). In addition, capsazepine was less effective at inhibiting specific [^{3}H]RTX binding in sensory neurons than in inhibiting the functional responses (calcium uptake) to RTX and capsaicin (85,94). Interestingly, RTX produced potent desensitization of subsequent Ca^{2+} uptake at low concentrations, corresponding to an action by the high-affinity R-site. Because this site was not associated with neural activation or calcium accumulation, desensitization may be due to an intracellular metabolic mechanism. Thus, the R-receptor has also been considered as a metabotropic-signaling mechanism while C-type receptor activation an ionotropic mechanism. The properties of hypothetical C- and R-type receptor subtypes are summarized in Table 4.

A vanilloid receptor, VR1 has recently been cloned (95) and was found exclusively in small sensory neurons as an integral part of the nerve cell membrane. The receptor showed properties similar to those seen in earlier studies of cultured sensory neurons when characterized

Table 4 Properties of C-Type and R-Type Vanilloid Receptors and Comparison with Cloned VR1

	VR1	C-type	R-type
Capsaicin (K_d)	316 nM	270 nM	4900 nM
Resiniferatoxin (K_d)	1.3 nM	1 nM	0.04 nM
Cooperativity (Hill slope)	1.0	0.9–1.2	1.5–2.0
Capsazepine	300 nM	290 nM	4000 nM
Ruthenium red (IC_{50})	10 μM	800 nM	14 nM
Ca^{2+} uptake	Yes	Yes	No
Desensitization	Yes	Yes	Yes
Toxicity	Yes	Yes	No

Source: Refs. 95, 98.

with capsaicin, RTX, capsazepine, and ruthenium red. These characteristics suggest that VR1 is similar to the C-receptor subtype described earlier (see Table 4). As with the native receptor, VR1 undergoes desensitization when repeatedly challenged with capsaicin, and cell neurotoxicity was observed only in cells expressing VR1 (95).

The availability of the VR1 clone offers the opportunity for a larger chemical-screening effort to detect new molecules with affinity at VR1. It is likely that other nonvanilloids, such as polygodial and isovaleraldahyde (isovaleral) (see Fig. 2) will also provide novel chemical leads to characterize the "vanilloid receptor." On the other hand, vanilloids also affect cell types other than sensory neurons. Thus, earlier molecular-cloning work (96) indicated that the RTX-binding protein occurred in nonneural or vanilloid-insensitive neural tissues. More recent studies have indicated that capsaicin and RTX can interact with nonneuronal tissue, particularly mast cells (97) and C6 glioma cells (98), in a way similar to sensory neurons. However, in keeping with recent studies on sensory neurons (99), comparisons of RTX binding and agonistic activity (calcium accumulation) also indicate significant differences. Thus, capsaicin and RTX-induced Ca^{2+} uptake was attenuated by capsazepine and ruthenium red. However, no high-affinity RTX binding could be detected and the potency of RTX to produce selective desensitization of Ca^{2+} uptake corresponded to the classification of this site as a C-type receptor rather than an R-type (98) (see Table 4). The presence of receptors on cell types other than sensory neurons offers alternative methods for ligand-screening programs. Although highlighting receptor and mechanistic heterogeneity these studies also suggest that vanilloid effects on nonneural tissues should be taken into account when considering the selectivity of therapeutic action or, indeed, opportunities for other therapeutic interventions.

E. An Endogenous Vanilloid Ligand?

By analogy with other receptor systems, a natural ligand for the vanilloid-binding protein may exist. Protons have been proposed because they activate sensory neurons by a mechanism similar to that of capsaicin (100,101). Interestingly, protons are produced abundantly in pathological conditions, such as ischemia and inflammation, in which nociceptors may be activated or sensitized. However, it is now clear that there is only partial overlap between sensory fiber sensitivity to protons and to capsaicin (102–104). In addition, the mechanism of action differs because there was little evidence for cross-desensitization even though both protons and capsaicin increased intracellular calcium which was important for desensitization (104,105). Finally, application of protons to the cloned VR1 receptor was itself ineffective (95), but the effect of capsaicin was significantly potentiated, and protons lower the threshold for heat-induced activation of VR1 (106). These data suggest chemical synergies may be important for pain signaling in a pathological setting (107).

There are, however, also striking similarities between capsaicin-induced activation of the cloned VR1 receptor and the effects of heat stimuli, suggesting that the vanilloid receptor may also be a transducer of noxious heat (95,106). This may be a trivial explanation for the burning quality of capsaicin-containing foods and capsaicin-induced pain. However, these findings are difficult to reconcile with earlier observations that heat responsiveness remains unchanged following capsaicin desensitization and that capsazepine may selectively abolish capsaicin-induced sensory fiber activation without affecting heat-induced activation (45).

VI. SUMMARY AND CONCLUSIONS

Significant progress has been made toward characterizing the plastic changes that occur in nociceptive pathways during chronic pain conditions. This has caused a fundamental shift in the way that pain therapy and analgesic drug development are being approached. Mechanistic and molecular studies have highlighted a variety of new targets, ranging from inhibitors of inflammatory mediators and growth factors, to selective blockers of afferent fiber functions. Focusing the discovery and development effort toward peripheral mechanisms is strategically self-evident considering the primary importance that peripheral nerve fibers have in the generation of pain signals and in the regulation of central excitability. Ultimately, new types of analgesics with therapeutic and safety profiles superior to present compounds will become available. Amongst these compounds are likely to peripherally directed opioids and new compounds that selectively block sensory fibers through action on the vanilloid receptor. Clearly, the discovery of VR1 and the likelihood of other specific receptor subtypes offer increasing opportunities to understand and control pain signaling, neurogenic inflammation, and pruritus.

REFERENCES

1. Dray A. Tasting the inflammatory soup: the role of peripheral neurones. Pain Revi 1994; 1:153–171.
2. Rang HP, Bevan SJ, Dray A. Nociceptive peripheral neurones: cellular properties. In: Wall PD, Melzack R, eds. Textbook of Pain. Edinburgh: Churchill Linvingstone, 1994:57–78.
3. Levine JD, Fields HL, Basbaum AI. Peptides and the primary afferent nociceptor. J Neurosci 1993 13:2273–2286.
4. Gracely RH, Lynch SA, Bennett GJ. Painful neuropathy: altered central processing maintaining dynamically by peripheral input. Pain 1992; 51:175–194.
5. Woolf CJ, Doubell TP. The pathophysiology of chronic pain—increased sensitivity to low threshold Aβ-fibre inputs. Curr Biol 1994; 4:525–534.
6. Bennett GJ. Neuropathic pain. In: Wall PD, Melzack R, eds. Textbook of Pain. Edinburgh: Churchill Livingstone, 1994:210–224.
7. Devor M. The pathophysiology of damaged peripheral nerves. In: Wall PD, Melzack R, eds. Textbook of Pain. 3rd ed. Edinburgh: Churchill Livingstone, 1994:79–100.
8. McLachlan EM, Janig W, Devor M, Michaelis M. Peripheral nerve injuries triggers noradrenergic sprouting within dorsal root ganglia. Nature 1993; 363:543–546.
9. Chen Y, Michaelis M, Janig W, Devor M. Adrenoreceptor subtype mediating sympathetic–sensory coupling in injured sensory neurons. J Neurophysiol 1996; 76:3721–3730.
10. Dray A. Pharmacology of peripheral afferent terminals. In: Yaksh TL, et al., eds. Anesthesia. Biologic Foundations. Philadelphia: Lippincott–Raven, 1997:543–556.

11. Dray A, Urban L. New pharmacological strategies for pain relief. Annu Rev Pharmacol Toxicol 1996; 36:253–280.
12. Yaksh TL, Rudy TA. Narcotic analgesics: CNS sites and mechanisms of action as revealed by intracerebral injection techniques. Pain 1978; 4:299–359.
13. Arvidsson U, Riedl M, Chakabarti S, et al. Distribution and targeting of μ-opiod receptor (MOR-1) in brain and spinal cord, J Neurosci 1995; 15:3328–3341.
14. Arvidsson U, Dado RJ, Riedl M, et al. δ-Opioid receptor immunoreactivity; distribution in brainstem and spinal cord, and relationship to biogenic amines and enkephalin. J Neurosci 1995; 15:1215–1235.
15. Bess D, Lombard MC, Besson JM. Autoradiographic distribution targeting of μ, δ, and κ opioid binding sites in the superficial dorsal horn, over the rostrocaudal axis of the rat spinal cord. Brain Res 1991; 548:287–291.
16. Zhang Q, Schafer M, Elde R, Stein C. Effects of neurotoxins and hindpaw inflammation on opioid receptor immunoreactivities in dorsal root ganglia. Neuroscience 1998; 85:281–291.
17. Coggeshall RE, Zhou S, Carlton SM. Opioid receptors on peripheral sensory axons. Brain Res 1997; 764:126–132.
18. Hassan AHS, Ableiter A, Stein C, Herz A. Inflammation of the rat paw enhances axonal transport of opioid receptors in the sciatic nerve and increases their density in the inflamed tissue. Neuroscience 1993; 55:185–195.
19. Stein C, Hassan AHS, Przewlocki R, Gramsch C, Peter K, Hertz A. Opioids from immunocytes interact with receptors on sensory nerves to inhibit nociception in inflammation. Proc Natl Acad Sci USA 1990; 87:5935–5939.
20. Mansour A, Fox CA, Burke S, Akil H, Watson SJ. Immunohistochemical localization of the cloned mu opioid receptor in the rat CNS. J Chem Neuroanat 1995; 8:283–305.
21. Kosterlitz HW, Wallis DI. The action of morphine-like drugs on impulse transmission in mammalian nerve fibres. Br J Pharmacol 1964; 22:499–510.
22. Yuge O, Matsumoto M, Kitahata LM, Collins JG, Senami M. Direct opioid application to peripheral nerves does not alter compound action potentials. Anesth Analg 1985; 64:667–671.
23. Raja SN, Meyer RA, Campbell JN, Khan AA. Narcotics do not alter the heat response of unmeylinated primary afferents in monkeys. Anesthesiology 1986; 65:468–473.
24. Senami M, Aoki M, Kitahata LM, Collins JG, Kumeta Y, Murata K. Lack of opiate effects on cat C polymodal nociceptive fibers. Pain 1986; 27:81–90.
25. Jurna T, Grossmann W. The effect of morphine on mammalian nerve fibres. Eur J Pharmacol 1977; 44:339–348.
26. Kayser V, Gobeaux D, Lombard MC, Guilbaud G, Besson JM. Potent and long lasting antinociceptive effects after injection of low doses of a mu-opioid receptor agonist, fentanyl, into the brachial plexus sheath of the rat. Pain 1990; 42:215–225.
27. Frank GB, Sudha TS. Effects of enkephalin, applied intracellularly, on action potentials in vertebrate A and C nerve fibre axons. Neuropharmacology 1987; 26:61–66.
28. Antonijevic I, Mousa SA, Schafer M, Stein C. Perinurial defect and peripheral opioid analgesia during inflammation. J Neurosci 1995; 15:165–172.
29. Schafer M, Carter L, Stein C. Interleukin-1β and corticotrophin releasing factor inhibit pain by releasing opioids from immune cells in inflamed tissue. Proc Natl Acad Sci USA 1994; 91:4219–4223.
30. Stein C, Millan MJ, Shippenberg TS, Peter K, Herz A. Peripheral opioid receptors mediating antinociception in inflammation. Evidence for involvement of mu, delta, and kappa receptors. J Pharmacol Exp Ther 1989; 248:1269–1275.
31. Burton MB, Gebhart GF. Effects of kappa-opioid receptor agonists on responses to colorectal distension in rats with and without acute colonic inflammation. J Pharmacol Exp Ther 1998; 285:707–715.
32. Levine JD, Taiwo YO. Involvement of the mu-opiate receptor in peripheral analgesia. Neuroscience 1989; 32:571–575.

33. Hong Y, Abbott FV. Peripheral opioid modulation of pain and inflammation in the formalin test. Eur J Pharmacol 1995; 277:21–28.
34. Ko MC, Butelman ER, Wood JH. The role of peripheral mu opioid receptors in the modulation of capsaicin-induced thermal nociception in rhesus monkeys. J Pharmacol Exp Ther 1998; 286:150–156.
35. Andreev N, Urban L, Dray A. Opioids suppress spontaneous activity of polymodal nociceptors in rat paw skin induced by ultraviolet irradiation. Neuroscience 1994; 58:793–798.
36. Kinnman E, Nygards EB, Hansson P. Peripherally administered morphine attenuates capsaicin-induced mechanical hypersensitivity in humans. Anesth Analg 1997; 84:595–599.
37. Stein C. Peripheral analgesic actions of opioids. Pain Symp Manage 1991; 6:119–124.
38. Barber A, Gottschlich R. Opioid agonists and antagonists: An evaluation of their peripheral actions in inflammation. Med Res Rev 1992; 12:525–562.
39. Negus SS, Gatch MB, Zhang X, Rice K. Behavioral effects of the delta-selective opioid agonist SNC80 and related compounds in rhesus monkey. J Pharmacol Exp Ther 1998; 286:362–375.
40. Sengupta JN, Su X, Gebhart GF. kappa, But not mu or delta, opioid attentuate responses to distension of afferent fibres innervating the rat colon. Gastroenterology 1996; 111:968–980.
41. Su X, Sengupta JN, Gebhart GF. Effects of opioids on mechanosensitive pelvic nerve afferent fibres innervating the urinary bladder of the rat. J Neurophysiol 1997; 77:1566–1580.
42. Barber A, Bartoszyk GD, Bender HM, et al. A pharmacological profile of the novel, peripherally-selective κ-opioid receptor agonist, EMD 61753. Br J Pharmacol 1994; 113:1317–1327.
43. Read NW, Abitbol JL, Bardhan KD, Whorwell PJ. Efficacy and safety of peripheral kappa agonist fedotozine versus placebo in the treatment of functional dyspepsia. Gut 1997; 41:664–668.
44. Dapoigny M, Abitbol JL, Fraitag B. Efficacy of peripheral kappa agonist fedotozine versus placebo in treatment of irritable bowel syndrome: a multicenter dose–response study. Dig Dis Sci 1995; 40:2244–2249.
45. Dray A, Bettany J, Forster P. Actions of capsaicin on peripheral nociceptors of the neonatal rat spinal cord–trial in-vitro: dependence of extracellular and independence of second messengers. Br J Pharmacol 1990; 101:727–733.
46. Winter J, Dray A, Wood JN, Yeats JC, Bevan S. Cellular mechanism of action of resiniferatoxin: a potent sensory neuron excitotoxin. Brain Res 1990; 520:131–140.
47. Dray A. Neuropharmacological mechanisms of capsaicin and related substances. Biochem Pharmacol 1992; 44:611–615.
48. Campbell EA, Bevan S, Dray A. Clinical applications of capsaicin and its analogues. In: Wood J N, ed. Capsaicin in the Study of Pain. London: Academic Press, 1993:255–272.
49. Winter J, Bevan S, Campbell EA. Capsaicin and pain mechanisms. Br J Anaesth 1995; 75:157–168.
50. Simone DA, Baumann TK, Lamotte RH. Dose-dependent pain and mechanical hyperalgesia in humans after intradermal injection of capsaicin. Pain 1989; 38:99–107.
51. Magnusson BM, Koshinen LO. Effects of topical application of capsaicin to human skin: a comparison of effects evaluated by visual assessment, sensation registration, skin blood flow and cutaneous impedance measurements. Acta Derm Venereol 1996; 76:129–132.
52. Lamotte RH, Shian CN, Simone DA, Tsai E-Fun P. Neurogenic hyperalgesia: psychophysical studies of underlying mechanisms. J Neurophysiol 1991; 66:190–211.
53. Schmelz M, Schmidt R, Ringkamp M, Handwerker HO, Torebjork HE. Sensitization of intensive branches of C nociceptors in human skin. J Physiol 1994; 480:389–394.
54. Sang CN, Gracely RH, Max MB, Bennett GJ. Capsaicin-evoked mechanical allodynia and hyperalgesia cross nerve territories. Evidence for a central mechanism. Anesthesiology 1996; 85:491–496.
55. Beydoun A, Dyke DB, Morrow TJ, Casey KL. Topical capsaicin selectively attenuates heat pain and A delta fiber-mediated laser-evoked potentials. Pain 1996; 65:189–196.
56. Anand P, Bloom SR, McGregor GP. Topical capsaicin pretreatment inhibits axon reflex vasodilation caused by somatostatin and vasoactive intestinal peptide in human skin. Br J Pharmacol 1983; 78: 665–669.

57. Bjerring P, Arendt–Nielsen L. Inhibition of histamine skin flare reaction following repeated topical application of capsaicin. Allergy 1990; 45:121–125.
58. Kenins P. Response of single nerve fibres to capsaicin applied to the skin. Neurosci Lett 1982; 29: 83–88.
59. Carter RB, Francis WR. Capsaicin desensitisation to plasma extravasation evoked by antidromic C-fiber stimulation is not associated with antinocieption in the rat. Neurosci Lett 1991; 127:49–52.
60. Lynn B, Ye W, Cotsell B. The actions of capsaicin applied topically to the skin of the rat on C-fibre afferents, antidromic vasodilatation and substance P levels. Br J Pharmacol 1992; 107:400–406.
61. McMahon SB, Lewin G, Bloom SR. The consequences of long-term topical capsaicin application in the rat. Pain 1991; 44:301–310.
62. Lazzeri M, Beneforti P, Benaim G, Maggi CA, Lecci A, Turini D. Intravesical capsaicin for treatment of severe bladder pain: a randomized placebo controlled study. J Urol 1996; 156:947–952.
63. Chandiramani VA, Peterson T, Duthie GS, Fowler CJ. Urodynamic changes during therapeutic intravesical instillations of capsaicin. Br J Urol 1996; 77:792–797.
64. Brand L, Berman E, Schwen R, et al. NE-19550: a novel, orally active anti-inflammatory analgesic. Drugs Exp Clin Res 1987; 13:259–265.
65. Sietsema WK, Berman EF, Farmer RW, Maddin CS. The antinociceptive effect and pharmacokinetics of olvanil following oral and subcutaneous dosing in the mouse. Life Sci 1988; 43:1385–1391.
66. Dray A, Dickenson A. Systemic capsaicin and olvanil reduce the acute algogenic and the late inflammatory phase following formalin injection into rodent paw. Pain 1991; 47:79–83.
67. Yang JM, Wu BN, Chen IJ. Depressor response of sodium nonivamide acetate: a newly synthesised non-pungent analogue of capsaicin. Asia Pac J Pharmacol 1992; 7:95–102.
68. Chen IJ, Yang JM, Yeh JL, Wu BN, Lo YC, Chen SJ. Hypotensive and antinociceptive effects of ether-linked and relatively non-pungent analogues of *N*-nonanoyl vanillylamide. Eur J Med Chem 1992; 27:187–192.
69. Davis KD, Meyer RA, Turnquist JL, Fillon TG, Pappagallo M, Campbell JN. Cutaneous pretreatment with the capsaicin analog NE-21610 prevents the pain to a burn and subsequent hyperalgesia. Pain 1995; 62:373–378.
70. Petersen M, Lamotte RH. Relationship between capsaicin sensitivity of mammalian sensory neurons, cell size and type of voltage gated Ca-current. Brain Res 1991; 561:20–26.
71. Seno N, Dray A. Capsaicin induced activation of fine afferent fibres from rat skin in vitro. Neuroscience 1993; 55:563–569.
72. Liu W, Simon SA. Capsaicin and nicotine both activate a subset of rat trigeminal ganglion neurons. Am J Physiol 1996; 270:1807–1814.
73. Wood JN, Docherty R. Chemical activators of sensory neurons. Annu Rev Physiol 1997; 59:457–482.
74. Lynn B. Capsaicin: actions on C fibre afferents that may be involved in itch. Skin Pharmacol 1992; 5:9–13.
75. McMahon SB, Kotzenburg M. Itching for an explanation. Trends Neurosci 1992; 15:497–501.
76. Docherty RJ, Robertson B, Bevan S. Capsaicin causes prolonged inhibition of voltage-activated calcium currents in adult rat dorsal root ganglion neurons in culture. Neuroscience 1991; 40:513–521.
77. Bleakman D, Brorson JR, Miller RJ. The effects of capsaicin on voltage-gated calcium currents and calcium signals in cultured root ganglion cells. Br J Pharmacol 1990; 101:423–431.
78. Dray A, Hankins MW, Yeats JC. Desensitization and capsaicin-induced release of substance P like immunoreactivity (SPLI) from the guinea pig ureter in vitro. Neuroscience 1989; 31:479–483.
79. Dickenson AH, Ashwood N, Sullivan AF, James I, Dray A. Antinociception produced by capsaicin: spinal or peripheral mechanism? Eur J Pharmacol 1990; 187:225–233.
80. Holzer P. Capsaicin: cellular targets, mechanisms of action, and selectivity for thin sensory neurons. Pharmacol Rev 1991; 43:143–201.
81. Szolcsányi J, Jancsó–Gábor A. Sensory effects of capsaicin congeners. I. Relationships between

chemical structure and pain producing potency of pungent agents. Arzneimittelforschung/Drug Res 1975; 25:1877–1881.
82. Walpole CSJ, Wrigglesworth R, Bevan S, et al. Analogues of capsaicin with agonist activity as novel analgesic agents; structure–activity studies. 1. The amide bond "B-region." J Med Chem 1993; 36:2373–2380.
83. Walpole CSJ, Wrigglesworth R, Bevan S, et al. Analogues of capsaicin with agonist activity as novel analgesic agents; structure–activity studies. 1. The hydrophobic side-chain "C-region." J Med Chem 1993; 36:2381–2389.
84. Walpole CSJ, Wrigglesworth R, Bevan S, et al. Analogues of capsaicin with agonist activity as novel analgesic agents; structure–activity studies. 1. The hydrophobic side-chain "C-region." J Med Chem 1993; 36:2362–2372.
85. Szállási A. The vanilloid (capsaicin) receptor: receptor types and species differences. Gen Pharmacol 1994; 25:223–243.
86. Acs G, Palkovits M, Blumberg PM. [^{3}H]Resiniferatoxin binding by the human vanilloid (capsaicin) receptor. Brain Res Mol Brain Res 1994; 23:185–190.
87. Blumberg PM, Szallasi Z, Acs G. Resiniferatoxin—an ultrapotent capsaicin analogue. In: Wood JN, ed. Capsaicin in the Study of Pain. London: Academic, 1993:45–62.
88. Bevan SJ, Hothi S, Hughes GA, et al. Capsazepine: a competitive antagonist of the sensory neurone excitant, capsaicin. Br J Pharmacol 1992; 197:544–552.
89. Franco–Cereceda A, Lundberg JM. Capsazepine inhibits low pH—and lactic acid evoked release of calcitonin gene-related peptide from sensory nerves in guinea-pig heart. Eur J Pharmacol 1992; 221:183–184.
90. Wardle KA, Ranson J, Sange GJ. Pharmacological characterization of the vanilloid receptor in the rat dorsal spinal cord. Br J Pharmacol 1997; 121:1012–1016.
91. Peterson M, Lamotte RH, Klusch A, Kniffki KD. Multiple capsaicin-evoked currents in isolated rat sensory neurons. Neuroscience 1996; 75:495–505.
92. Liu L, Simon SA. Capsaicin-induced currents with distinct desensitization and Ca^{2+} dependence in rat trigeminal ganglion cells. J Neurophysiol 1996; 754:1503–1514.
93. Dray A, Patel IA, Naeem S, Rueff A, Urban L. Studies with capsazepine on peripheral nociceptor activation by capsaicin and low pH: evidence for a dual effect of capsaicin. Br J Pharmacol 1992; 107:236P.
94. Acs G, Palkovits M, Blumberg PM. Comparision of [^{3}H] resiniferatoxin binding by the vanilloid (capsaicin) receptor in dorsal root ganglia, spinal cord, dorsal vagal complex, sciatic and vagal nerve and urinary bladder of the rat. Life Sci 1996; 55:1017–1026.
95. Caterina MJ, Schumacher MA, Tominaga M, Rosen TA, Levine JD, Julius D. The capsaicin receptor: a heat-activated ion channel in the pain pathway. Nature 1997; 389:816–824.
96. Ninkina NN, Willoughby JJ, Beech MM, Coote PR, Wood JN. Molecular cloning of a resiniferatoxin-binding protein. Brain Res Mol Brain Res 1994; 22:39–58.
97. Biro T, Maurer M, Modarres S, et al. Characterization of functional vanilloid receptors expressed by mast cells. Blood 1998; 91:1332–1340.
98. Biro T, Brodie C, Modarres S, Lewin NE, Acs P, Blumberg PM. Specific vanilloid responses in C6 rat glioma cells. Mol Brain Res 1998; 56:89–98.
99. Acs G, Biro T, Acs P, Modarres S, Blumberg PM. Differential activation and desensitization of sensory neurons by resiniferatoxin. J Neurosci 1997; 17:5622–5628.
100. Bevan S, Geppetti P. Protons: small stimulants of capsaicin-sensitive sensory nerves. Trends Neurosci 1994; 17:509–512.
101. Bevan S, Winter J. Nerve growth factor differentially regulates the chemosensitivities of cultured adult rat dorsal root ganglion neurons. J Neurosci 1995; 15:4918–4926.
102. Steen KH, Reeh PW, Anton F, Handwerker HO. Protons selectively induce lasting excitation and sensitization to mechanical structure of nociceptors in rat skin in vitro. J Neurosci 1992; 12:86–95.
103. Baumann TK, Burchiel KJ, Ingram SL, Martenson ME. Responses of adult human dorsal root ganglion neurons in culture to capsaicin and low pH. Pain 1996; 65:31–38.

104. Chen X, Belmonte C, Rang HP. Capsaicin and carbon dioxide act by distinct mechanisms on sensory nerve terminal in the cat cornea. Pain 1997; 70:23–29.
105. García-Hirschfeld J, López-Briones LG, Belmonte C, Valdeolmillos M. Intracellular free calcium responses to protons and capsaicin in cultured trigeminal neurons. Neuroscience 1995; 67:235–243.
106. Tominaga M, Caterina MJ, Malmberg AB, et al. The cloned capsaicin receptor integrates multiple pain-producing stimuli. Neuron 1998; 21:531–543.
107. Vyklicky L, Knotkova-Urbancova H, Vitaskova Z, Vlachova V, Kress M, Reeh PW. Inflammatory mediators at acidic pH activate capsaicin receptors in cultured sensory neurons from newborn rats. J Neurophysiol 1998; 79:670–676.
108. Hautkappe M, Roizon MF, Toledano A, Roth S, Jeffries JA, Ostermeir AM. Review of the effectiveness of capsaicin for painful cutaneous disorders and neural dysfunction. Clin J Pain 1998; 14:97–106.

10

Neuroimaging of Pain

Possibilities of Objective Measurements of Analgesic Actions in Human Subjects

David Borsook, Lino Becerra, Alison Comite, Gil Gonzalez, and Hans Breiter
Massachusetts General Hospital and Harvard Medical School, Boston, Massachusetts, U.S.A.

I. INTRODUCTION

A major pursuit in neurobiology is to understand the mechanism by which the organism reacts to sensory information. Central nervous system (CNS) regions, from peripheral nerve to cortex, activated by painful stimuli can be defined using electrophysiological recordings or markers of activity, such as the immediate early gene *fos* (Hunt et al., 1987). Animal studies are limited because it is difficult to quantify affective responses to pain, and they may not completely model the human experience. Recent advances in neuroimaging techniques offer tools to understand integrative neuronal processing in acute and chronic pain. Plastic changes producing alterations in sensory processing in patients with neuropathic pain (Flor et al., 1994; Borsook et al., 1998), the potential objective measurement of the chronic pain state (Iadarola et al., 1995), and the objective response to analgesic actions are potential areas of investigation.

Positron emission tomography (PET), and more recently, functional magnetic resonance imaging (fMRI), have produced some exciting insights into human brain function (Friston, 1998; Breiter et al., 1997). In clinical conditions of chronic pain, we have been limited in our ability to understand a particular patient's problem because of the lack of objective tests for pain. Furthermore, we are unaware of possible CNS changes that may take place over time in patients with chronic pain either as a natural process or as a result of pharmacological or other therapeutic interventions. Examples include repeated headaches producing a chronic headache syndrome; the onset and offset of painful conditions, such as phantom pain: and possible changes in the brain state associated with pain, such as depression. All these conditions have an underlying neurobiological basis, which we are only beginning to understand. Objective measurements of pain in human subjects, as determined by mapping patterns of neural activation, may provide novel insights into the state of the brain in pain.

II. IMAGING OF PAIN

A. Imaging Acute Pain

Imaging the CNS during a noxious stimulus is a relatively new area of research. Nevertheless, the value of exploring alterations of CNS function in human subjects is evident owing to significant contributions already made. For example, functional imaging has helped resolve the debate over such issues as whether or not the somatosensory cortex (SI) contributes to pain perception, and the role of the cingulate cortex in pain or unpleasantness. The first PET imaging of pain was reported in 1990. Two groups independently published PET data on CNS activation following a noxious thermal stimulus (Talbot et al., 1991; Jones et al., 1991). The only area showing common CNS activation in these two studies was the anterior cingulate cortex, (ACC) a region that has been implicated in pain suffering in clinical studies (Hurt and Ballantyne, 1974). Many CNS regions known from anatomical and physiological studies to be involved in pain processing (Willis et al., 1985) have been now shown in PET studies to be activated in various acute pain paradigms (Talbot et al., 1991; Coghill et al., 1994; Rainville et al., 1997).

Following initial reports of patterns of activation in regions such as the cingulate and somatosensory cortex, further studies were designed to try to understand the specificity of this activation. Do these regions activate only to noxious painful stimuli, or are they part of a generalized pattern of CNS activation following a stressor? Two reports have addressed this issue. The first, by Bushnell and colleagues at the Montreal Institute, showed that some regions, such as the insula, are specifically activated by pain when compared with vibration (Coghill et al., 1994). The second showed differences in pain intensity versus pain unpleasantness (the latter is thought to correlate in some manner with suffering) (Rainville et al., 1997). Levels of activation in the anterior cingulate cortex are greater with increased perceived levels of pain unpleasantness, but there is little change in levels of pain intensity in regions of the cortex (SI) that should correlate with pain intensity. In both cases, these novel approaches to investigating the pain system contribute to our knowledge of patterns of activation that may be specific to clinically related conditions, such as suffering or the specificity of CNS regions activated by pain.

B. Imaging Chronic Pain

Chronic pain of neuropathic origin results from damage to the peripheral or central nervous system. There is evidence of altered neural processing of sensory information following certain painful conditions, such as phantom pain (Flor et al., 1994; Ramachandran et al., 1992, 1995). One of the problems with functional imaging is the measurement of basal pain levels in patients with pain because of the requirement for a comparative baseline (i. e., an "on" state and an "off" state). In other words, the paradigm requires either the removal of the pain with an analgesic or exacerbation of the pain to compare alterations in cerebral blood flow (CBF). With use of PET, paired comparisons of rCBF were made between the patient's habitual pain state and the pain-alleviated state following a nerve block with lidocaine (Hsieh et al., 1995). Neuropathic pain, as determined by this approach, resulted in activation of bilateral anterior insula, posterior parietal, lateral inferior prefrontal, and posterior cingulate cortices, as well as the posterior sector of the right anterior cingulate cortex, regardless of the side of the pain. In addition, a reduction in rCBF was noted in the contralateral posterior thalamus, as seen in Iadarola's study. However, no significant change of rCBF was detected in the somatosensory areas (SI and SII), but there was preferential activation of the right ACC, regardless of the side of the pain's origin, which suggests that affective–motivational circuitry can be defined in chronic ongoing neuropathic pain.

Central pain or the "centralization of neuropathic pain" is not completely understood (see Birbaumer et al., 1995). Putative theories such as CNS hyperactivity or disinhibition have been described (Dejerine and Roussy, 1906; Head and Holmes, 1911; Flor et al., 1994). In attempts to understand what may be taking place in the CNS in human subjects, PET-imaging techniques have been used in patients with chronic neuropathic or cancer pain (Cesaro et al., 1991; Hirato et al., 1991, 1993, 1994; Derbyshire et al., 1994; Chabriat et al., 1992; DeSalles and Bittal, 1994; Iadarola et al., 1995; Hsieh et al., 1995). These early PET studies in patients with central pain have provided interesting data. Perhaps the most interesting contribution neuroimaging has made to the pain field (from a clinical point of view) comes from two studies of patients with neuropathic pain showing that there is a decrease in activity of the contralateral thalamus in these conditions (Iadarola et al., 1996; Hsieh et al., 1996). Such specificity of CNS patterns of activation in a clinical condition is one of the major focal points of future imaging of pain. Clearly, these early papers show that reliable results can be obtained with PET; therefore, similar findings should be easily demonstrated in fMRI.

There are a limited number of magnetoencephalographic (MEG) studies on chronic pain in humans. Despite the paucity of studies, one group has provided evidence for significant cortical reorganization (plasticity) in patients with amputation phantom arm pain using MEG recordings (Flor et al., 1995, 1997). In amputees who did not have phantom pain, no cortical reorganization was evident. The study suggests the possibility that phantom pain might be a consequence of plastic changes in the somatosensory cortex. Similar results were seen in animal studies revealing massive cortical reorganization after sensory deafferentation in adult macaques (Pons et al., 1991). It raises the question whether chronic neuropathic pain states share a pathophysiology linked to a common CNS plasticity (e.g., loss of inhibitory circuitry). None of these PET studies have yet demonstrated alterations in CNS regions that may be involved in altered behaviors (e.g., depression, reward circuitry) that are obvious targets of drug action. However, MEG studies have clearly demonstrated reversal of plasticity of cortical representation following peripheral blockade (Birbaumer et al., 1997).

At a neurobiological level, little is known about the plasticity of central reorganization (owing to sprouting, altered synaptic strength, or new connections) outside the spinal cord, although recent work has shown interesting changes in the thalamus (Davis et al., 1998). Presumably, events similar to those demonstrated in the spinal cord may take place all along the neuraxis. However, we have seen changes based on methods reported by Ramachandran and colleagues (Ramachandran et al., 1992, 1995). Such changes appear to be present immediately after amputation (Borsook et al., 1998); furthermore, blockade of pain in such patients reverses the cortical plasticity (Flor et al., 1997). CNS "neural plasticity" in neuropathic pain is not well understood and may be common to all patients with neuropathic pain.

III. PET IMAGING OF ANALGESIC DRUG ACTION

Opioids have been used in at least two PET studies in which subjects were given a single dose of either morphine (Jones et al., 1991) or fentanyl (Firestone et al., 1994). Morphine both decreases cerebral blood flow (Matsumiya and Dohi, 1983) or increases blood flow in specific CNS regions (Koskinen and Bill, 1983) in experimental animal models. More recent work has demonstrated that morphine produces a decrease in metabolic activity in rats in limbic structures such as the diagonal band of Broca, lateral septum, bed nucleus of the stria terminalis, horizontal limb of the diagonal band, habenular complex, and medial amygdala (Gescuk et al., 1994). In one study on the effects of fentanyl on CNS activity using PET, a significant increase in regional cerebral blood flow, consistent with regional neuronal activation, was shown in both cingulate and orbitofrontal and medial prefrontal cortices, as well as caudate nuclei, and decreases were found bilaterally in frontal and temporal areas and the cerebellum (Firestone et al., 1995).

Naloxone, a specific μ-antagonist, has no effect on normal subjects, but may have some effect on patients or animal models of neuropathic pain (Desmeules et al., 1993). However, naloxone reduces placebo-induced analgesia (Levine et al., 1978). Naloxone fails to produce any changes in cerebral metabolism in rats (Fanelli et al., 1988).

PET allows examination of chemical neurotransmission in the brain. Of key importance for PET research on neuroreceptors is the development of suitable radiolabeled tracers (ligands). A large problem in drug discovery is to find relevant in vitro or in vivo animal models and to be able to extrapolate the results to humans. Drug research now benefits from the fast development of imaging technologies that trace radiolabeled molecules directly in the human brain. PET and allied techniques use molecules that are labeled with short-lived radioisotopes and injected intravenously. The most straightforward approach is to radiolabel a new potential drug and then to trace its anatomical distribution and binding in the brain. An indirect approach is to study how the unlabeled drug inhibits specific radioligand binding. The demonstration of quantitative relations between drug binding in vivo and drug effects in patients is used to validate targets for drug action and to optimize clinical treatment (Farde, 1996).

Recently, it has been possible to quantify opioid receptors in vivo, as appropriate radioligands have been synthesized for PET studies. In rhesus monkeys, regional distribution of [^{11}C]pethidine showed high levels in the thalamus, a region known to have high levels of μ-opioid receptors; other areas involved in pain modulation were not investigated (Hartvig et al., 1990). The opioid ligands [^{11}C]diprenorphine (Jones et al., 1994) and [^{11}C]carfentanil (Titlier et al., 1989) have been used to image opioid receptor distribution in the human brain. In such studies, receptor density, affinity, and occupancy have been measured and, therefore, delineate direct pharmacological access to the endogenous opioid system in the human CNS. Few studies have looked at altered receptor binding in subjects with pain (Jones et al., 1994). In one such study, opioid receptors binding in four patients with rheumatoid arthritis were studied with and without pain. Increases in [^{11}C]diprenorphine binding was seen in association with the reduction of pain, suggesting that there are increases in binding during inflammatory pain.

IV. ISSUES WITH fMRI METHODOLOGIES

Magnetic resonance imaging (MRI) has now evolved to measure changes CNS activity, and it has an increasingly higher resolution, as more powerful magnets are available. MRI captures CNS anatomy in exquisite detail. Current limitations of magnetic field strength and correlation of vascular changes with neuronal activity still require further exploration. However, fMRI is available in most medical centers and there are no issues of ionizing radiation. Therefore, it is an ideal method to measure CNS changes over time.

fMRI uses blood oxygenation level-dependent (BOLD) image contrast (De Yoe et al., 1994). This measurement depends on the properties of hemoglobin to measure changes in blood flow, volume, or oxygenation in regions of the CNS activated by a particular paradigm. Only recently has a model been proposed to interpret fMRI signal changes in terms of these changes (VanZijl et al., 1998). During fMRI acquisition, the magnetic field aligns dipoles of protons of water that induces a static magnetization parallel to the magnetic field. A pulsed magnetic field is then introduced into the plane perpendicular to the static field. Following the pulse, the magnetization relaxes back to the static magnetic field and a changing magnetic flux is measured and spatially encoded. Because there are differences in relative water content of regions of the CNS,

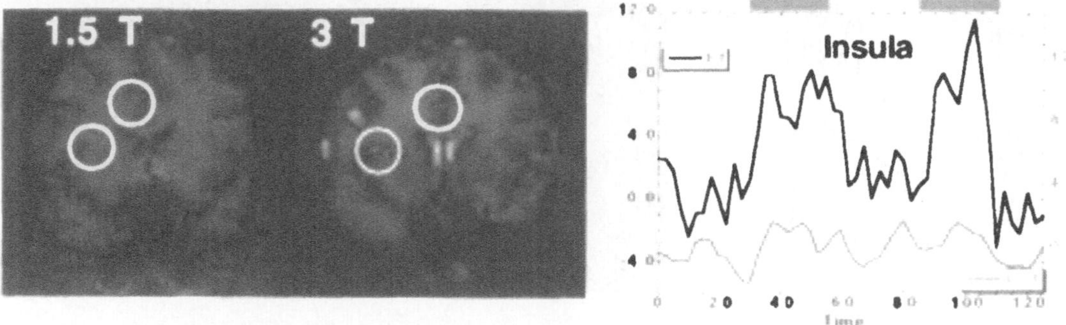

Figure 1 Differences in activation in insula and cingulate cortex following painful electrical stimulation to the forearm in the same individual at the same intensity (VAS 7/10 on a visual analog scale).

structures can be spatially mapped. There are two relaxation rates: the first is the rate of equilibrium toward the static field, and the second is the loss of magnetization from the pulsed field. It is the sensitivity of the second relaxation rate that is the basis of BOLD, which can measure physiological changes in blood (which has magnetic properties). Neurons induce focal increases in blood flow and volume, and this is measured on the foregoing basis.

Current measurement of fMRI signal changes are small (1–4%). In early fMRI responses to visual or acoustic stimuli (e.g., Bandettini et al., 1992), a clear correlation between the magnitude of the response and stimulus intensity was demonstrated. This is why many fMRI paradigms use repeated stimuli that may improve the sensitivity.

Stronger magnets are currently available and it is clear that the signal/noise ratio is improved, permitting greater resolution in fMRI experiments. Subjects who experience the same experimental paradigm at both 1.5 and 3 tesla show increased signal changes and greater resolution at 3 T. Figure 1 shows these changes in image and also in the percentage of signal change for the paradigm.

A. fMRI Studies of Pain

1. fMRI of Acute (Experimental) Pain

There are only a few reports of the use of fMRI in acute models of pain (Davis et al., 1995, 1997; Becerra et al., 1998). The first fMRI report of pain, used electrical stimulation, and demonstrated activation in the cingulate cortex and the somatosensory cortex (Davis et al., 1995). We have completed studies in two cohorts of male subjects on the effects of noxious (46°C) and nonnoxious (41°C) heat on regional CNS activation (Becerra et al., 1998). We demonstrate, with a separate cohort, that the results obtained are reliable, consistent, and show similar regional activation in the CNS to noxious heat as previously demonstrated in PET studies (Coghill et al., 1994; Casey et al., 1994, 1996). The results suggest that fMRI may be used for individual subjects.

2. fMRI of Chronic Pain

There is now a single fMRI defining changes in the CNS associated with chronic pain. There is a single report on the use of fMRI in evaluation of a particular therapeutic approach (Kiriakopoulos et al., 1997).

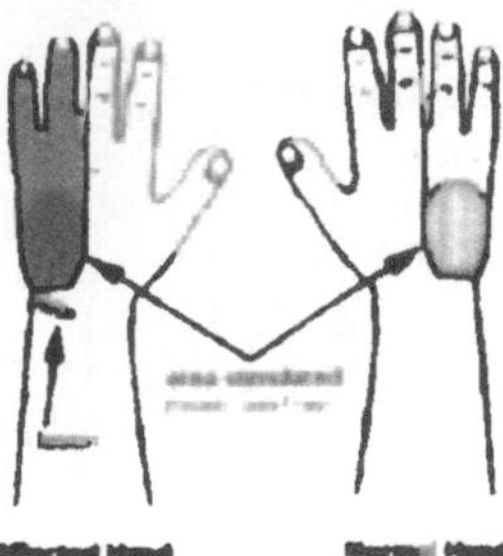

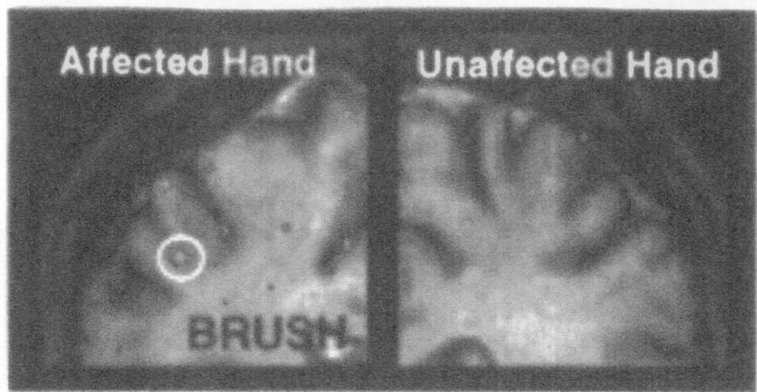

Figure 2 Activation by brush and von Frey hair in the SI cortex of patient with neuropathic pain of left hand. The left panel shows the area of neuropathic pain in the affected left-hand (dark) used to produce allodynia and the corresponding region used for parallel stimuli of brush and von Frey hairs. MRI images show activation in the SI for the affected hand following allodynia produced by brush. Note the activation in the cortex (white circle) representing the affected hand and not on the normal side. Even more profound activation was present following von Frey hair activation ($\rho = 8.3 \times 10^{-5}$) compared with activation of the unaffected hand ($\rho = 7.4 \times 10^{-3}$). Note that this data has not been tailaraiched and the sagittal localizing image shown identifies the slice that samples the SI cortex (black line and arrows).

3. Imaging Individual Patients with Neuropathic Pain: Is This Possible?

Currently, fMRI and PET analyses require averaging of data across subjects. One of the problems with imaging patients with clinical pain is that no two patients are alike and averaging data may distort the issue. We have begun studies to examine this problem, and the following example provides some insight into imaging individuals in pain (e.g., neuropathic pain of the hand). In a single patient with a neuropathic lesion of the dorsum of his left hand following a laceration wound involving nerve proximal to the wrist: brush and von Frey-induced hyperalgesia (allodynia; VAS = 8/10) was produced during fMRI recording. Before the fMRI scan the patient had undergone a careful neurological examination, sensory mapping, and sensory testing using brush and von Frey hairs. The sequences of activation was as follows: (1) right hand brush (stimulating the mirror region of the involved left hand); (2) left hand brush; (3) right hand von Frey hairs (again, stimulating the mirror area to show that he had neuropathic pain in his left hand); (4) left hand von Frey hairs. Figure 2 shows activation in SI contralateral to stimulation of the left hand, with no activation in the contralateral SI following stimulation of the intact hand. The data demonstrates our ability to image a patient with severe neuropathic pain involving the hand and, furthermore, that allodynia induced by von Frey hair or brush produces significant activation in the somatotopic region of the SI cortex. One of our objectives is to correlate activation seen following hyperalgesia and allodynia in neuropathic pain patients and demonstrate similarity in the circuits activated. Clearly, this would then allow us to determine the efficacy of analgesics on central pain processing in neuropathic pain conditions. In further support of the possible use of fMRI to determine analgesic action in single patients, we have recently shown that we can image the perceptual limb (i.e., the "representation of the phantom arm") in a single patient (Borsook et al., 1998).

B. fMRI Activation of CNS Regions by Analgesics: Proof of Concept for a Particular Drug

The ability to image the effectiveness of an analgesic action may provide an objective means of measuring analgesic action in various pain conditions. The nervous system generally responds to persistent drug-induced perturbations with compensatory adaptations. The precise adaptations to chronic stimulant administration, which might produce dependence, remain unknown. However, it has been hypothesized that the motivational components of drug dependence and withdrawal are produced by adaptations within the brain reward circuitry itself (Koob and Nestler, 1997; Nestler and Aghajanian, 1997). Drugs, such as morphine, that can induce physical dependence and withdrawal, are hypothesized to produce those effects in different regions of the CNS (when compared with cocaine, for example), including locus caeruleus (LC) neurons (Aghajanian, 1978; Rasmussen et al., 1990), hypothalamic neurons (Borsook et al., 1994), and their glutamatergic afferents (Akaoka and Aston–Jones, 1991) which appear to be the critical substrates of physical withdrawal from opiates. Finally, there is extensive literature on neuropathic pain responsiveness and nonresponsiveness to opioids (Dellemijn and Vanneste, 1997), but little is known about differences in CNS circuitry, if any, involved in these conditions (e.g., is there more activation of limbic circuitry versus somatotopic circuitry?).

1. Technical Issues in Measuring Drug Action Using fMRI

Our group has begun to define analgesic drug actions in acute and chronic pain using fMRI. Issues that need to be addressed relating to the action of a particular analgesic drug on CNS activation, include:

Drug Action on Cerebral Blood Flow (CBF). BOLD scanning uses venous oxygenation as an indirect marker of neuronal activation. Drugs may affect the CNS vessels directly or indirectly (e.g., owing to changes in heart rate and peripheral vascular resistance). Analgesics may act via neurotransmitters that have potent effects on vascular beds, including the CNS. Narcotic analgesics, such as morphine, affect blood flow. Infusions of drugs may produce a global decrease in CBF (Hoehner et al., 1993). CBF changes may alter the fMRI signal; however, a recent paper from our center has shown that a drug that clearly alters cerebral blood flow does not obscure regional activation using fMRI (Gollub et al., 1998).

Duration of Drug Action. Systemically injected narcotic analgesics have a relatively quick onset of action (within minutes of intravenous administration) and peak at near 10–15 min. The optimum time to measure analgesic effects becomes a paradigm problem. Here, fMRI has some advantages over PET, in that repeated-imaging samples may be performed over hours. However, novel analgesics that would be ideal to test in this environment may not have well-defined kinetics.

Measuring Analgesic Action Versus Nonspecific Effects. Differentiating analgesia versus other potential effects of a drug (e.g., euphoria) may be difficult to control for.

Correlation of Biological Effects. We also see that significant biological effects correlate with the clinical perception: a decrease in pain intensity scores follows analgesic administration. Analgesics may produce large signal changes in the brain stem as a result of increases in $ETco_2$ (hypercapnia produces midbrain activation) (Gozal et al., 1994).

Physiological Monitoring of Subjects. Continuous physiological monitoring of heart rate, systolic and diastolic blood pressure, and expired CO_2 can be performed utilizing the MRI compatible in vivo monitor for subject safety and interpretation of global arousal or anxiety.

Psychophysical Measurements of Painful Stimuli. The Verbal Analog Score (VAS) from 0–10 can be used to quantitate the subjective response to painful stimuli (Price et al., 1983; see also Price, 1994). Currently, we have found that it is difficult to obtain subject's response while the scan is in progress, but it is suitable to collect data immediately following fMRI acquisition.

Pulse Oximetry and Heart Rate. Heart rate has been routinely used as a measure of sympathetic response to noxious stimuli during anesthesia and surgery. In our preliminary studies we observed no correlation between heart rate and CBF changes, which coincides with previous PET studies (Coghill et al., 1994). Heart rate, using a specialized gated ECG monitor designed for use in MRI can be used, thereby eliminating the risk of interference and potential burns. Routine pulse oximetry monitoring, designed to be used in the magnet (Patteson et al., 1992), can also be used in studies of opioid action for which the risk of hypoxemia exists (Neil et al., 1987).

V. CONCLUSIONS

Once we have a more stringent method of evaluating activation of the normal nervous system to pain, we will be in a position to determine the efficacy of pharmacological agents in both normal volunteers by using surrogate models of painful conditions (e.g., capsaicin-induced hyperalgesia). Furthermore, the ability to provide objective evidence of a particular action of a drug will allow us to evaluate drugs with a small patient population (10–20 individuals). Such testing can take place in subjects with a variety of acute or chronic pain states, including arthritis, hyperalgesia, and central or peripheral neuropathic pain. This will be particularly so if a specific signature for pain is confirmed (e.g., hypoactivity in the thalamus).

REFERENCES

Aghajanian GK. Tolerance of locus coeruleus neurons to morphine and suppression of withdrawal response by clonidine. Nature. 1978; 276:186–188.

Akaoka H, Aston-Jones G. Opiate withdrawal-induced hyperactivity of locus coeruleus neurons is substantially mediated by augmented excitatory amino acid input. Neurosci 1991; 11:3830–3839.

Ballantine HTJr, Cassidy WL, Flanagan NB, Marino R Jr. Stereotaxic anterior cingulotomy for neuropsychiatric illness and intractable pain. Neurosurg 1967; 26:488–495.

Becerra LR, Breiter HC, Stojanovic M, Fishman S, Edwards A, Comite AR, Gonzalez RG, Borsook D. Human brain activation under controlled thermal stimulation and habituation to noxious heat: an fMRI study. Magn Reson Med 1999; 41:1044–1057.

Birbaumer N, Lutzenberger W, Montoya P, Larbig W, Unertl K, Topfner S, Grodd W, Taub E, Flor H. Effects of regional anesthesia on phantom limb pain are mirrored in changes in cortical reorganization. J Neurosci 1997; 17:5503–5508.

Birbaumer N, Flor H, Lutzenberger W, Elbert T. The corticalization of chronic pain. In: Bromm B, Desmedt DJ, eds. Advances in Pain Research and Therapy. Vol. 22. Pain and The Brain from Nociception to Cognition. New York. Raven Press, 1996:331–343.

Borsook D, Becerra L, Fishman S, Edwards A, Jennings CL, Stojanovic M, Papanicolas L, Ramachandran VS, Gonzalez RG, Breiter H. Acute plasticity in the human somatosensory cortex following amputation. Neuroreport 1998; 9:1013–1017.

Borsook D, Falkowski O, Rosen H, Comb M, Hyman SE. Opioids modulate stress-induced proenkephalin gene expression in the hypothalamus of transgenic mice: a model of endogenous opioid gene regulation by exogenous opioids. J Neurosci 1994; 14:7261–71.

Breiter HC, Gollub RL, Weisskoff RM, Kennedy DN, Makris N, Berke JD, Goodman JM, Kantor HL, Gastfriend DR, Riorden JP, Mathew RT, Rosen BR, Hyman SE. Acute effects of cocaine on human brain activity and emotion. Neuron 1997; 19:591–611.

Casey KL, Minoshima S, Berger KL, Kloeppe RA, Morrow TJ, Frey KA. Positron emission tomographic analysis of cerebral structures activated specifically by repetitive noxious heat stimuli. J Neurophysiol 1994; 71:802–807.

Casey KL, Minoshima S, Morrow TJ, Koeppe RA. Comparison of human cerebral activation patterns during cutaneous warmth, heat pain, and deep cold pain. J Neurophysiol 1996; 76:571–581.

Cesaro P, Mann MW, Moretti JL, Defer G, Rouldes B, Nguyen JP, Degos JD. Central pain and thalamic hyperactivity: a single photon emission computerized tomographic study. Pain 1991; 47:329–336.

Coghill RC, Talbot JD, Evans AC, Meyer E, Gjedde A, Bushnell MC, Duncan GH. Distributed processing of pain and vibration by the human brain. J Neurosci 1994; 14:4095–4108.

Davis KD, Wood ML, Crawley AP, Mikulis DJ. fMRI of human somatosensory and cingulate cortex during painful electrical nerve stimulation. Neuroreport 1995; 7:321–325.

Davis KD, Taylor SJ, Crawley AP, Wood ML, Mikulis DJ. Functional MRI of pain- and attention-related activations in the human cingulate cortex. J Neurophysiol 1997; 77:3370–3380.

Dejerine J, Roussy G. Le syndrome thalamique. Rev Neurol (Paris) 1906; 14:521–532.

Dellemijn PL, Vanneste JA. Randomized double-blind active–placebo-controlled crossover trial of intravenous fentanyl in neuropathic pain. Lancet 1997; 349:753–758.

Derbyshire SW, Jones AK, Devani P, Friston KJ, Feinmann C, Harris M, Pearce S, Watson JD, Frackowiak RS. Cerebral responses to pain in patients with atypical facial pain measured by positron emission tomography. J Neurol Neurosurg Psychiatry 1994; 57:1166–1172.

DeSalles AA, Bittar GT Jr. Thalamic pain syndrome: anatomic and metabolic correlation. Surg Neurol 1994; 41:147–151.

DeYoe EA, Bandettini P, Neitz J, Miller D, Winans P. Functional magnetic resonance imaging (fMRI) of the human brain. J Neurosci Methods 1994; 54:171–187.

Farde L. The advantage of using positron emission tomography in drug research. Trends Neurosci 1996; 19:211–214.

Firestone LL, Gyulai F, Mintun M, Adler LJ, Urso K, Winter PM. Human brain activity response to fentanyl imaged by positron emission tomography. Anesth Analg 1996; 82:1247–1251.

Friston KJ. Imaging neuroscience: principles or maps? Proc Nati Acad Sci USA 1998; 95:796–802.

Flor H, Elbert T, Knecht S, Wienbruch C, Pantev C, Birnbaumer N, Larbig W, Taub E. Phamtom-limb pain as a perceptual correlate of cortical reorganization following arm amputation. Nature 1995; 375:482–484.

Flor H, Braun C, Elbert T, Birbaumer N. Extensive reorganization of primary somatosensory cortex in chronic back pain patients. Neurosci Lett 1997; 224:5–8.

Gesuk B, Lang S, Porrino LJ, Kornetsky C. The local cerebral metabolic effects of morphine in rats exposed to footshock. Brain Res 1997; 663:303–311.

Gollub RL, Breiter HC, Kantor H, Kennedy D, Gastfriend D, Mathew RT, Makris N, Guimaraes A, Riorden J, Campbell T, Foley M, Hyman SE, Rosen B, Weiskoff R. Cocaine decreases cerebral blood flow, but does not obscure regional activation in functional magnetic resonance imaging in human subjects. J Cereb Blood Flow Metab 1998; 18:724–734.

Gozal D, Hathout GM, Kirlew KAT, Tang H, Woo MS, Zhang J, Lufkin RB, Harper R. Localization of putative neural respiratory regions in the human by functional magnetic resonance imaging. J Appl Physiol 1994; 76:2076–2083.

Hartvig P, Eckernas SA, Lindberg BS, Lundqvist H, Antoni G, Rimland A, Langstrom B. Regional distribution of the opioid receptor agonist *N*-(methyl-^{11}C) pethidine in the brain of the rhesus monkey studied with positron emission tomography. Pharmacol Toxicol 1990; 66:37–40.

Head H, Holmes G. Sensory disturbances from central lesions. Brain 1911; 34:102–254.

Hirato M, Kawashima Y, Shibazaki T, Shibasaki T, Ohye C. Pathophysiology of central (thalamic) pain: a possible role of the intralaminar nuclei in superficial pain. Acta Neurochir Suppl 1992; 52:133–136.

Hirato M, Horikoshi S, Kawashima Y, Satake K, Shibasaki T, Ohye C. The possible role of the cerebral cortex adjacent to the central sulcus for the genesis of central (thalamic) pain—a metabolic study. Acta Neurochir Suppl 1993; 58:141–144.

Hirato M, Watanabe K, Takahashi A, Hayase N, Horikoshi S, Shibasaki T, Ohye C. Pathophysiology of central (thalamic) pain: combined change of sensory thalamus with cerebral cortex around central sulcus. Stereotact Funct Neurosurg 1994; 62:300–303.

Holcomb HH, Cascella NG, Thaker GK, Medoff DR, Dannals RF, Tamminga CA. Functional sites of neuroleptic drug action in the human brain: PET/FDG studies with and without haloperidol. Am J Psychiatry. 1996; 153:41–49.

Hoehner PJ, Whitson JT, Kirsch JR, Traystman RJ. Effect of intracarotid and intraventricular morphine on regional cerebral blood flow and metabolism in pentobarbital-anesthetized dogs. Anesth Analg 1993; 76:266–273.

Hsieh JC, Belfrage M, Stone–Elander S, Hansson P, Ingvar M. Central representation of chronic ongoing neuropathic pain studied by positron emission tomography. Pain 1995; 63:225–236.

Hsieh JC, Stahle–Backdahl M, Hagermark O, Stone–Elander S, Rosenquist G, Ingvar M. Traumatic nociceptive pain activates the hypothalamus and periaqueductal gray: a positron emission tomography study. Pain 1996; 64:303–314.

Hurt RW, Ballantine HT Jr. Stereotactic anterior cingulate lesions for persistent pain: a report on 68 cases. Clin Neurosurg 1974; 21:334–351.

Iadarola MJ, Max MB, Berman KF, Byas–Smith MG, Coghill RC, Gracely RH, Bennett GJ. Unilateral decrease in thalamic activity observed with positron emission tomography in patients with chronic neuropathic pain. Pain 1995; 63:55–64.

Jones AK, Brown DW, Friston KJ, Qi LY, Frackowizk RS. Cortical and subcortical localization of response to pain in man using positron emission tomography. Proc R Soc Lond Ser B Biol Sci 1991a; 244: 39–44.

Jones AK, Liyi Q, Cunningham VV, Brown DW, Ha-Kawa S, Fujiwara T, Friston KF, Silva S, Luthra SK, Jones T. Endogenous opiate response to pain in rheumatoid arthritis and cortical and subcortical response to pain in normal volunteers using positron emission tomography. Int J Clin Pharmacol Res 1991b; 11:2–6.

Jones AK, Qi LY, Fujirawa T, Lutra SK, Ashburner J, Bloomfield P, Cunningham VJ, Itoh M, Fukuda H, Jones T. In vivo distribution of opioid receptors in man in relation to the cortical projections of the medial and lateral pain systems measured with positron emission tomography. Neurosci Lett 1991c; 126:25–28.

Jones AK, Cunningham VJ, Ha-Kawa SK, Fujiwara T, Liyii Q, Luthra SK, Ashburner J, Osman S, Jones T. Quantitation of [^{11}C]diprenorphine cerebral kinetics in man acquired by PET using presaturation, pulse–chase and tracer-only protocols. J Neurosci Methods 1994a; 51:123–134.

Jones AK, Cunningham VJ, Ha-Kawa S, Fujiwara T, Luthra SK, Silva S, Derbyshire S, Jones T. Changes in central opioid receptor binding in relation to inflammation and pain in patients with rheumatoid arthritis. Br J Rheumatol 1994b; 33:909–916.

Kiriakopoulos ET, Tasker RR, Nicosia S, Wood ML, Mikulis DJ. Functional magnetic resonance imaging: a potential tool for the evaluation of spinal cord stimulation: technical case report. Neurosurgery 1997; 41:501–504.

Koob GF, Nestler EJ. The neurobiology of drug addiction. J Neuropsychiatry Clin Neurosci 1997; 9:482–497.

Nestler EJ, Aghajanian GK. Molecular and cellular basis of addiction. Science 1997; 278:58–63.

Matsumiya N, Dohi S. Effects of intravenous or subarachnoid morphine on cerebral and spinal cord hemodynamics and antagonism with naloxone in dogs. Anesthesiology 1983; 59:175–181.

Neil SG, Lam AM, Turnbill KW, Tremper KK. Monitoring of oxygen. Can J Anesthesiol 1987; 34:56–63.

Patteson SK, Chesney JT. Anesthetic management for magnetic resonance imaging: problems and solutions. Anesth Analg 1992; 74:121–128.

Pons T, Garraghty PE, Ommaya AK, Kaas JH, Taub E, Mishkin M. Massive cortical reorganization after sensory deafferentation in adult macaques. Science 1991; 252:1857–1860.

Price DD, Hu JW, Dubner R, Gracely RH. Peripheral suppression of first pain and central summation of second pain evoked by noxious heat pulses. Pain 1997; 3:57–68.

Price DD, McGrath PA, Rafni A, Buckingham B. The validation of visual analogue scales as ratio scale measures for chronic and experimental pain. Pain 1983; 17:45–56.

Rainville P, Duncan GH, Price DD, Carrier B, Bushnell MC. Pain encoded in human anterior cingulate but not somatosensory cortex. Science 1997; 277:968–971.

Ramachandran VS, Rogers–Ramachandran D, Stewart M. Perceptual correlates of massive cortical reorganization Science 1992; 258:1159–1160.

Ramachandran VS, Rogers–Ramachandran D, Cobb S. Touching the phantom limb Nature 1995; 377: 489–490.

Rasmussen K, Beitner–Johnson DB, Krystal JH, Aghajanian GK, Nestler EJ. Opiate withdrawal and the rat locus coeruleus: behavioral, electrophysiological, and biochemical correlates. J Neurosci 1990; 10:2308–2317.

Talbot JD, Marret S, Evans AC, Meyer E, Bushnell MC, Duncan GH. Multiple representations of pain in human cerebral cortex. Science 1991; 251:1355–1358.

Titeler M, Lyon RA, Kuhar MJ, Frost JF, Dannals RF, Leonhardt S, Bullock A, Rydelek LT, Price DL, Struble RG. mu Opiate receptors are selectively labelled by [^{3}H]carfentanil in human and rat brain. Eur J Pharmacol 1989; 167:221–228.

Van Zijl PCM, Eleff SM, Ulatowski JA, Oja JME, Ulug AM, Traystman R, Kauppinen R. Quantitative assessment of blood flow, blood volume and blood oxygenation effects in functional magnetic resonance imaging. Nat Med 1998; 4:159–167.

Willis WD Jr. The Pain System. Basel: Karger, 1985.

11
Surrogate Models of Pain

G. C. Preston
Glaxo Wellcome Research and Development,
Greenford, Middlesex, England

I. INTRODUCTION

In the context of drug development, the term *surrogate* has come to mean an indirect measure that predicts the efficacy or safety of drugs in a clinical population. Surrogates may be developed for use in patients (e.g., the use of an imaging measure in place of subjective ratings in a study of clinical pain), but the focus of this chapter is on surrogates of efficacy based on pain models in healthy subjects.

Pain models in healthy volunteer subjects have traditionally been used to bridge the gap between animal models and clinical trials. The advantages of such studies are ethical and scientific—they allow the painful stimulation to be controlled and limited, experimental manipulations to be studied, and can employ sophisticated measures of subjects' responses (1,2). Pain models have contributed much to the understanding of pain physiology and psychophysics, but their use as predictors of analgesia in a clinical setting has tended to be disappointing.

One hindrance to the use of surrogates in pain research is the current system for classification of pain. Pain syndromes are currently identified anatomically, by duration (i.e., acute or chronic) and by the disease causing the pain (e.g., diabetic neuropathy). A system of surrogates designed to map onto clinical pain states defined in this way would be huge and redundant. In contrast, a mechanism-based classification of pain would point to a small, manageable set of mechanistic surrogates (e.g., features of nociception, pain arising from tissue injury, and pain arising from nervous system injury) (3). Candidate surrogates are given in Table 1. The mechanistic surrogates then need to be linked back to clinical pain states (e.g., for postoperative pain it would be necessary to know the relative contributions of nociception, pain arising from tissue damage, or other such).

There are several potential values of surrogates in the pain area. They can be used to explore mechanism of drug action and to investigate interactions between physiological systems. They can be used for investigating analgesic action (e.g., mechanistic comparisons between drugs, or between doses of an individual drug). The most important role potentially is in providing the basis for decision making. This is linked to the concept of surrogate validity discussed in the following.

Table 1 Candidate Mechanistic Surrogates

Mechanism	Candidate model
Nociceptive pain	Thermal pain
	Cold-pressor pain
	Pressure pain
	Ischemic pain
	Electrical stimulation
Pain and hypersensitivity arising from peripheral tissue damage	Heat burn
	Cold burn
	(Dental pain)
Pain arising from central sensitization	Capsaicin
	Mustard oil

II. SURROGATE VALIDITY

The term *validity* has several meanings, ranging from simple face validity to construct validity (4), but the key requirement for a surrogate is *predictive* validity (i.e., the extent to which the outcome of a manipulation in the surrogate model predicts an outcome in the clinical situation).

In its simplest form this relation can be expressed as a contingency table.

Effect in surrogate model	Effect in clinical condition	
	Negative	Positive
Negative	Correct rejection	Miss
Positive	False positive	Hit

To describe a surrogate as ''valid'' or ''not yet validated'' is an oversimplification, and it is more realistic to view validation as a continuous process, rather than a step in model development. The reason for this can be seen from the foregoing contingency table; specifically, new information will constantly be modifying the individual cells, and not all the cells will be well investigated. For example, compounds or manipulations that are negative in the surrogate model may not survive to be tested further in the clinic (this problem is more acute for the animal models that are used to select potential drugs for development). Similarly, except for placebo, agents that are *expected* to be negative are unlikely to be tested at all. Consequently, the true predictive validity can never be known.

There are several implications of this:

1. Any decisions based on a surrogate model should take this uncertainty surrounding the predictive power into account.
2. Models should continually be reevaluated, and a decision made whether the false-positive and miss rates are acceptable.
3. Inclusion of control compounds expected to be inactive should be encouraged (e.g., ''active placebos'' used in some studies to produce similar subjective effects to test agents without their analgesic properties) (5,6).

The value of surrogates, therefore, can best be realized under two circumstances:

1. For agents from an established pharmacological class, for which clinical data already exist, the models can be used to make comparisons against an established drug, and to evaluate dose–or concentration–effect relations, onset, or duration of action. For example, a cold-pressor pain model could reasonably be used in place of a clinical trial for the initial evaluation of a novel opioid.
2. For agents from a novel pharmacological class, models could be used to modify subsequent drug development programs. For example, if the result of (say) a cold-pressor study conducted early in development is positive, then this could provide sufficient confidence to take the drug into a full clinical trial program. If the result is negative, then an exploratory clinical study could be conducted instead. This approach, in effect, gives different weight to positive and negative results, in that a positive result expedites further investigation, but a negative result has no such effect.

In either event, surrogates can provide valuable information to guide subsequent decisions and potentially help in the mechanistic understanding of the molecule.

III. RECENT DEVELOPMENTS IN SURROGATES IN PAIN RESEARCH

A. Physiological Pain

Pain models can be characterized by three main variables: the method of producing the pain, the means of measuring the subjects' responses, and the psychophysical procedure linking the two. Gracely's excellent reviews of this area (1,2) summarize the approaches that have been used to date. Historically, a variety of procedures have been used to induce pain (e.g., mechanical pressure, ischemic pain, cold-pressor pain, and heat pain). Gracely (2) set out a series of criteria defining an ideal pain stimulus. These included a rapid onset and offset, repeatability with minimal temporal effects, and specificity to a restricted group of primary afferents. These criteria are excellent for ensuring that the system to be studied corresponds to the physiological system dedicated to the transmission of nociceptive information. This method is most successful at detecting the analgesic effects of opioids (5), but is inappropriate for detecting effects of nonsteroidal anti-inflammatory drugs (NSAIDs) or agents such as antiepileptic drugs that have efficacy in neuropathic pain states. The method is, therefore, restricted to a narrow class of pain, and is probably unsuitable for detecting nonopioid agents.

B. Clinical Pain

Clinical pain has three general features (7): There is spontaneous pain (dull, burning, or stabbing); hyperalgesia (increased response to painful stimuli); and allodynia (pain produced by stimuli that are not usually painful; e.g., touch). These features can be produced by either inflammatory pain (arising from tissue injury) or neuropathic pain (arising from damage to the nervous system). Inflammatory pain can result in peripheral sensitization, in which release of local inflammatory mediators in the periphery reduces the threshold for nociceptors, or central sensitization in which changes in the sensitivity of spinal cord neurons produce hyperalgesia and allodynia. Neuropathic pain can also potentially produce central sensitization. Recent models have sought to mimic these general mechanisms, and agents for treating pain in the future are likely to be directed toward treating these hypersensitivity states as much as treating the pain itself.

These hypersensitivity models do not fit in well with the classification of an ideal pain stimulus provided by Gracely (2). In particular, the painful or hypersensitive state is of slow onset and offset, repeated painful stimuli produce an enhancement of the response (wind-up), and a wider variety of afferents become capable of eliciting pain sensation (e.g., warmth or touch). For an excellent review of hyperalgesia models see Petersen (8). The list of models here is not exhaustive; for example, there is a body of work by Arendt–Neilsen that investigates the effects of agents on temporal summation (9). Two classes of model are discussed in the following.

C. Capsaicin Model

One of the most influential models to date has been based on capsaicin, the agent found in chilli peppers. Note that similar results may be obtained using mustard oil as the primary stimulus (10). Administration of capsaicin has been found to reliably produce pain, hyperalgesia (mainly to heat), and secondary hyperalgesia/allodynia to punctate mechanical stimuli, or touch/brush. The effects of capsaicin are thought to be mediated by the vanilloid VR1 receptor, which is proposed to be a natural detector of noxious heat (11), and that can also be modulated by acidic conditions occurring during inflammation or ischemia (12). The nociceptive neurons activated by capsaicin release neurotransmitters (including substance P in the spinal cord), mimicking the effect of chronic painful stimulation.

Key studies using the capsaicin model are given in Table 2. As can be seen, several procedures have been used. The agent may be given either topically or by intradermal injection across a range of doses; into either the forearm, the dorsum of the foot, or elsewhere; and the measurement may be either pain ratings to stimuli directed to the areas of hypersensitivity or measurement of the size of the areas themselves. Some generalities are beginning to emerge. Intradermal administration is more painful but produces more short-lived effects than topical application. The methods tend to produce data with high between-subject and within-subject variability. Liu (13) performed a study to compare the variability associated with different methods, and found that intradermal administration with clamping of skin temperature tended to produce the most robust model.

The pharmacological specificity of the capsaicin model is also beginning to be defined. Opioids (alfentanil and morphine) reduce pain, hyperalgesia, and allodynia. The *N*-methyl-D-aspartate (NMDA) antagonist ketamine attenuates pain and hyperalgesia, but weaker agents acting at the NMDA receptor (dextromethorphan or amitriptyline) have not.

Table 2 The Capsaicin Model in Man

Study	Model/manipulation	Key findings	Ref.
Simone et al., 1989	Intradermal capsaicin (0.01, 0.1, 1, 10, 100 μg, arm).	Dose-effect relation for intradermal capsaicin.	16
La Motte et al., 1991	Intradermal capsaicin (100 μg, arm).	Investigated peripheral and central mechanisms. Local anaesthetic blocked spread of hyperalgesia.	17
Koltzenburg et al., 1992	Topical capsaicin (1%, arm) or mustard oil. Effect of cooling and nerve block.	Defined static and dynamic components. Pain and allodynia abolished by skin cooling.	10

Table 2 Continued

Study	Model/manipulation	Key findings	Ref.
Torebork et al., 1992	Intradermal capsaicin (100 μg). Effects of nerve compression and intraneural microstimulation.	Establish fiber types responsible for initial pain, heat, and mechanical hyperalgesia.	18
Park et al., 1995	Intradermal capsaicin (250 μg, arm). Effect of ketamine, alfentanil, midazolam IV before/after capsaicin.	Ketamine and alfentanil reduce pain and pinprick hyperalgesia. Alfentanil reduced area of brush allodynia. No effect of midazolam. Preemptive study unsuccessful.	6
Kilo et al., 1995	Topical capsaicin (1%, arm). Comparison with freeze injury.	No effect of ibuprofen on peripheral or central effects of capsaicin.	19
Liu et al., 1995	Topical capsaicin (1%, arm) vs. intradermal (250 μg, arm), ± skin temperature clamping.	Quantify variability of methods. ID + temperature clamping produced least variability.	13
Andersen et al., 1996	Topical capsaicin (1%, foot). Effect of ketamine.	Ketamine reduced pain of electrical or laser heat stimuli in primary hyperalgesic area, and reduced temporal summation.	20
Liu et al., 1996	Intradermal capsaicin (100 μg, foot). Effect of α-antagonist phentolamine.	Phentolamine reduces allodynia, but not hyperalgesia.	21
Kinman et al., 1997	Intradermal capsaicin (50 μg, 2 arms). Effect of subcutaneous morphine.	No effect of morphine on spontaneous pain; morphine reduced area of mechanical hyperalgesia.	22
Kinman et al., 1997	Intradermal capsaicin (300 μg, arm). Effect of 90 mg dextromethorphan PO.	No effect of dextromethorphan.	23
Eisenach et al., 1997	Intradermal capsaicin (100 μg, arm or calf, repeated 4× within day). Effects of midazolam, amitriptyline, alfentanil.	Reduction of allodynia and hyperalgesia by alfentanil. No effects of amitriptyline (but different predrug baseline).	24
Wallace et al., 1997	Intradermal capsaicin (100 μg, arm). Effect of IV lidocaine.	Small effects of lidocaine on secondary hyperalgesia	25
Iadorola et al., 1998	Intradermal capsaicin (250 μg, arm). Regional cerebral blood flow using PET.	Investigation of brain areas activated by capsaicin pain, hyperalgesia and allodynia.	26
Magerl et al., 1998	Intradermal capsaicin (40 μg, arm).	Different mechanisms for secondary hyperalgesia/allodynia and temporal summation (windup).	27
Sang et al., 1998	Intradermal capsaicin (250 μg, arm).	AMPA/kainate antagonist reduces spontaneous pain and area of brush allodynia.	28

Table 3 Heat and Cold Injury Models in Man

Study	Model/manipulation	Key findings	Ref.
Dahl et al., 1993	Effects of pre- and postinjury lidocaine on burn injury.	Preemptive lidocaine produced short-lasting reduction in hyperalgesia.	14
Ilkjaer et al., 1996	Effects of ketamine on heat-burn pain.	Ketamine reduced primary and secondary hyperalgesia without affecting heat pain perception in normal skin.	29
Warnke et al., 1996	Effects of morphine or ketamine on temporal summation after burn injury.	Ketamine produced brief reduction in secondary hyperalgesia and temporal summation. No effect of morphine.	30
Ilkjaer et al., 1997	Effects of dextromethorphan (60, 120 mg PO) on heat-burn pain.	Dextromethorphan reduced pinprick hyperalgesia, but not brush allodynia.	31
Petersen et al., 1997	Effect of ibuprofen 600 mg on burn injury or finger-web mechanical stimulation.	Ibuprofen reduced brush-evoked pain and finger-web pain. No effect on area of allodynia or hyperalgesia after burn injury.	32
Pedersen et al., 1998	Heat injury. Investigation of temporal summation versus secondary hyperalgesia.	Secondary hyperalgesia has different mechanism to temporal summation of stimuli.	33
Kilo et al., 1994	Properties of freeze injury model.	Model produces mechanical hyperalgesia without brush allodynia. Inflammation has slow onset.	19
Kilo et al., 1995	Effect of ibuprofen on hyperalgesia produced by freeze injury.	Ibuprofen reduces freeze-induced hyperalgesia; no effect on capsaicin allodynia.	15

D. Heat or Cold Burn Models

Another class of model of clinical pain makes use of natural noxious stimulation (heat burn or cold burn produced by skin freezing) to produce tissue damage which, in turn, produces inflammation, primary and secondary hyperalgesia. These models are summarized in Table 3.

There are several methods for producing heat injury. For example, ultraviolet light may be used to produce mild injury similar to sunburn, whereas other investigators have used contact thermodes to produce more intense injury (14). Cold injury can be induced by briefly freezing a patch of skin (15). Heat injury produces reasonably long-lasting mechanical hyperalgesia and brush allodynia, whereas cold injury does not seem to produce brush allodynia. The pharmacological specificity of these models is similar to the capsaicin model (i.e., positive effects for opioids and ketamine, but no consistent effects of NSAIDs).

IV. FUTURE DIRECTIONS

The development of pain surrogates is currently at a very interesting point. On the one hand, there exist several well-established models in which a variety of agents have been tested (e.g., cold pressor pain). Broadly, these are models of physiological or nociceptive pain that have been developed empirically, rather than being based on theory. They do not obviously reflect processes that are engaged in chronic clinical pain conditions. They are mainly useful for detecting strong opioid-like analgesics. For these models to be maximally useful in future work is required to understand the underlying physiology.

A second set of models is being developed that is more firmly based on a mechanistic understanding of clinical pain. These seek to mimic phenomena such as peripheral and central sensitization. However, individual academic groups have developed variants of the models that differ in major details to the extent that it is difficult to determine whether different outcomes are due to genuine differences between agents or are just procedural differences. The models are also not optimized for testing analgesic agents (e.g., the time course may be inappropriate, or the variability unacceptably high).

For these newer models to be useful in the future there must be first some narrowing of experimental conditions, so that, for example, the "capsaicin models" used by all groups are reasonably equivalent. This would require the elimination of variants of the models that produce excessive variability or inconsistent outcomes, and the choice of outcome measures that are a good compromise between robustness and sensitivity to change. The next stage would be the systematic testing of a range of agents in the models and in clinical pain states to generate an understanding of the real predictive validity of the models. The ideal model would provide robust hypersensitivity lasting about 6 h, suitable either for testing agents preemptively or for testing agents' ability to abolish established hypersensitivity, and would produce no lasting tissue damage. A model that is able to reliably detect the analgesic effects of NSAIDs would also be useful.

Within the next few years, it will be possible to see to what extent surrogate models in the pain area really do form a useful bridge between animal and clinical data.

ACKNOWLEDGMENT

I would like to thank all the colleagues with whom I have worked on pain models—in particular Chris Lines, Kate Dawson, Nigel Baber, Chas Bountra, Joe Mercer, Janet Liptrot, Bob Lamb, John Posner, Steve Quessy, Paul Rees, Phil Barrington, Frank Hoke, and Judith Maconochie.

REFERENCES

1. Gracely RH. Methods of testing pain mechanisms in normal man. In: Wall PD, Melzack R, eds. Textbook of Pain. 2nd ed. Edinburgh: Churchill Livingstone, 1989:257–268.
2. Gracely RH. Studies of pain in normal man. In: Wall PD, Melzack R, eds. Textbook of Pain. 3rd ed. Edinburgh: Churchill Livingstone, 1994:315–336.
3. Woolf CJ, Bennett GJ, Doherty M, Dubner R, Kidd B, Koltzenburg M, Lipton R, Loeser JD, Payne R, Torebjork E. Towards a mechanism-based classification of pain. Pain 1998; 77:227–229.
4. Parrott AC. Performance tests in human psychopharmacology (1): test reliability and standardization. Hum Psychopharmacol 1991; 6:1–9.
5. Posner J. A modified submaximal effort tourniquet test for evaluation of analgesics in healthy volunteers. Pain 1984; 19:143–151.
6. Park KM, Max MB, Robinovitz E, Gracely RH, Bennett GJ. Effects of intravenous ketamine, alfentanil, or placebo on pain, pinprick hyperalgesia, and allodynia produced by intradermal capsaicin in human subjects. Pain 1995; 63:163–172.
7. Woolf CJ. A new strategy for the treatment of inflammatory pain. Prevention or elimination of central sensitization. Drugs 1994; Supp 5:1–9.

8. Petersen KL. Experimental cutaneous hyperalgesia in humans. IASP Newslett 1997; Nov/Dec.
9. Arendt–Nielsen L, Petersen-Felex S, Fischer M, Bak P, Bjerring P, Zbinden AM. The effect of *N*-methyl-D-aspartate antagonist (ketamine) on single and repeated nociceptive stimuli: a placebo-controlled experimental study. Anesth Analg 1995; 81:63–68.
10. Koltzenburg M, Lundberg LER, Torebjork HE. Dynamic and static components of mechanical hyperalgesia in human hairy skin. Pain 1992; 51:207–219.
11. Caterina MJ, Schumacher MA, Tominaga M, Rosen TA, Levine JD, Julius D. The capsaicin receptor: a heat-activated ion channel in the pain pathway. Nature 1997; 389:816–824.
12. Tominaga M, Caterina MJ, Malmberg AB, Rosen TA, Gilbert H, Skinner K, Raumann BE, Basbaum AI, Julius D. The cloned capsaicin receptor integrates multiple pain-producing stimuli. Neuron 1998; 21:531–543.
13. Liu M, Max MB, Robinovitz E, Bennett GJ. Capsaicin-evoked allodynia: a study of 3 methods. Anaesthesiology 1995; 83:A863
14. Dahl JB, Brennum J, Arendt–Neilsen L, Jensen TS, Kehlet H. The effect of pre- versus post injury infiltration with lidocaine on thermal and mechanical hyperalgesia after heat injury to the skin. Pain 1993; 53:43–51.
15. Kilo S, Forster C, Geisslinger G, Brune K, Handwerker HO. Inflammatory models of cutaneous hyperalgesia are sensitive to effects of ibuprofen in man. Pain 1995; 62:187–193.
16. Simone DA, Baumann TK, LaMotte RH. Dose-dependent pain and mechanical hyperalgesia in humans after intradermal injection of capsaicin. Pain 1989; 38:99–107.
17. LaMotte RH, Shain CN, Simone DA, Tsai EF. Neurogenic hyperalgesia: psychophysical studies of underlying mechanisms. J Neurophysiol 1991; 66:190–211.
18. Torebjork HE, Lundberg LER, LaMotte RH. Central changes in processing of mechanoreceptive input in capsaicin-induced secondary hyperalgesia in humans. J Physiol 1992; 448:765–780.
19. Kilo S, Schmelz M, Koltzenburg M, Handwerker HO. Different patterns of hyperalgesia induced by experimental inflammation in human skin. Brain 1994; 117:385–396.
20. Andersen OK, Felsby S, Nicolaisen L, Bjerring P, Jensen TS, Arendt–Neilsen L. The effect of ketamine on stimulation of primary and secondary hyperalgesic areas induced by capsaicin: a double blind placebo-controlled, human experimental study. Pain 1996; 66:51–62.
21. Liu M, Max MB, Parada S, Reowan JS, Bennett GJ. The sympathetic nervous system contributors to capsaicin-evoked mechanical allodynia but not pinprick hyperalgesia in humans. J Neurosci 1996; 16:7331–7335.
22. Kinnman E, Nygards EB, Hansson P. Peripheral alpha-adrenoreceptors are involved in the development of capsaicin induced ongoing and stimulus evoked pain in humans. Pain 1997; 69:79–85.
23. Kinnman E, Nygards EB, Hansson P. Effects of dextromethorphan in clinical doses on capsaicin-induced ongoing pain and mechanical hypersensitivity. J Pain Symp Manage 1997; 14:195–201.
24. Eisenach JC, Hood DD, Curry R, Tong C. Alfentanil, but not amitriptyline, reduces pain, hyperalgesia, and allodynia from intradermal injection of capsaicin in humans. Anesthesiology 1997; 86:1279–1287.
25. Wallace MS, Laitin S, Licht D, Yaksh TL. Concentration–effect relations for intravenous lidocaine infusions in human volunteers: effects on acute sensory thresholds and capsaicin-evoked hyperpathia. Anesthesiology 1997; 86:1262–1272.
26. Iadarola MJ, Berman KF, Zeffiro TA, Byas–Smith MG, Gracely RH, Max MB, Bennett GJ. Neural activation during acute capsaicin-evoked pain and allodynia assessed with PET. Brain 1998; 121: 931–947.
27. Magerl W, Wilk SH, Treede RD. Secondary hyperalgesia and perceptual wind-up following intradermal injection of capsaicin in humans. Pain 1998; 74:257–268.
28. Sang CN, Hostetter MP, Gracely RH, Chappell AS, Schoepp DD, Lee G, Whitcup S, Caruso R, Max MB. AMPA/kainate antagonist LY293558 reduces capsaicin-evoked hyperalgesia but not pain in normal skin in humans. Anesthesiology 1998; 89:1060–1067.
29. Ilkjaer S, Petersen KL, Brennum J, Wernberg M, Dahl JB. Effect of systemic *N*-methyl-D-aspartate receptor antagonist (ketamine) on primary and secondary hyperalgesia in humans. Br J Anaesth 1996; 76:829–834.

30. Warncke T, Stubhaug A, Jorum E. Ketamine an NMDA receptor antagonist suppresses spatial and temporal properties of burn-induced secondary hyperalgesia in man: a double blind, cross-over comparison with morphine and placebo. Pain 1997; 72:99–106.
31. Ilkjaer S, Dirks J, Brennum J, Wernberg M, Dahl JB. Effect of systemic *N*-methyl-D-aspartate receptor antagonist (dextromethorphan) on primary and secondary hyperalgesia in humans. Br J Anaesth 1997; 79:600–605.
32. Petersen KL, Brennum J, Dahl JB. Experimental evaluation of the analgesic effect of ibuprofen on primary and secondary hyperalgesia. Pain 1997; 70:167–174.
33. Pedersen JL, Andersen OK, Arendt–Nielsen L, Kehlet H. Hyperalgesia and temporal summation of pain after heat injury in man. Pain 1998; 74:189–197.

12
Acute Trauma and Postoperative Pain

Lesley M. Bromley
University College London School of Medicine, London, England

I. INTRODUCTION

The response of the nervous system to acute tissue injury is a sensitization of the tissues including and surrounding the injury. This permits recuperation and recovery because it produces behavior that avoids contact with all external stimuli. This response is common to all animals with a nervous system and is present in humans. Clearly, this response has a survival advantage, but evolution has not anticipated the development of the "controlled injury" in the form of surgery. In the context of modern surgical techniques and practice the sensitization that leads to pain and inactivity is no longer desirable. The rational management of acute pain is designed to anticipate and suppress this defense mechanism, and postoperative pain gives us the opportunity to plan analgesia from before the injury occurs.

The management of pain after surgery has become a more important issue in the last two decades for several reasons. The understanding of the basic science of the tissue injury—sensitization mechanisms at a peripheral and spinal level—has become much clearer in that time. Anesthetic and surgical techniques have developed to a point where surgical mortality is very low, patient expectations have changed such that survival is the norm and pain has become a more pressing issue for the patient. A number of reports from the United Kingdom and United States, published in the early part of the 1990s suggested that acute pain management was uniformly badly managed in hospitals, and that this was unnecessary with the level of knowledge and technology available (1,2). Indeed some surgeons felt that the use of analgesia would "mask" important physical signs in a surgical patient and should be withheld. The *British Medical Journal* published a paper entitled "Safety of early pain relief for acute abdominal pain" in 1992, suggesting that many surgical patients were expected by their doctors to experience pain, and a trial randomizing patients in acute pain to either morphine or saline was considered ethical (3).

II. CURRENT TECHNIQUES IN ACUTE PAIN MANAGEMENT

To assess the effectiveness of any pain management strategy, some form of reproducible and reliable pain measurement tool was needed. In general, in the 10-cm visual analogue scale (VAS) has been used, in research studies, but in the day-to-day measurement of pain in surgical wards, a simple verbal scale of 1, no pain, up to 4 or 5 as severe pain is more common. This latter form of assessment is really too crude to do more than display trends. Education of staff in understanding pain and its assessment helps produce more accurate data, and the introduction of regular pain assessment as part of routine postoperative observations has been an important part of improving postoperative pain management. Audit data of surgical patients receiving traditional postoperative analgesia of intramuscular opiates given every 4 h, as required, show median VAS scores at rest of 4.5 cm, and on movement of 7.9 cm after major surgery (4). This is clearly unacceptable, and many clinicians have taken on the challenge of improving on this type of audit result.

Many claims have been made for improved postoperative analgesia in addition to the humanitarian aspects of pain relief. It has been suggested that good postoperative analgesia can also reduce postoperative complications, mortality, and reduce hospital stay (5,6). Some analgesic techniques, for example, epidural infusion of local anesthetics, improve respiratory mechanics in the postoperative periods (7,8), and even reduce the incidence of deep vein thrombosis (9).

Our understanding of the basic science of acute tissue injury, the peripheral inflammatory mechanisms, and trauma-induced states in the spinal cord has now reached the point where the complexity of these mechanisms indicates that no one single drug is going to effectively abolish postoperative pain. In addition, there is still as much to be discovered and understood about the central modification of nociceptor input in acute pain as there is in nonacute pain. The role of adaptation and the stress response also remain to be elucidated. The rational approach to acute pain management must be to use this knowledge, and many clinical studies have been carried out to establish the optimum regimen for the management of acute pain.

Not withstanding this approach, the mainstay of postoperative pain for major surgery and trauma remains the use of the opiate drugs, either based on morphine or synthetic opioids, such as meperidine (pethidine) and its related compounds. New technology has allowed us to give these drugs in a more satisfactory manner, and evidence exists to suggest that the order and timing of the drug delivery is important. In addition, the use of weaker opioid agonists, nonsteroidal anti-inflammatory drugs (NSAIDs), and the simple analgesics, particularly acetaminophen (paracetamol) are used as acute pain abates. The intra-muscular injection of morphine every 4 h has been largely replaced by patient-controlled analgesia systems (PCA) that allow the patient to safely self-administer small boluses of intravenous opiates following major surgery. Intramuscular morphine has been retained, but with a better appreciation of the pharmacokinetics, allowing dosage intervals of less than 4 h as necessary, for intermediate and minor surgery.

The use of the epidural space to deliver both opiates and local anesthetics to the spinal cord has grown enormously in the last decade. Drugs are given into the epidural space through a catheter and can be given by intermittent bolus, continuous infusion, or by PCA. Epidural anesthesia or analgesia may be used as part of the anesthetic technique and continued into the postoperative period. This method requires specialist skills for placement of catheters, specialized equipment, and specialized nursing skills. These limitations confine the use of epidural techniques for pain relief to those with the resources to provide this.

None of the currently available analgesic drugs are without unwanted effects. The challenge of rational acute pain management with the drugs presently available is to produce optimal analgesia, with the minimum of unwanted effects. These unwanted effects may have a considerable influence on the experience the patient has of postoperative care. In particular the nausea and vomiting associated with opiates limits the use of PCA intravenous morphine. Patients report that some pain is acceptable to avoid the nausea. This is an important issue in interpreting clinical studies in acute pain management. In general, the use of PCA morphine has become the tool of measurement of the effectiveness of the analgesic intervention. Timing of administration of drugs perioperatively, use of different combinations of drugs perioperatively, and the timing and use of local anaesthetic blocks are all judged for their effectiveness by the amount of PCA morphine used in the postoperative period. This, with the VAS score, is used as a key outcome measure. An intervention is deemed effective if, in a randomized, controlled trial, a treatment reduces the use of PCA morphine to reach a VAS score equivalent to that of the untreated group. This can be only a crude measure of effectiveness as the use of PCA morphine can be influenced by factors other than pain.

III. APPLYING BASIC SCIENCE TO CLINICAL ACUTE PAIN MANAGEMENT

A. Peripheral mechanisms

Despite our increasing knowledge of the chemical basis of the acute inflammatory response and the numerous chemicals involved in sensitizing peripheral nociceptor endings, our only therapeutic tool for this area is the use of the nonsteroidal anti-inflammatory agents (NSAIDs). These agents inhibit the production of prostaglandins by inhibiting cyclooxygenase. Animal studies have shown that the use of NSAIDs given before the formalin test reduced the behavioral response characteristic of facilitated processing produced by formalin (10).

When introduced into clinical practice, it became clear that this group of drugs was not as potent as morphine, but if given in combination with opiates, they had a morphine-sparing effect (11,12). The use of NSAIDs has reduced the use of PCA morphine by between 40 and 60%, depending on the type of surgery (13,14). The incidence of opiate side effects is also reduced as a consequence of this reduction in opiate use. In intermediate types of surgery, the opiate-sparing effect is less marked, and the evidence for effective use of NSAIDs from clinical studies is less favorable (15). In some forms of minor surgery, NSAIDs may be the only analgesia required.

Intraoperative opiate requirements can also be reduced by the concurrent use of NSAIDs. Here the evidence is greater for major surgery than for intermediate and minor surgery. Attempts to demonstrate any advantage of preemptive action with NSAIDs have been unsuccessful (16).

NSAIDs have several unwanted effects that lead to some reservations about their use. The reduction of platelet function has led to anxiety about the potential for increased perioperative bleeding, although there are few clinical reports of problems in this area. The second unwanted effect that is more serious is the effect on renal blood flow. The reduction in renal blood flow produced by NSAIDs can lead to renal failure. This is compounded by the potential for prerenal failure associated with intraoperative blood loss, and many have counseled that NSAIDs should not be used intraoperatively for major surgery for this reason. The Royal College of Anaesthetists has recently issued guidelines on the use of NSAIDs in the perioperative period with the following recommendations: these drugs should not be used in renally compromised patients, renal function should be monitored regularly in all patients receiving NSAIDs after major surgery, and NSAIDs should be discontinued at the first sign of renal impairment (17).

The next generation of NSAIDs are designed to inhibit only the inducible form of cyclooxygenase; therefore, they should largely avoid the unwanted effects seen in the older drugs.

B. Mechanisms Involving the Spinal Cord

1. Nociceptive Input

If nociceptive input to the spinal cord can be blocked, then perception of pain will be absent. In practice, it appears to be very difficult to block all sensory input to the spinal cord by practical anesthetic methods. General anesthesia with opiate analgesia is certainly relatively ineffective. With epidural analgesia combined with general anesthesia, the density of epidural block required to produce absence of surgical nociceptive input cannot be obtained without profound cardiovascular depression. The use of a subarachnoid block with an awake patient produces the densest sensory block and, subsequently, the least postoperative pain. These techniques are only applicable to surgery in the lower abdomen and lower limbs (18).

Where general anesthesia with opiate analgesia is the only practical anesthetic for the surgery, the timing of opiate administration can influence the effectiveness of the analgesia. As demonstrated in animal studies, the spinal cord responses of secondary hyperalgesia and allodynia are produced by expansion of receptive fields and changes in central neuronal excitability following nociceptive input to the cord, which is a basic phenomenon called neuroplasticity. These effects in animals can be reduced by the administration of preinjury morphine, or by a local anesthetic block. Preemptive analgesia is more effective than a postemptive dose.

Professor Patrick Wall introduced the concept of preemptive analgesia to clinicians in his editorial in the journal *Pain* in 1988 (19). Subsequent to this editorial, many studies have been performed using different analgesic drugs and techniques. A number of the earlier papers compared preoperative analgesia using various analgesics, with a placebo pretreatment (20,21). In some studies the authors demonstrated long-lasting analgesia after preemptive treatment, but this is not a consistent finding (22,23).

Several studies have been conducted using opioid administration as the analgesic strategy to demonstrate preemptive analgesia. Katz et al. produced clinical evidence of preemptive analgesia in a study (24) that compared the effects of giving fentanyl by an epidural catheter before or 15 min after a surgical incision. They found that the postoperative consumption of morphine from a PCA was significantly less between 12 and 24 h in the preemptive group (24). Opioid drugs given intravenously have been examined for a preemptive effect in several studies, and there appears to be a different effect with different opioid analgesics. Alfentanil, a synthetic opioid with a rapid onset and offset, has been used in two studies (25,26). In these studies, the effect of alfentanil given either at induction or 1 min after skin incision was examined. No difference in postoperative analgesic consumption was demonstrated. These studies serve to illustrate some of the problems of clinical studies in preemptive analgesia that are discussed in an editorial by Kissin (27).

Two other studies evaluated the use of morphine, which has a longer duration of action than alfentanil. The timing of the morphine administration was either at the induction of anesthesia or at the very end of the surgery. Richmond et al. (28) demonstrated a significant reduction in morphine consumption in a group of women undergoing abdominal hysterectomy, who received a single dose of 10 mg of morphine intravenously at induction compared with the same dose given at the end of the surgery. This paper demonstrated the confounding effect of an opiate premedication. They had a third group of patients who were given 10 mg of morphine IM at approximately 1 h before the surgery. This group had no further opiate during surgery, and their morphine consumption postoperatively was intermediate between the preemptive and postoperative group. Undoubtedly, some of these patients had received a preemptive dose of morphine and others did not, as the timing of the premedication was anything from 1 h to 5 min before surgery. This study has two additional interesting findings. The authors tested the skin around the wound for touch and pain sensitivity using Von Frey hairs. The nonpreemptive patients were demonstrated to have an area of hyperalgesia not present in the preemptive group. This is strong clinical evidence that a phenomenon seen in basic science experiments of preemptive analgesia, prevention of central sensitization, is also a feature of clinical preemptive analgesia. The authors also measured pain scores at 24 h, after free access to morphine and at 48 h with only simple analgesics for the second 24 h.

A second paper by Mansfield et al. (29) compared two different doses of morphine preemptively with a postemptive dose given at the end of an abdominal hysterectomy. They were unable to demonstrate a difference between pre- and posttreatment in the lower dose group, but they showed a significant difference with the higher dose. In contrast Collis et al. (30) doubled the preemptive dose, but could not demonstrate any difference in postoperative morphine consumption. In this paper the authors note a very high incidence of nausea and vomiting in the patients.

Clearly, there can be a preemptive effect with morphine, although it has not been demonstrated with the synthetic short-acting opioids. The extent of the preemptive effect with opioids is perhaps less dramatic than that shown with effective local anesthetic block (31). This may be related to the duration of the nociceptive input after a surgical procedure, wherein the initial postoperative period is characterized by an acute inflammatory reaction which itself generates nociceptive input. The preemptive treatment needs to be maintained into the postoperative period to ensure that significant nociceptive input does not reach the spinal cord, which is preemptive analgesia in its broader sense. When local anesthetic blocks that are sufficiently dense to prevent conduction in C fibers are established before surgery, a clinically significant preemptive effect can be demonstrated (18). This led to attempts to demonstrate preemptive effects with a balanced or multimodal approach to analgesia (32). Unfortunately, this has been unsuccessful.

Both Katz et al. and Richmond et al. found that pain in the preemptive group was higher in the second 24 h after the injury. This may be accounted for partly by the observation that pretreatment with morphine acts indirectly to reduce the stimulation-evoked expression of preproenkephalin in response to nociceptive input. Effective continuous preemptive analgesia may overcome this phenomenon.

In addition to the preemptive effects of opiates, attention has been given to the role of the *N*-methyl-D-aspartate (NMDA) receptor in acute pain. There have been several clinical studies examining the use of NMDA receptor antagonists in the treatment of postopertative pain using ketamine or dextromethorphan. Ketamine has a number of actions in addition to its noncompetitive anti-NMDA receptor action which can be shown at low doses. Unfortunately its mixed action leads to many unwanted effects that have limited its widespread introduction as part of the acute pain management strategy. In clinical studies, low-dose ketamine given before surgical incision in combination with opioids produced a 60% reduction in PCA morphine use postoperatively (34). The use of ketamine also reduces the area of secondary hyperalgesia surrounding surgical wounds. The identification of a potent NMDA receptor antagonist without unwanted effects will be required to develop this application (35).

2. Descending Pathways

Nociceptive input can be modified in the dorsal horn by activation of descending α_2-noradrenergic pathways. This has led to attempts to modify acute pain using α_2-agonists. The only drug available in this class is clonidine, which is not a highly selective α_2-agonist. A number of studies have attempted to show a benefit from combining clonidine with local anesthetics or with local anesthetics and opiates in the epidural space (36,37). These studies have shown enhanced analgesia, or at least a morphine-sparing effect. The effect of clonidine in combination with opiates in the epidural space seems to be to produce an earlier onset and a longer duration of analgesia than with opiates alone. It has been suggested that clonidine given preemptively decreased postoperative pain and analgesia consumption in pediatric patients (38). However, the unwanted effects of clonidine, particularly sedation, bradycardia, and hypotension, have made it a difficult technique to apply widely.

Dexmedetomidine, a more selective α_2-agonist, currently used in veterinary anesthesia, is about to be introduced to human practice and may be more useful than clonidine.

Tramadol, an analgesic with combined opioid agonist and monoamine reuptake-blocking properties, did not improve acute postoperative pain following epidural administration in one study (38).

3. Other Modifiers of Spinal Nociceptive Input

Adenosine analogues produce analgesia after intrathecal administration in animals (39) through the A_1 adenosine receptor. Initial use of adenosine in volunteer experiments has confirmed its antinociceptive action (40), and one clinical study has shown that a low-dose infusion of adenosine during surgery can reduce the intraoperative use of anesthetic agents and the postoperative use of opiate analgesia (41).

Neostigmine has been used intrathecally in animal experiments and produces an analgesic effect, but its use in human volunteers produced a wide range of unacceptable side effects in the doses that produced analgesia (42). Recently, the combination of neostigmine and clonidine intrathecally has demonstrated synergistic analgesic effects in the lower limbs of volunteer patients (43). However, persistent nausea and motor weakness have made this technique impractical in the clinical setting.

C. Higher Centers

Opiate receptors in the brain stem, midbrain, and cortex are also activated following systemic use of opiate drugs in the management of acute pain. The exact contribution of spinal cord and central mechanisms to the overall analgesic effect is unknown.

IV. CONCLUSION

Undoubtedly the perception of pain is complex and can be modified both by pharmacology and by the brain's intrinsic activity. As yet there is no clinical strategy for reducing or modifying pain *perception* as opposed to pain *transmission* other than with opiate drugs. Acute, posttraumatic pain, is in general a short-lived phenomenon that resolves rapidly over time. This knowledge undoubtedly influences attitude and perception of pain in the individual, and since pain memory is poor, individuals may submit themselves to painful procedures such as childbirth more than once in a lifetime.

REFERENCES

1. Royal College of Surgeons of England, College of Anaesthetists. Commission on the provision of surgical services. Report of the working party on pain after surgery. London: Royal College of Surgeons, 1990.
2. Owen H, McMillan V, Rogwki D. Post operative pain therapy: a survey of patients expectations and their experiences. Pain 1990; 41:303–307
3. Gould TH, Crosby DL, Harmer M, Lloyd SM, Lunn JN, Rees GAD, Robers DE, Webster JA. Policy for controlling pain after surgery: effect of sequential changes in management. Br Med J 1992; 305: 1187–1193.
4. Attard AR, Corlett MJ, Kinder NJ, Leslie AP, Fraser IA. Safety of early pain relief for acute abdominal pain. Br Med J 1992; 305:554–556.
5. Wasylak TJ, Abbott FV, English MJM, Jeans M–E. Reduction of postoperative morbidity following patient controlled morphine. Can J Anaesth 1990; 37:726–731.

6. Moiniche S, Hansen BL, Christensen S–E, Dhal BJ, Kehlet H. Activity of patients and duration of hospitalisation following hip-replacement surgery with balanced treatment of pain and early mobilisation. Ugeskrift Laeger 1992; 154:1495–1499.
7. Jay C, Thomas H, Ray A, Farhat F, Lasser P, Bourgain J–L. Postoperative pulmonary complications. Epidural analgesia using bupivacine and opioids versus peripheral opioids. Anesthesiology 1993; 78:666–676.
8. Rawal N, Sjostrand U, Christofferson E, Dahlstrom B, Arvill E, Rydman H. Comparison of intramuscular and epidural morphine for post operative analgesia in the grossly obese: influence on postoperative ambulation and pulmonary function. Anesth Analg 1984; 63:592.
9. Tuman KJ, McArthy RJ, March RJ, DeLaria GA, Patell RV, Ivankovich AD. Effects of epidural anesthesia and analgesia on coagulation and outcome after major vascular surgery. Anesth Analg 1991; 73:696–704.
10. Coderre TJ, Vaccarino AL, Melzack R. Central nervous system plasticity in the tonic pain response to subcutaneous formalin injection. Brain Res 1990; 535:155–158.
11. Brown CR, Moodie JE, Wild VM, Bynum LJ. Comparison of intravenous ketorolac tromethamine and morphine sulphate in the treatment of post operative pain. Pharmacotherapy 1990; 10:116S–121S.
12. Pierce R, Fragen RJ, Pemberton DM. Intravenous ketorolac tromethamine versus morphine sulphate in the treatment of immediate post operative pain. Pharmacotherapy 1990; 10:111S–115S.
13. Kinsella J, Patrick JA, McArdle CS, Moffat AC, Prentics JW, Kenny GN. Ketorolac tromethamine for post operative analgesia after orthopaedic surgery. Br J Anaesth 1992; 69:19–22.
14. Gillies GWA, Kenny GNC, Bullingham RES, McArdle CS. The morphine sparing effects of ketorolac tromethamine: a study of a new parenteral non-steroidal anti-inflammatory agent after abdominal surgery. Anaesthesia 1987; 42:727–731.
15. Sevarino FB, Sinatra RS, Paige D, Ning T, Brull SJ, Silverman DG. The efficacy of intramuscular ketorolac in combination with intravenous PCA morphine for post operative pain relief. J Clin Anaesth 1992; 4:285–288.
16. Vanlersberghe C, Lauwers MH, Camu F. Pre-operative ketorolac administration has no pre-emptive analgesic effect for minor orthopaedic surgery. Acta Anaesthesiol Scand 1996;40:948–952.
17. The Royal College of Anaesthetists. Guidelines for the use of non-steroidal anti-inflammatory drugs in the perioperative period. Jan 1998.
18. Shir Y, Raja SN, Frank SM. The effect of epidural versus general anaesthesia on postoperative pain and analgesia requirements in patients undergoing radical prostatectomy. Anesthesiology 1994;80: 49–56.
19. Wall PD. The prevention of post operative pain. Pain 1988;32:289–290.
20. McQuay HJ, Carroll D, Moore RA. Postoperative orthopaedic pain—the effect of opiate premedication and local analgesic blocks. Pain 1988; 33:291–295.
21. Koskinen R, Tigerstedt I, Tammisto T. The effect of peroperative alfentanil on the need for immediate postoperative pain relief. Acta Anaesth Scand 1991; 35(suppl 96).
22. Johansson B, Glise H, Hallerback B, Dalman P, Kristoffersson A. Preoperative local infiltration with ropivacaine for postoperative pain relief after cholecystectomy. Anaesth Analg 1994; 78:210–214.
23. Harrison CA, Morris S, Harvey JS. Effect of illio-inguinal and illio-hypogastric block and wound infiltration with 0.5% bupivacaine on post operative pain after inguinal hernia repair. Br J Anaesth 1994; 72:691–693.
24. Katz J, Kavanagh BP, Sandler AN, Nierenberg H, Boylan JF, Friedlander M, Shaw BF. Pre-emptive analgesia: clinical evidence of neuroplasticity contributing to post operative pain. Anaesthesiology 1992; 77:429–446.
25. Wilson RJT, Leith S, Jackson IJB, Hunter D. Preemptive analgesia from intravenous administration of opioids. Anaesthesia 1994; 49:591–593.
26. Mansfield M, Meikle R, Miller C. A trial of pre-emptive analgesia Anaesthesia 1994; 49:1091–93.
27. Kissin I. Preemptive analgesia, why its effect is not always obvious. Anesthesiology 1996; 84:1015–1019.

28. Richmond CE, Bromley LM, Woolf CJ. Properative morphine pre-empts postoperative pain. Lancet 1993; 342:73–75.
29. Mansfield MD, James KS, Kinsella J. Influence of dose and timing of administration of morphine on postoperative pain and analgesic requirements Br J Anaesth 1996; 76:358–361.
30. Collis R, Brandner B, Bromley LM, Woolf CJ. Is there any clinical advantage in increasing the pre-emptive dose of morphine or combining pre-incisional with postincisional morphine administration? Br J Anaesth 1995; 74:396–399.
31. Kavanagh BP, Katz J, Sandler AN, Nierenberg H, Roger S, Boylkan JF, Laws AK. Multimodal analgesia before thoracic surgery does not reduce post operative pain. Br J Anaesth 1994; 73:184–189.
32. Crosby G, Marota JJA, Goto T, Uhl GR. Subarachnoid morphine reduces stimulation induced but not basal expression of propreenkephalin in rat spinal cord. Anesthesiology 1994; 81:1270–1276.
33. Deleted in proof.
34. Tverskoy M, Yuval O, Isakson A, Finger J, Bradley EL, Kissin I. Preemptive effect of fentanyl and ketamine on postoperative pain and wound hyperalgesia. Anaesth Analg 1994; 78:1–5.
35. Stubhaug A. Breivik H, Kreunen M, Foss A. Mapping of punctate hyperalgesia around a surgical incision demonstrates that ketamine is a powerful suppressor of central sensitisation to pain following surgery. Acta Anaesthesiol Scand 1997; 41:1124–1132.
36. Grace D, Bunting H, Milligan KR, Fee JP. Post operative analgesia after co-administration of clonidine and morphine by the intrathecal route in patients undergoing hip replacement. Anaesth Analg 1995; 80:86–91.
37. Rockemann MG, Seeling W, Brinkman A, Goertz AW, Hauber N, Junge J, Georgieff M. Analgesic and haemodynamic effects of epidural clonidine, clonidine/morphine and morphine after pancreatic surgery—a double blind study. Anaesth Analg 1995; 80:869–874.
38. Mostsch J, Bottinger BW, Bach A, Bohrer H, Skoberne T, Martin E. Caudal clonidine and bupivacaine for combined epidural and general anaesthesia in children. Acta Anaesthesiol Scand 1997; 41: 877–883.
38. Wilder–Smith CH, Wilder–Smith OH, Farschtschian M, Naji P. Preoperative adjuvant epidural tramadol: the effect of different doses on postoperative analgesia and pain processing. Acta Anaesthesiol Scand 1998; 42:299–305.
39. Nakamura I, Ohta Y, Kemmotsu O. Characterisation of adenosine receptors mediating spinal sensory transmission related to nociceptive information in the rat. Anaesthesiology 1997; 87:577–584.
40. Segerdhal M, Ekblom A, Sollevi A. The influence of adenosine, ketamine and morphine on experimentally induced ischaemic pain in healthy volunteers. Anesth Analg 1994; 79:787–791.
41. Segerdhal M, Ekblom A, Sandelin K, Wickham M, Sollevi A. Peroperative adenosine infusion reduces the requirements for isoflurane and postoperative analgesics. Anesth Analg 1995; 80:1145–1149.
42. Eisenach JC, Hood DD, Curry R. Phase I human safety assessment of intrathecal neostigmine containing methyl- and propyl parabens. Anesth Analg 1997; 85:842–846.
43. Hood D, Mallak KA, Eisenach JC, Tong C. Interaction between intrathecal neostigmine and epidural clonidine in human volunteers. Anaesthesiology 1996; 85:315–325.

13

Effectiveness of Needling Techniques with Special Reference to Myofascial Pain Syndromes

Andreas G. Erdmann and Rajesh Munglani
University of Cambridge and Addenbrooke's Hospital, Cambridge, England

C. Chan Gunn
Gunn Pain Clinic, Vancouver, British Columbia, Canada, and University of Washington School of Medicine, Seattle, Washington, U.S.A.

I. INTRODUCTION

The therapeutic use of needles to treat disease and pain has a long and venerated history. From the earliest literary references to acupuncture more than 2000 years ago, until the present day, acupuncture and other forms of dry needling have undergone steady development—in technique and in the conceptual understanding of the neurobiology of needling.

With its origins in the East, the vast majority of work was done in China and Japan, with little interest from the West until the early part of the 19th century. A relatively brief period of activity in Europe and America was followed by a gradual decline toward the end of that century. The 1950s saw a revival by a few practitioners, but it is only during the last 30 years that an increase in media and public interest has facilitated some basic research and allowed a wider acceptance of clinical acupuncture practice.

One major reason for the initial lack of acceptance by the scientific community is that acupuncture lacks a Western scientific and rational basis, having been based on the more philosophical tenets of Chinese medicine. However, recent years have seen the burgeoning of "scientific acupuncture," with emphasis on the anatomical and neurophysiological principles well known to Western medicine. A scientific understanding of the mechanisms of acupuncture pain relief is thus only beginning to emerge. Much well-designed research work is still required, in the basic sciences as well as in the clinical arena, and the numerous current theories are likely to undergo further change and modification. This review aims to provide a background and general appraisal of the effectiveness of acupuncture and other needling in chronic pain, followed by a consideration of current theoretical advances and presentation of the theory of radiculopathy (or neuropathy) and its application to myofascial pain.

A. Evidence for Acupuncture Efficacy

There is a considerable amount of literature that discusses the shortcomings of many studies in acupuncture research (1,2). The main problems concern the lack of

1. Study design and methods
2. Reproducibility
3. Outcome measures
4. Long-term follow-up
5. Placebo controls
6. Double-blinding

The additional problems of vastly different traditional Chinese medical diagnoses and therapies, as well as ethical, language, and cultural barriers, have also contributed to the stormy course of much of acupuncture research. Further consideration of the significant effect of the doctor–patient relationship and individual belief systems add complexity to this challenging area of research.

However, numerous attempts have been made to demonstrate the effects of acupuncture in the chronic pain setting. A large systematic review of 51 criteria-based acupuncture studies has placed particular emphasis on scientific and statistical quality (1). This comprehensive review showed that only 11 out of 51 trials scored more than 50 points out of a possible 100 relative to weighted quality variables. Of these more rigorous trials, five demonstrated positive results and six negative. It is also interesting that a high proportion of positive trials showed poor methodology, and treatment success is less commonly reported in well-designed studies. The authors further stated that no studies of high quality seem to exist. The conclusion made was that no definitive conclusions about the efficacy of acupuncture could be drawn.

By contrast, a prior metanalysis of the existing trials had suggested that pooling of some subgroup data provided significance in favor of acupuncture (3). However, little emphasis was placed on study design and methods in this analysis, which weakens its conclusive power considerably.

Further recent studies have also failed to show convincing evidence for the use of acupuncture in chronic pain. A prospective study investigating the effect of acupuncture on opioid-resistant chronic idiopathic pain demonstrated that only 2 out of 12 patients felt a substantial benefit in pain reduction after 8 months (4). Another investigation into chronic nociceptive back pain evaluated the effect of different modes of acupuncture stimulation (5). A sample of 30 persons was treated with manual needle stimulation, low-frequency electrical stimulation, or high-frequency electrical stimulation. Significant improvement was noted after 6 weeks in three out of four outcome measures in all groups, and improvement at 6 months was sustained in the low-frequency stimulation group only. However, longer-term data were not available.

Overall, data remain conflicting. High placebo effect rates of 30–35% frequently overwhelm other minor group differences. In the treatment of chronic back pain, for example, short-term effects appear to be positive, but rates vary from 26 (6) to 79% (7). This wide variation reflects differing measures and outcome criteria. Long-term effects are even harder to determine with follow-up periods from 40 h to 10 months posttreatment. This pattern of short-term improvement (averaging 50–80%), with minimal evidence for long-term benefit, is a common feature of many acupuncture trials treating various pain disorders. Important contributory factors to this wide variation of effect include differences in acupuncture technique and in the duration and number of treatment episodes. Site of needle insertion, timing of intervention, and type of stimulation are also parameters that should be controlled.

Interestingly, a recent study (1998) into the use of acupuncture in pain clinics in the United Kingdom revealed that a surprisingly high percentage (84%) offered acupuncture therapy (8). The clinical impression is, therefore, that acupuncture is valued, despite the lack of definitive well-presented evidence. Acupuncture is used in this context as another technique of peripheral sensory stimulation, which is already established as an effective pain therapy targeting endogenous pain modulation. However, acupuncture should not be seen as a panacea, but rather, as a useful additional tool in the treatment of some forms of chronic pain. Further rigorous research will be required to define its role more precisely.

II. MYOFASCIAL PAIN SYNDROMES

Myofascial pain syndrome is characterized by localized myalgia in one region of the body (contrasting with the more generalized muscle pain of fibromyalgia), in the absence of abnormalities in hematology, biochemistry, histology, or serology investigations. The muscles and their connective tissue attachments may be affected in any part of the body. Although relatively resistant to a wide range of treatment options, there is growing interest in the use of therapeutic needling techniques, which appear to offer considerable benefit in many patients.

The wide variety of musculoskeletal sites affected have resulted in frequently confusing nomenclature—usually corresponding to the site involved. Terms such as ''lateral epicondylitis,'' ''frozen shoulder,'' or even ''low back pain,'' are frequently used in situations where no other cause for pain can be found and in the absence of obvious injury or inflammation.

A. Pathophysiology

There is considerable ongoing debate focusing on the postulated mechanisms for the development and treatment of myofascial pain syndrome. Trauma, however, plays a central and uncontested role. Direct injury or muscle ''overloading'' is usually a factor, but repeated minor injuries (repetitive strain injury) are also increasingly considered as important. Initial theories have focused on the local effects of trauma and microtrauma, but there is also some evidence to support a neuropathic model. A discussion of the current theories will be followed by a review of the clinical assessment and treatment of the condition.

B. Nociceptive Theory

The basis of this theory depends on the activation and sensitization of nociceptors within muscle tissue. In the same way as the skin has Aδ-mechanothermal and C polymodal nociceptors, the corresponding nociceptors in muscle tissue are termed group III and group IV nociceptors, respectively. The characteristic quality of pain generated by activation of the Aδ (sharp) and C (dull) nociceptors in the skin is not, however, necessarily the same as that following activation of the corresponding muscle nociceptors (9).

Despite this, it might be reasonable to assume that if the quality of myofascial muscle pain is similar to that following skin C nociceptor activation, it is likely that group IV muscle nociceptors are responsible. Evidence that supports this hypothesis comes from clinical research that shows that myofascial pain can be reduced by stimulation of the superficial Aδ fibers, which block both skin and muscle C fiber spinal cord input by inhibitory interneurons in the dorsal horn (lamina I/II boundary). This may occur by a direct pathway from the Aδ fibers to spinal dorsal horn inhibitory neurons. Alternatively, indirect effects may be obtained through pathways in the periaqueductal gray matter linking the ascending spinothalamic tract to the descending inhibitory system (10).

Clinically, the main implication of this theory is that superficial dry needling, directly overlying painful trigger points, is all that is required to achieve pain relief (11). However, this does not explain why pain relief may last for weeks or months, and further attention to the long-term neural mechanisms is still required for a more satisfactory explanation.

C. The Theory of Radiculopathy or Neuropathy

The observation that pain is not necessarily associated with tissue injury has led to the concept that abnormal neural function may be responsible for a proportion of pain syndromes. A recent study has demonstrated that a considerable proportion (over 60%) of cancer patients with myofascial pain had symptoms and signs of neuropathic pain (12). The dysfunction of the nervous system may occur peripherally or centrally, leading to neuropathic pain; where pain may arise from a nonnoxious stimulus, or as a result of a pathophysiological functional disturbance in neuronal processing. As a result of this nerve dysfunction, which may be termed neuropathy, structural changes, such as muscle shortening and trophic changes, develop. Neuropathy is also generally associated with the following other features:

Pain unrelated to tissue damage
Delay in onset
Hyperalgesia
Dysesthesia
Allodynia
"Neuralgic" shooting or stabbing pain (neuropathic pain)
Summation and "afterreaction"

One may observe from this that neuropathic pain may be one component of neuropathy or radiculopathy.

1. Peripheral Mechanisms

Peripheral sensitization is usually perceived as the first process of a developing neuropathy. The nociceptors become increasingly sensitive to stimuli following surrounding inflammation or direct damage. However, the nerve may be damaged more proximally, at the root level. It is here that all the modalities served by the peripheral nerve may be affected; that is,

Motor nerve dysfunction (muscle shortening)
Autonomic changes (vasoconstriction, hyperhydrosis, trophedema)
Trophic alterations (hair loss, collagen degradation)

Minor damage at the proximal (root) level is not obvious clinically, but electrophysiological changes of spontaneous activity, exaggerated response to stimuli, and catecholamine sensitivity can be demonstrated. Work originally done by Cannon and Rosenblueth in the 1940s demonstrated that all innervated structures are dependent on incoming nerve impulses to provide a trophic (regulatory) effect. This input comprises both axoplasmic flow and electrical stimuli, and when input ceases, the innervated structures become highly sensitive and irritable (law of denervation) (13). All structures may develop supersensitivity following denervation. These include skeletal and smooth muscle, spinal neurons, sympathetic ganglia, sweat glands, and neuroglia.

It is important to note that complete denervation is not necessary to produce supersensitivity—a partial reduction in neuronal traffic for a time period is sufficient to cause "disuse" supersensitivity in the supplied structures (14,15). As a result, overreaction to many different stimuli occurs, and spontaneous electrical activity may promote pain or involuntary muscle activity. Increased sensitivity to chemical transmitters, including nerve growth factors, occurs along the whole length of the neuron; subsequent sprouting of neural fibers can lead to new connections with autonomic or sensory fibers.

The clinical relevance of the peripheral nerve injury model can be demonstrated in discussion of the development of spondylotic radiculopathy. Of the many causes of nerve damage, spondylosis (chronic attrition of intervertebral disk) is the most common factor affecting the vulnerably positioned spinal nerve root. Repeated major and minor injuries to the root area accumulate to form an "injury pool," explaining the increase in spondylosis-derived pain with age (16). The slow and chronic-relapsing nature of the disease frequently goes unnoticed, until an apparently minor incident provokes painful symptoms. Minor stimulation of a nerve rendered neuropathic by previous multiple insults can cause a sustained discharge and thereby persistent pain (17).

Nerve dysfunction manifests with motor, sensory, and autonomic changes. Motor changes frequently occur early, and consequent muscle shortening results from effects on the large-diameter motor neurons and myelinated afferents. Pain results from involvement of the nociceptive pathway and is not a universal feature. Collagen degradation also occurs secondary to neuropathy and can accelerate further structural weakness and degeneration (18).

2. Central Mechanisms

The interaction of peripheral and spinal mechanisms is central to the understanding of neuropathic pain and hypersensitivity. Central sensitization can occur following damage to a peripheral nerve or repetitive C-fiber nociceptor input. The following changes are associated with sensitization:

Increased dorsal horn spontaneous activity
Reduction in threshold for activation
Expansion of receptive field size
Increased response to afferent input
Prolonged afterdischarge

Molecular mechanisms responsible for these changes include *N*-methyl-D-aspartate (NMDA) channel activation, an increase in intracellular calcium, and wide dynamic range (WDR) neuron sensitization.

Central sensitization is maintained by ongoing afferent input or altered neural circuitry, or both. Increased recruitment of WDR neurons occurs (due to their large receptive field), as well as prolonged WDR discharge following stimulation because the normal inhibitory effects of Aβ fibers on Aδ and C activity are lost. The normal synaptic response to acute injury is mediated by AMPA and neurokinin acting on NK1 receptors, causing brief depolarization. Windup results from prolonged input by Aδ and C fibers, causing NMDA activation. This occurs when the AMPA and neurokinin receptor-mediated depolarization is of sufficient duration and magnitude to remove the Mg^{2+} block of the NMDA channel (19).

III. CLINICAL ASSESSMENT

A. Diagnosis

The diagnosis of radiculopathic pain and dysfunction is not always straightforward and requires considerable skill and practice. As the history is often noncontributory, extensive reliance on a careful and thorough physical examination is paramount. Further investigations are generally unhelpful, including thermography, nerve conduction studies, and electromyography.

Signs of neuropathy, as opposed to total denervation, are frequently subtle. Close inspection for motor, sensory, and autonomic changes in the skin and muscles is necessary. Vasoconstriction, increased sweating, and a hyperactive pilomotor reflex may be present. Pain may also provoke autonomic signs, and conversely, a stimulus causing autonomic activity may produce pain. "Trophedema" secondary to increased capillary permeability, although nonpitting to digital pressure, can be demonstrated with the "matchstick test."

Examination of the muscles, however, appears to offer the most reliable clinical indication of neuropathy. Increased muscle tone, tender points, palpable muscle contracture bands, and a restricted range of joint movement remain consistent features on assessment. Therefore, it is incumbent on the examiner to master in detail the anatomy of the muscles and their nerve supply.

Striated muscle contracture is an important feature of supersensitivity secondary to neuropathy (18). Owing to newly formed extrajunctional receptors, supersensitive muscle fibers develop tension in the absence of action potentials, and the resultant strain on connected tissues will give rise to pain (20). Muscle overreactivity to a wide variety of insults, both physical and chemical, also predominates in the clinical picture.

B. Treatment

1. Pharmacological

Treatment for myofascial pain syndrome is multifaceted, and a wide variety of drugs have been used with varying success. The presence of nerve dysfunction, or neuropathy, has led to attempts to target nerves pharmacologically. These have included the use of anticonvulsants, antidepressants, local anesthetics, ketamine, clonidine, mexilitine, capsaicin, magnesium, ketanserin, calcitonin, phentolamine, guanethidine, reserpine, and benzodiazepines. In a recent study, for example, intravenous lidocaine (lignocaine) has been used successfully in the treatment of fibromyalgia, demonstrating that the sodium channel is a potentially useful target for treatment (21). The current evidence suggests that antidepressants as well as anticonvulsants are effective in relieving neuropathic pain (22,23). Comparisons of tricyclic antidepressants showed no significant differences between them, although they were more effective than benzodiazepines (24).

Topical capsaicin cream also improves painful symptoms (25). There is limited further support given to the use of other pharmacological agents, but overall, no long-term data on analgesic effectiveness are available.

2. Physical

Physical forms of therapy are widely used as first-line treatment for peripheral neuropathic pain. The use of electrical stimulation has experimentally reversed the effects of supersensitivity (26). By temporarily increasing nerve traffic with stimulation, the reduction in impulse flow following neuropathy can be overcome. The innervated organ is "exercised," and the trophic effect is maintained. Pain is relieved, pending nerve recovery. Most injuries are minimal and resolve spontaneously without treatment, but minor injuries can be effectively treated in the short-term.

Physical stimulation techniques use this concept to achieve a similar effect. Examples include massage, activating pressure receptors; exercise, manipulation, and needling, stimulating muscle spindles; and heat and cold, affecting thermal receptors. Receptor stimuli are then transduced into nerve impulses that travel to the dorsal horn in the spinal cord.

Intramuscular stimulation (IMS) is a particular technique of dry needling that has been used successfully since 1985 to target muscle contracture that is secondary to neuropathy. Diagnosis and treatment, as well as progress, is determined according to the physical signs of neuropathy. Detailed knowledge of the anatomy and neurophysiology is, therefore, a prerequisite for effective application of IMS.

It is necessary to diagnose and treat the cause of spondylotic radiculopathy, and the numerous conditions causing impingement or entrapment of the nerve root need to be considered. Further investigations may be indicated and possible surgical options discussed. Initial local treatment may start with simple massage to tender and shortened muscles, followed by dry-needling techniques if appropriate.

The success of IMS depends on the skill and experience of the operator. Fine, flexible solid needles are used to find and release contractures, which are invisible to imaging techniques and clinically beyond the finger's reach. The needle transmits important feedback information as it traverses the tissues. "Needle-grasp," or the "Deqi response" confirms the remarkable cramp-like response of entering shortened and neuropathic muscle. The patient perceives a peculiar cramp-like quality of pain, which eases after a few minutes, together with the original symptoms, as the muscle shortening is released.

The contribution of specific nerve fibers to myofascial pain is still unclear, but research into progressive tactile hypersensitivity has provided some noteworthy results. Progressive tactile hypersensitivity is different from C-fiber–mediated sensitization, and demonstrates that Aβ-afferents also have the ability to induce wind-up. Therefore, it may be possible for other large proprioceptive afferent fibers in the muscle to contribute to myofascial pain. Future study should help clarify these issues.

The chronic situation is more complex. Fibrosis is often a dominant feature of the muscle contracture and requires more frequent and extensive needling. The response to dry needling is also less dramatic. Rarely, it may occur that a totally fibrotic muscle will not respond, but perseverance in most cases is rewarded with some improvement. Continued pain also occurs owing to shortened paraspinal muscles, which perpetuates compression and entrapment at the nerve root. Treatment to this area, therefore, is indicated.

IV. CONCLUSION

Myofascial pain syndromes are frequently difficult to manage, and the contribution of the radiculopathic model is significant to the understanding of this condition. Importantly, pain is only one of the possible manifestations of neuropathy and is not an invariable feature.

The cause of the radiculopathy needs to be targeted first. Given that spondylosis is the most common cause of radiculopathy, symptoms of myofascial pain are segmental and found in dermatomes, myotomes, and sclerotomes. Spinal examination is, therefore, essential, even with distal symptomatology. Subtle signs of neuropathy must also be actively sought. The proprioceptive component of neuropathy remains fundamental, and muscle shortening is a universal feature.

It should be noted that neuropathy may be an unexpected cause of various other conditions (e.g., tension headache, "frozen shoulder," and low back pain). Pain syndromes may thus not respond to conventional treatment and further treatment can be usefully directed within this neuropathic framework, with consideration for the use of intramuscular stimulation. Studies investigating IMS have shown a significant therapeutic benefit in a number of different conditions, such as low back pain, "tennis elbow," and hip pain (27–29). Further detailed and well-designed studies are required to establish the role of intramuscular stimulation as an effective and recognized treatment of choice for specific pain conditions, in line with encouraging anecdotal evidence.

REFERENCES

1. ter Riet G, Kleijnen J, Knipschild P. Acupuncture and chronic pain: a criteria-based meta-analysis. J Clin Epidemiol 1990; 43:1191–1199.
2. Richardson PH, Vincent CA. Acupuncture for the treatment of pain: a review of evaluative research. Pain 1986; 24:15–40.
3. Patel MS, Gutzwiller F, Paccaud F, et al. A meta-analysis of acupuncture for chronic pain. Int J Epidemiol 1989; 18:900–906.
4. Thomas M, Arner S, Lundeberg T. Is acupuncture an alternative in idiopathic pain disorder? Acta Anaesthesiol Scand 1992; 36:637–642.
5. Thomas M, Lundberg T. Importance of modes of acupuncture in the treatment of chronic nociceptive low back pain. Acta Anaesthesiol Scand 1994; 38:63–69.
6. Mendelson G, Selwood TS, Kranz H, et al. Acupuncture treatment of chronic back pain, a double-blind placebo-controlled trial. Am J Med 1983; 74:49–55.
7. Coan RM, Wong G, Su Liang Ku, et al. The acupuncture treatment of low back pain: a randomised controlled study. Am J Chin Med 1980; 8:181–189.
8. Woollam CHM, Jackson AQ. Acupuncture in the management of chronic pain. Anaesthesia 1998; 53:589–603.
9. Raja S, Meyer JN, Meyer RA. Peripheral mechanisms of somatic pain. Anaesthesiology 1988; 68: 571–590.
10. Bowsher D. Physiology and pathophysiology of pain. Acupunct Med 1990; 7:17–20
11. Macdonald AJR, Macrae KD, Master BR, et al. Superficial acupuncture in the relief of chronic low-back pain. Ann R Coll Surg Engl 1987; 65:44–46.
12. Loitman JE, et al. Myofascial pain syndrome in cancer patients with neuropathic pain. Abstr Am Acad Neurol Meet Minneapolis, Minnesota April–May 1998.
13. Cannon WB, Rosenblueth A. The Supersensitivity of Denervated Structures. New York: Macmillan, 1949.
14. Wall PD, Waxman S, Basbaum AI. Ongoing activity in peripheral nerve injury discharge. Exp Neurol 1974; 45:576–589.
15. Sharpless SK. Sensitivity-like phenomena in the central nervous system. Fed Proc 19; 34:1990–1997.
16. Thomas PK. Symptomatology and differential diagnosis of peripheral neuropathy: clinical features and differential diagnosis. In: Dyck PJ, et al., eds. Peripheral Neuropathy. Vol. 2. Philadelphia: WB Saunders, 1984;1169–1190.
17. Dyck PJ, Lambert EH, O'Brien PC. Pain in peripheral neuropathy related to rate and kind of fibre degeneration. Neurology 1976; 26:466–471.
18. Klein L, Dawson MH, and Heiple KG. Turnover of collagen in the adult rat after denervation. J Bone Joint Surg 1977; 59A:1065–1067.
19. Hudspith MJ. Glutamate: a role in normal brain function, anaesthesia, analgesia and CNS injury. Br J Anaesth 1997; 78:731–747.
20. McCain G. Fibromyositis. Clin Rev 1983; 38:197–207.
21. Sorenson J, Bengtsson A, Backman E, et al. Pain analysis in patients with fibromyalgia. Effects of intravenous morphine, lidocaine and ketamine. Scand J Rheumatol 1995; 24:360–365.
22. McQuay HJ, Carroll D, Jadad AR, et al. Anticonvulsant drugs for the management of pain—a systematic review. Br Med J 1995; 311:1047–1052.
23. McQuay HJ, Moore RA. Antidepressants and chronic pain. Br Med J 1997; 314:763–764.
24. McQuay HJ, Moore RA, eds. Antidepressants in neuropathic pain. In: An Evidence-Based Resource for Pain Relief. London: Oxford University Press, 1998.

25. Zhang WY, Li Wan Po A. The effectiveness of topically applied capsaicin: a meta-analysis. Eur J Clin Pharmacol 1994; 46:517–522.
26. Lomo T. The role of activity in the control of membrane and contractile properties of skeletal muscle. In: Thesleff S, ed. Motor Innervation of Muscle. New York: Academic Press, 1976:289–315.
27. Gunn CC, Milbrandt WE, Little AS, et al. Dry needling of muscle motor points for chronic low-back pain. Spine 1980; 5:279–291.
28. Gunn CC, Milbrandt WE. Tennis elbow and the cervical spine. Can Med Assoc J 1978; 114:803–809.
29. Gunn CC, Milbrandt WE. "Bursitis" around the hip. Am J Acupunct 1977; 5:53–60.

14
Advances in the Management of Spinal Pain and Radiofrequency Techniques

Andreas G. Erdmann and Rajesh Munglani
University of Cambridge and Addenbrooke's Hospital, Cambridge, England

I. INTRODUCTION

In the past two decades our understanding of the mechanisms of chronic pain have advanced tremendously. In particular, there is clear evidence for the role of the spinal cord and spinal cord structures in both initiation and maintenance of chronic pain. They not only give good explanations for clinically puzzling scenarios, such as complex spinal pain, but also provide a better scientific foundation for therapy of such conditions. A short introduction to the clinically relevant neurobiology of chronic pain will be followed by a section outlining the diagnosis and treatment of spinal pain.

II. BASIC SCIENCE CONCEPTS

A. Persistent Spinal Cord Changes Following Peripheral Inflammation or Nerve Injury

Damage to a peripheral nerve (such as compression of a nerve root by a prolapsing disk) or peripheral tissue inflammation (e.g., in arthritis) leads to an initiation of a cascade of molecular events within the peripheral nerve as well as in the spinal cord. Tissue inflammation is known to sensitize peripheral nerves so that they respond much more dramatically to stimulation. This partly explains, for example, the painful joint movement associated with arthritis.

However it is also well recognized that inflammation or peripheral nerve injury produce dramatic changes in the spinal cord. These events involve the release of neurotransmitters such as glutamate, substance P, neurokinin A, and calcitonin gene-related peptide (CGRP). This is followed by activation of certain receptors, such as the *N*-methyl-D-aspartate (NMDA) channel, which in turn, initiate a further cascade of events within neurons. This includes the activation of second messengers (including calcium, prostaglandins, and nitric oxide) and also expression of particular genes, such as c-*fos*. The amount of protein product of the c-*fos* gene in the spinal cord seems to correlate with the magnitude of the initial stimulus, yet it also mediates some of the adaptive responses of the spinal cord (see later).

Neuropeptide levels in the spinal cord also change. The levels of γ-aminobutyric acid (GABA; a profoundly inhibitory neuropeptide) fall and the levels of cholecystokinin (CCK), a neuropeptide with antiopioid actions, increase dramatically with peripheral nerve injury. An increased production of novel sodium channels mediated by nerve injury and nerve growth factors adds further to excess spinal cord excitability. The overall effect is a state of spinal cord disinhibition and increased receptivity to incoming stimuli.

Profound changes in neuronal phenotype occur, following nerve injury and inflammation. Large-diameter primary afferent neurons (which transmit nonnoxious stimuli) begin to express substance P (SP). As substance P is associated with only small-diameter neurons (which give rise to C-fibers and transmit pain and temperature) and transduction of noxious information, this may lead to misinterpretation of light touch and proprioception by the spinal cord and brain. Sprouting of the Aβ nerves within the spinal cord may also occur, with new contacts formed between the Aβ (laminae 3–4) and C-fibers (superficial laminae). This may form the basis of chronic pain and allodynia (1), and the subsequent reported reduction of neuronal sprouting with resolution of hyperalgesia is illustrative of remarkable spinal cord plasticity.

B. Neuropathic Pain Is Associated with the Loss of Opiate Sensitivity

Nerve injury in particular, induces various changes that diminish the action of opioids. At least three factors have been identified:

1. Loss of presynaptic opioid receptors
2. De novo production of opioid antagonistic neuropeptides (e.g., CCK) (2)
3. Opioid receptor tolerance owing to NMDA receptor activation (3)

Thus, chronic pain has to be managed in a radically different way than acute pain or postoperative pain where, for example, opioids are the mainstay of treatment. Opioids do have some effect in chronic nerve injury pain, but it is likely to be mediated in the brain, rather than spinally (4).

C. Sympathetic Nervous System Involvement

Peripheral nerve injury has been associated with

1. Sprouting of dorsal root ganglionic sympathetic fibers (5,6)
2. Adrenergic receptor expression causing sensitization to circulating norepinephrine

Despite often scant evidence of autonomic dysfunction (swelling, color or temperature change) there is increasing recognition given to the contribution of the sympathetic system in pain states, such as back pain.

All these changes outlined in the foregoing have profound functional implications leading to long-lasting changes in the processing of information entering the spinal cord. NMDA receptor or second-messenger activation and neuropeptide level changes lead to the heightened response of the spinal cord to further peripheral stimulation (*central sensitization*), giving rise to *allodynia* (the interpretation of previously innocuous sensation as if it was noxious) and *hyperalgesia* (a heightened response to noxious stimulation). The cascade of events initiated by a single insult may go on for weeks or months, and neuropeptide and c-*fos* expression persists well after resolution of the initial injury (7,8). These permanent plastic changes may be akin to a memory trace and may fundamentally and perhaps permanently alter the way the nervous system handles information. If these changes were indeed permanent, it would be appropriate to give attention to cortical mechanisms that have a powerful influence at the spinal cord as well as on the brain. This may include the use of antidepressants and pain management programs.

D. Prevention of Chronic Pain

Preemptive analgesia as a means of preventing chronic pain has been an area of considerable recent interest. Animal studies show a correlation between a phase 2 (delayed) pain response and the activation of spinal cord NMDA receptors. The activation of the NMDA receptor has, in other studies, also been shown to mediate sensitization of individual spinal cord neurons (including windup) and also to mediate enhancement of spinal cord reflexes (9).

However, conventional anesthesia does not reliably suppress phase 2 responses. Studies investigating isoflurane, intrathecal morphine, barbiturates, benzodiazepines, and opioids have shown only weak benefits (10). Clinically accepted doses have, at best, only moderate effects on afferent input, spinal cord sensitization, and modification of long-term pain perception.

As indicated by the expression of c-*fos* (early genomic expression), noxious stimuli still enter the spinal cord during apparently adequate anesthesia. It is not surprising, therefore, that clinical studies also fail to show an effect (11). The use of adjuncts to anesthesia (e.g., α_2-agonists, NMDA antagonists), which are able to suppress c-*fos* expression, have been shown experimentally to alter long-term pain behavior dramatically (12). Of interest is that the use of intrathecal local anesthesia, and intrathecal morphine, has actually caused excitation at low doses, and increased Fos expression (13). Comparative studies have also shown intrathecal local anesthesia to be less effective than sciatic nerve blockade in preventing development of chronic pain-related behavior (14). As a result, we cannot suggest that lack of perioperative pain behavior will imply reduced afferent input, or reduce its consequences. It is necessary to separate anesthesia from the processes involved in postinjury facilitation, enabling further thought to be given to the goals of the perioperative period.

Peripheral nerve blockade using local anesthetics is able to decrease pain perception over a wider area than expected (15). In addition, maintenance of the neurochemical changes in the central nervous system (CNS) is facilitated by continued peripheral input, which need not be abnormal. As a result, it can be suggested that continued peripheral input is important in maintaining central sensitization. The implications of this extend to the clinical practice of nerve blockade, in which a global reduction in nerve traffic allows the system to "wind down." The details of this are unclear, but it appears as if the electrical potential of the receiving neuron is critical in determining sensitization or adaptation (16). This has allowed a concept of a sensitive system to emerge, in which the addition of local anesthetic could "flip" a system from hypersensitivity to adaptation. In addition, the administration of agents that further antagonize the up-regulation of spinal cord second messengers (epidural steroids, NMDA antagonists, and α_2-agonists) also help reduce the level of central sensitization.

E. Predisposing Factors in Chronic Pain

The role of Fos protein is central to the mediation of spinal cord analgesic responses. The administration of antisense c-*fos* causes a progressive increase in hyperalgesia, indicating that Fos protein may have a low-level role in normal sensory transduction. Supraspinal adaptive responses also exist and these activate descending inhibitory pathways. There is some evidence to show that this balance between adaptive and sensitization mechanisms has a genetic component (17). Further studies in neuropathic pain have shown that hyperalgesia disappears before resolution of the nerve injury (18). The spinal cord changes discussed previously are likely to modify the effects of initial nerve injury and help resolution of hyperalgesia. If these adaptive mechanisms fail, the development of chronic pain is considered more likely (19). Interestingly, spinal magnetic resonance imaging (MRI) studies in asymptomatic patients have shown a potentially surgically treatable condition in one-third of the general population (20). This demonstrates the concept that a nociceptive source may not translate into cognitive pain, and that adaptive changes and cognitive elements may be an important final determinant of the clinical picture.

III. EPIDEMIOLOGY OF BACK PAIN

Back pain is an extremely common, almost universal, condition, affecting up to 90% of persons at some time in their life. Disability associated with low back pain also affects some 2–5% of the at-risk population and is reflected in millions of days lost each year in the workplace. Estimates of the financial burden resulting from back pain are staggering. The total cost in the United States was estimated at 60 billion dollars in 1990, which includes a figure of 35 billion dollars for working days lost (21). In the United Kingdom, the yearly average for back pain-related days of sickness is 33 million days/year, or approximately 2% of the workforce sick-listed per year. The time of life at which back pain is judged to have the greatest social and financial impact is in the middle working years, peaking at about 40 years of age. However, mechanical back pain is common from the early 20s until the late 50s, followed by a gradual decline in incidence (22). This decline may also reflect an increased focus on other emerging health problems. Following initial resolution of symptoms in the majority, a small proportion of patients will begin to show a pattern of chronicity. Identification of this group at an early stage would be ideal, but unfortunately is still proving an elusive goal.

Despite the common nature of back pain, treatment options are variable in their effectiveness. The vast majority (up to 90%) of acute back pain attacks will resolve in about 6 weeks, irrespective of the type of treatment (Fig. 1) (24). The crucial time for improvement appears to be between 2 and 12 weeks. However, persistent pain and disability highlight the frequent inadequacies felt when dealing with back pain that appears unresponsive to treatment. Difficulties in diagnosis and patient variability add to the complexities of management, and finding reliable, appropriate, and practical therapies can prove remarkably difficult.

Low-back disability is increasing and it would appear that this is a phenomenon of Western

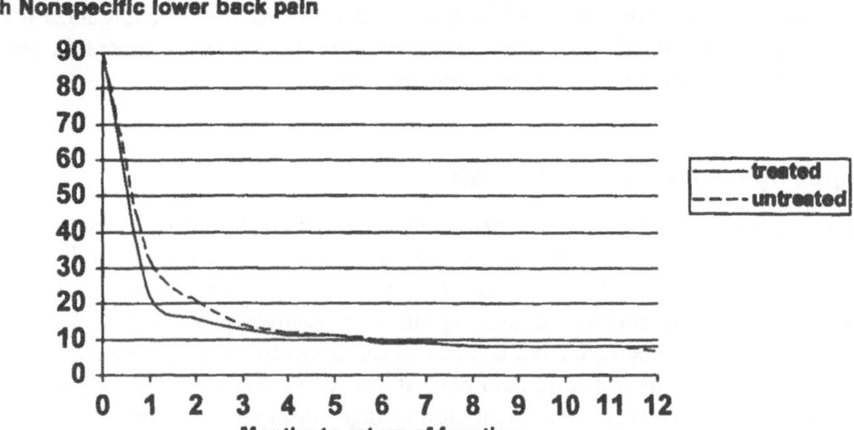

Figure 1 The return to function (in months after injury) of patients with acute nonspecific back pain: The treated group shows an earlier return to function when compared with the untreated group, but no significant difference is seen after 3–6 months. (From Ref. 24.)

society. Other developing nations report high incidences of back pain, but it is unusual for this result in a significant impairment to daily living (23). The context in which disability occurs is important, and a biopsychosocial model is frequently used to highlight the multifactorial nature of the condition.

The overall influence of back pain and disability is undeniably huge, and future success will hinge on effectively targeted prevention and well-researched clinical therapies.

IV. CLINICAL MANAGEMENT

The management of back pain can be divided up into two phases, according to the duration of the complaint and the response to treatment:

1. An early ("acute or subacute") phase, in which the early treatment options are considered, and efforts made to establish a diagnosis and exclude serious conditions requiring urgent attention. In this phase, the degree of pain is frequently proportional to the injury or illness and response to treatment is generally predictable. In general, this phase may last up to 2 years following presentation.
2. A late ("chronic") phase, in which, until recently, the diagnosis was frequently by exclusion and treatment response was unpredictable. The degree of pain and disability may appear out of proportion to the precipitating factors. Treatment is frequently in specialist clinics and usually commences after the initial diagnostic and treatment phase, usually after approximately 2 years.

A. Early (Acute or Subacute) Phase

Management of acute back pain will include the following:

1. History
2. Examination
3. Investigation
4. Diagnosis
5. Initial treatment

1. History

A full and thorough assessment of the clinical history is of great value in the diagnostic procedure. It is important to inquire about previous episodes of back pain at an early stage in the interview. The following information may be of further diagnostic value:

1. Nature of onset
2. Nature of pain–periodicity
3. History of trauma
4. Sudden onset in elderly (metastatic disease)
5. Occupation
6. Postural relief (may indicate mechanical cause)
7. Radicular pain (possible disk herniation)
8. Numbness, aggravated by Valsalva (disk herniation)
9. Improvement with exercise (inflammatory; c.f., mechanical)
10. Associated heat or cold changes (sympathetic influences)
11. Extent of disability; litigation factors
12. Psychological factors and social environment

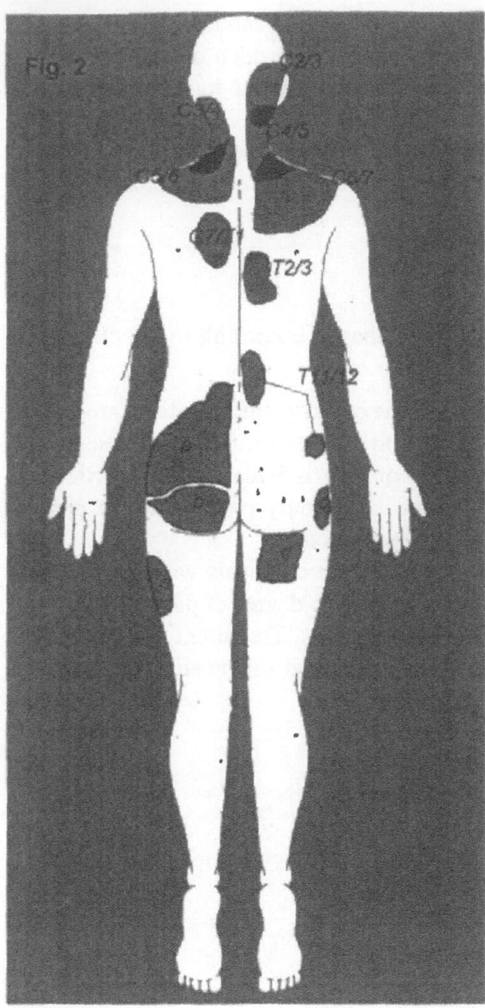

Figure 2 The more common pain referral patterns seen following stimulation of the zygapophyseal joints and dorsal rami in the cervical, thoracic, and lumbar regions in volunteers. a, lumbar region; b, gluteal region; c, trochanteric region; d, lateral thigh region; e, posterior thigh region. The lumbar patterns of referral are detailed in Table 1.

The pattern of pain radiation and localization is of some limited benefit in making a diagnosis. Pain "maps" have been drawn that attempt to correlate symptoms and localized pathology, using evoked pain. Unfortunately, there appears to be considerable overlap between areas, and the pattern of local pain referral remains only a rough guide to the specific origin of the pain stimulus (Fig. 2: Table 1).

2. Examination

Examination of a patient with back pain needs to be systematic and complete. The back needs to be inspected and palpated and the range of motion of the spine determined. It is particularly important to assess areas of increased or evoked pain, as valuable clues to the diagnosis may be forthcoming. Further examination of the neurological system is then undertaken, to delineate

Table 1 Regions of Pain Referral Following Stimulation of Facet Joints or Medial Branches

	Lumbar spinal region	Gluteal region	Trochanteric region	Lateral thigh region	Posterior thigh region
L1/2	100%	—	—	—	—
L2/3	100%	8%	17%	8%	—
L3/4	80%	40%	10%	20%	20%
L4/5	100%	27%	8%	15%	8%
L5/S1	78%	68%	16%	32%	5%

Source: Ref. 65.

neurological compromise and to alert the examiner to urgent conditions requiring immediate referral ("red flags") (Table 2) (24).

1. Inspection: poor posture, pelvic asymmetry, inflammation, gait abnormalities, poor vertebral alignment, loss of lumbar lordosis
2. Palpation: (1) of bony structures (pain may suggest fracture or infection); (2) of soft tissue.

Bony palpation causing pain over the vertebral spines may be helpful in infective conditions or traumatic fractures. Soft-tissue palpation should include all the muscles of the back and buttocks, but is rather nonspecific and unreliable. The presence or absence of trigger point pain

Table 2 "Red flags": Potentially Serious Conditions

Possible fracture	Possible tumor or infection	Possible cauda equina syndrome
Major trauma: vehicle accident or fall from height	Age over 50 or under 20	Saddle anesthesia
	History of cancer	Recent onset bladder dysfunction (urinary retention, increased frequency, overflow incontinence)
Minor trauma or strenuous lifting in older patients		
	Constitutional symptoms (fever, weight loss, chills)	
		Severe, progressive distal neurological deficit
	Risk factors: recent bacterial infection (example, UTI), IV drug use, immunosuppression (steroids, HIV, transplant)	
	Pain worse when supine, severe nighttime pain	
		Anal sphincter laxity
		Perineal or perianal sensory loss
		Major motor weakness (quadriceps, ankle flexors, evertors, dorsiflexors)

Source: Ref. 24.

and associated radicular symptoms may be useful in excluding myofascial pain. However, interobserver variation has been demonstrated to be extremely variable (25). Muscle spasm may also be difficult to distinguish from discrete painful areas.

The range of motion of the spine may also be helpful in diagnosis. Diminished lumbar flexion is nonspecific; however, radicular pain on flexion may suggest disk herniation. Pain on extension, rotation and lateral bending are possible indicators that facet joint involvement is present.

Neurological screening should focus on evidence of nerve root impairment, or spinal cord dysfunction. As most herniated disks cause root involvement at the L5 or S1 level, examination here is of particular importance. As a principle, dermatomal involvement is the key to a successful diagnosis and the motor findings are more specific than the more variable sensory findings.

Muscle weakness should be tested for specifically. Toewalking (S1) and heelwalking [L5/(4)], are useful, as is squatting [L4/(5)], dorsiflexion of toe [L5/(4)], ankle eversion (L5/S1), and toe flexion (S1). Muscle wasting can be measured by circumferential comparison with the other side. Ankle reflexes reflect the S1 root, and the knee jerk the L4 root (no L5 reflex). The plantar response may also indicate an upper motor neuron lesion. Sensory testing to pinprick and touch in the lumbar and sacral dermatomes is indicated, although it is sometimes difficult to interpret in the absence of other findings. Awareness of nondermatomal distributions of sensory loss is also important.

The straight leg-raising test may be useful to determine likely irritation of the L4/5/S1 nerve roots. This needs to elicit radicular pain in the appropriate distribution to be positive, and back pain or posterior thigh pain is considered a negative result.

Examination, therefore, plays an essential role in the diagnostic process. Differentiation of organic from nonorganic pathology is possible, and indications for further investigation are usually provided.

3. Investigation

This will be guided by the history and examination findings. Imaging techniques combined with laboratory evaluation will aid diagnosis in well-selected patients and serve as a useful baseline for future use.

Imaging Techniques

1. Radiography
2. Computed tomography (CT)
3. MRI
4. Myelography (with or without CT)
5. Diskography

Routine lumbar spine films have not shown any major benefits. Over 75% of patients have normal or insignificant films and the use of oblique radiographs adds information in only 3% of patients. If selection criteria are applied, for example, in suspected malignant disease and traumatic fractures, their usefulness increases significantly. CT and MRI are expensive procedures and relative difficulty in interpretation is frequently encountered. Up to 20% of asymptomatic patients show evidence of disk herniation or spinal stenosis (26). Nerve root pathology may be better seen using myelography, with or without CT, but carries the low risk of arachnoiditis. Diskography can be useful to detect smaller lesions not seen by MRI or CT, and if care is taken in the interpretation of the test, potentially unnecessary surgery may be avoided (i.e., if injection into the apparently abnormal disk does not evoke pain [negative test]).

Table 3 The Diagnostic Value of Different Techniques

Technique	Identify physiologic insult	Identify anatomical insult
History	+	+
Physical examination		
Circumference	+	+
Reflexes	++	++
Straight-leg raising	++	+
Motor	++	++
Sensory	++	++
Laboratory studies (ESR)	++	0
Bone scan	+++	++
EMG	+++	++
X-ray	0	+
CT	0	++++
MRI	0	++++
Myelo-CT	0	++++
Myelography	0	++++

Source: Ref. 24.

Laboratory Evaluation

1. ESR/CRP
2. Full blood count
3. HLA-B27
4. Autoantibodies
5. Prostate-specific antigen (PSA)

These test may be performed in selected patients when indicated (i.e., high suspicion of rheumatological disorders, infection, or ankylosing spondylitis).

4. Diagnosis

The diagnostic process in the initial stages of back pain has to involve the combination of often diverse findings on history, examination, and investigation. The careful selection of appropriate tests is essential to avoid overinvestigation and unnecessary expense, but signs and symptoms suggestive of more serious disease need to be fully and urgently investigated. Table 3 suggests the relative usefulness of individual aspects of history, examination, and investigation.

There is no ideal classification of conditions causing back pain. According to individual perspective, these may be based on anatomical areas, physiological changes, organ systems, degree or duration of complaint, urgency, or ranked according to frequency. The majority of clinicians would exclude urgent conditions first, and then determine the probable origin of the pain, using information from the history and examination to suggest further investigations. A clinical picture suggestive of a particular condition is likely to emerge, and appropriate treatment will follow.

A broad classification of back pain includes (27) the following:

1. Mechanical or activity-related: Mechanical-type back pain is by far the largest group, and includes a diverse number of conditions in which mechanical and activity factors

play a role. This group includes mechanical low back pain of nonspecific origin, as well as that due to demonstrable anatomical changes.

2. Neurological syndromes: These will include myelopathy (from intrinsic and extrinsic causes), neuropathy, plexopathy, mononeuropathy, and myopathy.
3. Systemic disorders: Systemic diseases, such as malignancy and infection, as well as inflammatory arthropathy, metabolic bone disease, and vascular disorders need exclusion.
4. Referred pain: Pain may also be referred, and common sites of origin will include gynecological, genitourinary, and gastrointestinal disorders, as well as hip pathology and abdominal aortic aneurysms.
5. Psychosocial factors: Somatoform disorders, psychiatric disorders, and psychosocial factors may present with back pain, and attendance from drug- or benefit-seeking individuals is occasionally seen.

To obtain a relatively precise diagnosis from the available information, it is helpful to consider the more common conditions that may be included in the mechanical-type group.

Mechanical low back pain includes a number of different conditions, but is essentially a nonspecific diagnosis, and is characterized by relatively localized pain, with radiation of pain a noncontributory finding. Good improvement of symptoms is frequently seen in the first 4 weeks, with 90% resolution by 6 months, and chronicity is a feature in less than 5% of patients.

Facet joint arthropathy has been a controversial diagnosis in the past, probably owing to operator inconsistency in performing diagnostic blockade. The facet joint is richly innervated and there is little doubt that derangements of the joint do cause pain.

Degenerative disk disorders have also been inconsistent in producing pain. Degeneration of the disks occurs in the 20s, and only a few will cause significant pain and disability. However, injection will provoke pain and radicular symptoms in many sufferers and extensive innervation is also seen.

Myofascial pain syndrome has been described in all large muscular groups in the body. A characteristic pattern of referral is seen, and confusingly radicular symptoms can also occur. As the muscles of the lower back are under particular stress, the incidence of pain is higher here than elsewhere. However, patients with genuine nerve root pathology may also describe muscle tenderness, making differentiation from myofascial pain difficult.

Herniation of the vertebral nucleus pulposus occurs predominantly at L4-5 and L5-S1 levels. Pain is referred in the root distribution in a proportion of patients only. This is due to mechanical and chemical irritation of the respective nerve roots involved. L4/L5 irritation causes pain from the buttocks down the anterolateral part of the leg to the medial foot and great toe. L5/S1 pain will also include distal involvement of the lateral foot and toes. However, clinical findings may not correlate with radiographic signs and another cause for back pain may be present.

Spondylolisthesis, or the displacement of one vertebral body on the next, usually occurs in an anterior direction, but may occasionally displace posteriorly. Pain in the acute phase usually originates from the stretched longitudinal ligaments, and marked slippage may produce radicular symptoms and cauda equina compression. Stability is thought to be maintained in the large majority of patients and the risk of progression is small, even in younger patients (less than 10%). However, surgical stabilization may be required if progression of symptoms continues.

Spinal stenosis may also cause back pain, which is usually progressive in the elderly, and may require surgical decompression to relieve pressure on the cauda equina or nerve roots. Relief of leg pain with resting and flexion is common, and a long, variable clinical course is usual.

Postsurgical back pain conditions form another large group. Pain may be due to arachnoiditis with scarring and fibrosis of the meninges producing nerve root irritation. Direct trauma, inadequate decompression, recurrent disk herniation, and instability are also implicated in pain following back surgery. Patient selection is critical in preventing further postsurgical morbidity.

A precise diagnosis following an episode of acute back pain may not be straightforward, but the prognosis is usually very good. Once urgent and serious conditions have been excluded, approximately 90% of patients will recover within the first 6 weeks. It is only in a small minority of patients that symptoms persist and in whom further diagnostic testing and intervention is required.

5. Initial Treatment

The evidence concerning the use of a wide variety of treatment options for acute back pain has been recently reviewed by the Clinical Standards Advisory Group (CSAG) (28). The majority of patients improve, regardless of the type of treatment given. However, the evidence was in favor of the following:

1. Bed rest, if required, for no more then 2 days
2. Trial of analgesics
3. Trial of antidepressants
4. Physical therapy

Despite the appropriate treatment of patients in the early stages, treatment appears to have little effect on the long-term outcome of back pain. It may shorten the duration and severity of the acute phase, but does not affect the chronicity or severity of chronic back pain. It becomes clear that there appears to be an intractable core of patients at approximately 6 months who remain disabled with back pain, and if they remain off work for more than 12 months are very unlikely to return to good functional status.

There is a vast amount of literature on the comparative merits of back pain treatments. Table 4 suggests the relative value of specific treatments in back pain. In the past, long periods of bed rest have been advocated, with limited evidence of significant benefit. Recent evidence has now shown that a period of 2–7 days of bed rest is actually worse than placebo or ordinary activity in relief of pain, rate of recovery, and return to normal function (29). Studies looking at the effects of prolonged rest have shown a loss of muscle strength at the rate of 3%/day, as well as the demineralization of bone, and prolongation of recovery is inevitable. Return to normal

Table 4 Proof of Treatment Effectiveness for Nonspecific Lower Back Pain

Duration of pain (days)	<7	7–42	43–90	>90
Bed rest <2 days	Conclusive	Conclusive	Low	Low
Bed rest <7 days	None	None	None	Negative
Acetaminophen/NSAID	Conclusive	Conclusive	Low	Low
Manipulation	Low	High	Low	None
Exercise	None	Low	Conclusive	Low
Facet injection	N/A	Negative	Negative	Negative
Surgery	N/A	None	None	None
Facet radiofrequency	N/A	N/A	N/A	Conclusive
Epidural steroid	N/A	N/A	None	None
Pain management program	N/A	N/A	N/A	Conclusive

Source: Ref. 24.

activity as soon as possible lessens the recovery time, and a short period of bed rest (less that 2 days) is not considered as treatment per se, but as a method of reducing pain in the short-term.

Nonsteroidal anti-inflammatory drugs (NSAIDs) have also been effective in reducing back pain (30). Regular dosing regimens are recommended, and acetaminophen (paracetamol) can be substituted with NSAIDs or acetaminophen–weak opioid compounds. In addition small doses of muscle relaxants (benzodiazepines or baclofen) may be useful in the short-term. The administration of low-dose antidepressants, such as amitriptyline (at an early stage) also improves recovery and pain.

A large number of exercise programs have been devised for use in the acute phase of back pain. Techniques from simple mobilization and gentle exercise, up to and including, intensive dynamic strength routines have been studied. The overwhelming evidence from these studies is that activity is beneficial in reducing pain and sick leave (23). The common misconception that exercise may be harmful applies to the most extreme programs only, and there is no doubt that the physical and psychological benefits of physical therapy play an extremely important role in the recovery from acute back pain.

Physiotherapy, and chiropractic manipulation, in particular, has been the subject of intense recent interest, possibly as a result of relatively low treatment success rates with conventional treatment. Although long-term studies have shown no benefits, there is some evidence that significant symptomatic relief can be achieved in the first 6 weeks (31,32). Selected patients who appear to require additional help or who are not returning to usual activities should be considered for manipulative therapy. Increased patient satisfaction and reduced pain is maximal in the first 2 weeks, but there is no difference evident after 4 weeks or in the long-term.

In the occasional patient, a diagnosis may be difficult to establish, or there is pain not responsive to treatment, and a longer process of diagnosis and treatment unfolds. The patient is usually investigated in some depth, and reviewed by specially teams. Surgery may be indicated or further medical management directed at a related disease. Relapsing back pain may also become continuous, and a chronic pattern of disease begins to emerge. In a minority of patients, disabling chronic back pain becomes a feature of their lives, despite extensive prior medical consultation, and the challenge of treating chronic back pain is presented.

B. Late (Chronic) Phase

Chronic spinal pain has a number of important features that distinguish it from acute back pain. Of these, perhaps the most important is that a growing consensus now considers chronic pain as a disease per se, rather than purely as a symptom. This enables the fundamental importance of the nonphysical elements of pain to be taken into account. The integration of the physical dimensions of pain with the psychological and social factors, which are inextricably linked together, allows a significant and deliberate move away from traditional Cartesian dogma. This is illustrated in Fig. 3. As a result, treatment of one area alone may not result in improvement at other levels, and the complexity of human suffering is a challenge that needs a multifaceted approach.

The approach to therapy for chronic back pain has been variably indefinite, in the absence of significant evidence favoring one specific treatment over another. In particular, evidence has been lacking concerning the longer-term effect of some procedures that may appear to be highly effective in the short term. With recent increasing interest in metanalysis, there is now a slowly growing body of evidence that can be used to guide appropriate therapy. When this evidence is integrated with knowledge of the anatomical and pathophysiological nature of back pain, it

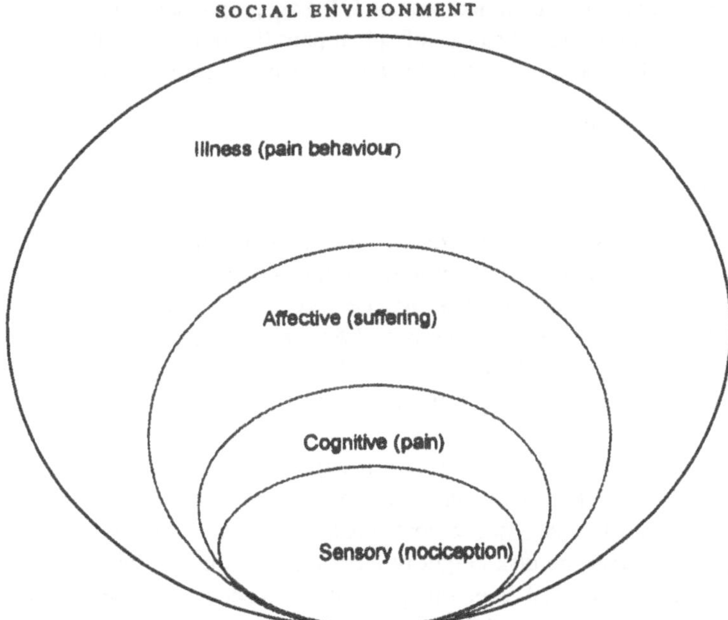

Figure 3 Biosocial model of pain. The consequences of pain are evident at many levels: Treatment of the nociceptive element alone may not lead to the resolution of other levels in the chronic situation. The importance of integrated and concurrent pain management programs (including cognitive behavioral therapy) must be emphasized, and should not be considered as merely a solution only if all else fails. (From Ref. 23.)

becomes possible to formulate a rational and logical treatment plan and to decide on the direction of treatment.

1. Anatomy and Pathophysiology

Studies on the causes of back pain in the 1930s directed major attention to the concept of disk herniation impinging on the nerve root (33). However, work had been done earlier, and subsequently, that suggested that spinal structures other than the spinal cord might also give rise to back and referred pain (34). These sources become more significant in chronic spinal pain. Provocation studies show that spinal cord structures, previously insensitive, can give rise to pain after moderate injury. The following structures have well-defined innervation (35):

1. Lumbar disk: sinuvertebral nerve, ventral nerve, gray rami communicantes
2. Posterior longitudinal ligament: sinuvertebral nerve
3. Anterior longitudinal ligament: gray rami communicantes
4. Iliocostalis lumborum/longissimus thoracis: lateral/intermediate dorsal rami branches
5. Facet joints/multifidus/interspinous ligament: medial branch of the dorsal rami

The two main causes of nonneuropathic pain are lumbar zygapophyseal joint arthritis (facet joint) and internal disk disruption (IDD) (36). IDD is not the same as disk protrusion. Disk protrusion can be seen on an MRI scan. In contrast, IDD does not show up well on MRI scans and is demonstrated best by disk stimulation and CT diskography. There is a high degree of correlation between the degree of annular disruption seen on CT diskography and pain experienced by disk stimulation (37,38). The principal causes of spinal pain (in patients with pain of more than 2 years duration and with unhelpful MRI and CT scan results) are the following:

1. Lumbar internal disk disruption pain (39%)
2. Lumbar facet joint pain (15–40%)
3. Sacroiliac joint pain (30%)

In the neck-pain population, cervical facet joint disease accounts for 50% of nonspecific causes of pain. This includes a large percentage of "whiplash" injuries persisting for more than 2 years. The other (specific) causes of lumbar back pain include disk herniation (2%), vertebral compression (4%), spondylolisthesis (3%), spinal stenosis (1%), spinal malignancy (0.7%), spondylitis (0.03%), and infection (0.001%) (39). By using placebo-controlled diagnostic blockade, up to 75% of patients with previously nonspecific back pain can be characterized in a specialized pain clinic.

The increasing acceptance of facet joint-derived pain is supported by studies that have shown that, once arthritic, nearly 50% of the body weight may pass through these joints (40,41). In addition to this, disk degeneration can cause further joint loading. Diurnal variation in facet joint-derived pain is common, given that the disk height reduces through the day, with subsequent increased facet joint loading. Postsurgical facet joint pain may also occur from mechanical disruption and diskectomy (with loss of disk height).

Electrophysiological and clinical studies have also shown that lumbar facet joint pain may radiate down the leg (42,43). This occurs because the posterior rami that supply the facet joint are branches of the same nerve that supplies sensation to the leg. In a similar manner, cervical facet joint disease frequently radiates to the occipital region and between the shoulder blades as well as into the upper limbs. Migraine ("cervicogenic") and atypical facial pain and may also originate from cervical joint disease through the so-called cervicotrigeminal link.

2. Treatment

The management of the patient with chronic back pain is multifactorial. As suggested previously, attention needs to be given to all elements of the complex nature of chronic pain. It is also worth noting that despite extensive prior investigation, it is possible that patients may develop new signs of acute disease: therefore, vigilance for these possibilities needs to be maintained.

Drug Therapy. The vast majority of patients who present to a chronic pain clinic with a history of back pain will be taking a number of different drugs and report varying levels of efficacy. Frequently, multiple changes of dosing and medication will have been attempted and benefits are often not felt to be significant. The central aim of drug therapy in chronic back pain is to provide a reasonable benefit within the limits of tolerance and safety. This is often difficult to achieve, and optimization may take some time and effort. Despite lack of evidence that medication alters the outcome of chronic back pain, it is clear that both symptom relief and improved activity can be achieved in some groups of patients. However, side effects may be troublesome and addiction and psychological dependence may be difficult problems to solve. Careful prescription and regular follow-up of patients is essential to enable optimization of frequently complex drug regimens.

Nonsteroidal anti-inflammatory drugs (NSAIDs). NSAIDs have enjoyed popularity in the chronic pain setting for some considerable time, predominantly because of their low addiction potential. However, the side effects of NSAIDs are considerable and easily underestimated. In particular, gastrointestinal bleeding and renal toxicity are common enough to cause concern. The use of modern, more specific (cyclooxygenase; Cox-2) agents (such as etodolac and meloxicam) appear to confer only a relative improvement in side effects. The marginal benefits obtained from of NSAIDs in many patients means that close monitoring of benefits and risks needs to be ongoing and attention given to patient education.

The anti-inflammatory mechanism of action of NSAIDs is at odds with the noninflammatory nature of most chronic pain. However, in conditions with an inflammatory component, or after activities likely to cause inflammation, consideration should be given to the use of NSAIDs, because it is in these groups of patients in whom the benefits are likely to be maximal.

Opioids. Controversy about the use of opioids in chronic back pain has revolved around the issue of addiction and the lack of evidence for any long-term benefit. If careful patient selection is employed, it is probably appropriate to prescribe opioid analgesia in situations when little else can be offered. The use of opioids can prove very effective in allowing certain patients to engage in rehabilitation programs and return to a reasonable level of function. Some studies have shown significant improvement in pain relief in chronic nonmalignant pain (44) and no decline in mood or cognition with long-term use of long-acting opioids (45).

A firmly structured prescription policy, with patient involvement, will go some way toward improving the difficulties some patients encounter with management of opioid use. The psychological background of individual patients will, largely, determine the potential for dose escalation or addiction, and awareness of opioid-seeking behavior is helpful in minimizing inappropriate use.

The question of which opioid to use is not altogether straightforward. Varying potencies will be appropriate for different patients and agents with longer-dosing intervals are usually preferred. Controlled dose-release agents are widely used and clinically reduce dose escalation and addiction. Evidence to suggest a benefit of one agent over another is beginning to emerge. Methadone has been extensively used in chronic pain, and patients who are responsive to low doses (20–30 mg/day) would appear less likely to require dose escalation. Recent studies also show that methadone, in addition to being a (predominantly) μ-opioid receptor agonist, also has NDMA receptor antagonistic activity (46). This suggests the probability of an additional mode of analgesic action. Buprenorphine also shows stability of dosing in the long-term and is another agent worth considering.

Antidepressants. Depression and its coexistence with chronic pain have evoked much interest in this interrelationship over recent years. Numerous studies on the effect of antidepressants on back pain have shown conflicting results (47). As a result no conclusions can yet be drawn on the efficacy of antidepressant medication in chronic back pain, and larger well-controlled studies are awaited.

The mechanism of action of antidepressant drugs in chronic pain is also incompletely understood. The principal question asked is whether antidepressants have direct analgesic action, or whether they are simply mood elevators. It can be seen clinically that the effects of antidepressant are seen at lower-dose ranges and are quicker in onset than those seen when treating depression. In addition, antidepressants show serotonin-uptake inhibition, and this suggests an effect on the descending inhibitory serotonergic pain pathways. However, serotonergic antidepressants show no pain relief benefit over noradrenergic antidepressants, suggesting that noradrenergic systems may also be involved in pain.

Nerve membrane stabilizers. The use of antiepileptic medication has been widespread in the chronic pain setting, usually secondary to nerve injury. The principal use in chronic back pain is in patients with documented nerve injury, and dose titration to the desired effect is recommended, with maximum effect expected at 2–4 weeks. The first agents to be successfully introduced as adjunctive therapy were carbamazepine and phenytoin, but the occurrence of side effects limits their use in some patients. This has led to the search for less toxic and more tolerable drugs. A recently introduced antiepileptic, gabapentin (up to 2400 mg/day), in early trials has shown initial promise in the treatment of neuropathic pain states (48). Another new agent, topiramate, is also expected to offer efficacy and good tolerability.

Other Drugs. As the knowledge of the mechanisms and mediators of chronic pain increases, so the opportunities for intervening at different receptor sites become available. There is a multitude of therapies available, all of which demonstrate the complexity of the pain cascade. Although the mechanisms leading to wind-down are still poorly understood, it would appear that ways of reducing central sensitization have an important role to play. NMDA activation can be reduced by the use of NMDA antagonists such as ketamine. Epidural steroids, NSAIDs, and ketamine reduce the sensitization of spinal cord neurons. GABA agonists, anticonvulsants, and some antidepressants may prevent spinal cord loss of inhibition. Neuronal sprouting in the spinal cord can be influenced by NMDA antagonists, neurotropins and cytokines. The release of tachykinins, such as substance P and NK-A, could in theory be prevented by neurokinin 1 and 2 antagonists, which are now undergoing phase 1 and 2 clinical trials. Sodium channel blockers, such as lidocaine (lignocaine) infusions and oral mexilitine or lamotrigine reduce increased excitability. The factors maintaining central sensitization can be depressed by the use of nerve blockade (with or without steroids), quanethidine blockade, α-agonists, and NSAIDs. The use of these additional agents needs to be individually tailored, and it is often only by following a process of trial and error that some success may be achieved.

Physical Therapy. The use of physical methods of therapy has been an important cornerstone in the overall management of chronic back pain. A plethora of different treatments have been advocated, all using varying degrees of activity and manipulation, and substantial differences between modalities have not been definitively demonstrated.

As in acute back pain, the use of manual therapy for chronic back pain has enjoyed recent interest. These techniques include soft tissue manipulation, massage, manual traction, corsets, joint manipulation, and joint mobilization. The considerable numbers of studies published to date have been hampered by poor study design and lack of controls, and have failed to demonstrate any comparative significant benefits in long-term chronic back pain patients (31,49,52). Some studies show a relatively rapid response to manipulation or chiropractic therapy in a small subgroup of unidentifiable patients, but the long-term results are not significant (50). Combined therapies are frequently used, which makes the effect of specific treatments hard to judge. It is common for activity-based exercises to run concurrently as well as subsequently, and in selected patients a case can be made for the use of combination physical therapy.

Physical exercise and physiotherapy have also been recommended, and they form the basis of a continuing program of physical rehabilitation. The methods in use vary from isometric exercise to intensive aerobic conditioning, but beneficial results from studies have been relatively limited over the past years. However, the majority of research indicates that regular gentle exercise of any kind is helpful in improving back status in the long-term, for as long as the training program is maintained (51). However, improved pain relief and greater muscle strength have not been shown reliably to improve activity or lifestyle and highlight the considerable difficulties in the treatment of chronic back pain. It is also of note that even if long-term outcome is uncertain, short-term improvements may allow the involvement in other beneficial activities.

Transcutaneous electrical nerve stimulation (TENS) has also enjoyed some popularity in the chronic pain setting. Despite the advantages of simplicity and considerable enthusiasm for its use, no well-designed trials have shown any advantage over placebo in the treatment of chronic back pain.

The overall impression obtained from the evidence now available is that patients benefit from active physical therapy, rather than passive therapy, and that long-term improvements are linked to compliance with a daily routine—an ideal often difficult to achieve.

Epidural Steroids. The use of epidural steroids is currently under considerable debate. A scientific rationale for their use is frequently lacking, and despite this, widespread use is evident. The argument for their use is in documented cases of acute nerve irritation or inflammation that presents clinically with characteristic radicular (not somatic) pain. However, significant evidence for their usefulness in chronic back pain is lacking, perhaps reflecting the reduced role that perineural inflammation plays in the chronic situation. Interestingly, one study has shown that methylprednisolone has a direct reversible inhibitory action on nociceptive axons, much like a local anesthetic (51). A recent large systematic review concludes that some short-term benefit may be achieved in patients with sciatica, but that long-term studies fail to demonstrate any benefit (53).

Facet Joint Blockade and Denervation. The increasing acceptance of facet joint-derived pain, and the "facet joint syndrome," has allowed the identification of another useful avenue in the management of chronic back pain. The extensive innervation of the facet joint from the medial branch of the sinuvertebral nerve allows the option of a direct injection into the facet joint or blockade of the supplying nerves. The injection of local anesthetic agents, with or without corticosteroids, allows the operator to identify if the joints are indeed a source of pain, without a permanent effect. This diagnostic procedure, if positive, can provide pain relief outlasting the duration of action of the injected agent, but should not be considered as treatment. Several studies have reported the relative ments of using local anesthetics, corticosteroids, or saline in terms of efficacy and duration of relief, with conflicting results (55,56). These would appear to miss the point of the usefulness of diagnostic blockade in finding a source for the patient's pain, which is able to add unique information to the diagnostic process, as well as being useful medicolegally and for patient reassurance. Further consideration can also be given to a placebo control and this will also assist in making the diagnosis more certain.

The long-term treatment of facet joint-derived pain is not always as straightforward as the diagnosis. A small proportion of patients might be candidates for surgical lumbar stabilization. However, the majority who have failed to respond to conservative measures would be suitable for permanent joint denervation procedures. A number of methods have been used and include cryotherapy, neurolytic agents, and radiofrequency thermocoagulation. Agents such a phenol have been used successfully for neurolysis, but the overwhelming evidence is currently in favor of thermocoagulation (57–64). Results show that approximately 50% of patients will have dramatic reductions in pain scores as well as significant reductions in disability and analgesic consumption. These improvements appear to be still sustained after 5 years in many patients, and show thermocoagulation to be a very effective treatment in selected groups of patients.

Intervertebral Diskography and Disk Denervation. The technique of provocation diskography has also been the subject of considerable controversy. Despite improved-imaging techniques using CT and MRI, diskography remains the only valid technique to assess whether pain is related directly to a disk. It is well recognized that minimally abnormal and normal images of disk anatomy frequently do not exclude disk-derived pain, and in these situations, diskography may still demonstrate pain from an apparently normal disk. The rich innervation of the outer one-third of the annulus explains the nociceptive origins of disk pain, and in normal diskography, injection within the inner third of the disk should provoke no more than sensation of mild pressure. However, if there is annular disruption, then substances impinging on the outer nociceptive fibers will cause pain. Further confirmation of disk-derived pain is evident if local anesthetic injected subsequently relieves the pain. The innervation of the anterior disk is not as segmental as the posterior portion, and frequently radiation into unexpectedly high dermatomes may occur from a lower lumbar lesion (i.e., inguinal pain (L1/L2) from L5 disk) (65).

It is important that diskography is interpreted in the light of previous clinical and radiographic findings. Patients who obtain no definitive diagnosis from prior efforts may be referred for diskography, and depending on the outcome, may proceed to diskectomy and vertebral body fusion, or may benefit from permanent disk denervation. The latter is achieved by the use of radiofrequency thermocoagulation and has an as yet uncertain success rate of between 33 and 60% over a 2-year period, as reported in one study (66).

Sympathetic Blockade. Some patients will not be fortunate enough to fall into the category of those responding well to facet joint or disk blockade. The disks and other surrounding spinal structures have significant sympathetic innervation, and this allows the operator to block the sympathetic pathways to establish the role of this system. Diagnostic blockade is usually performed at the L2 level, below which the lumbar sympathetic chain innervates numerous spinal structures (67). Lumbar sympathetic blockade has been also used to treat diskogenic pain, and the sympatholytic action of epidurals is self-evident (68). The fact that these blocks may be made permanent, usually by the use of neurolytic agents, has heightened interest in this area. Thermocoagulation of specific communicating rami (with their sympathetic components) has also been proposed for site-specific forms of disk-derived pain (69).

Pulsed Radiofrequency. Radiofrequency lesioning has been used for over 30 years in the treatment of numerous chronic pain complaints. The initial hypothesis was that the mode of action was presumed to be the destruction of nervous tissue by heat. However, that an electromagnetic field surrounds the tip of the electrode has led to speculation that a clinical effect may be related to this field. As the high temperatures (90°C) are seen at only the very tip of the needle and there is a rapid decrease in temperature away from the tip (especially in nonhomogeneous tissue), the possibility of an alternative mechanism has to be borne in mind. New techniques of pulsed radiofrequency (PRF) have now been developed in which the radiofrequency is applied for only 20 or 30 ms/s (pulsed), rather than continuously. In this way the electrode tip reaches a maximum heat of only 42°C. Studies show no signs of anatomical destruction of tissue or neuritis (70). The mechanism of action is as yet unclear, but PRF may act by stimulating spinal and supraspinal analgesic mechanisms, thereby reducing pain perception.

The efficacy and duration of relief obtained from PRF have yet to be widely quantified. However, initial reports and studies show very promising and dramatic results. The evidence thus far favors the use of PRF in neuropathic pain where the absence of neurological damage is desirable, and some patients have reported complete or nearly complete resolution of symptoms (71). The likely duration of pain relief has not yet been fully elucidated, but ongoing reports suggest that about 30–50% of patients will achieve between 6 months and 1 year of relief (Table 5; Fig. 4). The use of PRF is an exciting new area that shows great promise and may hold an important place in the therapeutic armamentarium in the future.

Spinal Cord Stimulation and Implantable Devices. There remains a core of patients who continue to suffer from severe chronic back pain despite intensive investigation and treatment, particularly in the post–back-surgery population. For these patients, diagnosed with failed back surgery syndrome (FBSS), treatment options are severely reduced and a difficult pain challenge is presented. The development of implantable spinal cord stimulators, however, has allowed a proportion of these patients to achieve a reasonable degree of pain relief and improve their function. Although the response to stimulation is quite variable, and there are risks and complications associated with the procedure, spinal column stimulation remains a useful option in treating such patients. A large survey of the literature concluded that approximately 50–60% of patients achieved 50% pain relief on long-term follow-up (72). However, a large proportion of patients did express that they would not choose spinal column stimulation again, demonstrating the considerable uncertainty about their use. Careful patient selection is recommended and patients

Table 5 Symptom Complex and Response to Pulsed Radiofrequency of Patients Who Showed Temporary Responses to Test Blocks with Local Anesthetic and Steroid

Subject no.	Type of pain	Response
1	Neuropathic back pain	Responded
2	Neuropathic chest pain	Responded
3	Neuropathic leg pain	Responded
4	Neuropathic leg pain	Responded
5	Neuropathic leg pain	Responded
6	Neuropathic chest pain	Responded
7	Peripheral neuroma	Responded
8	Peripheral neuroma	Responded
9	Back pain	No response
10	Back pain	No response
11	Back pain	No response
12	Back pain	No response
13	Back pain	No response
14	Neuropathic back pain	No response

with remediable conditions, major psychological illness, or secondary monetary gain issues should not receive stimulators.

Other methods of providing pain relief in intractable cases include the use of implantable devices. Here an extradural or intraspinal catheter may be implanted and attached to a small infusion system. Commonly, opioids or local anesthetics are slowly infused to provide more or less continuous pain relief. Again, the hazards of the procedure and of the infused drugs need to be realized and regular follow-up ensured (73).

Pain Management Programs. The treatment of chronic back pain needs to be directed at many levels, throughout the course of the illness. Early management of the cognitive and affective elements should be instituted, with an awareness of the fundamental importance of the psychosocial factors in chronic pain. Disability, more than actual pain, is inextricably linked to cognition and emotion, and efforts to reduce this have to include addressing these issues as well. Much has been written about the complexity of the pain response, and the physical manifestations on one hand and behavioral and cognitive changes on the other may well be two sides of the same coin. Recent evidence also shows that patients in pain have very differing central representation patterns as shown by positron emission tomography (PET) scanning (74).

The tendency is for many pain specialists to divide into two groups: those seeking a nociceptive source, and those looking for cognitive or behavioral explanations. The temptation to explore in one direction is strong, but it is only by addressing all aspects that a complete and holistic therapeutic intervention can be achieved.

The introduction of pain management programs (PMP) has proved an effective way to address the complexities of intractable chronic pain. The more intensive programs, involving multidisciplinary teams and extensive retraining have proved to be very effective in encouraging patients to regain control over the pain and their lives. The PMPs involve the patient during a committed period in reexploring the many levels of the pain experience. During this time, patients report a gradually increasing level of self-confidence and reduction in disability, with active physical therapy addressing the somatic aspect. Results show that patients have an increased quality of life and a reduced reliance on health care services that is evident at 6 months

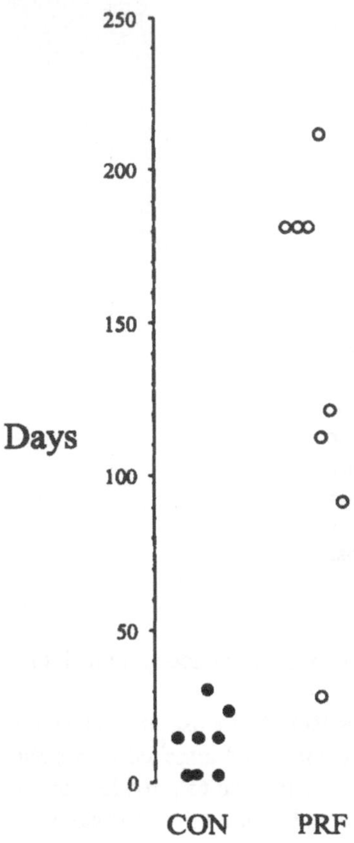

Figure 4 A pilot comparison of pulsed radiofrequency (PRF) with injection of steroid in patients with neuropathic pain who failed to respond to a range of other treatments: The effect of PRF outlasts that of the steroid group significantly. (From unpublished pilot data.)

after treatment and frequently continues for years (75–77). Although PMPs are expensive, the cost of back pain in unemployment and other benefits to the state is much greater.

V. CONCLUSION

The problem of chronic back pain is continuing to provide a substantial challenge to pain management teams and their resources. We suggest here a flowchart for the management of chronic back pain that has been unresponsive to initial treatment (see Fig. 5). Rapid advances in knowledge and novel therapies are adding to our understanding of the multifaceted nature of this condition, and much research still needs to be done to enable rational and effective management decisions to be taken. However, it is clear that an isolated approach with the sole emphasis on one or other aspect of the back pain problem is unlikely to bring satisfactory long-term improvement. Multidisciplinary pain teams, who address the physical and interventional therapy aspects, as well as the cognitive, behavioral and psychosocial factors, remain the ideal framework in which to bring about the most effective results. Human illness should be emphasized as a global entity and management needs to encompass all the relevant factors.

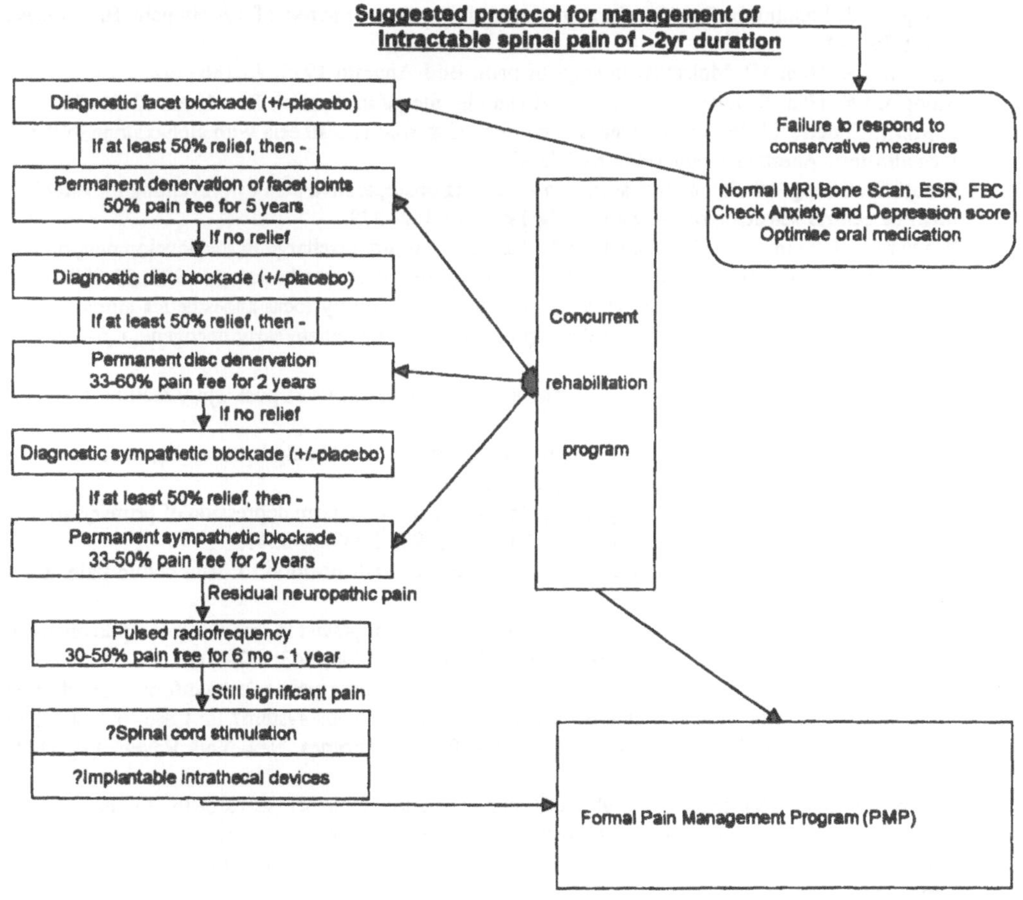

Figure 5 A suggested protocol for the management of intractable spinal pain of more than 2 yr duration, based on current evidence.

Note in proof: Since this chapter was written, the technique of intradiscal electrotherapy has been validated as a procedure for the treatment of discogenic pain.

REFERENCES

1. Woolf CJ, Shortland P, Coggeshall RE. Peripheral nerve injury triggers central sprouting of myelinated afferents. Nature 1992; 355:75–78.
2. Hokfelt T, Zhang X, Wiesenfeld–Hallin Z. Messenger plasticity in primary sensory neurons following axotomy and its functional implications. Trends Neurosci 1994; 17:22–30.
3. Mao J, Price DD, Mayer DJ. Mechanisms of hyperalgesia and morphine tolerance: a current view of their possible interactions. Pain 1995; 62:259–274.
4. Roud Mayne C, Hudspith MJ, Munglani R. Efficacy of opioids in neuropathic pain [letter]. Anaesthesia 1996; 51:1190.
5. Chung K, Kim HJK, Park MJ, et al. Abnormalities of sympathetic innervation in the area of an injured peripheral nerve in a rat model of neuropathic pain. Neurosci Lett 1993; 162:85–88.
6. McLachlan EM, Janig W, Devor M, et al. Peripheral nerve injury triggers noradrenergic sprouting within dorsal root ganglia. Nature 1993; 363:543–545.

7. Munglani R, Fleming B, Hunt SP. Remembrance of times past: the role of c-*fos* in pain. Br J Anaesth 1996; 76:1–4.
8. Munglani R, Hunt SP. Molecular biology of pain. Br J Anaesth 1995; 75:186–192.
9. Munglani R, Hunt S, Jones JG. Spinal cord and chronic pain. Anaesth Rev 1996; 12:53–76.
10. Gilron I, Coderre TJ. Pre-emptive analgesic effect of steroid anaesthesia with alphaxalone in the rat formalin test. Anesthesiology 1996; 84:572–579.
11. Woolf CJ, Chong MS. Preemptive analgesia—treating postoperative pain by preventing the establishment of central sensitization. Anesth Analg 1993; 72:362–379.
12. Yamamoto T, Shimoyama N, Mizuguchi T. Role of the injury discharge in the development of thermal hyperaesthesia after sciatic nerve constriction in the rat. Anaesthesiology 1993; 79:993–1002.
13. Nivarthi RN, Grant GJ, Turndorf H, et al. Spinal anaesthesia by local anaesthetics stimulates the enzyme protein kinase C and induces the expression of an immediate early oncogene, c-*fos*. Anesth Analg 1996; 83:542–547.
14. Abram SE, Yaksh TL. Morphine but not inhalational anesthesia blocks post injury facilitation. Anesthesiology 1993; 78:713–721.
15. Gracely RH, Lynch SA, Bennett GJ. Painful neuropathy: altered central processing maintained dynamically by peripheral input. Pain 1992; 51:175–194.
16. Randic M, Jiang MC, Cerne R. Long term potentiation and long term depression of primary afferent neurotransmission in the rat spinal cord. J Neurosci 1993; 13:5228–5241.
17. Devor M, Raber P. Experimental evidence of a genetic predisposition to neuropathic pain. Eur J Pain 1991; 12:65–68.
18. Munglani R, Harrison S, Smith G, et al. Neuropeptide changes persist in spinal cord despite resolving hyperalgesia in a rat model of mononeuropathy. Brain Res 1996; 743:102–108.
19. Zimmerman M. Central nervous system mechanisms modulating pain-related information: do they become deficient after lesions of the peripheral or central nervous system? In: Casey KL, ed. Pain and Central Nervous System Disease: The Central Pain Syndromes. New York:Raven, 1991;183–199.
20. Boden SD, Davis DO, Dina TS, et al. Abnormal magnetic resonance scans of the lumbar spine in asymptomatic subjects. A prospective investigation. J Bone Joint Surg 1990; 72A:403–408.
21. Frymoyer JW. Quality. An international challenge to the diagnosis and treatment of disorders of the lumbar spine. Spine 1993; 18:2147–2152.
22. Bombardier C, Kerr MS, Shannon HS, et al. A guide to interpreting epidemiological studies on the etiology of back pain. Spine 1994; 19(18S):2047S–2056S.
23. Waddell G. A new clinical model for the treatment of low-back pain. Spine 1987; 12:632–644.
24. Fordyce WE. Back Pain in the Workforce. Seattle: IASP Press, 1995.
25. Nice DA, Riddle DL, Lamb RL, et al. Intertester reliability of judgements of the presence of trigger points in patients with low back pain. Arch Phys Med Rehabil 1992; 73:893–898.
26. Jensen MC, Brant–Zawadski MN, Obuchowski N, et al. Magnetic resonance imaging of the lumbar spine in people without back pain. N Engl J Med 1994; 331:69.
27. Wheeler AH. Diagnosis and management of low back pain and sciatica. Am Fam Phys 1995; 52: 1333–1341.
28. Rosen M. The Clinical Standards Advisory Group (CSAG) Report on Back Pain. London: HMSO, 1994.
29. Malmivaara A, Hakkinen U, Aro Heinrichs ML, et al. The treatment of acute low back pain: bed rest, exercises or ordinary activity? N Engl J Med 1995; 332:351–355.
30. Koes BW, Scholten RJP, Mens JMA, et al. Efficacy of NSAIDs for low back pain: a systematic review of randomised controlled trials of 11 interventions. In: Low Back Pain in Primary Care: Effectiveness of Diagnostic and Therapeutic Interventions; Institute for Research in Extramural Medicine, 1996:171–190.
31. Shekelle PG, Adams AH, Chassin MR, et al. Spinal manipulation for low back pain. Ann Intern Med 1992; 117:590–598.
32. Koes BW, Assendelft WJJ, van der Heiden GJMG, et al. Spinal manipulation and mobilisation for back and neck pain: a blinded review. Br Med J 1991; 303:1298–1303.

33. Mixter WJ, and Barr JS. Rupture of the intervertebral disc with involvement of the spinal canal. N Engl J Med 1934; 211:210–215.
34. Goldwait JE. The lumbosacral articulation: an explanation of many cases of lumbago, sciatica and paraplegia. Boston Med Surg J 1911; 164:365–372.
35. Bogduk N. The innervation of the lumbar spine. Spine 1983; 8:286–293.
36. Schwarzer AC, Aprill CN, Derby R, et al. The relative contributions of the disc and zygapophyseal joint in chronic low back pain. Spine 1994; 19:801–806.
37. Moneta GB, Videman T, Kaivanto K, et al. Reported pain during lumbar discography as a function of anular ruptures and disc degeneration: a re-analysis of 833 discograms. Spine 1994; 19:1968–1974.
38. Schwarzer AC, Aprill CN, Derby R, et al. The prevalence and clinical features of internal disc disruption in patients with chronic low back pain. Spine 1995; 20:1878–1883.
39. Deyo RA. Understanding the accuracy of diagnostic tests. In: Weistein JN, Rydevik BL, Sonntag VKH, eds. Essentials of the Spine. New York: Raven, 1995:55–71.
40. Yang KH, King AI. Mechanism of facet load transmission as a hypothesis for low-back pain. Spine 1984; 9:557–565.
41. Lewinnek GE, Warfield CA. Facet joint degeneration as a cause of low back pain. Clin Orthop Relat Res 1986; 213:216–222.
42. Gillette RG, Kramis RC, Roberts WJ. Characterisation of spinal somatosensory neurons having receptive fields in lumbar tissues of cats. Pain 1993; 54:85–98.
43. Mooney V, Robertson J. The facet syndrome. Clin Orthop 1976; 115:49–156.
44. Zenz M, Strumpf M, Tryba M. Long-term oral opioid therapy in patients with chronic nonmalignant pain. J Pain Sympt Manage 1992; 7:69–77.
45. Haythornthwaite JA, Menefee LA, Quatrano–Piacentini AL, et al. Outcome of chronic opioid therapy for non cancer pain. J Pain Sympt Manage 1998; 15:185–194.
46. Morley JS, Makin MK. The use of methadone in cancer pain poorly responsive to other opioids. Pain Rev 1998; 5:51–58.
47. Turner JA, Denny MC. Do antidepressant medications relieve chronic low back pain? J Fam Pract 1993; 37:545–553.
48. Rosenberg JM, et al. The effect of gabapentin on neuropathic pain. Clin J Pain 1997; 13:251–255.
49. Pope MH, Phillips RB, Haugh LD, et al. A prospective randomised three-week trial of spinal manipulation, transcutaneous muscle stimulation, massage and corset in the treatment of subacute low back pain. Spine 1994; 19:2571–2577.
50. Doran DML, Newell DJ. Manipulation in treatment of low back pain: a multicentre study. Br Med J 1975; 2:161–164.
51. Manniche C, Lundberg E, Christensen I, et al. Intensive dynamic exercises for chronic low back pain: a clinical trial. Pain 1991; 47:53–63.
52. Koes BW, Assendelft WJJ, van der Heijden GJMG, et al. Spinal manipulation and mobilisation for back and neck pain: a blinded review. Br Med J 1991; 303:1298–1303.
53. Johansson A, Hao J, Sjolund B. Local corticosteroid application blocks transmission in normal nociceptive C-fibres. Acta Anaesthesiol Scand 1990; 34:335–338.
54. Koes BW, Scholten RJPM, Mens JMA, et al. Efficacy of epidural steroid injections for low-back pain and sciatica: a systematic review of randomised clinical trials. Pain 1995; 63:279–288.
55. Jackson RP, Jacobs RR, Montesano PX. Facet joint injections in low back pain; a prospective clinical study. Spine 1988; 13:966–971.
56. Lippitt AB. The facet joint and its role in spinal pain. Management with spinal joint injections. Spine 1984; 9:746–750.
57. Mehta M, Sluijter ME. The treatment of chronic back pain. A preliminary survey of the effect of radiofrequency denervation of the posterior vertebral joints. Anaesthesia 1979; 34:768–775.
58. Ignelzi RJ, Cummings TW. A statistical analysis of percutaneous radiofrequency lesions in the treatment of chronic low back pain and sciatica. Pain 1980; 8:181–187.
59. Bogduk N, Marsland A. The cervical zygapophysial joints as a source of neck pain. Spine 1988; 13:610–617.

60. Silvers HR. Lumbar percutaneous facet rhizotomy. Spine 1990; 15:36–40.
61. Bogduk N, Aprill C. On the nature of neck pain, discography and cervical zygapophysial joint blocks. Pain 1993; 54:213–217.
62. Gallagher JP, Petriccione Di Vadi L, Wedley JR, et al. Radiofrequency facet joint denervation in the treatment of low back pain: a prospective controlled double-blind study to assess its efficacy. Pain Clin 1994; 7:193–198.
63. North RB, Han M, Zahurak M, et al. Radiofrequency lumbar facet denervation: analysis of prognostic factors. Pain 1994; 57:77–83.
64. Lord SM, Barnsley L, Wallis BJ, et al. Percutaneous radio-frequency neurotomy for chronic cervical zygopophyseal joint pain. N Engl J Med 1996; 335:1721–1726.
65. Morinaga T, Takahashi K, Yamagata M, et al. Sensory innervation of the anterior portion of the lumbar intervertebral disc. Spine 1996; 21:1848–1851.
66. Kleef M, Barendse GA, Wilmnik JT, et al. Percutaneous intradiscal radio-frequency thermocoagulation in chronic non-specific low back pain. Pain Clin 1996; 9:259–268.
67. Takahashi H, Yanagida H, Morita S. Analysis of the underlying mechanism of sympathetically maintained pain in the back and leg due to lumbar impairment: pain relieving effect of lumbar chemical sympathectomy. Pain Clin 1996; 9:251–258.
68. Nakamura SI, Takahashi K, Takahashi Y, et al. The afferent pathways of discogenic low-back pain. Evaluation of L2 spinal nerve infiltration. J Bone Joint Surg 1996; (B)78:606–612.
69. Sluijter ME. The use of radiofrequency lesions for pain relief in failed back patients. Int Disabil Stud 1988; 10:37–43.
70. Sluijter ME, van Kleef M. Characteristic and mode of action of radiofrequency lesions. Curr Rev Pain 1998; 2:143–150.
71. Munglani R. The longer term effect of pulsed radiofrequency for neuropathic pain. Pain 1999; 80: 437–439.
72. Turner JA, Loeser JD, Bell KD. Spinal cord stimulation in low back and leg pain: a systematic literature synthesis. Neurosurgery 1995; 35:1088–1095.
73. Krames ES. Intraspinal opioids for nonmalignant pain. Curr Rev Pain 1997; 1:198–212.
74. Hsieh JC, Belfrage M, Stone-Elander S, et al. Central representation of chronic ongoing neuropathic pain studied by positron emission tomography. Pain 1995; 63:225–236.
75. Harkapaa K, Mellin G, Jarvikoski A, et al. A controlled study on the outcome of inpatient and outpatient treatment of low back pain. Part III. Long-term follow-up of pain, disability, and compliance. Scand J Rehabil Med 1990; 22:181–188.
76. Moffett JAK, Chase SM, Portek I, et al. A controlled, prospective study to evaluate the effectiveness of a back school in the relief of chronic low back pain. Spine 1986; 11:120–122.
77. Bendix AF, Bendix T, Ostenfeld S, et al. Active treatment programs for patients with chronic low back pain: a prospective, randomized, observer-blinded study. Eur Spine J 1995; 4:148–152.

15

Pulsed Radiofrequency Treatment of Chronic Neck, Back, Sympathetic, and Peripheral Neuroma–Derived Pain

Rajesh Munglani and Kathrin A. Stauffer
University of Cambridge and Addenbrooke's Hospital, Cambridge, England

I. INTRODUCTION

The use of radiofrequency (RF) lesions in the treatment of chronic pain has a long history. It has been presumed that the mode of action of the technique is due to the heating effect caused by the current. However, as Sluijter et al. (1) have recently pointed out, after heat lesioning of the dorsal root ganglia (DRG), the pain relief may outlast the perceived sensory loss, indicating that there may be other analgesic effects of the technique. Slappendel (2) reported that for the treatment of benign cervicobrachialgia, they could not distinguish between a 67°C lesion and a 40°C heat lesion. Furthermore, Sluijter et al. (1) also reported in two small studies that pulsed radiofrequency (PRF) provided better and longer-lasting analgesia than either a low-temperature continuous radiofrequency or a simple local anesthetic and steroid block.

We recently reported our initial experience of PRF, which seemed to show greatest efficacy for the treatment of neurographic pain (3). In this chapter we present our findings with PRF in radicular neuropathic pain, sympathetic pain, and in the treatment of pain that may be emanating from peripheral neuromas.

II. METHODS

In this open study, patients offered PRF were outpatients at pain clinics in Cambridge, England. Patients were suffering from chronic pain with strong neuropathic features of at least 18 months standing, but more typically with pain histories going back between 5 and 60 years. The patients had typically tried multiple drug therapies, including trials of antidepressants, anticonvulsants including gabapentin, nonsteroidal anti-inflammatory drugs (NSAIDs), and long-term opioid therapy, without success. In addition, patients would also have had multiple interventional pain procedures such as epidurals, diagnostic DRG blocks, sympathetic blocks, diagnostic or permanent lumbar or cervical zygapophyseal joint blocks, without long-term success.

Criteria for administration of PRF included a significant, but short-lived, analgesic response to a block to either dorsal root ganglion, lumbar sympathetic chain, or the site of a peripheral neuroma, performed with local anesthetic and steroid. Responders to diagnostic sympathetic blockade were offered PRF to the sympathetic chain if it was judged inadvisable to perform a phenolic block of the sympathetic chain (4).

All patients who received PRF treatment over a period of about 10 months were included in the survey, with the exception of two cancer patients, one of whom had died at the time of the survey, and one further patient who was judged to be unable to understand the questions.

The PRF procedure was performed as follows. Under midazolam sedation and x-ray control, the skin was anesthetized by the injection of up to 2 mL 1% local anesthetic (LA). Using a modified RDG radiofrequency generator (RDG Medical, 429 Brighton Road, South Croydon, Surrey, UK), PRF to the DRG was performed under x-ray control using a 20–30 ms/s pulse at a frequency of 2 Hz for 180 s, with the temperature rising at the probe tip to no more than 42°C. Up to 2 mL of 0.5% LA and up to 20 mg of corticosteroid was then injected at each DRG thereafter (i.e., identical to that received previously and to which the patient had only a short-lasting response). The positioning of the probes near the lumbar DRG used a standard tunnel vision approach, with the tip advanced no farther than the midfacet line. In the cervical region, the tip was originally placed on the cervical root, rather than the DRG, but on the later patients, it was placed nearer the DRG using a tunnel vision approach.

PRF to the lumbar sympathetic nerves was performed using conventional approaches as described in the literature (4). PRF to local neuromas was performed by placing the tip at the site of maximum tenderness.

Typically, 3 months posttreatment, and in some cases up to 6 months posttreatment, patients were sent a questionnaire. The questionnaire consisted of the following:

1. Three visual analog pain scores (VAS) of 100-mm length each, for pain pretreatment, pain in the first weeks posttreatment, and pain at the time of assessment.
2. One question about how long the benefit of the treatment lasted (later converted to weeks).
3. One question about medication pretreatment and posttreatment.
4. A series of questions about improvement in disability posttreatment as compared with pretreatment. Two versions of this section were prepared, one for back pain consisting of 18 items [taken from Roland and Morris (5)] and one for neck pain consisting of 13 items [following the items used by the Neck Disability Index (6)].
5. Two questions about changes in locus and quality of the pain.
6. One question about the patient's overall judgment of the experience.
7. One question about side effects and any other comments.

Pain scores were measured in millimetres (0–100). The duration of improvement was expressed in weeks on a scale from 0 to 13, with durations given as "a few days" scored as 1 week, and durations of more than 3 months scored as 13 weeks or longer. Medication was scored as either "less or weaker," "more or stronger," or "no change." Disability improvement was expressed as a percentage, with 0% being no improvement and 100% being maximally improved to normal function. Quality and locus of pain were scored as either "change" or "no change." The last two questions about the patient's personal experience were not entered in the database.

The data were entered into a database using Filemaker Pro (Claris Works) and analyzed using Statview 4 (Abacus Concepts) on a PowerMac 7200/90.

III. RESULTS

Sixty questionnaires were sent out to patients treated with PRF. Of these, 42 (70%) were completed and returned. In addition, three patients responded by letter without completing the questionnaire and were not included in the analysis. Their responses would not change any of our conclusions.

Depending on the treatment received, the patients who returned completed questionnaires were broken down into the following categories:

A. Lumbar DRG

Twenty-nine patients whose predominant complaint was of neuropathic-type sciatica, and whose pain had previously been temporarily abolished with local anesthetic and steroid to the DRG site. L5 location was the largest subgroup in this category. Fourteen of them had previous spinal surgery for back pain and sciatica.

B. Cervical DRG

The cervical DRG category contained six patients. Three of the patients in this category presented with neck pain, and two presented with cervicogenic headaches. These five patients had suffered prior whiplash-type events. The sixth patient presented with phantom pain after upper limb amputation. The cervical DRG patients were sent the questionnaire containing the neck disability items; all others were sent the questionnaire containing the back pain disability questions.

C. Local Neuroma

One patient was suffering from Morton's neuroma between the metatarsal heads (a previous neuroma in another metatarsal interspace had been removed surgically with complications; hence, this wish to try a more conservative approach). Another patient had a peripheral neuroma on the lateral aspect of the right knee which six previous explorations had failed to cure. A third patient suffered from intense neuropathic pain on the lateral aspect of the fifth finger occurring after a golfing injury, for which repeated surgical exploration had been unsuccessful. In all cases, prior block with a small dose of local anesthetic and steroid had temporarily and completely removed the pain.

D. Lumbar Sympathetic Chain

In this category, there were four patients, two of them suffering from low back pain, one suffering from rectal pain, and one suffering from abdominal pain. In all cases, the pain was shown to have a major sympathetic element by prior diagnostic lumbar sympathetic blockade with local anesthetic and steroid.

Of the total of 42 responses, 33 (79%) reported less pain after the treatment. In 19 cases (45%), the improvement lasted to the time of the survey, that is at least 13 weeks (Fig. 1). Six patients (15%) benefited for between 4 and 13 weeks, and 10 patients (22%) experienced relief of their pain lasting for 3 weeks or less. Thus, we concluded that 24 patients, or 58%, showed a response to PRF that lasted beyond 3 weeks. Of these "long-term responders," 14 were in the lumbar DRG category, 4 in the cervical DRG category, and 3 each in the neuroma and sympathetic categories (Table 1).

Figure 2 shows the amount of benefit experienced by patients. Long-term responders scored a reduction in pain scores from 79.6 (SE 3.7) to 37.0 (SE 5.8), or from 100 to 46% ($p < 0.0001$). Short-term responders experienced a transient reduction in pain scores from 81.8 (SE 4.9) to 52.3 (SE 10.8), before returning to 85.3 (SE 3.6) ($p = 0.003$). Nonresponders typically reported a slight, statistically nonsignificant, increase in pain scores from 76.9 (SE 3.8) to 83.1

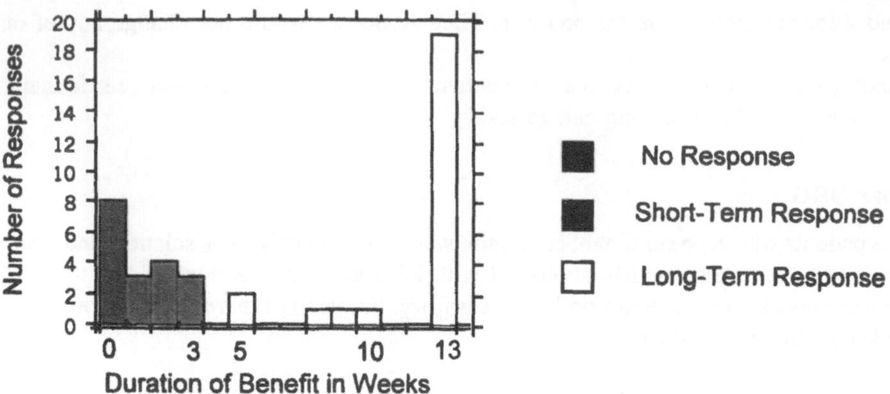

Figure 1 Histogram showing the duration of benefit after PRF treatment ($N = 42$): Durations indicated by patients were converted into weeks; time spans of a few days were scored as 1 week; benefit still persisting at the time of the survey (at least 3 months posttreatment, and in some cases more than 6 months posttreatment) was scored as 13 weeks or longer.

(SE 3.9) in the first weeks posttreatment, which subsequently returned to 72.4 (SE 9.9) ($p = 0.28$). The slightly lower final pain scores of this group were due to two patients having their medication increased following the unsuccessful procedure.

Figure 3 shows the amount of pain relief experienced by the long-term responders broken down into the different treatment categories. Patients in the neuroma category experienced the most dramatic improvement, reducing average pain scores from 74.3 (SE 9.9) to 14.3 (SE 3.2) ($p < 0.02$). Cervical patients ended up with less than half their pain pretreatment, from 82.0 (SE 7.2) to 33.2 (SE 15.9) ($p < 0.02$). Lumbar patients reduced their pain scores from 80.9 (SE 5.2) to 42.1 (SE 7.8) ($p = 0.0002$). Improvement in sympathetic patients was smallest and statistically least significant, with pain scores reducing from 75.3 (SE 13.0) to 41.0 (SE 19.7) ($p = 0.45$).

There was no correlation between the duration of pretreatment pain and either the duration or the amount of the benefit they experienced (data not shown). A study of the patients' clinical notes revealed that there were no discernible traits that either responders or nonresponders had in common, other than chronic pain with neuropathic or sympathetic elements.

Table 1 Responses to PRF in Patient Categories[a]

Treatment category	No response	Short-term response	Long-term response
Lumbar DRG	7 (24%)	8 (28%)	14 (48%)
Cervical DRG	1 (17%)	1 (17%)	4 (66%)
Lumbar sympathetic chain	0	1 (17%)	3 (75%)
Neuroma	0	0	3 (100%)
Total	8 (19%)	10 (24%)	24 (57%)

[a] Number of responses reporting no benefit, short-term (3 weeks or less) benefit, or long-term (between 5 weeks and 9 months) benefit after PRF treatment. The responses are divided into categories according to pain locus and treatment locus (see text for details). Note that the total number of responses is 42, as one patient received PRF to two different loci with different responses.

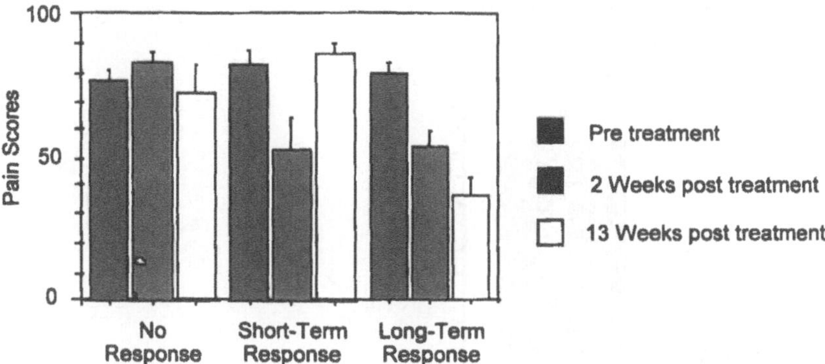

Figure 2 Pain scores: ANOVA of pain experienced by patients treated with PRF, as self-reported in pain 100-mm VAS. The graph shows the mean ± 1 standard error of mean (SEM) of patients' pain pretreatment, 3 weeks posttreatment, and 13 weeks posttreatment. The patients are separated into nonresponders, short-term responders, and long-term responders. All pain scores are drawn to scale.

Disability improvements were highest in the long-term responders group, scoring an average of 51.9% (SE 7.0) improvement (Fig. 4). Short-term responders scored a small improvement of 9.1% (SE 5.9) ($p = 0.0009$). All nonresponders scored zero. Four patients in the short-term responders group scored disability improvements whereas five scored none. With one exception, all long-term responders scored disability improvements.

Thirteen patients (32%) were able to reduce their medication as a consequence of the PRF treatment, in four cases stopping oral medication altogether (Table 2). Twelve of these were long-term responders, and one fell into the short-term responders group. Five patients (three long-term responders, one short-term responder, and one nonresponder) indicated that they did not take any medication before the treatment, and therefore scored "no change." Two nonre-

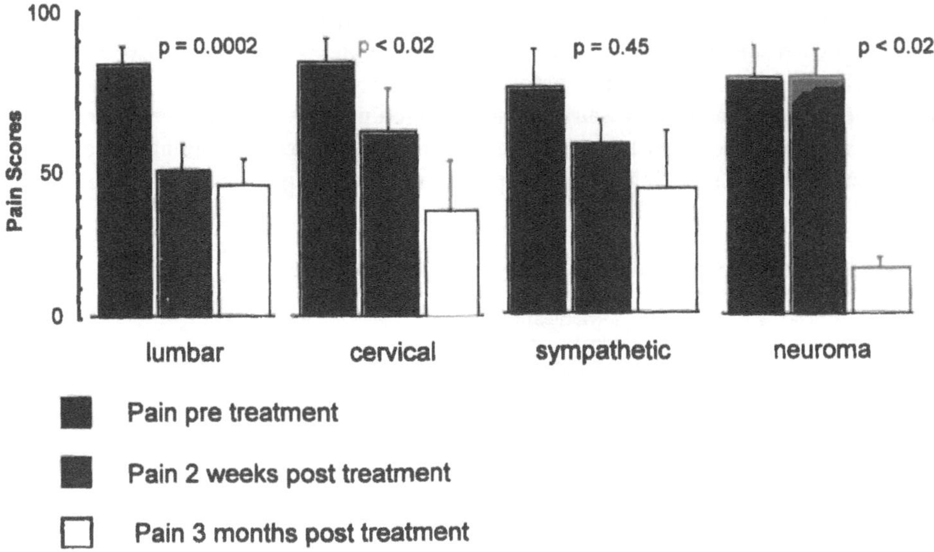

Figure 3 Pain scores of long-term responders by patient category: ANOVA of pain scores of long-term responders by treatment location. Mean VAS scores/100 with SEM bars.

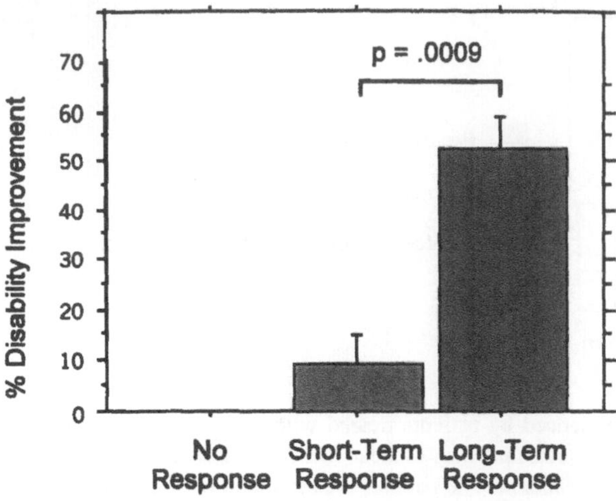

Figure 4 Disability improvements: The effects of PRF treatment on disability improvements in percent (mean ± SEM), with 0% being no improvement, and 100% being improvement in all items listed. Patients are separated into nonresponders, short-term responders, and long-term responders.

sponders, one short-term responder, and two long-term responders reported an increase in medication at the time of the survey. One patient did not answer the question.

The answers to the questions after pain locus and character made it clear that no new pains had occurred in the time between the treatment and the survey to confound results, except in one patient whose condition was exacerbated by reinjury a short time after the treatment, and who, as a consequence, was classified as a short-term responder. There did not appear to be any consistent way in which the treatment changed the character of patients' pain (data not shown).

It was expected that patients would experience some initial soreness as a result of the treatment. Indeed, nine patients (22%) reported an initial exacerbation of their pain. In five of these the pain improved subsequently, in two it returned to the previous level, and two felt they were in more pain after the treatment than before.

Mild side effects appeared to be fairly common: three patients reported headaches, one patient reported sweating, one patient reported nausea, and one patient reported nausea as well as increased micturition and sweating. A further patient reported weight gain that was not ex-

Table 2 Changes in Consumption of Analgesic Drugs[a]

	Medication		
Patient groups	Less/weaker	Same	More/stronger
Nonresponders	0	6	2
Short-term responders	1	7	1
Long-term responders	12	10	2

[a] Self-report of patients' consumption of analgesic medication before and after PRF treatment. Changes were scored as "less/weaker," "no change," or "more/stronger." Responses were separated into no response, short-term response, and long-term response. Patients who did not take any medication for their pain pretreatment scored "no change" (three long-term responders, one short-term responder, one nonresponder). One patient did not answer the question.

plained. Two of the patients reporting headaches had been treated with PRF to the cervical DRG. No serious side effects occurred in the study population.

Patients generally commented very favorably on the relative noninvasiveness of the PRF treatment and on the minimal amount of pain involved. A single patient felt that the treatment was more painful than previous ones. Several responders emphasized the need for patience while waiting up to several weeks for the treatment to have its beneficial effect.

IV. DISCUSSION

A. Response of Patients

Initial experiences with PRF are extremely encouraging. Even though the patients seen were typically suffering from long-standing pain and had histories of previous unsuccessful treatments, including, in some cases, multiple neurosurgical interventions, PRF to the DRG seemed to have an analgesic effect in a large proportion of these patients. There was also a lasting analgesic effect in the chronic whiplash patients, who had failed to respond to other treatments, including conservative therapy and diagnostic or permanent facet joint blocks.

One main difficulty in assessing the benefit of PRF was to separate out the effect of the concomitant steroid injections. The decision to give concomitant local anesthetic and steroids was made based on an earlier pilot study that suggested that mechanical provocation of the DRG by the tip of the PRF needle caused pain and soreness for a number of weeks before the effect of the PRF was felt. We found that this initial period of discomfort was reduced if local anesthetic and steroid were injected after the PRF was performed through the same cannula. Since all the patients in this study had previously had local anesthetic and steroid blocks alone, with effects that lasted for less than 3 weeks, we concluded that those patients who benefited for longer than 3 weeks in this study (long-term responders) were likely to be "true" PRF responders. As the histogram in Fig. 1 shows, the duration of the benefit that patients experienced appears indeed to be clustered in two time ranges: one range of up to about 3 weeks, and one range of 3 months and more. The assumption that the shorter time range represents the benefit from local anesthetic plus steroid injections, and the longer time range represents benefit from the PRF treatment proper, seems reasonable.

The fact that the survey presented here was conducted by the treating physician and his research associate means that in this open study, we cannot exclude a strong placebo, novelty, or charisma effect. This means that our preliminary results probably represent a rather optimistic estimate of the benefits of PRF. Thus, the figure of 57% responders who experienced approximately 50% pain relief is likely high. However, all the patients had also previously received other unsuccessful treatments, some of them by the same physician, and were therefore a group of patients capable of delivering negative feedback to the physician.

The effect of patients' condition reverting to mean is unlikely to distort our results because of the length of the waiting lists (up to 1 year), which means that patients treated in the chronic pain clinics are not selected for exacerbations of a chronic condition. It is also possible that the effect of PRF may be explained by some natural resolution or undulation in the chronicity of the patients' condition. However, these patients were chosen because they had severe unremitting pain that had not responded to other forms of treatment, including invasive treatments.

B. Changes in Pain and Disability Scores

The results of the pain scores make it clear that the PRF treatment did not remove pain completely. On average, patients still scored 37/100 on the VAS. This conforms to expectations about any treatment of long-standing chronic pain. It is also an encouraging result in terms of the ability of the patients in the survey to quantify their own pain, and the realism with which they appear able to view their own situation.

The variations in pain scores between the different treatment categories appear comparatively small. Given the small sample sizes in all the categories except lumbar DRG, it seems premature to conclude that PRF is particularly effective if applied topically or to the cervical DRG.

Disability improvements were surprisingly high. It is clear that a 100% disability improvement could be experienced only by someone whose previous functioning was impaired in 100% of the items listed in the survey; therefore, the survey would have tended to score lower improvement rates for mildly disabled patients than for more strongly disabled patients. This is the "basement" effect, with more available room to move up. The finding of nearly 50% improvement in the responders group therefore suggested that some moderately to severely disabled patients had experienced improvements in a wide range of activities, consistent with a profound change in patients' perception of their own ability to perform everyday tasks. Compared with the reported improvements in disability, the reduction in consumption of analgesic medication seemed rather small. Presumably, this reflected the fact that even responders to PRF treatment still experienced a certain amount of residual pain.

C. Mechanism of Action of PRF

Sluijter et al. (1) described a possible electric field effect for PRF, with an estimated field strength at the probe tip of 2.8×10^4 V/m and current density of possibly 2×10^4 A/m^2. However, little is known about the clinical effects of such fields on living tissue. In electrophysiological experiments, the lower frequencies are similar to those that may induce long-term depression within the spinal cord (7–9). The observation that this technique may work on peripheral nerves, sympathetic nerves, and spinal roots, suggests that a particular signal stimulates peripheral nerves that subsequently activate central pain mechanisms, in a fashion akin to some of the possible actions of a TENS machine, including enhancement of the descending control systems and production of endogenous opioids (10). The observation that the effect of PRF is not instantaneous suggests that time is required for activation of complex and hitherto unknown analgesic systems.

V. CONCLUSIONS

It is clear that PRF seems a very promising treatment for a number of conditions, including chronic radicular neuropathic pain, sympathetic pain, and pain from peripheral neuroma. The treatment is performed in an outpatient setting. It is relatively noninvasive, produces no apparent irreversible structural changes or sensory loss, and can be repeated when the benefit wears off. Side effects appear to be minor, so far, and transient. However it is clear, now that there appears to be a beneficial effect, more studies have to be carried out to quantify the success rate more realistically, including double-blinded, randomized control studies with a sham PRF option. This is currently underway. Also more research is needed to elucidate the exact mode of action of PRF.

ACKNOWLEDGMENT

The authors would like to thank the clinical staff for their help with patient treatments.

REFERENCES

1. Sluijter ME, Cosman ER, Rittman WB, Van Kleef M. The effects of PRF fields to the DRG—a preliminary report. Pain Clin 1998; 11:109–117.
2. Slappendel R, Crul BJP Braak GJJ, Geurts JWM, Booij LHDJ, Voerman VF, Boo T. The efficacy of radiofrequency lesioning of the cervical DRG in a double blind randomized study: no difference between 40°C and 67°C treatments. Pain 1997; 73:159–163.
3. Munglani R. The longer term effect of PRF for neuropathic pain. Pain 1999; 80:437–439.
4. Munglani R, Hill R. Other drugs including sympathetic block. In: Wall PD, Melzack R, eds. Textbook of Pain. Edinburgh: Churchill Livingstone: 1999.
5. Roland M, Morris R. A study of the natural history of back pain, part 1: development of a reliable and sensitive measure of disability in low back pain. Spine 1983; 8:1141–1144.
6. Vernon H, Mior S. The neck disability index: a study of reliability and validity. J Manipulative Physiol Ther 1991; 14:409–415.
7. Randic M, Jiang MC, Cerne R. Long term potentiation and long term depression of primary afferent neurotransmission in the rat spinal cord. J Neurosci 1993; 13:5228–5241.
8. Sandkuler J, Chen GJ, Cheng G, Randic, MJ. Low-frequency stimulation of afferent A delta fibers induce long term depression at primary afferent synapses with substantia gelatinosa neurones in the rat. J Neurosci 1997; 17:6483–6491.
9. Pockett S. Spinal cord plasticity and chronic pain. Anesth Analg 1995; 80:173–179.
10. Bowsher D. Mechanisms of acupuncture. In: Filshie J, White A, eds. Medical Acupuncture. Edinburgh: Churchill Livingstone, 1998:69–82.

16
Spinal Cord Stimulation

Y. Michael A. Tai
Wexham Park Hospital, Slough, Berkshire, England

Julie A. Payne
Royal Albert Edward Infirmary, Lancashire, England

I. INTRODUCTION

Spinal cord stimulation (SCS) is a nondestructive, nonmedicated, reversible neuromodulation technique for the management of intractable neuropathic pain conditions. It is recognized as a valuable additional tool to the pain specialist's armamentarium. Clinical evidence is now accumulating to suggest that, when used appropriately in a multidisciplinary pain setting, SCS has an important and special role in the treatment of certain pain subgroups who would otherwise remain untreatable. For example, the patient often would have tried all modalities of treatment, ranging from pharmacological manipulation, interventional nerve block or destructive lesioning, to psychological counseling, and complementary therapy, before undergoing SCS with spectacular results.

II. HISTORICAL BACKGROUND

Although the use of electricity in pain management was well known to the ancient Greeks and to the Romans, the main force for the development of implantable electrical stimulation for pain relief has been the gate control theory of Melzack and Wall (1). Inspired by the concept and the initial success in stimulating peripheral nerves, Shealy and his co-workers (2) demonstrated that dorsal column stimulation in cats blocked both the prolonged small C-fibers after discharge and the behavioral response to acute pain. Thus encouraged, the first dorsal column stimulator targeting the ascending collaterals of the large Aβ-fibers was performed in March 1967 (3). Although dorsal column stimulation was first used, subsequent studies failed to show any difference in pain control when either the dorsal or ventral spinal cord was stimulated. Nowadays the term *spinal cord stimulation* should be considered as synonymous with dorsal column stimulation.

During the early days, SCS had a rather checkered and undistinguished career. That was mainly due to the inappropriate selection of patients because the concept of neuropathic pain was not then widely appreciated. The problem was further compounded by a much higher rate of equipment failure. It is perhaps not surprising that relatively poor and disappointing results were reported in the early period of SCS, which very nearly led to its demise. Recent improvements in hardware have resulted in a resurrection of the enthusiasm of SCS. This, coupled with better understanding of the clinical indications and more robust patient selection, has undoubtedly underpinned its renaissance (4–8).

III. CLINICAL INDICATIONS

It is recognized that SCS has no place in the management of nocigenic pain conditions (e.g., arthritic pain). It is effective in neuropathic pain where there is established deafferentation accompanied by autonomic disturbance. The following list of complex chronic pain syndromes may be thought of as worthy of consideration for SCS:

1. Failed back surgery syndrome (FBSS) (9–11)
2. Complex regional pain syndromes [i.e., reflex sympathetic dystrophy (12) ($CRPS_1$) and causalgia (13) ($CRPS_2$)]
3. Vasospastic disorders (e.g., Raynaud's disease) (14,15)
4. Angina pectoris (16–18)
5. Peripheral vascular disease (PVD) (19–22)
6. Postamputation phantom and stump pain (23–25)
7. Nerve and nerve root lesion [e.g., diabetic neuropathy (26), postherpetic neuralgia (27), brachial plexus avulsions (28)]
8. Craniofacial pain [e.g., occipital neuralgia (29), trigeminal neuralgia (30)]

Although SCS is thought to produce its analgesic effect through targeting the ascending collaterals of the large Aβ-fibers, the precise mechanisms by which SCS affects the perception of pain is still virtually unknown. In spite of some evidence suggesting that SCS causes release of endorphins and inhibits the transmission of noxious stimuli, naloxone does not appear to prevent SCS-induced pain relief (31). Biochemical and pharmacological studies have contributed relatively little. Animal studies by Linderoth and his colleagues have identified the release of neurotransmitters centrally and the sympathetic mediation of peripheral vasodilation by SCS (32,33). The antisympathetic activity of SCS is possibly through releasing segmental spinal reflexes and inhibiting sympathetic fiber discharge (20,34). Naver and his colleagues in Sweden have suggested in a more recent paper that the marked vasodilation is mediated by sympathetic vasomotor fibers, by modulation of central neuronal circuits involved in the regulation of skin sympathetic discharge (35). The beneficial effects of SCS in PVD caused by microcirculatory changes have been demonstrated by Jacobs et al. (36,37). In another paper by Galley et al. an increase in transcutaneous oxygen tension has also been demonstrated (38). Thus, the benign effects on angina, Raynaud's disease, and CRPSs may become apparent. Even so, we still do not know for certain whether pain relief is secondary to reduced ischemic changes or whether the apparent antisympathetic effect is secondary to pain relief, or both.

IV. PATIENT SELECTION

Although there is no hard and fast rule to decide which patient is suitable or not to undergo SCS, a successful outcome probably depends more on careful case selection than on any other factor. That, in turn, very much relies on the individual expertise and experience accumulated within a particular implant center.

It is commonly acknowledged that chronic pain sufferers do unavoidably develop associated behavioral problems. Thus, depression, anxiety, obsession with a sense of hopelessness, and low social self-esteem are common denominators in a chronic pain syndrome. However, although very few pain specialists would deny the relevance of psychological factors in pain management, the interpretation of their significance to implant or not may often be flawed. Long et al. (39) subjected their patients to a battery of psychological tests before implant, but 7 years later half were considered to have been unsuitable. Burton (40) similarly came to the conclusion that 8–10% of his patients were unsuitable retrospectively, in spite of an extensive and comprehensive preoperative screening process. Therefore, it may not be simply a question of identifying psychological factors for exclusion, but one of assessing their relevant importance to the case (e.g., cognitive, affective, and personality aspects) in relation to the severity of the physical pain and disability. More recently, North and his co-workers (41) have come to the conclusion that psychological testing is of modest value and explains little of the observed variance in outcome. They have found little evidence for selecting patients for SCS on the basis of psychological testing. No doubt, the usefulness or otherwise of psychological screening will continue as a controversial topic among some of the major implant centers.

In certain centers, the application of transcutaneous electrical nerve stimulation (TENS) would be considered an essential part of the screening program for SCS, so that the lack of response to TENS would be considered as unsuitable. Others may feel that any failure to TENS does not indicate that SCS will fail. Indeed in FBSS, some workers have been unable to establish any significant correlation between the responses to TENS and to SCS (11). In general terms, it is now accepted that TENS is not a useful predictor of outcome for SCS.

Trial cord stimulation is another method often considered to be part of the treatment protocol (42–44). The aim may be either simply the confirmation of parasthesia(e) to cover the painful area(s) following the insertion and placement of the electrodes' lead epidurally, or the keeping of the electrodes in place, tunneled subcutaneously, and connected to an external trial screener, sometimes for days or even weeks, to ascertain if the patient experiences adequate pain relief. Because there is always the possibility of a placebo response, a longer trial would, in theory, be expected to reduce the number of false-positive reactions. However, the advantages in doing so can often be outweighed by the disadvantages (e.g., infection, electrodes migration, or false-negative reactions), as it has been known that patients sometimes may not achieve adequate pain control at first, but if implanted will then progress to achieving good symptomatic relief later on (45,46). Although there are many protagonists, trial cord stimulation has never proved to be as successful a screening test as many would have hoped. Indeed the question one very frequently hears being asked is: "If only those who responded to a trial stimulation were implanted, why was the success rate not 100%?" In the series by Nielson et al., in spite of screening 221 patients and rejecting nearly half, the success rate after permanent implant was only 40% (47). Likewise, Siegfried and Lazorthes rejected more than half in a large group of patients with FBSS, but the success rate at 1 year had already fallen to near 50% (48). A similar failure rate has been reported also by several other workers (9,49). The reason for that may be due to the more special nature of FBSS, possibly encompassing both nocigenic and neuropathic pain components. Paradoxically, the reported success rate of other neuropathic conditions, such as CRPSs, phantom pain, brachial plexus avulsion, PVD, and angina is much higher and more encouraging. In our practice, we have now moved away from the concept of prolonged trial cord stimulation, preferring instead the shorter period of demonstrable parasthesia(e) in targeted area(s) in an awake patient during the first stage of the procedure, preceded by trial in-patient epidural catheterization.

V. IMPLANT TECHNIQUE

The SCS system comprises three parts: the electrodes' lead, the extension cable, and the power source. The lead has four or more electrodes and is of two varieties. One form of lead can be

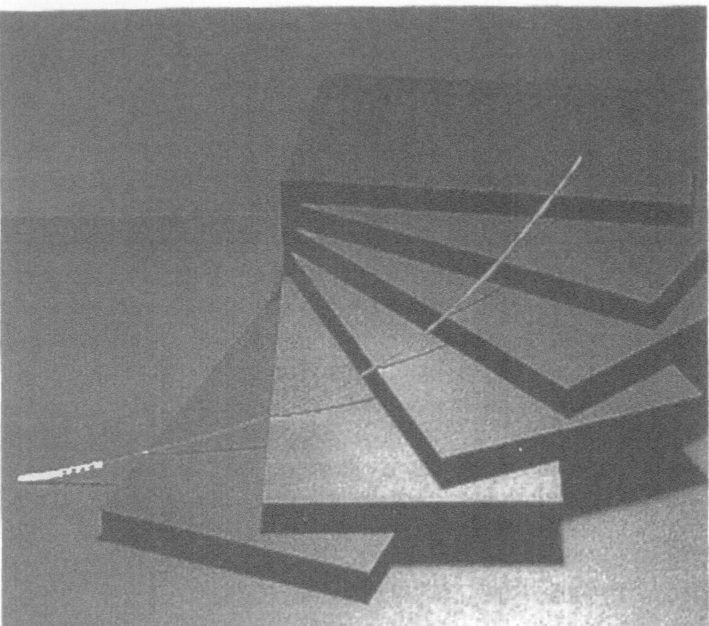

Figure 1 Quad lead for epidural insertion percutaneous.

inserted through a Tuohy needle percutaneously (Fig. 1). The other is a flat plate that requires an open laminotomy operation for its insertion (Fig. 2). Both have their advantages and disadvantages. Thus, the flat plate is inserted with the patient fully anesthetized without trial stimulation, is more surgically traumatic, but is more securely placed to avoid the possibility of migration. The electrodes' lead, on the other hand, is inserted percutaneously under a local anesthetic and can be tested to ensure correct placement in an awake patient, but is more prone to migration. The extension cable is a conduction wire that carries the electrical impulses from the power source to the electrodes. The power source can be a totally internalized pulse generator run by an in-built lithium battery (Fig. 3), or an external radiofrequency (RF)-coupled receiver–transmitter powered by rechargeable batteries (Fig. 4). The former has the aesthetic appeal of being unobtrusive and uncluttered, whereas the latter can be considered by some as cumbersome. However, the major difference between the two is the likely recurring costs to replace the former every few years on exhaustion of the lithium battery.

To achieve successful stimulation, the correct placement of the lead electrodes epidurally, be that percutaneously using fluoroscopy (Fig. 5) or surgically under direct vision (Fig. 6), must be considered paramount in the whole concept of SCS implant. Electrodes are placed rostral above the level of the pain, and ipsilateral for unilateral pain. For bilateral pain, it is essential to aim at having the electrodes placed dead-center over the midline of the cord, or, in certain instances, by the insertion of two lead electrodes placed centrally in parallel. The mapping of successfully stimulating different anatomical areas has been analyzed extensively by Barolat and his colleagues (50). In our experience, we would advise T7–L1 for the lower limb (buttock to foot), T1–T4 for angina, C5–C7 for the upper limb, C2–C4 for the neck and shoulder, and C1–C2 for craniofacial areas. If the electrodes are too lateral, stimulation of the dorsal root fibers would predominate. This would explain the uncomfortable "tight band" sensation round

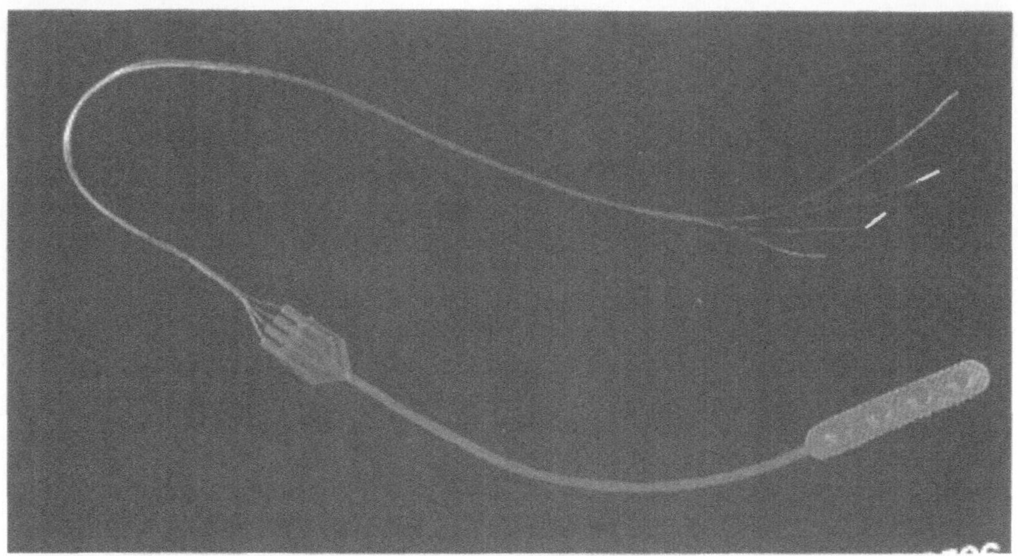

Figure 2 Resume lead for epidural placement via a laminotomy.

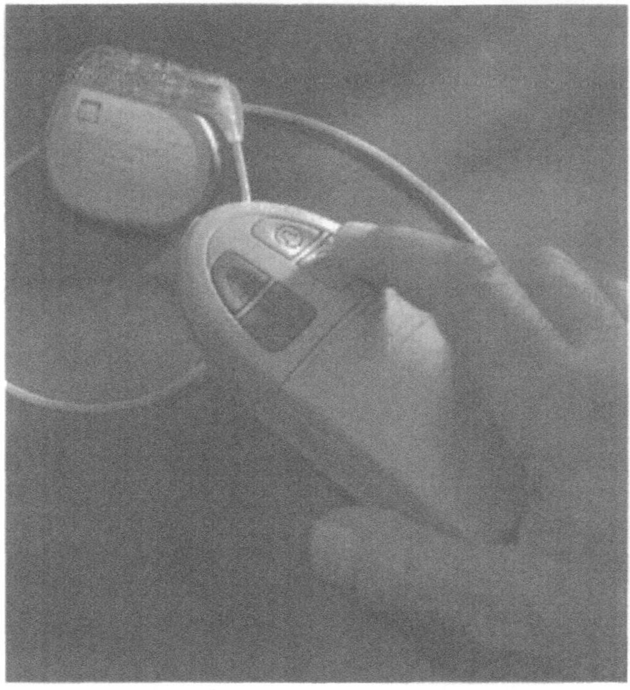

Figure 3 Itrel internalized pulse generator and a patient-controlled hand-held programmer.

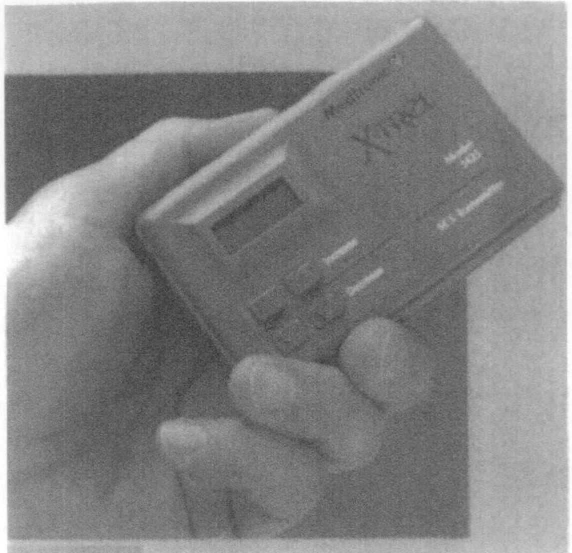

Figure 4 Xtrel external transmitter.

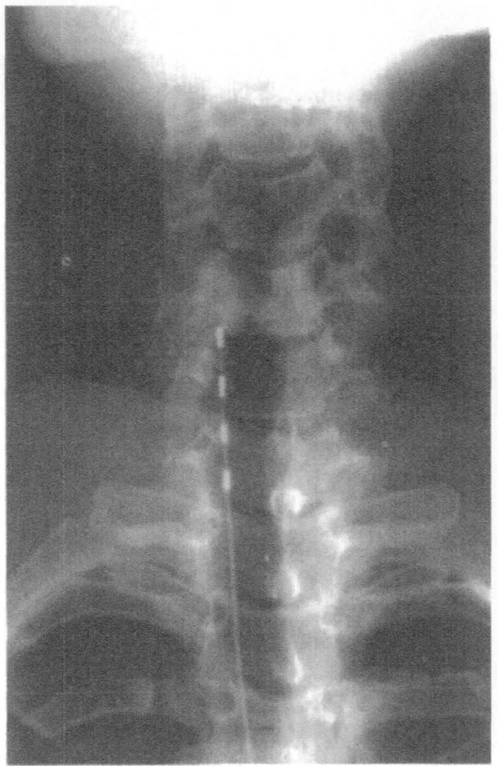

Figure 5 Quad lead in the cervical epidural space.

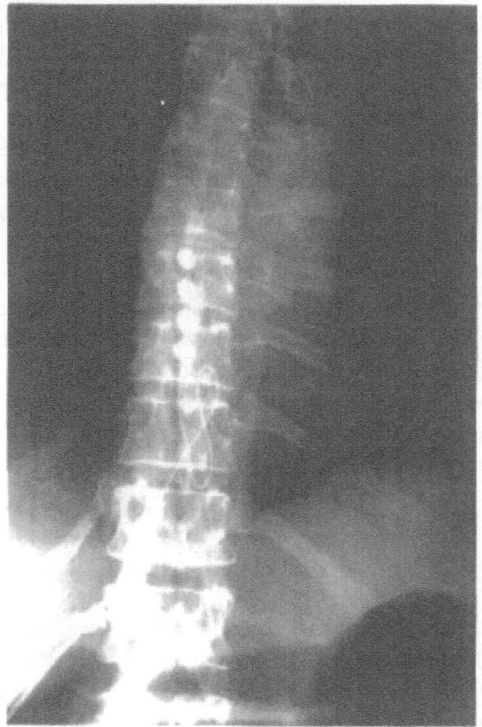

Figure 6 Resume lead in the thoracic epidural space.

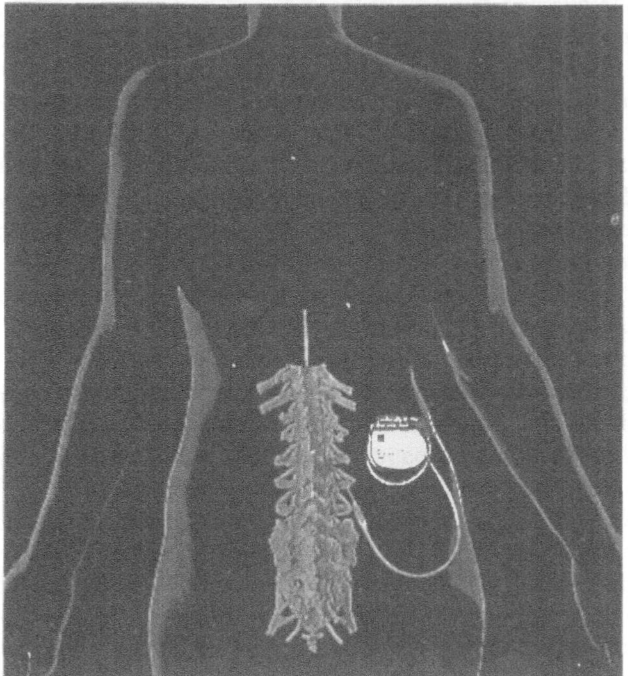

Figure 7 A totally internalized spinal cord stimulation system.

the waist or in the anterior abdominal wall during insertion for low back pain. Certain areas, such as the center of the back, the perineum, and the face, are notoriously difficult to target selectively. The degree of stimulation may also be influenced by the distance between the electrodes and the spinal cord at different levels, or between standing upright and lying down. Following the correct placement of the electrodes, the second stage of the implant procedure is then completed by joining them to the pulse generator or receiver, housed in a subcutaneous pocket, through the extension cable tunneled subcutaneously (Fig. 7). It is customary to carry out the whole procedure under broad-spectrum antibiotic cover.

Most of the complications experienced by the authors nowadays are of a minor nature. Because of newly developed and improved hardware, and a rigid postimplant regimen to be adhered to, complications, such as migration of electrodes, lead fracture, or dislodgement, are of rare occurrence. The accumulation of serous fluid in the subcutaneous pocket housing the pulse generator or receiver can occasionally happen, requiring diligent and meticulous lookout so that emptying by aspiration in an aseptic environment can be arranged. With antibiotic cover using ceftazedime and vancomycin, infection is very rarely a problem.

VI. IMPLANT COORDINATOR

The proper education of a patient (i.e., advice and counseling) should commence immediately on recruitment into the implant program. This important aspect of patient management lies within the role of a clinical nurse specialist in chronic pain management, acting as the implant coordinator. As an important team player (51–53), preferably having already attended a course and acquired the diploma in pain management, she would be expected to be in possession of good communication and organizational skills, together with a sound practical knowledge of neuromodulation implantation technology for pain control. It is expected that many hours will be spent in educating the patient and relatives throughout the pre- and postimplant periods, reiterating information, offering support, and answering queries, ideally by a telephone help line.

Before the SCS implant, a good rapport is established between the pain nurse, the patient, and the family. Any information provided must be plain and straightforward, with clear objectives. Thus, the patient is told that SCS is not a cure, not for getting rid of the pain, and that an achievable 50% reduction would be deemed a success. It is the usual practice to interview the patient and a member of the family together initially, as whatever the patient experiences later on has a consequence on the rest of the family. The two stages of the implant procedure are explained and, for percutaneous insertion of the lead, the importance of patient cooperation while awake during the first stage of the procedure is emphasized. The patient is allowed to see and handle the model of the pulse generator or receiver–transmitter, so that there is full understanding of the device and the proposed subcutaneous pocket site to house it. A patient needs to be made aware of all the pitfalls and complications of SCS. Last but not least, and to reiterate what has already been told in the clinic, the patient is provided with an information leaflet detailing all the implications of SCS, together with postimplant instructions.

Following an implant, it is the role of the pain nurse to liaise closely with the ward staff. During the first 24 h the patient is nursed lying flat in bed. Thereafter, mobilization should be gradual and gentle, from lying to sitting in bed, and finally standing and walking under trained nurse supervision before discharged home on the third or the fourth day after the implant. By then the patient would have been fully taught, either the use of his portable telemetry handset for the internalized pulse generator, or the application of external transmitter over the implanted RF receiver. All patients are advised to avoid lifting, bending, twisting, or stretching movements

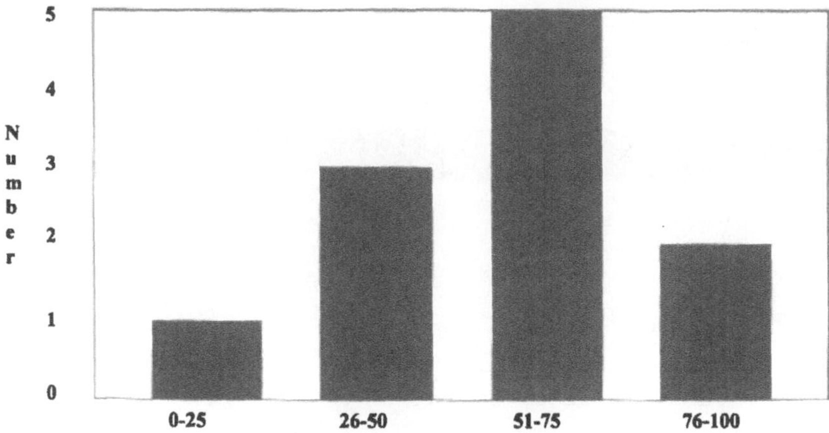

Figure 8 Reduction of pain intensity following SCS: 7 of 11 patients (64%) are experiencing >50% pain reduction [measured on visual analog scale (VAS)].

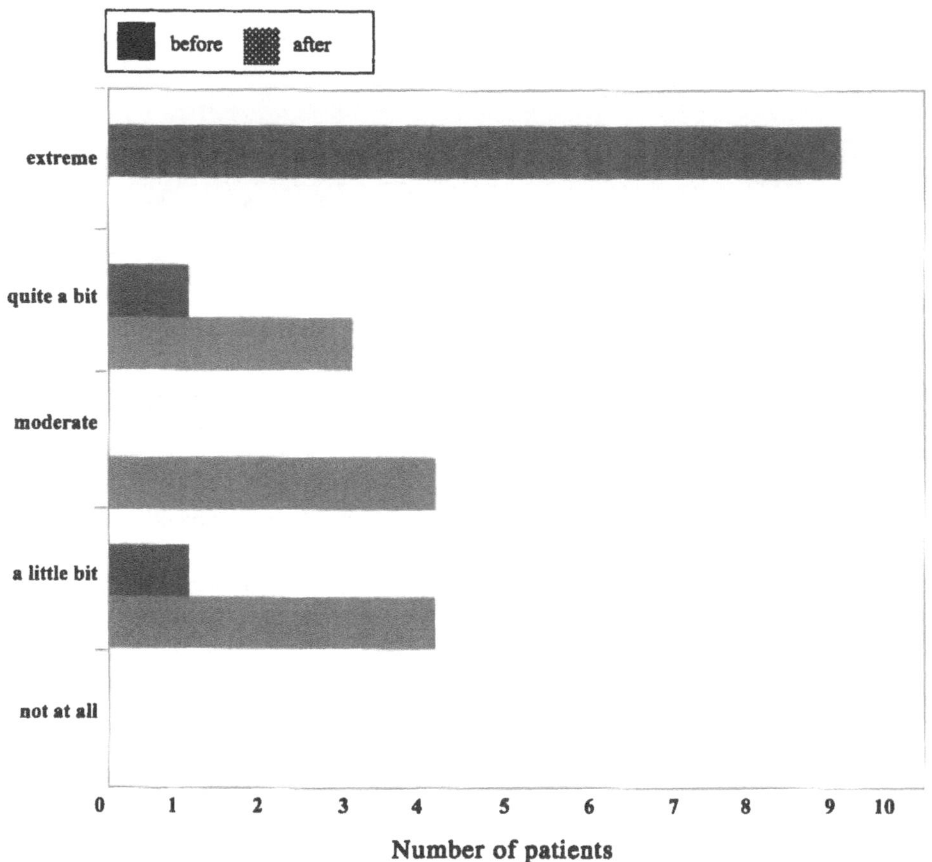

Figure 9 Pain interference with "work": ability to "work" seems improved.

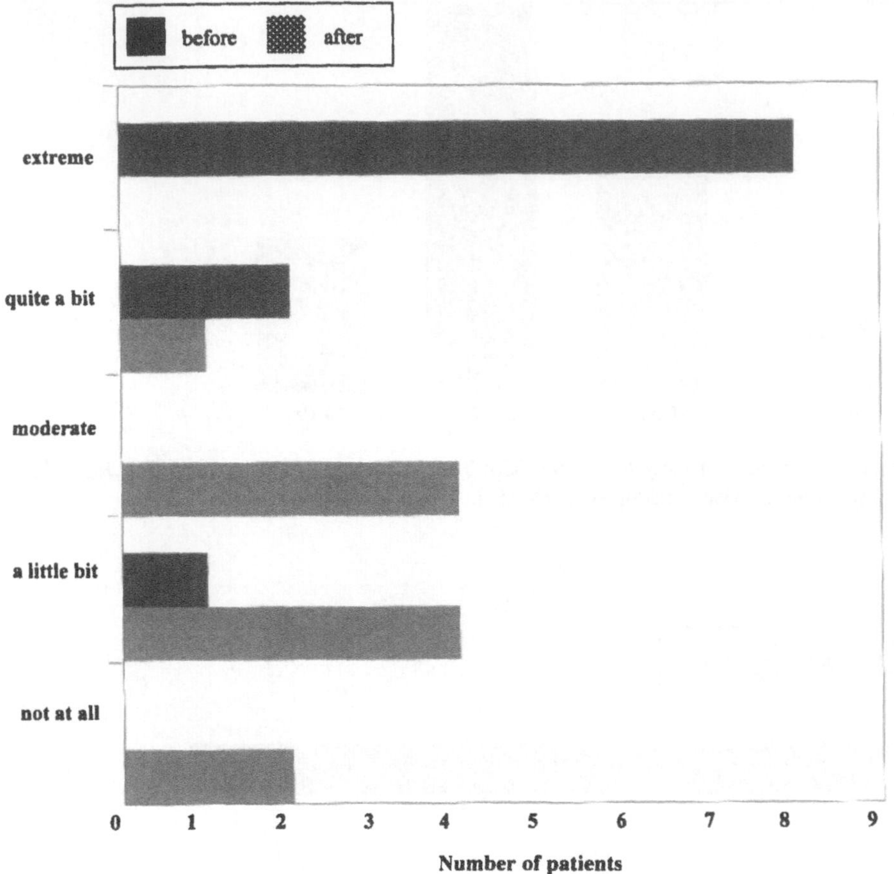

Figure 10 Pain interference with social life: quality of social life seems improved.

for 6 weeks to prevent the electrodes' lead migration or dislodgement. The patient is given an appointment to return to the clinic 2 weeks later for wound inspection, sutures removal, and if need be fine-tuning to the SCS.

As an implant coordinator, it is also the role of the pain nurse to assist during the percutaneous insertion of the electrodes lead and to perform the process of trial screening using the external screener. She is there to support the awake patient during the first stage of the implant and to assess the stimulation outcome of the screening process. The pain nurse is responsible for the ordering of the SCS hardware and storage. Registration of the device with the manufacturer, record keeping, troubleshooting, and periodic fine-tuning of the SCS are other important functions of her role. There is no doubt in our view that an efficient implant coordinator is an asset in keeping down the incidences of the so-called late implant failures.

VII. COST EFFECTIVENESS AND AUDIT

By the time they are considered for SCS, usually as a last resort, most patients would have experienced multiple treatment failures, taking a large amount of drugs, and paying frequent visits to doctors and specialists. As a consequence of that, many of them would have lost confi-

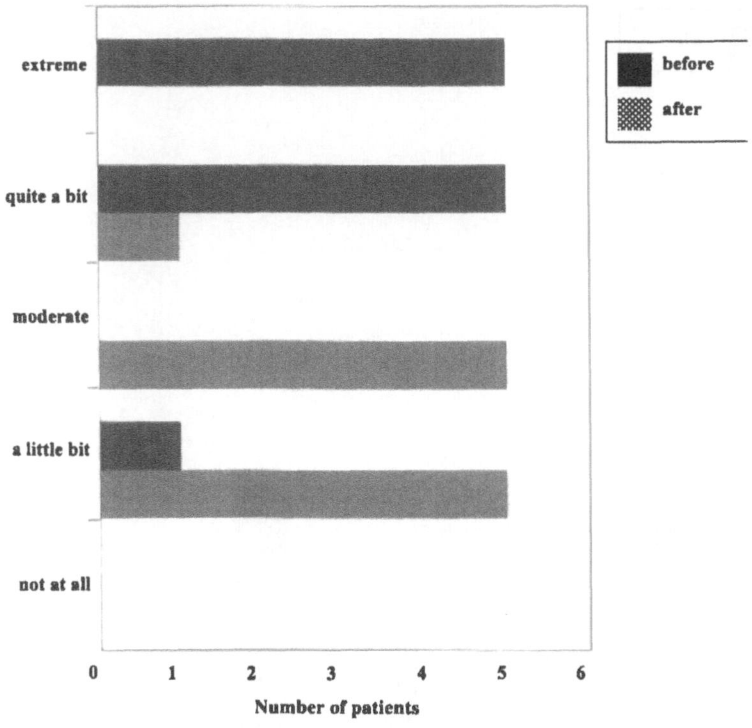

Figure 11 Pain interference with sleep: obvious reduction of sleep disturbance by pain.

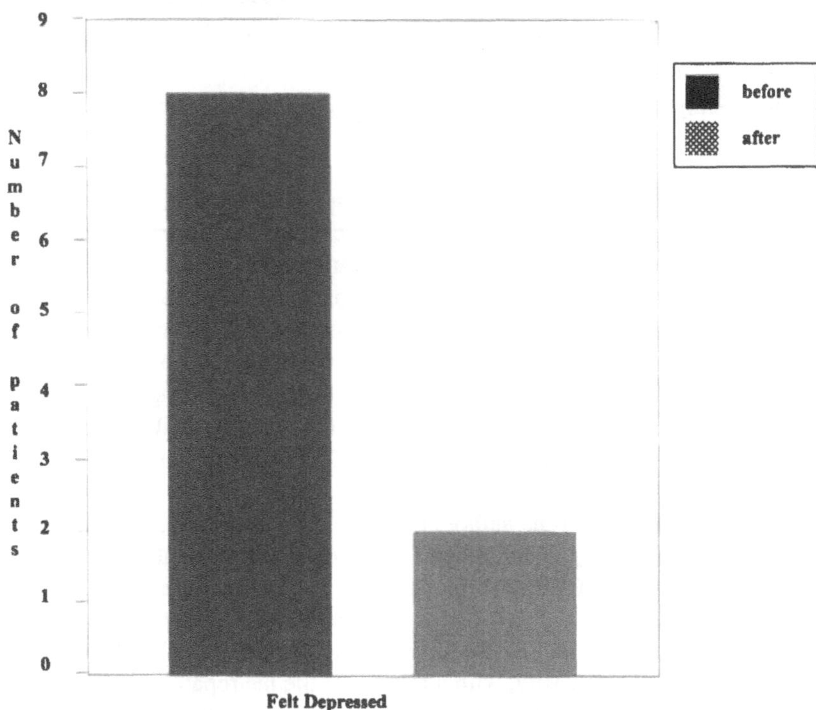

Figure 12 Number of patients feeling depressed reduced from eight to two following spinal cord stimulation.

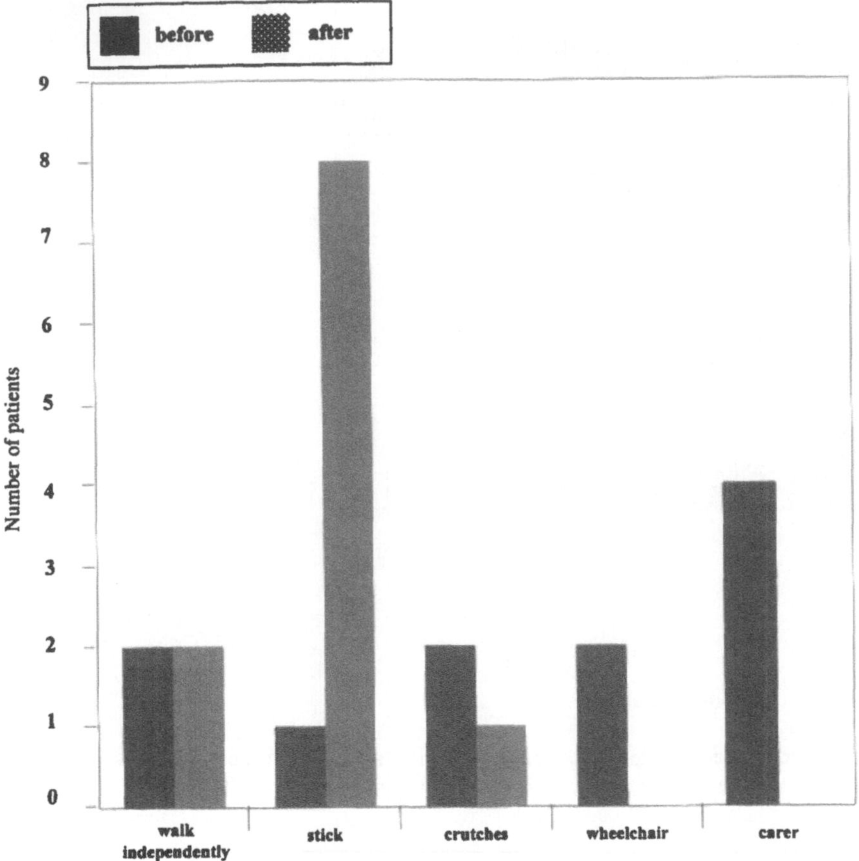

Figure 13 Reliance on mobility aids: increased level of mobility after spinal cord stimulation.

dence in the medical profession, become unemployable, and displayed outward signs of psychological disorder, including the lowering of mood and self-esteem. An overall improved quality of life following a successful implant (e.g., a reduction in drug intake, a lowering of the frequency of physician's surgery visits or hospital admissions, an increase in the activity level, and a better family or social lifestyle) is the best indicator for assessment of the cost effectiveness in SCS (54). By and large, it is unrealistic to use "return to work" as one of the criteria to assess, as failure to do so is very much dependent on other factors, including age, physical disability, labor market force, and the socioeconomic climate of the locality. All such considerations should be weighed against the high initial cost of SCS, and for an internalized pulse generator, the recurring costs.

An internal audit was carried out by the authors in 1997 on 11 patients who had received SCS implants. Eight patients had FBSS, 2 were diagnosed brachial plexus avulsion injury and 1 patient reflex sympathetic dystrophy ($CRPS_1$) in the left foot. A questionnaire was sent to the patients with questions concerning pre- and postimplant pain intensity, interference with daily life activity, sleep disturbance, mobility, and mood. Seven of the 11 patients (64%) experienced 50% or more in the reduction of pain intensity, with a change of the neuropathic characteristics of pain, such as shooting and burning, to a much more bearable sensation of dull-ache (Fig. 8). Pain interference with the ability to "work" (Fig. 9) and with the social life (Fig. 10) became less. Sleep had improved (Fig. 11) and the number of patients who admitted that they were depressed beforehand was markedly reduced from 8 down to 2 (Fig. 12). In term of mobility, 9 of 11 patients before the implant were very disabled, relying on stick, crutches, wheelchair, or a carer to get about, whereas all those 9 patients had become more independent afterward, with 8 reversing to just the use of walking sticks (Fig. 13).

Clearly there is a need to instigate some form of cost analysis and audit in the United Kingdom of SCS in relation to individuals, purchasers, and the society as a whole. With better methods of outcome assessment and patient selection in the major implant centers, it should result in more awareness and wider acceptance of the efficacy of this treatment. We hope that, in turn, there will be more patients, who otherwise would be suffering from some of the most intractable and untreatable complex chronic pain syndromes, also obtaining the benefits of this form of treatment.

REFERENCES

1. Melzack R, Wall PD. Pain mechanism: a new theory. Science 1965; 150:971–979.
2. Shealy CN, Taslitz N, Mortimer JT, Becker DP. Electrical inhibition of pain: experimental evaluation. Anesth Analg 1967; 46:299–304.
3. Shealy CN, Mortimer JT, Reswick JB. Electrical inhibition of pain by stimulation of the dorsal columns: preliminary clinical report. Anesth Analg 1967; 46:489–491.
4. Meglio M, Cioni B, Rossi GF. Spinal cord stimulation in management of chronic pain: a 9 year experience. J Neurosurg 1989; 70:519–524.
5. Simpson BA. Spinal cord stimulation in 60 cases of intractable pain. J Neurol Neurosurg Psychiatry 1991; 54:96–199.
6. Kumar K, Nath R, Wyant GM. Treatment of chronic pain by epidural spinal cord stimulation: a 10 year experience. J Neurosurg 1991; 75:402–407.
7. North RB, Kidd DH, Zahurak M, et al. Spinal cord stimulation for chronic, intractable pain: experience over two decades. Neurosurgery 1993; 32:384–394.
8. Watkins ES, Koeze TH. Spinal cord stimulation and pain relief. Br Med J 1993; 307:462.
9. North RB, Ewend MG, Lawton MT, et al. Failed back surgery syndrome: 5 year follow-up after spinal cord stimulator implantation. Neurosurgery 1991; 28:692–699.
10. De La Porte C, Van de Kelft E. Spinal cord stimulation in failed back surgery syndrome. Pain 1993; 52:55–61.
11. Le Doux MS, Langford KH. Spinal cord stimulation for the failed back syndrome. Spine 1993; 18: 191–194.
12. Barolat G, Schwartzman RJ, Woo R. Epidural spinal cord stimulation in the management of reflex sympathetic dystrophy. Stereotact Funct Neurosurg 1989; 53:29–39.
13. Broseta J, Roedan P, Gonzales-Darder J, et al. Chronic epidural dorsal column stimulation in the treatment of causalgic pain. Appl Neurophysiol 1982; 45:190–194.
14. Robina FJ, Dominguez M, Diaz M, et al. Spinal cord stimulation for relief of chronic pain in vasospastic disorders of the upper limbs. Neurosurgery 1989; 24:63–67.
15. Francaviglia N, Silvertro C, Maiello M, et al. Spinal cord stimulation for the treatment of progressive systemic scleroris and Raynaud's syndrome. Br J Neurosurg 1994; 8:567–571.
16. Mannheimer C, Augustinsson L–E, Carlsson CH, et al. Epidural spinal electrical stimulation in severe angina pectoris. Br Heart J 1988; 59:56–61.
17. Sanderson JE, Brooksby P, Waterhouse D, et al. Epidural spinal electrical stimulation for severe angina: a study of its effects on symptoms, exercise tolerance and degree of ischaemia. Eur Heart J 1992; 13:628–633.
18. Mannheimer C, Eliasson T, Andersson B, et al. Effects of spinal cord stimulation in angina pectoris induced by pacing and possible mechanisms of action. Br Med J 1993; 307:477–480.
19. Tallis RC, Illis LS, Sedgwick EM, et al. Spinal cord stimulation in peripheral vascular disease. J Neurol Neurosurg Psychiatry 1983; 46:478–484.
20. Augustinsson LE, Holm J, Carlsson CA, Jivegard L. Epidural electrical stimulation in severe limb

ischaemia: evidence of pain relief increased blood flow and a possible limb-saving effect. Ann Surg 1985; 202:104–110.
21. Jacobs MJHM, Slaaf DW, Reneman RS. Dorsal column stimulation in critical limb ischaemia. Vasc Med Rev 1990; 1:215–220.
22. Horsch S, Claeys L. Epidural spinal cord stimulation in the treatment of severe peripheral arterial occlusive disease. Ann Vasc Surg 1994; 8:468–474.
23. Miles JB, Lipton S. Phantom limb pain treated by electrical stimulation. Pain 1987; 5:373–382.
24. Krainick JU, Thoden U, Riechert T. Pain reduction in amputees by long-term spinal cord stimulation (five year study). J Neurosurg 1980; 52:346–350.
25. Van Dongen VCP, Liem AL. Phantom limb and stump pain and its treatment with spinal cord stimulation. J Rehabil Sci 1995; 8:110–114.
26. Tesfaye S, Watt J, Benbow SJ, et al. Electrical spinal-cord stimulation for painful diabetic peripheral neuropathy. Lancet 1996; 348:1698–1701.
27. Meglio M, Cioni B, Prezioso A, Talamonti G. Spinal cord stimulation (SCS) in the treatment of post herpetic pain. Acta Neurochir Suppl 1989; 46:65–66.
28. Bennett MI, Tai YMA. Cervical dorsal column stimulation relieves pain of brachial plexus avulsion. J R Soc Med 1994; 87:5–6.
29. Tai YMA. Dorsal column implant for the management of cranio-facial pain. 2nd International Congress of the International Neuromodulation Society, Gothenburg, Sweden, 1994.
30. Barolat G, Knobler RL, Lublin FD. Trigeminal neuralgia in a patient with multiple scleroris treated with high cervical spinal cord stimulation: case report. Appl Neurophysiol 1988; 51:333–337.
31. Freeman TB, Campbell JN, Long DM. Naloxone does not affect pain relief induced by electrical stimulation in man. Pain 1983; 17:189–195.
32. Linderoth B, Stiller C–O, Gunasekera L, et al. Release of neurotransmitters in the CNS by spinal cord stimulation: survey of present state of knowledge and recent experimental studies. Stereotact Funct Neurosurg 1993; 61:157–170.
33. Linderoth B, Herrogodts P, Meyerson BA. Sympathetic mediation of peripheral vasodilatation induced by spinal cord stimulation: animal studies of the role of cholinergic and adrenergic receptor subtypes. Neurosurgery 1994; 35:711–719.
34. Meglio M, Cioni B. Effect of spinal cord stimulation on heart rate. In: Lazorthes Y, Upton ARM, eds. Neurostimulation: an Overview. New York: Futura, 1985:185–189.
35. Navar H, Augustinsson L–E, Elam M. The vasodilating effect of spinal dorsal column stimulation is mediated by sympathetic nerves. Clin Autonom Res 1992; 2:41–45.
36. Jacobs MJHM, Jorning PJG, Joshi SR, et al. Epidural spinal cord electrical stimulation improves microvascular blood flow in severe limb ischaemia. Ann Surg 1988; 207:179–183.
37. Jacobs MJHM, Jorning PJG, Beckers RCY, et al. Foot salvage and improvement of microvascular blood flow as a result of epidural spinal cord electrical stimulation. J Vasc Surg 1990; 12:354–360.
38. Galley D, Rettori R, Boccalon H, et al. Electric stimulation of the spinal cord in arterial diseases of the legs: a multicenter study of 244 patients. J Mal Vasc 1992; 17:208–213.
39. Long DM, Erikson D, Campbell J, North R. Electrical stimulation of the spinal cord and peripheral nerves for pain control: a 10-year experience. Appl Neurophysiol 1981; 44:207–217.
40. Burton C. Dorsal column stimulation: optimization of application. Surg Neurol 1975; 4:171–176.
41. North RB, Kidd DH, Wimberly RL, Edwin D. Prognostic value of psychological testing in patients undergoing spinal cord stimulation: a prospective study. Neurosurgery 1996; 39:301–310.
42. Hosobuchi Y, Adams JE, Weinstein PR. Preliminary percutaneous dorsal column stimulation prior to permanent implantation: technical note. J Neurosurg 1972; 37:242–245.
43. Miles J, Lipton S, Hayward M, et al. Pain relief by implanted electrical stimulators. Lancet 1974; 1:777–779.
44. Erickson DL. Percutaneous trial of stimulation for patient selection for implantable stimulating devices. J Neurosurg 1975; 43:440–444.
45. Sweet WH, Wepsic JG. Stimulation of the posterior column of the spinal cord for pain control: indications, technique and results. Clin Neurosurg 1974; 21:278–310.
46. Simpson BA. Spinal cord stimulation. Pain Rev 1994; 1:199–230.

47. Nielson KD, Adams JE, Hosbuchi Y. Experience with dorsal column stimulation for relief of chronic intractable pain: 1968–1973. Surg Neurol 1975; 4:148–152.
48. Siegfied J, Lazorthes Y. Long-term follow-up of dorsal cord stimulation for chronic pain syndrome after multiple lumbar operations. Appl Neurophysiol 1982; 45:201–204.
49. Kupers RC, Van den Oever R, Van Houdenhove B, et al. Spinal cord stimulation in Belgium: a nation-wide survey on the incidence, indications and therapeutic efficacy by the health insurer. Pain 1994; 56:211–216.
50. Barolat G, Massaro F, He J, et al. Mapping of sensory responses to epidural stimulation of the intraspinal neural structures in man. J Neurosurg 1993; 78:233–239.
51. Gilbert M, Counsell CM, Martin P, Snively C. Spinal cord stimulation for chronic intractable pain: nursing implications. J Neurosci Nurs 1994; 26:347–351.
52. Forrest DM. Practical points: spinal cord stimulator therapy. J Perianesth Nurs 1996; 11:349–352.
53. Ronk LL. Spinal cord stimulation for chronic, non-malignant pain. Orthop Nurs 1996; 15:53–58.
54. Bel S, Bauer BL. Dorsal column stimulation (DCS): cost to benefit analysis. Acta Neurochir Suppl 1991; 52:121–123.

17

Spinal Endoscopy

Its Current Status and Role in Lumbosacral Radiculopathy

Jonathan Richardson
Bradford Royal Infirmary, Bradford, West Yorkshire, England

I. INTRODUCTION

Chronic back pain is devouring medical resources at an exponential rate, with trends showing all developed countries to be affected. Eighty percent of populations will suffer back pain and, although most of these episodes settle, in many patients they recur. Following acute severe back pain with radicular symptoms, up to 30% of patients still have pain, a reduced capacity for work, and a restriction in leisure activities at 1 year (1).

The outlook for these patients is not good; severe radicular pain is difficult to manage. Pharmacotherapy entails unlicensed drug use; it is often only partially effective and it can be expensive. Spinal cord stimulation is suitable for only a proportion of patients; it is expensive in terms of hardware purchase and medical time and may require repeat interventions. Met-analysis has concluded that placement of epidural steroids may be beneficial for only up to 6 months (2). Surgery has a substantial morbidity that includes a pain recurrence rate estimated to lie between 15 and 50% (3). The *failed back surgery syndrome* (FBSS) is a descriptive term for these patients, defined as a combination of severe nociceptive and neuropathic pains that become more associated with psychosocial behavioral disabilities as treatments fail and time goes on. The accurate diagnosis and the effective management of severe radicular pain is a great challenge.

II. DIAGNOSIS

Trying to accurately diagnose back pain is difficult. Radiological-imaging techniques provide superbly detailed views, but their diagnostic usefulness for benign disease can be very disappointing. Multiple gross disk prolapses can be entirely asymptomatic. Likewise, it is not at all unusual for a patient complaining of well-localized severe radicular pain, easily confused with a repeat disk prolapse, to have no specific changes on computed tomographic (CT) or magnetic resonance (MRI) scanning. A major drawback of all investigations is that they cannot distinguish the causes of pain from abnormalities related to trauma and ageing.

Spinal endoscopy is different. It is a minimally invasive, interactive method of examining the spinal canal. Examination of the contents of the dural sac is easy, as they are suspended in

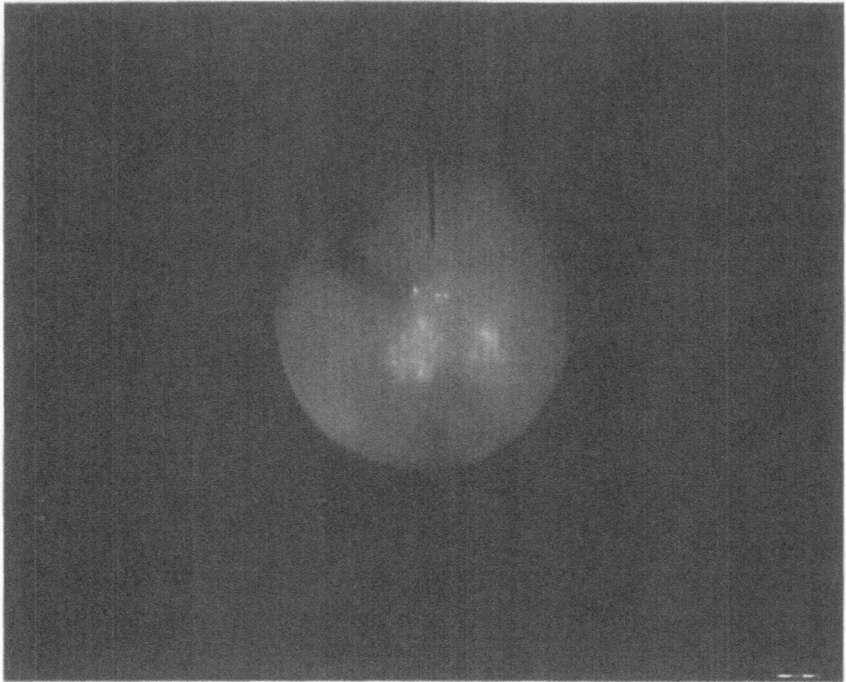

Figure 1 A healthy nerve root.

clear cerebrospinal fluid (CSF). With recent advances in instrumentation, especially involving fully steerable, flexible instruments, along with a saline delivery system, a multilevel detailed examination of the epidural space (epiduroscopy) can now be satisfactorily achieved. In color and in four dimensions, high-quality views aid the examiner in exactly identifying the nerve roots that are implicated in pain generation.

Noninflamed healthy nerve roots appear as white or slightly pink structures, with blood vessels running across their surface (Fig. 1), and they transmit a marked pulsation from the dural sac. Inflamed nerve roots, on the other hand, are red and edematous. Multiple adhesions may obscure the nerve (Fig. 2), but nevertheless the area often remains very pain-sensitive. Pathological nerve roots, probably because of the surrounding adhesions, can be avascular structures (i.e., devoid of surface vessels) and nonpulsatile. Through interaction with the patient, by gently probing with the tip of the endoscope, the response elicited is diagnostically useful with the patient reporting if his or her typical pain has been reproduced. Noninflamed nerve roots elicit a nonpainful response when contacted. Spinal endoscopy and MRI scanning have different attributes, and it is apparent that they are complementary (Table 1).

III. INSTRUMENTATION

Spinoscopy is not a new concept. The first instrument is thought to have been built in 1935 by Elias Stern in the United States (4), following an idea by Michael S. Burman (5). He never used it himself in patients, but spinoscopy (looking mainly into the intrathecal space) was avidly taken up by Pool, a neurosurgeon, in New York (6). Remarkably, by 1942 he had published a case series of 400 patients (7).

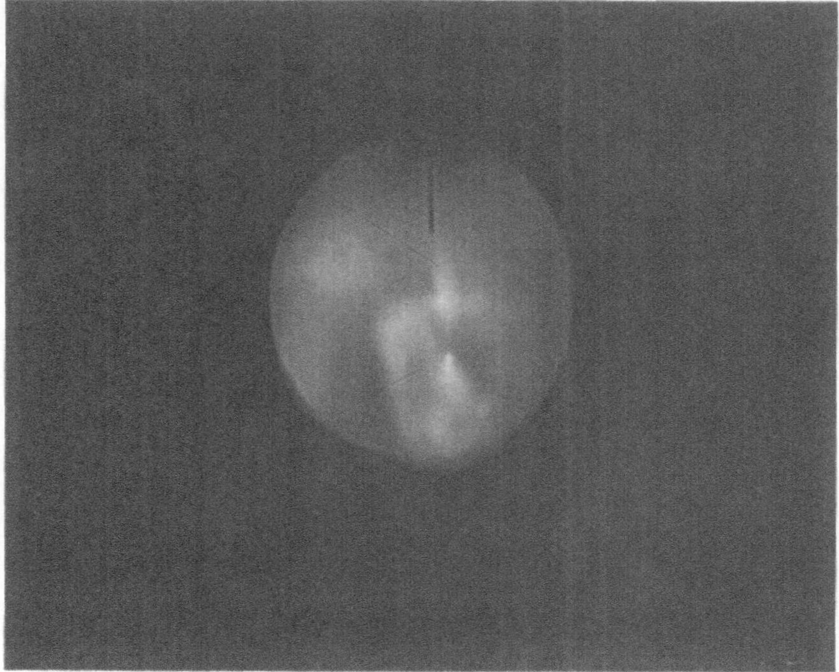

Figure 2 A tethered S1 nerve root: Note the sling of fibrous tissue around its origin.

The first instruments were large and rigid and had poor light sources (Fig. 3). They were inserted between spinous processes and allowed the examination of a single spinal level. The usefulness and safety of this procedure would have been limited, but nevertheless, in the 1940s when soft-tissue–imaging techniques were both invasive and relatively crude, Pool found the technique of sufficient benefit in some patients to obviate the need for iodized oil (Lipiodol) myelography and exploratory surgery (7).

Ooi in Japan introduced flexible light sources and later flexible endoscopes (8,9). For examination of the epidural space (as opposed to the intrathecal space), a clear optical medium has to be

Table 1 Suggested Comparison of Spinal Endoscopy with MRI Scanning for the Diagnosis and Management of Back Pain with Radiculopathy

	Spinal endoscopy	MRI scanning
Nerve root anatomy	+(Close up views only possible)	++
Nerve root vascularity	++	–
Nerve root inflammation	++	+/–
Nerve root sensitivity	++	–
Diagnostic localization of pain	++	–
Identification of fibrous tissue	++	+
Disk prolapse identification	+/– (Anterior structure)	++
Assessment of spinal canal size	+	++
Exclusion of serious pathology	+(Biopsy possible)	++
Therapeutic aspects	++	–

++, very helpful; +, helpful; –, not helpful.

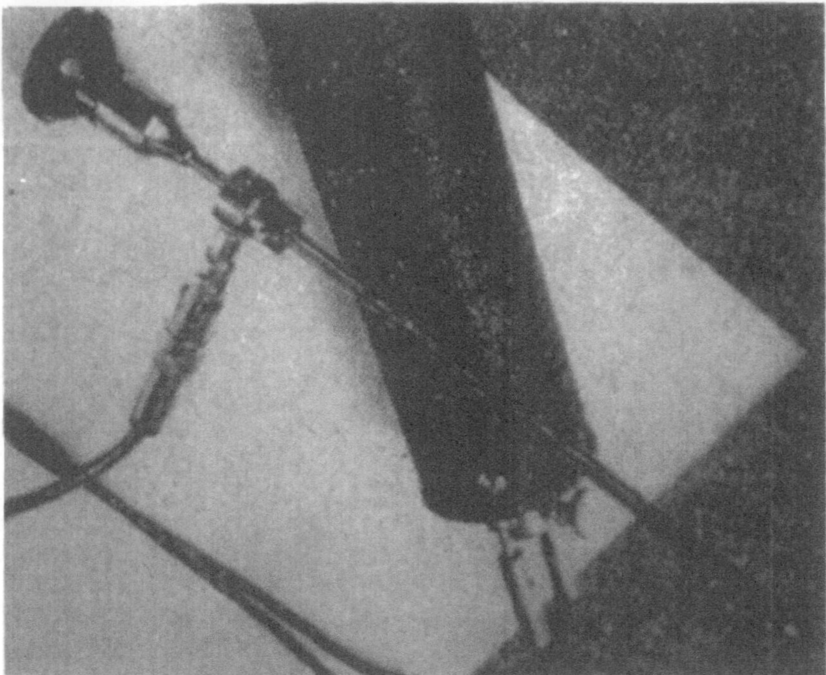

Figure 3 Early instruments were large, rigid, and had poor light sources.

introduced so that tissues are far enough away from the lens to be focused on. Air or saline can be used. Shimoji in Japan circumvented this problem as recently as 1990 by deliberately making holes in the dura to leak CSF (10). By 1994 saline delivery systems were available (11).

Modern precision instruments are of various sizes and contain many thousands of optical fibers along with a number of light bundles (Fig. 4). An outside diameter of 0.9 mm is in common use. Image quality is remarkable. They are flexible, which facilitates the examination of a number of spinal levels and allows the instrument to be introduced away from the proposed site of pathology. Some manufacturers have separated the steering facility from the endoscope itself, which requires a separate disposable outer steering sheath (video-guided catheter).

IV. TECHNIQUE

Spinal endoscopy can be performed anywhere: in an operating room, or in an endoscopy or a radiology suite. A limited examination can be done simply by insertion of a naked spinal endoscope through a Tuohy needle. For more precise examinations of several spinal levels, a larger instrument with steering capability is usually inserted through the sacral hiatus using a Seldinger technique. The patient's pain and its approximate dermatomal level should be known to the operator so that the examination can be focused in that area.

V. DIAGNOSTIC USEFULNESS OF SPINAL ENDOSCOPY

From the outset, the conditions for which spinal endoscopy was diagnostically useful included herniation of the nucleus pulposus, hypertrophy of the ligamentum flavum, chronic adhesive

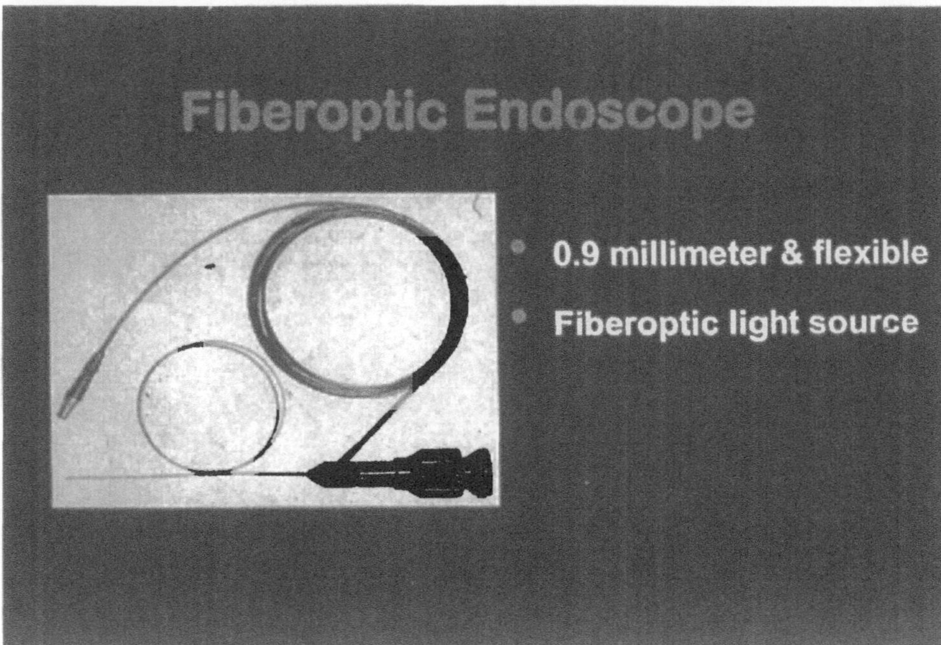

Figure 4 A typical modern instrument: It is small (outside diameter 0.9 mm), flexible, has clear optics, with high resolution, and good light-carrying capabilities. (Courtesy of Myelotec Inc., Rosswell, GA).

arachnoiditis, granulations, benign tumors, lipoidosis, varicosities of the dura, arteriosclerosis of the spinal cord, metastatic neoplasms, and differentiation of operable from nonoperable lesions of the cauda equina (6–10). The author uses the technique for identification of nerve roots involved in pain generation (12).

VI. THERAPEUTIC OPTIONS

A. Adhesiolysis

Once the nerve roots involved in pain generation are identified, if adhesions are present (see Fig. 2), they can be mobilized by sweeping the tip of the instrument back and forth. This must be carried out with great gentleness in a cooperative and sensible (albeit lightly sedated) patient. With a report of paresthesias, it is essential to stop immediately. Additional room around the nerve root can be created hydrostatically by the saline flow. A marked improvement in symptoms has been reported, partly or entirely, through this mechanism (7,9,10,12–14). The success of this procedure can be evaluated by pre- and postprocedure epidurography (Figs. 5 and 6).

B. Targeted Therapy

Targeted pharmacotherapy is a valuable aspect of spinal endoscopy. Traditionally, deposition of steroids and other epidural medications usually takes place a long way from their desired site of action. Large filling defects are frequently seen on epidurography in patients with radiculopathies (often caused by epidural fibrosis), and it is likely that medication injection broadly takes a similar path. The amounts reaching the adhesion-encased nerve root in question will

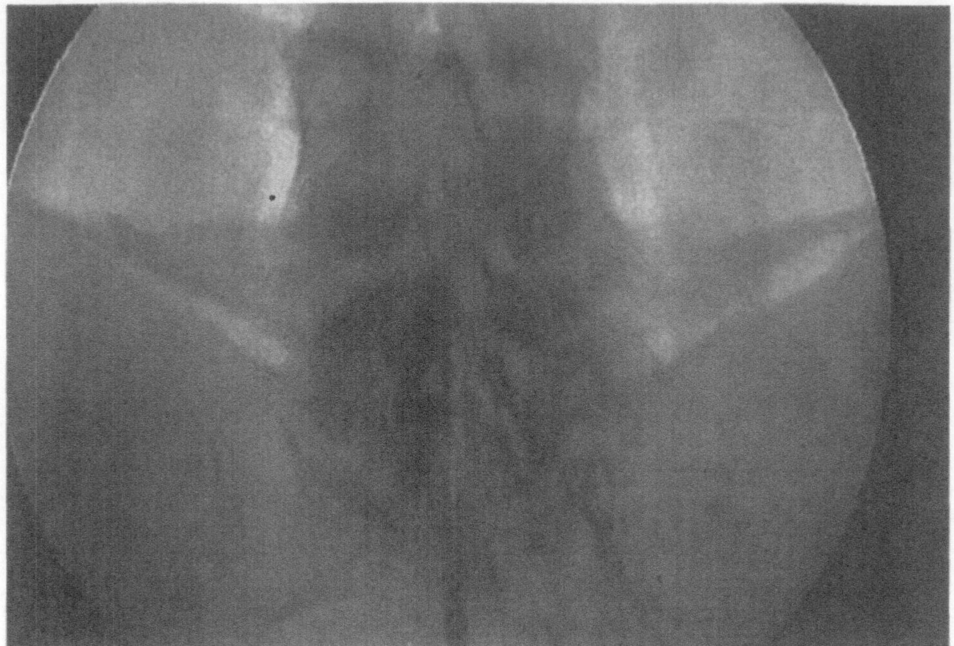

Figure 5 A preoperative epidurogram of a 50-year-old woman who had undergone two previous diskectomies: She re-presented with right-sided radiculopathic symptoms and signs, predominently in the S1 distribution. Note the poor flow contrast of the intervertebral foramina on the right.

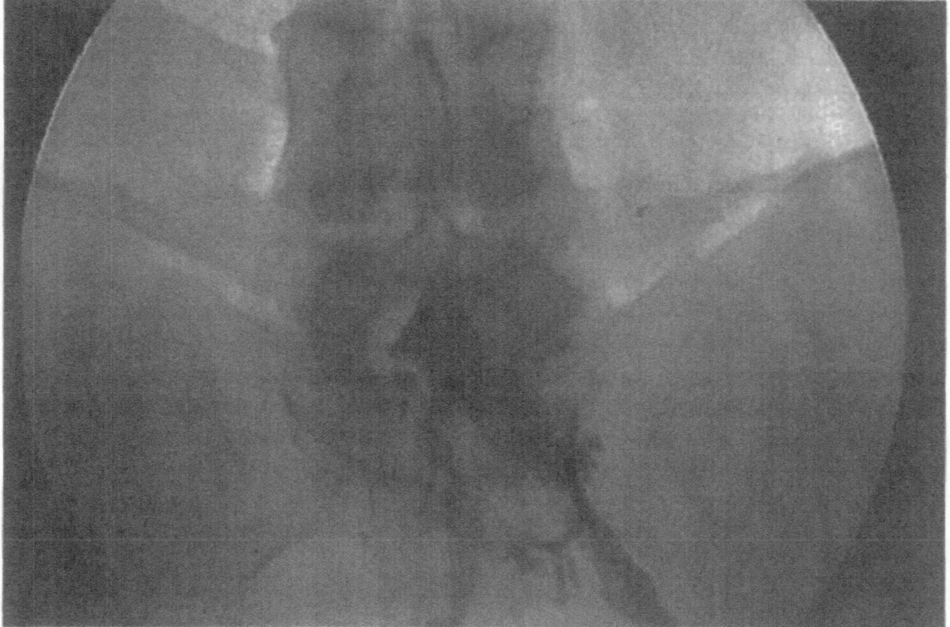

Figure 6 Postprocedure repeat epidurography in the same patient demonstrated that an effective right-sided adhesiolysis (neuroplasty) had been carried out, with good flow of contrast through the S1 nerve root.

Table 2 Patient Characteristics (n = 31)

Age	Sex	Symptom duration (yrs)	Radiculopathy[a]	Intervertebral disk disease	Previous back surgery	Disk lesion still present on CT/MRI
48 (SD 13.6)	16 m 15 f	10.3 (±SE 2.3) (range 2–26)	20	27	18	17

[a] Numbness, paresthesias weakness.

probably be very small. Direct vision allows medication to be deposited very accurately in high local concentrations, while avoiding the risk of inadvertent intrathecal administration, an important safety feature (15).

VII. OUTCOME STUDIES

There are no systematic outcome studies on the usefulness or otherwise of spinal endoscopy in patients with back pain and radiculopathies, although several case reports and series have made mention of good improvements (7,9,10,12–14). In our institution, I have been involved with this technique for over 2 years. Our results are presented here.

A. Case Series

All patients over a 12-month period (April 1998 to April 1999) with chronic low back pain and a radiculopathic element, who had had a poor response to other analgesic modalities and had consented to undergo spinal endoscopy, were studied. The procedure was carried out with minimal sedation so that cooperation could be assured. Thirty-one patients with pain duration of 2–26 years (mean of 10.3), 18 of whom had a failed back surgery syndrome (3), completed treatment. The ratio of males to females was 16:15 and the age at presentation ranged from 28 to 78 years with a mean of 47.7 years (Table 2).

It was possible to steer the instrument to what the patient described as the exact epidural site of origin of back pain and leg pain, which was found in all cases to be a nerve root(s). The location of this structure had been suggested by history and abnormal epidurographic filling defects corresponding with the estimated site of pain in 27 of 31 patients. Contact with noninflamed nerve roots was reported as nonpainful, a finding that has previously been reported (16,17a). Fibrous adhesions around the nerve root were clearly seen in all patients, irrespective of previous back surgery, and these were very dense in 13 (42%) (Table 3). With movement

Table 3 Procedure Data (n = 31)

Matching of preprocedure epidurogram filling defects with symptoms	Epiduroscopy findings	Duration	Postprocedure epidurogram	Intraoperative complications
27	Identification of pain generator in 29; adhesions in 31; dense fibrosis in 13; disk prolapse in 1.	52 min (Range 44–80)	Performed in 16; improved in 12	Nil

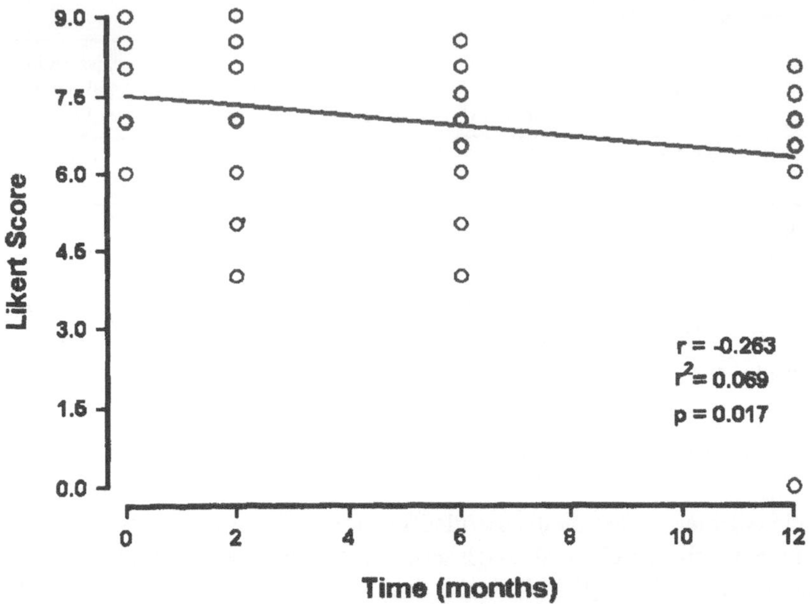

Figure 7 The solid squares represent the mean pain scores at each time point with 95% confidence intervals. Improvements in mean pain scores were maintained at all time periods ($p < 0.05$).

of the instrument to examine this area, along with a constant saline flow, mobilization of adhesions away from the nerve root (neuroplasty) was directly observed, and in some patients, an increase in transmitted nerve root pulsation was seen. Postprocedure epidurography showed contrast flow through previously blocked intervertebral foramina in 12 of 16 patients in whom it was performed (75%) (see Figs. 5, 6, and Table 3). The neuroplasty effectively formed a pocket for the subsequent placement of bupivacaine, dexamethasone, and clonidine. The mean duration of the procedure was 52 min (range 44–80), following which the patient was kept supine for at least 1 h and discharged from hospital the same day.

Baseline pain scores (0 representing no pain; 10 representing the worst pain imaginable) and total functional scores (0 representing virtual immobility; 9 representing very good function) (17b) were 8.2 ± 0.28 (2 standard errors of the mean) and 1.35 ± 0.42, respectively. Subsequent measures at 2, 6, and 12 months were compared using Kruskal–Wallis one-way analysis of variance (ANOVA). Statistically significant improvements in mean pain scores were found which were maintained at all time periods ($p < 0.05$) (Fig. 7). Total function scores also showed marked improvements at all time periods ($p < 0.05$) (Fig. 8). Neither pain nor function score improvement were related to symptom duration.

Two patients had nonpersistent paresthesias of the lower limb. All patients had some nonpersistent postoperative low back discomfort and two had 2-day fluid leaks of saline from the sacral hiatus (the site of instrument insertion). No dural tap headache occurred.

B. Discussion

Investment of nerve roots by connective tissue may exacerbate any compression, leading to an increase in permeability of the endoneural capillaries, promoting endoneural edema formation (18,19). The resulting increase in the intraneural fluid pressure leads to an impairment of the

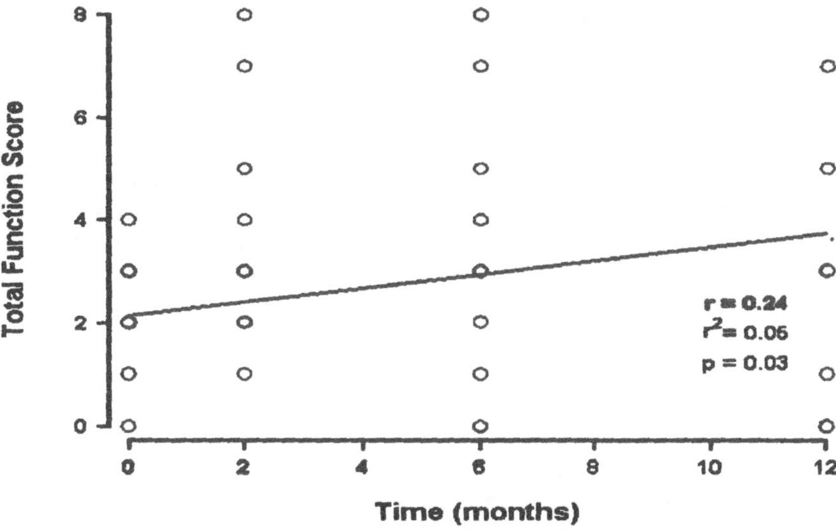

Figure 8 The solid squares represent the mean total function score at each time point with 95% confidence intervals. Marked improvements were found at all time periods ($p < 0.05$).

nutritional transport to the nerve root, as nutrition depends on diffusion of nutrients from the CSF, the blood supply being relatively poor (18–20). In disease states, especially with adhesive arachnoiditis, nutrition becomes critical (19). Intraneural edema and venous stasis promote fibroblast invasion, thereby exacerbating excessive connective tissue formation (18,19,21) with worsening nerve root adhesions and fibrosis.

A striking finding of this case series is that all patients were found to have scar tissue involving granulations and adhesions between the nerve root, the dura, and the ligamentum flavum, with dense fibrosis in 42% (see Fig. 2). This suggests that gadolinium-enhanced MRI scanning, currently the investigation of choice for epidural fibrosis (22), produces a large underestimate of its incidence and severity.

It is possible that endoscopic adhesiolysis leads to an improvement in venous drainage and, hence, a reduction in intraneural edema. CSF nutrition may therefore improve and the stimulus to fibroblastic activity may decline. Additionally, a restoration in CSF nerve growth factor delivery (necessary for maintenance of the integrity of myelin sheaths) (23), may lead to a reduction in mechanical sensitivity and, hence, radicular pain.

Dilution or "washingout" of phospholipase A_2 and synovial cytokines, which leak from damaged intervertebral disks and zygoapophyseal joints and result in local and nerve root inflammation (24), may also contribute to an improvement in symptoms. This mechanism may explain the improvement that has been found in saline injection control groups in studies of epidural steroids (25,26).

Spinal endoscopy permits the accurate placement of epidural medications, in this case series, methylprednisolone (Depo-medrone), bupivacaine, and clonidine. The ensuing mechanical and hydrostatic adhesiolysis effectively forms a pocket for the solution (see Figs. 5 and 6). Delivery of medication into this pocket facilitates the optimum possible benefit that can be derived from these medications.

Further mechanisms explaining our positive results include analgesia, resulting from the use of clonidine, and a placebo response. It could also be argued that a natural improvement would have occurred anyway without any form of intervention, although the duration of symptoms, a mean of 10.3 (range 2–26) years, would not suggest this.

C. Summary

Spinal endoscopy is probably the method of choice for the diagnosis of epidural fibrosis. It is a safe technique that holds great promise for a reduction in pain and disability. These results need to be confirmed, randomized controlled trials are required, and the mechanisms for improvement need to be studied.

VIII. THE FUTURE

Spinal anatomy both in the normal situation and in disease states needs to be studied. Igarashi in Japan has made a commendable start on the former (27–30).

The physiology of the spinal nerve root deserves special study in view of its role in pain generation and its unique structural, vascular, and nutritional weaknesses (compared with the peripheral nerve) (19). Our ignorance of the in situ pathophysiology of disease and the effects of therapy is profound.

Therapeutic options include surgery, the recovery of foreign bodies (e.g., sheered epidural catheter), and targeted destructive lesions for the management of terminal (e.g., cancer) pain.

IX. CONCLUSION

Spinal endoscopy with modern equipment has great diagnostic, teaching, research, and therapeutic potential (12). It holds great promise for the improved diagnosis and management of long-term chronic radicular pain and disability. With care it is a safe procedure. Systematic studies are required.

REFERENCES

1. Weber H, Holme I, Amlie E. The natural course of acute sciatica with nerve root symptoms in a double-blind, placebo controlled trial evaluating the effect of piroxicam. Spine 1993; 18:1433–1438.
2. Koes BW, Scholten RJ, Mens JM, Bouter LM. Efficacy of epidural steroid injections for low-back pain and sciatica: a systematic review of randomized clinical trials. Pain 1995; 63:279–288.
3. Follet KA, Dirkes BA. Etiology and evaluation of the failed back surgery syndrome. Neurosurg Q 1993; 3:40–59.
4. Stern EL. The spinascope: a new instrument for visualizing the spinal canal and its contents. Med Rec (NY) 1936; 143:31–32.
5. Burman MS. Myeloscopy or the direct visualisation of the spinal canal and its contents. J Bone Joint Surg 1931; 13:695–696.
6. Pool JL. Myeloscopy: intraspinal endoscopy. Surgery 1942; 11:169–182.
7. Pool JL. Direct visualisation of dorsal nerve roots of the cauda equina by means of a myeloscope. Arch Neurol Psychiatry 1938; 39:1308.
8. Ooi Y, Morisaki N. Intrathecal lumbar endoscope. Clin Orthop Surg (Jpn) 1969; 4:295–297.
9. Ooi Y, Satoh Y, Hirose K, Mikanagi K, Morisaki N. Myeloscopy. Acta Orthop Belg 1978; 44:881–894.
10. Shimoji K, Fujioka H, Onodera M, Hokari T, Fukuda S, Fujiwara N, Hatori T. Observation of spinal

canal and cysternae with the newly developed small-diameter, flexible fiberscopes. Anesthesiology 1991; 75:341–344.

11. Heavner JE, Chokhavatia S, Kizelshteyn G. Percutaneous evaluation of the epidural and subarachnoid space with a flexible fiberscope. Reg Anesth 1991; 15(S):85.
12. Richardson J. Realising visions. Br J Anaesth 1999; 83:369–371.
13. Saberski LR, Kitahata LM. Direct visualization of the lumbosacral epidural space through the sacral hiatus. Anesth Analg 1995; 80:839–840.
14. Saberski LR, Brull SJ. Epidural endoscopy-aided drug delivery: a case report. Yale J Biol Med 1995; 68:17–18.
15. Abram SE. Treatment of lumbosacral radiculopathy with epidural steroids. Anesthesiology 1999; 91:1937–1941.
16. Kuslich SD, Ulstrom CL, Michael CJ. The tissue origin of low back pain and sciatica: a report of pain response to tissue stimulation during operation on the lumbar spine using local anesthesia. Orthop Clin North Am 1991; 22:181–187.

17a. Smyth MJ, Wright V. Sciatica and the intervertebral disc. An experimental study. J Bone Joint 1958; 40A:1401–1418.

17b. Waddell G, Main CJ. Assessment of severity in lowback disorders. Spine 1984; 9:204–208.

18. Olmarker K, Rydevik B. Pathophysiology of sciatica. Orthop Clin North Am 1991; 22:223–234.
19. Hasue M. Pain and the nerve root. An interdisciplinary approach. Spine 1993; 18:2053–2058.
20. Rydevik B, Holm S, Brown MD, Lundborg G. Diffusion from the cerebrospinal fluid as a nutritional pathway for spinal nerve roots. Acta Physiol Scand 1990; 138:247–248.
21. Cooper RG, Mitchell WS, Illingworth KJ, Clair Forbes WS, Gillespie JE, Jayson MIV. The role of epidural fibrinolysis in the persistence of postlaminectomy back pain. Spine 1991; 16:1044–1048.
22. Wilkinson LS, Elson E, Saifuddin A, Ransford AO. Defining the use of gadolinium enhanced MRI in the assessment of the postoperative lumbar spine. Clin Radiol 1997; 52:530–534.
23. Devor M. Neuropathic pain and the injured nerve: peripheral mechanisms. Br Med Bull 1991; 47: 619–630.
24. Olmarker K, Rydevik B, Nordborg C. Autologous nucleus pulposus induced neurophysiologic and histologic changes in porcine cauda equina nerve roots. Spine 1993; 18:1425–1432.
25. Evans W. Intrasacral epidural injection in the treatment of sciatica. Lancet 1930; 1:1225–1229.
26. Snoek W, Weber H, Jörgensen B. Double-blind evaluation of extradural methylprednisolone for herniated nucleus pulposus. Acta Orthop Scand 1977; 48:635–641.
27. Igarashi T, Hirabayashi Y, Shimizu R, Mitsuhata H, Saitoh K, Fukuda H, Konishi A, Asahara H. Inflammatory changes after extradural anaesthesia may affect the spread of local anaesthetic within the extradural space. Br J Anaesth 1996; 77:347–351.
28. Igarashi T, Hirabayashi Y, Shimizu R, Saitoh K, Fukuda H, Mitsuhata H. The lumbar extradural structure changes with increasing age. Br J Anaesth 1997; 78:149–152.
29. Igarashi T, Hirabayashi Y, Shimizu R, Saitoh K, Fukuda H. Thoracic and lumbar extradural structure examined by extraduroscope. Br J Anaesth 1998; 81:121–125.
30. Igarashi T, Hirabayashi Y, Shimizu R, Saitoh K, Fukuda H. The epidural structure changes during deep breathing. Can J Anesth 1999; 46:850–855.

18
Cancer Pain Treatment

Margaret Saunders
Papworth Hospital, Cambridge, England

Sarah Booth
Addenbrooke's Hospital, Cambridge, England

I. INTRODUCTION

This chapter will consider the recent advances in the use of some well-established drugs together with some newer drugs that have become available to manage cancer pain. The current controversies in the use of opioids will be reviewed. New therapies that have emerged and are emerging for neuropathic cancer pain will be considered. Bone pain and incident pain remain difficult areas for the clinician and current strategies are discussed in some detail. Both authors are palliative medicine physicians working in general hospitals, but with a hospice background.

It is important to realize that cancer pain is almost always a complex phenomenon. The pathophysiology of cancer pain is commonly mixed: for example, a patient with a malignant epidural mass will often experience bony, nociceptive, and neuropathic pain concurrently. Each component will require separate identification and treatment. The nature and reputation of the disease itself, with all the attending folklore, will provoke fear in many patients and their families. Coincident pain may also occur from nonmalignant conditions. Careful, thorough assessment is vital to achieve good pain relief.

II. EXTENT OF THE PROBLEM

The past two decades have seen tremendous advances in both our understanding and treatment of cancer pain. Despite this, the fear of pain remains the greatest anxiety for many of those in whom cancer has been diagnosed.

There are over 5 million cancer deaths worldwide per year—about 3 million of these are in developing countries. This number is predicted to increase rapidly over the next few years as a consequence of increasing longevity (1). It is estimated that at least 80% of cancer patients experience pain at some time during their illness and that the prevalence of pain increases as the disease advances (2).

III. WORLD HEALTH ORGANIZATION

Since 1980 the World Health Organization (WHO) has worked to promote palliative care and cancer pain relief. The WHO guidelines on "cancer pain relief" were first made available in

---

* This chapter was submitted to editors in 1999.

1986 (3), and when implemented, they provide effective control of pain in 80–90% of cancer patients. The second, updated edition of the guidelines was published in 1996. The guidelines advocate a simple "analgesic ladder" approach to cancer pain and have subsequently been assessed and shown to work in over 30,000 patients (4,5). WHO has promoted the use of oral drugs and has collaborated with the International Narcotics Control Board to ensure the regulated availability of opioids worldwide (6).

Through their handbook *National Cancer Control Programmes: Priorities and Managerial Guidelines*, WHO has provided the information necessary to formulate governmental policies, to initiate education programs, and to ensure opioid availability at a national level. Over 60 countries have adopted cancer pain and palliative care as a priority as part of their national cancer control program (7,8).

IV. TREATMENT OPTIONS

A. Opioids

It is encouraging that there has been a documented increase, year by year, in the use of morphine throughout both the developed and developing world. Education resulting in an improved understanding of pain mechanisms and the continuum of opioid responsiveness should lead to targeted use of opioids for appropriate pains, in appropriate doses, with the addition of secondary analgesia. Recent research has led to the introduction of new strong opioids and novel methods of drug delivery. This opens up the possibility that alternative strong opioids may need to be used when it is not possible to overcome the adverse effects of morphine—a technique that has become known as "opioid rotation" (although this can be a misleading term) (9). The awareness of the need to elicit and actively address adverse effects of morphine has been facilitated by the development of some newer opioids with differing receptor activity and an altered spectrum of unwanted effects.

B. Transdermal Fentanyl

It has now been demonstrated that there is a lower incidence of constipation and nausea and vomiting with transdermal fentanyl than with morphine (10,11). Patients troubled by these symptoms with morphine, in spite of adequate treatment, may benefit from a switch to this preparation. Guidelines on switching preparation are easily available (12): it is important to warn patients about possible short-lived withdrawal phenomena associated with the change (11–13). Short-acting oral transmucosal and intranasal preparations of fentanyl are currently being evaluated—pain relief occurs within 5 min of administration. A remaining drawback with the use of transdermal fentanyl is that another short-acting opioid needs to be used for "breakthrough" or rescue medication because effective analgesia is reached with the transdermal preparation only after 12–16 h. The results from these trials of short-acting fentanyl preparations are awaited with interest, for they may fill a gap in currently available drugs for cancer pain (14).

V. TYPES OF PAIN

A. Nonopioid Responsive Pain

Widespread acceptance and use of opioids has in some instances led to the expectation that all pain will respond to opioids if given in sufficient quantities. This expectation is not borne out either by clinical practice or by the recently developed scientific models of pain. Pain that is found to be only partially responsive to opioid medication or indeed nonresponsive to opioid medication often falls into one of the categories of either neuropathic pain, bone pain, incident pain, or total pain.

B. Total Pain

The psychological state of the patient with cancer will be intrinsically linked to their experience of pain, and successful treatment of pain will often be dependent on addressing both psychological and physical needs. This is nowhere more clearly exemplified than in the situation of "total pain" (15), of which there is a growing awareness.

When a patient has total pain, somatic manifestations may appear to be the most important. Patients often demand or appear to need extensive investigation or intervention (including pain blocks). Many of the usual pharmacological measures appear useless, or pain may be relieved in one part of the body only to appear somewhere else. (Total pain has also been characterized as "opioid-irrelevant pain" by Dr. John Hinton, consulting psychiatrist to St. Christopher's Hospice). Frequently patients will deny any anxiety or psychological distress, but will manifest their distress physically. This distress will also be transferred to the team caring for the patient. The patient may need frequent admission to the hospital or hospice and will "demand" continual nursing attention.

Pain is always an experience of the mind and the body and a "holistic" approach to the patient, taking into account the physical, psychological, spiritual, and social dimensions of pain, is the key to achieving any control, particularly in the patient with advanced cancer. When the patient has total pain both he or she and frequently the family feel overwhelmed by the experience and can find no relief. Advanced nursing care is vital to achieving good pain control. Radiotherapists, medical oncologists, pain specialists, palliative care physicians, orthopedic surgeons, and psychiatrists are among the many disciplines who may need to be involved in controlling any cancer pain. For a patient in total pain, other professionals who may be central to care include social workers, psychologists, chaplains, physiotherapists, and occupational therapists. All the resources of hospice are often needed, including inpatient care, day care, and complementary therapies, such as art or music therapy, as well as respite for the family. Indeed, opioid-irrelevant pain in cancer is the most taxing of the difficult pains that are encountered by specialists. The pain is frequently not "controlled" but "contained," the aim being to achieve the best relief possible without lasting psychological sequelae in those left after the patient has died. Bereavement support is often needed for the surviving family. Patients with total pain can split both hospital and community teams and this can be avoided only if there is a recognition that the patient's distress is spilling over and that the focus of care needs to embrace all aspects of pain. Specialist palliative care is usually central to the care of these patients.

C. Neuropathic Pain

Neuropathic pain is caused by pathological change or dysfunction in either the peripheral or central nervous system. When associated with cancer, it may be defined as "pain in an area of abnormal or absent sensation" (17). Other terms used to describe this entity include neurogenic pain (18), deafferentation pain (19), and dysesthetic pain. The word neuropathic is becoming the accepted term as it encompasses change in *function* as well as damage to a nerve as possible causes of pain. Its exact incidence is unknown, but in one series of 2118 cancer patients referred to a specialist pain service (5,20), 34% had neuropathic pain.

Neuropathic pain in cancer is not one pathophysiological entity; for example, it may include sympathetically maintained pain (20). It has also been demonstrated that many cancer patients have more than one pain (21), and that each pain may have more than one cause, so that thorough evaluation requires a detailed history of each component of a patient's pain and an understanding of the disease status in that individual.

The clinical features associated with neuropathic pain in cancer include *dysesthesia* (i.e., the "unpleasant" and unusual qualities that allow it to be distinguished from nociceptive pain). Many words used in medical literature to describe neuropathic pain are not used by patients themselves. Clinicians should ask directly about abnormal sensations associated with the pain, such as "electric shocks," shooting, pricking, tingling, burning, and "vice-like" or pressure feelings. Particular features include the following:

Allodynia: when pain is provoked by a normally innocuous stimulus that would usually produce the sensation of pressure or temperature change. Many patients will describe severe pain from the lightest touch of bedclothes or garments on their skin.

Hyperalgesia: in which there is an increased response to a stimulus that is normally painful (i.e., the pain threshold is normal but the pain felt is abnormally severe).

Hyperpathia: defined as a painful syndrome characterized by an exaggerated response to a stimulus, especially a repeated stimulus in an area that is relatively anesthetic (i.e., when the pain threshold is raised). Other features of hyperpathia include imperfect localization and identification of the stimulus, delay, and aftersensation.

Assessment of the patient with neuropathic pain is discussed in detail elsewhere in this volume, but it is important that relevant neurological examination is carried out. Signs of sudomotor and vasomotor dysfunction are often detected in areas of neuropathic pain. It should also be remembered that patients with advanced cancer often have several symptoms and that pain may not be the most distressing one. Pain and psychological distress are almost always inextricably linked, and a full pain assessment will involve evaluating the patient as a person and the patient's concerns and aims, in addition to deciding on likely physical causes for the pain.

Our understanding of neuropathic pain has increased over the past decade with the realization that the nervous system is not a "hard-wired, line-labeled system" (22), but one that demonstrates "plasticity" so that the function and structure of the system alters with continuing development, experience, or the effects of injury. The nervous system seems to hold a "memory of pain"—induction of the c-*fos* gene by prolonged peripheral input leads to structural change and may explain this. In addition it has now been demonstrated in the laboratory that injury may induce a hyperexcitable state in the dorsal horn neurons, called ***windup***, in which continued peripheral input causes increasing central activity. Windup can be reduced or abolished by *N*-methyl-D-aspartate (NMDA) antagonists, which has lead to some advances in the therapy of this predictably "difficult" pain.

D. Treatment of Neuropathic Pain

The best treatment can be given only when there is an understanding of the likely cause of the pain. Pain may result from the cancer itself (e.g., direct infiltration or compression of a nerve by tumor), from cancer treatment (e.g., postmastectomy pain), or from a coexisting nonmalignant condition (e.g., diabetic neuropathy), all of which have been extensively reviewed (23). An important feature of cancer-related neuropathic pain is that it is not "pure": an epidural mass can cause pressure on nerves, giving pain with features of autonomic dysfunction and dysesthesia. Bony pain may also be present.

There is no universally accepted clinical algorithm for the treatment of neuropathic pain in cancer. Antitumor treatment should always be considered, as this may help pain relief. It was traditionally taught that neuropathic pain could be distinguished from nociceptive pain by the "lack of analgesic effect of opioids" (24), but this has been superseded by the idea that neuropathic pain shows a continuum of response to opioids (25), and that opioid-responsiveness is a very complex phenomenon (26) related to the individual patient, the pain itself and the opioid being used. The differing metabolic pathways of the newer synthetic opioids may influence their effect in neuropathic pain. It may be that morphine is the least effective opioid in this condition.

It is now common practice to give a trial of opioids for neuropathic pain, but not to persist with dose escalation if there is no early sign of response. Other authorities (27) also advise that nonsteroidal anti-inflammatory agents (NSAIDs) should be used judiciously with other conventional treatments for neuropathic pain (e.g., antidepressants), particularly as cancer-related neuropathic pain is so seldom a "pure" phenomenon. When and if first-line treatments fail there are no straightforward, universally accepted guidelines about what should be used next, and again, the severity of the pain, assessed in the context of the patient's personal agenda, the patient's other problems, and the stage of the patient's cancer, will provide some guidance to possible other treatments. There are no randomized controlled trials to guide practice in resistant cancer-related neuropathic pain, and further treatment is often related to local expertise and practice.

1. Methadone

There are some theoretical reasons to offer a trial of methadone. This drug is an NMDA receptor antagonist as well as a powerful μ-receptor agonist, and in recent years has been reclaimed for the treatment of nociceptive and neuropathic cancer pain (28). It fell into disuse in the developed world because of its unpredictable, sometimes extremely prolonged half-life (8–80 h) which led to some fatalities from respiratory depression. As used by experienced clinicians with a thorough understanding of its pharmacodynamic and pharmacokinetic properties, it is becoming an accepted tool in the management of difficult neuropathic pain, although there are no randomized, controlled data to guide its use.

2. Ketamine

Ketamine, best known as an anesthetic drug producing dissociative anesthesia, is also a nonselective NMDA receptor antagonist that is now becoming used in the management of both nonmalignant and malignant neuropathic pain (29,30). There are no prospective placebo-controlled studies using ketamine in cancer-related neuropathic pain, but there are a number of case reports and open studies that describe benefit in patients with previously resistant pain (31). After the likely response to ketamine for an individual has been tested by a bolus dose (typically 5–10 mg) given intravenously or subcutaneously (s.c.), it can be continued by s.c. infusion. The doses used are much smaller than those used in anesthetic practice. Recommended dosing regimens vary (32). In some centers a starting dose of 0.01 mg/kg/h is used; in others, lower doses of 100 mg/day are given initially and the dose increased by 100 mg/day to 500–600 mg daily (31). Dysphoric effects may be prevented by prescribing a low dose of benzodiazepine or haloperidol. If the patient is taking a regular opioid, the opioid dose should be reduced by about 50% (with "as required" doses available) when ketamine is started, because opioid toxicity may occur if ketamine treatment is effective.

3. Gabapentin

Gabapentin is a new anticonvulsant that has been used in neuropathic pain, both malignant and nonmalignant, when other therapies have failed (33). Its mode of action is uncertain: it is structurally related to γ-aminobutyric acid (GABA), but it is thought to interact with an as yet unknown receptor in the CNS. It is generally better tolerated than older anticonvulsants (e.g., carbamazepine), but it can cause dizziness and sedation. A usual dose is 100–300 mg t.i.d. The dose should be reduced in patients with renal impairment.

4. Sympathetic Blockade

An element of sympathetically maintained pain should be suspected if symptoms of neuropathic pain are accompanied by signs of local autonomic dysfunction, such as abnormal sweating, vasomotor instability, or swelling. A sympathetic block may be used, first diagnostically, then, if beneficial, for treatment in conjunction with other therapy for neuropathic pain (34).

5. Epidural Opioids and Local Anesthetics

Where other treatments have failed, a combination of an opioid with a low concentration of local anesthetic, administered by the epidural route, may succeed. This technique is no bar to domiciliary care and is increasingly used where local expertise allows.

6. Additional Treatments

These include the use of transcutaneous nerve stimulation (TENS) machines and other techniques, such as massage, heat and cold application, hypnosis, and visualization. There is no evidence to guide clinicians as to when these methods may be most effective. Again a careful assessment of the person and the likely causes of pain will help. Some patients do not like the feeling that the TENS machine produces, but others are pleased to have something they can use when they choose and that does not affect their level of consciousness. Hypnosis and visualization are useful for those who can cooperate with these techniques, but some persons are frightened of them. Massage may be particularly useful for patients who are anxious or very tense, but have difficulty expressing these feelings in words. In all these cases, these techniques are part of care, not the whole treatment.

E. Incident Pain

Incident pain can be defined as pain related to a specific activity such as weight-bearing or coughing. There is still controversy about the definition, classification, and possible subsets of this type of pain, and no randomized controlled data are available to guide the clinician in treatment (35). In general, the patient's pain is well-controlled while at rest, but it is very severe, albeit short-lived, when activity is carried out. If the overall analgesic dose is increased so that the patient becomes pain-free with activity, then he or she may suffer adverse effects when at rest because the patient may now be relatively "overdosed." Incident pain may be neuropathic or nociceptive in origin. Pain on weight-bearing may be associated with pathological fractures, and internal fixation and radiotherapy are then the treatments of choice. If the patient is too ill for operative treatment, an epidural can allow comfortable nursing care and greatly improve quality of life. Epidurals and nerve blocks are the best option currently available for incident pain, but are not always appropriate or practical. Treatment is currently very difficult and often imperfect. A rapid-onset, short-acting analgesic would represent an advance for this distressing and disabling type of cancer pain.

F. Bone Pain

Pain arising from pathology in bone is a problem frequently encountered by all who work with cancer patients.

Three of the most prevalent cancers of the Western world (lung cancer, breast cancer, and prostatic cancer), all give rise to secondary spread in the bones. The incidence of bone metastases in breast and prostatic cancer is variably estimated at up to 85% at autopsy (36). Patients with breast or prostatic cancer even after diagnosis of bone metastases will have a long median survival, 17 and 20 months, respectively, with a 20% survival to 5 years in prostatic cancer (37). Thus, the morbidity associated with bone metastases—pain, pathological fracture, immobility, and impaired quality of life—all present a huge problem.

Extensive research has led to a better understanding of why skeletal metastases occur where they do (predominantly the axial skeleton), and of osteoclast activation, the initiating event in establishing metastatic growth in bone. Technical developments now provide a greater ability to accurately assess the extent of bone metastatic disease by radionuclide scanning, computed tomography, and magnetic resonance imaging.

However, there is still a lack of knowledge on why some metastatic lesions in bone are painful, whereas others are not, and why pain may be experienced in one area for several days then reduce or disappear, only to become evident in another area. A better understanding has been gained of some of the cytokine mediators involved in the process of ostoclast activation, osteolysis, and osteoblastic activity, but the ability to suppress cytokine activity remains limited (38,39). Prostaglandins that are active in the mediation of osteoclastic bone destruction have been identified and are thought to be responsible for stimulating pain receptors. Some of the pain caused by bone metastases can be attributed to nerve compression and muscle spasm, but the picture remains incomplete.

Initial assessment of any pain in cancer patients must include a detailed history, with examination and documentation of pain site or sites, pain character, and known aggravating and relieving factors. (It is important to remember that pain caused by arthritis can be as common in the cancer population as in the normal population.)

In the majority of cases, metastatic bone disease reflects a noncurable condition, such that the focus of treatment is on symptom control and disease containment. Much pain caused by metastatic bone disease will respond to nonsteroidal anti-inflammatory medication combined with low-dose opioid therapy.

When simple analgesic medication is insufficient, the mainstay of treatment for painful bone metastases remains external beam radiotherapy. Radiotherapy, frequently given as a single fraction to painful areas corresponding to radiologically demonstrable active disease, results in a 70–80% response rate (40). Reduction in pain may occur at any time from within hours of treatment to up to 3 weeks after treatment, and may be partial or complete. Longer fractionated courses of radiotherapy may be given to long bones in painful areas representing incipient fracture (with or without orthopedic stabilization) or to areas of the vertebral column to limit radiation to the spinal cord. In a smaller number of cases, other approaches (e.g., extensive orthopedic surgical procedures to stabilize the spine, chemotherapy for widespread disease, or hemibody irradiation) may be appropriate and can produce pain relief. When treating patients with incurable disease and a limited life expectancy, the benefits of any treatment must be balanced against the morbidity incurred and the requirement for hospitalization.

Problems arise for the physician when radiotherapy and simple analgesic combinations no longer produce effective pain relief. Modification and intensification of analgesic medication may be helpful, but alternative approaches may be necessary. In the past decade two forms of systemic therapy—radioactive isotope treatment and bisphosphonate therapy—have gained widespread acceptance but limited use.

1. Radioactive Isotope Treatment

Isotope treatment for bone metastases using radioactive strontium was first reported in the early 1940s (41), but was not developed until the 1970s.

Strontium is a calcium analogue. The strontium 89 isotope is an (almost) pure beta particle emitter. After injection, strontium 89 is taken up and retained in areas of osteogenesis (such as occur in bone metastases) producing prolonged radiation of metastatic lesions with minimal radiation to surrounding healthy tissue. Response rates, measured in terms of pain relief, vary, but partial pain relief is reportedly achieved in 80% patients with breast or prostatic carcinoma (42).

Advantages of this treatment are the ability to synchronously treat widespread lesions, on an outpatient basis, with minimal morbidity. Myelosuppresion is rarely severe, previous external local radiotherapy does not preclude treatment, and retreatment is possible after a period of 3 months (43). There is evidence that the requirement for further radiotherapy is reduced or delayed, but there is no survival advantage (44). Disadvantages reside in the high cost of treatment and the incomplete nature of pain relief. These disadvantages highlight the way forward for further development. Trials on alternative isotopes, combining radiosensitizing chemotherapy with radiopharmaceuticals, and intensifying treatment with bone marrow support have been suggested as areas of further study.

2. Bisphosphonates

Radiotherapy reduces bone pain by directly treating metastatic lesions within the bone. It is now widely accepted that a prerequisite for metastatic tumor growth in bone is that of osteoclast activation. Reduction of osteoclast activation can be brought about by systemic treatment with chemicals known as bisphosphonates. Bisphosphonates are synthetic analogues of pyrophosphate, with a strong affinity for hydroxyapatite crystals. After having entered the bone, bisphosphonates are directly toxic to osteoclasts, disrupt osteoclast formation from precursor cells, and inhibit osteoclast activity, but the mechanisms by which these effects are produced remain incompletely understood (45,46). Owing to very poor bioavailability after ingestion when used for the treatment of existing bone pain, bisphosphonates are best administered intravenously. The most commonly used bisphosphonates are sodium clodronate and pamidronate disodium. After administration of a bolus infusion, the palliative response, in the form of reduction of bone pain, may commence within a few days. The precise regimen for treatment remains uncertain, as does the response rate. Some patients are able to maintain the benefits of bisphosphonate infusion by continuing daily oral medication, but others require repeated bolus infusions at 3- to 4-week intervals. Bisphosphonates have a low toxicity and are generally well tolerated. Bisphosphonates do not treat the underlying malignant process, but they can provide a prolonged reduction in morbidity by reducing bone pain and reducing susceptibility to fracture.

Given the increasing number of patients surviving with extensive metastatic disease, the challenge to develop and improve our treatments for the prevention and reduction of bone pain is formidable. Research continues to find new and more effective radiopharmaceuticals, improved and more potent bisphosphonates, and to elucidate the role of other agents known to be active in bone disease (e.g., calcitonin). Perhaps the greatest challenge now lies in improving our understanding of why malignant disease metastasizes and grows in bone, and in discovering the etiology of the bone pain itself.

VI. SUMMARY

Many advances have been made in the treatment of cancer pain in both the developed and developing world. Increasing sophistication in the treatment of the cancers themselves must be matched by increased understanding and treatment of the pain and morbidity arising from these diseases.

Clinical care of patients with malignant pain could be greatly improved by the development of pharmacological agents:

1. For the treatment of neuropathic pain
2. That are powerful μ-agonists without the adverse effects of morphine, but with the same flexibility in modes of delivery
3. That are powerful analgesics with a very rapid onset of action, working as quickly as sublingual nitrates in angina
4. That are more effective in the treatment of bone pain, arising perhaps from current work to improve our understanding of the pathophysiology of this syndrome

REFERENCES

1. Stjernsward J. Palliative medicine–a global perspective. In: Doyle D, Hanks GWC, Macdonald N, eds. Oxford Textbook of Palliative Medicine. 2nd ed. London: Oxford University Press, 1997:805–816.
2. Foley KM. The treatment of cancer pain. N Engl J Med 1985; 313:84–94.
3. World Health Organization. Cancer pain relief. Geneva: World Health Organization, 1986.
4. Ventafridda V, Caraceni A, Gamba A. Field-testing of the WHO guidelines for cancer pain relief: summary report of demonstration projects. In: Bonica J, Foley KM, Ventafridda V, Callaway MV, eds. Second International Congress on Cancer Pain. New York: Raven, 1990:451–464.
5. Zech DFL, Grond S, Lynch J, Hertel D, Lehmann KA. Validation of WHO guidelines for cancer pain relief: a 10 year prospective study. Pain 1995; 68:65–76.
6. United Nations International Narcotics Control Board. Demand for and Supply of Opiates for Medical and Scientific Needs. New York: United Nations, 1989.
7. World Health Organization. National cancer control programmes. Policies and managerial guidelines. Geneva; World Health Organization, 1995.
8. World Health Organization. Cancer control programme. Introducing the national cancer control programmes. Cancer Care 1994; 1:1–5.
9. de Stoutz MD, Bruera E, Suarez–Almazor M. Opioid rotation for toxicity reduction in terminal care patients. J Pain Sympt Manage 1995; 10:5:378–384.
10. Payne R. Factors influencing quality of life in cancer patients: the role of transdermal fentanyl in the management of pain. Semin Oncol 1998; 25(3 suppl 7):47–53.
11. Ahmedzai S, Brooks D. Transdermal fentanyl versus sustained-release oral morphine in cancer pain: preference, efficacy, and quality of life. J Pain Sympt Manage 1997; 14:139–146.
12. Twycross R, Wilcock A, Thorp S, eds. Analgesics. In: Palliative Care Formulary. Radcliffe Medical Press, 1998:115–119.
13. Sloan PA, Moulin DE, Hays H. A clinical evaluation of transdermal therapeutic system fentanyl for the treatment of cancer pain. J Pain Sympt Manage 1998; 16:102–111.
14. Farrar JT, Clearly J, Rauck R, Busch M, Nordbock E. Oral transmucosal fentanyl citrate: randomised, double-blinded, placebo-controlled trial for treatment of breakthrough pain in cancer patients. J Natl Cancer Inst 1998; 900:611–616.
15. Saunders CM. The nature and nurture of pain control. In: The Management of Terminal Illness. London: Edward Arnold, 1967.
16. Kearney MK. Experience in a hospice with patients suffering cancer pain. In: Doyle D, ed. Opioids and the Treatment of Cancer Pain. Royal Society of Medicine Services, 1990:69–74.
17. Glynn C. An approach to the management of the patient with deafferentation pain. Palliat Med 1989; 3:13–21.
18. Bowsher D. Pathways and mechanism. In: Swerdlow M, Charlton JE, eds. Relief of Intractable Pain. 4th ed. Philadelphia: Lea & Febiger, 1989: 1484–1514.
19. Wall PD, Melzack R, eds. Textbook of Pain. 2nd ed. Edinburgh: Churchill Livingstone, 1989.
20. Martin LA, Hagen NA. Neuropathic pain in cancer patients: mechanisms, syndromes, and clinical controversies. J Pain Sympt Manage 1997; 14:99–117.
21. Twycross R, Fairfield S. Pain in far-advanced cancer. Pain 1982; 14:303–310.

22. McQuay HJ, Dickenson AH. Implications of nervous system plasticity for pain management. Anaesthesia 1990; 45:101–102.
23. Patt RB. Cancer pain syndromes. In: Patt RB, ed. Cancer Pain. Philadelphia: Lippincott, 1993.
24. Arner S, Meyerson BA. Lack of analgesic effect of opioids on neuropathic and idiopathic forms of pain. Pain 1988; 33:11–23.
25. Jadad AR, Carroll D, Glynn CJ, Moore RA, McQuay HJ. Morphine responsiveness of chronic pain: double blind randomised crossover study with patient-controlled analgesia. Lancet 1992; 339:1367–1371.
26. Portenoy RK, Foley KM, Inturrisi CE. The nature of opioid responsiveness and its implications for neuropathic pain: new hypotheses derived from studies of opioid infusions. Pain 1990; 43:273–286.
27. Dellemijn PL, Verbeist HB, Van Vliet JJ, Roos PJ, Vecht CJ. Medical theory of malignant nerve pain. A randomised double-blind exploratory trial with naproxen versus slow-release morphine. Eur J Cancer 1994; 30:1244–1250.
28. Ripamonti C, Zecca E, Bruera E. An update on the clinical use of methadone for cancer pain. Pain 1997; 70:109–115.
29. Meller ST, Ketamine: relief from chronic pain through actions at the NMDA receptor? Pain 1996; 68:435–436.
30. Luczak J, Dickenson AH, Aruga, Kotlinska–Lemieszek A. The role of ketamine an NMDA receptor antagonist in the management of pain. Prog Palliat Care 1995; 3:127–134.
31. Twycross R, Wilcock A, Thorp S, eds. Drugs used in anesthesia. In: Palliative Care Formulary. Radcliffe Medical Press, 1998:175–181.
32. Twycross R. Miscellaneous drugs. In: Twycross R. Pain Relief in Advanced Cancer. Edinburgh: Churchill Livingstone, 1994:455–486.
33. Rosner H. Gabapentin adjunctive therapy in neuropathic pain states. Clin J Pain 1996; 12:56–58.
34. Boas RA, Cousins MJ. Diagnostic neural blockade. In: Cousins MJ, Bridenbaugh PO, eds. Neural Blockade in Clinical Anaesthesia and Management of pain. 2nd ed. Philadelphia: Lippincott, 1988: 885–898.
35. McQuay HJ, Jadad AR. Incident pain. Cancer Surv 1994; 21:17–2.
36. Galasko CSB. The anatomy and pathways of skeletal metastases. In: Weiss L, Gilbert AH, eds. Bone Metastasis. Boston: GK Hall, 1981:49–63.
37. Rubens RD. The nature of metastatic bone disease. In: Rubens RD, Fogelman I, eds. Bone Metastases: Diagnosis and Treatment. New York: Springer-Verlag, 1991:1–9.
38. Garrett IR. Bone destruction in cancer. Semin Oncol 1993; 20(suppl 2):4.
39. Diel IJ, Solomayer E–F. Bisphosphonates in the anti-osteolytic therapy of metastatic bone cancer. Zentralbl Gynakol 1996; 118:10.
40. Needham PR, Hoskin PJ. Radiotherapy for painful bone metastases. Palliat Med 1994; 8:95–104.
41. Pecher C. Preliminary report on the use of radioactive strontium in the treatment of metastatic bone cancer. Univ Calif Pub Pharmacol 1942; 11:117–139.
42. Robinson RG, Preston DF, Schiefelbein M, Baxter KG. Strontium 89 therapy for the palliation of pain due to osseous metastases. JAMA 1995; 274:420–424.
43. McEwan AJB, Porter AT, Venner PM, Amyotte G. An evaluation of the safety and efficacy of treatment with strontium-89 in patients who have previously received wide field radiotherapy. Antibody Immunoconj Radiopharm 1990; 3:91–98.
44. Bolger JJ, Dearnley DP, Kirk D, Lewington VJ, Mason MD, Quilty PM, Reed NSE, Russell JM, Yardley J. Strontium-89 (Metastron) versus external beam radiotherapy in patients with painful bone metastases secondary to prostatic cancer: preliminary report of a multi centre trial. Semin Oncol 1993; 20(suppl 2):32–33.
45. Boonenkamp MP, Van der Wee-Pals LJA. Two modes of action of bisphosphonates on osteolytic resorption of mineralised bone matrix. Bone Miner 1986; 1:27–39.
46. Coleman RE, Purohit OP. Osteoclast inhibition for the treatment of bone metastases. Cancer Treat Rev 1993; 19:79–103.

19
Inflammatory Joint Disease and Pain

Sarah Greer and Brian L. Hazleman
Addenbrooke's Hospital, Cambridge, England

I. INTRODUCTION

It is important to remember that drug treatment is just one component in the total management of arthritis patients. Management must also include advice about rest and exercises, splintage, the provision of appliances designed to reduce dependence on others, and advice about employment. However, it is now clear that in well-organized studies using defined populations, usually patients with early disease, major differences can be achieved with several different therapies.

Drug regimens must be tailored to the need of the individual patient. Rheumatoid arthritis (RA) is sometimes badly treated. Patients are kept on anti-inflammatory drugs alone for long periods in the face of obvious deterioration, or corticosteroids are given early, with considerable immediate effect at the cost of complications later on. The inflammatory process can usually be suppressed with symptomatic improvement, better function, less stiffness, and considerable pain relief, but the disease cannot be cured. Hence, adequate patient education is required from the outset, stressing the importance of controlling the disease to help give the patient realistic expectations. The aims of the treatment are to reduce, inflammation, maintain function, and prevent deformities. Adequate suppression of chronic inflammation allows secondary manifestations, such as anemia to revert to normal.

Because these diseases are generally incurable and difficult to manage, there is a pressing need for novel approaches to their treatment.

II. PATHOGENESIS OF RHEUMATOID ARTHRITIS

Our understanding of the pathogenesis of rheumatoid arthritis has improved markedly in recent years. There are two main hypotheses, the macrophage–mesenchymal and the T cell, although the true cause remains elusive.

Macrophage and fibroblast products are predominant in the rheumatoid joint, in contrast to the paucity of T-cell products. There is little doubt to their importance in the final destructive phase of the disease. A rational therapeutic approach has been to inhibit proinflammatory macrophages producing cytokines, such as tumor necrosis factor-α (TNF-α) and interleukin (IL)1_{β}, and mesenchymal enzymes, such as metalloproteases (MMP). However it can be argued that treatments against cytokines, although beneficial are only short-lasting, as they treat only the final pathway of the inflammatory cascade, leaving the underlying immune process that drives the disease untouched.

The hypotheses are not mutually exclusive. For example, a T-cell–specific process might initiate RA and then become gradually less important as cytokine networks and autonomous synoviocytes develop. Continued low-level T-cell activation could help maintain the cytokine network.

III. CYCLOOXYGENASE RESEARCH

One of the targets for the activity of nonsteroidal anti-inflammatory drugs (NSAIDs) is cyclooxygenase, the enzyme responsible for forming prostaglandins (PGs) from arachidonic acid (1). With the discovery that there are two isoforms of cyclooxygenase the ultimate goal of preventive therapeutic efficacy combined with good tolerability seems to be within reach (2).

The constitutive isoform, cyclooxygenase-1 (COX-1), produces prostaglandins, such as PGE_2 and PGI_2, that are important in many physiological processes, notably in the kidney and stomach. Cyclooxygenase-2 (COX-2) activity was initially discovered in 1989. Undetectable in most tissues, COX-2 is expressed in response to stimuli, such as inflammatory cytokines or growth factors. Inducible expression of COX-2 occurs in various cell types, including macrophages and synoviocytes. Also COX-2 expression is up-regulated in response to a variety of physiological stimuli, including in the kidney in response to sodium and water deprivation, in the spinal cord following painful stimuli, in the ovary during ovulation, and in bone in response to parathyroid hormone.

The COX-1 isoform is constitutively expressed in a wider variety of tissues than COX-2 and is thought to perform "housekeeping" functions by producing prostaglandins that regulate normal cell activity (for example, gastric cytoprotection, platelet aggregation, and renal sodium and water balance). In most tissues, COX-1 levels are only slightly altered by physiological stimuli. However, COX-1 appears to be involved only in generating the prostanoid products that exert cytoprotective effects in the gastric mucosa, as well as those involved in platelet function. The clear demonstration that COX-1, but not COX-2, is expressed in the gastric mucosa and platelets implies that specific COX-2 inhibitors will not provoke the gastrointestinal bleeding and other side effects associated with current nonsteroidal anti-inflammatory drugs.

However, despite the degree to which they appear to affect COX-2, all current NSAIDs are associated with gastrointestinal bleeding. It appears that only specific (not selective) inhibition of COX-2, with no action on COX-1 function, will lead to clinical benefit with no risk of COX-1-related side effects. This is borne out by studies of celecoxib (a highly specific COX-2 inhibitor). When compared with meloxicam (a selective COX-2 inhibitor), gastrointestinal and renal injury did not occur with celecoxib (3). A pilot safety study in 128 healthy subjects demonstrated that no person receiving placebo or celecoxib, 100 or 200 mg twice daily for 7 days, developed endoscopically demonstrable gastric or duodenal ulcers, whereas 6 patients receiving naproxen, 500 mg twice daily, developed gastric ulcers (4).

Cyclooxygenase-2 inhibition by NSAIDs also appears to be an important mechanism of cancer chemoprevention. Inflammation of gastrointestinal organs is often associated with an increased risk of cancer, and COX-2 is an integral part of the inflammatory process. Evidence also exists that regular consumption of aspirin may reduce the risk of gastric and esophageal cancers (5).

IV. GENE THERAPY

In its broadest sense, gene therapy is the transfer to patients of a gene, or genes, for therapeutic purposes. Gene transfer provides the opportunity to deliver protein products, as well as therapeutic species of nucleic acids, such as antisense RNA, much more efficiently than traditional methods of drug therapy. In addition, sustained, in situ production of the gene products would eliminate the need for frequent administration. Gene therapy also has the ability to produce high, sustained concentrations of therapeutic macromolecules within a defined anatomical location.

Genes may be introduced into cells in situ; this is known as in vivo gene therapy. Or cells, may be removed from the patient, genetically modified, and then returned to the same individual; this is known as ex vivo gene therapy.

Vectors are usually used that facilitate the uptake and expression of genes by cells. Because viruses transfer genes to cells so efficiently, many vectors are derived from viruses that have been genetically disabled to prevent pathology without compromising infectivity. Vectors based on retroviruses, adenoviruses, and adenoassociated viruses are currently being used in human gene therapy trials. Also nonviral vectors, such as liposomes, are also being evaluated, but remain much less efficient than vectors based on viruses.

For the treatment of chronic conditions there is a need for vectors to either give long-term gene expression or to lend themselves to frequent readministration. Integrating viruses, such as retrovirus and adenoassociated virus, become established within the chromosomes of the host cells and provide the best prospects for long-term gene expression.

Data from preclinical studies in a variety of animal models permit guarded optimism about the future of gene therapy in autoimmune disorders. Most attention has been directed toward the treatment of rheumatoid arthritis; for instance an antiarthritic effect has been noted after transfer of genes encoding IL-1Ra to the synovium (6).

The first human trial of gene therapy for arthritis began in July 1996 at the University of Pittsburgh Medical Center. The investigation follows an ex vivo protocol in which a human IL-1Ra cDNA is transferred to the metacarpalphalangeal joints of postmenopausal women with rheumatoid arthritis. In a double-blind fashion, two joints received the IL-1Ra transgenes and two control joints did not. Gene transfer was performed 1 week before the joints were surgically removed and replaced with prostheses. Because this is the first application of gene therapy to a nonlethal disease, the overriding priority has been to establish that gene transfer is safe and feasible (7).

V. USE OF STEROIDS IN EARLY INFLAMMATION

Preservation of the articular surface in rheumatoid arthritis is a therapeutic priority, but success has been elusive. A fixed dose of 7.5 mg of prednisolone for 2 years will significantly reduce progression of disease, but on prednisolone withdrawal there is significant deterioration despite patients continuing on antirheumatoid treatment (8).

There is now convincing evidence from several studies that, in early disease, low-dose oral or parental corticosteroids successfully suppress disease activity until other therapy can take effect. However, no study has been able to induce lasting remission convincingly in the majority of patients. On the contrary, even with high-dose prednisolone, a sizeable proportion of patients show only a partial response.

VI. BIOLOGICAL AGENTS FOR THE TREATMENT OF INFLAMMATORY DISEASE

Since the development of techniques for monoclonal antibody (MAb) production have improved, the diversity and numbers of potential antibodies for therapy have grown almost out of all proportion. Autoimmune diseases, transplantation, and cancer treatments have proved to be natural targets for experimentation with MAbs. Rheumatoid arthritis is no exception, since the mid-1980s several different antibodies have been tested in the clinical setting, targeting cytokine production, adhesion molecules, and T cells. Success has been disappointing, with clinical benefits often lasting only a few months, often coupled with long-term lymphopenia, the implications of which are as yet uncertain. The targets for monoclonal antibody therapy in RA are the cells and cytokines (e.g., $CD4^+$ T cells and TNF-α) involved in the inflammatory process that can be so debilitating and painful in these patients.

The specificity of MAbs allows them to bind to any potential target with high affinity, this may lead to depletion of the target antigen or interference of its normal function by a "blocking" mechanism. Efficacy of the treatments are measured by the number of swollen and tender joints, as well a by systemic inflammatory markers such as C-reactive protein (CRP) in the same way as all RA drug therapies.

Although there is general agreement that the initial disease is T-cell–driven, the full pathogenesis of RA has not been determined. It is thought that the recognition of a joint antigen by the T cells results in their activation and proliferation, leading to up-regulation of the inflammatory cytokines IL-1, IL-6, and TNF-α. How the disease is maintained, however, is less clear. It may be that it remains T-cell–driven (9) and several therapeutic strategies have been directed toward regulation of these "rogue" T cells, such as the use of cyclosporine. There are some, however, who believe the importance of T cells diminishes in the more chronic disease, that inflammation and joint destruction do not necessarily correlate with each other, and that each must be addressed with a separate treatment strategy (10).

The first MAbs used in clinical trials were murine. These were inevitably immunogenic, causing a human antimouse antibody (HAMA) response restricting multiple treatments owing to the potential of anaphylaxis. Most antibodies now in use are either chimeric or humanized. Chimeric antibodies retain the mouse variable region, but this is then fused to a human constant region. Humanized antibodies go one step forward with retaining only the mouse complementary-determining regions, the rest of the antibody being human. Chimeric and humanized antibodies are less immunogenic and more suitable for multiple treatments or long-term therapy.

The first humanized antibody to be used in clinical trials was Campath-1H, an antibody directed against the CD52 antigen found on the cell surface of most lymphocytes, with a higher concentration found on B and T lymphocytes (11). Significantly, it is not found on the $CD34^+$ pluripotent stem cells, retaining the ability to regenerate depleted cell types.

The rationale behind the Campath-1H was to deplete the T cells that were driving the rheumatoid arthritis and sustaining the joint inflammation. The new T cells regenerated would not show the same autoimmune characteristics. Results from these studies show improvement in the number of tender and swollen joints, but made no impact on erythrocyte sedimentation rate (ESR) or CRP measurements (12). There was significant symptomatic relief in the majority of patients treated, but unfortunately, this was short-lived. The degree of symptom control did not correlate with the peripheral T-cell count: the patients remained profoundly lymphopenic long after their symptoms progressed, even up to 6 years posttreatment (unpublished). There is evidence that even though these patients are exhibiting a peripheral lymphopenia long-term, there is still a significant accumulation of T cells in the joint, indicating either a lack of penetration or efficacy of Campath-1H into the synovial tissue (13).

More disease-specific MAbs have also been studied, including MAbs against the CD4 antigen, found on so-called helper T lymphocytes, and monocytes. It is thought that $CD4^+$ T lymphocytes are the main subtype of T cell involved in the pathogenesis of rheumatoid arthritis, and the T cells found in the synovium are predominantly of this type (14).

Several groups have reported trials into the depleting CD4 MAb cM-T412. Similar to the Campath-1H, there was an initial improvement in swollen and tender joint counts, but the benefit rarely lasted more than 3 months (15). Results were variable, depending on the study type: placebo-controlled trials showing less benefit than open studies. In all cases, CD4 counts fell rapidly, within the first few hours, and although there was some initial improvement, there is evidence of a prolonged lymphopenia for a considerable time later, up to 5 years posttreatment (16). Similar to Campath-1H, benefit from treatment with cM-T412 did not correlate with peripheral $CD4^+$ T-cell count. It was, however, shown to penetrate the synovium, with the clinical improvement correlating with the percentage of coated synovial lymphocytes (17).

Treatment with higher doses of both Campath-1H and cM-T412 is restricted because of the peripheral lymphopenia. Recent follow-up reports suggest, however, that the peripheral lymphopenia is not associated with an increase in morbidity or mortality. A 5-year follow-up study of 33 patients treated with cM-T412 shows no unexpected infection or malignancies (16). This is mirrored in our own follow-up of patients up to 7 years after Campath-1H treatment (unpublished). It is possible that in the future these therapies may be revisited in higher doses, but for now they remain out of favor in the treatment of RA.

In animal models, tolerance can be affected in the absence of lymphocyte depletion (18). Two nondepleting CD4 MAbs are being studied, the humanized antibody 4162W94 (Glaxo Wellcome), and EDEC-CE9, a primatized antibody. Preliminary results are encouraging, those treated with 4162W94 show evidence of the antibody penetrating the synovial tissue and only a transient decrease in $CD4^+$ cell counts. Placebo-controlled trials with EDEC-CE9 have demonstrated significant improvement in tender and swollen joint counts (19). Further studies are underway.

Studies have also examined MAbs to CD7 and CD5 (20). There was no clinical improvement in patients treated with CD7 (which was later shown to be nonpathogenic in RA). Antibodies against CD5 gave encouraging results with initial open-labeled studies, but this was not repeated in a later placebo-controlled study.

The other main targets for MAb therapy are the cytokines involved in the inflammatory response. In particular, cytokines known to be up-regulated in RA are IL-6, IL-1, and TNF-α. Plasma levels of IL-6 correlate with disease activity, antibodies against IL-6 led to not only a reduction in disease activity, but also in inflammatory markers such as CRP levels. This is in contrast to T-cell–directed therapies that led to symptomatic control, but little measurable improvement in ESR or CRP. Symptomatic relief, however, similar to the T-cell therapies, was short-lived, averaging 2 months (21).

Interleukin-2 receptor (CD25) is up-regulated in activated T cells. Stimulation by the cytokine IL-2 leads to proliferation and stimulation of T cells. It is this pathway that is interrupted by cyclosporine. An early open-labeled study on three RA patients with Campath-6 (rat anti-CD25) showed a dramatic, but short-term, response lasting up to 2 months in two patients and just 1 month in one patient (22). The immunogenicity of the antibody excluded retreatment.

Antibodies against TNF-α are better studied, with significant responses seen in treated groups in double-blind studies. Symptomatic improvement was seen within 24 h of treatment, and a reduction in inflammatory markers was also demonstrated. Benefits lasted for up to 3 months, with subsequent treatments with TNF-α giving shorter response times.

The future for monoclonal antibody therapy in RA is uncertain. Certainly, the early trials with nondepleting CD4 antibodies and anti-TNF-α are encouraging but, until we have the results of larger studies, it is hard to predict their usefulness in routine treatment for RA. The cost of producing the antibodies is high, and the long-term effects of immune manipulation are only now beginning to be studied. However, antibody therapy may find its niche in treating acute disease flares, perhaps then moving on to more conventional disease-modifying drugs.

The cost implications may be dampened if a single treatment with a monoclonal antibody gives long-term benefit, for this it is possible that we need to look at a combination of antibody therapies (e.g., anti-CD4 and anti-TNF-α) (23).

VII. IMMUNOSUPPRESSIVE DRUGS

Immunosuppressive drugs are reserved for the treatment of severe RA and its complications, such as vasculitis, and for use in patients who have not responded to standard disease-modifying antirheumatic drug (DMARD) therapy. Azathioprine and cyclophosphamide are the drugs most commonly used.

The purine analogue azathioprine is effective and may be safely combined with parenteral gold. Bone marrow toxicity and the induction of lymphoma are rare, whereas nausea and hepatotoxicity are more common. Cyclophosphamide is often given if vasculitis is present, but it can cause bladder toxicity and permanent gonadal failure in men and women.

VIII. NEWER DRUGS IN RA TREATMENT: CYCLOSPORINE

Cyclosporine (Sandimmune) is a selective immunosuppressant that has recently been licensed for use in severe RA and should be used where other DMARDs are ineffective or inappropriate. Cyclosporine may cause a decrease in renal function or hypertension. Both effects are easily monitored.

IX. PROGNOSIS

The course of RA is variable, and it is often not possible to predict at onset those patients who will develop severe disease. In general, 25% remain fit for all normal activities, 40% have moderate impairment of function, 25% are quite badly disabled, and 10% become wheelchair patients.

A poor prognosis is indicated by a number of factors, as follows:

Extraarticular manifestations
Insiduous polyarticular onset
High titer of rheumatoid factor
Functional disability at 1 year
Presence of HLA-DR4
Early appearance of erosions on x-ray films

Patients who have remissions generally do better than those with continuous disease, and explosive onset is often associated with a good outcome.

REFERENCES

1. Vane JR. Inhibition of prostaglandin synthesis as a mechanism of action for the aspirin-like drugs. Nature 1971; 231:232–235.
2. Furst DE. Meloxicam: selective COX 2 inhibition in clinical practice. Semin Arthritis Rheum 1997; 26:21.7.
3. Maziasz T, Seibert K, Khan N, Paulson S, Isakson P. Preclinical pharmacology of celecoxib and demonstration of superior GI safety compared with NSAIDs in dogs. Arthritis Rheum 1997; 40(suppl):983a.
4. Lanza FL, Callison DA, Hubbard RC, Shawn SV, Talwalker S, Geis GS. A pilot endoscopic study

of the gastroduodenal effects of SC-58635, a COX-2 selective inhibitor. Arthritis Rheum 1997; 40(suppl):373a.
5. Farrow DC, Vaughan TL, Hansten PD, Stanford JL, Rische HA, Gammon MD. Use of aspirin and other non-steroidal anti-inflammatory drugs and risk of oesophageal and gastric cancer. Cancer Epidemiol Biomarkers Prev 1998; 7:97–102.
6. Bakker AC, Joosten LAB, Arntz OJ, Helsen MMA, Bendele AM, Van de Loo FAJ, van den Berg WB. Prevention of murine collagen-induced arthritis in the knee and ipsilateral paw by local expression of human interleukin-1 receptor antagonist protein in the knee. Arthritis Rheum 1997; 40:893–900.
7. Evans CH, Robbins PD, Ghivizzani SD, Herndon JH, Kang R, Bahnson AB. Clinical trial to assess the safety, feasibility, and efficacy of transferring a potentially anti-arthritic cytokine gene to human joints with rheumatoid arthritis. Hum Gene Ther 1996; 7:1261–1280.
8. Hickling P, Jacoby RK, Kirwan JR. Joint destruction after glucocorticoids are withdrawn in early rheumatoid arthritis. Br J Radiol 1998; 37:930–936.
9. Panayi GS. The immunopathogenesis of rheumatoid arthritis. Br J Rheumatol 1993; 32(suppl 1):4–14.
10. Zvaifler NJ, Firestein GS. Pannus and pannocytes. Arthritis Rheum 1994; 37:783–789.
11. Hale G, Xia MQ, Tighe HP, Dyer MJS, Waldmann H. The CAMPATH-1H antigen (CDw52). Tissue Antigens 1990; 35:118–127.
12. Isaacs JD, Watts RA, Hazleman BL, Hale G, Keogan MT, Cobbold SP, Waldman H. Humanised monoclonal antibody therapy for rheumatoid arthritis. Lancet 1992; 340:748–752.
13. Ruderman EM, Weinblatt ME, Thurmond LM, Pinkus GS, Gravallese EM. Synovial tişsue response to treatment with Campath-1H. Arthritis Rheum 1995; 38:254–258.
14. Poulter LW, Duke O, Panayi GS, Hobbs S, Raftery MJ, Janossy G. Activated T lymphocytes in the synovial membrane in rheumatoid arthritis and other arthropathies. Scand Immunol 1985; 22:683–690.
15. Choy EHS. Clinical pharmacology and therapeutic potential of monoclonal antibody treatment in rheumatoid arthritis. Drugs Aging 1998; 12:139–148.
16. Moreland LW, Bucy RP, Jackson B, James T, Koopman WJ. Long term (5 years) follow-up of rheumatoid arthritis patients treated with a depleting anti-CD4 monoclonal antibody, cM-T412 [abstr]. Arthritis Rheum 1996; 39(suppl):S244.
17. Choy EHS, Pitzalis C, Cauli A, Bijl JA, Schantz A, Woody J, Kingsley GH, Panayi GS. Percentage of anti-CD4 monoclonal antibody-coated lymphocytes in the rheumatoid joint is associated with clinical improvement. Implications for the development of immunotherapeutic dosing regimens. Arthritis Rheum 1996; 39:52–56.
18. Panayi GS, Choy EHS, Connolly DJA, Regan T, Manna VK, Rapson N, Kingsley GH, Johnston, JM. T cell hypothesis in rheumatoid arthritis (RA) tested by humanised non-depleting anti-CD4 monoclonal antibody (mAb): I. Suppression of disease activity and acute phase response [abstr]. Arthritis Rheum 1996; 39(suppl):S244.
19. Levy R, Weisman M, Wiesenhutter C, Yocum D, Schnitzer T, Goldman A, Schiff M, Breedveld F, MacDonald B. Results of a placebo controlled, multicenter trial using a primatized, non-depleting, anti-CD4 monoclonal antibody in the treatment of rheumatoid arthritis [abstr]. Arthritis Rheum 1996; 39(suppl):S122.
20. Choy EHS, Kingsley GH, Panayi GS. Monoclonal antibody therapy in rheumatoid arthritis. Br J Rheumatol 1990; 37:484–490.
21. Wendling D, Radacot E, Wijdeenes J. Treatment of severe rheumatoid arthritis by anti-interleukin 6 monoclonal antibody. J Rheumatol 1992; 19:22–25.
22. Kyle V, Coughlan RJ, Tighe H, Waldmann H, Hazleman BL. Beneficial effect of monoclonal antibody to interleukin 2 receptor on activated T cells in rheumatoid arthritis. Ann Rheum Dis 1989; 48:428–429.
23. Moreland LW, Heck LW, Koopman WJ. Biologic agents for treating rheumatoid arthritis concepts and progress. Arthritis Rheum 1997; 40:397–409.

20

Chronic Nonmalignant Visceral Pain Syndromes of the Abdomen, Pelvis, and Bladder and Chronic Urogenital and Rectal Pain

Ursula Wesselmann
Johns Hopkins University School of Medicine, Baltimore, Maryland, U.S.A.

I. INTRODUCTION

This chapter will discuss chronic, nonmalignant pain syndromes of the abdomen, pelvis, and bladder and pain syndromes of the urogenital floor. Pain syndromes of the abdomen, pelvis, and bladder belong to the category of visceral pain. The first symptoms of visceral disease are usually discomfort and pain. These are the symptoms that prompt most patients with visceral disease to seek medical care. In clinical practice much emphasis has been placed on finding a specific etiology and specific pathological markers for visceral disease. Surprisingly, however, little attention has been paid to the clinical management of pain in visceral disease. Several reasons might account for this. Patients have difficulty in being able to describe and localize visceral pain, and physicians and other health care providers have difficulty in being able to examine and measure (quantify) visceral pain. Furthermore, the differential diagnosis of visceral disease is usually quite complex because the symptoms are often diffuse and nonspecific. Most efforts of health care personnel are spent on identifying the underlying etiology because this is an area that they have been trained in during their medical education. While many guidelines have been published on diagnosing and treating nonmalignant and malignant visceral disease, no specific guidelines yet exist on the management of visceral pain, and physicians and other health care providers are left without any concepts on the approach to the patient with visceral disease who presents with pain.

Chronic urogenital and rectal pain syndromes are common, well-described, but poorly understood focal pain syndromes that can significantly impair the quality of life of the patient. Patients with these pain syndromes often suffer for many years, have seen numerous physicians in numerous subspecialties, and are frustrated and embarrassed. They are usually evaluated and treated by urologists, gynecologists, gastroenterologists, and internists. As in patients with visceral chronic pain syndromes, the focus is frequently on finding and treating the underlying etiology of the chronic pain syndrome, and these patients often undergo many diagnostic tests and procedures. However, in many cases the examination and workup remain unrevealing, and no specific cause of the pain can be identified. Although these patients are often depressed, rarely are these pain syndromes the only manifestation of a psychiatric disease. In these cases it is important to recognize that the patient is suffering from a chronic urogenital or rectal pain syndrome and to direct treatment strategies toward symptomatic pain management.

Despite the challenge inherent in the management of chronic visceral and urogenital or rectal pain, some pain relief can be offered to almost all patients (1–3). Effective treatment modalities are available to lessen the effect of pain and offer reasonable expectations of an improved functional status.

II. CHRONIC NONMALIGNANT VISCERAL PAIN SYNDROMES OF THE ABDOMEN, PELVIS, AND BLADDER

A. Neurobiology of Visceral Pain

The visceral structures that may give rise to pain in the abdomen, pelvis, or bladder belong to the gastrointestinal and genitourinary system and the associated blood vessels and lymphatic structures. Viscera in the abdominal and pelvic cavity receive afferent innervation by way of the autonomic nerve trunks. The visceral afferents that travel in the sympathetic nerve trunk have cell bodies in the thoracolumbar distribution, and those that travel with the parasympathetic fibers have cell bodies in the sacral dorsal ganglia. Both visceral sensory pathways are involved in visceral sensations and reflexes (Figs. 1 and 2). These neural structures comprise the first of numerous relays of sensory neurons that transmit painful sensations from the abdominal–pelvic cavity to the brain. Ascending visceral spinal pathways include the dorsal columns and the spinothalamic and spinoreticular tracts (4). Little is known about the destination of the dorsal column pathways for visceral pain. Recent research indicates that this pathway includes neurons in the nucleus gracilis and the ventral posterolateral nucleus of the thalamus (5).

The existence of visceral nociceptors has been debated for a long time. This is partially due to the difficulty of defining and applying physiologically relevant noxious stimuli to the viscera. Research in animal models of visceral pain has shown that several kinds of sensory receptors exist in most internal organs and that different pain states are mediated by different neurophysiological mechanisms (6). Acute, brief visceral pain, such as pain during acute colic, seems to be triggered initially by the activation of high-threshold visceral afferents and by the high-frequency bursts that these stimuli evoke in intensity-coding afferent fibers, which are afferents with a range of responsiveness in the innocuous and noxious ranges. However, more prolonged forms of visceral stimulation, including those leading to hypoxia and inflammation of the tissue, result in sensitization of high-threshold receptors and bringing into play previously unresponsive afferent fibers (silent nociceptors—see later discussion). This increased afferent activity enhances the excitability of central neurons and it is hypothesized that this leads to the development of persistent pain states. In addition, a special class of C-fiber nociceptors, mechanoinsensitive or "silent" nociceptors, has been found in nearly all tissues. They were first described in an animal model of experimental arthritis (7) and, subsequently, in animal models of visceral pain (8). Silent afferents are activated only in the presence of tissue damage or inflammation. Following release of injury products, these previously silent receptors are activated by a wide range of thermal and mechanical stimuli and may also have a background discharge.

Persistent pain of visceral origin is a much greater clinical problem than that from skin, but the overwhelming focus of experimental work on pain mechanisms relates to cutaneous sensation. Until relatively recently, it was often assumed that concepts derived from cutaneous studies could be transferred to the visceral domain. However, there are several reasons to believe that the neural mechanisms involved in pain and hyperalgesia of the skin are different from the mechanisms involved in painful sensations from the viscera (9,10).

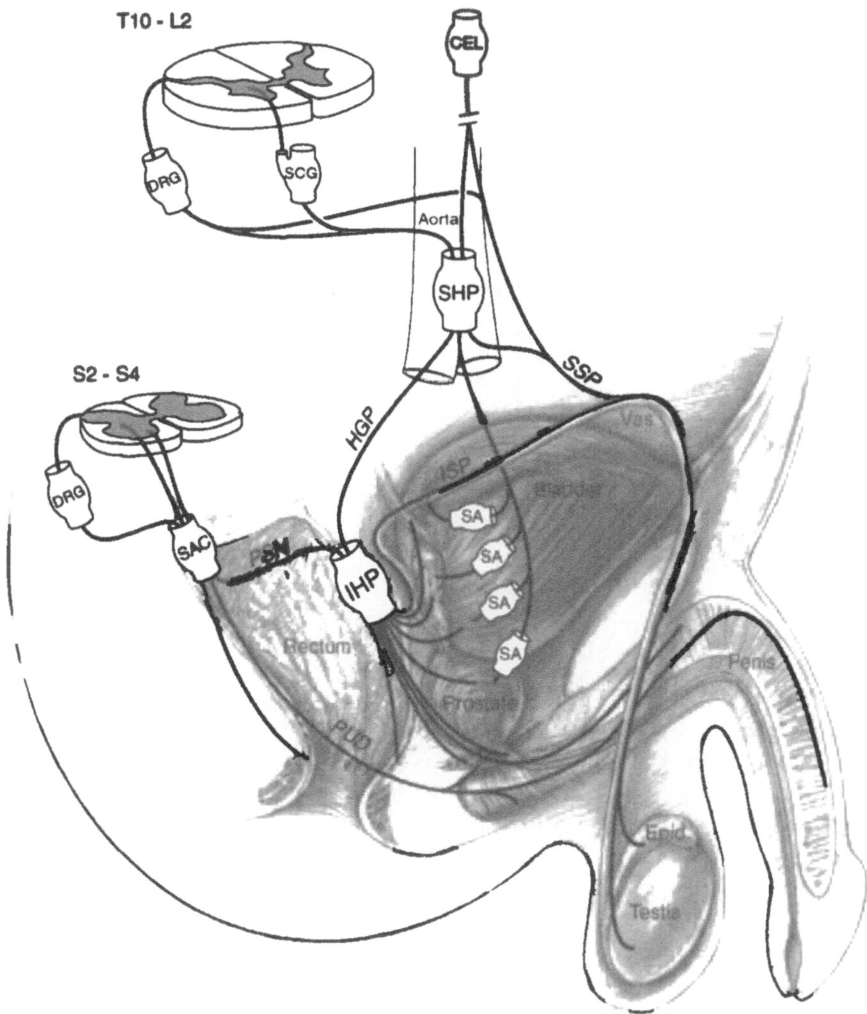

Figure 1 Schematic drawing showing the innervation of the urogenital and rectal area in males: Although this diagram attempts to show the innervation in humans, much of the anatomical information is derived from animal data. CEL, celiac plexus; DRG, dorsal root ganglion; HGP, hypogastric plexus; IHP, inferior hypogastric plexus; ISP, inferior spermatic plexus; PSN, pelvic splanchnic nerve; PUD, pudendal nerve; Epid, epididymis; SA, short adrenergic projections; SAC, sacral plexus; SCG, sympathetic chain ganglion; SHP, superior hypogastric plexus; SSP, superior spermatic plexus. (From Ref. 1 with permission.)

Visceral pain is a diffuse sensation that cannot be precisely localized. There are two components of visceral pain that were originally described more than 100 years ago (11): *true visceral pain*—deep visceral pain arising from inside the body; and *referred visceral pain*—pain that is referred to segmentally related somatic structures (muscle, subcutaneous tissue, skin). Secondary hyperalgesia usually develops at the referred site (12). Several explanations have been offered for the existence of referred pain (10). An initial model for interpreting referred pain was based on the idea of *viscerosomatic convergence* occurring in primary afferent fibers,

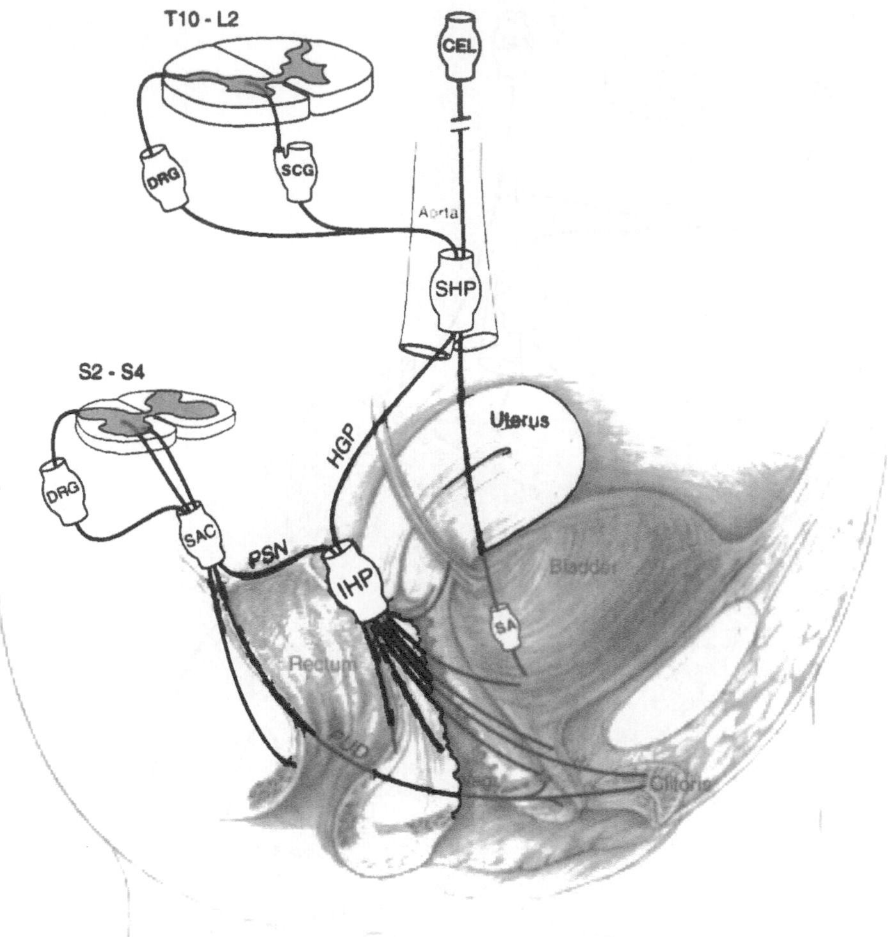

Figure 2 Schematic drawing showing the innervation of the urogenital and rectal area in females: Although this diagram attempts to show the innervation in humans, much of the anatomical information is derived from animal data. CEL, celiac plexus; DRG, dorsal root ganglion; HGP, hypogastric plexus; IHP, inferior hypogastric plexus; PSN, pelvic splanchnic nerve; PUD, pudendal nerve; SA, short adrenergic projections; SAC, sacral plexus; SCG, sympathetic chain ganglion; SHP, superior hypogastric plexus; Vag, vagina. (From Ref. 1 with permission.)

with multiple branches innervating both viscera and somatic structures. This hypothesis is unlikely, because few branching axons have been found in animal studies. Also the hypothesis does not explain the time delay in the evolution of referred pain. Another suggested mechanism for referred pain is that visceral and somatic primary neurons converge onto common spinal neurons. This is the *convergence–projection* theory. There is considerable experimental evidence for this hypothesis (13). It offers a ready explanation for the segmental nature of referred pain, but does not address explicitly the issue of hyperalgesia in the referred zone. To interpret "referred pain with hyperalgesia," two main theories have been proposed, which are not mutually exclusive. The first is known as *convergence–facilitation* theory. It proposes that the abnormal visceral input would produce an irritable focus in the relative spinal cord segment, thus facilitating messages from somatic structures. The second theory postulates that the *visceral afferent barrage* induces the activation of a reflex arc, the afferent branch of which is presented by visceral afferent fibers and the efferent branch by somatic efferents and sympathetic efferents toward the somatic structures (muscle, subcutis, and skin). The efferent impulses toward the periphery would then sensitize nociceptors in the parietal tissues of the referred area, thus resulting in the phenomenon of hyperalgesia.

When treating a patient with chronic visceral pain it is important to consider both aspects of the pain syndrome, including the pain deep in the abdominal–pelvic cavity and pain referred to somatic structures (muscle, subcutis, and skin). From a clinical standpoint it is important to be aware that a pain treatment strategy might have a positive effect on one component of the pain, whereas the other component persists, requiring additional interventions. It is, therefore, important to ask the patient about the effect of an intervention on all components of the pain.

Conventional diagnostic techniques, including surgical exploration, do not reveal any source for the chronic visceral pain syndrome in many patients. On the other hand, presence of abdominal, pelvic, or bladder pathology is not always related to the chronic pain syndrome, evidenced by the fact that removal of the pathological source often does not result in pain relief (14). Several psychophysical observations suggest that visceral inputs, similar to cutaneous inputs, are subject to sensitization (15). It has been proposed that patients with chronic abdominal–pelvic pain suffer from visceral hyperalgesia. Even though the end results of visceral hyperalgesia may be similar or indistinguishable, a wide variety of different mechanisms (infection, ischemia, obstruction, stress, or other major life events) may be responsible for sensitization in different parts of the abdominal–pelvic cavity (16). This hypothesis has allowed a more functional understanding of the chronic visceral pain syndromes and has shifted the focus from the unrevealing and never-ending search for organ pathology, to a physiological marker: visceral hyperalgesia. This concept will open new avenues for rational drug therapy for these disorders (17,18).

B. Clinical Characteristics and Treatment Strategies of Chronic Nonmalignant Visceral Pain Syndromes of the Abdomen and Pelvis

1. Definition of Chronic Abdominal and Pelvic Pain Syndromes

Definitions of chronic abdominal and pelvic pain are broadly based on duration, the anatomical–physical basis, or psychological characteristics of the pain (19). The International Association for the Study of Pain (IASP) defines *chronic abdominal pain syndromes* according to origin (neurological origin—intercostal neuralgia, 12th-rib syndrome, nerve entrapment; visceral origin—cardiac failure, gallbladder disease, postcholecystectomy syndrome, chronic gastric or duodenal ulcer, mesenteric ischemia, Crohn's disease, chronic constipation, irritable bowel syndrome, diverticular disease of the colon; generalized diseases—familial Mediterranean fever, abdominal migraine, porphyria). The IASP defines *chronic pelvic pain* without obvious pathology as chronic or recurrent pelvic pain that apparently has a gynecological origin, but for which no definitive lesion or cause is found (20).

However, the IASP definition for pelvic pain has not been widely used in the literature (14), and might need to be revised. This definition implies absence of pathology, which might not necessarily be true, and it also excludes cases in which pathology is present, although not necessarily the cause of pain. The relation of pain to the presence of pathology is often unclear in women with chronic pelvic pain. For example, a patient may have severe pelvic pathology, such as adhesions or endometriosis, with little or no pain. In contrast, another patient might have severe pain, but minimal pelvic pathology (21). In this chapter we will refer to chronic abdominal and pelvic pain as pain in the same location for at least 6 months (14,22).

2. Clinical Presentation, Evaluation, and Pain Treatment Strategies

More than half of the patients in gastroenterological clinics complain of abdominal symptoms, but conventional diagnostic tests show no demonstrable cause (23). For irritable bowel syndrome (IBS), it has been shown that 1.5–3% of the population suffers from IBS at any point in time (24). Chronic pelvic pain is a common problem among women. In a recent study in the United States including 5263 eligible women aged 18–50 years, 14.7% reported chronic pelvic pain (25). Fifteen percent of these women with chronic pelvic pain reported time lost from work and 45% reported reduced work productivity. In the United States, 10% of outpatient gynecological consultations are for chronic pelvic pain (26). Estimated medical costs for outpatient visits for chronic pelvic pain in the United States are 881.5 million dollars per year.

Patients with chronic abdominal or pelvic pain syndromes complain about deep pain in the abdominal or pelvic cavity that is unilateral, bilateral, or in the midline. The pain is often radiating to the back, anterior abdominal wall, buttocks, hips, perineal area, and legs (referred pain to somatic structures). Some patients present with "more than one abdominal–pelvic pain"; an example is the strong covariation of menstrual and bowel symptoms and the overlap in the diagnoses of dysmenorrhea and functional bowel disorders (27). The differential diagnosis is wide and includes basically every organ in the abdominal cavity as well as blood vessels and lymphatic structures. Other etiologies to be considered include the musculoskeletal system, a neurological problem, and psychiatric etiologies. Localization of the source of pain is often difficult or inaccurate, because of the overlapping innervation pattern of the visceral organs.

Because the diagnosis based on history and physical examination is often unrevealing, many patients undergo exploratory abdominal or pelvic surgery at some point. Laparoscopy serves three important diagnostic functions: diagnostic confirmation, histological documentation, and patient reassurance (28). Retrospective review of data of patients with chronic pelvic pain undergoing laparoscopic surgery has shown that fewer than 50% of patients are helped by diagnostic or therapeutic laparoscopy, implicating that laparoscopy is neither the ultimate investigation nor treatment for chronic pelvic pain (29). Similar retrospective studies on patients with chronic abdominal pain have not yet been reported.

The workup of the patient with chronic abdominal–pelvic pain is complex, given the wide diversity of possible etiologies and frequently the nonspecificity of the clinical presentation. It is important that no organic pathology is overlooked that can be treated in an etiological fashion to relieve the pain. This requires the concerted effort of different medical subspecialties. A thorough review of all previous consultations, and diagnostic and therapeutic interventions is imperative to decide whether further diagnostic workup is required and when to stop further diagnostic evaluations. These are very important clinical decisions, and require a lot of clinical experience in the field of chronic abdominal–pelvic pain. It is important that the physician is not impelled by the lack of findings to institute more invasive procedures in an effort to find a nonexistent pathological condition. The pain history focuses on the nature, intensity, temporal pattern, location, duration, and radiation of the pain, as well as precipitating and relieving factors. Areas of "true visceral pain" and "referred visceral pain" are documented. Associated changes in bowel or bladder motility should be evaluated. The physical evaluation is focused on the area of pain and includes a general physical, abdominal–pelvic, and musculoskeletal examination, as well as a neurological examination focusing on possible entrapment neuropathies and neuralgias. Procedures during the physical examination that provoke or exacerbate the pelvic pain are carefully noted. Areas of hyperalgesia and trigger points are documented. As in other chronic pain conditions, psychosocial and behavioral assessment is an essential part of the evaluation of chronic pelvic pain.

The management of chronic abdominal–pelvic pain, a multifacet disease, requires a multifacet approach, which may include pharmacological and psychological interventions, physical therapy, regional anesthesia techniques, and selected surgical interventions.

Surgical Management. Traditionally, surgical approaches toward the treatment of abdominal–pelvic pain were very common, often targeted at removal of the organ that was thought to have caused the chronic pain syndrome to begin with, such as surgical extirpation of all internal reproductive organs for chronic pelvic pain. However, review of the long-term success of surgical procedures for chronic abdominal–pelvic pain has shown that the results are often disappointing when pain is the only indication for surgery. The American College of Obstetricians and Gynecologists has recommended, therefore, that surgical therapy for chronic pain should be limited to the treatment of surgically correctable etiologies (22). It is often thought that when a surgically correctable etiology can be identified, its removal will result in a cure of the chronic pain syndrome. However, review of the outcome of surgical procedures in patients with chronic abdominal or pelvic pain show that the chronic pain syndrome may be improved, but also, it may be unchanged or worsened by the procedure (22). It is very important that the patient and the physician are aware of nonsurgical alternatives (30).

Neurosurgical Interventions. Splanchnicectomy has been advocated for intractable abdominal pain, specifically pain associated with chronic pancreatitis (31). Simplified thoracoscopic approaches have recently been described with excellent postoperative recovery and excellent pain relief (32,33). The efficacy of presacral neurectomy and amputation of the uterosacral ligaments in the treatment of chronic pelvic pain has been debated for decades since the early descriptions by Ruggi (34). As medical therapy was advancing, presacral neurectomy was replaced by pharmacological and hormonal approaches to the management of chronic pelvic pain. Recently, with the widespread use of laparoscopic surgery, there has been a new interest in pelvic denervation for chronic pelvic pain. Reports in the literature are controversial on the pain relief achieved with these procedures (35,36). Better characterization of the patients who respond and do not respond to these procedures might help identify patients who might benefit from the procedure. A diagnostic superior hypogastric plexus block might help predict the success of a surgical presacral neurectomy. Controlled studies are necessary to verify this concept.

Abdominal or pelvic surgery might result in ilioinguinal, iliohypogastric (groin pain), or genitofemoral nerve (lower abdominal and perineal pain) entrapment. Case reports have documented significant pain relief after neurectomy of these nerves (37). To identify patients who might benefit from surgical neurectomy for pain relief, local anesthetic nerve blocks of these nerves are recommended as a diagnostic procedure.

Recently, limited midline myelotomy has been advocated for the relief of pelvic cancer pain (5,38) based on very promising results in a limited number of cancer patients. The aim of this procedure is to interrupt ascending nociceptive signals from the pelvic organs traveling in the medial part of the posterior column. Notwithstanding these encouraging results in patients with cancer, several pain specialists have suggested that midline myelotomy cannot be recommended for the treatment of nonmalignant pelvic pain at this point, because the function of the dorsal column pathway and the long-term consequences of its surgical interruption are not yet understood (39,40).

Pharmacological Treatment. Despite that chronic abdominal–pelvic pain syndromes are very common, very little is yet known about effective pharmacological treatment. Several different pharmacological classes of medications have been demonstrated to be effective in alleviating pain in patients with chronic pain syndromes (2,41): NSAIDs, antidepressants, anticonvulsants, local anesthetic, antiarrhythmics, and opioids. Most of these pain medications have been evaluated for the treatment of chronic neuropathic pain, central pain, and back pain. Very few case reports or clinical trials have focused on the treatment of chronic abdominal or pelvic pain with pain medications (see Ref. 2 for discussion). These studies and clinical experience suggest that visceral pain syndromes can be successfully treated with medications commonly used to treat other chronic pain syndromes. However, further clinical and basic science research in this area is urgently needed to assess which class of pain medications might be most successful for a given clinical presentation of abdominal–pelvic pain. Currently, as in many other areas of chronic pain, pain medications are chosen on a trial and error basis, for we have no method to predict which drug is most likely to alleviate pain in a given individual patient. As different medications can have different and selective effects on certain aspects of pain, it is important that the effects on each aspect of pain are carefully monitored.

Regional Anesthesia Techniques. Regional anesthesia techniques have been advocated as diagnostic tools and therapeutic interventions for patients with chronic abdominal and pelvic pain (42). The celiac plexus innervates most of the abdominal viscera, including stomach, liver, biliary tract, pancreas, spleen, kidneys, adrenals, omentum, small bowel, and large bowel to the level of the splenic flexure. The superior hypogastric plexus (see Figs. 1 and 2), located just inferior to the aortic bifurcation, innervates the pelvic organs. There has been a new interest in neurolytic celiac and superior hypogastric plexus blocks for the treatment of chronic abdominal or pelvic pain associated with cancer (43–45). Anecdotal reports have also described these blocks in the setting of nonmalignant abdominal or pelvic pain, either with local anesthetic agents or neurolytic agents (42,46). Further controlled studies are necessary to assess the indications for nonmalignant pain, especially the use of neurolytic blocks. Analgesia after anesthetic or neurolytic blockade of these plexuses might be due to interruption of the sympathetic outflow to the abdominal or pelvic organs, similar to sympathetically maintained pain syndromes (47), or because of interruption of the afferent pathways.

Chronic pelvic pain may be due to entrapment of the ilioinguinal, iliohypogastric, genitofemoral, or pudendal nerves. Many patients presenting with nerve entrapments had abdominal surgery in the past, and the entrapment is due to scar tissue formed around these nerves. Often the chronic pain can be managed with repeated local anesthetic nerve blocks to these nerves spaced over time (42).

TENS, Physical Therapy, Trigger Point Injections, and Acupuncture. The use of transcutaneous electrical nerve stimulation therapy (TENS) can provide excellent pain relief for some patients without the side effects associated with pharmacological treatment. TENS has been used successfully in patients with primary dysmenorrhea and in patients with noncyclic chronic pelvic pain (42,48). Musculoskeletal dysfunction often contributes to the signs and symptoms of chronic abdominal and pelvic pain, because visceral pain is referred to somatic structures, including the musculature (see foregoing). Physical therapy can decrease musculoskeletal pain, helps to improve mobility, and is an important aspect of a multidisciplinary approach to the treatment of chronic pelvic pain (49). Myofascial pain has been shown to respond to trigger point injections. Slocumb has applied this technique to chronic pelvic pain and reported high rates of pain relief with local anesthetic injections into trigger points in the abdominal wall and sacral and vaginal areas (50). Acupuncture has not been systematically studied as a separate treatment component for chronic visceral pain. Anecdotal reports in which acupuncture has been used as part of a multidisciplinary treatment approach, indicate an effective role for the management of chronic pelvic pain (19).

Vascular Approaches for Chronic Pelvic Pain. Beard et al. (51) have shown that venous congestion is a common finding in patients with chronic pelvic pain. The mechanisms whereby pelvic congestion causes pelvic pain are poorly understood. Medroxyprogesterone acetate reduces pelvic pain and venous congestion in these patients (52); however, there was a high relapse rate after treatment was stopped. Bilateral oophorectomy combined with hysterectomy and hormone replacement therapy has been suggested by this group for women with chronic pelvic pain caused by pelvic congestion who have failed to respond to medical treatment (51). Transcatheter embolization of lumbo-ovarian varices has been described as a safe technique offering symptomatic relief in selected patients with chronic pelvic pain caused by pelvic congestion (53,54).

Psychological Aspects. As in other chronic pain syndromes, psychological treatment should be part of the multidisciplinary treatment plan. The literature examining psychological factors in abdominal pain and especially in pelvic pain has demonstrated several consistent findings. For example, a lifetime prevalence of depression in women with chronic pelvic pain has been reported at 64%, compared with 17% of gynecological controls, and a current incidence of depression for 28% of chronic pelvic pain patients versus 3% for gynecological controls (55). A history of sexual abuse has long been anecdotally associated with the development of a variety of medical symptoms, but that association appears to be particularly strong with chronic pelvic pain. Drossman (56) reported that there is a history of sexual or physical abuse in up to 44% of women with irritable bowel syndrome. As in other chronic pain patients, it is difficult to assume cause and effect between psychological history and the development of abdominal or pelvic pain retrospectively. Some studies have suggested that the psychological abnormalities often found in these patients are secondary to their patient status, rather than the primary factor causing the chronic pain syndrome (57). Psychological techniques include relaxation techniques, biofeedback, psychotherapy, and group therapy (58). Furthermore, psychological factors that might affect the success of any treatment should be discussed with the patient. Patients who have suffered from chronic pain for many years, and have been through many diagnostic tests and treatment failures, often remain anxious, are impatient, and have unrealistic expectations about a quick cure.

Dietary Modifications. Dietary modifications have been suggested in patients presenting with chronic gastrointestinal pain. There are no side effects associated with this approach, and therefore a dietary modification should be considered early on in the treatment plan. Much is gained if this approach is successful, and nothing is lost if this approach does not result in pain relief. The aggressive use of high-fiber diets and bulking agents has been reported to result in pain relief in 70% of patients with irritable bowel syndrome (59).

C. Clinical Characteristics and Treatment Strategies of Interstitial Cystitis

The urinary bladder receives a dual visceral afferent innervation which projects to sacral and thoracolumbar spinal segments (see Figs. 1 and 2). The sacral afferent innervation is the major pathway for all sensations, including pain, and for the regulation of micturition and continence. Little is known about the functional significance of the thoracolumbar afferents, although they are certainly involved in the generation of discomfort and pain elicited from the urinary bladder (60). Corresponding to the dual afferent innervation, the urinary bladder has two zones of referred pain, one in the dermatomes–myotomes of the lower thoracic and upper lumbar segments, and one in the dermatomes–myotomes of the sacral segments S2–S4.

Interstitial cystitis (IC) is a chronic, painful, and often debilitating disease of the urinary bladder (61,62), for which the etiology and pathophysiology are largely unknown (63–65). It is characterized by pelvic and suprapubic pain, urinary symptoms such as frequency and urgency, and in females often as dyspareunia that may be relieved by voiding. IC subdivides into an ulcerative and nonulcerative type as determined by cystoscopic findings of either Hunner's ulcer or glomerulations without ulcer on the bladder wall (65–68). The National Institutes of Health (NIDDK) have established research diagnostic criteria for IC (69,70). The NIDDK criteria require the identification of glomerulations or classic Hunner's ulcer on cystoscopic examination. To be diagnosed with IC according to the NIDDK criteria, patients must present with irritative voiding symptoms consisting of urinary frequency and urgency, along with pain symptoms referable to the lower urinary tract as outlined in the foregoing. The following criteria are stated to exclude the diagnosis of interstitial cystitis:

1. Bladder capacity greater than 350 mL on awake cystometry using either a gas- or a liquid-filling medium.
2. Absence of intense urge to void with the bladder filled to 100 mL gas or 150 mL water during cystometry, using a fill rate of 30–100 mL/min.
3. The demonstration of phasic involuntary contractions on cystometry using the filling rate described previously.
4. Duration of symptoms less than 9 months.
5. Absence of nocturia.
6. Symptoms relieved by antimicrobial, urinary antiseptics, anticholinergics, or antispasmodics.
7. A frequency of urination while awake of less than eight times a day.
8. A diagnosis of bacterial cystitis or prostatitis within a 3-month period.
9. Bladder or ureteral calculi.
10. Active genital herpes.
11. Uterine, cervical, vaginal, or urethral cancer.
12. Urethral diverticulum.
13. Cyclophosphamide or any type of chemical cystitis.
14. Tuberculous cystitis.
15. Radiation cystitis.
16. Benign or malignant bladder tumors.
17. Vaginitis.
18. Age less than 18 years.

Recent reports have raised concerns that the cystoscopic pathology, as required by the NIDDK criteria might be nonspecific (71).

Pain is a prominent characteristic of IC. Data from the ICDB study (72) show that 93.6% of the patients enrolled reported having some pain on some part of their body. Of the patients having pain, 80.4, 73.8, 65.7, and 51.5% reported having pain in their lower abdomen, urethra, lower back, and vaginal area, respectively. Types of pain varied with "pressure" and "aching" being the most common types.

IC has been reported to be associated with other chronic pain conditions, including either *systemic pain syndromes*—fibromyalgia, or *localized pain syndromes*—irritable bowel syndrome, vulvodynia, prostatodynia, and migraine headaches (73–77). It has been hypothesized that the somatic and visceral pain complaints in these patients are an expression of a generalized (central) lowering in pain thresholds (76).

It has been suggested that somewhere between 450,000 (62) and 1 million persons (78) in the United States suffer from IC or IC-like conditions. The most recent study on the epidemiology of IC used the Nurses' Health Study (NSH) I and II cohort as a study population and reported the prevalence of IC in NSH II as 67:100,000 and in NSH I as 52:100,000 (79). From the National Household Interview Survey (78), it was estimated that among IC patients the female/male ratio is 9:1. The majority of patients with IC reported in the epidemiological literature are white (72,80). IC tends to appear in young to middle-aged individuals. Simon et al. (72) reported on the demographic characteristics of patients with IC in the ICDB study sample: 27.8% were 18–34 years old, 50.2% were 35–54 years, and 21.9% were 55 years or older.

Etiologies that have been considered include infection (61,81,82), lymphatic or vascular obstruction (61), immunological deficiencies (61), glycosaminoglycan layer deficiency (61,83,84), presence of toxic urogenous substance (61), neural factors, and primary mast cell disorders (65,85,86). The fact that IC is rare in prepubertal children, and is most frequently diagnosed in women in their reproductive ages, and the observation that symptoms are exacerbated in many patients during menstruation, are consistent with an influence of changes in levels of estrogen and progesterone. Bladder mast cell expression of high-affinity estrogen receptors has been described in patients with interstitial cystitis, indicating a possible site of interaction (87).

The presentation of symptoms can be quite variable among patients with IC, leading several authors to propose that IC is a complex of diseases, rather than just one (88). Many authors believe that a combination of etiologies is likely (89). Interestingly, Baskin and Tanagho (90) reported several cases for whom removal of the bladder in IC patients did not lead to a resolution of pain, postulating that once the cause leading to the onset of IC has resolved, it may leave in its wake a chronic visceral pain syndrome. Since the etiology of IC remains unclear, it is difficult to direct treatment against its specific cause or causes.

A variety of oral, intravesical, surgical, local, and behaviorally based treatments have been suggested for the management of IC. Surgical approaches include removal or modification of the bladder (91). Local treatments include laser therapy (92), hydrodistension (91–94), and uretheral dilation (91), infusions of various materials into the bladder, such as dimethylsulfoxide (DMSO) (93,95–98), silver nitrate (93), heparin (93), chlorpactin (93), and hyaluronic acid (99). Oral medications include medications used for other chronic pain syndromes, such as amitriptyline (100,101) and calcium channel blockers (102). Hydroxyzine and other antihistamines (103,104) have been advocated for a presumed allergic etiology. Pentosan polysulfate sodium, a mild anticoagulant with properties of sulfated glycosaminoglycans and an affinity for mucosal membranes, has been used for treatment of IC based on the hypothesis that a defect in the glycosaminoglycan layer contributes to the pathogenesis (105). Nonmedical treatment strategies such as TENS (106), acupuncture (107), behavioral interventions (including the keeping of voiding diaries, pelvic floor muscle training), and acid-lowering diets have been advocated (108,109). Many reports on the treatment of IC are anecdotoal. Multicenter, controlled trials are necessary (and several are currently underway) comparing different treatment strategies for the management of IC to allow for improved—logical and systematic—treatment approaches.

Interstitial cystitis shares many features with other chronic nonmalignant visceral pain syndromes. As outlined earlier, not much emphasis has yet been placed on evaluating the neurophysiological mechanisms of pain in IC and on treating pain in patients with IC. Recognizing that a spectrum of insults to the bladder can result in IC and visceral pain symptoms associated with this disease might open an additional and new avenue for evaluating and understanding its pathophysiological mechanisms, and might result in the development of novel treatment strategies (17,18).

III. UROGENITAL AND RECTAL PAIN

A. Neurobiology of Urogenital and Rectal Pain

The pelvic floor is a highly specialized area of the body that is responsible for carrying out a host of basic biological functions, including defecation, micturition, copulation, and reproduction. The display of these diverse functions relies on precise nervous system control, coordinated with endocrine and other local control mechanisms. The complexity of this network has largely been considered to account for the slow progress in our understanding of the neurobiology of the urogenital tract as compared with other areas of the body. In addition, these areas of the body are often considered taboo in our society, and this might be another reason why there has been fairly little neuroanatomical, neurophysiological, and neuropharmacological research in this area. [A detailed review of the neurobiology of the urogenital tract is provided in Ref. (3)]. Briefly, the innervation of the pelvic floor involves both components of the autonomic nervous system, the sympathetic and parasympathetic divisions, as well as the somatic nervous systems (110–112) (see Figs. 1 and 2). Sensations from the urogenital tract are mainly conveyed by the sacral afferent parasympathetic system, with a far lesser afferent supply from afferents traveling with the thoracolumbar sympathetics (60). However, sensations of the testis and epididymis may predominantly involve thoracolumbar afferents (60). Neuropeptide release appears to account for perineal sensations (60).

B. Clinical Characteristics and Treatment Strategies of Chronic Urogenital and Rectal Pain Syndromes

1. Vulvodynia

Hyperesthesia of the vulva was apparently a well-described entity in American and European gynecological textbooks in the last century (113,114). However, despite these early reports the medical literature did not mention vulvar pain again until the early 1980s when a new interest in this chronic pain syndrome developed. *Vulvodynia* is defined as chronic vulvar discomfort and includes several subgroups: vulvar dermatosis, cyclic vulvovaginitis, vulvar vestibulitis, vulvar papillomatosis and essential vulvodynia (115).

The incidence or prevalence of vulvodynia is unknown. A recent survey of sexual dysfunction, analyzing data from the National Health and Social Life Survey, reported that 16% of women between the ages of 18 and 59 years living in households throughout the United States experience pain during sex (116). When these data were analyzed by age group, the highest number of women reporting pain during sex was in the 18–29 years age group. The location and etiology of pain was not analyzed in this study. It has been estimated that at least 200,000 women in the United States suffer from significant vulvar discomfort that greatly reduces their quality of life (117). The age distribution ranges from the 20s to late 60s (118). Goetsch (119) reported that 15% of all patients seen in her general gynecological private practice fulfilled the definition of vulvar vestibulitis, a major subgroup of vulvodynia. It is important to point out that these patients had not come for a gynecological evaluation because of vulvar pain. Fifty percent of these patients had always experienced entry dyspareunia and pain with inserting tampons, most since their teenage years. They had often wondered whether they were unique or had a hidden emotional aversion to sex.

Chronic vulvodynia is often characterized by an acute onset. Some patients recall frequent episodes of a vaginal infection, local treatments of the vulvar or vaginal area (application of steroid or antimicrobial cream, cryo- or laser surgery), or changes in the pattern of sexual activity before the onset of vulvodynia. These aspects are quite common events in the medical history of many women in their reproductive ages, and it is unclear why some women develop chronic vulvar pain after these events and others do not. Many women cannot recall any initiating event. The physical examination in patients with vulvodynia is usually normal, except for hyperalgesia in the vulvar area: pain can easily be elicited or exacerbated by a simple "swabtest": touching the vulvar area with a moist cotton swab results in sharp, burning pain (119). This "hyperalgesia" is similar to sensory findings in patients with painful neuropathies of the extremities. Recent histological studies of vaginal biopsy specimen reported vestibular neural hyperplasia in women with vulvar vestibulitis, which might provide a morphological explanation for the pain in vulvar vestibulitis syndrome (120,121).

To confirm the diagnosis of vulvodynia, excluding secondary causes such as dermatitis or gynecological infections, and to design a treatment plan, a multidisciplinary approach involving collaborations of gynecologists, dermatologists, neurologists, pain specialists, psychologists, and psychiatrists is important. Many patients can be helped with oral medications recommended for neuropathic pain management, including antidepressants, anticonvulsants, membrane-stabilizing agents, and opioids (1). In patients with vulvar vestibulitis, where a very localized small area is painful, topical treatment regimens, such as creams with local anesthetics, aspirin, steroids, or estrogen might reduce the pain. In an uncontrolled study, intralesional interferon-alfa injections into the vulvar vestibule were reported to reduce pain in about 50% of the patients (122). Glazer et al. (123) reported pain relief in over 80% of patients with vulvar vestibulitis using electromyographic biofeedback of the pelvic floor musculature. As this treatment is not associated with any side effects and given the high response rate reported in this study, a trial of this treatment modality should be considered. Surgical procedures have been advocated to remove the painful skin area in patients with vulvar vestibulitis (see review in Ref. 1). The most commonly used procedure is perineoplasty. Risks include general anesthesia, prolonged healing period, intraoperative bleeding, and disfigurement of the vulvar area (124). A simplified surgical revision, as an alternative to this extensive surgical intervention, has been suggested by Goetsch (124), where the painful area is excised under local anesthesia.

Many women with vulvodynia are in their reproductive ages and previously had satisfying sexual relationships. They often become depressed and anxious after suffering from chronic vulvar pain for months or years, without finding a cure. The involvement of a psychologist or psychiatrist trained in pain management early in the evaluation and treatment of patients with vulvodynia is recommended.

2. Orchialgia

Similar to women who suffer from pain syndromes of the reproductive organs, men with chronic orchialgia are often embarrassed to talk about it. Many patients cannot recall any precipitating event that led to the onset of the chronic pain syndrome. Secondary causes of chronic orchialgia include infection, tumor, testicular torsion, varicocele, hydrocele, spermatocele, trauma (bicycle accident), and previous surgical interventions (125,126). The differential diagnosis includes referred pain from the ureter, or the hip, or lumbar facet joints, and entrapment neuropathies of the ilioinguinal or genitofemoral nerve (127,128). Neuropathic testicular pain has also been attributed to diabetic neuropathy (129). Vasectomy has been reported to be a frequent cause of chronic testicular pain (130,131). There is usually no erectile or ejaculatory dysfunction associated with chronic orchialgia (125).

A careful history, physical examination, and urological evaluation will reveal most secondary causes of chronic testicular pain. Selected additional tests might include a gastroenterological evaluation to rule out referred pain from the lower pelvic organs or herniography to evaluate for an occult hernia. The neurological evaluation is directed toward the lumbosacral roots, the ilioinguinal, genitofemoral, and pudendal nerves, and the autonomic nerve supply to the testis. A vascular evaluation should be considered if an aneurysm is suspected. In many cases, however, the pain remains unexplained despite a very thorough diagnostic workup. Treatment of chronic orchialgia is directed toward the underlying etiology, if an underlying etiology can be identified. A hydrocele, varicocele, or spermatocele usually are not the cause of chronic orchialgia, but a coincidental finding (128).

Traditionally pain management for chronic orchialgia in the urology clinics consisted of a trial of antibiotics and NSAIDs with the aim of treating a possible occult inflammatory process. There is evidence from recent research that medical management including medications used for other chronic pain syndromes, such as low-dose antidepressants, anticonvulsants, membrane-stabilizing agents, and opiates are often effective for treatment of chronic orchialgia (129–132). Transcutaneous electrical nerve stimulation (TENS) might be helpful (131). In patients where a sympathetic component is suspected in the maintenance of chronic orchialgia, repeated lumbar sympathetic blocks with local anesthetic, oral sympatholytic drugs, or repeated infusions with phentolamine may result in marked pain relief (133). Drastic surgical procedures have been recommended for the treatment of chronic orchialgia, such as epididymectomy and orchiectomy (125,134). A priori, from a neuropathophysiological perspective it would be surprising, given the central aspects of chronic pain syndromes, if surgical removal of the testis or epididymis would result in pain relief. As an alternative to surgical removal of these organs, microsurgical denervation has been suggested (135,136).

3. Prostatodynia

Often the term *prostatitis* is used to describe any unexplained symptom or condition that might possibly originate from the prostate gland (137). In the United States approximately 25% of men presenting with genitourinary tract problems are diagnosed with prostatitis (138,139). Drach (140) defined four categories of prostatitis: (1) acute bacterial prostatitis, (2) chronic bacterial prostatitis, (3) nonbacterial prostatitis (including nonbacterial infections, allergic, and autoimmune prostatitis), and (4) prostatodynia. *Prostatodynia* is defined as persistent complaints of urinary urgency, dysuria, poor urinary flow, and perineal discomfort or pain, without evidence of bacteria or purulence in the prostatic fluid (140). Patients report pain in the perineum, lower back, suprapubic area, and groin, as well as pain on ejaculation. Prostatodynia accounts for approximately 30% of patients presenting with prostatitis (141). The age range is from 20 to 60 years of age (142).

Physical examination of the prostate is typically normal, without any signs of tenderness. A thorough urological evaluation is indicated including urinalysis, urine culture, urine cytology, and urethral cultures (143). Referred pain from the colon or rectum needs to be ruled out. Prostatodynia is a diagnosis of exclusion where it is assumed that the chronic pain syndrome is related to the prostate, but no inflammatory prostatic process can be identified.

The most frequently advocated treatment is antibiotics, despite that usually no infectious etiology can be found (143). Oral α-adrenergic blockers have been reported to improve the voiding abnormalities as well as pain. The most frequently used agents are prazosin, terazosin, and doxazosin; however, their use is often limited by side effects, most frequently hypotension (144). Pelvic floor relaxation techniques and muscle-relaxing agents have been reported to result in marked improvement of the symptomatology based on a muscular component to the chronic pain syndrome (142,145). As in other chronic pain syndromes of the pelvic floor, anecdotal clinical experience suggests that the pain can be relieved with medications (antidepressants, anticonvulsants, membrane-stabilizing agents, or opioids) commonly used to treat other chronic pain syndromes, but controlled clinical studies have not yet been performed.

4. Urethral Syndrome

Many women present to the urologist, gynecologist, or family physician with painful micturition, but no evidence of organic disease, and the urine culture is negative by standard techniques. To describe this problem, the term "urethral syndrome" was coined by Gallagher et al. in 1965 (146). The *urethral syndrome* describes a disease entity characterized by urinary urgency, frequency, dysuria and, at times, by suprapubic and back pain and urinary hesitancy, in the absence of objective urological findings. It has been estimated that the urethral syndrome accounts for as many as 5 million office visits a year in the United States (147). The urethral syndrome typically occurs in women during their reproductive years (148,149), but it has also been reported in children (149) and in men (150).

The etiology of the urethral syndrome is unclear. Several theories have been proposed, however, with little supporting evidence. One popular theory is that symptoms are caused by urethral obstruction and are thus surgically treatable (151,152). Although surgical procedures aimed at relieving a urethral obstruction claim excellent results, it has to be cautioned that diagnostic criteria were unfortunately poorly documented. Most importantly, there is rarely evidence to support an anatomically obstructive etiology. These procedures involve some risk of incontinence and are of uncertain and usually temporary efficacy (153). There is little support for an inflammatory or infectious etiology of the urethral syndrome (reviewed in Ref. 154). Urinary hesitance, which is often reported by patients with urethral syndrome, might be due to spasms of the external urethral sphincter. Several studies reported a staccato or prolonged flow phase during uroflowmetry and increased external sphincter tone detected on urethral pressure profilometry in patients with urethral syndrome (149,153,155). However, these urodynamic findings may also be produced voluntarily in a neurologically intact person; therefore, they are difficult to interpret (154). In contrast to other chronic nonmalignant pain genitourinary pain syndromes, the rates of spontaneous remission are very high in this patient population (156,157).

A thorough diagnostic evaluation is crucial. The symptoms of the urethral syndrome are indistinguishable from those caused by urinary infections, tumors, stones, interstitial cystitis, and many other entities, and these conditions have to be ruled out. Urethral syndrome is a diagnosis of exclusion. The evaluation begins with a thorough urological examination, including urine analysis, culture, and cytology. Radiographic studies, urodynamic studies, and cystoscopy are indicated in selected patients (154). In females, a gynecological problem needs to be ruled out. Systemic diseases affecting the innervation of the urogenital area, including multiple sclerosis, collagen diseases, and diabetes mellitus, have to be considered. A psychological evaluation should be part of the multidisciplinary evaluation to rule out a psychogenic etiology and to assess for symptoms of depression associated with the chronic pain syndrome.

Various invasive and medical treatment options have been suggested for patients with urethral syndrome (reviewed in Ref. 154): endoscopic and open surgical procedures have been advocated with the aim to eliminate a presumed urethral stenosis. Fulguration, scarification, resection, or cryosurgery have been reported to obliterate cystoscopically apparent urethritis. Bladder instillations with a variety of anti-inflammatory or cauterizing agents, and systemic therapy with anticholinergics, α-adrenergic blockers, and muscle relaxants have been considered. Electrical stimulation and biofeedback have been advocated to correct neurogenic causes. High rates of success were found with skeletal muscle relaxants or electrostimulation combined with biofeedback techniques (149,153). While exercising caution toward invasive and irreversible therapeutic procedures, a conservative approach is recommended, for this is usually as effective as surgery, less expensive, and most importantly, less subject to risk (156,158).

5. Rectal Pain

Pain in the rectal–anal area can occur as a constant pain—*proctodynia*—or as paroxysms of pain—*proctalgia fugax*.

Proctodynia is often caused by local disease of the anus or rectum, or it can be referred from the urogenital tract or the lumbosacral spine. It is important to initiate a comprehensive workup, because in most cases, the underlying etiology can be found. Intractable rectal pain has occasionally been associated with pudendal neuralgia, and has been treated successfully with neuropathic pain medications (159). Chronic idiopathic anal pain has been associated with abnormal anorectal manometric profiles, probably resulting from a dysfunction of the striated external anal sphincter. Biofeedback training has been effective in these cases (160).

Proctalgia fugax is characterized by sudden attacks of intense pain of short duration in the region of the internal anal sphincter and the anorectal ring. The incidence of proctalgia fugax has been reported as high as 14% in the general population, and as high as 33% in patients with gastrointestinal disease (161,162). The immediate cause of proctalgia fugax seems to be muscle spasms, but the etiology of this syndrome remains unclear (163). A consistent phenomenon in all studies seems to be gastrointestinal smooth-muscle dysfunction. As with many of the urogenital pain syndromes, in the majority of patients with proctalgia fugax the physical examination is normal, and common anorectal diseases, such as hemorrhoids and anal fissures, seem to be unrelated to the paroxysmal pain problem.

Simple and effective remedies have been suggested to end the acute pain attack associated with proctalgia fugax: immediate taking of food or drink, dilation of the anorectum (digital dilation, attempting a bowel movement, or inserting a tap-water enema) that can be done by the patient, hot sitz baths, and firm pressure to the perineum (164–166). A variety of drugs have been suggested in anecdotal reports: antispasmodics, nitroglycerin, nifedipine, carbamazepine, diltiazem, and albuterol (salbutamol) (rewiewed in Ref. 1). It is important to reassure the patient that the symptoms, although quite troublesome, are not signs of a life-threatening disease and may improve with time. Psychological assessment is important to rule out a depressive symptomatology contributing to the chronic pain syndrome.

IV. FUTURE DIRECTIONS

Although the chronic nonmalignant pain syndromes discussed in this chapter—abdominal pain, pelvic pain, urogenital pain, and rectal pain—are quite frequent, many of the patients suffering from these pain syndromes do not receive adequate pain management, and some patients do not receive any pain treatment at all. Frequently, the focus is on finding and possibly treating the underlying etiology. Pain, a prominent symptom, is often considered only as a symptom of the chronic disease, but not as a treatable entity of its own (17,18). In the future, novel treatment strategies might become available targeted specifically against the pathophysiological mechanisms of the chronic pain syndromes discussed here. Although these developments may be on the horizon, it is very important to realize what can now be done for patients who suffer from chronic pain syndromes of the abdomen, pelvis, bladder, and pelvic floor. Most currently available treatment options for these pain syndromes are empirical only. Although these pain syndromes can rarely be cured, some pain relief can be provided to almost all patients using a multidisciplinary approach, including pain medications (antidepressants, anticonvulsants, membrane-stabilizing agents, and opioids), local treatment regimens, nerve blocks, selected surgical procedures, physical therapy, and psychological support (1–3). Educating patients and their health care providers about currently available pain treatment strategies will be an important step forward, as many are not aware of options that currently already exist.

Further research is urgently needed to develop improved and more specific pain treatment strategies for these patients. A major issue that needs to be addressed is that many patients suffering from the pain syndromes discussed here are women in their reproductive ages. Many medical pain treatment modalities cannot be offered to these patients if they plan to become pregnant, because continuation of the medication would not be safe during pregnancy. Similar to other fields where chronic disease is treated in women throughout their reproductive years (e.g., epilepsy), algorithms will have to be developed to address this issue and special efforts will have to be devoted to design specific treatments for this patient population.

Progress in the treatment of the chronic pain syndromes of the abdomen, pelvis, bladder, and pelvic floor is likely to come from the combination of basic science and clinical research studies: (1) it is important to develop and study specific animal models of these chronic pain syndromes in which the peripheral and central processing of nociceptive information and its pharmacological manipulation can be evaluated; (2) clinical studies are necessary to assess the characteristics of pain in these patients and controlled clinical trials are important to study the effects of traditional analgesics and of new analgesics targeted against the pathophysiological pain mechanisms.

ACKNOWLEDGMENTS

Ursula Wesselmann is supported by NIH grants DA10802 (NIDA) and NS36553 (NINDS; Office of Research for Women's Health) and the Blaustein Pain Research Foundation.

REFERENCES

1. Wesselmann U, Burnett AL, Heinberg LJ. The urogenital and rectal pain syndromes. Pain 1997; 73:269–294.
2. Wesselmann U. Management of chronic pelvic pain. In: Aronoff GM, ed. Evaluation and Treatment of Chronic Pain. 3rd ed. Baltimore: Williams & Wilkins, 1998:269–279.
3. Wesselmann U, Burnett AL. Genitourinary pain. In: Wall PD, Melzack R, eds. Textbook of Pain. 4th ed. New York: Churchill Livingstone, 1999:689–709.
4. Willis WD, Coggeshall RE. Sensory Mechanisms of the Spinal Cord. New York: Plenum Press, 1991:456–459.
5. Hirshberg RM, Al-Chaer ED, Lawand NB, Westlund KN, Willis WD. Is there a pathway in the posterior funiculus that signals visceral pain? Pain 1996; 67:291–305.
6. Cervero F, Jänig W. Visceral nociceptors: a new world order? Trends Neurosci 1992; 15:374–378.
7. Schaible HG, Grubb BD. Afferent and spinal mechanisms of joint pain. Pain 1993; 55:5–54.
8. Häbler HJ, Jänig W, Koltzenburg M. A novel type of unmyelinated chemosensitive nociceptor in the acutely inflamed urinary bladder. Agents Actions 1988; 25:219–221.
9. Gebhart GF. Visceral nociception: consequences, modulation and the future. Eur J Anaesthiol 1995; 12:24–27.
10. McMahon SB, Dmitrieva N, Koltzenburg M. Visceral pain. Br J Anaesth 1995; 75:132–144.
11. Head H. On disturbances of sensation with special reference to the pain of visceral disease. Brain 1893; 16:1–113.
12. Giamberardino MA, Vecchiet L. Experimental studies on pelvic pain. Pain Rev 1994; 1:102–115.
13. Cervero F. Sensory innervation of the viscera: peripheral basis of visceral pain. Physiol Rev 1994; 74:95–138.
14. Campbell F, Collett BJ. Chronic pelvic pain. Br J Anaesth 1994; 73:571–573.
15. Ness TJ, Richter HE, Varner RE, Fillingim RB. A psychophysical study of discomfort produced by repeated filling of the urinary bladder. Pain 1998; 76:61–69.
16. Mayer EA, Raybould HE, eds. Basic and Clinical Aspects of Chronic Abdominal Pain. Pain Research and Clinical Management. Vol. 9. Amsterdam: Elsevier, 1993.
17. Wesselmann U. A call for recognizing, legitimizing, and treating chronic visceral pain syndromes. Pain Forum 1999; 8:146–150.
18. Wesselmann U. [Guest Editorial]: Pain—the neglected aspect of visceral disease. Eur J Pain 1999; 3:189–191.

19. Steege JF, Stout AL, Somkuti SG. Chronic pelvic pain in women: toward an integrative model. Obstet Gynecol Surv 1993; 48:95–110.
20. Merskey H, Bogduk N. Classification of Chronic Pain. Seattle: IASP Press, 1994.
21. Ryder RM. Chronic pelvic pain. Am Fam Phys 1996; 54:2225–2232.
22. ACOG Technical Bulletin: Chronic pelvic pain, number 223—May 1996. Int J Gynecol Obstet 1996; 54:59–68.
23. Azpiroz F. Sensitivity of the stomach and small bowel: human research and clinical relevance. In: Gebhart GF, ed. Visceral Pain. Seattle: IASP Press, 1995:391–428.
24. Sandler RS. Epidemiology of irritable bowel syndrome in the United States. Gastroenterology 1990; 99:409–415.
25. Mathias SD, Kuppermann M, Liberman RF, Lipschutz RC, Steege JF. Chronic pelvic pain: prevalence, health-related quality of life, and economic correlates. Obstet Gynecol 1996; 87:321–327.
26. Reiter RC. A profile of women with chronic pelvic pain. Clin Obstet Gynecol 1990; 33:130–136.
27. Moore J, Barlow D, Jewell D, Kennedy S. Do gastrointestinal symptoms vary with the menstrual cycle? Br J Obstet Gynaecol 1998; 105:1322–1325.
28. Parsons LH, Stovall TG. Surgical management of chronic pelvic pain. Obstet Gynecol Clin North Am 1993; 20:765–778.
29. Howard FM. The role of laparoscopy in chronic pelvic pain: promise and pitfalls. Obstet Gynecol Surv 1993; 48:357–387.
30. Carleson KJ, Miller BA, Fowler FJ Jr. The Maine Women's Health Study. II Outcomes of nonsurgical management of leiomyomas, abnormal bleeding, and chronic pelvic pain. Obstet Gynecol 1994; 83:566–572.
31. Stone HH, Chauvin EJ. Pancreatic denervation for pain relief in chronic alcohol associated pancreatitis. Br J Surg 1990; 77:303–305.
32. Kusano T, Miyazato H, Shiraishi M, et al. Thoracoscopic thoracic splanchnicectomy for chronic pancreatitis with intractable abdominal pain. Surg Laparosc Endosc 1997; 7:213–218.
33. Noppen M, Meysman M, D'Haese J, et al. Thoracoscopic splanchnicolysis for the relief of chronic pancreatitis pain: experience of a group of pneumonologists. Chest 1998; 113:528–531.
34. Ruggi C. La simpatectomia addominale utero-ovarica come mezzo di cura di alcune lesioni interne degli organi genitali della donna. Bologna: Zanichelli, 1899.
35. Zullo F, Pellicano M, DeStefano R, Mastrantonio P, Mencaglia L, Stampini A, Zupi E, Busacca M. Efficacy of laparoscopic pelvic denervation in central-type chronic pelvic pain: a multicenter study. J Gynecol Surg 1996; 12:35–40.
36. Lee RB, Stone K, Magelssen D, Belts RP, Benson WL. Presacral neurectomy for chronic pelvic pain. Obstet Gynecol 1986; 68:517–521.
37. Harms BA, DeHaas DR, Starling JR. Diagnosis and management of genitofemoral neuralgia. Neurosurgery 1987; 102:583–586.
38. Gildenberg PL, Hirshberg RM. Limited myelotomy for the treatment of intractable cancer pain. J Neurol Neurosurg Psychiatry 1984; 47:94–96.
39. Berkley KJ. On the dorsal columns: translating basic research hypotheses to the clinic. Pain 1997; 70:103–107.
40. Gybels JM. Commissural myelotomy revisited. Pain 1997; 70:1–2.
41. Galer BS. Neuropathic pain of peripheral origin: advances in pharmacologic treatment. Neurology 1995; 45:S17–S25.
42. McDonald JS. Management of chronic pelvic pain. Obstet Gynecol Clin North Am 1993; 20:817–838.
43. Eisenberg E, Carr DB, Chalmers TC. Neurolytic celiac plexus block for treatment of cancer pain: a meta-analysis. Anesth Analg 1995; 80:290–295.
44. Leon–Casasola OA, Kent E, Lema MJ. Neurolytic superior hypogastric plexus block for chronic pelvic pain associated with cancer. Pain 1993; 54:145–151.
45. Plancarte R, de Leon–Casasola OA, El-Helaly M, Allende S, Lema MJ. Neurolytic superior hypogastric plexus block for chronic pelvic pain associated with cancer. Reg Anesth 1997; 22:562–568.

46. Wechsler RJ, Maurer PM, Halpern EJ, Frank ED. Superior hypogastric plexus block for chronic pelvic pain in the presence of endometriosis. CT techniques and results. Radiology 1995; 196:103–106.
47. Wesselmann U, Raja SN. Reflex sympathetic dystrophy/causalgia. Anesth Clin North Am 1997; 15:407–427.
48. Milsom I, Hedner N, Mannheimer C. A comparative study of the effect of high-intensity transcutaneous nerve stimulation and oral naproxen on intrauterine pressure and menstrual pain in patients with primary dysmenorrhea. Am J Obstet Gynecol 1994; 170:123–129.
49. Baker PK. Musculoskeletal origins of chronic pelvic pain: diagnosis and treatment. Obstet Gynecol Clin North Am 1993; 20:719–742.
50. Slocumb JC. Neurological factors in chronic pelvic pain: trigger points and the abdominal pelvic pain syndrome. Am J Obstet Gynecol 1984; 149:536–543.
51. Beard RW, Kennedy RG, Gangar KF, Stones RW, Rogers V, Reginald PW, Anderson M. Bilateral oophorectomy and hysterectomy in the treatment of intractable pelvic pain associated with pelvic congestion. Br J Obstet Gynaecol 1991; 98:988–992.
52. Farquhar CM, Rogers V, Franks S, Pearce S, Wadsworth J, Beard RW. A randomized controlled trial of medroxyprogesterone acetate and psychotherapy for the treatment of pelvic congestion. Br J Obstet Gynaecol 1989; 96:1153–1162.
53. Sichlau MJ, Yao JST, Vogelzang RL. Transcatheter embolotherapy for the treatment of pelvic congestion syndrome. Obstet Gynecol 1994; 83:892–896.
54. Capasso P, Simons C, Trotteur G, Dindelinger RF, Henroteaux D, Gaspard U. Treatment of symptomatic pelvic varices by ovarian vein embolization. Cardiovasc Intervent Radiol 1997; 20:107–111.
55. Walker E, Katon W, Harrop–Griffiths J, et al. Relationship of chronic pelvic pain to psychiatric diagnoses and childhood sexual abuse. Am J Psychiatry 1988; 145:75–80.
56. Drossman DA, Leserman J, Nachman G, et al. Sexual and physical abuse in women with functional or organic gastrointestinal disorders. Ann Intern Med 1990; 113:823–833.
57. Kumar D, Pfeffer J, Wingate DL. Role of psychological factors in the irritable bowel syndrome. Digestion 1990; 45:80–87.
58. Rosenthal RH. Psychology of chronic pelvic pain. Obstet Gynecol Clin North Am 1993; 20:627–642.
59. Harvey RF, Mauad EC, Brown AM. Prognosis in the irritable bowel syndrome: a 5 year prospective study. Lancet 1987; 1:963–965.
60. Jänig W, Koltzenburg M. Pain arising from the urogenital tract. In: Maggi CA, ed. Nervous Control of the Urogenital System. Chur, Switzerland: Harwood Academic, 1993:525–578.
61. Ratliff TL, Klutke CG, McDougall EM. The etiology of interstitial cystitis. Urol Clin North Am 1994; 21:21–30.
62. Slade D, Ratner V, Chalker R. A collaborative approach to managing interstitial cystitis. Urology 1997; 49:10–13.
63. Ruggieri MR, Chelsky MJ, Rosen SI, Shickley TJ, Hanno PM. Current findings and future research avenues in the study of interstitial cystitis. Urol Clin North Am 1994; 21:163–176.
64. Toozs–Hobson P, Gleeson C, Cardozo L. Interstitial cystitis—still an enigma after 80 years. Br J Obstet Gynaecol 1996; 103:621–624.
65. Elbadawi A. Interstitial cystitis: a critique of current concepts with a new proposal for pathologic diagnosis and pathogenesis. Urology 1997; 49:14–40.
66. Johansson SL, Fall M. Pathology of interstitial cystitis. Urol Clin North Am 1994; 21:55–62.
67. Messing E, Pauk D, Schaeffer A, Nieweglowski M, Nyberg LM, Landis JR, Cook YLM, Simon LJ, ICDB Study Group. Associations among cystoscopic findings and symptoms and physical examination findings in women enrolled in the Interstitial Cystitis Data Base Study. Urology 1997; 49: 81–85.
68. Nigro DA, Wein AJ, Foy M, Parsons CL, Williams M, Nyberg LM, Landis JR, Cook YLM, Simon LJ, ICDB Study Group. Associations among cystoscopic and urodynamic findings for women enrolled in the Interstitial Cystitis Data Base Study. Urology 1997; 49:86–92.

69. Gillenwater JY, Wein AJ. Summary of the National Institute of Arthritis, Diabetes, Digestive and Kidney Diseases Workshop on Interstitial Cystitis, National Institutes of Health, Bethesda, Maryland, August 28–29, 1987. J Urol 1988; 140:203–206.
70. Wein AJ, Hanno PM, Gillenwater JY, Staskin DR, Krane RJ. Interstitial cystitis: an introduction to the problem. In: Hanno PM, ed. Interstitial Cystitis. London:springer-Verlag, 1990:3–5.
71. Hanno PM, Landis RJ, Matthews-Cook Y, Kusek J, Nyberg L, The Interstial Cystitis Database Study Group. The diagnosis of interstitial cystitis revisited: lessons learned from the National Institutes of Health Interstitial Cystitis Database. J Urol 1999; 161:553–557.
72. Simon LJ, Landis R, Erickson DR, Nyberg LM, the ICDB Study Group. The Interstitial Cystitis Data Base Study: concepts and preliminary baseline descriptive statistics. Urology 1997; 49(suppl 5A):64–75.
73. Fitzpatrick CC, Delancey JOL, Elkins TE, McGuire EJ. Vulvar vestibulitis and interstitial cystitis: a disorder of urogenital sinus-derived epithelium? Obstet Gynecol 1993; 81:860–862.
74. Miller JL, Rothman I, Bavendam TG, Berger RE. Prostatodynia and interstitial cystitis: one and the same? Urology 1995; 45:587–589.
75. Alagiri M, Chottiner S, Ratner V, Slade D, Hanno PM. Interstitial cystitis: unexplained associations with other chronic disease and pain. Urology 1997; 49(suppl 5A):52–57.
76. Clauw DJ, Schmidt M, Radulovic D, Singer A, Katz P, Bresette J. The relationship between fibromyalgia and interstitial cystitis. J Psychiatr Res 1997; 31:125–131.
77. Berger RE, Miller JE, Rothman I, Krieger JN, Muller CH. Bladder petechiae after cystoscopy and hydrodistension in men diagnosed with prostate pain. J Urol 1998; 159:83–85.
78. Jones CA, Nyberg LM. Epidemiology of interstitial cystitis. Urology 1997; 49(suppl 5A):2–9.
79. Curhan GC, Speizer FE, Hunter DJ, Curhan SG, Stampfer MJ. Epidemiology of interstitial cystitis: a population based study. J Urol 1999; 161:549–552.
80. Koziol JA. Epidemiology of interstitial cystitis. Urol Clin North Am 1994; 21:7–20.
81. Warren JW. Interstitial cystitis as an infectious disease. Urol Clin North Am 1994; 21:31–40.
82. Duncan JL, Schaeffer AJ. Do infectious agents cause interstitial cystitis? Urology 1997; 49:48–51.
83. Mobley DF, Baum N. Interstitial cystitis: when urgency and frequency mean more than routine inflammation. Postgrad Med 1996; 99:201–208.
84. Parsons CL. Epithelial coating techniques in the treatment of interstitial cystitis. Urology 1997; 49: 100–104.
85. Sant GR, Theoharides TC. The role of mast cell in interstitial cystitis. Urol Clin North Am 1994; 21:41–54.
86. Hofmeister M, He F, Ratliff TL, Mahoney T, Becich MJ. Mast cell and nerve fibers in interstitial cystitis: an algorithm for histological diagnosis via quantitative image analysis and morphometry. Urology 1997; 49:41–47.
87. Pang X, Cotreau-Bibbo MM, Sant GR, Theoharides TC. Bladder mast cell expression of high affinity oestrogen receptors in patients with interstitial cystitis. Br J Urol 1995; 75:154–161.
88. Koziol JA, Adams HP, Frutos A. Discrimination between the ulcerous and non-ulcerous forms of interstitial cystitis by non-invasive findings. J Urol 1996; 155:87–90.
89. Holm-Bentzen M, Nordlong J. Etiology: etiologic and pathogenetic theories in interstitial cystitis. In: Hanno MD, ed. Interstitial Cystitis. London: Springer-Verlag, 1990:63–77.
90. Baskin LS, Tanagho EA. Pain without pelvic organs. J Urol 1992; 147:683–686.
91. Irwin PP, Galloway NTM. Surgical management of interstitial cystitis. Urol Clin North Am 1994; 21:145–152.
92. Malloy TR, Shanberg AM. Laser therapy for interstitial cystitis. Urol Clin North Am 1994; 21: 141–144.
93. Sant GR, LaRock DR. Standard intravesical therapies for interstitial cystitis. Urol Clin North Am 1994; 21:73–84.
94. Zimmern PE. Hydrodistension in suspected interstitial cystitis patients: diagnosis and therapeutic benefits. Urology 1995; 153:290A.
95. Fowler JE. Prospective study of intravesical dimethyl sulfoxide in treatment of suspected early interstitial cystitis. Urology 1981; 18:21–26.

96. Barker SB, Matthews PN, Philip PF, Williams G. Prospective study of intravesical dimethyl sulphoxide in the treatment of chronic inflammatory bladder disease. Br J Urol 1987; 59:142–144.
97. Childs SJ. Dimethyl sulfone in the treatment of interstitial cystitis. Urol Clin North Am 1994; 21: 85–88.
98. Parkin J, Shea C, Sant GR. Intravesical dimethyl sulfoxide (DMSO) for interstitial cystitis—a practical approach. Urology 1997; 49:105–107.
99. Morales A, Emerson L, Nickel JC. Intravesical hyaluronic acid in the treatment of refractory interstitial cystitis. Urology 1997; 49:111–113.
100. Hanno PM. Diagnosis of interstitial cystitis. Urol Clin North Am 1994; 21:63–66.
101. Pranikoff K, Constantino G. The use of amitriptyline in patients with urinary frequency and pain. Urology 1998; 51(suppl 5A):179–181.
102. Fleischmann J. Calcium channel antagonists in the treatment of interstitial cystitis. Urol Clin North Am 1994; 21:107–112.
103. Simmons JL, Bunce PL. On the use of antihistamine in the treatment of interstitial cystitis. Am J Surg 1958; 24:664–667.
104. Theoharides TC, Sant GR. Hydroxyzine therapy for interstitial cystitis. Urology 1997; 49:108–110.
105. Jepsen JV, Sall M, Rhodes PR, Schmid D, Messing E, Bruskewitz RC. Long-term experience with pentosanpolysulfate in interstitial cystitis. Urology 1998; 51:381–387.
106. Fall M, Lindstrom S. Transcutaneous electrical nerve stimulation in classic and nonulcer interstitial cystitis. Urol Clin North Am 1994; 21:131–139.
107. Geirsson G, Wang YG, Lindstrom S, Fall M. Traditional acupuncture and electrical stimulation of the posterior tibial nerve. A trial in chronic interstitial cystitis. Scand J Urol Nephrol 1993; 27:67–70.
108. Chaiken DC, Blaivas JG, Blaivas ST. Behavioral therapy for the treatment of refractory interstitial cystitis. J Urol 1993; 149:1445–1448.
109. Whitmore KE. Self-care regimens for patients with interstitial cystitis. Urol Clin North Am 1994; 21:121–130.
110. Morrison JFB. Role of higher levels of the central nervous system. In: Torrens M, Morrison JFB, eds. The Physiology of the Lower Urinary Tract. London: Springer-Verlag, 1987:237–274.
111. De Groat WC, Booth AM, Yoshimura N. Neurophysiology of micturition and its modification in animal models of human disease. In: Maggi CA, ed. Nervous Control of the Urogenital System. Chur, Switzerland: Harwood Academic, 1993:227–290.
112. De Groat WC. Neurophysiology of the pelvic organs. In: Rushton DN, ed. Handbook of Neuro-Urology. New York: Marcel Dekker, 1994:55–93.
113. Thomas TG, ed. Practical Treatise on the Diseases of Woman. Philadelphia: Henry C, Lea's Son, 1880:145–147.
114. Pozzi SJ. Traite de Gynecologie Clinique et Operatoire. Paris: Masson, 1897.
115. McKay M. Burning vulva syndrome. J Reprod Med 1984; 29:457.
116. Laumann EO, Paik A, Rosen RC. Sexual dysfunction in the United States. Prevalence and predictors. JAMA 1999; 281:537–544.
117. Jones KD, Lehr ST. Vulvodynia: diagnostic techniques and treatment modalities. Nurse Pract 1994; 19:34–46.
118. Lynch PJ. Vulvodynia: a syndrome of unexplained vulvar pain, psychologic disability and sexual dysfunction. J Reprod Med 1986; 31:773–780.
119. Goetsch MF. Vulvar vestibulitis: prevalence and historic features in a general gynecologic practice population. Am J Obstet Gynecol 1991; 164:1609–1616.
120. Bohm–Starke N, Hilliges M, Falconer C, Rylander E. Increased intraepithelial innervation in women with vulvar vestibulitis syndrome. Gynecol Obstet Invest 1998; 46:256–260.
121. Westrom LV, Willen R. Vestibular nerve fiber proliferation in vulvar vestibulitis syndrome. Obstet Gynecol 1998; 91:572–576.
122. Marinoff SC, Turner ML, Hirsch RP, Richard G. Intralesional alpha interferon cost effective therapy for vulvar vestibulitis syndrome. J Reprod Med 1993; 38:19–24.
123. Glazer HI, Rodke G, Swencionis C, Hertz R, Young AW. Treatment of vulvar vestibulitis syndrome

with electromyographic biofeedback of pelvic floor musculature. J Reprod Med 1995; 40:283–290.
124. Goetsch MF. Simplified surgical revision of the vulvar vestibule for vulvar vestibulitis. Am J Obstet Gynecol 1996; 174:1701–1707.
125. Davis BE, Noble MJ, Weigel JW, Foret J, Mebust WK. Analysis and management of chronic testicular pain. J Urol 1990; 143:936–939.
126. Costabile RA, Hahn M, McLeod DG. Chronic orchialgia in the pain prone patient: the clinical perspective. Am Urol Assoc 1991; 146:1571–1574.
127. Bennini A. Die Ilioinguinalis- und Genitofemoralisneuralgie. Schweiz Rundsch Med 1992; 81: 1114–1120.
128. Hagen NA. Sharp, shooting neuropathic pain in the rectum or genitals: pudendal neuralgia. J Pain Sympt Manage 1993; 8:496–501.
129. Holland JM, Feldman JL, Gilbert HC. Phantom orchalgia. J Urol 1994; 152:2291–2293.
130. McMahon AJ, Buckley J, Taylor A, Lloyd SN, Deane RF, Kirk D. Chronic testicular pain following vasectomy. Br J Urol 1992; 69:188–191.
131. Hayden LJ. Chronic testicular pain. Aust Fam Phys 1993; 22:1357–1365.
132. Wesselmann U, Burnett AL, Heinberg LJ. Chronic testicular pain—a neuropathic pain syndrome: diagnosis and treatment [abstr]. 8th World Congress on Pain 1996:256.
133. Wesselmann U, Burnett AL, Campbell JN. The role of the sympathetic nervous system in chronic visceral pain. Soc Neurosci Abstr 1995; 21:1157.
134. Chen TF, Ball RY. Epididymectomy for post-vasectomy pain: histological review. Br J Urol 1991; 68:407–413.
135. Levine LA, Matkov TG, Lubenow TR. Microsurgical denervation of the spermatic cord: a surgical alternative in the treatment of chronic orchialgia. J Urol 1996; 155:1005–1007.
136. Heidenreich A, Zumbe J, Martinez F, Grozinger K, Engelmann UH. Die mikrochirurgisché testikuläre Denervierung als Therapieoption der chronischen Testalgie. Urologe A 1997; 36:177–180.
137. Nickel JC. Prostatitis—myths and realities. Urology 1998; 51:363–366.
138. Lipsky BA. Urinary tract infections in men. Ann Intern Med 1989; 110:138.
139. Meares EMJ. Prostatitis and related disorders. In: Walsh PC, Retik AB, Stanley TA, Vaughan EDJ, eds. Campbell's Urology. 6th ed. Philadelphia: WB Saunders, 1992:807–822.
140. Drach GW, Fair WR, Meares EM, Stamey TA. Classification of benign diseases associated with prostatic pain: prostatitis or prostatodynia? J Urol 1978; 120:266.
141. Brunner H, Weidner W, Schiefer HC. Studies on the role of *Ureaplasma urealyticum* and *Mycoplasma hominis* in prostatitis. J Infect Dis 1983; 126:807–813.
142. Moul JW. Prostatitis: sorting out the different causes. Postgrad Med 1993; 94:191–194.
143. de la Rosette JJMCH, Hubregtse MR, Karhaus HFM, Debruyne FMJ. Results of a questionnaire among Dutch urologists and general practitioners concerning diagnostics and treatment of patients with prostatitis syndrome. Eur Urol 1992; 22:14–19.
144. Barbalias GA, Nikiforidis G, Liatsikos EN. Alpha-blockers for the treatment of chronic prostatitis in combination with antibiotics. J Urol 1998; 159:883–887.
145. Segura JW, Opitz JL, Greene LF. Prostatosis, prostatitis or pelvic floor tension myalgia? J Urol 1979; 122:168–169.
146. Gallagher DJA, Montgomerie JZ, North JDK. Acute infections of the urinary tract and the urethral syndrome in general practice. Br Med J 1965; 1:622–626.
147. Peters–Gee JM. Bladder and urethral syndromes. In: Steege JF, Metzger DA, Levy BS, eds. Chronic Pelvic Pain. Philadelphia: WB Saunders, 1998:197–204.
148. Carson CC, Osborne D, Segura JW. Psychological characteristics of patients with female urethral syndrome. J Clin Psychol 1979; 35:312–315.
149. Kaplan WE, Firlit CF, Schoenberg HW. The female urethral syndrome: external sphincter spasm as etiology. J Urol 1980; 124:48–49.
150. Barbalias GA. Prostatodynia or painful male urethral syndrome? Urology 1990; 36:146–153.
151. Davis DM. Vesicle orifice obstruction in women and its treatment by transurethral resection. J Urol 1955; 73:112–117.

152. Bergman A, Karram M, Bhatia NN. Urethral syndrome: a comparison of different treatment modalities. J Reprod Med 1989; 34:157–160.
153. Schmidt RA, Tanagho EA. Urethral syndrome or urinary tract infection? Urology 1981; 18:424–427.
154. Messinger EM. Urethral syndrome. In: Walsh PC, Retik AB, Stanley TA, Vaughan EDJ, eds. Campbell's Urology. 6th ed. Philadelphia: WB Saunders, 1992:997–1005.
155. Raz S, Smith RB. External sphincter spasticity syndrome in female patients. J Urol 1976; 115:443–446.
156. Carson CC, Segura JW, Osborne DM. Evaluation and treatment of the female urethral syndrome. J Urol 1980; 124:609–610.
157. Zufall R. Ineffectiveness of treatment of urethral syndrome in women. Urology 1978; 12:337–339.
158. Bodner DR. The urethral syndrome. Urol Clin North Am 1988; 15:699–704.
159. Ger GH, Wexner SD, Jorge JM, Lee E, Amaranath A, Heyman S, Nogueras JJ, Jagelman DG. Evaluation and treatment of chronic intractable rectal pain—a frustrating endeavor. Dis Colon Rectum 1993; 36:139–145.
160. Grimaud JC, Bouvier M, Naudy B, Guien C, Salducci J. Manometric and radiologic investigations and biofeedback treatment of chronic idiopathic anal pain. Dis Colon Rectum 1991; 38:690–695.
161. Thompson WG, Heaton KW. Proctalgia fugax. J R Coll Phys (Lond) 1980; 14:247–248.
162. Thompson WG. Proctalgia fugax in patients with the irritable bowel, peptic ulcer, or inflammatory bowel disease. Am J Gastroenterol 1984; 79:450–452.
163. Karras JD, Angelo G. Proctalgia fugax. Am J Surg 1951; 82:616–625.
164. Ewing MR. Proctalgia fugax. Br Med J 1953; 9:1083–1085.
165. Penny RW. The doctor's disease: proctalgia fugax. Practitioner 1970; 204:843–845.
166. Rockefeller R. Digital dilatation for relief of proctalgia fugax. Am Fam Phys 1996; 54:72.

21
Nerve Injury Pain

Gudarz Davar
Brigham and Women's Hospital and Harvard Medical School, Boston, Massachusetts, U.S.A.

I. INTRODUCTION

Pain that arises from disease in which damage to, or disease involving, peripheral sensory nerves remains one of the most difficult clinical problems faced by physicians. Despite advances in our understanding of what might cause this pain, fully effective treatment evades us. Much of this difficulty is due both to a lack of understanding of the diverse origins of this type of pain and the specific mechanisms that apply in each instance. Although the development of clinically relevant models of nerve injury pain has improved our understanding of the possible causes of this pain, additional research will be needed to establish the importance of these findings for humans.

In this chapter, we will review what is known about the prevalence and diagnostic features of nerve injury pain, and then describe recent developments in our understanding of the pathophysiology, and current and future directions for the treatment of this pain.

Portions of this chapter are adapted from an article recently published in *Neurologic Clinics of North America* (1).

II. EPIDEMIOLOGY

The overall incidence and prevalence of nerve injury pain are unknown. This is largely due to the relatively recent recognition of this type of pain as a specific diagnostic entity, and the absence of studies that have examined the epidemiology of nerve injury pain. Several studies have estimated the prevalence of certain types of pain in which nerve injury may play a role (e.g., cancer, AIDS, spinal cord injury, low back pain), whereas other studies have examined the prevalence of pain in conditions associated with direct injury to sensory nerves (e.g., varicella zoster neuralgia, postsurgical pain, painful diabetic neuropathy). In patients with cancer, prospective assessments suggest that as many as 34% of those referred to a pain service will have nerve injury pain (2), while in AIDS patients, at least 28% will experience painful polyneuropathy (3). Similarly, for those with varicella zoster neuralgia, about 10–15% will develop persistent pain (postherpetic neuralgia), although the incidence rises with increasing age of the patient and may be as high as 80% in those older than the age of 80 years (4). Prevalence rates of close to 30% for postmastectomy pain (5) and between 13 and 60% for painful diabetic neuropathy (6,7) support the idea that nerve injury pain is a frequent consequence of medical and neurological disease. Although we can obtain a fairly accurate picture of the prevalence of pain in these specific instances, variability in pain symptoms between diseases and our lack of understanding of what nerve injury pain is, or what causes it, make generalization from these studies to overall prevalence rates difficult. As we understand more about nerve injury pain, we may be able to devise instruments that can accurately assess the overall incidence and prevalence of this condition.

III. DIAGNOSIS

We have elected to use the more generic term of "nerve injury pain" in this chapter, because recent evidence has suggested the possibility of diverse origins for this pain (see following Sec. IV) that include both abnormal neuronal excitability and signaling to sensory afferents from within the normal or disturbed (e.g., reactive Schwann cells, tumor cells) microenvironment of a peripheral nerve. It has been assumed in the past, perhaps partly because of the nature of the symptoms and evidence of neurophysiological changes after nerve injury, that this type of pain had its origin within nerves and was thus called "neuropathic pain." At present, there are no scientifically validated clinical or diagnostic criteria that can be used to establish the presence of nerve injury pain. However, the International Association for the Study of Pain has established a definition of *neuropathic pain* as, "any pain syndrome in which the predominating mechanism is a site of aberrant somatosensory processing in the peripheral or central nervous system." (8) Aspects of this definition are incorporated into generally accepted diagnostic features for nerve injury pain of nonmalignant origin (9) that include a history of nerve injury with evidence of sensory loss; persistent pain that is burning or sharp and shooting in quality; and a poor response to standard analgesics. Diagnostic criteria have not been established for nerve injury pain that is due to malignancy, although many of these same clinical features are observed.

The recent development of methods for the semiquantitative asessment of cutaneous sensory loss, or abnormalities of sensory response, to noxious and nonnoxious stimuli (quantitative sensory testing) may eventually improve our ability to diagnose nerve injury pain (10). This method uses a computer-driven program of thermal stimuli to establish the threshold at which an individual will respond to noxious and nonnoxious thermal stimuli. Lowering of the threshold may suggest the presence of hyperresponsiveness (e.g., allodynia or hyperalgesia), whereas an increase in the threshold suggests the possibility of cutaneous sensory loss. Although this is a subjective assessment, response reliability can be assessed to improve confidence in the results. Furthermore, this sensory testing method examines the function of small-caliber sensory afferents that cannot be effectively studied by any other existing technology.

IV. PATHOPHYSIOLOGY OF NERVE INJURY PAIN

A. Evidence from Studies in Animals

1. Animal Models

In the past, our understanding of the causes of nerve injury pain has been hindered by the absence of appropriate animal models for this condition. However, within the last 5–10 years several animals models have been described that approximate the pathology and some of the symptoms observed in humans with nerve injury pain. Most of these models involve complete or partial injury to the rat sciatic (11–17) or spinal (18) nerves, and spinal dorsal horn (19).

This type of injury usually leads to the development of both spontaneous and stimulus-evoked behaviors that suggest that the animal is suffering from experimental nerve injury pain.

Behavioral signs of pain can also be observed in animals with systemic illnesses that cause nerve injury pain in humans. For example, in the nonobese diabetic (NOD) mouse, an animal model of type 1 insulin-dependent diabetes in humans (20–23), pain behaviors are observed both in diabetic animals and in their nondiabetic siblings (24). Although the cause of this pain behavior is unknown, this unexpected observation suggests that pain and sensory disturbances in diabetic animals, or diabetic humans, might be the result of a preexisting abnormality in somatosensory pathways. In addition to suggesting the presence of heritable factors that might affect the development of pain, animal models such as the NOD mouse might have advantages over the existing models for studying pain mechanisms because they may more closely resemble human disease. Additional clinically relevant animal models of nerve injury pain that have recently been developed include the induction of local neural inflammation, and tissue implantation of tumor cells to induce pain behavior in rodents (25,26). Exogenous application of mediators made by tumor cells that might contribute to pain in patients with cancer (27) have also been used to induce pain behavior and activation of nociceptive afferents in rodents (28–30,30a). Evidence that these mediators cause pain behavior when secreted at physiologically relevant concentrations by experimentally implanted tumors remains to be determined.

The exact mechanism underlying pain behavior in these diverse animal models remains uncertain, but several candidate pathways have been examined in detail and will be discussed in the following. It should be remembered that despite what these animal models have taught us about the possible origins of nerve injury pain, the importance of these factors for nerve injury pain in humans remains to be established.

2. Physiological and Pharmacological Studies

The establishment of reliable animal models of nerve injury pain led directly to studies of the pathophysiology of pain behavior in these models. Early interest, based on evidence for glutamate as a fast-excitatory neurotransmitter at the primary afferent synapse and on its known neurotoxic effects, led to the examination of this neurotransmitter in the pathogenesis of nerve injury pain. Similarly, the electrophysiological identification of abnormal spontaneous activity in nociceptive and nonnociceptive afferents after nerve injury, and the known importance of ion channels in maintaining neuronal excitability and contributing to the propagation of neuronal impulses, have led to an investigation of known and novel sodium channel-dependent mechanisms in the animal models. Cell surface receptors that modulate excitability of sensory neurons might also contribute to the development of abnormal spontaneous activity in nociceptive neurons in these models. More recently, consistent with a focus on the initiating events surrounding nerve injury, the importance of proinflammatory mediators released at the site of nerve injury has become an area of intense investigation into the cause of this type of pain. Hopefully, some or all of these potential neurobiological mechanisms will prove to be critical for the pathogenesis of nerve injury pain, and thereby, lead to the development of therapeutic targets useful for the prevention or treatment of this disabling consequence of trauma or illness (1).

Glutamate/NMDA–Receptor Mechanisms. Experimental studies support the idea that the neurotransmitter glutamate, or its receptors, may mediate the development or maintenance of nerve injury pain. For example, the preemptive systemic administration of the noncompetitive *N*-methyl-D-apartate (NMDA) receptor (NMDAR) antagonist, dizocilpine (MK-801), completely blocks the development of thermal noxious stimulus-evoked pain behavior in rats with experimental nerve injury (31), whereas intrathecal administration of MK-801 reduces pain be-

Table 1 Examples of Types of Nerve Injury Pain and Pharmacological Agents That May Be Useful for Their Treatment

Type of pain	Agent	Refs.
Postherpetic neuralgia (PHN)	NMDA receptor antagonists	84
	Local anesthetics	94, 95
	Gabapentin	113
	Opioids	116, 117
Painful diabetic neuropathy	Mexilitene	92
	Tricyclic antidepressants	114
Posttraumatic pain with allodynia	NMDA receptor antagonists	85
Phantom limb pain	NMDA receptor antagonists	87

havior in this same model (32–34) (Table 1). NMDAR antagonists also reduce touch-evoked mechanical hyperresponsiveness (allodynia) in animals with experimental nerve injury (35,36).

Ion Channel-Based Mechanisms. Never injury pain might also result from increased primary afferent excitability that develops secondary to changes in the distribution or expression of sodium channels involved in the maintenance and propagation of impulses in sensory afferents (37,38). The voltage-sensitive Na^+ channel is an ion channel that is essential for the maintenance and propagation of impulses in afferent neurons (39). It has already been shown by computer simulations that the threshold for neuronal firing is highly sensitive to Na^+ channel density at the site of impulse initiation (electrogenesis), and that a small addition of Na^+ channels can shift an afferent fiber into a state of hyperexcitability, and even yield spontaneous discharge (40). It has also been shown using immunocytochemical methods, ethylenediamine tetrodotoxin (en-TTX) binding, and intramembrane particle analysis, that Na^+ channels accumulate in the axon membrane at sites of nerve injury. Consistent with this putative mechanism of injury-induced, enhanced neuronal hyperexcitability, pain behavior and the accompanying hyperexcitability are transiently suppressed by a range of Na^+ channel antagonists after nerve injury (41,42). Although the regulation of Na^+ channel synthesis and membrane insertion is only poorly understood at present, this is now an area of intense investigation in pain research. Evidence already exists that mRNA for brain type III Na^+ channel gene appears to be up-regulated in primary sensory neurons following peripheral nerve injury in adult rats (43). Recently, it has also been shown that a peripheral nerve-specific type of Na^+ channel gene appears to be translocated to the site of injury in an animal model of experimental nerve injury pain (44,44a).

Pharmacological studies and clinical results also support a role for Na^+ channel-mediated events in nerve injury pain. For example, agents that are used with some degree of success to treat this pain, such as the local anesthetics, or the anticonvulsants sodium phenytoin and carbamazepine, are known to have pharmacological actions on this ion channel and can (for local anesthetics; LAs) suppress ectopic activity in sensory afferents at serum levels well below those required to block normal peripheral nerve conduction (27,45,46). Similarly, in the animal models of nerve injury pain, comparable doses of systemic lidocaine cause a prolonged suppression of tactile allodynia (47).

Cell Surface Receptors. The primary target of research into cell surface receptor-mediated mechanisms has been the adrenergic receptors. Although there are no currently available adrenergic receptor antagonists that have been shown to be clearly effective for nerve injury pain, experimental evidence is accumulating that may implicate adrenergic pathways (48) or adrenergic receptors in sensory ganglia in the initiation or maintenance of such pain (49–51).

Some classes of α-adrenergic receptors are present on DRG neurons (52) and DRG satellite cells and may be up-regulated after partial nerve injury (53,50). Consistent with these reports, Northern blot analyses of DRG ipsilateral to injury in animals with an experimental painful neuropathy reveals the presence of a previously undetected adrenergic receptor-like mRNA that appears to be regulated by this injury (54). These results suggest a possible role for adrenergic receptors in the pathogenesis of nerve injury pain. Existing agents, or compounds in development that target known or novel adrenergic receptors, might eventually be shown to have efficacy for the treatment of nerve injury pain.

Inflammatory Mechanisms. Several recent reports suggest the potential pathophysiological importance of inflammation for nerve—injury-induced pain (55–57). For example, signs of inflammation that develop following trauma to the rat sciatic nerve in the experimental models are well described (58–62). Chronic constrictive injury of the rat sciatic nerve (CCI) (12) causes perineurial edema and damage, wallerian degeneration, and infiltration of the endoneurium by macrophages (63,64). The time course of macrophage infiltration approximately parallels the development of pain behavior that peaks at about 7–10 days after nerve injury (12). These macrophages are known to contain many proinflammatory mediators and enzymes that participate further in the recruitment of inflammatory cells and in the development of the inflammatory response. These substances (e.g., the proinflammatory cytokines) may also participate directly in the pain symptoms that follow nerve injury (60,65–68). For instance, a proinflammatory cytokine expressed by Schwann cells, macrophages, mast cells, fibroblasts, and endothelium (by 7 days) after CCI (68), tumor necrosis factor (TNF-α), contributes to the accumulation and activation of leukocytes at sites of local inflammation, and to the further local secretion of other cytokines (69). A role for TNF-α in the pathogenesis of nerve injury pain is supported by recent observations that exogenous local TNF-α administered to the sciatic nerve produces pain behavior and activation of primary afferents in rats (8,28). Consistent with a role for this cytokine in nerve injury pain, preemptive systemic administration of the hypnotic, thalidomide (a putative inhibitor of TNF-α release from macrophages), reduces both injury-induced vascular changes and endoneurial TNF-α 5 days after a CCI in rats, whereas postoperative administration diminishes pain behavior for the period between 5 and 9 days after nerve injury (67,70). Also, local administration of IL-10, an endogenous anti-inflammatory peptide that functionally inhibits TNF-α, reduces pain behavior in this model of experimental nerve injury pain (71). Efforts aimed at blocking inflammation might also target the recruitment of inflammatory cells to the site of nerve injury. Blockade of the recruitment and activation of macrophages with both broad-spectrum (e.g., glucocorticoids) and more specific (e.g., complement inhibitors) anti-inflammatory agents could result in a reduction of the cellular response and, consequently, in a reduction of pain. Consistent with this possibility, systemic administration of a glucocorticoid, dexamethasone (DEX), decreases both pain behavior and inflammation in CCI (72–74). Because this effect of DEX might be due to a direct inhibition of injured primary afferents, more specific blockers of the macrophage response, such as selective agents against an initiator of the inflammatory response, complement, might help establish which of these mechanisms is important (75–77). Blockers of complement, an important activator of the macrophage response, may be useful for inhibiting inflammation after nerve injury without causing inhibition of primary afferent activity. Complement activation and deposition are increased in peripheral nerve injury, and complement is a potent chemoattractant and activator of macrophages, presumed to be the primary cell type contributing to the initiation and elaboration of the inflammatory response in peripheral nerve (76).

Other Mechanisms. Several other mechanistic targets have been examined as possible causes of nerve injury pain, including nitric oxide (NO), the diffusible, endogenous neurotransmitter and mediator of vascular and inflammatory responses. No has been recently implicated in the pathophysiology of nerve injury pain based on reductions in pain behavior produced by the local or intrathecal administration of nitro-L-arginine methyl ester (L-NAME) (an NO synthase blocker) (78,79). L-NAME also inhibits ongoing activity originating in dorsal root ganglia caused by peripheral nerve injury (80). Despite this experimental evidence, a critical role for this neurotransmitter in this condition remains to be established.

B. Evidence from Studies of Neurons in Culture

In vitro studies of the physiological processes of sensory neurons in culture can allow us to examine cellular events that might ultimately influence the experience of pain in a highly controlled fashion. For example, dorsal root ganglion (DRG) neurons can be isolated from rats and studied in vitro, where the extracellular and intracellular milieu can be controlled, allowing detailed analysis of their electrophysiological properties. By using this method, evidence of abnormal hyperexcitability in DRG neurons has been obtained that can be correlated with behavioral signs of pain in animals with nerve injury (81). When DRG neurons were isolated from the nerve-injured side after sciatic nerve injury, they were observed to have a significantly higher incidence of spontaneous action potentials than DRG neurons from the uninjured side. Most importantly, this difference was most evident in the small- to medium-size DRG neurons, which include nociceptive neurons giving rise to Aδ- and C-fibers. These findings demonstrate that excitability changes induced by nerve injury at or near the DRG in experimental models of nerve injury pain, and may underlie pain behavior observed in this model, can be maintained in a dissociated cell preparation. This highly reductionistic system, while not representative of events in the whole animal, could allow for a more mechanistic examination of the origins of nerve injury-induced abnormal excitability of sensory afferents (82).

Animal models, and to some degree in vitro models, have provided a foundation for the clinical investigation and validation of rational targets to be used in the development of new drugs to treat nerve injury pain. The results of these investigations, for several classes of neuropharmacological targets, will be discussed next.

V. APPROACHES TO TREATMENT

A. Glutamate/NMDA Receptor Antagonists

Consistent with the results observed in animals, several double-blind, placebo-controlled trials have demonstrated the effectiveness of ketamine, a noncompetitive NMDAR antagonist, in patients with nerve injury pain. These studies showed effectiveness with either a single bolus dose (1–250 μg/kg) or a continuous infusion (mean dose 58 ± 5 mg/2 h) intravenous (IV) ketamine, at subanesthetic concentrations, on both spontaneous pain measured by a visual analog scale (VAS), and on mechanically, but not thermally, evoked pain sensation (83–87). In one of these studies, ketamine reduced the pain from postherpetic neuralgia (PHN), but morphine did not, when compared with saline. However, the results with ketamine and morphine were no different when these treatments were compared. This lack of difference could be due to the low dosages of morphine used (0.075 mg/kg), whereas it has been suggested that high doses of opioids may be required for analgesia in nerve injury pain (88). Alternatively, the small numbers of patients described in this study may have limited the opportunity to observe potential differences between these two treatments.

Despite these early, promising results with ketamine, dose-limiting side effects characteristic of this dissociative anesthetic in adults (e.g., nausea, dizziness, and central nervous system signs of disturbed consciousness) were observed in all studies. Although these side effects might be reduced by long-term administration of oral ketamine, the safety and efficacy of this approach is not yet established (89). Other, orally available, NMDAR antagonists, such as dextromethorphan, have also been tried for nerve injury pain, but have not yet shown analgesic efficacy in controlled, randomized, double-blind crossover trials (90). Nevertheless, given the absence of effective alternatives, other clinically available NMDAR antagonists (e.g., amantadine, memantine, magnesium sulfate) might be effective and should be considered both for controlled clinical study and for the treatment of nerve injury pain.

B. Sodium Channel Antagonists

Systemic (parenteral) LAs in humans (e.g., lidocaine) can also reduce the symptoms of nerve injury pain, but their long-term use is often precluded by tachyphylaxis and dose-related toxic effects. Orally administered lidocaine-like antiarrhythmics, such as mexilitene, may be an alternative to parenteral LAs, and have reduced nerve injury pain in several controlled clinical trials (91,92). Topical application of lidocaine is reported to be effective for some forms of nerve injury pain (PHN) (94,95), and may offer distinct advantages because side effects are minimal and plasma concentrations stay well below toxic levels.

Anticonvulsants also reduce the symptoms of nerve injury pain (91,92), possibly partly by suppressing ectopic activity in sensory neurons (45,46,98–102). Although this effect is believed to be mediated by the central nervous system, a peripheral nervous system site of action may be involved as well. Some of the new generation anticonvulsants that are thought to act on sodium channels, such as lamotrigine, decrease high-frequency repetitive firing of voltage-dependent sodium action potentials under conditions of sustained neuronal depolarization (103), and thus, they might be effective either by this mechanism or through their capacity to prevent the release of glutamate from sensory afferents (104).

C. Other Anticonvulsants

Although the antiepileptic gabapentin has been reported to be effective in animals with behavioral signs of nerve injury pain (105–107) and in some patients with nerve injury pain, including postherpetic neuralgia (108–113), the mechanism of action of this drug has not been established. Therefore, both the development of additional agents that target a putative receptor, or derivatives of gabapentin that have improved efficacy may be hindered. Further discussion of this agent's possible efficacy for nerve injury pain can be found in Chapter 65.

D. Antidepressants

Although antidepressant medications have been clearly shown to ameliorate nerve injury pain, the mechanism underlying their analgesic effect remains unclear. Greater efficacy of norepinephrinergic agents over serotoninergic ones might suggest the importance of the former pathways over the latter in the pathogenesis of nerve injury pain, but this remains speculative (114). A larger discussion of the use of antidepressants for nerve injury pain is addressed in Chapter 46.

E. Anti-Inflammatory Agents

Anti-inflammatories represent a relatively underexamined option for the treatment of nerve injury pain. This is largely the result of the apparent poor efficiacy of NSAIDs, and other low-potency anti-inflammatory agents, in patients with a variety of persistent pain states caused by nerve injury. However, an emerging understanding of the complex and likely critical importance of inflammatory mediators (see foregoing) in the pathogenesis of nerve injury pain should lead to an increasingly prominent role of anti-inflammatories for the treatment of nerve injury pain. Also, recently developed anti-inflammatory agents that can be used to treat inflammation-associated pain with possibly lower risks of gastrointestinal irritation or othe side effects, such as the cyclooxygenase-2 (COX-2) inhibitors, might also be useful for the prevention of treatment of nerve injury pain (115).

F. Opioids

Despite longstanding concerns by physicians about the use of opioids for nerve injury or other types of persistent pain, opioids agonists (predominantly μ-agonists) have clear efficacy in the treatment of some forms of nerve–injury-associated pain such as postherpetic neuralgia (PHN) (116,117). Although the mechanism of pain in PHN remains unclear, these data support a closer examination of the effectiveness of opioids for other types of nerve injury pain.

VI. NOVEL PHARMACOLOGICAL APPROACHES

A. Cellular and Molecular Approaches to Gene Therapy for Pain

Nerve injury pain is often localized to the dermatomes supplied by an injured nerve, and the adjacent dermatomes. Targeted treatments that provide localized analgesia could provide an alternative to systemically administered agents. For instance, with genetically engineered viral vectors containing "analgesic" genes, treatment could be directed to the site of injury, or within pain pathways, to induce analgesia without systemic side effects (118,119). Transplantation of progenitor or adult cells that secrete analgesic substances may represent another viable alternative for localized treatment of nerve injury pain (120). Effective treatment with such gene- or cell-based approaches could reduce the requirement for repeated or long-term administration of systemic analgesics in patients with nerve injury pain.

B. Analgesic Viral Vectors

Virus vectors represent one potentially intriguing method for the delivery of analgesic genes to treat pain (119). Viral vectors have been successfully used to deliver a variety of functional genes to rodent sensory neurons (121–125). Most recently, exciting evidence has emerged showing that replication-defective herpes simplex virus (HSV) vectors can be used to deliver analgesic neuropeptides to peripheral sensory neurons in which they could alter the physiology of these neurons involved in pain transmission (118,119). Although analgesic effects observed in rodents by Wilson et al. (118) with an enkephalin-containing herpes virus were likely due to the release of enkephalin from transfected cells, this has not been fully established. Also, although potentially useful, herpes vectors are not without risks (e.g., the potential for recombination events with wild-type virus) in humans. Thus, their initial use will likely be restricted to patients with an end-of-life illness for whom all other options have been exhausted. Recent studies suggest that adenoviral vectors may provide another method for gene delivery to the spinal cord to alleviate some forms of persistent nerve injury pain (119).

C. Cell and Tissue Transplants for Pain

Several tissue types have been transplanted into the nervous system to treat experimental pain in animals (120). Unfortunately, these tissues secrete rather low levels of potentially analgesic substances, such as catecholamines and enkephalins. Furthermore, the risks associated with autologous tissue (e.g., adrenal medulla) transplantation, and poor availability of supplies of heterologous tissues may further restrict the use of this approach. Genetically modified cells that oversecrete analgesic genes might enhance this potential method of pain treatment. For example, clonal cell lines can be transfected with coding sequences for analgesic neuropeptides and then transplanted into spinal sites where they are capable of inducing antinociceptive effects in normal animals (126,127). In one such study, the antinociceptive potential of AtT-20 cells (a pituitary tumor cell line), transfected with the human proenkephalin gene (*hENK*) was examined after transplantation into the intrathecal space of mice (127). Although acute antinociceptive effects were not observed with this treatment alone, the administration of isoproterenol (thought to stimulate the release of opioids from these cells) induced naloxone-reversible antinociception. In addition, mice that had received also showed reduced tolerance to the effects of acutely administered morphine. Although mice in these studies had normal weight gains, suggesting the ability to thrive, 10% of animals developed hindlimb paralysis 3 weeks after cell implantation. The use of growth-arrested or differentiated, clonally derived cells that stably express analgesic genes in vivo may address this complication of tumor cell implantation. Although speculative, the delivery of clonal cells to sites of injury in the peripheral nervous system might also reduce central nervous system complications, while still providing analgesia.

Despite our lack of understanding about what causes nerve injury pain, gene-based vectors and genetically modified cells that express analgesic substances might improve our ability to deliver analgesia without systemic side effects in these patients.

VII. CONCLUSIONS

The severity, and relative refractoriness to treatment, of nerve injury pain have led to recent intensive efforts to identify causes and more effective treatments for this type of pain. However, our continued lack of understanding about what actually causes this pain in humans challenges us to establish better preclinical models of nerve injury pain that reflect the diverse pathophysiology observed in human nerve injury pain states. Such in vivo and in vitro models may subsequently enable the development of more effective, targeted treatments for nerve injury pain.

REFERENCES

1. Hans G, Davar G. Recent advances in the pharmacology of nerve injury pain. Neurol Clin North Am 1998; 951–965.
2. Grond S, Zech D, Diefenbach C, Radbruch L, Lehmann KA. Assessment of cancer pain: a prospective evaluation in 2266 cancer patients referred to a pain service. Pain 1996; 64:107–114.
3. Hewitt DJ, McDonald M, Portenoy RK, Rosenfeld B, Passik S, Breitbart W. Pain syndromes and etiologies in ambulatory AIDS patients. Pain 1997; 70:117–123.
4. Ragozzino MW, Melton LJ 3d, Kurland LT, Chu CP, Perry HO. Population-based study of herpes zoster and its sequelae. Medicine (Baltimore) 1982; 61:310–316.
5. Stevens PE, Dibble SL, Miaskowski C. Prevalence, characteristics, and impact of postmastectomy pain syndrome: an investigation of women's experiences. Pain 1995; 61:61–68.
6. O'Hare JA, Abuaisha F, Geoghegan M. Prevalence and forms of neuropathic morbidity in 800 diabetics. Ir J Med Sci 1994; 163:132–135.
7. Veves A, Manes C, Murray HJ, Young MJ, Boulton AJ. Painful neuropathy and foot ulceration in diabetic patients. Diabetes Care 1993; 16:1187–1189.

8. Classification of chronic pain. In: Merskey H, Bogduk N, eds. IASP Task Force on Taxonomy. 2nd ed. Seattle: IASP Press, 1994:209–214.
9. Fields HL. Pain. New York: McGraw Hill, 1987.
10. Zarlansky R, Yarnitsky D. Clinical applications of quantitative sensory testing. J Neurol Sci 1998; 153:215–238.
11. Attal N, Jazat F, Kayser V, Guilbaud G. Further evidence for "pain-related" behaviours in a model of unilateral peripheral mononeuropathy. Pain 1990; 41:235–251.
12. Bennett GJ, Xie YK. A peripheral mononeuropathy in rat that produces disorders of pain sensation like those seen in man. Pain 1988; 33:87–107.
13. Coderre T, Grimes RW, Melzack R. Deafferentation and chronic pain in animals: an evaluation of evidence suggesting autotomy is related to pain. Pain 1986; 26:61–84.
14. DeLeo JA, Coombs DW, Willenbring S, Colburn RW, Fromm C, Wagner R, Twitchell BB. Characterization of a neuropathic pain model: sciatic cryoneurolysis in the rat. Pain 1994; 56:9–16.
15. Lombard MC, Nashold BS, Albe-Fessard D. Deafferentation hypersensitivity in the rat after dorsal rhizotomy: possible animal model for chronic pain. Pain 1979; 6:163–174.
16. Seltzer Z, Dubner R, Shir Y. A novel behavioral model of neuropathic pain disorders produced in rats by partial sciatic nerve injury. Pain 1990; 43:205–218.
17. Wall PD, Devor M, Inbal R, Scadding JW, Schonfeld D, Seltzer Z, Tomkiewicz MM. Autotomy following peripheral nerve lesions: experimental anaesthesia dolorosa. Pain 1979; 7:103–113.
18. Kim SH, Chung JM. An experimental model for peripheral neuropathy produced by segmental nerve ligation in the rat. Pain 1992; 50:355–363.
19. Wiesenfeld Z, Lindblom U. Behavioral and electrophysiological effects of various types of peripheral nerve lesions in the rat: a comparison of possible models for chronic pain. Pain 1980; 8:285–298.
20. Harada M, Makino S. Biology of the NOD mouse. Annu Rep Shionogi Res Lab 1992; 42:70–99.
21. Hattori M, Buse JB, Jackson RA, et al. The NOD mouse: recessive diabetogenic gene in the major histocompatibility complex. Science 1986; 231:733–735.
22. Hattori M, Matsumoto E, Itoh N. Modifier gene for enhancing glomerulosclerosis in BC1[(NOD × *Mus spretus*)F1 × NOD] mice. Diabetes 1994; 43:106A.
23. Karasik A, Hattori M. Use of animal models in the study of diabetes. In: Weir G, Kahn CR, eds. Joslin's Diabetes Mellitus. 13th ed. Philadelphia: Lea & Febiger, 1994:318–350.
24. Davar G, Waikar S, Eisenberg E, Hattori M, Thalhammer JG. Behavioral evidence of thermal hyperalgesia in non-obese diabetic mice with and without insulin-dependent diabetes. Neurosci Lett 1995; 190:171–174.
25. Eliav E, Herzburg U, Ruda MA, Bennett GJ. Neuropathic pain from an experimental neuritis of the rat sciatic nerve. Pain 1999; 83:169–182.
26. Wacnik PW, Stone LS, Laughlin TM, Kitto KF, Ramnaraine MLR, Mantyh PW, Beitz AJ, Wilcox GL. A practical model of cancer pain: comparing different hind limb sites of melanoma implantation. Soc Neurosci Abstr 1998; 247.2.
27. Carducci MA, Bowling MK, Rogers T, Leahy TL, Janus TJ, Padley RJ, Nelson JB. Endothelin receptor antagonist, ABT-627, for prostate cancer: initial trial results. American Association for Cancer Research Meeting, Indian Wells, CA, December 1998. [Abstr C-24].
28. Sorkin LS, Xiao WH, Wagner R, Myers RR. Tumour necrosis factor-alpha induces ectopic activity in nociceptive primary afferent fibres. Neuroscience 1997; 81:255–262.
29. Wagner R, Myers RR. Endoneurial injection of TNF-alpha produces neuropathic pain behaviors. Neuroreport 1996; 7:2897–2901.
30. Davar G, Hans G, Fareed MU, Sinnott C, Strichartz G. Behavioral signs of acute pain produced by application of endothelin-1 to rat sciatic nerve. Neuroreport 1998; 9:2279–2283.
30a. Fareed MU, Hans G, Atanda A, Strichartz G, Davar G. Pharmacologic characterization of acute pain behavior produced by application of endothelin-1 to rat sciatic nerve. J Pain 1999; 1:46–53.
31. Davar G, Hama A, Deykin A, Vos B, Maciewicz RJ. MK-801 blocks the development of thermal hyperalgesia in a rat model of experimental painful neuropathy. Brain Res 1991; 553:327–330.

32. Coderre TJ. The role of excitatory amino acid receptors and intracellular messengers in persistent nociception after tissue injury in rats. Mol Neurobiol 1993; 7:229–246.
33. Mao J, Price DD, Mayer DJ, Lu J, Hayes RL. Intrathecal MK-801 and local nerve anesthesia synergistically reduce nociceptive behaviors in rats with experimental peripheral mononeuropathy. Brain Res 1992; 576:254–262.
34. Yamamoto T, Yaksh TL. Comparison of the antinociceptive effects of pre- and posttreatment with intrathecal morphine and MK801, an NMDA antagonist, on the formalin test in the rat. Anesthesiology 1992; 77:757–763.
35. Qian J, Brown SD, Carlton SM. Systemic ketamine attenuates nociceptive behaviors in a rat model of peripheral neuropathy. Brain Res 1996; 715:51–62.
36. Yaksh TL. Behavioral and autonomic correlates of the tactile evoked allodynia produced by spinal glycine inhibition: effects of modulatory receptor systems and excitatory amino acid antagonists. Pain 1989; 37:111–123.
37. Devor M, Basbaum AI, Bennett GJ, Blumberg H, Campbell JN, Dembowsky KP, Guilbaud G, Janig W, Koltzenberg M, Levine JD, Otten UH, Portenoy RK. Mechanisms of neuropathic pain following peripheral injury. In: Basbaum AI, Besson JM, eds. Towards a New Pharmacology of Pain. Dahlem Konferenzen. Chichester: Wiley. 1991:417–440.
38. Devor M, Govrin–Lippmann R, Angelides K. Na^+ channel immunolocalization in peripheral mammalian axons and changes following nerve injury and neuroma formation. J Neurosci 1993; 13: 1976–1992.
39. Hille B. Ionic Channels of Excitable Membranes. 2nd ed. Sunderland, MA: Sinauer, 1992.
40. Matzner O, Devor M. Na^+ conductance and the threshold for repetitive neuronal firing. Brain Res 1992; 597:92–98.
41. Devor M. The pathophysiology of damaged peripheral nerves. In: Wall PD, Melzack R, eds. Textbook of Pain, 3rd ed. London: Chruchill Livingstone, 1994:79–100.
42. Matzner O, Devor M. Hyperexcitability at sites of nerve injury depends on voltage-sensitive Na^+ channels. J Neurophysiol 1994; 72:349–359.
43. Waxman SG, Kocsis JD, Black JA. Type III sodium channel mRNA is expressed in embryonic but not adult spinal sensory neurons, and is reexpressed following axotomy. J Neurophysiol 1994; 72:466–470.
44. Novakovic SD, Tzoumaka E, McGivern JG, Haraguchi M, Sangameswaran L, Gogas KR, Eglen RM, Hunter JC. Distribution of the tetrodotoxin-resistant sodium channel PN3 in rat sensory neurons in normal and neuropathic conditions. J Neurosci 1998; 18:2174–2187.
44a. Tzoumaka E, Novakovic SD, Haraguchi M, Sangameswaran L, Wong K, Gogas KR, Hunter JC. PN3 sodium channel distribution in the dorsal root ganglia of normal and neuropathic rats. Proc West Pharmacol Soc 1997; 40:69–72.
45. Devor M, Wall PD, Catalan N. Systemic lidocaine silences ectopic neuroma and DRG discharge without blocking nerve conduction. Pain 1992; 48:261–268.
46. Tanelian DL, MacIver MB. Analgesic concentrations of lidocaine suppress tonic A-delta and C fiber discharges produced by acute injury. Anesthesiology 1991; 74:934–936.
47. Sinnott CJ, Garfield JM, Strichartz GR. Differential efficacy of intravenous lidocaine in alleviating ipsilateral versus contralateral neuropathic pain in the rat. Pain 1999; 80:521–533.
48. McLachlan EM, Janig W, Devor M, Michaelis M. Peripheral nerve injury triggers noradrenergic sprouting within dorsal root ganglia. Nature 1993; 363:543–545.
49. Birder LA, Perl ER. Upregulation of α_{2A} adrenergic receptor subtype after peripheral nerve injury. Soc Neurosci Abstr 1996; 709.3.
50. Nishiyama K, Brighton BW, Bossut DF, Perl ER. Peripheral nerve injury enhances α_2-adrenergic receptor expression by some DRG neurons. Soc Neurosci Abstr 1993; 19:499.
51. Sato J, Perl ER. Adrenergic excitation of cutaneous pain receptors induced by peripheral nerve injury. Science 1991; 251:1608–1610.
52. Nicholas AP, Pieribone V, Hokfelt T. Distributions of mRNAs for alpha-2 adrenergic receptor subtypes in rat brain: an in situ hybridization study. J Comp Neurol 1993; 328:575–594.
53. Cho HJ, Kim DS, Lee NH, Kim JK, Lee KM, Han KS, Kang YN, Kim KJ. Changes in the alpha

2-adrenergic receptor subtypes gene expression in rat dorsal root ganglion in an experimental model of neuropathic pain. Neuroreport 1997; 8:3119–3122.

54. Fareed MU, Lee DH, Noh HR, Chung JM, Davar G. Identification and increased expression of a novel alpha-2 adrenoreceptor mRNA in a rat model of experimental painful neuropathy. In: Jensen TS, Turner JA, Wiesenfeld–Hallin Z, eds. Proceedings of the 8th World Congress on Pain (Progress in Pain Research and Management). Seattle: IASP Press, 1997; 8:539–546.

55. Hafer–Macko CE, Sheikh KA, Li CY, Ho TW, Cornblath DR, McKhann GM, Asbury AK, Griffin JW. Immune attack on the schwann cell surface in acute inflammatory demyelinating polyneuropathy. Ann Neurol 1996; 39:625–635.

56. Schmidt B, Toyka KV, Kiefer R, Full J, Hartung H–P, Pollard J. Inflammatory infiltrates in sural nerve biopsies in Guillain–Barre syndrome and chronic inflammatory demyelinating neuropathy. Muscle Nerve 1996; 19:474–487.

57. Swartz NG, Beck RW, Savino PJ, Sergott RC, Bosley TM, Lam BL, Drucker M, Katz B. Pain in anterior ischemic optic neuropathy. Neuroophthalmology 1995; 15:9–10.

58. Avellino AM, Hart D, Daily AT, MacKinnon M, Ellegala D, Kliot M. Differential macrophage responses in the peripheral and central nervous system during wallerian degeneration of axons. Exp Neurol 1995; 136:183–198.

59. Dahlin L. Prevention of macrophage invasion impairs regeneration in nerve grafts. Brain Res 1995; 679:274–280.

60. Danielsen N, Dahlin LB, Thomsen P. Inflammatory cells and mediators in the silicone chamber model for nerve regeneration. Biomaterials 1993; 14:1180–1185.

61. Monaco S, Gehrmann J, Raivich G, Kreutzberg GW. MHC-positive, ramified macrophages in the normal and injured rat peripheral nervous system. J Neurocytol 1992; 21:623–634.

62. Perry VH, Brown MC, Gordon S. The macrophage response to central and peripheral nerve injury. A possible role for macrophages in regeneration. J Exp Med 1987; 165:1218–1223.

63. Sommer C, Galbraith JA, Heckman HM, Myers RR. Pathology of experimental compression neuropathy producing hyperesthesia. J Neuropathol Exp Neurol 1993; 52:223–233.

64. Sommer C, Lalond A, Heckman HM, Rodrigues M, Myers RR. Quantitative neuropathology of a focal nerve injury causing hyperalgesia. J Neuropathol Exp Neurol 1995; 67:635–643.

65. Lindholm D, Heumann R, Meyer M, Thoenen H. Interleukin-1 regulates synthesis of nerve growth factor in non-neuronal cells of rat sciatic nerve. Nature 1987; 330:658–659.

66. Rotshenker S, Aamar S, Barak V. Interleukin-1 activity in lesioned peripheral nerve. J Neuroimmunol 1992; 39:75–80.

67. Sommer C, Myers RR. Vascular changes in a model of painful neuropathy. Exp Neurol 1996; 141: 113–119.

68. Wagner R, Myers RR. Schwann cells produce tumor necrosis factor alpha: expression in injured and non-injured nerves. Neuroscience 1996; 73:625–629.

69. Watkins LR, Maier SF, Goehler LE. Immune activation: the role of pro-inflammatory cytokines in inflammation, illness responses and pathological pain states. Pain 1995; 63:289–302.

70. Sommer S, Marziniak M, Myers RR. The effect of thalidomide treatment on vascular pathology and hyperalgesia caused by chronic constriction injury of rat nerve. Pain 1998; 74:83–90.

71. Wagner R, Janjigan M, Myers RR. Anti-inflammatory interleukin-10 therapy in CCU neuropathy decreases thermal hyperalgesia, macrophage recruitment, and endoneurial TNF-α expression. Pain 1998; 74:35–42.

72. Clatworthy AL, Illich PA, Castro GA, Walters ET. Role of peri-axonal inflammation in the development of thermal hyperalgesia and guarding behavior in a rat model of neuropathic pain. Neurosci Lett 1995; 184:5–8.

73. Hama AT, Fareed MU, Kral MG, Xiong Z, Study RE, Davar G. Suppression of hyperalgesia but not spontaneous activity in dorsal root ganglion neurons with dexamethasone in rats with a chronic constriction injury. Soc Neurosci Abstr 1997; 71.9.

74. Johansson A, Bennett GJ. Effect of local methylprednisolone on pain in a nerve injury model. A pilot study. Reg Anesth 1997; 22:59–65.

75. Bruck W, Friede RL. Anti-macrophage CR3 antibody blocks myelin phagocytosis by macrophages in vitro. Acta Neuropathol (Berl) 1990; 80:415–418.
76. Griffin JW, George R, Ho T. Macrophage systems in peripheral nerves. A review. J Neuropathol Exp Neurol 1993; 52:553–560.
77. Johansson A, Hao J, Sjolund B. Local corticosteroid application blocks transmission in normal nociceptive C-fibres. Acta Anaesthesiol Scand 1990; 34:335–338.
78. Thomas DA, Ren K, Besse D, Ruda MA, Dubner R. Application of nitric oxide synthase inhibitor, *N*-omega-nitro-L-arginine methyl ester, on injured nerve attenuates neuropathy-induced thermal hyperalgesia in rats. Neurosci Lett 1996; 210:124–126.
79. Meller ST, Pechman PS, Gebhart GF, Maves TJ. Nitric oxide mediates the thermal hyperalgesia produced in a model of neuropathic pain in the rat. Neuroscience 1992; 50:7–10.
80. Wiesenfeld–Hallin Z, Hao JX, Xu XJ, Hokfelt T. Nitric oxide mediates ongoing discharges in dorsal root ganglion cells after peripheral nerve injury. J Neurophysiol 1993; 70:2350–2353.
81. Study RE, Kral MG. Spontaneous action potential activity in isolated dorsal root ganglion neurons from rats with a painful neuropathy. Pain 1996; 65:235–242.
82. Kajander KC, Wakisaka S, Bennett GJ. Spontaneous discharge originates in the dorsal root ganglion at the onset of a painful neuropathy in the rat. Neurosci Lett 1992; 135:225–228.
83. Backonja M, Arndt G, Gombar KA, Check B, Zimmermann M. Response of chronic neuropathic pain syndromes to ketamine: a preliminary study. Pain 1994; 56:51–57.
84. Eide PK, Jorum E, Stubhaug A, Bremmes J, Breivik H. Relief of post-herpetic neuralgia with the *N*-methyl-D-aspartic acid receptor antagonist: a double-blind, cross-over comparison with morphine and placebo. Pain 1996; 58:347–354.
85. Felsby S, Nielsen J, Arendt–Nielsen L, Jensen TS. NMDA receptor blockade in chronic neuropathic pain: a comparison of ketamine and magnesium chloride. Pain 1995; 64:283–291.
86. Max MB, Byas–Smith MG, Gracely RH, Bennett GJ. Intravenous infusion of the NMDA antagonist, ketamine, in chronic posttraumatic pain with allodynia: a double-blind comparison to alfentanil and placebo. Clin Neuropharmacol 1995; 18:360–368.
87. Nikolajsen L, Hansen CL, Nielsen J, Keller J, Arendt–Nielsen L, Jensen TS. The effect of ketamine on phantom pain: a central neuropathic disorder maintained by peripheral input. Pain 1996; 67:69–77.
88. Portenoy RK, Foley KM, Inturrisi CE. The nature of opioid responsiveness and its implications for neuropathic pain: new hypotheses derived from studies of opioid infusions. Pain 1990; 43:273–286.
89. Klepstad P, Borchgrevink PC. Four years' treatment with ketamine and a trial of dextromethorphan in a patient with severe post-herpetic neuralgia. Acta Anaesthesiol Scand 1997; 41:422–426.
90. McQuay HJ, Carroll D, Jadad AR, Glynn CJ, Jack T, Moore RA, Wiffeh PJ. Dextromethorphan for the treatment of neuropathic pain: a double-blind randomised controlled crossover trial with integral n-of-1 design. Pain 1994; 59:127–133.
91. Chabal C, Jacobson L, Mariano A, Chaney E, Britell CW. The use of oral mexiletine for the treatment of pain after peripheral nerve injury. Anesthesiology 1992; 76:513–517.
92. Dejgard A, Petersen P, Kastrup J. Mexiletine for treatment of chronic painful diabetic neuropathy. Lancet 1992; 2:9–11.
93. Stracke H, Meyer UE, Schumacher HE, Federlin K. Mexiletine in the treatment of diabetic neuropathy. Diabetes Care 1992; 15:1550–1555.
94. Rowbotham MC, Davies PS, Fields HL. Topical lidocaine gel relieves postherpetic neuralgia. Ann Neurol 1995; 37:246–253.
95. Rowbotham MC, Davies PS, Verkempinck C, Galer BS. Lidocaine patch: double-blind controlled study of a new treatment method for post-herpetic neuralgia. Pain 1996; 65:39–44.
96. Swerdlow M. Anticonvulsant drugs and chronic pain. Clin Neuropharmacol 1984; 7:51–82.
97. Swerdlow M. Review: the use of local anaesthetics for relief of chronic pain. Pain Clin 1988; 2: 3–6.

98. Burchiel KJ. Carbamazepine inhibits spontaneous activity in experimental neuromas. Exp Neurol 1988; 102:249–253.
99. Chabal C, Russell LC, Burchiel KJ. The effect of intravenous lidocaine, tocainide, and mexiletine on spontaneously active fibers originating in rat sciatic neuromas. Pain 1989; 38:333–338.
100. Wall PD, Gutnick M. Properties of afferent nerve impulses originating from a neuroma. Nature 1974; 248:740–743.
101. Wall PD, Gutnick M. Ongoing activity in peripheral nerves: the physiology and pharmacology of impulses originating from a neuroma. Exp Neurol 1974; 43:580–593.
102. Yaari Y, Devor M. Phenytoin suppresses spontaneous ectopic discharge in rat sciatic nerve neuromas. Neurosci Lett 1985; 58:117–122.
103. Xie X, Lancaster B, Peakman T, Garthwaite J. Interaction of the antiepileptic drug lamotrigine with recombinant rat brain type IIA Na^+ channels and with native Na^+ channels in rat hippocampal neurones. Pflugers Arch Eur J Physiol 1995; 430:437–446.
104. McGeer EG, Zhu SG. Lamotrigine protects against kainate but not ibotenate lesions in rat striatum. Neurosci Lett 1990; 112:348–351.
105. Gillin S, Sorkin LS. Gabapentin reverses the allodynia produced by the administration of anti-GD_2 ganglioside, an immunotherapeutic drug. Am J Med 1995; 103:111–116.
106. Hunter JC, Gogas KR, Hedley LR, Jacobson LO, Kassotakis L, Thompson J, Fontana DJ. The effect of novel anti-epileptic drugs in rat experimental models of acute and chronic pain. Eur J Pharmacol 1997; 324:153–160.
107. Hwang JH, Yaksh TL. Effect of subarachnoid gabapentin on tactile-evoked allodynia in a surgically induced neuropathic pain model in the rat. Reg Anesth 1998; 22:249–256.
108. Houtchens MK, Richert JR, Sami A, Rose JW. Open label gabapentin treatment for pain in multiple sclerosis. Multiple Sclerosis 1997; 3:250–253.
109. Rosenberg JM, Harrell C, Ristic H, Werner RA, de Rosayro AM. The effect of gabapentin on neuropathic pain. Clin J Pain 1997; 13:251–255.
110. Rosner H, Rubin L, Kestenbaum A. Gabapentin adjunctive therapy in neuropathic pain states. Clin J Pain 1996; 12:56–58.
111. Samkoff LM, Daras M, Tuchman AJ, Koppel BS. Amelioration of refractory dysesthetic limb pain in multiple sclerosis by gabapentin. Neurology 1997; 49:304–305.
112. Sist TC, Filadora VA 2nd, Miner M, Lema M. Experience with gabapentin for neuropathic pain in the head and neck: report of ten cases. Reg Anesth 1997; 22:473–478.
113. Rowbotham M, Harden N, Stacey B, Bernstein P, Magnus–Miller L. Gabapentin for the treatment of postherpetic neuralgia: a randomized controlled trial. JAMA 1998; 280:1837–1842.
114. Max MB, Lynch SA, Muir J, Shoaf SE, Smoller B, Dubner R. Effects of desipramine, amitriptyline, and fluoxetine on pain in diabetic neuropathy. N Engl J Med 1992; 326:1250–1256.
115. Geis GS. Update on clinical developments with celecoxib, a new specific COX-2 inhibitor: what can we expect? J Rheumatol 1999; 26(suppl 56):31–36.
116. Rowbotham MC, Reisner–Keller LA, Fields HL. Both intravenous lidocaine and morphine reduce the pain of postherpetic neuralgia. Neurology 1991; 41:1024–1028.
117. Watson CP, Babul N. Efficacy of oxycodone in neuropathic pain: a randomized trial in postherpetic neuralgia. Neurology 1998; 50:1837–1841.
118. Wilson SP, Yeomans DC, Bender MA, Lu Y, Goins WF, Glorioso JC. Antihyperalgesic effects of infection with a preproenkephalin-encoding herpes virus. Proc Natl Acad Sci USA 1999; 96:3211–3216.
119. Finegold AA, Mannes AJ, Iadarola MJ. A paracrine. Paradigm for in vivo gene therapy in the central nervous system: treatment of chronic pain. Hum Gene Ther 1999; 10:1251–1258.
120. Czech KA, Sagen J. Update on cellular transplantation into the CNS as a novel therapy for chronic pain. Prog Neurobiol 1995; 46:507–529.
121. Davar G. Gene therapy for pain. In: Chiocca EA, Breakefield XO, eds. Gene Transfer and Therapy for Neurological Disorders. Totowa, NJ: Humana Press, 1997:419–426.
122. Davar G, Kramer MF, Garber D, Roca AL, Andersen JK, Bebrin W, Coen DM, Kosz–Vnenchak

M, Knipe DM, Breakefield XO, Isacson O. Comparative efficacy of expression of genes delivered to mouse sensory neurons with herpes virus vectors. J Comp Neurol 1994; 339:3–11.

123. Dobson AT, Sederati F, Devi–Rao G, Flanagan WM, Farrell MJ, Stevens JG, Wagner EK, Feldman LT. Identification of the latency-associated transcript promoter by expression of rabbit beta-globin mRNA in mouse sensory nerve ganglia latently infected with a recombinant herpes simplex virus. J Virol 1996; 63:3844–3851.
124. Dobson AT, Margolis TP, Sedarati F, Stevens JG, Feldman LT. A latent, nonpathogenic HSV-1-derived vector stably expresses β-galactosidase in mouse neurons. Neuron 1990; 5:353–360.
125. Ho DY, Mocarski ES. β-Galactosidase as a marker in the peripheral and neural tissues of the herpes simplex virus-infected mouse. Virology 1988; 167:279–283.
126. Saitoh Y, Taki T, Arita N, Ohnishi T, Hayakawa T. Cell therapy with encapsulated xenogeneic tumor cells secreting B-endorphin for treatment of peripheral pain. Cell Transplantation 1995; 4(S1):S13–S17.
127. Wu HH, Wilcox GL, McLoon SC. Implantation of AtT-20 or genetically modified AtT-20/hENK cells in the mouse spinal cord induced antinociception and opioid tolerance. J Neurosci 1994; 14: 4806–4814.

22
Sympathetically Maintained Pain

Ralf Baron and Wilfrid Jänig
Christian–Albrechts University, Kiel, Germany

I. INTRODUCTION

A. Definition of Sympathetically Maintained Pain

Interruption of the sympathetic nerve supply to the affected extremity has been used to treat certain pain syndromes for many years. These syndromes include reflex sympathetic dystrophy (RSD), causalgia, posttraumatic neuralgia, phantom limb pain, and to a certain extent, acute herpes zoster. Two therapeutical techniques to block sympathetic nerves are currently used: (1) injections of local anesthetic around sympathetic paravertebral ganglia that project to the affected body part (sympathetic ganglion blocks), and (2) regional intravenous application of guanethidine, bretylium, or reserpine (which all deplete norepinephrine in the postganglionic axon) to an isolated extremity blocked with a tourniquet (intravenous regional sympatholysis).

In particular, in RSD and causalgia, clinical experience and uncontrolled studies in hundreds of patients show a beneficial effect of these sympatholytic procedures. Therefore, many authors believe that a sympathetic component of the pain is a characteristic feature of these syndromes and, therefore, a successful symptomatic blockade was used as a necessary element for the diagnosis of RSD and causalgia (1,2).

On the other hand, many authors do not support the concept that the sympathetic nervous system is actively involved in the generation of pain, and they propose, that the role of the sympathetic nervous system has to be reconsidered or even completely discarded (3,4). They claim that interventions that block sympathetic activity lack specificity and argue that the techniques and results of sympathetic blockade have rarely been adequately evaluated and are usually not placebo controlled (5).

Recently, a consensus conference discussed this issue. On the basis of experience and recent clinical studies, the following was agreed: Neuropathic pain patients presenting with exactly the same clinical signs and symptoms can clearly be divided into two groups by the negative or positive effect of sympathetic blockade (6,7). The pain component that is relieved by specific sympatholytic procedures is considered *sympathetically maintained pain* (SMP). Thus, SMP is now defined to be a *symptom* and *not a clinical entity*. The positive effect of a sympathetic blockade is not essential for the diagnosis of RSD or causalgia. On the other hand, the only possibility to differentiate between SMP and "sympathetically independent pain" (SIP) is the efficacy of a correctly applied sympatholytic intervention (8).

Furthermore, a new terminology was suggested by the consensus conference participants. It was agreed that the term reflex sympathetic dystrophy is not appropriate as a clinical designation because it has been used to describe a much more extensive range of clinical presentations than originally intended. Moreover, because the pathophysiological mechanisms underlying these syndromes are poorly understood it is probably premature to use terms such as "reflex" and "sympathetic." Therefore, the new terminology is based entirely on elements of history, symptoms, and findings on clinical examination, with no implied pathophysiological mechanism (8). According to the International Association for the Study of Pain (IASP), *Classification of Chronic Pain*, reflex sympathetic dystrophy and causalgia are now called *complex regional pain syndromes* (CRPS). In CRPS type I (reflex sympathetic dystrophy) minor injuries at the limb or lesions in remote body areas precede the onset of symptoms. CRPS type II (causalgia) develops after injury of a major peripheral nerve (9).

II. CLINICAL CHARACTERISTICS OF SELECTED PAIN SYNDROMES WITH SMP

A. CRPS Type II (Causalgia)

As defined by the American Civil War physician, S. Weir Mitchell (10), *causalgia* is burning pain that develops in the distal extremity following traumatic partial peripheral nerve injury. Mitchell had a vast experience with peripheral nerve injury. Among his patients, about 10% had a dramatic clinical syndrome that consisted of prominent distal burning pain. In addition to spontaneous pain, patients reported exquisite hypersensitivity of the skin to light mechanical stimulation. Furthermore, movement, loud noises, or strong emotions could trigger their pain. In addition to sensory abnormalities, Mitchell observed distal extremity swelling, smoothness, and mottling of the skin, and in some cases, acute arthritis. In most cases, the limb was cold and sweaty. Mitchell was emphatic that the sensory and trophic abnormalities spread beyond the innervation territory of the injured peripheral nerve and were often remote from the site of injury. The nerve lesions giving rise to this syndrome were always partial; complete transection never caused it in his patients.

Fifty years after Mitchell, Leriche (11) reported that sympathectomy dramatically relieves causalgia. This notion was confirmed in several large clinical series, primarily in wounded soldiers. In his exhaustive 1967 centennial review, Richards describes the clinical features of causalgia and the effect of sympatholytic interventions in hundreds of cases (12). He was very emphatic about the dramatic response of causalgia to sympathetic blockade. The classic syndrome causalgia, as described by Mitchell, is now included in the term CRPS II.

B. Posttraumatic Neuralgia

It is important to recognize that many posttraumatic neuropathy patients have pain, but do not have the full clinical picture of causalgia. In these cases, in contrast to causalgia patients, the pain is located largely within the innervation territory of the injured nerve (13). Although these patients often describe their pain as burning, they exhibit a less complex clinical picture than patients with causalgia and do not show marked swelling or a tendency for progressive spread of symptoms (see foregoing). The cardinal symptoms are spontaneous burning pain, hyperalgesia, and mechanical and cold allodynia. These sensory symptoms are confined to the territory of the affected peripheral nerve, although allodynia may extend beyond the border of nerve territories to a certain degree. Spontaneous and evoked pain are felt superficially and not deeply inside the extremity, and the intensity of both is not dependent on the position of the extremity. The patients occasionally obtain relief with sympatholytic procedures, although much less often than those with causalgia.

Following the IASP classification it is possible to use the name *neuralgia* for this type of neuropathic pain (pain within the innervation territory of a lesioned nerve; i.e., posttraumatic neuralgia). However, the new definition of CRPS II includes the statement that symptoms may also be limited to the territory of a single peripheral nerve. Therefore, the term CRPS II provides space to include these localized posttraumatic neuropathies. An inherent weakness of this definition of CRPS II is that different syndromes with different underlying mechanisms are obviously included.

C. CRPS Type I (Reflex Sympathetic Dystrophy)

The concept that sympathetic outflow can influence pain was extended to a group of patients without overt nerve injury. These patients develop asymmetrical distal extremity pain and swelling. The disorder was first described by Paul Sudeck early in the century (14). Precipitating events include particularly fracture or minor soft tissue trauma, and more rarely low-grade infection, frostbite, or burns, as well as stroke and myocardial infarction. The swelling and pain often develop at a site remote from the inciting injury, and there is no obvious local tissue damaging process at the site of pain and swelling (15). Because vasomotor (altered skin color and temperature) and sudomotor abnormalities (altered sweat production) are common, the pain and swelling are often spatially remote from the inciting injury, and patients typically obtain dramatic relief with sympathetic block. This syndrome was named *reflex sympathetic dystrophy* (RSD) by Evans in 1946 (16). According to the IASP *Classification of Chronic Pain* (9) reflex sympathetic dystrophy is now called *complex regional pain syndromes* (CRPS) type I. Patients with CRPS I are much more common than those with CRPS II.

CRPS I patients often report a *burning spontaneous pain* (17) felt deeply inside the distal part of the affected extremity. It is characteristically of disproportionate intensity to the inciting event. The pain usually increases when the extremity is in a dependent position. Stimulus-evoked pains are a striking clinical feature. They include mechanical and thermal hyperalgesia. These sensory abnormalities appear earliest and are most pronounced distally and have no consistent spatial relations to individual nerve territories or to the site of the inciting lesion (18,19). Typically, the pain can be elicited by movements and pressure at the joints, even if these are not directly affected by the inciting lesion. In addition, somatosensory deficits may be present.

Autonomic abnormalities include swelling and changes of sweating and skin blood flow (20–24). At normal room temperature the skin temperature of the limbs shows a systematic side difference in about 80% of the patients (i.e., the affected extremity is either warmer or colder). In the acute stages of CRPS I, the affected limb is more often warmer than the contralateral limb. Sweating abnormalities are present in nearly all CRPS I patients. Either hypohidrosis or, more frequently, hyperhidrosis is present, most frequently at the palmar side of the hand or plantar side of the foot (20,21,25,26).

It is possible that there is an inflammatory component of CRPS I in the acute phase. This is based on the observation that in the acute phase all classic signs and symptoms of inflammation—rubor, color, dolor, tumor, and functio laesa—are present. The acute distal swelling of the affected limb depends very critically on aggravating stimuli. Because it often diminishes after sympathetic blocks, it is likely that it is maintained by sympathetic activity (2).

Trophic changes such as abnormal nail growth, increased or decreased hair growth, fibrosis, thin glossy skin, and osteoporosis may be present, particularly in chronic stages. Restrictions of passive movement are often present in long-standing cases and may be related to both functional motor disturbances and trophic changes of joints and tendons. *Weakness* of all muscles of the affected distal extremity is often present although this is difficult to interpret because of pain with effort. Small accurate movements of the affected distal extremity are characteristically impaired (2). Nerve conduction and electromyography studies are normal, except in patients in very chronic and advanced stages. Therefore, the peripheral motor neuron and the neuromuscular junction are unlikely to contribute to the motor dysfunction. About half of the patients have a postural or action tremor that represents an increased physiological tremor (27). In about 10% of cases dystonia of the affected hand or foot develops (28,29).

III. THE EXPERIMENTAL AND CLINICAL BASIS FOR A PATHOLOGICAL INTERACTION OF SYMPATHETIC AND AFFERENT NEURONS

A. Animal Studies

Under physiological conditions, primary afferent nociceptors do not have catecholamine sensitivity and their activity is unaffected by sympathetic outflow (30). However, under pathological conditions a sympathetic–afferent interaction is established, such that the sympathetic efferents can enhance primary afferent nociceptor activity. Two categories of influence of the sympathetic neurons on afferent neurons can be distinguished. This distinction seems to be related to whether the coupling between afferent and sympathetic neurons develops after *traumatic nerve damage* or after *peripheral tissue inflammation* associated with nociceptor sensitization. Traumatic nerve injuries may be used as a model for causalgia and posttraumatic neuralgias in humans, whereas animal models of inflammatory pain may share mechanisms with human reflex sympathetic dystrophy.

1. Influence of Sympathetic Activity and Catecholamines on Primary Afferents After Nerve Damage

After complete nerve injury in experimental animals, surviving cutaneous afferents may develop noradrenergic sensitivity (Fig. 1A). Myelinated and unmyelinated afferents innervating the stump neuroma can be excited by epimephrine or by stimulation of sympathetic efferents that have regenerated into the neuroma (31–34). In mature neuromata the catecholamine sensitivity is much less pronounced (33,35). However, as late as 1 year after complete section and reanastomosis of peripheral nerves, electrical stimulation of the sympathetic trunk remains capable of activating regenerated C fibers, probably of nociceptor function (36). Within 2 weeks of a partial nerve lesion, electrical stimulation of the sympathetic trunk and injections of catecholamines can activate or sensitize C nociceptors in the partially injured nerve, including those in continuity with their peripheral targets (37–39) (see Fig. 1B).

In addition to the peripheral interaction, coupling of sympathetic and afferent neurons may also occur within the dorsal root ganglion (DRG; see Fig. 1A). After a complete nerve lesion, some DRG somata with Aβ-fibers and a few with C fibers develop ectopic activity. Electrical stimulation of sympathetic efferents innervating the DRG may lead to an α_2-adrenoceptor-mediated increase of this spontaneous activity (40–42). This increased adrenergic sensitivity is paralleled by morphological changes within the DRG (see Fig. 1A). After the nerve lesion, sympathetic postganglionic fibers that normally innervate blood vessels within the DRG sprout to form basket-like terminals around large primary afferent somata that project into the

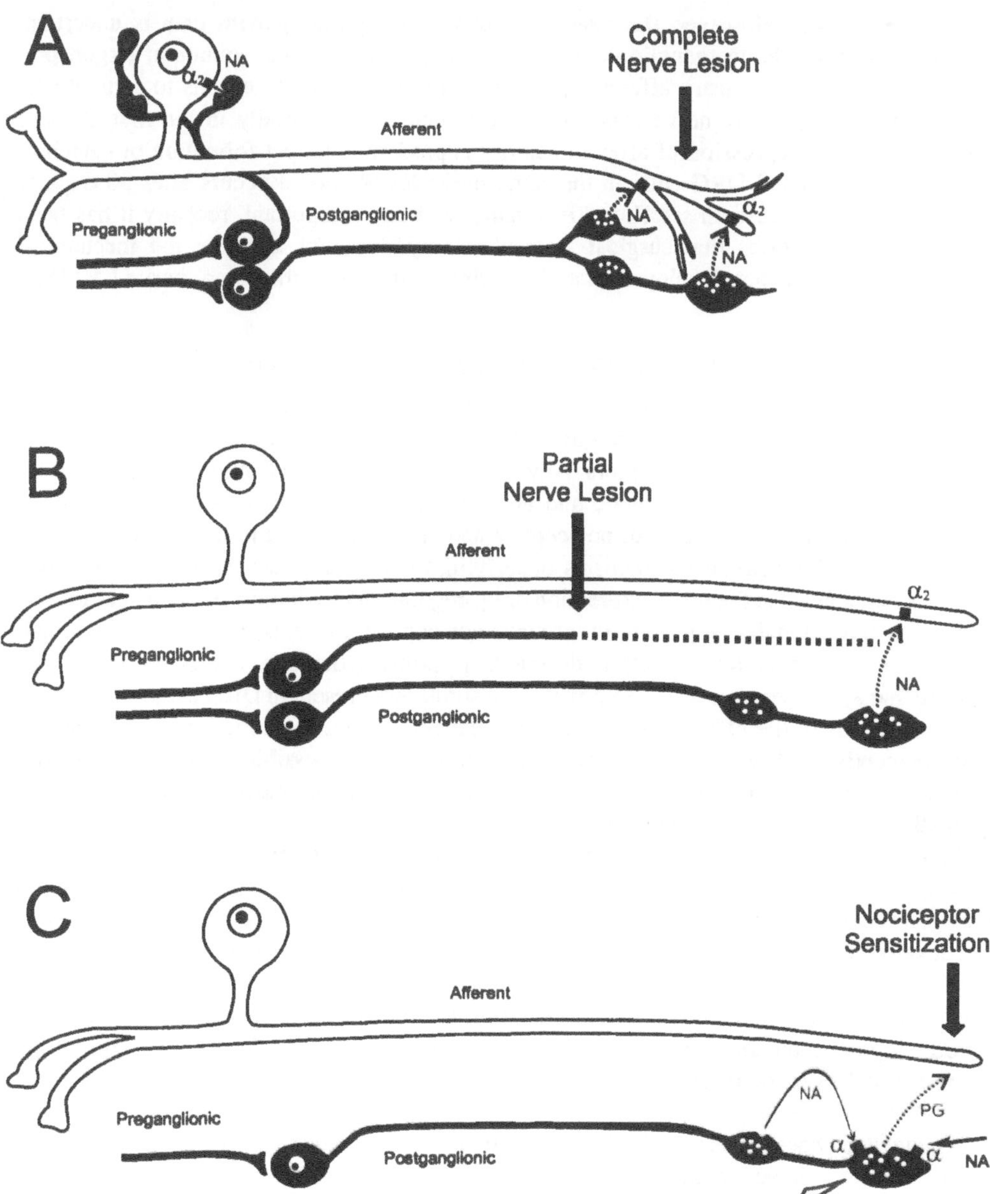

Figure 1 Influence of sympathetic activity and catecholamines on primary afferent neurons: (A) Complete nerve lesion: The sympathetic–afferent interaction is located in the neuroma and in the dorsal root ganglion. It is mediated by norepinephrine (NA) released from postganglionic neurons and a_2-adrenoceptors expressed at the plasma membrane of afferent fibers. (B) Partial nerve lesion: Partial nerve injury is followed by a decrease of the sympathetic innervation density (stippled postganglionic neuron). This induces an up-regulation of functional a_2-adrenoceptors at the membrane of intact nociceptive fibers. (C) After tissue inflammation, intact but sensitized primary afferents acquire nonepinephrinie sensitivity. Norepinephrine is not acting directly on afferents but induces the release of prostaglandins (PG) from sympathetic terminals that sensitize the afferents. In turn bradykinin- and nerve growth factor (NGF)-induced nociceptor sensitization is also mediated by the release of prostaglandins from postganglionic fibers. (From Ref. 74.)

injured nerve (43–45). However, the relation of this DRG sprouting with pain is uncertain. Sprouting of sympathetic postganglionic terminals is largely around the somata of larger, presumably nonnociceptive primary afferents (43). Activation of afferent neurons to sympathetic stimulation following sciatic nerve lesion in the rat occurs preferentially in the first 20 days after lesion, but later depression of afferent activity is predominant, yet formation of catecholaminergic baskets around DRG cells in the same nerve lesion model occurs after 30 days or more (for extensive discussion see Ref. 30). Finally, and most important, recently it has been shown in two laboratories that surgical sympathectomy does not alleviate the mechanical allodynia-like behavior that develops in rats following lesioning of the spinal nerve L5 (46).

2. Adrenoceptors Involved in Chemical Sympathetic–Afferent Coupling

The excitation and depression of axotomized dorsal root ganglion cells and the excitation of afferent terminals in neuromas generated by activation of the sympathetic innervation are suggested to be mediated by α-adrenoceptors. Any hypothesis about this chemical norepinephrine-mediated coupling between sympathetic and afferent neurons has to explain how functional adrenoceptors appear on the surface of nociceptive and other afferent neurons as a consequence of a nerve lesion. The cellular mechanisms underlying the increased sensitivity are unknown. An obvious explanation is the novel expression or up-regulation of adrenoceptors. Alternatively, the receptors may normally be present on primary nociceptive afferents, but not be functional; they may become uncovered and effective during the response to damage. This is consistent with the finding that adrenoceptor mRNA is normally constitutively present in DRG cells (47,48). The affinity for ligands or the effectiveness of the subsequent cellular transduction may change in injured nociceptive and nonnociceptive afferent neurons. These possibilities are not mutually exclusive, and it is possible that several mechanisms contribute simultaneously to the expression of sympathetically mediated afferent excitation.

Perl and co-workers (37,49) suggest, on the basis of their experiments on polymodal nociceptors following partial nerve lesion, that the expression or up-regulation of adrenoceptors in primary afferent neurons is related to the sympathetic denervation of the target tissue, analogous to the development of the so-called denervation supersensitivity that is observed in effector tissues following their denervation (50). This is supported by their recent experimental observation that cutaneous nociceptive C fibers in the rabbit ear may develop adrenoceptor sensitivity following surgical sympathectomy (51). However, the percentage of afferents excited and the number of impulses in the responding afferents to close-arterial injection of norepinephrine are small.

Knowledge about the subtypes of α-adrenoceptor(s) involved in the sympathetic–afferent coupling following nerve trauma is important for an understanding of the underlying neural mechanism, and may be useful in the design of more specific treatment modalities for neuropathic pain conditions involving sympathetic efferent activity. Sato and Perl (37) have shown that excitation and sensitization of polymodal nociceptors in the rabbit ear skin generated by electrical stimulation of the sympathetic supply or by norepinephrine after partial lesion of the auricular nerve is largely mediated by α_2-adrenoceptors. Investigation of sympathetic–sensory coupling at the site of experimental nerve injury in neuromas and at the cell bodies of axotomized afferent neurons using type-selective agonists and antagonists have shown that this transmission is also largely mediated by α_2-adrenoceptors (41). In normal (uninjured) DRG neurons, mRNA for α_{2A}- and particularly α_{2B}-adrenoceptors are present, whereas mRNA for α_1-adrenoceptors is either absent or at a very low level (48). These results were obtained in rats. Caution is required to generalize these results. There may exist species differences as far as the expression of adrenoceptors following trauma is concerned.

3. Influence of Sympathetic Activity and Catecholamines on Primary Afferents After Tissue Inflammation (Intact but Sensitized Primary Afferents)

Animal studies demonstrate that catecholamines can activate primary afferent C nociceptors after thermal (52) and chemical (53,54) sensitization. The sympathetic–primary afferent interaction is mediated by α_2-adrenoceptors (55). After chronic sensitization with chloroform, norepinephrine enhances behavioral responses to nociceptive stimulation (56). Interestingly, surgical sympathetomy prevents the sensitizing effect of injected norepinephrine. These findings indicate that norepinephrine acts indirectly on afferents through the sympathetic postganglionic neuron. Norepinephrine may induce the release of other substances (e.g., prostaglandins; PG) from sympathetic terminals that sensitize the afferents (see Fig. 1C).

Sensitization of nociceptive primary afferents by such proinflammatory mediators as bradykinin and nerve growth factor (NGF) also depends on an intact sympathetic nervous system (57–59). Surgical removal of the postganglionic neurons, but not interruption of the preganglionic axons (decentralization), decreases the sensitizing effect of these substances (60). These results indicate that the sensitizing effect of these substances depends on the anatomical integrity of the postganglionic fibers, rather than sympathetic activity or norepinephrine release. It has been proposed (60) that bradykinin, similar to norepinephrine, acts indirectly on nociceptor terminals by inducing the release of prostaglandins from sympathetic fibers (see Fig. 1C).

It has to be emphasized that most of the evidence to support these conclusions is based on behavioral experiments and the effects of pharmacological interventions. It is tacitly assumed that the behavioral changes reflect sensitivity changes of nociceptors. A direct neurophysiological demonstration for the proposed presynaptic action on postganglionic fibers by bradykinin or norepinephrine that precipitate the sensitization of nociceptive afferents does not yet exist.

However, this concept is of particular interest because of the evidence that, in its early phase, RSD might have an inflammatory component. If this mechanism does contribute significantly to pain, then reducing sympathetic postganglionic neural activity would not be effective, compared with surgical postganglionic sympathectomy. Furthermore, pain relief should occur only days after surgical (postganglionic) sympathectomy if this mechanism were to operate, because it takes days for the sympathetic terminals to degenerate after removal of their cell bodies.

4. Indirect Coupling Between Noradrenergic Nerve Terminals and Nociceptors in the Periphery via the Vascular Bed

The possibility for an indirect coupling between sympathetic and afferent nerve terminals should not be discarded. Dramatic changes may occur in vascular perfusion of the micromilieu surrounding the nociceptors after nerve trauma. These changes are related to the consequences of denervation and reinnervation by postganglionic vasoconstrictor neurons and afferent nociceptive neurons and the development of hyperreactivity of blood vessels (61,62). Whether these changes lead indirectly to sensitization of nociceptors awaits experimental proof. This topic has been discussed in detail (63).

B. Human Experimental Studies

1. Activation of Sympathetic Neurons and Application of Catecholamines

Clinical studies support the idea that nociceptors develop catecholamine sensitivity after complete or partial nerve lesions. Long after limb amputation, injection of norepinephrine around a stump neuroma is reported to be intensely painful (64). Furthermore, intraoperative stimulation of the sympathetic chain induces an increase of spontaneous pain in patients with causalgia

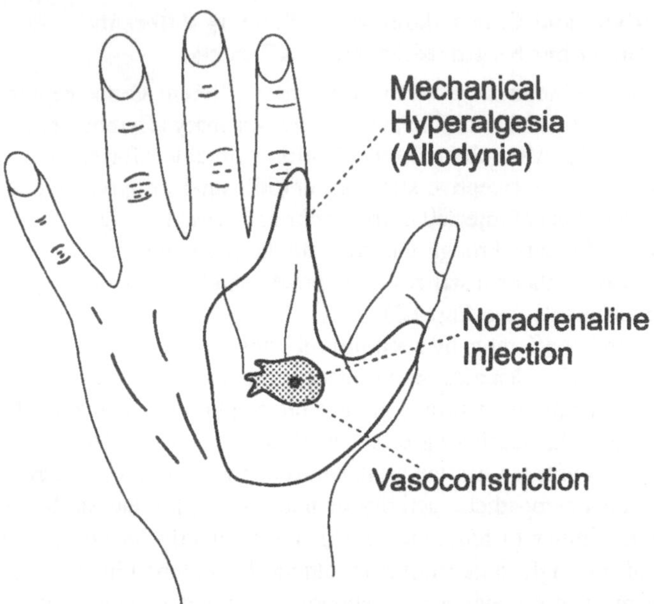

Figure 2 Effect of intracutaneous application of norepinephrine in patients with posttraumatic neuralgias. Application of norepinephrine into a symptomatic skin area was capable of rekindling spontaneous pain and dynamic mechanical hyperalgesia (allodynia) after they had been relieved by sympathetic blockade. This confirms the noradrenergic sensitivity of human cutaneous nociceptors after partial nerve lesion. (From Ref. 67.)

(65,66). In posttraumatic neuralgias, intracutaneous application of norepinephrine into a symptomatic area rekindles spontaneous pain and dynamic mechanical hyperalgesia that had been relieved by sympathetic blockade, confirming the noradrenergic sensitivity of human nociceptors after partial nerve lesion (Fig. 2) (67). In postherpetic neuralgia, spontaneous pain and mechanical hyperalgesia may be enhanced after injection of epinephrine or phenylephrine (68).

Cutaneous application of capsaicin, the purified active ingredient of chili peppers, causes neurogenic inflammation by activating and sensitizing nociceptors. Consistent with animal experiments, an adrenergic effect on sensitized cutaneous nociceptors was recently described in this model in human subjects. Topical capsaicin application followed by norepinephrine iontophoresis increased and prolonged hyperalgesia to heat (69). Moreover, application of phentolamine, an α-adrenoceptor antagonist, reduced pain and mechanical hyperalgesia in capsaicin-sensitized skin (70,71). However, sympathetic cutaneous vasoconstrictor activity modulated in its physiological range by thermoregulatory reflexes was reported not to influence capsaicin-induced pain and mechanical hyperalgesia (72). Furthermore, activation of skin sympathetic vasoconstrictor neurons did not change the mustard oil-induced discharge of single microneurographically recorded cutaneous C nociceptors (73).

IV. CONCLUSION

Animal research and studies in humans have provided extensive evidence in favor of an abnormal coupling between sympathetic and afferent neurons under pathophysiological conditions. Consistent with this idea, clinical experience and uncontrolled studies in hundreds of patients with RSD and causalgia show a beneficial effect of sympatholytic procedures. However, alternative mechanisms for the pain in these syndromes should be addressed and studied under experimental conditions. Furthermore, controlled studies testing the efficacy of sympatholytic procedures are desperately needed to prove that activity in the sympathetic nervous system causes pain in patients with neuropathic pain states.

ACKNOWLEDGMENTS

This work was supported by the Wilhelm Sander–Stiftung (RB), the Alexander von Humboldt–Stiftung (RB), the German Research Foundation (WJ and RB), and the German Israeli Foundation (WJ).

REFERENCES

1. Fields HL. Pain. New York: McGraw Hill, 1987.
2. Blumberg H, Jänig W. Clinical manifestation of reflex sympathetic dystrophy and sympathetically maintained pain. In: PD Wall Melzack eds. Textbook of Pain. New York Churchill Livingstone, 1994:685–697.
3. Schott GD. Visceral afferents: their contribution to "sympathetic dependent" pain. Brain 1994; 117: 397–413.
4. Verdugo RJ, Ochoa JL. "Sympathetically maintained pain." I. Phentolamine block questions the concept. Neurology 1994; 44:1003–1010.
5. Price DD, Long S, Wilsey B, Rafii A. Analysis of peak magnitude and duration of analgesia produced by local anesthetics injected into sympathetic ganglia of complex regional pain syndrome patients. Clin J Pain 1998; 14:216–226.
6. Amér S. Intravenous phentolamine test: diagnostic and prognostic use in reflex sympathetic dystrophy. Pain 1991; 46:17–22.
7. Raja SN, Treede RD, Davis KD, Campbell JN. Systemic alpha-adrenergic blockade with phentolamine: a diagnostic test for sympathetically maintained pain. Anesthesiology 1991; 74:691–698.
8. Stanton–Hicks M, Jänig W, Hassenbusch S, Haddox JD, Boas R, Wilson P. Reflex sympathetic dystrophy: changing concepts and taxonomy. Pain 1995; 63:127–133.
9. Merskey H, Bogduk N. Classification of Chronic Pain: Descriptions of Chronic Pain Syndromes and Definition of Terms Seattle: IASP Press, 1995.
10. Mitchell SW. Injuries of Nerves and their Consequences. New York: Dover, 1865.
11. Leriche R. De la causalgie envisagée comme une névrite du sympathique et de son traitement par la dénudation et l'excision des plexus nerveux péri-artériels. Presse Med 1916; 24:178–180.
12. Richards RL. Causalgia. A centennial review. Arch Neurol 1967; 16:339–350.
13. Baron R, Jänig W. Pain syndromes with causal participation of the sympathetic nervous system. Anaesthesist 1998; 47:4–23.
14. Sudeck P. Über die akute (trophoneurotische) Knochenatrophie nach Entzündungen und Traumen der Extremitäten. Detch Med Wochenschr 1902; 28:336–342.
15. Veldman PHJM. Clinical aspects of reflex sympathetic dystrophy. Dissertation, Nijmegen 1995.
16. Evans JA. Reflex sympathetic dystrophy. Surg Clin North Am 1946; 26:435–448.
17. Galer BS, Jensen MP. Development and preliminary validation of a pain measure specific to neuropathic pain: the Neuropathic Pain Scale. Neurology 1997; 48:332–338.
18. Price DD, Bennett GJ, Rafii A. Psychophysical observations on patients with neuropathic pain relieved by a sympathetic block. Pain 1989; 36:273–288.
19. Price DD, Long S, Huitt C. Sensory testing of pathophysiological mechanisms of pain in patients with reflex sympathetic dystrophy. Pain 1992; 49:163–173.
20. Chelimsky TC, Low PA, Naessens JM, Wilson PR, Amadio PC, O'Brien PC. Value of autonomic testing in reflex sympathetic dystrophy. Mayo Clin Proc 1995; 70:1029–1040.

21. Baron R, Maier C. Reflex sympathetic dystrophy: skin blood flow, sympathetic vasoconstrictor reflexes and pain before and after surgical sympathectomy. Pain 1996; 67:317–326.
22. Baron R, Blumberg H, Jänig W. Clinical characteristics of patients with complex regional pain syndromes in Germany with special emphasis on vasomotor function. In: Jänig W, Stanton–Hicks M, eds. Progress in Pain Research and Management. Vol 6. Reflex Sympathetic Dystrophy—a Reappraisal. Seattle: IASP 5, 1996.
23. Birklein F, Riedl B, Neundörfer B, Handwerker HO. Sympathetic vasoconstrictor reflex pattern in patients with complex regional pain syndrome. Pain 1998; 75:93–100.
24. Wasner G, Heckmann K, Maier C, Baron R. Vascular abnormalities in acute reflex sympathetic dystrophy (CRPS I)—complete inhibition of sympathetic nerve activity with recovery. Arch Neurol 1999; 56:613–620.
25. Low PA, Amadio PC, Wilson PR, McManis PG, Willner CL. Laboratory findings in reflex sympathetic dystrophy: a preliminary report. Clin J Pain 1994; 10:235–239.
26. Birklein F, Sittle R, Spitzer A, Claus D, Neundörfer B, Handwerker HO. Sudomotor function in sympathetic reflex dystrophy. Pain 1997; 69:49–54.
27. Deuschl G, Blumberg H, Lücking CH. Tremor in reflex sympathetic dystrophy. Arch Neurol 1991; 48:1247–1252.
28. Bhatia KP, Bhatt MH, Marsden CD. The causalgia–dystonia syndrome. Brain 1993; 116:843–851.
29. Marsden CD, Obeso JA, Traub MM, Rothwell JC, Kranz H, La Cruz F. Muscle spasms associated with Sudeck's atrophy after injury. Br Med J (Clin Res Edit.) 1984; 288:173–176.
30. Jänig W, Levine JD, Michaelis M. Interactions of sympathetic and primary afferent neurons following nerve injury and tissue trauma. Prog Brain Res 1996; 113:161–184.
31. Devor M, Jänig W. Activation of myelinated afferents ending in a neuroma by stimulation of the sympathetic supply in the rat. Neurosci Lett 1981; 24:43–47.
32. Scadding JW. Development of ongoing activity, mechanosensitivity, and adrenaline sensitivity in severed peripheral nerve axons. Exp Neurol 1981; 73:345–364.
33. Blumberg H, Jänig W. Discharge pattern of afferent fibers from a neuroma. Pain 1984; 20:335–353.
34. Burchiel KJ. Spontaneous impulse generation in normal and denervated dorsal root ganglia: sensitivity to alpha-adrenergic stimulation and hypoxia. Exp Neurol 1984; 85:257–272.
35. Jänig W. Activation of afferent fibers ending in an old neuroma by sympathetic stimulation in the rat. Neurosci Lett 1990; 111:309–314.
36. Häbler HJ, Jänig W, Koltzenburg M. Activation of unmyelinated afferents in chronically lesioned nerves by adrenaline and excitation of sympathetic efferents in the cat. Neurosci Lett 1987; 82:35–40.
37. Sato J, Perl ER. Adrenergic excitation of cutaneous pain receptors induced by peripheral nerve injury. Science 1991; 251:1608–1610.
38. Shyu BC, Danielsen N, Andersson SA, Dahlin LB. Effects of sympathetic stimulation on C-fibre response after peripheral nerve compression: an experimental study in the rabbit common peroneal nerve. Acta Physiol Scand 1990; 140:237–243.
39. O'Halloran KD, Perl ER. Effects of partial nerve injury on the responses of C-fiber polymodal nociceptors to adrenergic agonists. Brain Res 1997; 759:233–240.
40. Devor M, Jänig W, Michaelis M. Modulation of activity in dorsal root ganglion neurons by sympathetic activation in nerve-injured rats. J Neurophysiol 1994; 71:38–47.
41. Chen Y, Michaelis M, Jänig W, Devor M. Adrenoreceptor subtype mediating sympathetic–sensory coupling in injured sensory neurons. J Neurophysiol 1996; 76:3721–3730.
42. Michaelis M, Devor M, Jänig W. Sympathetic modulation of activity in dorsal root ganglion neurons changes over time following peripheral nerve injury. J Neurophysiol 1996; 76:753–763.
43. McLachlan EM, Jänig W, Devor M, Michaelis M. Peripheral nerve injury triggers noradrenergic sprouting within dorsal root ganglia. Nature 1993; 363:543–546.
44. Chung K, Lee BH, Yoon YW, Chung JM. Sympathetic sprouting in the dorsal root ganglia of the injured peripheral nerve in a rat neuropathic pain model. J Comp Neurol 1996; 376:241–252.
45. Chung K, Yoon YW, Chung JM. Sprouting sympathetic fibers form synaptic varicosities in the dorsal root ganglion of the rat with neuropathic injury. Brain Res 1997; 751:275–280.

46. Ringkamp M, Eschenfelder S, Grethel EJ, Häbler H–J, Meyer RA, Jänig W, Raja SN. Lumbar sympathectomy failed to reverse mechanical allodynia- and hyperalgesia-like behavior in rats with L5 spinal nerve injury. Pain 1999; 79:143–153.
47. Nicholas AP, Pieribone V, Hökfelt T. Distributions of mRNAs for alpha-2 adrenergic receptor subtypes in rat brain: an in situ hybridization study. J Comp Neurol 1993; 328:575–594.
48. Pieribone VA, Nicholas AP, Dagerlind A, Hökfelt T. Distribution of alpha 1 adrenoceptros in rat brain revealed by in situ hybridization experiments utilizing subtype-specific probes. J Neurosci 1994; 14:4252–4268.
49. Perl ER. A reevaluation of mechanisms leading to sympathetically related pain. In: Fields HL, Liebeskind JC, eds. Pharmacological Approaches to the Treatment of Chronic Pain: New Concepts and Critical Issues. Progress in Pain Research and Management. Seattle: IASP, 1994:129–150.
50. Fleming WW, Westfall DP. Adaptive supersensitivity. In: Trendelenburg U, Weiner N, eds. Handbook of Experimental Pharmacology Vol 90/I. Catecholamines. New York: Springer Verlag, 1988: 509–559.
51. Bossut DF, Shea VK, Perl ER. Sympathectomy induces adrenergic excitability of cutaneous C-fiber nociceptors. J Neurophysiol 1996; 75:514–517.
52. Roberts WJ, Elardo SM. Sympathetic activation of A-delta nociceptors. Somatosens Res 1985; 3: 33–44.
53. Nakamura M, Ferreira SH. A peripheral sympathetic component in inflammatory hyperalgesia. Eur J Pharmacol 1987; 135:145–153.
54. Hu SJ, Zhu J. Sympathetic facilitation of sustained discharges of polymodal nociceptors. Pain 1989; 38:85–90.
55. Sato J, Suzuki S, Iseki T, Kumazawa T. Adrenergic excitation of cutaneous nociceptors in chronically inflammed rats. Neurosci Lett 1993; 164:225–228.
56. Levine JD, Taiwo YO, Collins SD, Tam JK. Noradrenaline hyperalgesia is mediated through interaction with sympathetic postganglionic neurone terminals rather than activation of primary afferent nociceptors. Nature 1986; 323:158–160.
57. Andreev N, Dimitrieva N, Koltzenburg M, McMahon SB. Peripheral administration of nerve growth factor in the adult rat produces a thermal hyperalgesia that requires the presence of sympathetic postganglionic neurones. Pain 1995; 63:109–115.
58. Woolf CJ, Ma QP, Allchorne A, Poole S. Peripheral cell types contributing to the hyperalgesic action of nerve growth factor in inflammation. J Neurosci 1996; 16:2716–2723.
59. Khasar SG, Miao FJ, Jänig W, Levine JD. Vagotomy-induced enhancement of mechanical hyperalgesia in the rat is sympathoadrenal-mediated. J Neurosci 1998; 18:3043–3049.
60. Khasar SG, Miao FJ–P, Jänig W, Levine JD. Modulation of bradykinin-induced mechanical hyperalgesia in the rat skin by activity in the abdominal vagal afferents. Eur J Neurosci 1998; 10:435–444.
61. Jobling P, McLachlan EM, Jänig W, Anderson CR. Electrophysiological responses in the rat tail artery during reinnervation following lesions of the sympathetic supply. J Physiol (Lond) 1992; 454: 107–128.
62. Koltzenburg M, Häbler HJ, Jänig W. Functional reinnervation of the vasculature of the adult cat paw pad by axons originally innervating vessels in hairy skin. Neuroscience 1995; 67:245–252.
63. Jänig W, McLachlan EM. The role of modifications in noradrenergic peripheral pathways after nerve lesions in the generation of pain. In: Fields HL, Liebeskind JC, eds. Pharmacological Approaches to the Treatment of Pain: New Concepts and Critical Issues. Progress in Pain Research and Mangement. Seattle: IASP, 1994:101–128.
64. Chabal C, Jacobson L, Russell LC, Burchiel KJ. Pain response to perineuromal injection of normal saline, epinephrine, and lidocaine in humans. Pain 1992; 49:9–12.
65. Walker AE, Nulsen F. Electrical stimulation of the upper thoracic portion of the sympathetic chain in man. Arch Neurol Psychiatry 1948; 59:559–560.
66. White JC, Sweet WH. Pain and the Neurosurgeon. Springfield, IL: Charles C Thomas, 1969.
67. Torebjörk E, Wahren L, Wallin G, Hallin R, Koltzenburg M. Noradrenaline-evoked pain in neuralgia. Pain 1995; 63:11–20.

68. Choi B, Rowbotham MC. Effect of adrenergic receptor activation on post-herpetic neuralgia pain and sensory disturbances. Pain 1997; 69:55–63.
69. Drummond PD. Noradrenaline increases hyperalgesia to heat in skin sensitized by capsaicin. Pain 1995; 60:311–315.
70. Liu M, Max MB, Parada S, Rowan JS, Bennett GJ. The sympathetic nervous system contributes to capsaicin-evoked mechanical allodynia but not pinprick hyperalgesia in humans. J Neurosci 1996; 16:7331–7335.
71. Kinnman E, Nygards EB, Hansson P. Peripheral alpha-adrenoreceptors are involved in the development of capsaicin induced ongoing and stimulus evoked pain in humans. Pain 1997; 69:79–85.
72. Baron R, Wasner GL, Borgstedt R, Hastedt E, Schulte H, Binder A, Kopper F, Rowbotham M, Levine JD, Fields HL. Effect of sympathetic activity on capsaicin evoked spontaneous pain, hyperalgesia and vasodilatation. Neurology 1999; 52:923–932.
73. Elam M, Skarphedinsson JO, Olhausson B, Wallin BG. No apparent sympathetic modulation of single C-fiber afferent transmission in human volunteers. In: Abstracts of the 8th World Congress on Pain Vancouver: IASP 1996:398.
74. Baron R. The infuence of sympathetic nerve activity and catecholamines on primary afferent neurons. IASP Newslett May/June 1998; 3–8.

23

Headache

Basic Anatomy and Physiology of the Trigeminovascular System

Peter J. Goadsby
The National Hospital for Neurology and Neurosurgery, London, England

I. INTRODUCTION

Common to any medical problem, understanding emerging treatments or proposing new strategies is facilitated by a grasp of the anatomy and physiology of the relevant body systems. Pain is an excellent example of this principle, and headache a typical case in which basic information can greatly enhance therapeutic understanding. Newer therapies are covered elsewhere in this volume (see Chap. 61), so here I will concentrate on a neurobiological framework for these treatments. Fuller descriptions of the basic issues (1) and the clinical picture have been recently published (2,3). To set the issues in context it is appropriate to outline very briefly the clinical problem and then deal with the anatomy and physiology that can explain much of what is seen in practice.

II. HEADACHE: A CLINICAL PROBLEM

Headache can broadly be considered as being either primary or secondary (4). This distinction is helpful clinically and has biological implications. *Secondary headaches* are headaches caused by some recognized cause, such as infection, blood in the subarachnoid space, or a brain tumor, whereas *primary headaches* are headaches in which the headache is the disease itself and is not caused by any overt structural problem. Although attractive, the tenet of structural normality seems to be incorrect, at least for a rare form of primary headache called cluster headache in which there is activation in the gray matter of the posterior hypothalamic region (5) and structural change with an increase in the size of that region compared with noncluster headache brains (6). Furthermore, the general implication is that secondary headache can be understood in terms of the anatomy and physiology of the cranial pain pathways and their normal central nervous system (CNS) control mechanisms, whereas primary headache requires a further permission or generation system to coherently explain the clinical manifestation. The common primary and secondary headaches are listed in the Table 1, along with their population prevalence. These data illustrate how common headache is and thus the interest in developing headache treatments.

Migraine is the most common of the disabling primary headaches. Migraine is, in essence, an episodic headache with certain associated features (Table 2), and it is these features that give

Table 1 Common Causes of Headache

Primary Headache		Secondary Headache	
Type	Prevalence (%)	Type	Prevalence (%)
Migraine	16	Systemic infection	63
Tension-type	69	Head injury	4
Cluster headache	0.1	Subarachnoid hemorrhage	<1
Idiopathic stabbing	2	Vascular disorders	1
Exertional	1	Brain tumor	0.1

Source: Ref. 79.

Table 2 IHS Features of Migraine

Episodic headache (4–72 h) with the following features:	
Any two of:	Any one of:
Unilateral	Nausea/vomiting
Throbbing	Photophobia and phonophobia
Worsened by movement	
Moderate or severe	

Source: Ref. 4.

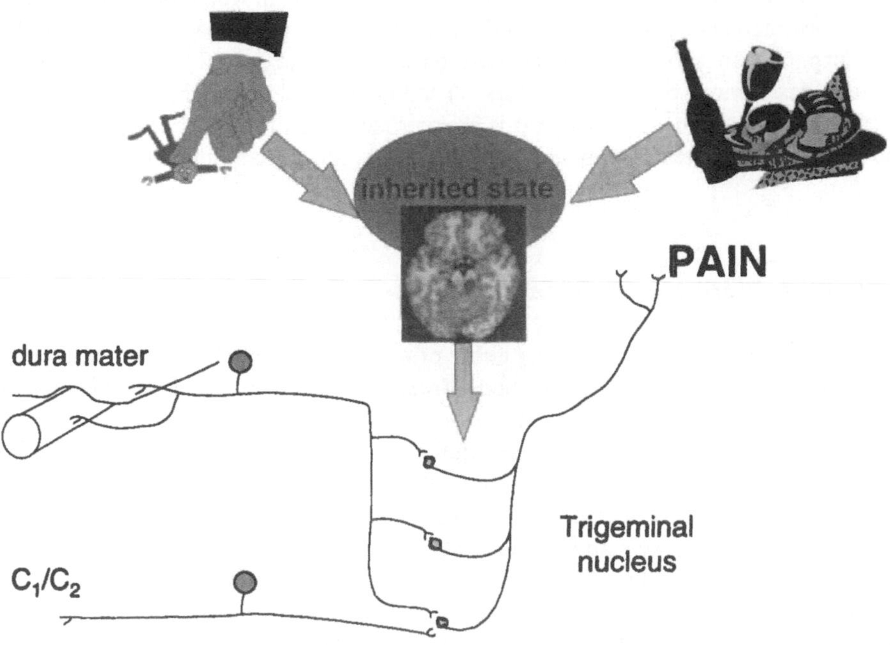

Figure 1 Migraine is an inherited state of the central nervous system that, when challenged by certain triggers such as stress or foodstuffs, results in dysfunction of pain and other sensory control systems that reside in the brain stem or diencephalon. The example of activation in the midbrain from the work of Diener's group is illustrated. Dysfunction in these gating systems allows an excess of afferent information that is perceived as pain, sensitivity to light, sound, or movement. The pivotal information for pain traverses the trigeminal nucleus caudalis with input from intracranial pain-producing structures, such as the large vessels and dura mater, and high cervical structures. This overlap accounts for the pattern of pain in migraine, which does not respect cutaneous innervation patterns. (From Ref. 70.)

the clues to its pathophysiology. Tension-type headache is headache without features. It is my view that both types of primary headache have episodic and chronic forms, but this issue is hotly debated (7,8). The biology of migraine will serve as a template for understanding headache anatomy and physiology (Fig. 1). Migraine is the best-studied form of primary headache, and the fundamental messages concerning trigeminal anatomy and physiology are likely to apply across many forms of headache.

III. BASIC NEUROBIOLOGY OF MIGRAINE

The essential elements to be considered in understanding migraine are the following:

1. Anatomy of head pain, particularly that of the trigeminovascular system.
2. Physiology and pharmacology of activation of the peripheral branches of the ophthalmic branch of the trigeminal nerve as marked by plasma protein extravasation and neuropeptide release.
3. Physiology and pharmacology of the trigeminal nucleus, in particular its caudal most part, the trigeminocervical complex.
4. Brain stem and diencephalic modulatory systems that control trigeminal pain processing

A. Anatomy

1. The Trigeminal Innervation of Pain-Producing Intracranial Structures

Surrounding the large cerebral vessels, pial vessels, large venous sinuses, and dura mater is a plexus of largely unmyelinated fibers that arise from the ophthalmic division of the trigeminal ganglion and in the posterior fossa from the upper cervical dorsal roots. Trigeminal fibers innervating cerebral vessels arise from neurons in the trigeminal ganglion that contain substance P and calcitonin gene-related peptide (CGRP) (9), both of which can be released when the trigeminal ganglion is stimulated either in humans or cats (10). Stimulation of the cranial vessels, such as the superior sagittal sinus (SSS), is certainly painful in humans (11). Human dural nerves that innervate the cranial vessels largely consist of small-diameter–myelinated and unmyelinated fibers that almost certainly subserve a nociceptive function.

What then is the source of pain in migraine? It must be borne in mind that the pain process is likely to be a combination of direct factors (i.e., activation of the nociceptors of pain-producing intracranial structures); in concert with a reduction in the normal functioning of the endogenous pain control pathways that normally gate that pain (12). Certainly, if the carotid artery is occluded ipsilateral to the side of headache in migraineurs, then two-thirds will experience relief, although this does not at all account for the other one-third (13). Moreover, distension of major cerebral vessels by balloon dilation leads to pain referred to the ophthalmic division of the trigeminal nerve (14).

B. Activation of the Trigeminovascular System—Peripheral Connections

1. Plasma Protein Extravasation

Moskowitz (15) has provided an elegant series of experiments to suggest that the pain of migraine may be a form of sterile neurogenic inflammation. Neurogenic plasma extravasation can be seen during electrical stimulation of the trigeminal ganglion in the rat (16). Plasma extravasation can be blocked by ergot alkaloids, indomethacin, acetylsalicylic acid, and the serotonin

(5HT)-1-like agonist, sumatriptan. The pharmacology of the new abortive antimigraine drugs has been recently reviewed in detail (17). In addition, there are structural changes seen in the dura mater that are seen with trigeminal ganglion stimulation, and these include mast cell degranulation (18) and changes in postcapillary venules, including platelet aggregation (18). Although it is generally accepted that such changes, and particularly the initiation of a sterile inflammatory response, would cause pain, it is not clear whether this is sufficient of itself, or if it requires other stimulators or promoters. Some recent clinical data demanding that the role of plasma protein extravasation be reexamined. Moreover, although the plasma extravasation in the retina seen after trigeminal ganglion stimulation in experimental animals can be blocked by sumatriptan, no extravasation is seen with retinal angiography during acute attacks of migraine or cluster headache (19). From these observations and the lack of success of endothelin antagonists (20), conformationally restricted sumatriptan, CP-122,288 (21), and zolmitriptan, 4991W93 (22), analogues, neurosteroids (23), and substance P (neurokinin 1) antagonists (24–27), it can be concluded that blockade of neurogenic plasma protein extravasation is not completely predictive of antimigraine efficacy in humans.

2. Neuropeptide Studies

Electrical stimulation of the trigeminal ganglion in both humans and the cat leads to increases in extracerebral blood flow and local release of both CGRP and SP (10). In the cat, trigeminal ganglion stimulation also increases cerebral blood flow by a pathway traversing the greater superficial petrosal branch of the facial nerve (28), again releasing a powerful vasodilator peptide, vasoactive intestinal polypeptide (VIP) (29). Interestingly, the VIP-ergic innervation of the cerebral vessels is predominantly anterior, rather than posterior, and this may contribute to this region's vulnerability to spreading depression and partly explain why the aura is so very often seen to commence posteriorly. Stimulation of the more specifically vascular pain-producing superior sagittal sinus increases cerebral blood flow (30) and jugular vein CGRP levels (31). Human evidence that CGRP is elevated in the headache phase of migraine (32,33), cluster headache (34,35), and chronic paroxysmal hemicrania (36) supports the view that the trigeminovascular system may be activated in a protective role in these conditions.

3. Clinical Observations of the Trigeminovascular System

Drummond and Lance (13) have shown that in at least one-third of patients there is a significant extracerebral vascular component to the headache. The level of CGRP is elevated in the external jugular vein blood of migraineurs during headache (32), clearly demonstrating some activation of trigeminovascular neurons during migraine, with or without aura. These data have been confirmed in adolescent migraineurs (33). Whether the activity is peripherally generated is again uncertain, although it is clear that such changes partly can be seen in both man and cat with direct stimulation of the trigeminal ganglion (10). The release of these peptides offers the prospect of a marker for migraine that can be readily determined from a simple venous blood sample.

C. Central Processing of Trigeminovascular Pain: the Trigeminocervical Complex

The sites within the brain stem that are responsible for craniovascular pain have begun to be mapped. By using Fos immunohistochemistry (a method for looking at activated cells). Fos production is reported in the trigeminal nucleus caudalis (37), after meningeal irritation with blood whereas Fos-like immunoreactivity is seen in the trigeminal nucleus caudalis and in the dorsal horn at the C1 and C2 levels after stimulation of the superior sagittal sinus in the cat (38) and monkey (39), and in the middle meningeal artery in both species (40). These latter findings are in accord with similar data using 2-deoxyglucose measurements with superior sagittal sinus stimulation (41) and contribute to our view of the trigeminal nucleus extending beyond the traditional nucleus caudalis to the dorsal horn of the high cervical region in a functional continuum that includes a cervical extension, a trigeminal nucleus cervicalis. To complete the anatomical loop, we have recently seen that stimulation of a branch of C2, the greater occipital nerve, increases metabolic activity in the same regions—the trigeminal nucleus caudalis and C1/2 dorsal horn—as is seen with sagittal sinus stimulation (42). Thus, the same group of cells has input from both supratentorial clearly trigeminally innervated structures and from branches of the nerve roots of the high cervical spinal cord, thus accounting for the referral of pain to the neck that is seen so commonly in the clinic. The group of cells could be considered functionally as the *trigeminocervical* complex.

These data demonstrate that a substantial portion of the trigeminovascular nociceptive information comes by way of the most caudal cells. This concept provides an anatomical explanation for the referral of pain to the back of the head in migraine. Moreover, experimental pharmacological evidence suggests that some abortive antimigraine drugs, such as ergots (43), acetylsalicylic acid (44), sumatriptan after blood–brain barrier disruption (45,46), naratriptan (47,48), alniditan (49), eletriptan (50), rizatriptan (51), and zolmitriptan (52) can have actions at these second-order neurons that reduce cell activity and suggest a further possible site for therapeutic intervention in migraine. Furthermore, nitric oxide synthesis inhibition which can inhibit the pain of both migraine (53) and chronic tension-type headache (54) will also attenuate transmission in the trigeminocervical complex (55). If we consider postsynaptic transmission, it is again clear in the experimental animal that activation of *N*-methyl-D-aspartate (NMDA) and α-amino-3-hydroxy-5-methylisoxazole-4-proprionic acid (AMPA) can play a role at this nucleus (56–60).

Thalamic processing. Following transmission in the caudal brain stem and high cervical spinal cord, information is relayed in a group of fibers (the quintothalamic tract) to the thalamus. Processing of vascular pain in the thalamus occurs in the ventroposteromedial thalamus, medial nucleus of the posterior complex, and in the intralaminar thalamus (61). By application of capsaicin to the superior sagittal sinus, Zagami (62) has shown that trigeminal projections with a high degree of nociceptive input are processed in neurons, particularly in the ventroposteromedial thalamus and in its ventral periphery. These findings have been substantiated by evidence in humans in cluster headache and in short-lasting unilateral neuralgiform headaches, with conjunctival injection and tearing (SUNCT) for contralateral thalamic activation using positron-emission tomography (PET) (5) and BOLD contrast fMRI (63). The properties and further higher center connections of these neurons are the subject of ongoing studies that will allow us to build up a more complete picture of the trigeminovascular pain pathways (Table 3).

D. Central Modulation of Trigeminal Pain

In the experimental animal stimulation of a discrete nucleus in the brain stem, the nucleus locus caeruleus (the main central noradrenergic nucleus), reduces cerebral blood flow in a frequency-dependent manner (64) through an α_2-adrenoceptor–linked mechanism (65). This reduction is maximal in the occipital cortex (66). Although a 25% overall reduction in cerebral blood flow is seen, extracerebral vasodilation occurs in parallel (66,67). In addition, the main serotonin-containing nucleus in the brain stem, the midbrain dorsal raphe nucleus, can increase cerebral blood flow when activated (12). Raskin (68) has reported that stimulation of humans in the region of the periaqueductal gray matter can induce a headache indistinguishable from migraine,

Table 3 Neuroanatomical Processing of Vascular Head Pain

Target innervation	Structure	Comments
Cranial vessels Dura mater	Ophthalmic branch of trigeminal nerve	
1st	Trigeminal ganglion	Middle cranial fossa
2nd	Trigeminal nucleus (quintothalamic tract)	Trigeminal n. caudalis and C1/C2 dorsal horns
3rd	Thalamus	Ventrobasal complex Medial n. of posterior group Intralaminar complex
Final	Cortex	Insulae Frontal cortex Anterior cingulate cortex Basal ganglia

and this report has been substantiated (69). These human observations and the animal studies can be viewed with renewed interest given the description in humans of activation of the rostral brain stem in PET studies during migraine without aura (70). These areas are active immediately after successful treatment of the headache, but are not active interictally. Recently, we have demonstrated the activation of neurons in the periaqueductal gray matter with stimulus of the superior sagittal sinus (71), and these neurons can inhibit trigeminal neuronal activation that arises from superior sagittal sinus stimulation (72), reinforcing the importance of understanding brain stem modulatory centers in migraine.

1. Migraine and the Blood–Brain Barrier

Some very compelling data from a clinical study of aura raises the possibility that the blood–brain barrier may not be normal in migraine. In a well-conducted study of patients with migraine with aura, the effect of sumatriptan on the aura was examined. The drug was administered at the onset of aura in a placebo-controlled, double-blind parallel groups study as a 6-mg–subcutaneous injection, thus assuring absorption. In this setting, sumatriptan neither shortened nor lengthened the aura when compared with placebo. The most fascinating aspect of the study was that the incidence of headache in the placebo and the treated group was the same, so that despite having good delivery and a suitable drug level, with the mean length of the aura being 20 min, headache still occurred. What is further and perhaps even more remarkable is that the developed headache responded to a further sumatriptan injection (73). These data suggest that sumatriptan does not have access to a crucial receptor site during aura and that the interaction of the drug concentration and rate of absorption, along with access to the appropriate site are the elements of the equation required to terminate the attack.

What site in the body does sumatriptan not have access to readily? The obvious suggestion is a site behind the blood–brain barrier, which opens up the very exciting possibility that the blood–brain barrier may not be normal in the headache phase of migraine. Indeed, better access to sites within the CNS may be advantageous in drug development, rather than a drawback. Results from clinical studies with newer, more brain-penetrant 5-$HT_{1B/1D}$ agonists, such as eletriptan (74), naratriptan (75), rizatriptan (76), and zolmitriptan (77) indicate that such access to central nervous system sites may confirm an advantage, although more head-to-head comparisons are needed (78).

IV. SUMMARY

An understanding of the basic anatomy and physiology of the cranial circulation facilitates the assessment and management of patients with headache, particularly neurovascular headaches, such as migraine. At the very least, all pain is perceived and processed in the brain. Indeed, with migraine it is likely that the fundamental problem and its clinical expression are driven by the CNS, and thus its study relative to headache is warranted. As therapy evolves, such an understanding will be necessary as new and highly specific receptor-targeted compounds allow us to treat and to improve headache control in our many patients.

ACKNOWLEDGMENTS

The author acknowledges the valuable collaboration of L Edvinsson, KL Hoskin, YE Knight, A May, A Bahra, RJ Storer, J Classey, S Akerman, P Hammond, and M Lasalandra in the conduct of many of the experiments described here. The work of the author's reviewed herein has been supported by the Wellcome Trust and the Migraine Trust. PJG is a Wellcome Senior Research Fellow.

REFERENCES

1. Goadsby PJ, Silberstein SD, eds. Headache. New York: Butterworth-Heinemann, 1997. (Asbury A, Marsden CD, ed. Blue Books in Practical Neurology; vol 17).
2. Lance JW, Goadsby PJ. Mechanism and Management of Headache. (6th ed.) London: Butterworth-Heinemann, 1998.
3. Silberstein SD, Lipton RB, Goadsby PJ. Headache in Clinical Practice. Oxford: ISIS Medical Media, 1998.
4. Goadsby PJ, Olesen J. Diagnosis and management of migraine. Br Med J 1996; 312:1279–1282.
5. May A, Bahra A, Buchel C, et al. Hypothalamic activation in cluster headache attacks. Lancet 1998; 351:275–278.
6. May A, Ashburner J, Buchel C, et al. Correlation between structural and functional changes in brain in an idiopathic headache syndrome. Nat Med 1999; 5:836–838.
7. Silberstein SD, Lipton RB, Sliwinski M. Classification of daily and near-daily headaches: a field study of revised IHS criteria. Neurology 1996; 47:871–875.
8. Olesen J, Rasmussen BK. The International Headache Society classification of chronic daily or near daily headaches: a critque of the criticism. Cephalalgia 1996; 16:407–411.
9. Uddman R, Edvinsson L, Ekman R, et al. Innervation of the feline cerebral vasculature by nerve fibers containing calcitonin gene-related peptide: trigeminal origin and co-existence with substance P. Neurosci Lett 1985; 62:131–136.
10. Goadsby PJ, Edvinsson L, Ekman R. Release of vasoactive peptides in the extracerebral circulation of man and the cat during activation of the trigeminovascular system. Ann Neurol 1988; 23:193–196.
11. Feindel W, Penfield W, McNaughton F. The tentorial nerves and localisation of intracranial pain in man. Neurology 1960; 10:555–563.
12. Goadsby PJ, Zagami AS, Lambert GA. Neural processing of craniovascular pain: a synthesis of the central structures involved in migraine. Headache 1991; 31:365–371.
13. Drummond PD, Lance JW. Extracranial vascular changes and the source of pain in migraine headache. Ann Neurol 1983; 13:32–37.
14. Nichols FT, Mawad M, Mohr JP, et al. Focal headache during balloon inflation in the vertebral and basilar arteries. Headache 1993; 33:87–89.

15. Moskowitz MA. Basic mechanisms in vascular headache. Neurol Clin 1990; 8:801–815.
16. Markowitz S, Saito K, Moskowitz MA. Neurogenically mediated leakage of plasma proteins occurs from blood vessels in dura mater but not brain. J Neurosci 1987; 7:4129–4136.
17. Cutrer FM, Limmroth V, Waeber C, et al. New targets for antimigraine drug development. In: Goadsby PJ, Silberstein SD, eds. Headache. Philadelphia: Butterworth-Heinemann, 1997:59–72.
18. Dimitriadou V, Buzzi MG, Moskowitz MA, et al. Trigeminal sensory fiber stimulation induces morphological changes reflecting secretion in rat dura mater mast cells. Neuroscience 1991; 44:97–112.
19. May A, Shepheard S, Wessing A, et al. Retinal plasma extravasation can be evoked by trigeminal stimulation in rat but does not occur during migraine attacks. Brain 1998; 121:1231–1237.
20. May A, Gijsman HJ, Wallnoefer A, et al. Endothelin antagonist bosentan blocks neurogenic inflammation, but is not effective in aborting migraine attacks. Pain 1996; 67:375–378.
21. Roon K, Diener HC, Ellis P, et al. CP-122,288 blocks neurogenic inflammation, but is not effective in aborting migraine attacks: results of two controlled clinical studies. Cephalalgia 1997; 17:245.
22. Giles H, Honey A, Edvinsson L, et al. Preclinical pharmacology of 4991W93, a potent inhibitor of neurogenic plasma protein extravasation. Cephalalgia 1999; 19:402.
23. Data J, Britch K, Westergaard N, et al. A double-blind study of ganaxolone in the acute treatment of migraine headaches with or without an aura in premenopausal females. Headache 1998; 38:380.
24. Goldstein DJ, Wang O, Saper JR, et al. Ineffectiveness of neurokinin-1 antagonist in acute migraine: a crossover study. Cephalalgia 1997; 17:785–790.
25. Diener HC. Substance-P antagonist RPR100893-201 is not effective in human migraine attacks. In: Olesen J, Tfelt–Hansen P, eds. Proceedings of the 7th-International Headache Seminar. New York: Lippincott–Raven, 1996.
26. Connor HE, Bertin L, Gillies S, Beattie DT, Ward P, The GR205171 Clinical Study Group. Clinical evaluation of a novel, potent, CNS penetrating NK_1 receptor antagonist in the acute treatment of migraine. Cephalalgia 1998; 18:392.
27. Norman B, Panebianco D, Block GA. A placebo-controlled, in-clinic study to explore the preliminary safety and efficacy of intravenous L-758,298 (a prodrug of the NK1 receptor antagonist L-754,030) in the acute treatment of migraine. Cephalalgia 1998; 18:407.
28. Goadsby PJ, Duckworth JW. Effect of stimulation of trigeminal ganglion on regional cerebral blood flow in cats. Am J Physiol 1987; 253:R270–R274.
29. Goadsby PJ, Macdonald GJ. The effect of infusion of various peptide antisera on vasodilatation in the cat common carotid vascular territory. Clin Exp Neurol 1985; 21:115–121.
30. Lambert GA, Goadsby PJ, Zagami AS, et al. Comparative effects of stimulation of the trigeminal ganglion and the superior sagittal sinus on cerebral blood flow and evoked potentials in the cat. Brain Res 1988; 453:143–149.
31. Zagami AS, Goadsby PJ, Edvinsson L. Stimulation of the superior sagittal sinus in the cat causes release of vasoactive peptides. Neuropeptides 1990; 16:69–75.
32. Goadsby PJ, Edvinsson L, Ekman R. Vasoactive peptide release in the extracerebral circulation of humans during migraine headache. Ann Neurol 1990; 28:183–187.
33. Gallai V, Sarchielli P, Floridi A, et al. Vasoactive peptides levels in the plasma of young migraine patients with and without aura assessed both interictally and ictally. Cephalalgia 1995; 15:384–390.
34. Goadsby PJ, Edvinsson L. Human in vivo evidence for trigeminovascular activation in cluster headache. Brain 1994; 117:427–434.
35. Fanciullacci M, Alessandri M, Figini M, et al. Increases in plasma calcitonin gene-related peptide from extracerebral circulation during nitroglycerin-induced cluster headache attack. Pain 1995; 60: 119–123.
36. Goadsby PJ, Edvinsson L. Neuropeptide changes in a case of chronic paroxysmal hemicrania—evidence for trigemino-parasympathetic activation. Cephalalgia 1996; 16:448–450.
37. Nozaki K, Boccalini P, Moskowitz MA. Expression of c-*fos*-like immunoreactivity in brainstem after meningeal irritation by blood in the subarachnoid space. Neuroscience 1992; 49:669–680.
38. Kaube H, Keay K, Hoskin KL, et al. Expression of c-*fos*-like immunoreactivity in the trigeminal nucleus caudalis and high cervical cord following stimulation of the sagittal sinus in the cat. Brain Res 1993; 629:95–102.

39. Goadsby PJ, Hoskin KL. The distribution of trigeminovascular afferents in the non-human primate brain *Macaca nemestrina*: a c-*fos* immunocytochemical study. J Anat 1997; 190:367–375.
40. Hoskin KL, Zagami A, Goadsby PJ. Stimulation of the middle meningeal artery leads to bilateral Fos expression in the trigeminocervical nucleus: a comparative study of monkey and cat. J Anat 1999; 194:579–588.
41. Goadsby PJ, Zagami AS. Stimulation of the superior sagittal sinus increases metabolic activity and blood flow in certain regions of the brainstem and upper cervical spinal cord of the cat. Brain 1991; 114:1001–1011.
42. Goadsby PJ, Hoskin KL, Knight YE. Stimulation of the greater occipital nerve increases metabolic activity in the trigeminal nucleus caudalis and cervical dorsal horn of the cat. Pain 1997; 73:23–28.
43. Hoskin KL, Kaube H, Goadsby PJ. Central activation of the trigeminovascular pathway in the cat is inhibited by dihydroergotamine: a c-*Fos* and electrophysiology study. Brain 1996; 119:249–256.
44. Kaube H, Hoskin KL, Goadsby PJ. Intravenous acetylsalicylic acid inhibits central trigeminal neurons in the dorsal horn of the upper cervical spinal cord in the cat. Headache 1993; 33:541–550.
45. Kaube H, Hoskin KL, Goadsby PJ. Sumatriptan inhibits central trigeminal neurons only after blood–brain barrier disruption. Br J Pharmacol 1993; 109:788–792.
46. Shepheard SL, Williamson DJ, Beer MS, et al., Hargreaves RJ. Differential effects of 5-$HT_{1B/1D}$ receptor agonists on neurogenic dural plasma extravasation and vasodilation in anaesthetized rats. Neuropharmacology 1997; 36:525–533.
47. Goadsby PJ, Knight YE. Naratriptan inhibits trigeminal neurons after intravenous administration through an action at the serotonin ($5HT_{1B/1D}$) receptors. Br J Pharmacol 1997; 122:918–922.
48. Cumberbatch MJ, Hill RG, Hargreaves RJ. Differential effects of the $5HT_{1B/1D}$ receptor agonist naratriptan on trigeminal versus spinal nociceptive responses. Cephalalgia 1998; 18:659–664.
49. Boers PM, Donaldson C, Zagami AS, et al. 5-HT(1A) and 5-HT (1B/1D) receptors are involved in the modulation of the trigemino vascular system of the cat: a microiontophoretic study. Neuropharmacology 2000; 39:1833–1847.
50. Goadsby PJ, Hoskin KL. Differential effects of low dose CP122,288 and eletriptan on Fos expression due to stimulation of the superior sagittal sinus in the cat. Pain 1999; 82:15–22.
51. Cumberbatch MJ, Hill RG, Hargreaves RJ. Rizatriptan has central antinociceptive effects against durally evoked responses. Eur J Pharmacol 1997; 328:37–40.
52. Goadsby PJ, Hoskin KL. Inhibition of trigeminal neurons by intravenous administration of the serotonin (5HT)-1-D receptor agonist zolmitriptan (311C90): are brain stem sites a therapeutic target in migraine? Pain 1996; 67:355–359.
53. Lassen LH, Ashina M, Christiansen I, et al. Nitric oxide synthesis inhibition in migraine. Lancet 1997; 349:401–402.
54. Ashina M, Lassen LH, Bendtsen L, et al. Effect of inhibition of nitric oxide synthase on chronic tension-type headache. Lancet 1999; 353:287–289.
55. Hoskin KL, Bulmer DCE, Goadsby PJ. Fos expression in the trigeminocervical complex of the cat after stimulation of the superior sagittal sinus is reduced by L-NAME. Neurosci Lett 1999; 266:173–176.
56. Mitsikostas DD, Sanchez del Rio M, Waeber C, et al. The NMDA receptor antagonist MK-801 reduces capsaicin-induced c-*fos* expression within rat trigeminal nucleus caudalis. Pain 1998; 76: 239–248.
57. Mitsikotas DD, Sanchez del Rio M, Waeber C, et al. Non-NMDA glutamate receptors modulate capsaicin induced c-*fos* expression within trigeminal nucleus. Br J Pharmacol 1999; 127:623–630.
58. Storer RJ, Goadsby PJ. Trigeminovascular nociceptive transmission involves NMDA and non-NMDA glutamate receptors. Neuroscience 1999; 90:1371–1376.
59. Classey JD, Knight YE, Goadsby PJ. MK-801 reduces Fos-like immunoreactivity in trigeminocervical complex of cat. Cephalalgia 1999; 19:394.
60. Goadsby PJ, Classey JD. Blood flow responses in trigeminocervical complex involve glutamate. Cephalalgia 1999; 19:315.
61. Zagami AS, Goadsby PJ. Stimulation of the superior sagittal sinus increases metabolic activity in

cat thalamus. In: Rose FC, ed. New Advances in Headache Research: 2. London: Smith-Gordon & Co, 1991:169–171.
62. Zagami AS, Lambert GA. Craniovascular application of capsaicin activates nociceptive thalamic neurons in the cat. Neurosci Lett 1991; 121:187–190.
63. May A, Bahra A, Buchel C, et al. Functional magnetic resonance imaging in spontaneous attacks of SUNCT: short-lasting neuralgiform headache with conjunctival injection and tearing. Ann Neurol 1999; 46:791–794.
64. Goadsby PJ, Lambert GA, Lance JW. Differential effects on the internal and external carotid circulation of the monkey evoked by locus coeruleus stimulation. Brain Res 1982; 249:247–254.
65. Goadsby PJ, Lambert GA, Lance JW. The mechanism of cerebrovascular vasoconstriction in response to locus coeruleus stimulation. Brain Res 1985; 326:213–217.
66. Goadsby PJ, Duckworth JW. Locus coeruleus stimulation leads to reductions in regional cerebral blood flow in the cat. J Cereb Blood Flow Metabol 1987; 7:S221.
67. Goadsby PJ, Lambert GA, Lance JW. Effects of locus coeruleus stimulation on carotid vascular resistance in the cat. Brain Res 1983; 278:175–183.
68. Raskin NH, Hosobuchi Y, Lamb S. Headache may arise from perturbation of brain. Headache 1987; 27:416–420.
69. Veloso F, Kumar K, Toth C. Headache secondary to deep brain implantation. Headache 1998; 38: 507–515.
70. Weiller C, May A, Limmroth V, et al. Brain stem activation in spontaneous human migraine attacks. Nat Med 1995; 1:658–660.
71. Hoskin KL, Bulmer D, Lasalandra M, et al. Fos expression in the periaqueductal gray following stimulation of the superior sagittal sinus (SSS) in both the cat and the monkey. Cephalalgia 1998; 18:402.
72. Knight YE, Goadsby PJ. Brainstem stimulation inhibits trigeminal neurons in the cat. Cephalalgia 1999; 19:315.
73. Bates D, Ashford E, Dawson R, et al. Subcutaneous sumatriptan during the migraine aura. Neurology 1994; 44:1587–1592.
74. Goadsby PJ, Ferrari MD, Olesen J, et al. Eletriptan in acute migraine: a double-blind, placebo-controlled comparison to sumatriptan. Neurology 2000; 54:156–163.
75. Dahlof C, Hogenhuis L, Olesen J, et al. Early clinical experience with subcutaneous naratriptan in the acute treatment of migraine: a dose-ranging study. Eur J Neurol 1998; 5:469–477.
76. Tfelt-Hansen P, Teall J, Rodriguez F, et al. Oral rizatriptan versus oral sumatriptan: a direct comparative study in the acute treatment of migraine. Headache 1998; 38:748–755.
77. Palmer KJ, Spencer CM. Zolmitriptan. CNS Drugs 1997; 7:468–478.
78. Goadsby PJ. A *Triptan* too far. J Neurol Neurosurg Psychiatry 1998; 64:143–147.
79. Rassmussen BK. Epidemology of headache. Cephalalgia 1995; 15:45–68.

24

Psychological Factors in Measurement of Pain

Maria Koutantji and Shirley Pearce
University of East Anglia, Norwich, England

I. INTRODUCTION

Pain experience is a result of physiological, psychological, and behavioral processes (1), and it achieves meaning within a cultural context (2,3). The need to measure pain arises in a variety of situations in both clinical and research settings, and more than one of these domains should be sampled to adequately assess the multidimensional nature of pain (4,5). A variety of measures have been developed to assess each component of the pain experience. These include subjective self-report of the sensory and hedonic motivational properties of pain, measures of pain behaviors, measurements of the physiological component of pain experience (6), including magnetic resonance imaging (MRI) technology (7), which are more widely used in experimental work.

In discussing psychological factors in the measurement of pain, we will consider the measures that have been developed for the various aspects of the pain experience, as well as the influence that psychological factors have on the accuracy and reliability of pain measurements. We shall present a brief outline of the most widely used measures to assess subjective psychological and behavioral aspects of pain, and continue with a discussion of the evidence on the effect of psychological factors on pain assessment. Issues specific to measurement of pain in children (8), and the elderly and cognitively impaired people (9) are considered beyond the scope of this chapter.

II. ASSESSING THE PSYCHOLOGICAL/SUBJECTIVE COMPONENT OF PAIN

A. Rating Scales

Rating scales in various forms (verbal, numeric, and visual) have been used extensively in acute, clinical, and experimental pain. Verbal-rating scales range from 5-point scales (e.g., none . . . mild . . . moderate . . . severe . . . unbearable) to 15-point scales, with anchors ranging from extremely weak to extremely intense, with verbal gradations in between 0 or 0-00, with the instruction that 0 represents one end of the pain continuum and the higher number represents the other extreme. Visual analog scales involve asking patients to put a mark on a horizontal line (usually 10 cm in length) with anchors at each end representing the range of pain experience.

All of these measures have been used extensively in both clinical and research settings, and the relative strengths of each have been described (10).

Considerable attention has been given to identifying the most reliable and effective of the various scales (11–14). There is some evidence suggesting that numeric-rating scales are better than visual analog scales in terms of ease of administration and scoring, and elderly people find them easier to complete (11). The 101-point–rating scale has received widespread support in terms of reliability, validity, and patient acceptability. Numeric rating scales, such as the 101-point scale may be more reliable owing to the effects of different verbal anchors on a patient's ratings for both pain intensity and affect scales (5). For example, an anchor "worst pain imaginable" may have a different effect on the patient's perception of the scale space than the anchor "extremely bad pain." Which ever of the rating scales are chosen, they will be limited because they measure only one dimension of the pain experience; hence, it is a limited measure of the total pain experience, which involves the associated mood and behavior. Rating scales are also limited in the sense that, although they appear to have the qualities of ratio scales, they are, in fact, not. For example, the distance between 3 and 4 on the scale may not be the same as the distance between 4 and 5. Hence, the data emerging from the scales should not be subjected to many of the statistical analyses that often are applied to them. Despite these limitations, rating scales are an important part of the assessment of pain and, provided they are used conservatively and with careful interpretation, they will form a core part of the assessment battery.

B. Questionnaires

Alternatives or additions to rating scales are the pain questionnaires. The McGill Pain Questionnaire (MPQ) (15) has been the most widely used pain descriptor questionnaire, and consists of pain adjectives describing sensory, affective, and evaluative qualities of pain. It made a significant contribution in the field, as it drew attention to the affective and evaluative qualities of the pain experience, in addition to sensory attributes. It had been subjected to rigorous psychometric evaluation with equivocal results (3,16). A top-down approach was used in its development in which scientists' and clinicians' language for pain was used to determine the items, as opposed to using patient-derived descriptors. Despite this, it is a useful and widely used measure of the qualitative aspects of pain experience.

Since the development of MPQ there have been a proliferation of self-report questionnaires assessing a variety of pain-related domains. The measures that follow are chosen on the basis of their widespread use or to illustrate the range of domains that are considered of interest to evaluate.

The Fear of Pain Questionnaire (17) and the Pain Anxiety Symptoms Scale (18) are examples of measures developed to assess aspects of mood associated with pain. They need to be used more widely to demonstrate that there are valid and reliable measures for different pain populations and useful predictors of psychological adjustment. They represent an important development, for the earlier measures of mood in pain have focused on depression, rather than anxiety, and have used general measures that have been developed to assess low mood in psychiatric populations [e.g., the Beck Depression Inventory (19)], rather than pain-specific measures. This makes interpretation of scales by pain patients difficult because many of the items covering somatic aspects of depression (e.g., difficulty sleeping) may be scored positively because of their pain experience, rather than depressed mood. This problem of the overlap between pain and somatic symptoms of depression have been discussed (20). An attempt to develop a specific measure of negative pain affect is the Pain Discomfort Scale (21), which may become a useful adjunct to the intensity-rating scales.

Table 1 Some of the Questionnaires Used to Assess Psychological Aspects of Pain

Heightened body awareness
Modified Somatic Perception Questionnaire (23)
Pain-related cognitions
The Pain Cognitions Questionnaire (24)
The Pain Beliefs and Perceptions Inventory (25)
The Pain Beliefs Questionnaire (26)
Coping
The Chronic Pain Coping Inventory (27)
Coping Strategies Questionnaire (28,29)
The Ways of Coping Questionnaire (30): a widely used generic measure of coping that has been extensively used with chronic illness populations
Perceived control over pain and perceived helplessness
The Locus of Control Measure (31)
The Multidimensional Locus of Pain Control Questionnaire (MLPC) (32)
The Arthritis Helplessness Index (33): a disease-specific measure

In recognition of the broad nature of pain experience and the role of cognitions and coping style in adjustment to pain, considerable attention has been devoted in recent years to the development of measures to assess pain beliefs and coping. These are reviewed elsewhere (22) with an outline of the theoretical background to the cognitive behavioral model of pain that has been so influential in the development of pain coping management programs. The main measures and references for their details are provided in Table 1, but at present it is difficult to recommend any specific measure for general use, as many of the measures have been used only on relatively limited populations.

1. Quality of Life Measures

When assessing the severity of chronic pain, an evaluation of its influence on the patient's general life experience is an essential addition to the assessment of the sensory and affective qualities of the pain, because this is the aspect of the chronic pain problem that is most likely to respond to intervention.

A good example of a pain-specific quality of life measure is the West Haven–Yale Multidimensional Pain Inventory (MPI) (34), which has been widely used in chronic pain research to evaluate treatment outcome for psychological pain management studies. It assesses pain severity, interference, control, distress, spouse support, and type of spousal response to pain (e.g., solicitous, distracting, or punishing), and activity (e.g., household, outdoor, away from home, or social).

C. Assessing Pain Behaviors

Pain behavior, or the things people do when in pain, and the limitations on behavior associated with pain experience have attracted attention because they are among the few objectively quantifiable aspects of the pain experience; issues and methods used to date are described elsewhere (35).

Observational methods in which certain behaviors are recorded by trained observers over specified time periods are the most reliable, but may be time-consuming and influenced by routine clinical practice. Self-report measures of pain behavior (e.g., The Phillips Pain Behavior Checklist; 36), are more practical, but less reliable.

Most clinical assessments of pain, especially chronic pain, require patients to recall pain intensity and distress over previous days or weeks. It is assumed that a patient's recall is reasonably accurate, and yet recent research has identified several factors that influence the accuracy of patients' recall and might, therefore, inappropriately influence treatment decisions.

III. THE EFFECT OF PSYCHOLOGICAL FACTORS ON PAIN ASSESSMENT

Current pain levels appear to influence patients' recall of previous pain. For example, Eich et al. (37) compared hourly pain diaries with ratings of minimum, maximum, and usual levels of previous pain completed by headache patients. They found that patients overestimated their prior pain levels when their current pain intensity was high and vice versa, presenting evidence that pain distorts current self-report measures. Similar effects were observed by Smith and Safer (38) when they compared pain ratings and medication use (recorded on an electronic diary) to self-report pain ratings, for the previous day and week, obtained by a group of chronic pain patients before receiving physical therapy (PT), and another group who gave their ratings after physical treatment. Current pain intensity influenced chronic pain patients' recall for both pain levels and medication use. Patients' ratings obtained before PT significantly overestimated pain levels and medication, and patients' ratings received after PT significantly underestimated them. Further confirmation of a pain report bias effect owing to current pain levels was reported by Bryant (39) who studied chronic pain patients before and after a pain management program; patients who reported increased pain or depression over the duration of the program overestimated their pretreatment levels of pain and depression.

Being in pain is also associated with an increased recall of autobiographical memories involving pain. Eich et al. (40), who used an autobiographical memory task in female students, compared retrieval of real-life events when the subjects were experiencing menstrual pain and when they were pain-free. They found that pain promoted recall of unpleasant events when it was associated with depressed mood.

Morley (41) investigated the effects of memories for pain events and non-pain events in medical students. Pain event memories were rated as more surprising, inducing more negative emotional change and provoking greater change in ongoing activity than no-pain event memories. Ratings of intensity and sensory quality were associated with the reported vividness of the pain event memory. None of the subjects reported sensory re-experiencing pain, and 41% of the sample were unable to recall the sensory quality of the pain event. It seems that the memory for a pain event is easily accessible, whereas the elements of the pain experience, such as its sensory and affective qualities, and its somatosensory component are affected by the specific qualities of the pain event. This has also been demonstrated for patients with chronic pain. Wright and Morley (42) show that chronic pain status is also associated with increased recall of autobiographical memories involving chronic pain. Hence, it is reasonable to conclude that current pain intensity levels systematically distort past pain report with low intensity, resulting in underestimation of past pain levels and high pain intensity in overestimation of them.

In summary, the purpose of the pain assessment, the context and setting of the assessment, the type of pain, the developmental stage and cognitive abilities of the patients or participants, and the availability of valid, reliable, and feasible measurements should all guide the selection of pain measurements. There is no one "correct" or "perfect" measure of pain. In interpreting pain ratings we should consider the potential circumstantial and cognitive biases operating, and we should try to minimize these by employing more than one pain measure and selecting the ones that have been shown to be influenced the least. Recent years have seen a great growth in measures of all aspects of pain and, as information grows about their strengths and weaknesses, we should be able to distill a set of measures that goes some way toward Gracely's (43) quest for the ideal pain measure that is sensitive to change, bias-free, and able to discriminate the sensory from the motivational, behavioral, and coping aspects of pain.

REFERENCES

1. Melzack R, Wall PD. The Challenge of Pain. Penguin Books, 1988.
2. Bates MS, Edwards WT, Anderson KO. Ethnocultural variations in chronic pain perception. Pain 1993; 52:101–112.
3. Skevington SM. Psychology of Pain. Wiley, 1995.
4. Turk CD, Melzack R. The measurement of pain and the assessment of people experiencing pain. In: Turk CD, Melzack R, eds. Handbook of Pain Assessment. New York: Guildford, 1992:3–12.
5. Williams AC de C. Pain measurement in chronic pain management. Pain Rev 1995; 2:39–63.
6. Flor H, Miltner W, Birbaumer N. Psychophysiological recording methods. In: Turk CD, Melzack R, eds. Handbook of Pain Assessment. New York: Guildford, 1992:169–190.
7. Talbot JD, Marrett S, Evans AC, Meyer E, Bushnell MC, Duncan GH. Multiple representations of pain in human cerebral cortex. Science 1991; 251:1355–1358.
8. McGrath PJ, Unruh AM. Measurement and assessment of paediatric pain. In: Wall PD, Melzack R, eds. Textbook of Pain. 3rd ed. Edinburgh: Churchill Livingstone, 1994:303–313.
9. Weiner D, Pieper C, McConnell E, Martinez S, Keefe F. Pain measurement in elders with chronic low back pain: traditional and alternative approaches. Pain 1996; 67:461–467.
10. Jensen MP, Karoly P. Self-report scales and procedures for assessing pain in adults. In: Turk CD, Melzack R, eds. Handbook of Pain Assessment. New York: Guildford, 1992:135–151.
11. Jensen MP, Karoly P, Braver S. The measurement of clinical pain intensity: a comparison of six methods. Pain 1986; 27:117–126.
12. Jensen MP, Turner JA, Romano JM. What is the maximum number of levels needed in pain intensity measurement? Pain 1994; 58:387–392.
13. Collins SL, Moore RA, McQuay HJ. The visual analogue pain intensity scale: what is moderate pain in millimetres? Pain 1997; 72:95–97.
14. Jensen MP, Turner LR, Turner JA, Romano JM. The use of multiple-item scales for pain intensity measurement in chronic pain patients. Pain 1996; 67:35–40.
15. Melzack R. The McGill Pain Questionnaire: major properties and scoring methods. Pain 1975; 1: 277–299.
16. Melzack R, Katz J. The McGill Pain Questionnaire: appraisal and current status. In: Turk CD, Melzack R, eds. Handbook of Pain Assessment. New York: Guildford, 1992:152–168.
17. McNeil DW, Rainwater AJ III. Development of the Fear of Pain Questionnaire-III. J Behav Med 1998; 21:389–410.
18. McCracken LM, Zayfert C, Cross RT. The Pain Anxiety Symptoms Scale: development and validation of a scale to measure fear of pain. Pain 1992; 50:76–83.
19. Beck AT, Ward CH, Mendelson M, Mock J. An inventory measuring depression. Arch Gen Psychiatry 1961; 4:561–571.
20. Williams AC de C, Richardson PH. What does the BDI measure in chronic pain? Pain 1993; 55: 259–266.
21. Jensen MP, Karoly P, Harris P. Assessing the affective component of chronic pain: development of the Pain Discomfort Scale. J Psychosom Res 1991; 35:149–154.

22. DeGood DE, Shutty MS Jr. Assessment of pain beliefs, coping and self-efficacy. In: Turk CD, Melzack R, eds. Handbook of Pain Assessment. New York: Guildford, 1992:214–234.
23. Main CJ. The Modified Somatic Perception Questionnaire (MSPQ). J Psychosom Res 1983; 52:157–168.
24. Boston K, Pearce S, Richardson PH. The Pain Cognitions Questionnaire. J Psychosom Res 1990; 34:103–109.
25. Williams DA, Thorn BE. An empirical assessment of pain beliefs. Pain 1989; 36:351–358.
26. Edwards LC, Pearce SA, Turner–Strokes L, Jones A. The Pain Beliefs Questionnaire: an investigation of beliefs in the causes and consequences of pain. Pain 1992; 51:276–282.
27. Jensen MP, Turner JA, Romano JM, Storm SE. The Chronic Pain Coping Inventory: development and preliminary validation. Pain 1995; 60:203–216.
28. Rosenstiel AK, Keefe FJ. The use of coping strategies in chronic low back pain patients: relationship to patient characteristics and current adjustment. Pain 1983; 17:33–44.
29. Swartzman LC, Gwadry FG, Shapiro AP, Teasell RW. The factor structure of the Coping Strategies Questionnaire. Pain 1994; 57:311–316.
30. Folkman S, Lazarus RS. The Ways of Coping Questionnaire. Consulting Psychologists Press, Mind Garden, 1988.
31. Skevington SM. A standardised scale to measure beliefs about controlling pain (BPCQ): a preliminary study. Psychol Health 1990; 4:221–232.
32. Ter Kuile MM, Linssen ACG, Spinhoven P. The development of the Multidimensional Locus of Pain Control Questionnaire (MLPC): factor structure, reliability, and validity. J Psychopathol Behav Assess 1993; 15:387–404.
33. Nicassio PM, et al. The measurement of helplessness in rheumatoid arthritis. The development of the Arthritis Helplessness Index. J Rheumatol 1985; 12:462–467.
34. Turk RD, Kerns DC, Rudy TE. The West-Haven Yale Multidimensional Pain Inventory (WHYMPI). Pain 1985; 23:245–256.
35. Keefe FJ, Williams DA. (1992). Assessment of pain behavior. In: Turk CD, Melzack R, eds. Handbook of Pain Assessment. New York: Guildford, 1992:275–291.
36. Philips HC. Avoidance behaviour and its role in sustaining chronic pain. Behav Res Ther 1987; 25: 273–279.
37. Eich E, Reeves JL, Jaeger B, Graff–Radford SB. Memory for pain: relation between past and present pain intensity. Pain 1985; 23:375–379.
38. Smith WB, Safer MA. Effects of present pain level on recall of chronic pain and medication use. Pain 1993; 55:355–361.
39. Bryant RA. Memory for pain and affect in chronic pain patients. Pain 1993; 54:347–351.
40. Eich E, Rachman S, Lopatka C. Affect, pain and autobiographical memory. J Abnorm Psychol 1990; 99:174–178.
41. Morley S. Vivid memory for "everyday pains." Pain 1993; 55:55–62.
42. Wright J, Morley S. Autobiographical memory and chronic pain. Br J Clin Psychol 1995; 34:255–265.
43. Gracely RH. Pain language and ideal pain assessment. In: Melzack R, ed. Pain Measurement and Assessment. New York: Raven Press, 1983:71–78.

25

Challenges and Pitfalls of Clinical Trials

Evaluating Novel Analgesics for Neuropathic Pain

Christine Nai-Mei Sang
Massachusetts General Hospital and Harvard Medical School, Boston, Massachusetts, U.S.A.

I. INTRODUCTION

The first one or two clinical trials evaluating the efficacy of a novel drug have a direct effect on the future of that drug, and sometimes the future of that class of drugs. Following phases Ia, Ib, and IIa studies, a critical decision must be made: to pursue or not to pursue further clinical development. When treatment differences are found to be large, the concerns over trial design tend to melt away and decisions to proceed are relatively easy. However, results of trials with various classes of analgesics in neuropathic pain have thus far demonstrated that treatment differences are modest, at best (1). Therefore, design choices must be tailored to both the aims of the individual study, as well as to the longer-range goals of drug development. For example, duplicate treatment versus placebo studies, with no regard for dose–effect, would be of little use in guiding the future direction.

Dose selection in the patient population from which the study groups will be chosen is a critical decision point in clinical development. Dose–response relationships should be emphasized early, which would allow for more accurate adjustments of dose in the larger comparative studies. After preliminary evidence of efficacy has been obtained and the dose range has been established, the pharmaceutical sponsor should be able to make a decision about undertaking full development and begin to formulate a New Drug Application (NDA) plan.

The design of controlled clinical trials follows a basic set of principles and guidelines that have been widely reviewed in many books, chapters, and journal articles (2–4). This chapter will consider several pitfalls and explore innovations in the design and analyses of early pivotal comparative clinical trials, particularly those concerning dose-ranging studies and the difficulty of choosing appropriate doses for comparative studies. It will not specifically address other concerns related to the larger comparative therapeutic trials, which occur later in clinical development (i.e., phase III).

II. THE DESIGN

Innovative clinical trial designs are needed to define clinical issues, such as therapeutic window. The discovery of new selective agents to target specific mechanisms has been rapid, but even the development of these agents has been confounded by narrow therapeutic ratios for virtually every potential analgesic class that has undergone clinical development thus far. The potential for toxicity of each new drug in humans differs from that in animals, because of differences in drug metabolism, elimination or binding; schedule dependency owing to exposure time differences; and target cell sensitivity (5). The empiric jump from animal toxicity data to analogous studies in humans largely ignores these inherent differences between species, and animal pharmacological studies provide merely guidance for determining the best starting drug regimens that will maximize the chance of demonstrating efficacy in the absence of toxicity.

The first studies addressing the question of efficacy should consider using flexible-dosing schemes that incorporate doses high enough to be accompanied by some degree of toxicity, rather than fixed-dose study designs. The choice of fixed doses is usually based on the available phase I data in normal volunteers, but are often poorly estimated. First, the maximum dose determined in phase I studies is, in fact, the mean maximum dose tolerated by every patient, who have low and high drug clearances alike (6). Second, on average, patients tolerate higher doses of compounds than human volunteers (7,8). Finally, inadequate doses (unlikely to be associated with side effects) in comparative studies are often chosen to avoid attrition of subjects (9). The incorrect choice of a dose in later comparative trials may partly account for many of the negative studies evaluating potential analgesics. Missing the finding of efficacy in an inadequate dose range when higher doses may demonstrate benefit would adversely affect the clinical development of a potentially useful compound. Doses chosen to be too high may result in unacceptable toxicities that may unfairly halt development of that compound. After such studies are performed, early phase II studies in patients should be performed that incorporate two dose levels: the dose at which patients are expected to benefit, and the dose beyond which toxicity develops (10).

A. Innovations in Late Phase I Trials

In addition to evaluating toxicity, phase I single-blind dose-escalation studies may address not only more sophisticated pharmacokinetics and metabolism, bioavailability, and bioequivalence, and drug interaction studies, but also the question of analgesic efficacy. Although limited by fewer subjects, single-blinding, and a time–treatment interaction, these data would allow for the best-choice doses for later placebo-controlled efficacy studies evaluating the same compound. Because the selection of close ranges are based on results from toxicology studies in at least two animal species, this step is often bypassed because of issues of cost and time, but may potentially risk the future of the drug of interest. Incorporating efficacy outcomes would also be valuable in the case of a steep dose–toxicity curve, or when there is concern that a critical concentration at the target site may be attained (such as penetration of the blood brain barrier).

After these first studies are completed, systematically characterizing a new analgesic's dose–response curve would determine the slope and ceiling of the analgesic effect, which are useful data for the design of subsequent efficacy studies using fixed doses. In addition to choosing several doses of the test drug to establish a dose–response, the use of placebo and one or more standard drugs would have the additional advantage of helping determine the clinical significance of the effect, if an effect is demonstrated. The use of graded doses of the treatment and graded doses of the standard would further allow the determination of the equianalgesic dose levels, as well as the side effect profiles (and, hence, the therapeutic ratios) of the treatment and the standard, and permit future relative potency assays. The doses of the test drug chosen need to be sufficiently wide to result in an effect that approximates the relative potency of the standard.

B. Use of Human Experimental Pain Models

The use of experimental pain models would allow early dose-finding studies in healthy volunteers to incorporate questions of efficacy. These human studies may differentiate between effects on various types of experimental pain stimuli, such as thermal thresholds and heat pain intensity during suprathreshold stimuli (11–13) or various components of models from which we can infer sensitization of central nervous system neurons, such as capsaicin-evoked allodynia (14,15). Because pain syndromes are complex with complicated mechanisms, psychophysical components of experimental pain models may provide the human correlate to behavioral assays in animal pain models for which the pharmacology is being elucidated. Late phase I experimental pain studies in human volunteers may attempt to determine the ascending portion of the sigmoid dose–response curve, such as the use of maximal-tolerated dose and 33% of maximal-tolerated dose (13). However, data generated using these models must be interpreted with caution. There are still no publications that demonstrate the value of treating symptoms associated with these experimental pain methods to predict success in treating chronic neuropathic pain in patients.

C. Systematic Assessment of Dose–Response in Proof of Concept Trials

Dose–response relationships may be evaluated using parallel or crossover designs using randomly assigned fixed doses. Titration schemes may be incorporated, as long as final doses remain fixed. Parallel dose–response studies, however, are limited by group information and a group dose–response curve to determine patient-specific dose–response relations. When the natural history of the pain syndrome is relatively stable, without the expectation of spontaneous improvement or worsening of the primary outcome of interest, a within-patient design, such as the crossover dose–response study may provide individual dose–response curves, as long as spontaneous change may be assessed and separated from the response to an increased dose. However, potential sources of bias such as carryover effects, inadequate washout periods, inconsistent baseline levels of pain intensity, and period effects, may limit the utility of the crossover design. The number of subjects needed for such a study can be minimized by enrolling responders only (16). Unfortunately, such "enrichment" designs may also may limit internal validity by breaking the treatment blind, as each subject has been previously exposed to the treatment being evaluated (17). Moreover, limiting the study group to responders only would reduce the generalizability of the data.

D. Titration Schemes in Multiple Dose Analgesic Regimens

The design of clinical trials using multiple dose regimens should consider drug characteristics in the consideration of dosing schedules, titration schedules, and potential pharmacokinetic interactions with concurrent drugs. Dosing intervals that are too long may result in lower treatment efficacy because of inadequate drug levels. Aggressive titration schedules may increase the risk of serious adverse events that could potentially influence the future of the study drug.

Dose–response relationships are often obscured by titration schemes that titrate to a tolerance or effectiveness endpoint (16). This is because titration may proceed preferentially in those patients who do not respond to the lower dose. Patients who respond to low doses would tend to stay at low doses; patients without benefit at low doses would tend to titrate to higher doses. Unless titration takes place the same way in every patient, it would result in an inability to compare each dose with other doses or with placebo. If the dose–response curve is relatively flat, patients on larger doses may be found to have smaller effects than patients on lower doses, resulting in an overestimate of the dose for future studies. Moreover, because of the possibility of spontaneous change in pain intensity over time, any notable effect may be the result of time and not of an increased dose (16). Therefore, it is advisable to ensure that each subject be titrated at specified intervals, not dependent on response; otherwise, dose will no longer remain an independent variable. Dose changes should occur at the exact time for all subjects, and enough time must be allowed at each dose for the full effect of the drug to take effect. Then, the drug–placebo difference could be compared for each dose level, thereby demonstrating a dose–response relation (16), despite a potential time–treatment interaction. Traditionally, titration to a defined endpoint is a typical method of selecting a dose of analgesic in the clinical setting.

Failure to pick up a treatment effect may be due to an incorrect length of the study period. Many compounds require 4–6 weeks until treatment effects may be detected, whereas other compounds may lose effectiveness over time, as with the development of tolerance. Therefore, the duration of each treatment's maintenance period should carefully consider efficacy data in animal models for each test drug.

E. Phase II Designs

The most commonly used crossover design is the 2 × 2 Latin square design (A-B, B-A; where A and B represent two treatments). Sources of confounding and bias in such designs include inconvenience to patients because of the longer study period, patient withdrawals, unstable disease, sequence (order) effect, period (time) effect, and pharmacological and psychological carryover effects. Paired analyses must account for these effects. Even parallel-designed studies may not be free of potential carryover effects from analgesics received before study entry (18). If we could assume no carryover or period effect, it would be possible to allocate patients to any sequence; in reality, it is necessary to ensure that known and unknown patient variables, which may influence treatment outcome, are equally distributed among treatment groups, and sequences chosen need to be balanced (every treatment is represented in every period with the same frequency). In studies evaluating morphine in chronic cancer pain patients, these include age, race, baseline pain intensity, character and site of pain (19).

U.S. Food and Drug Agency (FDA) statisticians have been reluctant to accept the standard 2 × 2 crossover design. Unlike crossover designs involving three or more treatments, the 2 × 2 Latin square design dose not allow for a valid estimate of carryover effect (persistent effect of the treatment into the next treatment period, such as analgesic effect, rebound pain, or withdrawal), period effect, or sequence effect (treatment-by-period interaction, the influence of time on the outcome of interest) (20). In patients assigned to the sequence B-A, it is possible to observe only how treatment A behaves when it is preceded by treatment B. If treatment A has a different effect during period 2, it is impossible to decide whether the difference is due to an order (sequence) effect or to the treatment period. For example, period 1 estimates are made without having experienced the placebo, in contrast to period 2. Because it follows treatment with active drug, the placebo may be judged less effective during period 2 than if it had been administered during period 1 (20). When there are two treatments with the limitation of two periods, the design A-B, B-A, A-A, B-B is the best compromise in the presence of carryover effects (21). Unfortunately, four times as many patients are required as the traditional A-B, B-A design to achieve the same precision if no carryover effects existed. Designs that allow assessments of potential confounders such as treatment, period, and sequence effect require (1) longer study periods (i.e., A-B-B, B-A-A, A-B-B-A, B-A-A-B,...), or (2) larger numbers of subjects (as mentioned earlier, A-B, B-A, A-A, B-B), and are often no more efficient than parallel group designs. Hence, they are often discouraged by the pharmaceutical sponsor because of increased cost and potentially higher dropout rates in the first case, and a reliance upon between-group comparisons in the second case, for which the study is likely to be underpowered.

Still, crossover designs with three or more periods are frequently used. Williams squares are a variation on the traditional set of balanced Latin squares for which each treatment follows every other one once (if even numbers of treatments are evaluated) or twice (if odd numbers of treatments are evaluated). These require fewer subjects than a complete set of balanced Latin squares (22). Incomplete block crossover designs, in which the last period of a balanced set of sequences are removed, have also been used to assess analgesic efficacy (22). The sequence of treatments remains balanced for order.

The effect of prognostic variables based on symptoms, such as presence of allodynia, or based on mechanisms inferred from sensory findings [such as repeated painful electric shocks and repeated suprathreshold heat pulses (23)] on the response to treatment may be controlled by blocking or matching in parallel studies or stratifying in either parallel or crossover studies (24). In the randomized blocks design, treatments are randomly assigned to patients paired to form pairs or blocks matched by (for example) presence of mechanical allodynia. For example, one member of each pair is randomly assigned to receive treatment, while the other receives placebo or the comparator. Matching criteria must not be so tight that they result in an inability to match subjects with each other. The use of stratification also permits control of prognostic variables. Patients may be randomly assigned to treatment groups using a randomization schedule set up for each stratum by initial severity of pain, type of pain, or concurrent analgesics. In the analysis, it is important to evaluate a potential treatment-by-stratum interaction, to identify those patients for whom the treatment may be useful or have toxicity.

In the final analysis, it is necessary to weigh the advantages of the design and treatment options against the cost of running such trials (including the cost of negative results and, therefore, the potential to miss the further development of a potential winner).

F. Combination Studies

Combination therapy used in a fixed-dose ratio may provide a more robust analgesic effect by acting (theoretically) at different sites such that a critical threshold for toxicity for either site is not achieved. Such studies should not test treatments that target similar pain mechanisms (for example, two NMDA receptor antagonists). One would then predict an analgesic effect that is at least additive, and greater than the combined side effects. Designs that characterize synergism require several doses of many dose ratios involving the use of multiple doses of each drug and the combination (25,26). There are few if any controlled studies systematically evaluating analgesic synergism in humans (27), and we may look forward to future studies using new designs (28).

III. THE SUBJECTS

Selection bias is a common source of error in study design. Selection bias may occur if the treatments are assigned preferentially to one treatment group, leading to systematic error between treatment groups. Preferentially entering patients with prior exposure to an analgesic in the same drug class as the test compound, subjects who have responded in the past to one of the drugs under study, or subjects who have failed on a drug in the same class as the active control, may also potentially result in bias. It may be possible to stratify by these variables with enough power to provide answers that may aid in the design of subsequent comparative trials.

Poor selection of the study population by clinicians may result in bias. Contributing to this is disagreement among physicians over the diagnostic criteria critical to the selection of patients as subjects. Clinical findings may be simply wrong as compared with an independent standard of accuracy (29). Sources of variability include age, gender, liver disease, concurrent drugs (inducers and inhibitors of biotransformation or metabolism), and the capacity for drug metabolism.

IV. OTHER SOURCES OF SYSTEMATIC ERRORS AND BIAS

Treatment-related bias has the potential for either concealing a treatment difference when one exists, or claiming that one exists when it does not.

A. Inadequate Blinding

Unblinding can create an artificial treatment benefit. In a single-dose study of clonidine, versus codeine, versus ibuprofen, versus placebo, Max et al. (30) noted that for all treatments, especially for placebo, greater pain relief was reported during trials in which patients noted side effects. Moscucci et al. (31) assessed patients' blindedness to treatment at the end of a double-blind clinical trial evaluating an oral antiobesity drug versus inert placebo. There was a tendency for more side effects and better outcome in the subgroup of subjects who guessed that they were receiving active medication, including those receiving placebo (placebo responders). The only predictor of guessing active medication was the presence of adverse side effects. Therefore, an active placebo may be useful to mimic the side effects of the test drugs under study.

The study personnel's preference for treatment or the unblinding of treatment assignment by side effects may also influence the evaluation of the study drug. Noseworthy et al. (32) in a trial evaluating the efficacy of cyclophosphamide versus plasma exchange in alleviating symptoms of multiple sclerosis, demonstrated that the unblinded, but not the blinded, neurologists' scores showed efficacy of plasma exchange, and concluded that physician blinding prevented an erroneous conclusion about treatment efficacy (false-positive type 1 error).

B. Poor Compliance

Poor compliance is the most common cause of nonresponse to medication and can undermine the validity of clinical trials (33). In early-phase clinical trials, noncompliance may interfere with assessment of pharmacokinetics and toxicity of the drug, which may result in an inappropriate dose selection for later clinical studies. If compliance is low, results may demonstrate no treatment effect exists when, in fact, one exists, or underestimate the minimally effective dose or toxicities (34). Age, education, gender, intelligence, and race have a limited effect on compliance; in contrast, self-administered treatments and long-term treatments are associated with poor compliance (33). Manual pill counts, often used to assess compliance, are associated with significant intersubject and intrasubject variability, which is masked by long-term averages (34).

C. Use of Concomitant Analgesics

Multiple concomitant analgesics are frequently used in the treatment of neuropathic pain, many of which are continued at stable doses during the clinical trial. Concurrent analgesics during the trial may result in potential drug interactions involving the cytochromes P450 1A2, 2D6, and 3A3/4 isoenzymes, and may be predictable based on the knowledge of which compounds induce, inhibit, or are metabolized by the specific cytochrome P450 enzymes. For example, genes encoding P450 2D6 exhibit polymorphism leading to clinical phenotypes showing extensive or poor drug metabolism (35). Substrates include codeine, methadone, oxycodone, tricyclic antidepressants (amitriptyline, nortriptyline), SSRIs (fluoxetine, paroxetine), antipsychotics (haloperidol), sodium channel blockers (mexiletine), and dextromethorphan (36). Inhibitory interactions may lead to elevated test drug levels, whereas inductive interactions may lead to inadequate test drug levels, resulting in an increased risk of either developing toxicity or dosing that is inadequate. On the other hand, if the study drug itself induces or inhibits hepatic metabolism, any treatment effect may be attributed to alterations in blood levels of concomitant analgesics, rather than to the test drug itself (37). Such effects should be considered when choosing dose ranges for subsequent trials. Post hoc stratification by the effect of concurrent medications on hepatic metabolism (enzyme induction versus inhibition) may be useful in the analysis, but is unlikely to be adequately powered. Although concentration-controlled trials attempt to minimize pharmacokinetic variability, they may not address pharmacodynamic differences in response (6).

V. THE ANALYSIS

Bias may be introduced during the analysis phase of a trial. The following are a few common statistical pitfalls.

Sheiner (38) cited a study by McQuay et al. (39) as one example of an interesting result not fully appreciated because an inappropriate analysis was performed in an otherwise commendable study. McQuay et al. evaluated 5, 10, and 25 mg of oral bromfenac compared with acetaminophen and placebo in a double-blind parallel group study. They concluded that no significant distinction was achieved between the 10- and 25-mg bromfenac doses, using pairwise comparisons of the mean response over time between the two doses. In fact, Sheiner argues, because a regression analysis was not performed, a dose–response relation was missed that would have demonstrated that a ceiling effect had not been reached.

Patients are often excluded in the analysis because they have not fully complied with the treatment regimen or were later deemed ineligible. If eligibility criteria are reevaluated, then analysis should be performed and presented for each subgroup of patients, as well as an analysis of all patients enrolled in the study (intent-to-treat analysis). The intent-to-treat analysis may lack power and dilute out a treatment effect, as variable compliance results in an increase in type II error for the original test (38). On the other hand, an interpretation of the analysis based on completers alone may introduce significant bias because compliance itself may represent an outcome (based on tolerability or side effects) (40). It is, therefore, usually preferable to perform both analyses, particularly in small clinical trials that address not only efficacy but also mechanisms.

If outcome data are missing for reasons associated with the treatment (e.g., if a patient drops out because of a good or poor response to the treatment), then this may bias the results. If the endpoint is measured over a finite range (e.g., visual analog scale), the data can be analyzed first using the lowest possible value for the missing point, then with the highest possible value. If the two analyses result in the same overall conclusion, then they may be presented (24). Independent analyses of the subgroup of dropouts should also be performed.

The validity of peeking at the data without intending to change plans to stop or continue based on the result, is a hotly debated topic (3). Among analgesic trials without stopping rules, interim analyses are common. For any individual analysis, the greater the number of significance tests that are performed, the greater the chance of finding significance where none exists. Moreover, when a test of significance is performed at various points over the course of a study, the probability of obtaining a significant result approaches unity (3). Therefore, unless strict stopping rules with adjusted p values are enforced, interim analyses should be avoided.

VI. SUMMARY

Late phase I and early phase II randomized controlled comparative trials of novel analgesics serve as the pivotal step in the decision to go forward to phase III trials, which are designed to identify treatment effect of a clinically appropriate size. Time spent up front during exploratory development to establish dose–response values for analgesia would allow the determination of optimizing the clinical doses used in later clinical development.

ACKNOWLEDGMENTS

I would like to thank Dr. Abraham Sunshine for his critical review of the manuscript.

REFERENCES

1. Kingery WS. A critical review of controlled clinical trials for peripheral neuropathic pain and complex regional pain syndromes. Pain 1997; 73:123–139.
2. Max MB. Neuropathic pain syndromes. In: Max MB, Portenoy RK, Laska EM, eds. The Design of Analgesic Clinical Trials. New York: Raven Press, 1991:193–219.
3. Meinert CL. Clinical Trials: Design, Conduct, and Analysis. New York: Oxford University Press, 1986:212.
4. Friedman L. Fundamentals of Clinical Trials. 2nd ed. Littleton: PSG Publishing, 1985.
5. Collins JM, Zaharko DS, Dedrick RLC, Habner BA. Potential roles for preclinical pharmacology in phase I clinical trials. Cancer Treat Rep 1986; 70:73–80.
6. Johnston A, Holt DW. Concentration-controlled trials: what does the future hold? Clin Pharmacokinet 1995; 28:93–99.
7. Sramek JJ, Hurley DJ, Warley TS, Satterwhite JH, Hourani J, Dies F, Cutler NR. The safety and tolerance of xanomeline tartrate in patients with Alzheimer's disease. J Clin Pharmacol 1996; 35: 800–806.
8. Leppik IE, Marinenau KJ, Graves NM, Rask CA. MK-801 for epilepsy: a pilot study. Neurology 1988; 38:405.
9. Schmidt R. Dose-finding studies in clinical drug development. Eur J Clin Pharmacol 1988: 34:15–19.
10. Maxwell C. The dose response relationship and clinical trials. In: Lasagna L, Erill S, Naranjo CA, eds. Dose–Response Relationships in Clinical Pharmacology. Amsterdam: Elsevier Science, 1989: 1131–1140.
11. Beecher HK. The measurement of pain. Pharm Rev 1957; 9:59–209.
12. Chapman CR, Casey KL, Dubner R, Foley KM, Gracely RH, Reading AE. Pain measurement: an overview. Pain 1985; 22:1–31.
13. Sang C, Hostetter MP, Gracely RH, Chappell AS, Schoepp DD, Lee G, Whitcup S, Caruso R, Max MB. AMPA/kainate antagonist LY293558 reduces capsaicin-evoked hyperalgesia but not pain in normal skin in humans. Anesthesiology 1998; 89:1060–1067.
14. Simone DA, Baumann TK, LaMotte RH. Dose-dependent pain and mechanical hyperalgesia in humans after intradermal injection of capsaicin. Pain 1989; 38:99–107.

15. Sang CN, Gracely RH, Max MB, Bennett GJ. Capsaicin-evoked mechanical allodynia and hyperalgesia cross nerve territories. Evidence for a central mechanism. Anesthesiology 1996; 85:491–496.
16. Temple R. Dose–response and registration of new drugs. In: Lasagna L, Erill S, Naranjo CA, eds. Dose–Response Relationships in Clinical Pharmacology. Amsterdam: Elsevier Science, 1989:145–167.
17. Leber PD, Davis CS. Threats to the validity of clinical trials employing enrichment strategies for sample selection. Contr Clin Trials 1998; 19:178–187.
18. Beaver WT. Measurement of analgesic efficacy in man. Adv Pain Res Ther 1983; 5:411–434.
19. Kaiko RF, Wallenstein SL, Rogers AG, Houde RW. Sources of variation in analgesic responses in cancer patients with chronic pain receiving morphine. Pain 1983; 15:191–200.
20. Woods JR, Williams JG, Tavel M. The two period crossover design in medical research. Ann Intern Med 1989; 110:560–566.
21. Laska E, Meisner M, Kushner HB. Optimal crossover designs in the presence of carryover effects. Biometrics 1983; 39:1087–1091.
22. Jones D, Kenward MG. Design and Analysis of Cross-Over Trials. London: Chapman & Hall, 1989.
23. Price DD, Mao J, Frenk H, Mayer DJ. The *N*-methyl-D-aspartate receptor antagonist dextromethorphan selectively reduces temporal summation of second pain in man. Pain 1994; 59:165–74.
24. Fleiss JL. The Design and Analysis of Clinical Experiments. New York: John Wiley & Sons, 1986.
25. Laska E, Meisner M, Siegel C. Simple designs and model-free tests for synergy. Biometrics 1994; 50:834–841.
26. Berenbaum MC. What is synergy? Pharmacol Rev 1989; 41:93–141.
27. Sethna NF, Liu M, Gracely R, Bennett GJ, Max MB. Analgesic and cognitive effects of intravenous ketamine–alfentanil combinations versus either drug alone after intradermal capsaicin in normal subjects. Anesth Analg 1998; 86:1250–1256.
28. Plummer JL, Short TG. Statistical modeling of the effects of drug combinations. J Pharmacol Methods 1990; 23:297–309.
29. Koran LM. The reliability of clinical methods, data and judgments. N Engl J Med 1975; 293:642–646.
30. Max MB, Schafer SC, Culnane M, Dubner R, Gracely RH. Association of pain relief with drug side effects in postherpetic neuralgia: a single-dose study of clonidine, codeine, ibuprofen, and placebo. Clin Pharmacol Ther 1988; 43:363–371.
31. Moscucci M, Byrne L, Weintraub M, Cox C. Blinding, unblinding, and the placebo effect: an analysis of patients' guesses of treatment assignment in a double-blinded clinical trial. Clin Pharmacol Ther 1987; 41:259–265.
32. Noseworthy JH, Ebers GC, Vandervoort MK, Farquhar RE, Yetisir E, Roberts R. The impact of blinding on the results of a randomized, placebo-controlled multiple sclerosis clinical trial. Neurology 1994; 44:16–20.
33. Boudes P. Drug compliance in therapeutic trials: a review. Contr Clin Trials 1998; 19:257–268.
34. Rudd P, Byyny RL, Zachary V, LoVerde ME, Titus C, Mitchell WD, Marshall G. The natural history of medication compliance in a drug trial: limitations of pill counts. Clin Pharmacol Ther 1989; 46:169–176.
35. Cholerton S, Daly AK, Idle JR. The role of individual human cytochromes P450 in drug metabolism and clinical response. Trends Pharmacol Sci 1992; 13:434–439.
36. Virani A, Mailis A, Shapiro LE, Shear NH. Drug interactions in human neuropathic pain pharmacotherapy. Pain 1997; 73:3–13.
37. Levy RH, Mattson RH, Meldrum BS, eds. Antieptileptic Drugs. 4th ed New York: Raven Press, 1995:1063–1070.
38. Sheiner LB. The intellectual health of clinical drug evaluation. Clin Pharmacol Ther 1991; 50:4–9.
39. McQuay HJ, Carroll D, Frankland T, Harvey M, Moore A. Bromfenac, acetaminophen, and placebo in orthopedic postoperative pain. Clin Pharmacol Ther 1990; 47:760–766.
40. Buyse ME. Analysis of clinical trial outcomes: some comments on subgroup analyses. Controlled Clin Trials 1989; 10(4 suppl):187S–194S.

26
Molecular Approaches to the Study of Pain

Richard A. Newton, C. Patrick Case and Sally N. Lawson
University of Bristol, Bristol, England

Sharon Bingham, Philip Davey, Andrew D. Medhurst, Val Piercy, Pravin Raval, Andrew A. Parsons, and Gareth J. Sanger
SmithKline Beecham Pharmaceuticals, Harlow, Essex, England

I. INTRODUCTION

Both tissue injury and peripheral nerve damage cause barrages of impulses along primary afferent nociceptive neurons. Both the primary afferent neurons and spinal cord neurons in nociceptive pathways can become sensitized, leading to chronic pain. Insights into the molecular changes accompanying the development of abnormal sensation may be gained by monitoring changes in gene expression in these neurons. It is, therefore, necessary to have an effective means of identifying those genes that are differentially expressed among the approximately 15,000 expressed in a particular cell (1). Widely used approaches are the selection of known candidate genes for analysis, and screening methods to search for those genes for which expressions are changed. In contrast to candidate gene strategies, screening methods identify both known and novel genes and are not susceptible to prior assumptions. This chapter will, therefore, describe the application of screening methods to pain research.

Gene expression can be studied by monitoring mRNA levels, with several different screening strategies in existence for identifying and isolating those mRNAs that differ in abundance under altered conditions. The emerging oligonucleotide array technologies (2) will potentially provide the most rapid and comprehensive screen for differential gene expression; however, they are currently restricted to known genes and require specialized and expensive imaging equipment. The techniques of differential hybridization and subtractive hybridization provide two major approaches for distinguishing mRNAs in comparative studies, and both have been successfully applied to the identification of genes involved in peripheral nerve injury (3) and nociceptor function (4). A third, more recent and sensitive technique is mRNA differential display (5), and the intent of this chapter is to describe the application of this technique to the search for previously undetected alterations in gene expression in primary afferent neurons using a model of neuropathic pain. Initially, however, the essential features of the more commonly used differential and subtractive hybridization techniques will be summarized.

II. DIFFERENTIAL HYBRIDIZATION

As with the other screening techniques, it is necessary to synthesize a DNA copy of the mRNA population using the enzyme reverse transcriptase (RT). This DNA that has been reverse transcribed from RNA, is known as complimentary DNA (cDNA). In differential hybridization, cDNA synthesis is carried out in the presence of a labeled deoxynucleotide so that the labeled cDNA is a complex probe derived from all the mRNAs. Probes generated with RNA isolated from two experimental conditions are used to screen a cDNA library previously prepared from the tissue in which differential expression is being examined. For example, differential hybridization has been used to examine the expression of mRNAs in dorsal root ganglia (DRG) following injury to the peripheral axons of the DRG (3). A cDNA library was constructed with RNA extracted from DRG 3 days after sciatic nerve crush. Probes derived from RNA isolated from DRG either ipsilateral or contralateral to the injury were then used to screen small aliquots of this library. Comparison of replicate membranes of the library hybridized with the two sets of probes identifies clones of mRNAs with reduced or increased hybridization signals, which are potentially differentially expressed. Following their studies, De Leon et al. reported the increased expression of 0.15% of the clones screened, and they identified and confirmed the induction in damaged neurons of a fatty acids binding protein, DA11.

Although the technique is technically straightforward, its use is limited to the detection of high-abundance mRNAs because the cDNAs derived from rare mRNAs will have only a very small fraction of radioactivity present in the complex probe.

III. SUBTRACTIVE HYBRIDIZATION

There are several different subtractive hybridization techniques, including recent ones based on the polymerase chain reaction (PCR) (6). Here, we shall give a brief description of a commonly used approach similar to that applied to the isolation of peripheral nervous system-specific genes such as the SNS sodium channel (7). A large amount of RNA from a control sample is photobiotinylated and hybridized to a smaller amount of single-stranded cDNA from the experimental sample. The biotinylated mRNA:cDNA hybrids represent sequences expressed in both conditions, which are removed by the addition of avidin, followed by phenol–chloroform extraction. The nonbiotinylated, single-stranded cDNAs remaining in aqueous solution can then be inserted into a vector to generate a library of potentially up-regulated sequences. Although the technique can detect rare RNAs, the presence of residual, noninduced clones following subtraction presents a significant problem. These false-positives can be reduced by increasing the amount of control sample RNA; however, it will also result in only strongly induced mRNAs being detected. The technique also allows assessment of changes in only a single direction.

IV. DIFFERENTIAL DISPLAY

This PCR-based technique has several advantages over the previous methods for isolating differentially expressed genes including:

1. The ability to simultaneously analyze multiple samples
2. The simultaneous detection of decreased and increased expression
3. High sensitivity, which allows detection of low-copy number mRNAs
4. Low quantity of mRNA required

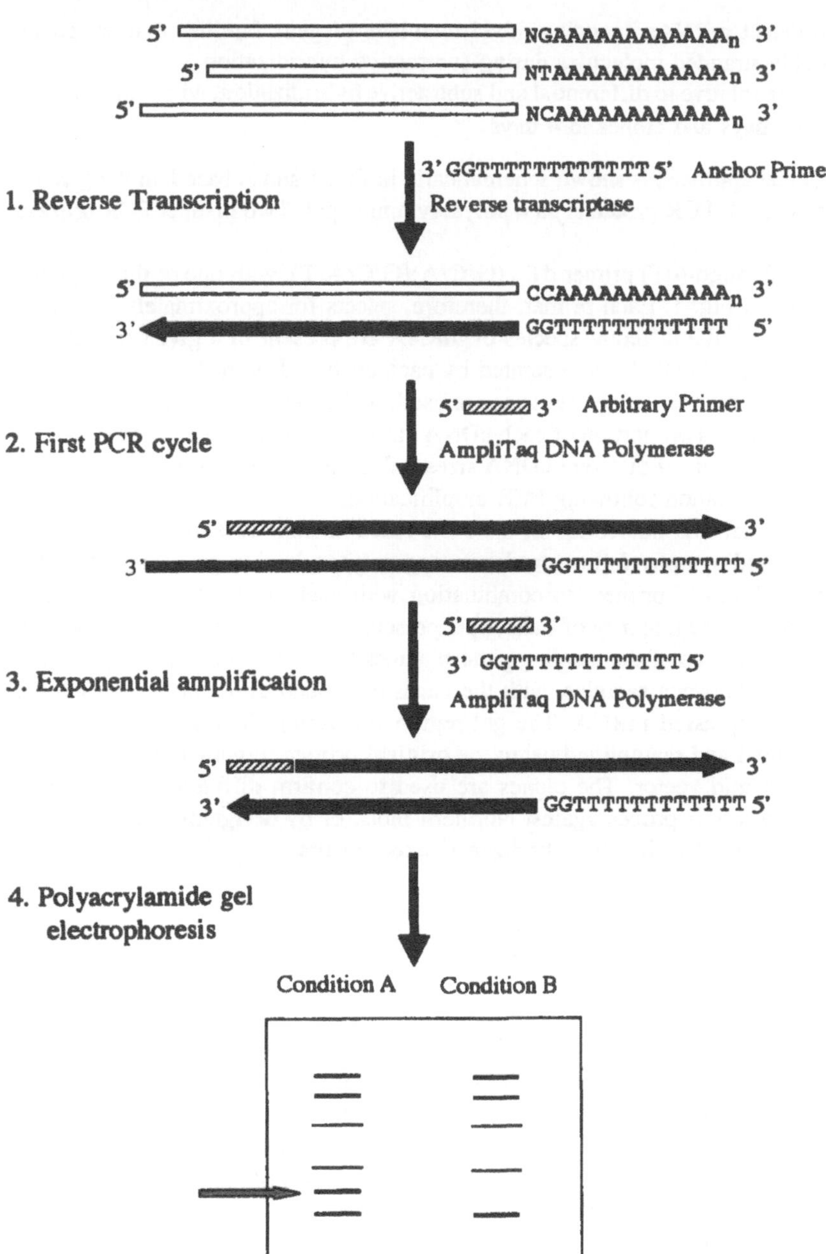

Figure 1 Schematic representation of differential display: (1) Each cDNA synthesis uses a primer that anchors to the two nucleotides upstream from the poly-A tail of mRNAs. The primer $dT_{12}GG$ represents one of 12 possible two-base anchored primers which, following reverse transcription, creates one of the 12 possible cDNA pools. (2) In the first PCR cycle, an upstream primer of arbitrary sequence hybridizes to a proportion of the cDNAs at different positions in different cDNAs. Primer extension by Taq polymerase then creates a double-stranded cDNA. (3) Exponential amplification in the presence of a radiolabeled nucleotide generates sufficient product for visualization by gel electophoresis and autoradiography. A differentially expressed band is indicated by the arrow.

5. Ability to detect mRNAs encoding novel members of gene families that are easily lost as double-stranded molecules during subtractive hybridization
6. Fast procedure relative to differential and subtractive hybridization, with band patterns obtained in 2 days and clones in 4 days

The general experimental approach is shown schematically in Fig. 1 and is based on the generation of subpopulations of RT-PCR products on a polyacrylamide gel. Two distinct PCR primers are utilized:

1. An anchored 3′ oligo-(dT) primer dT_{12} (G/C/A)(G/C/A/T), with one of the 12 possibilities, dT_{12}GG, shown in Fig. 1. Each primer, therefore, selects for approximately 1/12th of the mRNA. Since about 15,000 different species of mRNA are present in a given cell, then a subset of approximately 1,250 cDNAs is generated by each anchored primer.

2. A 5′ arbitrary primer of defined sequence is used, which, at an appropriate annealing temperature, will hybridize to a proportion of each cDNA subset at a region of varying distances from their 3′ end: 50–100 bands of different cDNA sizes will be generated for a given arbitrary and anchored primer combination following PCR amplification.

Inclusion of a radiolabeled nucleotide in the PCR reaction mixture allows the products to be visualized by autoradiography following denaturing polyacrylamide gel electrophoresis. The use of different arbitrary 5′ primers in combination with each of the twelve 3′ primers should lead to the display of the majority of transcripts present in a cell. Differential expression is assessed by visual comparison of the banding pattern across lanes. The vast majority of PCR products will be identical between samples, with the occasional band differences representing a putative differentially expressed mRNA. The gel region containing the differential band is excised, the DNA is eluted and reamplified using the original primer combination, and then is finally cloned into a plasmid vector. The clones are used to confirm differential expression, either by using them directly as probes against Northern blots, or by designing specific oligonucleotides for use in RT-PCR or in situ hybridization experiments.

V. APPLICATION OF DIFFERENTIAL DISPLAY TO THE STUDY OF NEUROPATHIC PAIN

Differential display has previously been successfully used to identify genes expressed in regenerating motor and sensory neurons following crush injury of the sciatic nerve (8). We wanted to identify genes associated with painful neuropathy, particularly relative to diabetic neuropathy, one of the major complications of diabetes. Therefore, we used an animal model of neuropathic pain based on a unilateral partial injury of the sciatic nerve (9) and applied it to Zucker Diabetic Fatty (ZDF) rats in addition to lean (LN) nondiabetic rats. Differential display was then used to assess changes in gene expression in ipsilateral and contralateral L4 and L5 DRG. The presence of diabetes may augment or depress expression of injury-related genes and change expression of novel genes. A similar experimental design was used to examine expression of growth-associated proteins following crush injury in control and streptozocin-induced diabetic rats (10).

VI. EXPERIMENTAL DESIGN

Withdrawal latencies to a noxious thermal stimulus, applied separately to each foot, were measured, and a mean baseline withdrawal was calculated. Approximately half the left sciatic nerve was unilaterally ligated at thigh level, and 14 days after surgery, thermal hyperalgesia was tested in LN and hyperglycemic ZDF rats. Animals were used for differential display only if they showed both guarding of the ipsilateral paw, and a ratio of latency at day 14/presurgery baseline latency for the ipsilateral side that was less than 0.8. L4 and L5 DRG were isolated from the ipsilateral (L) and contralateral (R) side of hyperalgesic and sham-operated rats and total RNA prepared. DRG from several hyperalgesic animals were also retained for in situ experiments. Differential display analysis was performed using the Hieroglyph mRNA Profile System (Genomyx Corporation).

Probably the major disadvantage reported with differential display is a potentially high false-positive rate, where clones isolated from differential bands on a gel subsequently fail to replicate the expression pattern in confirmation experiments. Therefore, we incorporated several strategies to diminish this possibility:

1. RNA isolations were processed as a batch to increase standardization between animals then aliquots of RNA pooled as detailed in the following.
2. For both ZDF and LN hyperalgesic rats, the animals were divided into two pools (A and B) which both had similar mean levels of hyperalgesia. This gave eight RNA sample lanes:

POOL A		POOL B		POOL A		POOL B	
ZDF (L)	ZDF (R)	ZDF (L)	ZDF (R)	LN (L)	LN (R)	LN (L)	LN (R)

Only changes that were replicated between the independent pools were considered for further analysis.

3. Sham ZDF and sham LN controls were included to give a further four lanes:

Sham ZDF (L)	Sham ZDF (R)	Sham LN (L)	Sham LN (R)

4. Extended sequencing gels were run on the GenomyxLR DNA sequencer to maximize resolution of bands and, thereby, to avoid cloning similarly migrating sequences.
5. Long anchor and arbitrary primers were used. Following low-stringency annealing for the first few cycles of PCR, these could be used under stringent conditions for subsequent cycles, thereby preventing mispriming during the amplification process.
6. RNA samples to which no reverse transcriptase was added were also used as a template to check for the presence of DNA contamination from the RNA isolation procedure.

VII. VALIDATION OF EXPERIMENTAL MODEL AND TECHNIQUE

Targeted differential display is a variation on the standard technique that uses a 5′ primer for which the sequence is designed to match a known gene, rather than being of an arbitrary nature. If the sequence of the 3′-untranslated (UTR) region is known, then the appropriate anchor primer can be selected and the size of the product predicted. We designed a 5′ primer for a message that is known to be induced following rat sciatic nerve injury; vasoactive intestinal peptide (VIP)

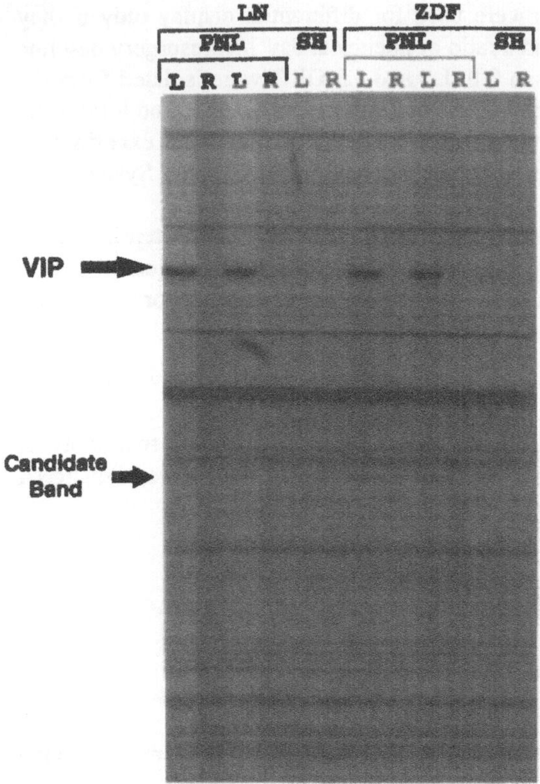

Figure 2 Autoradiogram showing a section of a differential display gel: Lanes show cDNAs obtained from mRNA from ipsilateral (L) and contralateral (R) DRG of ZDF and LN rats following unilateral partial nerve ligation (PNL) or sham (SH) surgery. A 5′ primer homologous to an upstream region of the VIP gene was used in combination with the $dT_{12}GC$ anchor and gave rise to the approximately 1-kb band indicated. A differential band of much lower intensity that was unrelated to VIP is also visible. It can be seen that both bands are present only in the ipsilateral side of nerve-injured animals.

mRNA (11). The 3′ UTR region of VIP mRNA ends . . . $TTGCA_n$; hence, a $dT_{12}GC$ anchor was used in combination with a 5′ primer homologous to a region approximately 1-kb upstream. A product of this expected size was clearly evident and was present in only the ipsilateral lanes of hyperalgesic animals (Fig. 2). The identity of the band as VIP was confirmed following cloning and sequencing. Since in differential display the initial primer annealing is carried out at low stringency, many transcripts unrelated to VIP are also amplified. Indeed, a second differential band of lower intensity is also indicated in Fig. 2. Subsequent cloning and sequencing revealed that it was unrelated to the glucagon polypeptide family; therefore, the VIP primer was also functioning as an arbitrary primer. The two bands of Fig. 2 also illustrate the range of band intensities seen, which may reflect either the initial relative abundance of their mRNAs or differences in primer homology and thus priming efficiency.

VIII. EXPERIMENTAL RESULTS AND DISCUSSION

We utilized 22 different arbitrary primers that can be used in combination with the 12 anchored primers to give a possible 264 primer combinations. Because 50–100 bands are observed per gel, this number of combinations would display close to 20,000 mRNAs, the approximate number in a cell. However this does not take into account the inevitable redundancy of the displays (i.e., some mRNAs will be displayed more than once, whereas others, particularly rare messages, will not be detected). Despite incomplete coverage of the mRNA population with such primer combinations, the technique still provides an excellent chance of detecting important changes in gene expression under conditions for which the number of genes differentially expressed is fairly high. So far, the use of 104 primer combinations in our experiments has identified 18 bands that are differentially expressed between ipsilateral and contralateral DRG of hyperalgesic animals: 17 represented bands that were up-regulated ipsilaterally and 1 band was down-regulated in ipsilateral DRG. Each band has been cloned and, for each, confirmation is attempted by designing specific RT-PCR primers for the predominant clone of each band. Currently, five clones have undergone RT-PCR confirmation with four replicating the original expression pattern on the gel. Three of these confirmed clones show a similar level of ipsilateral induction in LN and ZDF rats, whereas the other clone demonstrated a greater induction in the DRG of ZDF than in LN rats.

The majority of clones isolated so far fail to match those deposited in any sequence databases. This could be due to the mRNA identified being novel, or it may be a consequence of the 3′ UTR targeting inherent with differential displays and, therefore, represents the 3′ UTR of a characterized mRNA for which the sequence in this region is unknown. This latter possibility is reduced in our system by the bands selected being between 0.4 and 1.8 kb, which increases the chance of obtaining sequence information in the coding region. The 5′ upstream sequence of the confirmed differential clones that appear novel are being determined using the 5′ RACE method (12).

An additional caveat alluded to previously is that the cloning of a band often gave rise to several different clones owing to comigrating DNA species in addition to the DNA of interest. Although initially representing a small percentage of the band, these comigrating species increase their proportion during reamplification and may also clone more efficiently. The clone we isolated that did not replicate the expression pattern may represent just such a species. This problem can be circumvented by purifying the eluted band on a single-strand conformation polymorphism gel before reamplification and cloning (13). A final note of caution is that, frequently, large differences seen on the gel are subsequently confirmed as much less dramatic changes demonstrating the essentially qualitative nature of the technique when a fixed number of PCR cycles are used (14).

The differential display procedure described here represents an excellent alternative to subtractive or differential hybridization techniques. The results demonstrate the ability of the technique to identify differentially expressed genes in a pain model when the appropriate experimental strategies are adopted. Correct application of the technique to various pain models should allow further elucidation of the molecular changes occurring during the development of aberrant sensation.

REFERENCES

1. Alberts B, Bray D, Lewis J, Raff M, Roberts K, Watson JD. Molecular Biology of the Cell. 2nd ed. New York: Garland, 1989.
2. Hoheisel JD. Oligomer-chip technology. Trends Biotechnol 1997; 15:465–469.
3. De Leon M, Welcher AA, Nahin RH, Liu Y, Ruda MA, Shooter EM, Molina CA. Fatty acid binding protein is induced in neurons of the dorsal root ganglia after peripheral nerve injury. J Neurosci Res 1996; 44:283–292.

4. Akopian AN, Abson NC, Wood JN. Molecular genetic approaches to nociceptor development and function. Trends Neurosci 1996; 19:240–246.
5. Liang P, Pardee AB. Differential display of eukaryotic messenger RNA by means of the polymerase chain reaction. Science 1992; 257:967–971.
6. Diatchenko L, Lau YF, Campbell AP, Chenchik A, Moqadam F, Huang B, Lukyanov S, Lukyanov K, Gurskaya N, Sverdlov ED, Siebert PD. Suppression subtractive hybridization: a method for generating differentially regulated or tissue-specific cDNA probes and libraries. Proc Natl Acad Sci USA 1996; 93:6025–6030.
7. Akopian AN, Wood JN. Peripheral nervous system-specific genes identified by subtractive cDNA cloning. J Biol Chem 1995; 270:21264–21270.
8. Livesey FJ, O'Brien JA, Li M, Smith AG, Murphy LJ, Hunt SP. A Schwann cell mitogen accompanying regeneration of motor neurons. Nature 1997; 390:614–618.
9. Seltzer Z, Dubner R, Shir Y. A novel behavioral model of neuropathic pain disorders produced in rats by partial sciatic nerve injury. Pain 1990; 43:205–218.
10. Mohiuddin L, Tomlinson DR. Impaired molecular regenerative responses in sensory neurones of diabetic rats. Diabetes 1997; 46:2057–2062.
11. Nielsch U, Keen P. Reciprocal regulation of tachykinin- and vasoactive intestinal peptide-gene expression in rat sensory neurones following cut and crush injury. Brain Res 1989; 481:25–30.
12. Frohman MA. Rapid amplification of complementary DNA ends for generation of full-length complementary DNAs: thermal RACE. Methods Enzymol 1993; 218:340–356.
13. Mathieu-Daude F, Cheng R, Welsh J, McClelland M. Screening of differentially amplified cDNA products from RNA arbitrarily primed PCR fingerprints using single strand conformation polymorphism (SSCP) gels. Nucleic Acids Res 1996; 24:1504–1507.
14. Bauer D, Muller H, Reich J, Riedel H, Ahrenkiel V, Warthoe P, Strauss M. Identification of differentially expressed mRNA species by an improved display technique (DDRT–PCR). Nucleic Acids Res 1993; 21:4272–4280.

27
Molecular Validation of Pain Targets

Simon Tate
Glaxo Wellcome Research and Development, Stevenage, Hertfordshire, England

I. INTRODUCTION

The explosion of information, which is now provided from the rapidly expanding field of molecular biology, has made a significant impression on pain research. Not only have several novel targets been identified, but also the molecular identity of many existing pain targets, previously characterized by their pharmacological properties, has been resolved. One can now obtain rapid distribution data on any target of interest using polymerase chain reaction (PCR) technology. More detailed distribution information can be gained from Northern-blotting protocols, ribonuclease (RNase) protection assays, and in situ and immunohybridization. These breakthroughs in distribution analysis now let the pain researcher correlate the time course of gene expression changes with measures of behavioral hyperalgesia in animal models of pain. (1,2). Perhaps the most significant influence of molecular biology on the field of pain research has been the cloning, expression, and functional analysis of genes thought to be involved in the underlying pathophysiology of pain. Examples of this include the cloning of the opioid receptor gene family (3–8), the cannabinoid receptors (9,10), the bradykinin receptors, B_1 and B_2 (11,12), the cholecystokinin (CCK)-B receptor (13), and the neurotrophin receptor family (14). Once cloned, the use of heterologous expression systems coupled with the ability to genetically manipulate the target amino acid sequence has permitted detailed structure–function relations to be determined (15–17). Additional information can be obtained from the combination of mRNA distribution using in situ hybridization with receptor autoradiography (18).

Two very powerful methods are now available for the determination of gene function: namely, the antisense gene knockdown approach and homologous recombination gene knockout technology. Both of these methods allow the systematic study of the molecular mechanisms underlying the pathology. The principal advantages of these techniques are that the primary genetic lesion will be known and that any pathology will occur in the context of the whole animal. Access to gene knockout technologies can provide useful target validation information, because selective pharmacological antagonists are often unavailable, especially when the target of interest is a novel gene product. For detailed reviews on antisense and knockout approaches, undertaken relative to pain research, the reader is referred to Fraser and Wahlestedt (19) and Mogil and Grisel (20).

The rest of this chapter focuses on two gene families that have recently been defined at the molecular level and have been of particular interest to the academic and industrial research communities. The elucidation of cycloxygenase-2 (COX-2) and the sensory neuronal-specific voltage-gated sodium channels as pain targets and the methods used to validate these genes in pain pathophysiology, will be discussed.

II. CYCLOOXYGENASE (COX)

Cyclooxygenase (COX), or prostaglandin G/H synthase (PGHS), catalyzes the rate-limiting step in the conversion of arachidonic acid to the bioactive prostaglandins and thromboxane (21). Two isoforms of cyclooxygenase have been cloned, termed COX-1 and COX-2 (22–27). COX-1 is expressed constitutively in a wide range of tissues and may account for the housekeeping role of cyclooxygenase. COX-2 however, is rapidly induced in response to a wide range of biological and inflammatory mediators (28–32). More recent evidence has suggested a role for COX-2 in the pathogenesis of both Alzheimer's disease and colorectal cancer (33,34). The disparate function of the two cyclooxygenase isoforms has led to the hypothesis that compounds that selectively inhibit COX-2 will provide the next generation of nonsteroidal anti-inflammatory drugs (NSAIDs). This class of compounds should have a reduced side effect profile, because COX-1 will retain biological activity and thus can perform its beneficial housekeeping role. The molecular experimentation that assisted in the development of this hypothesis is further outlined in the following.

Human COX-2 encodes a protein of 604 amino acids and shares 61% identity with the predicted amino sequence of human COX-1. COX-1 and COX-2 isoforms have been cloned from several species including, sheep, chicken, mouse, and rat (35–41). The tissue distribution of COX-2 and COX-1 has been investigated using reverse transcriptase (RT)–PCR, RNase protection assay, and Northern blotting (40,42,43). COX-1 was constitutively expressed in most tissues, although with a differing abundance of transcript levels. However, by probing a Northern blot with a specific probe, we have shown that human (h)COX-2 mRNA can be detected only in a subset of tissues as shown in Fig. 1. COX-2 transcripts were present at high levels in the prostate gland and peripheral blood leukocytes; at moderate levels in the small intestine and placenta; and at low levels in the colon and ovary. In itself, this distribution data would not be sufficient to validate COX-2 as a pain target. Indeed, when one looks farther into the distribution profiles of the cyclooxygenase isoforms in different species, there are significant differences. For example, COX-2 appears to be expressed as a constitutive enzyme in rat brain, and it was expressed at very low basal levels in most tissues tested (44). By contrast, only low levels of basal COX-2 have been reported in human brain by RT–PCR studies (43), and the transcript was not detected in human brain by Northern blotting, as shown in Fig. 1. These species differences serve to highlight the importance of studying the human enzyme, which has been made possible by molecular technology.

COX-2 mRNA and protein can be rapidly induced in response to certain biological mediators such as proinflammatory cytokines, lipopolysaccharides (LPS) and phorbol esters (29–32). The COX-2 mRNA and protein have been localized to the endoplasmic reticulum, contiguous with the nuclear membrane, whereas the COX-1 mRNA and protein appear to be largely present in the cytoplasmic regions of the cell (42). We used a human skin fibroblast cell line (HSF-9) to investigate the basal levels of hCOX-1 and hCOX-2 mRNA transcripts and their regulation following addition of interleukin-1 (IL-1). We isolated mRNA from HSF-9 cells, which had either been supplemented or starved of serum, or following addition of IL-1. We employed an RNA slot-blot approach to visualize the mRNA transcripts using ^{32}P-labeled probes specific for either hCOX-1 or hCOX-2. COX-1 mRNA was found in all three lanes, with little or no induction by IL-1, although the presence of fetal calf serum (FCS) does appear to increase the levels of hCOX-1 transcript. hCOX-2 mRNA was absent in serum-starved cells and also in the presence

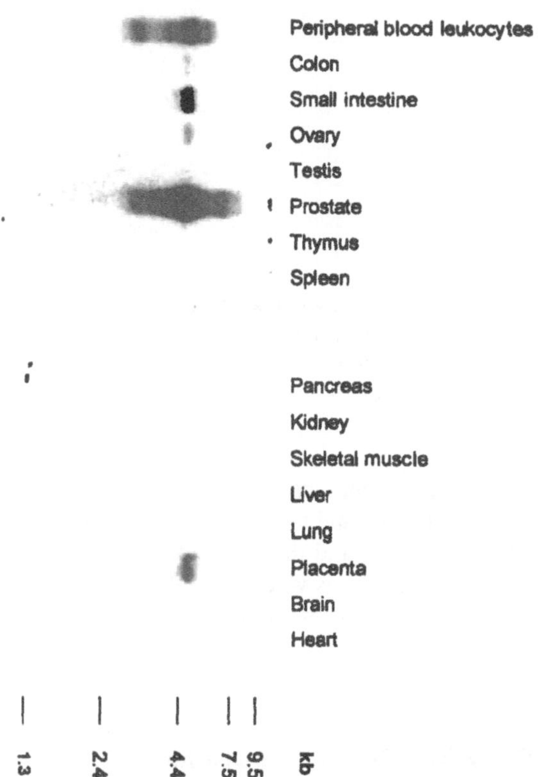

Figure 1 Human multiple tissue Northern blots (Clontech) hybridized with a ^{32}P-labeled hCOX-2-specific probe. Note the intense 4.8-kb transcript present in peripheral blood leukocytes and prostate gland, and the less intense, but specific, signals in placenta, small intestine, ovary, and colon.

of 10% FCS; however, addition of IL-1 caused a rapid and substantial induction of the hCOX-2 transcript (Fig. 2). A similar induction of hCOX-2 mRNA with IL-1 has been demonstrated in cultured rheumatoid synoviocytes (45). IL-1 is a proinflammatory cytokine that can be produced by both synovial fibroblasts and macrophages. Experimentally, injection of IL-1 into joints produces an inflammation of the synovium, and the level of IL-1 found in plasma has been correlated to the symptomatology of rheumatoid arthritis (RA) (46,47).

Taken together these data suggest a role for COX-2 in the inflammatory processes that occur in chronic inflammatory pain states, such as RA. Many pharmaceutical companies have now exploited mammalian cell expression technology to identify small-molecule inhibitors that show a preference for hCOX-2 over hCOX-1 (48–50). The first generation of these so called COX-2 selective molecules were first prescribed at the beginning of 1999, fewer than 7 years after the enzyme was first cloned.

Embryonic stem cell technology was employed to generate homozygous COX-1 and COX-2 null mice (51–53); however, these studies were not able to further define the individual roles of the two enzymes. Surprisingly, mice lacking COX-2 displayed normal responses to inflammatory mediators and have severely underdeveloped kidneys. By complete contrast, mice lacking the COX-1 gene develop normally, have a decreased inflammatory response to arachidonic acid and are more resistant to indomethacin-induced gastric ulceration. One may speculate

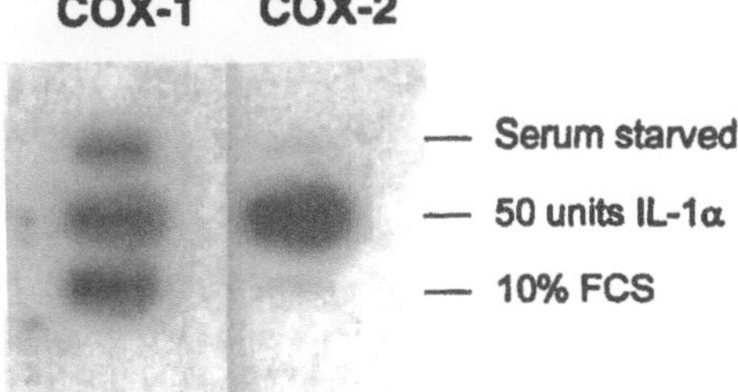

Figure 2 Slot-blot analysis of RNA prepared from HSF-9 cells, hybridized with hCOX-1 and hCOX-2-specific, ^{32}P-labeled probes. COX-2 mRNA was detected only when the cells were grown in the presence of Il-1. COX-1 mRNA was expressed in serum-starved cells and cells treated with IL-1. Expression of COX-1 was increased when cells were grown in the presence of 10% FCS.

that, had COX-2 been an orphan gene of unknown function, these knockout studies would not have served to validate it as a target. A cautionary note should be added at this point, for both of these genes were knocked out throughout development and the ideal knockout experiment would only remove the function of COX-2 in the adult. This is where the inducible and conditional knockout animals will present a more reliable and valuable tool for the determination of gene function in such studies (54).

III. SENSORY NEURONAL SPECIFIC VOLTAGE-GATED SODIUM CHANNELS

Voltage-gated sodium channels (VGSCs) are responsible for the rising phase of the action potential and play a key role in mediating electrical activity in excitable tissues. The channels comprise a multisubunit complex consisting of a large (230- to 270-kDa), highly glycosylated α-subunit and one or two smaller β-subunits (β_1 and β_2) (55). The α-subunits are part of a multigene family, with at least ten members, discovered so far in mammals (56–62). Structurally they consist of four homologous domains (DI–IV), each containing six potential α-helical transmembrane segments (S_1–S_6) making up the pore-forming region.

A potent blocker of VGSCs is the puffer fish toxin, tetrodotoxin (TTX). Although most VGSCs are TTX-sensitive and are inhibited by low nanomolar concentrations of TTX, three channels have now been cloned that are inhibited only by micromolar concentrations of TTX. These are the TTX-resistant (TTX-R), major cardiac channel h1/SKM2, and the sensory neuron-specific channels SNS/PN3 (hereafter referred to as SNS1) (55,60,61) and NaN/SNS2 (hereafter referred to as SNS2) (63,64). Molecular technology, which initially led to the isolation of these channels based on their sequence homology with the other members of the VGSC gene family, has permitted further validation of these channels as pain targets.

The sensory neuron-specific sodium channels, SNS1 and SNS2 are, as their name suggests, found in only dorsal root ganglion (DRG) neurons (Fig. 3). We studied the distribution profiles of both genes by probing multiple tissue Northern blots with specific SNS1 and SNS2 probes. Across a range of rat tissues, including DRG, spinal cord, brain, adrenal gland, heart, and PC12 cells plus and minus nerve growth factor (NGF), a single transcript of approximately 8 kb for SNS1 and 7.5 kb for SNS2 was detected in the dorsal root ganglia (DRG) lane, with no hybridization evident for the other tissues, even following long exposure times. Similarly, no hybridization

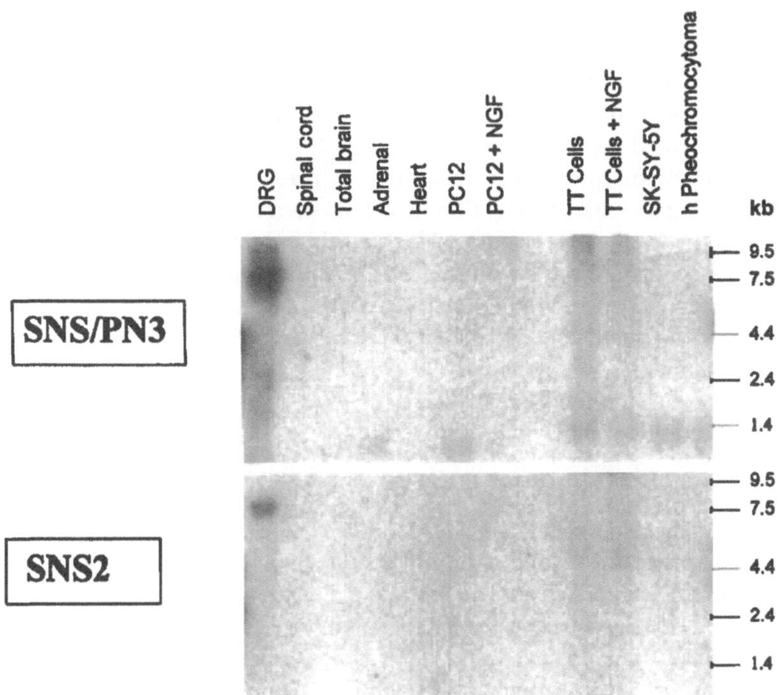

Figure 3 A multiple tissue Northern blot, showing that SNS/PN3 and SNS2 mRNA expression is confined to DRG neurons.

was observed with human pheochromocytoma cells, a human neuroendocrine cell line (TT), or a neuroblastoma cell line (SK-SH-5Y). RT–PCR experiments have demonstrated the existence of both SNS1 and SNS2 in human DRG mRNA (data not shown).

We generated type-specific antipeptide antibodies for SNS1 and SNS2 for use in target validation studies. With use of immunohistochemical technology, we noted labeling of the small-diameter population of DRG fibers with both SNS1 and SNS2 antibodies (Fig. 4). Double-labeling for SNS1 mRNA and SNS2 protein in the same section showed colocalization only in small-diameter neuronal cell bodies. Co-localization in only small neurons was also apparent when double-labeling experiments were performed with SNS2 mRNA and SNS1 protein (64). Large neurons have been observed with a signal for SNS1 mRNA or protein where SNS2 protein

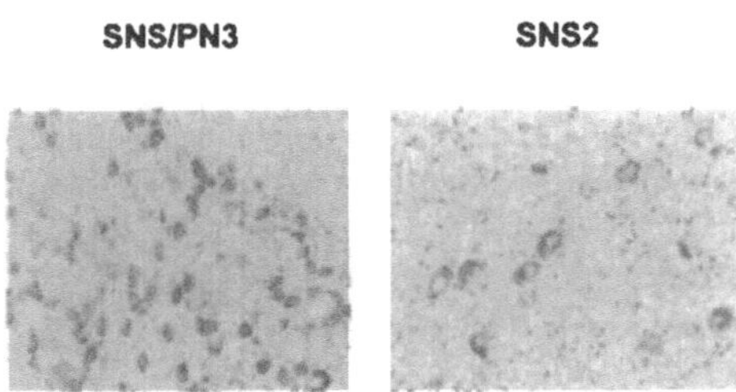

Figure 4 Photomicrographs showing SNS/PN3 and SNS2 immunohistochemical staining in 20-μm sections of L4 and L5 dorsal root ganglion. The specific antibodies raised against SNS/PN3 and SNS2 show labeling in predominantly small neurons.

or mRNA was absent (64). Both the P2X3 receptor (65,66) and the recently cloned capsaicin receptor VR1 are also selectively distributed on small-diameter sensory neurones (67,68).

Dorsal root ganglion (DRG) neurons are a functionally heterogeneous group of sensory cells, highly specialized to transduce either low- or high-intensity peripheral stimuli and transmit the sensory information to the central nervous system (CNS) (69,70). Small-diameter neurons, most of which are high-threshold nociceptors, coexpress a rapidly inactivating fast TTX-sensitive current and a slowly activating and inactivating TTX-R sodium current. The larger-diameter cells express only a TTX-sensitive sodium current (71–73). Molecular distribution studies have suggested that these sodium currents are the result of the differential expression of different VGSCs, the TTX-S current being mediated by PN1, rSCP6/PN4, rBI, rBII, or rBIII, which are found in large and small sensory neurons and the TTX-R current by SNS1 and SNS2, which are found in small and medium-sized DRG neurons (74–76).

The TTX-R sodium current in the DRG is of interest because its differential expression in small neurons offers the possibility of blocking activity only in these pain-signaling neurons. The TTX-R current is, moreover, augmented by inflammatory mediators and, therefore, may contribute to the sensitization of nociceptor terminals after inflammation (77–79). Following chronic constriction injury of the sciatic nerve, SNS1 protein translocates from the cell body to the peripheral axons accumulating at the site of injury (80). Together, this implies a key role for TTX-R in the activation of nociceptors in inflammatory and neuropathic pain. The TTX-R current recorded from isolated DRG neurons, appears to be relatively heterogeneous, displaying different kinetic properties in different neurons (81–83). We can now postulate that two distinct VGSC α-subunits, SNS2 and SNS1 are responsible for the TTX-R current in small-diameter DRG neurons. Given the selective distribution and discrete functional properties of SNS2, these findings indicate the need to target both SNS1 and SNS2 and in the search for selective analgesics directed toward the TTX-R sodium current.

REFERENCES

1. Lanteri-Minet M, De Pommery J, Herdegen T, Weil-Fugazza J, Bravo R, Menetrey D. Differential time course and spatial expression of Fos, Jun and Krox-24 proteins in spinal cord in rats undergoing subacute or chronic somatic inflammation. J Comp Neurol 1993; 333:223–235.
2. Hunt SP, Pini A, Evan G. Induction of c-*fos*-like protein in spinal cord neurons following sensory stimulation. Nature 1987; 328:632–634.
3. Kieffer BL, Befort K, Gaveriaux-Ruff C, Hirth CG. The delta-opioid receptor: isolation of a cDNA by expression cloning and pharmacological characterization. Proc Natl Acad Sci USA 1992; 89: 12048–12052.
4. Evans CJ, Keith DE Jr, Morrison H, Magendzo K, Edwards RH. Cloning of a delta opioid receptor by functional expression. Science 1992; 258:1952–1955.
5. Chen Y, Mestek A, Liu J, Hurley JA, Yu L. Molecular cloning and functional expression of a mu-opioid receptor from rat brain. Mol Pharmacol 1993; 44:8–12.
6. Yasuda K, Raynor K, Kong H, Breder CD, Takeda J, Reisine T, Bell GI. Cloning and functional comparison of kappa and delta opioid receptors from mouse brain. Proc Natl Acad Sci USA 1993; 90:6736–6740.
7. Raynor K, Kong H, Chen Y, Yasuda K, Yu L, Bell GI, Reisine T. Pharmacological characterization of the cloned κ-, δ- and μ-opioid receptors. Mol Pharmacol 1993; 45:330–334.
8. Reisine T, Bell GI. Molecular biology of opioid receptors. Trends Neurosci 1993; 16:506–510.
9. Munro S, Thoma KL, Abu-Shaar M. Molecular characterization of a peripheral receptor for cannabinoids. Nature 1993; 365:61–65.
10. Matsuda LA, Lolait SJ, Brownstein MJ, Young AC, Bonner TI. Structure of a cannabinoid receptor and functional expression of the cloned cDNA. Nature 1990; 346:561–564.

11. McEachern AE, Shelton ER, Bhakta S, Obernolte R, Bach C, Zuppan P, Fujisaki J, Aldrich RW, Jarnagin K. Expression cloning of a rat B_2 bradykinin receptor. Proc Natl Acad Sci USA 1991; 88: 7724–7728.
12. Menke JG, Borkowski JA, Bierilo KK, MacNeil T, Derrick AW, Schneck KA, Ransom RW, Strader CD, Linemeyer DL, Hess JF. Expression cloning of a human B_1 bradykinin receptor. J Biol Chem 1994; 269:21583–21586.
13. Denyer J, Gray J, Wong M, Stolz M, Tate S. Molecular and pharmacological characterization of the human CCK-B receptor. Eur J Pharmacol 1994; 268:29–41.
14. Shelton DL, Sutherland J, Gripp J, Camerato T, Armanini MP, Phillips HS, Carroll K, Spencer SD, Levinson AD. Human *trks*: molecular cloning, tissue distribution, and expression of extracellular domain immunoadhesins. Neuroscience 1995; 15:477–491.
15. Zukin RS, Bennett MVL. Alternatively spliced isoforms of the NMDARI receptor subunit. Trends Neurosci 1995; 18:306–313.
16. Yang N, George AL, Horn R. Molecular basis of charge movement in voltage-gated sodium channels. Neuron 1996; 16:113–122.
17. Tallent M, Dichter MA, Reisine T. Differential regulation of the cloned kappa and mu opioid receptors. Neuroscience 1998; 85:873–885.
18. Mansour A, Fox CA, Akil H, Watson SJ. Opioid-receptor mRNA expression in the rat CNS: anatomical and functional implications. Trends Neurosci 1995; 18:22–29.
19. Fraser GL, Wahlestedt C. Antisense approaches in the study of pain. Mol Neurobiol pain. Progr Pain Res Manage 1997; 9:319–336.
20. Mogil JS, Grisel JE. Transgenic studies of pain. Pain 1998; 77:107–128.
21. DeWitt DL. Prostaglandin endoperoxide synthase: regulation of enzyme expression. Biochim Biophys Acta 1991; 1083:121–134.
22. Kujubu DA, Fletcher BS, Varnum BC, Lim RW, Herschman HR. TIS10, a phorbol ester tumor promoter-inducible mRNA from Swiss 3T3 cells, encodes a novel prostaglandin synthase/cyclooxygenase homologue. J Biol Chem 1992; 266:12866–12872.
23. Ryseck RP, Raynoschek C, Macdonald-Bravo H, Dorfman K, Mattei MG, Bravo R. Identification of an immediate early gene, ***pghs-b***, whose protein product has prostaglandin synthase/cyclooxygenase activity. Cell Growth Differ 1992; 3:443–450.
24. Yokoyama C, Tanabe T. Cloning of human gene encoding prostaglandin endoperoxide synthase and primary structure of the enzyme. Biochem Biophys Res Commun 1989; 165:888–894.
25. Hla T, Farrell M, Kumar A, Bailey JM. Isolation of the cDNA for human prostaglandin H synthase. Prostaglandins 1986; 32:829–845.
26. Funk CD, Funk LB, Kennedy ME, Pong AS, Fitzgerald GA. Human platelet/erythroleukemia cell prostaglandin G/H synthase: cDNA cloning, expression, and gene chromosomal assignment. FASEB J 1991; 5:2304–2312.
27. Hla T, Neilson K. Human cyclooxygenase-2 cDNA. Proc Natl Acad Sci USA 1992; 89:7384–7388.
28. Hla T, Ristimaki A, Appleby S, Barriocanl JG. Cyclooxygenase gene expression in inflammation and angiogenesis. Ann N Y Acad Sci 1993; 696:197–204.
29. Pritchard KA, O'Banion MK, Miano JM, Vlasic N, Bhatia UG, Young DA, Stemerman MB. Induction of cyclooxygenase-2 in rat vascular smooth muscle cells in vitro and in vivo. J Biol Chem 1994; 269:8504–8509.
30. Hemel SL, Monick MM, Hunninghake GW. Lipopolysaccharide induces prostaglandin H synthase-2 protein and mRNA in human alveolar macrophages and blood monocytes. J Clin Invest 1994; 93: 391–396.
31. O'Sullivan MG, Huggins EM, Meade EA, DeWitt DL, McCall CE. Lipopolysaccharide induces prostaglandin H synthase-2 in alveolar macrophages. Biochem Biophys Res Commun 1992; 187(2): 1123–1127.
32. Lee SH, Soyoola E, Chanmugam P, Hart S, Sun W, Zhong H, Liou S, Simmons D, Hwang D. Selective expression of mitogen-inducible cyclooxygenase in macrophages stimulated with lipopolysaccharide. J Biol Chem 1992; 267(6):25934–25938.
33. Schnabel J. Alzheimer's disease: arthritis of the brain? New Sci 1993; 138:22–26.

34. Sano H, Kawahito Y, Wilder RL, Hashiramoto A, Mukai S, Asai K, Kimura S, Kato H, Kondo M, Hla T. Expression of cyclooxygenase-1 and -2 in human colorectal cancer. Cancer Res 1995; 55: 3785–3789.
35. Reed DW, Bradshaw WS, Xie W, Simmons DL. In vivo and in vitro expression of a non-mammalian cyclooxygenase-1. Prostaglandins 1996; 52:269–284.
36. DeWitt DL, Smith WL. Primary structure of prostaglandin G/H synthase from sheep vesicular gland determined from the complementary DNA sequence. Proc Natl Acad Sci USA 1988; 85:1412–1416.
37. Zhang V, O'Sullivan M, Hussain H, Roswit WT, Holtzman MJ. Molecular cloning, functional expression, and selective regulation of ovine prostaglandin H synthase-2. Biochem Biophys Res Commun 1996; 227:499–506.
38. Meade EA, Smith WL, DeWitt D. Expression of the murine prostaglandin (PGH) synthase-1 and PGH synthase-2 isozymes in cos-1 cells. J Lipid Mediat 1993; 6:119–129.
39. Sirois J, Richards JS. Purification and characterization of a novel, distinct isoform of prostaglandin endoperoxide synthase induced by human chorionic gonadotropin in granulosa cells of rat preovulatory follicles. J Biol Chem 1992; 267:6382–6388.
40. Feng L, Sun W, Xia Y, Tang WW, Chanmugam P, Soyoola E, Wilson CB, Hwang D. Cloning two isoforms of rat cyclooxygenase: differential regulation of their expression. Arch Biochem Biophys 1993; 307:361–368.
41. Kennedy BP, Chan CC, Culp SA, Cromlish WA. Cloning an expression of rat prostaglandin endoperoxide synthase (cyclooxygenase)-2 cDNA. Biochem Biophys Res Commun 1993; 197:494–500.
42. Regier MK, DeWitt DL, Schindler MS, Smith WL. Subcellular localization of prostaglandin endoperoxide synthase-2 in murine 3T3 cells. Arch Biochem Biophys 1993; 301:439–444.
43. O'Neill GP, Ford-Hutchinson AW. Expression of mRNA for cyclooxygenase-1 and cyclooxygenase-2 in human tissues. FEBS Lett 1993; 330:156–160.
44. Yamagata K, Andreasson KI, Kaufmann WE, Barnes CA, Worley PF. Expression of a mitogen-inducible cyclooxygenase in brain neurons: regulation by synaptic activity and glucocorticoids. Neuron 1993; 11:371–386.
45. Crofford LJ, Wilder RL, Ristimaki AP, Sano H, Remmers EF, Epps HR, Hla T. Cyclooxygenase-1 and -2 expression in rheumatoid synovial tissues. J Clin Invest 1994; 93:1095–1101.
46. Andreis M, Stastny P, Ziff M. Experimental arthritis produced by mediators of delayed sensitivity. Arthritis Rheum 1974; 17:537–551.
47. Eastgate JA, Symons JA, Wood NC, Grinlinton FM, di Giovine FS, Duff GW. Correlation of plasma interleukin 1 levels with disease activity in rheumatoid arthritis. Lancet 1988; 2:706–709.
48. O'Neill GP, Mancini JA, Kargman S, Yergey J, Kwan MY, Falgueyret JP, Abramovitz M, Kennedy BP, Ouellet M, Cromlish W, Culp S, Evans JF, Ford-Hutchinson AW, Vickers PJ. Overexpression of human prostaglandin G/H synthase-1 and -2 by recombinant vaccinia virus: inhibition by nonsteroidal anti-inflammatory drugs and biosynthesis of 15-hydroxyeicosatetraenoic acid. Mol Pharmacol 1993; 45:245–254.
49. Seibert K, Zhang Y, Leahy K, Hauser S, Masferrer J, Perkins W, Lee L, Isakson P. Pharmacological and biochemical demonstration of the role of cycooxygenase 2 in inflammation and pain. Proc Natl Acad Sci USA 1994; 91:12013–12017.
50. Cromlish WA, Payette P, Culp SA, Ouellet M, Percival MD, Kennedy BP. High-level expression of active human cyclooxygenase-2 in insect cells. Arch Biochem Biophys 1994; 314:193–199.
51. Langenbach R, Morham SG, Tiano HF, Loftin CD, Ghanayem BI, Chulada PC, Mahler JF, Lee CA, Goulding EH, Kluckman KD, Kim HS, Smithies O. Prostaglandin synthase 1 gene disruption in mice reduces arachidonic acid-induced inflammation and indomethacin-induced gastric ulceration. Cell 1995; 83:483–492.
52. Dinchuk JE, Car BD, Focht RJ, Johnston JJ, Jaffee BD, Covington MB, Contel NR, Eng VM, Collins RJ, Czerniak PM, Gorry SA, Trzaskos JM. Renal abnormalities and an altered inflammatory response in mice lacking cyclooxygenase II. Nature 1995; 378:406–409.
53. Morham SG, Langenbach R, Loftin CD, Tiano HF, Vouloumanos N, Jennette JC, Mahler JF, Kluckman KD, Ledford A, Lee CA, Smithies O. Prostaglandin synthase 2 gene disruption causes severe renal pathology in the mouse. Cell 1995; 83:473–482.

54. Chen J, Kelz MB, Zeng G, Sakai N, Steffen C, Shockett PE, Picciotto MR, Duman RS, Nestler EJ. Transgenic animals with inducible, targeted gene expression in brain. Mol Pharmacol 1998; 54:495–503.
55. Goldin AL. Ligand and Voltage-Gated Ion Channels. Vol 2. Boca Raton, FL: CRC Press, 1994.
56. Catterall WA. Cellular and molecular biology of voltage-gated sodium channels. Physiol Rev 1992; 72:S15–S48.
57. Fish LM, Sangameswaran L, Delgado SG, Koch BD, Jakeman, LB, Kwan J, Herman RC. Cloning of a sodium channel α-subunit (PN-1) from rat dorsal root ganglia. Soc Neurosci Abstr 1995; 21: 1824.
58. Klugbauer N, Lacinova L, Flockerzi V, Hofmann F. Structure and functional expression of a new member of the tetrodotoxin-sensitive voltage-gated sodium channel family from human neuroendocrine cells. EMBO J. 1995; 14:1084–1090.
59. Mandel G. Tissue-specific expression of the voltage-sensitive sodium channel. J Membr Biol 1992; 125:193–205.
60. Akopian AN, Sivilotti L, Wood J. A tetrodotoxin-resistant voltage gated sodium channel expressed by sensory neurons. Nature 1996; 379:257–262.
61. Sangameswaran L, Delgado SG, Fish LM, Koc BD, Jakeman LB, Stewart GR, Sze P, Hunter JC, Eglen RM, Herman RC. Structure and function of a novel voltage-gated, tetrodotoxin-resistant sodium channel specific to sensory neurons. J Biol Chem 1996; 271:5953–5956.
62. Toledo–Aral JJ, Moss BL, He Z, Koszowski AG, Whisenand T, Levinson SR, Wolf JJ, Silos–Santiago I, Halegoua S, Mandel G. Identification of PN-1, a predominant voltage-dependent sodium channel expressed principally in peripheral neurons. Proc Natl Acad Sci USA 1997; 94:1527–1532.
63. Dib-Hajj SD, Tyrrell L, Black JA, Waxman SG. NaN, a novel voltage-gated Na channel, is expressed preferentially in peripheral sensory neurons and down-regulated after axotomy. Proc Natl Acad Sci USA 1998; 95:8963–8968.
64. Tate S, Benn S, Hick C, Trezise T, John V, Mannion R, Costigan M, Plumpton C, Grose D, Gladwell Z, Kendall G, Dale K, Bountra C, Woolf C. Two sodium channels contribute to the TTX-R sodium current in primary sensory neurones. Nat Neurosci 1998; 1:653–655.
65. Chen CC, Akopian AN, Sivilotti L, Colquhoun D, Burnstock G, Wood JN. A P2X purinoceptor expressed by a subset of sensory neurons. Nature 1995; 377:428–431.
66. Lewis C, Neidhart S, Holy C, North RA, Buell G, Surprenant A. Coexpression of P2X2 and P2X3 receptor subunits can account for ATP-gated currents in sensory neurons. Nature 1995; 377:432–435.
67. Caterina MJ, Schumacher MA, Tominaga M, Rosen TA, Levine JD, Julius D. The capsaicin receptor: a heat-activated ion channel in the pain pathway. Nature 1997; 389:816–824.
68. Tominaga M, Caterina MJ, Malmberg AB, Rosen TA, Gilbert H, Skinner K, Raumann BE, Basbaum AI, Julius D. The cloned capsaicin receptor integrates multiple pain-producing stimuli. Neuron 1998; 21:531–543.
69. Fitzgerald M. The course and termination of primary afferent fibres. In: Textbook of Pain. Wall PD, Melzack R, eds. Churchill Livingstone, 1984; 34–48.
70. Perl ER. Function of dorsal root ganglion neurons: an overview. In: Scott SA, ed. Sensory Neurons. New York: Oxford University Press, 1992; 2–23.
71. Caffrey JM, Eng DL, Black JA, Waxman SG, Kocsis JD. Three types of sodium channels in adult rat dorsal root ganglion neurons. Brain Res 1992; 592:283–297.
72. Elliott AA, Elliott JR. Characterization of TTX-sensitive and TTX-resistant sodium currents in small cells from adult rat dorsal root ganglia. J Physiol 1993; 463:39–56.
73. Roy ML, Narahashi T. Differential properties of tetrodotoxin-sensitive and tetrodotoxin-resistant sodium channels in rat dorsal root ganglion. J Neurosci 1992; 12:2104–2111.
74. Waxman SG, Kocsis JD, Black JA. Type III sodium channel mRNA is expressed in embryonic but not adult spinal sensory neurons, and is re-expressed following axotomy. J Neurophysiol 1994; 72: 466–470.
75. Black JA, Dib-Hajj S, Mcnabola K, Jeste S, Rizzo MA, Kocsis JD, Waxman SG. Spinal sensory neurons express multiple sodium channel α-subunit mRNAs. Mol Brain Res 1996; 43:117–131.

76. Black JA, Waxman SG. Sodium channel expression: a dynamic process in neurons and non-neuronal cells. Dev Neurosci 1996; 18:139–152.
77. Aguayo LG, White G. Effects of nerve growth factor on TTX and capsaicin-sensitivity in adult rat sensory neurons. Brain Res 1992; 570:61–67.
78. England S, Bevan S, Docherty RJ. PGE_2 modulates the tetrodotoxin-resistant sodium current in neonatal rat dorsal root ganglion neurons via the cyclic AMP-protein kinase A cascade. J Physiol 1996; 495:429–440.
79. Gold MS, Reichling DB, Shuster MJ, Levin JD. Hyperalgesic agents increase a tetrodotoxin-resistant Na^+ current in nociceptors. Proc Natl Acad Sci USA 1996; 93:1108–1112.
80. Novakovic SD, Tzoumaka E, McGivern JG, Haraguchi M, Sangameswaran L, Gogas KR, Eglen RM, Hunter JC. Distribution of the tetrodotoxin-resistant sodium channel PN3 in rat sensory neurons in normal and neuropathic conditions. J Neurosci 1998; 18:2174–2187.
81. Rizzo MA, Kocsis JD, Waxman SG. Slow sodium conductances of dorsal root ganglion neurons: intraneuronal homogeneity and interneuronal heterogeneity. J Neurophysiol 1994; 72:2796–2815.
82. Haper AA, Lawson SN. Conduction velocity is related to morphological cell type in rat dorsal root ganglion neurons. J Physiol 1985; 359:31–46.
83. Scholz A, Appel N, Vogel W. Two types of TTX-resistant and one TTX-sensitive Na^+ channel in rat dorsal root ganglion neurons and their blockade by halothane. Euro J Neurosci 1998; 10:2547–2556.

28
Genetics of Pain

Philippe Sanseau and Karen Lewis
GlaxoSmithKline, Stevenage, Hertfordshire, England

I. INTRODUCTION

For the past 50 years it has been known that sensitivity to pain and responses to analgesics are variable among people (1–3). This variability is due to a combination of genetic and environmental factors. These influences underlie the considerable clinical differences observed in pain-related syndromes. The finding of several endogenous receptor ligands is likely to be why the study of genetics of pain has been overlooked. This pharmacological approach has led to the discovery of detailed processes in pain transmission and modulation (4,5).

One main goal of genetics is to relate DNA sequence variation (genotype) to altered phenotype. Classic genetic techniques in organisms can be used to look at the heritability of a particular trait and determine if a genetic approach is feasible. If the heritability of a trait is partially genetic (i.e., not due to only environmental factors), the mode of inheritance could be determined. Obviously, this may be recessive or dominant.

Genetic methods have also been widely used to map disease traits onto particular genomic loci in many organisms, particularly human and mouse. Once a disease's genetic locus is identified by linkage analysis (6), genes can be isolated using a battery of gene-hunting techniques, such as sequencing, cDNA library hybridizations, exon trapping, or cDNA selection (7,8). Identifying new human genes is likely to become much easier in the immediate future with the availability of the complete human genome sequence (9). The physical-mapping approach (both linkage and association) has been particularly successful in cloning of single disease genes (10,11). However, it is well recognized that both linkage and association analysis are much more difficult for multigenic human disease (12).

A simple, but more empirical approach, is to analyze candidate genes for sequence variation. Candidate genes implicated in a particular disease pathway can be scanned to see whether a genotype correlates with a particular phenotype in a selected population. Many genotyping techniques are now available (13). Some exciting approaches are based on the use of DNA microarrays for high-throughput analysis. Moreover this candidate gene method can be used to analyze the genotype of patients exhibiting variations in drug response–efficacy, drug metabolism, or adverse side effects. By determining a patient genotype for a specific candidate gene, it may be possible to elucidate why certain patients demonstrate adverse drug reactions or respond differently to identical treatments. In addition, when DNA samples are available, it should be possible to perform retrospective genotyping analysis to reevaluate drugs that had previously failed clinical trials following efficacy or toxicity problems.

In this chapter, we will focus mainly on different applications of genetics to pain syndromes in humans and mice and on the heritability of pain traits.

Several studies have demonstrated that environmental influences, such as culture, attention state, and stress can significantly influence the perception of painful stimuli (14). The important role of genetic factors in the mediation of sensitivity to pain and pain inhibition between individuals is now much more apparent. Unfortunately, only a few genetic models for pain-relevant traits have been identified in humans.

For example, patients have different responses to opiate treatment. Profiling individuals based on genotype may help elucidate why they react differently to the same medication. It may also allow drug administrators to select a "most effective" course of treatment based on an understanding of an individual's genetic profile.

II. INDIVIDUAL SUSCEPTIBILITY TO PAIN STIMULI

Perceived intensity of pain is related to the intensity of the painful stimuli (15,16); however, individual variation in the threshold sensitivity has been well documented (15). Earlier work on the tolerance to various stimuli, such as heat, electrical current, and noxious pressure, has shown a high degree of individual variability in humans (1,2,17). More recent studies have confirmed the importance of interindividual variability to pain thresholds to various stimuli (18–20).

The response to opiate analgesics for inhibition to pain shows a significant degree of variability among individuals (21,22). The influence on the variability of the subject genotype has been highlighted in preclinical studies (23,24). There is also evidence of variability of the actions of morphine in dental extraction. Moreover, genetic studies in mice have identified loci for pain-related traits. For example, a locus on chromosome 10 that influences the analgesic effects of morphine has been described (25).

A. Heritability of Pain Traits in Humans

One important question for investigators interested in the genetics of pain is to distinguish between variability in environmental and genetic factors. Twin studies have been performed to help in the separation of these factors. In this type of analysis, one compares the concordance rate of pain-related traits between identical–monozygotic twins against fraternal–dizygotic twins. Estimations of the influence of genetic factors on the phenotypic variance have been reported: between 39–58% for migraine (26–28), 55% for menstrual pain (29), and 50% for back pain (30). Genetic analysis is certainly a feasible option for the pain-related traits with a high percentage of heritability.

B. Heritability of Pain Traits in Rodents

In mice, the heritability for nociceptive and analgesic sensitivity to pain could be as high as 78% (31–33). The identification of pain "disease" rodent genes may greatly help our understanding of the biological pathways. However, investigators should not make the assumption that the same set of genes are implicated in the pain networks of both mice and humans.

III. PAIN AND HUMAN STUDIES

A. Genetic Polymorphisms and Pain

1. Cytochrome P450

A genetic polymorphism with possible relevance to opiate sensitivity is found in about 8–10% of European and northern whites who are poor metabolizers of the liver isozyme P-450 IID6 (sparteine–debrisoquin). The absence of the isozyme is caused by mutations in the neuronal cytochrome P450IID6 (CYP2D6) gene (34). In poor metabolizers, this isozyme is absent from the liver (35). The *O*-demethylation of codeine (methylmorphine) to morphine by human liver microsomes requires this enzyme (36,37). In poor metabolizers of P-450 IID6, codeine is not activated into morphine, making codeine an inefficient analgesic for these individuals (38). The variable individual rates of codeine bioactivation may explain its poor efficacy for pain relief in some cancer patients (39).

2. μ- and δ-Opioid Receptors

Common allelic variants have been identified in the μ-opioid receptor. The A118G variant results in an Asn/Asp change and seems to be present in a lower proportion of opioid-dependent subjects compared with controls. The C17T polymorphism is more common in opioid-dependent subjects (40). In another study, four DNA sequence variants were analyzed, and no significant associations were identified between the alleles and the patients with alcohol-dependence diagnosis (41). No significant differences in the frequencies of two polymorphisms have been identified in a substance-abuse group and matched controls (42). However, a trend was noted for a higher frequency of one allele in the substance-abuse group ($p = 0.05$).

Interestingly, μ-receptors' densities are not identical among individuals, as shown by binding studies in postmortem brain samples (43). An understanding of these differences in gene expressions levels has driven the search for functional polymorphisms in the 5′-flanking sequences of the gene (44). Initial analyses have not identified human variants that can be involved in the function of the μ-receptor (41,44).

A polymorphism for the δ-opioid receptor has been identified in the coding region of the gene. The T307C variant does not result in an amino acid substitution. However, statistically, heroin addicts were significantly more likely to have the CC genotype, rather than the TT genotype (45). Although the reasons for the association are mysterious, it was concluded that individuals with the CC genotype were more susceptible to become heroin addicts. Therefore, the δ-receptor may have a functional role in the pathophysiology of opioid dependence.

B. Pain-Related Traits in Humans

1. Migraine

Migraine is one of the most common pain syndromes. Recently, a form of migraine, familial hemiplegic migraine, was associated with mutations in the P/Q-type calcium channel α_1-subunit gene or CACNL1A4 (46). Previous linkage studies have shown that the disease susceptibility gene is located on human chromosome 19p13 (47). The gene was cloned and four different missense point mutations were identified in affected individuals from diseased families. Interestingly, some mutations are also associated with episodic ataxia type-2.

It is likely that other genes (in addition to ion channels) contribute to migraine phenotypes (48). Recently, one publication (49) suggested the presence of familial migraine susceptibility loci on human chromosome X. This observation may explain the increased prevalence of migraine in females (49). Studies in the early 1990s indicate that migraine affects 18% of females, compared with only 6% of males (50,51). Moreover, these findings confirm that typical familial migraine is a heterogeneous disorder.

2. Congenital Insensitivity to Pain with Anhidrosis

Another interesting human pain model is that of individuals with congenital insensitivity to pain with anhidrosis (CIPA). CIPA is also described as hereditary sensory and autonomic neuropathy type IV or HSAN IV. This is an autosomal-recessive disorder affecting the peripheral and central nervous system (CNS). CIPA is characterized by onset manifestations in infancy with recurrent fever related to anhidrosis (absence of sweating); absence of reaction to noxious stimuli, resulting in repeated soft-tissue damage; painless fractures, and joint injuries (52). To date fewer that 40 cases have been described in the literature (53). Indo and co-workers identified the human gene based on the phenotypic similarities between CIPA and the null-mutant mice lacking the *Ntrk1* gene encoding the nerve growth factor (NGF)-specific tyrosine kinase receptor. Using a candidate gene approach, they identified three exonic mutations in the homologous human gene, *NTRK1* (known also as *TRKA*) (54). The *TRKA* receptor has been cloned from a human colon carcinoma and is expressed in the nervous system and phosphorylated in response to NGF (55). NGF induces neurite outgrowth and promotes survival of embryonic sensory and sympathetic neurons (56). The human *NTRK1* gene has been isolated and characterized. It spans close to 23 kb of genomic DNA, and it is split into 17 exons. The gene is located on human chromosome 1q32-41 (57). With this knowledge and modern biology techniques, the developmental and biological regulation of the *NTRK1* gene can be studied.

3. Other Human Pain Pathologies

CIPA is one of five hereditary sensory and automic neuropathies, all of which are characterized by sensory disturbances (58). Clinical and pathological similarities exist with familial dysautonomia also termed Riley–Day syndrome or HSAN III. The gene for this disorder has been mapped to chromosome 9q31-33 (59). Other syndromes in which pain sensation is impaired include Lesch–Nyhan syndrome (60), Tourette's syndrome (61), and De Lange's syndrome (62). The identification of such patients can be made easier by looking at patients genotypes. Gaining an insight into why patients with a diagnosis of such neuropathies do not experience pain can help in the future design of medicines for pain treatments.

IV. ANIMAL MODELS OF PAIN

A relatively large number of genetic models of pain have been developed in animals, especially in the mouse and rat. The assumption is that these models will shed light on the genetics of pain in humans.

Genetic differences in rodents are responsible for differences in the response to a variety of noxious stimuli. A number of animal models bearing genetic differences in response to these stimuli have been established in rodents using selective breeding, inbred strains, or mutations. Mouse models have also been used to assess individual variability in sensitization to the prolonged effect of cocaine (63). Increased locomotor activity was used as a behavioral model of sensitization.

A. Production of Animal Models

Animal models have been produced using various methods and technologies.

1. Inbred Strains

Such strains are established by repeated sibling matings (inbred strains) for at least 20 generations. Because strains have common ancestors, it is more likely for the offspring to have two copies of the same allele and, therefore, it is homozygous. Under the same experimental conditions, genetic factors, rather than environmental factors, are more likely to be responsible for the differences between inbred strains. Therefore, the identification of a particular trait is based on the comparison of responses in a panel of inbred strains.

2. Recombinant Inbred Strains

It is possible to develop more complex genetic models from inbred strains. Recombinant inbred (RI) strains are the descendants of an F_2 intercross between two inbred progenitor strains. One advantage of these RI strains is their use for linkage analysis with no more test crosses.

3. Spontaneous Mutants

Spontaneous mutants can also be used for the identification of pain-related genetic traits. For example, mutants have been identified in the B6 strain. These mutants display different sensitivities to opioid analgesia (64).

4. Transgenic Animals

Transgenic technology has been extensively used to relate gene function to phenotypes in rodents. Investigators are producing transgenic mice that either do not express or that overexpress pain candidate genes, such as various receptors (e.g., opioids, neurotrophins, TRKAs, or serotonins), pain mediators (e.g., interleukin-6 and enkephalins), or intracellular signal transduction molecules (e.g., nitric oxide, PKA, PKCγ). The knockout (KO) mouse construction has been the most widely used approach. It is based on the use of homologous recombination to introduce the DNA fragment of interest into a precise chromosomal location (65). Selection markers such as neomycin and thymidine kinase are introduced to allow the selection of homologous recombinations in a background of random integrations (66). Integration can be either within the targeted sequence or replacing it. Transgenic embryonic cells (ES) have also been used largely for microinjection in the blastocoele cavity of a mouse embryo. Blastocysts are implanted into the uterus of a pseudopregnant foster mother. Pluripotent mammalian ES cells would resume normal development and mix with host cells after implantation (67). The resulting transgenic mice are called chimeras. The use of transgenic technology has both advantages and limitations. These have been reviewed elsewhere (68). One major disadvantage is the difficulty of interpreting the phenotypes obtained. Results can be grouped into three categories:

1. Gene disruption could be lethal; however, this is relatively rare (69).
2. No change.
3. Change with wild-type animal.

Because genes are involved in complex and not linear biological pathways and the influence of environmental factors are unclear, the conclusions are not at all obvious. Moreover results from transgenic experiments have sometimes been controversial and difficult to interpret. The main advantage of transgenic approaches is the complete selectivity in knockout animals. In some examples, it has been possible to analyze the functional role of proteins involved in pain-related traits because other tools (pharmacological or immunological) are unavailable. Transgenics, similar to other technologies, is just another tool (although a powerful one) and should be used in combination with other approaches to yield useful results in the understanding of pain mechanisms.

B. Examples of Animal Models

1. CXBK Mouse

Several well-characterized RI strains have been used as genetic rodent models for pain. One of the most extensively studied models during the last 25 years is the CXBK mouse; this strain has a deficiency in morphine response (70,71). Compared with other strains of the CXB series, the CXBK strain had the lowest opiate-binding and the lowest analgesic response to morphine (72). CXBK mice seem to have normal levels of endogenous opioid peptides (73). A possible role for μ-receptors in opiate-binding deficiency has been postulated after binding and autoradiographic experiments (74).

2. HA/LA Mouse

Another popular model is the high-analgesia/low-analgesia (HA/LA) mouse (75). These mice have been selected by exposition to stressful external factors to create a sensation of pain. The swim stress-induced analgesia (SIA) test was used to breed an outbred population of mice for high and low analgesia resulting from a 3-min forced swim in 20°C water. HA/LA mice are considered an important genetic model for endogenous pain inhibition because of large differences in the SIA test. Binding studies with naloxone (76,77) have strongly suggested the importance of genes underlying opioid mechanisms of endogenous pain selection. Moreover a possible role of μ-receptors located in the thalamus has been postulated. HA mice had up-regulated opiate-binding density in the whole brain and a large increase in the medial thalamus, in comparison with the LA mice (78). To study which genes have been modified, test crosses using HA and LA mice have been performed. From this work it was concluded that a relatively few genetic loci are responsible for the levels of analgesia observed in the HA mice (79).

3. HAR/LAR Mouse

Different responses to the morphine congener levorphanol were used to breed selective mice and obtain the high-analgesic response (HAR)/low-analgesic response (LAR) mice (80). Sensitivity to a hot plate was monitored after injection of a single dose of levorphanol and tested again 2 days later after injection of a saline solution. Mice were scored for analgesia based on the ratio of levorphanol-treated versus saline-treated latencies. HAR and LAR mice were defined as the animals with the highest and lowest scoring quartiles. These lines have been used mainly for the identification of chemical compounds with a drug action similar to levorphanol. The results have shown that nonopioid and μ-, δ-, and κ-opioid receptor mechanisms are implicated (81,82). Following mendelian segregation analysis, it has been suggested that a genetic overlap may exist between the HA/LA and HAR/LAR mice (83).

4. HA/LA Rats

Other important animal pain models are the high-autotomy/low-autotomy (HA/LA) rats. *Autotomy* is defined as self-injury to a denervated limb and could be a model for human deafferentation (84). Devor and Raber started with the Sabra strain of rat and, after unilateral sectioning of the sciatic and saphenous nerves, they selected rats for high- or low-autotomy scores (85). Mendelian analysis has strongly suggested that a major recessive gene is responsible for the autotomy phenotype.

C. Pain-Related Genes in Animals

Various articles describing the identification of chromosomal loci for pain-related genes in mice have been published in which quantitative trait locus (QTL) approaches were used. For morphine analgesia, at least one "hot spot" has been confirmed with a lod score of 3.9 ($p < 0.00002$) on mouse chromosome 10 by using the hot-plate assay. The locus is located near the markers Mpmv5 and D10Mit51 and has a size of approximately 0–20 cM (25). Interestingly, the mouse μ-opioid receptor (*Orpm* gene) is a good candidate gene which lies in the locus. QTL has also been applied in an attempt to identify loci for stress-induced analgesia (SIA) in both males and females. A particular region, named Fsial on chromosome 8 with a lod score of 6.1 ($p = 0.000000112$), has been identified only in females ($p = 0.038$ in males). This QTL accounts for 17–26% of the overall variance of the trait in females (86). Such a result provides evidence for a sex-specific mechanism for SIA.

Another QTL-mapping analysis has revealed linkage to basal nociceptive sensibility by the hot-plate assay (87). The region with the highest lod score of 0.005 in males (only 0.085 in females) is relatively large (50–80 cM) and is located on the mouse chromosome 4 near the D4Mit71 marker. A good candidate gene has been mapped in the locus: the murine δ-opioid receptor or *Oprd1*. To test *Oprd1* as a candidate gene, the QTL mice strains were given doses of δ-, κ-, and μ-receptor–specific antagonists before the hot-plate assay. The δ-antagonist naltrindole (NTI; 5 mg/kg) lowered thermal nociception latencies.

These two QTL examples are important for illustrating the role of gender in the perception of pain.

V. CONCLUSION

The availability of the human genome sequence will greatly facilitate the identification of all human genes (9). The combination of the mapping of thousands of single nucleotide polymorphisms (SNPs) with the sequence information will provide very powerful tools for the positional cloning of human disease genes. Some of the transcripts identified are likely to be involved in pain-related traits, such as migraine. Investigators will be able to use these genes as research tools to understand a biological pathway, or maybe, directly as targets for new drugs.

Genomic technologies, particularly differential gene expression studies, are likely to provide very high-throughput methods not only for the identification of genes, but also for the understanding of biological pathways. Recently, cDNA microarrays (88) have been used to identify physiological gene expression patterns in different systems, such as yeast (89) and cultures of human fibroblasts (90). Clusters of genes that show similar patterns of gene expression are identified using various software and algorithms (91).

These results provide the first step toward the construction of biological or genetic networks (92) into which pain-related genes can be placed.

REFERENCES

1. Beecher HK. Quantification of the subjective pain experience. Proc Annu Meet Am Psychopathol Assoc 1965; 53:111–128.
2. Wolff BB, Kantor TG, Jarvik ME, Laska E. Response of experimental pain to analgesic drugs. 1. Morphine, aspirin, and placebo. Clin Pharmacol Ther 1966; 7:224–238.
3. Wolff BB. Measurement of human pain. Res Publ Assoc Res Nerv Ment Dis 1980; 58:173–184.
4. Basbaum AI, Fields HL. Endogenous pain control systems: brainstem spinal pathways and endorphin circuitry. Annu Rev Neurosci 1984; 7:309–338.
5. Terman GW, Shavit Y, Lewis JW, Cannon JT, Liebeskind JC. Intrinsic mechanisms of pain inhibition: activation by stress. Science 1984; 226:1270–1277.
6. Silver LE. Mouse Genetics: Concepts and Applications. New York: Oxford University Press, 1995.
7. Pribill I, Barnes GT, Chen JM, Church D, Buckler A, Baxendale S, Bates GP, Lehrach H, Gusella MJ, Duyao MP, Ambrose CM, Gusella JF, Macdonald ME. Exon trapping and sequence-based methods of gene finding in transcript mapping of human 4p 16.3. Somat Cell Mol Genet 1997; 23:413–427.
8. Rogner UC, Heiss NS, Kioschis P, Wiemann S, Korn B, Poustka A. Transcriptional analysis of the candidate region for incontinentia pigmenti (IP2) in Xq28. PCR Methods Appl 1996; 6:922–934.
9. Collins FS, Patrinos A, Jordan E, Chakravarti A, Gesteland R, Walters L. New goals for the US Human Genome Project: 1998–2003. Science 1998; 282:682–689.
10. Iannuzzi MC, Rybicki BA, Maliarik M, Popovich J. Finding disease genes—from cystic fibrosis to sarcoidosis. Chest 1997; 111:S70–S73.
11. Laan M, Paabo S. Demographic history and linkage disequilibrium in human populations. Nat Genet 1997; 17:435–438.
12. Gelbert LM, Gregg RE. Will genetics really revolutionize the drug discovery process. Curr Opin Biotechnol 1997; 8:669–674.
13. Hosking L, Au K, Sanseau P. Mutation detection. In: Foulkes WD, Hodgson SV, eds. Inherited Susceptibility to Cancer: Clinical, Predictive and Ethical Perspectives. London: Cambridge University Press, 1998; 134–149.
14. Chapman CR, Turner JA. Psychologic and psychosocial aspects of acute pain. In: Bonica JJ, ed. The Management of Pain. 2nd ed. Philadelphia: Lea & Febiger, 1990; 122–132.
15. Hardy JD, Wolff HG, Goodell H. Pain sensations and reactions. Baltimore, MD: Williams & Wilkins, 1952.
16. LaMotte RJ, Campbell JN. Comparison of responses of warm and nociceptive C-fiber afferents in monkey with human judgements of thermal pain. J Neurophysiol 1978; 41:509–517.
17. Woodrow KM, Friedman GD, Siegelaub AB, Collen MF. Pain tolerance: differences according to age, sex and race. Psychosom Med 1972; 34:548–556.
18. Brennum J, Kjeldsen M, Jensen K, Jensen TS. Measurements of human pressure–pain thresholds on fingers and toes. Pain 1989; 38:211–217.
19. Isselee H, De Laat A, Lesaffre E, Lysens R. Short-term reproducibility of pressure pain thresholds in masseter and temporalis muscles of symptom-free subjects. Eur J Oral Sci 1997; 105:583–587.
20. Jacobs JG, Geenan R, Van Der Heide A, Rasker JJ, Bijlsma JW. Are tender point scores assessed by manual palpation in fibromyalgia reliable? An investigation into the variance of tender point scores. Scand J Rheumatol 1995; 24:243–247.
21. Beaver WT, Feise G. Comparison of the analgesic effects of morphine, hydroxyzine, and their combination in patients with postoperative pain. In: Bonica JJ, Albe–Fessard D, eds. Advances in Pain Research and Therapy. New York: Raven Press, 1976:553–557.
22. Cooper SA, Beaver WT. A model to evaluate mild analgesics in oral surgery outpatients. Clin Pharmacol Ther 1976; 20:241–250.
23. Belknap JK, O'Toole LA. Studies of genetic differences in response to opioid drugs. In: Harris RA, Crabbe JC, eds. The genetic basis of alcohol and drug actions. New York: Plenum Press, 1992:225–252.
24. Mogil JS, Sternberg W, Marek P, Sadowski B, Belknap J, Liebeskind JC. The genetics of pain and pain inhibition. Proc Natl Acad Sci USA 1996; 93:3048–3055.

25. Belknap JK, Mogil JS, Helms ML, Richards SP, O'Toole LA, Bergeson SE, Buck KJ. Localization to chromosome 10 of a locus influencing morphine analgesia in crosses derived from C57BL/6 and DBA/2 strains. Life Sci 1995; 57:117–124.
26. Honkasalo ML, Kaprio J, Winter T, Heikkila K, Sillanpaa M, Koskenvuo M. Migraine and concomitant symptoms among 8167 adult twin pairs. Headache 1995; 35:70–78.
27. Larsson B, Bille B, Pedersen NL. Genetic influence in headaches: a Swedish twin study. Headache 1995; 35:513–519.
28. Ziegler DK, Hur YM, Bouchard TJ Jr, Hassanein RS, Barter R. Migraine in twins raised together and apart. Headache 1998; 38:417–422.
29. Treloar SA, Martin NG, Heath A. Longitudinal genetic analysis of menstrual flow, pain, and limitation in a sample of Australian twins. Behav Genet 1998; 28:107–116.
30. Bengtsson B, Thorson J. Back pain: a study of twins. Acta Genet Med Gemellol (Roma) 1991; 40: 83–90.
31. Kest B, Wilson SG, Mogil JS. Sex differences in supraspinal morphine analgesia are dependent on genotype. J Pharmacol Exp Ther 1999; 289:1370–1375.
32. Mogil JS, Wilson SG, Bon K, Lee SE, Chung K, Raber P, Pieper JO, Hain HS, Belknap JK, Hubert L, Elmer GI, Chung JM, Devor M. Heritability of nociception I: responses of 11 inbred mouse strains on 12 measures of nociception. Pain 1999; 80:67–82.
33. Mogil JS, Wilson SG, Bon K, Lee SE, Chung K, Raber P, Pieper JO, Hain HS, Belknap JK, Hubert L, Elmer GI, Chung JM, Devor M. Heritability of nociception. II. "Types" of nociception revealed by genetic correlation analysis. Pain 1999; 80:83–93.
34. Alvan G, Bechtel P, Iselius L, Gundert-Remy U. Hydroxylation polymorphisms of debrisoquine and mephenytonin in European populations. J Clin Pharmacol 1991; 39:533–537.
35. Zanger UM, Vilbois F, Hardwick J, Meyer UA. Absence of hepatic cytochrome P450 bufl causes genetically deficient debrisoquine oxidation in man. Biochemistry 1988; 27:5447–5454.
36. Yue QY, Svensson JO, Alm C, Sjoqvist F, Sawe J. Codeine *O*-demmethylation co-segregates with polymorphic debrisoquine hydroxylation. Br J Clin Pharmacol 1989; 28:639–645.
37. Chen ZR, Somogyi AA, Bocher F. Polymorphic *O*-demethylation of codeine. Lancet 1988; 2:914–915.
38. Desmeules J, Gascon M, Dayer P, Magistris M. Impact of environmental and genetic factors on codeine analgesia. Eur J Clin Pharmacol 1991; 41:23–26.
39. Ventrafrida Y, Tamburini M, Caraceni A. A validation study of the WHO method for cancer pain relief. Cancer 1987; 59:850–856.
40. Bond C, LaForge KS, Tian M, Melia D, Zhang S, Borg L, Gong J, Schluger J, Strong JA, Leal SM, Tischfield JA, Kreek MJ, Yu L. Single-nucleotide polymorphism in the human mu opioid receptor gene alters beta-endorphin binding and activity: possible implications for opiate addiction. Proc Natl Acad Sci USA 1998; 95:9608–9613.
41. Bergen AW, Kokoszka J, Peterson R, Long JC, Virkkunen M, Linnoila M, Goldman D. mu Opioid receptor gene variants: lack of association with alcohol dependence. Mol Psychiatry 1997; 2:490–494.
42. Berrettini WH, Hoehe MR, Ferraro TN, DeMaria PA, Gottheil E. Human μ opioid receptor gene polymorphisms and vulnerability to substance abuse. Addict Biol 1997; 2:303–308.
43. Pfeiffer A, Pasi A, Meraein P, Herz A. Opiate receptor binding sites in human brain. Brain Res 1982; 248:87–96.
44. Uhl GR, Sora I, Wang Z. The μ opiate receptor as a candidate gene for pain: polymorphisms, variations inexpression, nociception, and opiate responses. Proc Natl Acad Sci USA 1999; 96:7752–7755.
45. Mayer P, Rochlitz H, Rauch E, Rommelspacher H, Hasse HE, Schmidt S, Hollt V. Association between a delta opioid receptor gene polymorphism and heroin dependence in man. Neuroreport 1997; 8:2547–2550.
46. Ophoff RA, Terwindt GM, Vergouwe MN, Van Eijk R, Oefner PJ, Hoffman SMG, Lamerdin JE, Mohrenweiser HW, Bulman DE, Ferrari M, Haan J, Lindhout D, Van Ommen G-JB, Hofker MH, Ferrari MD, Frants RR. Familial hemiplegic migraine and episodic ataxia type-2 are caused by mutations in the Ca^{2+} channel gene CACNL1A4. Cell 1996; 87:543–552.

47. Joutel A, Bousser M–G, Biousse V, Labauge P, Chabriat H, Nibbio A, Maciazek J, Meyer B, Bach M–A, Weissenbach J, Lathrop GM, Tournier–Lasserve E. A gene for familial hemiplegia maps to chromosome 19. Nat Genet 1993; 5:40–45.
48. Peroutka SJ. Genetic basis of migraine. Clin Neurosci 1998; 5:34–37.
49. Nyholt DR, Dawkins JL, Brimage PJ, Goadsby PJ, Nicholson GA, Gryffiths LR. Evidence for an X-linked genetic component in familial typical migraine. Hum Mol Genet 1998; 7:459–463.
50. Stewart WF, Lipton RB, Celentano DD, Reed ML. Prevalence of migraine headache in the United States. JAMA 1992; 267:64–69.
51. Stewart WF, Linet MS, Celentano DD, Natta MV, Ziegler D. Age- and sex-specific incidence rates of migraine with and without visual aura. Am J Epidemiol 1991; 134:1111–1120.
52. Vital A, Fontan D, Julien J, Talon P, Heron B, Routon MC, Ponsat G, Vital C. Congenital insensitivity to pain with anhydrosis report of two unrelated cases. J Periph Nerv Syst 1998; 32:125–132.
53. Berkovitch M, Copeliovitch L, Tauber T, Vaknin Z, Lahat E. Hereditary insensitivity to pain with anhidrosis. Pediatr Neurol 1998; 19:227–229.
54. Indo Y, Tsuruta M, Hayashida Y, Karim MA, Ohta K, Kawano T, Mitsubuchi H, Tonoki H, Awaya Y, Matsuda I. Mutations in the TRKA/NGF receptor gene in patients with congenital insensitivity to pain with anhidrosis. Nat Genet 1996; 13:485–488.
55. Kaplan DR, Hempstead BL. The *trk* proto-oncogene product: a signal transducing receptor for nerve growth factor. Science 1991; 252:554–558.
56. Indo Y, Mardy S, Tsuruta M, Karim MA, Matsuda I. Structure and organisation of the human *TRKA* gene encoding a high affinity receptor for nerve growth factor. Jpn J Hum Genet 1997; 42:343–351.
57. Miozzo M, Pierotti MA. Human *TRK* proto-oncogene maps to chromosome 1q32-q41. Oncogene 1990; 5:1411–1414.
58. Berkovitch M, Copeliovitch L, Tauber T, Vaknin Z, Lahat E. Hereditary insensitivity to pain with anhidrosis. Pediatr Neurol 1998; 19:227–229.
59. Blumenfield. Localisation of the gene for familial dysautonomia of chromosome 9 and definition of DNA markers for genetic diagnosis. Nat Genet 1993; 4:160–164.
60. Shapira J, Zilberman Y, Becker A. Lesch–Nyhan syndrome: a nonextracting approach to prevent mutilation. Spec Care Dent 1985; 5:210–212.
61. Lowe O. Tourette's syndrome: management of oral complications. J Dent Child 1986; 53:456–460.
62. Shear CS, Nyhan WL, Kirman BH, Stem J. Self mutilative behavior as a feature of the de Lange syndrome. J Pediatr 1971; 78:506–509.
63. Elemer IE, Gorelick DA, Goldberg SR, Rothman RB. Acute sensitivity vs. context-specific sensitization to cocaine as a function of genotype. Pharmacol Biochem Behav 1996; 53:623–628.
64. Mathiasen JR, Raffa RB, Vaught JL. C57BL/6J-bgJ (beige) mice: differential sensitivity in the tail flick test to centrally administered mu- and delta-opioid receptor agonists. Life Sci 1987; 40:1989–1994.
65. Smithies O, Gregg RG, Boggs SS, Koralewski MA, Kucherlapati RS. Insertion of DNA sequences into the human chromosomal β-globin locus by homologous recombination. Nature 1985; 317:230–234.
66. Mansour SL, Thomas KR, Capecchi MR. Disruption of the proto-oncogene *int-2* in mouse embryo-derived stem cells: a general strategy for targeting mutations to non-selectable genes. Nature 1988; 336:348–352.
67. Bradley A, Evans M, Kaufman MH, Robertson EJ. Formation of germ-line chimaeras from embryo teratocarcinoma cell lines. Nature 1984; 309:255–256.
68. Mogil JS, Grisel JE. Transgenics studies of pain. Pain 1998; 77:107–128.
69. Sharstry BS. More to learn from gene knockouts. Mol Cell Biochem 1994; 136:171–182.
70. Bailey DW. Allelic forms of a gene controlling the female immune response to the male antigen in mice. Transplantation 1971; 11:426–428.
71. Shuster L, Webster GW, Yu G, Eleftheriou BE. A genetic analysis of the response to morphine in mice: analgesia and running. Psychopharmacologia 1975; 42:249–254.
72. Baran A, Shuster L, Eleftheriou BE, Bailey DW. Opiate receptors in mice: genetic differences. Life Sci 1975; 17:633–640.

73. Roy B, Cheng RSS, Phelan J, Pomeranz BE. Endogenous and exogenous opiate agonists and antagonists. In: Ware EL, ed. New York: Pergamon, 1979:297–300.
74. Moskowitz AS, Goodman RR. Autoradiographic analysis of mu1, mu2, and delta opioid binding in the central nervous system of C57BL/6BY and CXBK (opioid receptor-deficient) mice. Brain Res 1985; 360:108–116.
75. Panocka I, Marek P, Sadowski B. Inheritance of stress-induced analgesia in mice. Selective breeding study. Brain Res 1986; 397:152–155.
76. Panocka I, Marek P, Sadowski B. Differentiation of neurochemical basis of stress-induced analgesia in mice by selective breeding. Brain Res 1986; 397:156–160.
77. Panocka I, Sadowski B. Correlation between magnitude and opioid mediation of stress-induced analgesia: individual differences and the effect of selective breeding. Acta Neurobiol Exp (Warsz) 1990; 50:535–538.
78. Mogil JS, Marek P, O'Toole LA, Helms ML, Sadowski B, Liebeskind JC, Belknap JK. mu-Opiate receptor binding is up-regulated in mice selectively bred for high stress-induced analgesia. Brain Res 1994; 653:16–22.
79. Mogil JS, Marek P, Flodman P, Spence MA, Sternberg WF, Kest B, Sadowski B, Liebeskind JC. One or two genetic loci mediate high opiate analgesia in selectively bred mice. Pain 1995; 60:125–135.
80. Belknap JK, Haltli NR, Goebel DM, Lame M. Selective breeding for high and low levels of opiate-induced analgesia in mice. Behav Genet 1983; 13:383–396.
81. Belknap JK, Danielson PW, Laursen SE, Noordewier B. Selective breeding for levorphanol-induced antinociception on the hot-plate assay: commonalities in mechanism of action with morphine, pentazocine, ethylketocyclazocine, U-50488H and clonidine in mice. J Pharmacol Exp Ther 1987; 241: 477–481.
82. Belknap JK, Laursen SE. DSLET (D-ser2-leu5-enkephalin-Thr6) produces analgesia on the hot plate by mechanisms largely different from DAGO and morphine-like opioids. Life Sci 1987; 41:391–395.
83. Mogil JS, Flodman P, Spence MA, Sternberg WF, Kest B, Sadowski B, Liebeskind JC, Belknap JK. Oligogenic determination of morphine analgesic magnitude: a genetic analysis of selectively bred mouse lines. Behav Genet 1995; 25:397–406.
84. Wall PD, Devor M, Inbal R, Scadding JW, Schonfeld D, Seltzer Z, Tomkiewicz MM. Autotomy following peripheral nerve lesions: experimental anaesthesia dolorosa. Pain 1979; 7:103–111.
85. Devor M, Raber P. Heritability of symptoms in an experimental model of neuropathic pain. Pain 1990; 42:51–67.
86. Mogil JS, Richards SP, O'Toole LA, Helms ML, Mitchell SR, Kest B, Belknap JK. Identification of a sex-specific quantitative trait locus mediating nonopioid stress-induced analgesia in female mice. J Neurosci 1997; 17:7995–8002.
87. Mogil JS, Richards SP, O'Toole LA, Helms ML, Mitchell SR, Belknap JK. Genetic sensitivity to hot-plate nociception in DBA/2J and C57BL/6J inbred mouse strains: possible sex-specific mediation by delta2-opioid receptors. Pain 1997; 70:267–277.
88. Schena M, Shalon D, Davis RW, Brown PO. Quantitative monitoring of gene expression patterns with a complementary DNA microarray. Science 1995; 270:467–470.
89. DeRisi JL, Iyer VR, Brown PO. Exploring the metabolic and genetic control of gene expression on a genomic scale. Science 1997; 278:680–686.
90. Iyer VR, Eisen MB, Ross DT, Schuler G, Moore T, Lee JCF, Trent JM, Staudt LM, Hudson J Jr, Boguski MS, Lashkari D, Shalon D, Botstein D, Brown P. The transcriptional program in the response of human fibroblasts to serum. Science 1999; 283:83–87.
91. Eisen MB, Spellman PT, Brown PO, Botstein D. Cluster analysis and display of genome-wide expression patterns. Proc Natl Acad Sci USA 1998; 95:14863–14868.
92. Tavazoie S, Hughes JD, Campbell MJ, Cho RJ, Church GM. Systematic determination of genetic network architecture. Nat Genet 1999; 22:281–285.

29
Animal Models of Pain

Philip J. Siddall
University of Sydney and Royal North Shore Hospital, St Leonards, New South Wales, Australia

Rajesh Munglani
University of Cambridge and Addenbrooke's Hospital, Cambridge, England

I. INTRODUCTION

Animal models of pain have been invaluable tools in many of the advances in our understanding of pain mechanisms. Pain can broadly be divided into two types: nociceptive and neuropathic. Nociceptive pain refers to pain arising from direct stimulation of nociceptors, such as occurs with trauma or inflammation. Neuropathic pain refers to pain arising from damage to the nervous system. Nociceptive pain can be further divided into pain caused by a well-defined, short-lasting, noxious stimulus, and pain associated with the secondary changes associated with inflammation. Therefore, there are three main types of pain that appear to have distinct, although overlapping mechanisms. Animal models have been developed to explore the mechanisms and possible treatments for each of these different types of pain. This chapter briefly reviews the most commonly used animal models of acute nociceptive, inflammatory, and neuropathic pain.

II. NOCICEPTIVE PAIN MODELS

Several nociceptive models have been developed as assays of pain behavior and fall mainly into two categories: those that employ an acute nociceptive stimulus and that are concerned with short-term nociceptive responses, and those that are more concerned with the medium or long-term responses associated with inflammation. Historically, acute nociceptive tests have been the predominant means of pain assay. However, the increased interest in the long-term peripheral and central responses to inflammation and the importance of these processes to understanding chronic pain has led to an increased use of the inflammatory models.

A. Acute Nociceptive

1. Tail Flick

The tail-flick test was one of the first, and remains one of the most widely used, tests of acute nociception. It was described more than 50 years ago and consists of focusing a beam of radiant heat on the tail of the animal and measuring the time until the animal flicks the tail away from the beam (D'Amour and Smith, 1941). It is not blocked by spinal transection and, therefore, is a spinally mediated nociceptive reflex. Although a useful test, there are concerns about the interaction between temperature and skin blood flow and tail flick latency. This is an issue that must be considered in interpretation of results.

2. Tail Immersion

Tail immersion is similar to tail flick, but the tail is heated by immersion in hot water that is kept at a constant temperature.

3. Hot Plate Test

The hot plate test was initially described in 1944, and, with the tail-flick test, remains one of the most commonly used test of acute nociception (Woolfe and MacDonald, 1944). The test has been modified so that the animal is placed on the hot plate which is usually kept at a constant 50° or 55°C. The latency to behavioral responses times, including licking the paw, jumping, shaking the paw, or holding it against the body, are then measured as indicators of nociception.

The increasing temperature hot plate test uses the same basic design, but the initial temperature of the plate is set below the noxious threshold (42°–43°C) and is gradually increased until a response is observed or until the cutoff temperature (50°–52°C) is reached. The temperature of the plate when a response occurs (hindpaw licking), rather than latency, is used as the endpoint. This form of the test has been found to be more sensitive and less influenced by pretest skin temperature.

4. Radiant Heat and Laser Irradiation

In these tests, the animal is placed in a Plexiglas container or suitably restrained, and a focused radiant heat source or laser is used to heat the paw from underneath the floor, which is transparent. The beam is coupled to a movement detector switch that cuts out when the foot is removed from the heat source. Withdrawal latency is then used as a measure of nociception.

5. Paw Pressure and Tail Pinch

These tests use mechanical, rather than thermal, stimuli. An increasing pressure is applied to the paw or the tail, and the force is recorded when withdrawal or vocalization occurs (Randall and Selitto, 1957). Paw pressure is a measure of a nociceptive response, but is used with models of inflammatory and neuropathic pain.

6. Von Frey Hairs

Von Frey hairs are also used with inflammatory and neuropathic models. They comprise a number of graded and calibrated monofilaments which apply a known force to the skin. Filaments of varying force are applied to the skin until the threshold for vocalization or withdrawal is obtained.

7. Visceral Distension

The rectum and distal colon are distended with constant pressure by means of a balloon in an effort to reproduce the pain seen clinically following visceral distension.

8. Foot Shock

Foot shock is sometimes used as a measure of nociception, but because of the nature of the stimulus, there is some difficulty in interpretation and correlation with pain.

B. Inflammation

Although models of acute pain have been useful in understanding some facets of pain processing, their usefulness in examining the mechanisms of clinical pain conditions is limited. In the clinical situation, pain rarely takes the form of a brief, noxious, but nondamaging stimulus. More commonly, the changes associated with the inflammation directly affect the responsiveness of the nociceptive system both peripherally and centrally. Therefore, many more recent studies have employed animal models in which pain is associated with inflammation. These models use different agents that result in several specific changes that, nevertheless, share common features.

1. Topical Capsaicin

Capsaicin is applied to the skin and results in a neurogenic inflammatory response.

2. Skin Irradiation

Irradiation of the skin by ultraviolet light produces localized inflammation and hyperalgesia of the exposed area.

3. Subcutaneous Carrageenan and Brewer's Yeast

Injection of both of these agents subcutaneously into the paw results in localized inflammation and hyperalgesia with associated nociceptive behavior including licking and lifting and protection of the injected paw.

4. Subcutaneous Formalin

Diluted formalin is injected subcutaneously into a paw to induce inflammation. Two phases are observed: an early phase that commences immediately following injection and lasts for 5–10 min, and a late phase that lasts for 15–60 min following injection (Dubuisson and Dennis, 1977). The stimulus during the early phase is due to direct chemical activation of nociceptors, whereas the late phase has an inflammatory component and is dependent on central processing in the spinal cord. Similar to the tail-flick test, it has been demonstrated that blood flow changes may affect the late phase of the test.

5. Intramuscular Irritants

Intramuscular injection of bradykinin is believed to produce a nociceptive muscle stimulus, and experimental inflammation of the muscle can be induced by intramuscular injections of carrageenan.

6. Monoarthritis

Several agents, including carageenan, uric acid, and mustard oil, can be injected into the knee or ankle joint to induce a monoarthritis with behavioral changes that last several days. A more long-lasting monoarthritis can be produced by injection of complete adjuvant into the tibiotarsal joint of rats. The effects produced in this model are more pronounced and last approximately 6 weeks.

7. Polyarthritis

Injection of Freund's complete adjuvant (FCA) intradermally into the tail of rats results in polyarthritis that develops over weeks and last for several months. It appears to show many of the features and responds similarly to human arthritic conditions. Vocalization response and paw volume are used as measures.

8. Abdominal and Visceral Pain

Intraperitoneal injection of irritants induces a syndrome of "writhing," which consists of contractions of the abdomen, twisting and turning of the trunk, and extension of the hind limbs, and is sometimes known as the abdominal stretch assay. Several compounds are used including bradykinin, acetylcholine, acetic acid, and phenylquinone. There is wide variability of response in this test, including attenuation by drugs that have little analgesic action in humans.

Extensive animal studies have also been carried out using the bladder as a model of visceral pain (Janig and Koltzenburg, 1993). In this model, irritant chemicals are introduced into the bladder to produce inflammation, with little tissue destruction (Koltzenburg and McMahon, 1986).

C. Intrathecal Administration of Agents

Intrathecal injection of agents can be used to study a "painful" state in the absence of peripheral nociceptor stimulation. Intrathecal injection of glutamate and substance P results in biting and scratching that is directed toward the caudal region of the body. Other agents include capsaicin, and agents that act on *N*-methyl-D-aspartate (NMDA) and α-amino-3-hydroxy-5-methylisoxazole (AMPA) receptors. Intrathecal injection of strychnine results in mechanical allodynia in the dermatomes corresponding to the level of injection.

III. NEUROPATHIC PAIN MODELS

A. Introduction

Neuropathic pain can be broadly divided into central and peripheral neuropathic pain depending on whether the primary lesion or dysfunction is situated in the central or peripheral nervous system and may be due to mechanical trauma, ischemia, degeneration, or inflammation. The injury results in a broad range of pathologies. These range from a transient ischemia, which may result in a selective loss of specific neuronal type, to complete denervation.

These pathophysiological changes result in several features, including (1) unpleasant, spontaneous, abnormal sensations (dysesthesias) and pains that are often sharp, shooting, electric, or burning in quality; (2) attribution of the location of the pain to an area of sensory loss or disturbance; and (3) altered responsiveness of the tissues that are affected. These alterations in tissue responsiveness include pain in response to a stimulus that does not normally provoke pain (allodynia), an increased response to a stimulus that is normally painful (hyperalgesia), temporal and spatial summation, and after-sensation (hyperpathia). As well as the features described, sympathetic nervous system involvement is commonly seen in models of neuropathic pain. This may include vasomotor and sudomotor changes, abnormalities of hair and nail growth, and osteoporosis.

B. Peripheral Nerve Injury

Animal models of neuropathic pain have largely focused on peripheral nerve injury. Some of the models are quite specific to certain neuropathic pain conditions and include animal models of trigeminal neuralgia (Vos and Maciewicz, 1994), diabetic neuropathy (Burchiel et al., 1985), and vincristine neuropathy (Aley et al., 1996). However, most animal studies have been performed using models that are more generally related to peripheral nerve injury.

1. Neuroma Model

The neuroma model was one of the first models used to investigate pain following peripheral nerve injury (Wall et al., 1979). In this model, the sciatic and saphenous nerves are transected, the central end is tied off and 5 mm of the nerve distal to the transection is removed. This procedure completely denervates the hindpaw of the rat. It results in autotomy (self-mutilation of the limb) which is believed to be a sign of spontaneous pain. The neuroma model reflects the pain that occurs following complete nerve transection (anesthesia dolorosa) or the phantom pain that occurs following limb amputation.

Although the transection model was useful in helping understand the pain that occurs following complete deafferentation, it is still not certain that autotomy is due to pain and not to complete absence of sensation. Furthermore, many of the pain conditions seen following nerve injury are due to partial, rather than complete, nerve injury. Because of these constraints, several models of partial nerve injury have been developed. These include chronic constriction injury (Bennett and Xie, 1988), partial nerve ligation (Seltzer et al. 1990), the spinal nerve transection (Lombard et al., 1979) or ligation (Kim and Chung, 1992; Carlton et al., 1994), cryoneurolysis (Deleo et al., 1994) and sciatic nerve ischemia (Kupers et al., 1998). These models have the advantage that input is preserved and allows analysis of changes in mechanical and thermal thresholds in addition to the guarding and autotomy that are believed to be signs of spontaneous pain.

2. Chronic Constriction Injury

The chronic constriction injury model (Bennett and Xie, 1988) was the first of these neuropathic pain models to be developed. In this model, about 4–5 mm of sciatic nerve is exposed at the level of the thigh and is loosely ligated with four ligatures of 4-0 chromic catgut spaced about 1-mm apart. The ligatures are tied closely enough to cause slight constriction and swelling, but not enough to result in complete denervation. It results in severe damage to myelinated fibers and significant disruption and loss of unmyelinated axons. Similar to the transection model, this model results in autotomy but animals also exhibit features of guarding, thermal and mechanical hyperalgesia, thermal and mechanical allodynia, and sympathetic changes.

3. Sciatic Nerve Partial Ligation

In this model, the sciatic nerve on one side is partially (one-third to one-half) ligated with 8-0 silk. This procedure results in mechanical allodynia, thermal and mechanical hyperalgesia, guarding, but not autotomy, and signs of sympathetic involvement (Seltzer et al., 1990).

With the increasing interest in the investigation of molecular processes associated with neuropathic pain and the availability of transgenic mice, it has become necessary to develop mouse models of neuropathic pain. Tight ligation of one-half to one-third of the sciatic nerve with 9-0 silk suture in the mouse model similarly results in thermal and mechanical allodynia on the ligated side which is reduced by sympathetic blockade (Malmberg and Basbaum, 1998).

4. Spinal Nerve Ligation

This model involves tight ligation of the L5 and L6 spinal nerves with 3-0 silk. This results in signs of spontaneous pain, guarding, mechanical allodynia, and thermal hyperalgesia. The model was originally developed in the rat (Kim and Chung, 1992), but has also been used in primates (Carlton et al., 1994).

5. Cryoneurolysis

In this model, the sciatic nerve is injured proximal to the trifurcation using a cryoprobe cooled to −60°C. The probe is cooled for 30 s, thawed for 5 s, and recooled for 30 s. This injury results in signs of spontaneous pain, mechanical allodynia, and autotomy, but not thermal hyperalgesia. (Deleo et al., 1994).

6. Ischemic Injury

A model of ischemic nerve injury has been developed that produces features of neuropathic pain (Kupers et al., 1998). In this model, a photosensitizing dye is injected systemically and the exposed sciatic nerve is laser irradiated for up to 2 min. This results in axonal degeneration and demyelination of large fibers. Signs of mechanical and thermal allodynia and hyperalgesia and spontaneous pain (paw shaking, paw elevation, and "freezing" behavior) are present for up to 10 weeks following injury.

7. Diabetes

Streptozocin-induced diabetic rats have been used to investigate the abnormalities of sensation which can occur with diabetes mellitus (Burchiel et al. 1985). Strains of rats that spontaneously develop diabetes have also been used.

C. Spinal Cord Injury

Relatively few studies have used animal models to investigate the mechanisms or management of pain following damage to the central nervous system. Several animal models have been used to investigate pain following spinal cord injury and include a cord transection or partial transection model (Levitt and Levitt, 1981), an irradiation-induced cord ischemia model (Hao et al., 1991; Xu et al., 1992), an excitotoxic model using intraspinal injections of quisqualate (Yezierski and Park, 1993), and a contusion model that uses weight drop to produce mechanical trauma to the spinal cord (Siddall et al., 1995).

These animal models of spinal cord injury pain, while not producing identical features, nevertheless result in patterns of behavior that are similar among models. They all result in an increased sensitivity or reduced threshold to mechanical and, in one case, thermal stimuli in the dermatomes that correspond to the level of injury. Two of the models also result in autotomy (Levitt and Levitt, 1981; Xu et al., 1992).

Electrophysiological recordings in both the ischemic (Hao et al., 1992) and excitotoxic (Yezierski and Park, 1993) models demonstrate abnormal activity of spinal neurons adjacent to the lesion, with lowering of threshold, increased levels of background spontaneous discharge, and prolonged afterdischarges.

D. Sympathetic Nervous System

Studies that have investigated autonomic nervous system mechanisms have generally used existing models of peripheral nerve injury (Shir and Seltzer, 1990; Wakisaka et al., 1991; Chung et al., 1993; Bennett and Roberts, 1996). Features such as skin temperature changes, swelling, and redness of the skin have been observed in the CCI model (Bennett and Xie, 1988) and in other models (Seltzer et al., 1990; Kim and Chung, 1992). Therefore, it is difficult to distinguish animal models in which the pain has a sympathetic component from general models of peripheral nerve injury-induced neuropathic pain.

IV. CONCLUSIONS

There are several limitations associated with the use of animal models. These include trying to determine and correlate animal behavior with the human experience of pain, using a specific physiological response, such a spinal nociceptive reflex, as a measure of pain; accurately linking models to specific clinical pain syndromes; and transferring findings from animal studies to clinical use. Finally, it is extremely difficult to model the complex emotional, behavioral, and environmental factors that form part of the human pain experience. Therefore, it is not surprising that the predictive ability of animal models is sometimes poor. Nevertheless, animal models of pain have been extremely useful in helping understand the physiological processes involved in the development and maintenance of chronic pain, in exploring and developing new treatments, and in providing insights into clinical presentation.

REFERENCES

Aley KO, Reichling DB, Levine JD. (1996) Vincristine hyperalgesia in the rat—a model of painful vincristine neuropathy in humans. Neuroscience 73:259–265.

Bennett GJ, Roberts WJ. (1996) Animal models and their contribution to our understanding of complex regonal pain syndromes I and II. In: Janig W, Stanton–Hicks M, eds. Reflex Sympathetic Dystrophy: A Reappraisal. Prog Pain Res Manage 6:107–122.

Bennett GJ, Xie Y–K. (1988) A peripheral mononeuropathy in rat that produces disorders of pain sensation like those seen in man. Pain 33:87–107.

Burchiel KJ, Russell LC, Lee RP, Sima AAF. (1985) Spontaneous activity of primary afferent neurons in diabetic BB/Wistar rats. Diabetes 34:1210–1213.

Carlton SM, Lekan HA, Kim SH, Chung JM. (1994) Behavioral manifestations of an experimental model for peripheral neuropathy produced by spinal nerve ligation in the primate. Pain 56:155–166.

Chung K, Kim HJ, Na HS, Park MJ, Chung JM. (1993) Abnormalities of sympathetic innervation in the area of an injured peripheral nerve in a rat model of neuropathic pain. Neurosci Lett 162:85–88.

D'Amour FE, Smith DL. (1941) A method for determining loss of pain sensation. J Pharmacol 72:74–79.

Deleo JA, Coombs DW, Willenbring S, Colburn RW, Fromm C, Wagner R, Twitchell BB. (1994) Characterization of a neuropathic pain model—sciatic cryoneurolysis in the rat. Pain 56:9–16.

Dubuisson D, Dennis SG. (1977) The formalin test: a quantitative study of the analgesic effects of morphine, meperidine, and brain stem stimulation in rats and cats. Pain 4:161–174.

Hao JX, Xu XJ, Aldskogius H, Seiger A, Wiesenfeld–Hallin Z. (1991) Allodynia-like effects in rat after ischaemic spinal cord injury photochemically induced by laser irradiation. Pain 45:175–185.

Hao JX, Xu XJ, Yu YX, Seiger A, Wiesenfeld–Hallin Z. (1992) Transient spinal cord ischaemia induces temporary hypersensitivity of dorsal horn wide dynamic range neurons to myelinated, but not unmyelinated, fiber input. J Neurophysiol 68:384–391.

Janig W, Koltzenburg M. (1993) Pain arising from the urogenital tract. In: CA Maggi, ed. Nervous Control of the Urogenital System. Chur: Harwood: pp. 525–578.

Kim SH, Chung JM. (1992) An experimental model for peripheral neuropathy produced by segmental spinal nerve ligation in the rat. Pain 50:355–363.

Koltzenburg M, McMahon SB. (1986) Plasma extravasation in the rat urinary bladder following mechanical, electrical and chemical stimuli: evidence for a new population of chemosensitive primary sensory afferents. Neurosci Lett 72:352–356.

Kupers R, Yu W, Persson JKE, Xu XJ, Wiesenfeld-Hallin Z. (1998) Photochemically-induced ischemia of the rat sciatic nerve produces a dose-dependent and highly reproducible mechanical, heat and cold allodynia, and signs of spontaneous pain. Pain 76:45–59.

Levitt M, Levitt JH. (1981) The deafferentation syndrome in monkeys: dysaesthesias of spinal origin. Pain 10:129–147.

Lombard MC, Nashold BS, Albe–Fessard D. (1979) Deafferentation hypersensitivity in the rat after dorsal rhizotomy: a possible model of chronic pain. Pain 6:163–174.

Malmberg AB, Basbaum AI. (1998) Partial sciatic nerve injury in the mouse as a model of neuropathic pain—behavioral and neuroanatomical correlates. Pain 76:215–222.

Randall LO, Selitto JJ. (1957) A method for measurement of analgesic activity on inflamed tissue. Arch Int Pharmacodyn Ther 111:409–418.

Seltzer Z, Dubner R, Shir Y. (1990) A novel behavioral model of neuropathic pain disorders produced in rats by partial sciatic nerve injury. Pain 43:205–218.

Shir Y, Seltzer Z. (1990) A-fibers mediate mechanical hyperesthesia and allodynia and C-fibers mediate thermal hyperalgesia in a new model of causalgiform pain disorders in rats. Neurosci. Lett 115:62–67.

Siddall PJ, Xu CL, Cousins MJ. (1995) Allodynia following traumatic spinal cord injury in the rat. Neuroreport 6:1241–1244.

Vos BP, Maciewicz RJ. (1994) Behavioral evidence of trigeminal neuropathic pain following chronic constriction injury to rats' infraorbital nerve. J Neurosci 14:2708–2723.

Wakisaka S, Kajander KC, Bennett GJ. (1991) Abnormal skin temperature and abnormal sympathetic vasomotor innervation in an experimental painful peripheral neuropathy. Pain 46:299–313.

Wall PD, Devor M, Inbal R, Scadding JW, Schonfield D, Seltzer Z, Tomkiewicz MM. (1979) Autotomy following peripheral nerve lesions: experimental anesthesia dolorosa. Pain 7:103–113.

Woolfe G, MacDonald AD. (1944) The evaluation of the analgesic action of pethidine hydrochloride (Demerol). J Pharmacol Exp Ther 80:300–307.

Xu X–J, Hao JX, Aldskogius, H, Seiger A, Wiesenfeld–Hallin Z. (1992) Chronic pain-related syndrome in rats after ischemic spinal cord lesion: a possible animal model for pain in patients with spinal cord injury. Pain 48:279–290.

Yezierski RP, Park SH. (1993) The mechanosensitivity of spinal sensory neurons following intraspinal injections of quisqualic acid in the rat. Neurosci Lett 157:115–119.

30

An Overview of Current and Investigational Drugs for the Treatment of Acute and Chronic Pain

William K. Schmidt
Adolor Corporation, Exton, Pennsylvania, U.S.A.

I. INTRODUCTION

Pain is one of the most basic clinical symptoms seen by every physician and is often the primary reason that patients seek medical advice. Over 100 million patients experience acute or chronic pain annually in the United States caused by headache, muscle strains and sprains, arthritis, trauma, cancer, surgery, and back injuries, among others. Because pain impairs one's ability to carry out a productive life, pain in general and chronic pain in particular are serious health and economic problems.

It used to be thought that moderate-severe pain was reasonably well treated by narcotic analgesics and narcotic-aspirin or narcotic-acetaminophen combination products, many of which are available in the generic market and are relatively inexpensive to purchase. Starting with the discovery of purified morphine by the German chemist Sertürner in 1806, more than 16 other narcotic-related analgesics and one nonsteroidal anti-inflammatory drug (NSAID) product have been approved for treating postsurgical pain or moderate-severe acute or chronic pain (Fig. 1). All but one of these drugs share the property of interacting with the morphine μ opioid receptor in the brain to produce some or all of their analgesic effects. The only exception is ketorolac, first introduced as an injectable product for treating moderate-severe pain in 1990 and later as an oral product in 1991 (see below). The major change in this market segment has come with the introduction during the past decade of sustained-release preparations of opioid narcotic analgesics, but individual products that have even modest differentiation from existing drugs (e.g., tramadol, see below) have experienced explosive growth in use.

It also was once thought that the mild-to-moderate segment was reasonably well satisfied by aspirin, acetaminophen, ibuprofen, and other NSAID products, all of which have the potential for gastric ulceration and bleeding. The introduction of two COX-2 inhibitors in 1999 completely changed the way that many physicians think about treating acute or chronic pain in the mild-moderate category and revitalized the market for mild-moderate pain analgesics.

Oral opioids are frequently added to NSAIDs or COX-2 inhibitors for higher levels of pain relief, but these frequently cause drowsiness or dizziness and carry the added risk of narcotic-related side effects, tolerance and addiction liability, and toxicity by themselves or

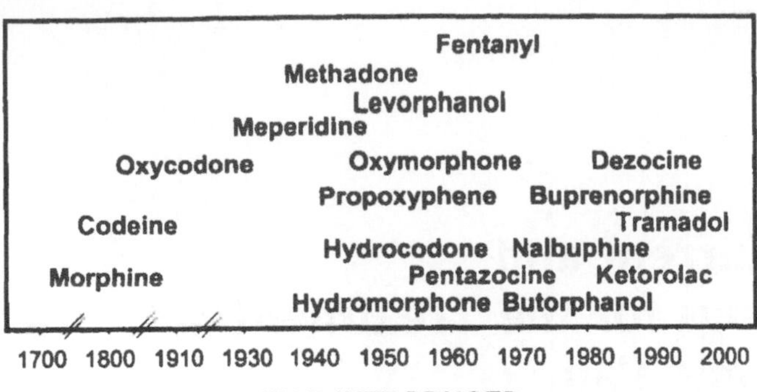

Figure 1 Analgesics for moderate-severe pain.

in combination with alcohol or other drugs. Patients with advanced cancer pain, osteoarthritis, rheumatoid arthritis, or neuropathic pain frequently do not achieve adequate relief of pain with existing drugs owing to sometimes-limited efficacy, tolerance development (to opioid narcotic analgesics), or intolerable side effects. Patients in European, Latin American, and Asian countries use minimal amounts of narcotics because of their abuse and addiction potential.

Hence, there is a significant unmet medical need for safer, nonabusable, nonaddicting, nonscheduled, and non-tolerance-producing oral and parenteral products for the treatment of mild-moderate and moderate-severe pain. Market statistics show a continuing unmet medical need for safer, easier-to-use, and more effective treatments for both acute and chronic pain. Some types of pain, such as neuropathic pain, visceral pain, and some types of centrally mediated pain, are not managed well with existing therapies and require new approaches to pain management.

A. Growth Factors in the Analgesic Market

There has been an increasing focus on pain management throughout the health care industry. Recently published guidelines of the World Health Organization and the U.S. Agency for Health Care Policy and Research have encouraged the use of more progressive analgesic therapy for treating cancer pain, acute pain, and chronic pain (1–6). In 1991, the American Board of Medical Specialties designated the treatment of pain as a recognized specialty for physicians. The number of physicians receiving specialty training in pain management increased from 446 in 1993, the first year in which certifications were granted, to a total of over 2500 in 2000 (Fig. 2). The American Board of Medicine began granting certifications in pain management in the year 2000 when they issued over 1300 certifications. As of 1999, all U.S. hospitals and health care facilities have been required to assess the adequacy of pain treatment for each patient on a daily basis to achieve accreditation by the Joint Commission on Accreditation of Healthcare Organizations. Hence, there has been greater emphasis on both the diagnosis and treatment of acute and chronic pain in recent years.

The other major driving forces for growth in the analgesic market can be summarized as follows:

Increasing recognition of the need for effective pain management and its therapeutic benefits;

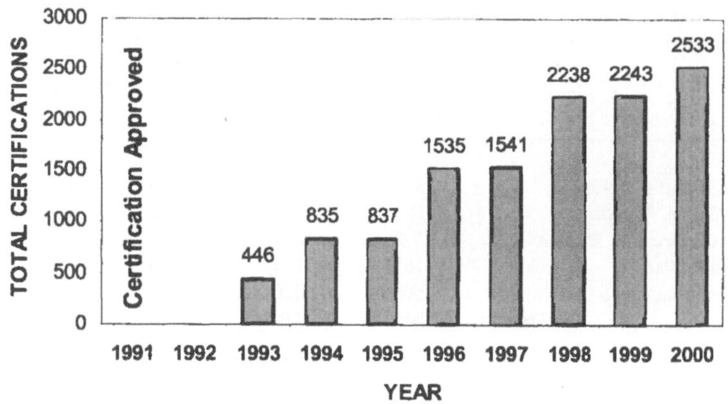

Figure 2 Certification in pain management. The American Board of Medicine provided 1335 additional certifications in the year 2000. (From American Board of Medical Specialties, 2000.)

Rapid market acceptance of new products with novel mechanisms of action;
Targeted markets that permit cost-effective selling and marketing; and
Growth in the aged population with an associated increased incidence of pain.

II. CURRENT PAIN MANAGEMENT MARKET

Growth in the pain management market has been significant in recent years and is expected to continue. Over the 7-year period 1994–2001, the market for prescription analgesic drugs increased more than 2.5× to $14.6 billion in the United States (Table 1). The rate of growth has increased in recent years; the prescription pain management market in the United States grew 6% per year from 1994 to 1998, and then grew 24% between May 1, 2000 and April 30, 2001. This growth has been fueled in part by increased demand following the release of World Health Organization and U.S. government guidelines for the treatment of pain, as mentioned above, but also by the introduction of newer nonnarcotic analgesics and sustained-release formulations of older opioid analgesics. These newer products have perceived efficacy or safety benefits and have expanded their market segments accordingly. The rapid acceptance of newly introduced products illustrates that there are still many unmet medical needs in the pain management market and that physicians are willing to prescribe new and improved products as they become available.

Individual new products introduced since 1995 (e.g., tramadol, newer sustained-release narcotic analgesics, COX-2 inhibitors) have provided growth rates within their product categories of 35–75% per year and the overall analgesic market has grown at a compound annual growth rate of 14% per year since 1994 (Table 1). This compares favorably with a 16% annualized growth rate previously reported by this author for the years 1992–1997 (7). Expected new product introductions over the next 2–5 years promise to keep the market growing at an annualized rate equal to or in excess of 14% per year.

The analgesic market segment can be divided into three major categories: *mild-to-moderate pain* ($6.7 billion, dominated in financial value by the newly introduced COX-2 inhibitors); *moderate-to-severe pain* ($4.9 billion, dominated by sustained-release opioids, tramadol, and hydrocodone-acetaminophen products); and topical pain, itch, and *special-purpose analgesic and anti-itch products* (nearly $3.0 billion, dominated by triptan-type antimigraine products,

Table 1 U.S. Analgesic Market (1994–2001)

Market segment	Representative brands	1994 U.S. sales ($MM)	1997 U.S. sales ($MM)	1999 U.S. sales ($MM)	2001 U.S. sales ($MM)
Moderate-to-severe pain					
Morphines	MS Contin, morphine	326	494	700	1,177
Codeines	OxyContin, Vicodin®	563	709	1,326	2,450
Synthetic narcotics	Talwin, Demerol, Darvon®	305	251	286	286
Synthetic nonnarcotic inj.	Toradol, Stadol®	161	148	119	91
Synthetic nonnarcotic oral	Ultram, Stadol NS	509	828	772	942
	Total	$1,864	$2,430	$3,203	$4,946
		Compound annual growth rate = 15%			
Mild-to-moderate pain					
Aspirin	Bayer, generics	315	339	197	196
Acetaminophen	Tylenol, generics	818	733	461	378
NSAIDs, oral	Motrin, Voltaren	1,800	1,901	1,551	1,423
COX-2 inhibitors	Celebrex, Vioxx	—	—	1,546	4,709
	Total	$2,933	$2,973	$3,755	$6,706
		Compound annual growth rate = 13%			
Topical pain, itch, and special-purpose analgesics					
Antimigraine	Imitrex, Zomig, Maxalt	302	851	1,171	1,666
Corticosteroids, dermal	Elocon, Synalar	510	590	640	747
Antipruritics, dermal	Caladryl, Calahist	58	56	38	43
Local anesthetics, dermal	Solarcaine, Lanacane	12	12	7	8
NSAIDs, ophthalmic	Acular, Voltaren	38	61	75	89
Special use products	Actiq, Synvisc, Lidoderm	3	29	173	401
	Total	$923	$1,599	$2,104	$2,951
		Compound annual growth rate = 18%			

Special use products = transmucosal fentanyl (Oralet, Actiq), hyaluronic acid (Hyalgan®), hylan (Synvisc), pentosan polysulfate (Elmiron), remifentanil (Ultiva), strontium-89 chloride (Metastron), samarium-153 EDTMP (Quadramet), clonidine (Duraclon), and lidocaine patch (Lidoderm)

Total analgesic market		1994	1997	1999	2001
Moderate-to-severe pain		1,864	2,430	3,203	4,946
Mild-to-moderate pain		2,933	2,973	3,755	6,706
Topical pain, itch, and special purpose analgesics		923	1,599	2,104	2,951
	Total	$5,720	$7,002	$9,062	$14,604
		Compound annual growth rate = 14%			
Total U.S. pharmaceutical market ($ millions)		$70,731	$94,082	$122,020	$185,667
	Compound annual growth rate, total U.S. pharma market = 15%				
Pain as % total U.S. pharma market		8.1%	7.4%	7.4%	7.9%

This table does not include sales of disease-modifying antiarthritic drugs (DMARDs), which are not used primarily for pain control.

Data source: IMS HEALTH © 1994, 1997, 1999, 2001, 2002 Retail and Provider Perspective. (IMS reports about 99% of the U.S. market including: chain and independent pharmacies, food stores w/pharmacies, mail order, HMOs, non-federal hospitals, federal facilities, clinics, long-term-care facilities, home health, and miscellaneous).

corticosteroids, and, more recently, viscosupplementation products to reduce arthritis pain in the knee).

Within the *mild-to-moderate* and *moderate-to-severe* market segments, newer products must compete with older products, many of which are now available in generic formulations, are undifferentiated, and are relatively inexpensive. Aside from the newly introduced products, the mild-moderate pain market has five over-the-counter (OTC) products (aspirin, acetaminophen, ibuprofen, ketoprofen, and naproxen), which are promoted extensively to consumers. In addition, more than 20 NSAIDS (including higher-strength or controlled-release formulations of ibuprofen, ketoprofen, and naproxen) and two COX-2 inhibitors are available for prescription use (see Appendix I).

Within the *moderate-to-severe* market segment, market differentiation is often by Drug Enforcement Agency (DEA) schedule (or lack thereof) and by immediate release (mostly older, generic products) versus newer sustained-release formulations. Most oral narcotic analgesic products containing oxycodone (C-II), hydrocodone or codeine (C-III), or propoxyphene or pentazocine (C-IV) are sold in combination with aspirin, acetaminophen, or ibuprofen (see Appendix I). Only a few products (tramadol, ketorolac, nalbuphine, dezocine, methotrimeprazine) are available as prescription products without DEA regulatory control.

Despite the widespread availability of *mild-to-moderate* and *moderate-to-severe* pain products, the data in Table 1 show that the fastest-growing segment of the analgesics market (more than 130× in 7 years, starting from a base of only $3 million in 1994), has come from a variety of newly introduced *special-use products* used to treat breakthrough-pain (Actiq), neuropathic pain (Lidoderm), interstitial cystitis (Elmiron), and the previously mentioned viscosupplementation products (Synvisc, Hyalgan). Other major market advances have come from the newer "triptan"-related antimigraine products (5-HT_{1d} or 5-$HT_{1d/1b}$ agonists; nearly 6× increase in market size over 7 years).

A. Growth of the Moderate-Severe Pain Market

Compared to similar surveys by this author in 1994–2000 (7–12), substantial growth in the moderate-severe pain market has been achieved by sustained-release oral morphine and oxycodone preparations and by the Duragesic transdermal fentanyl patch, all of which are indicated for chronic pain conditions and now comprise 48% of the market for moderate-severe pain. This is strikingly higher as a percentage of the moderate-severe pain market than sustained-release preparations had in 1994 (11%), 1997 (20%), and 1999 (35%) (7,10,12).

The shift in 1994–2001 market share for products in the moderate-severe pain market is shown graphically in Figure 3; the growth in sustained-release narcotic analgesics is shown in Figure 4.

Within the moderate-severe pain category, the significant growth has also occurred with nonnarcotic analgesics indicated for moderate-severe pain. Tramadol (Ultram), a nonnarcotic analgesic introduced to the U.S. market in April 1995, achieved $663 million sales in 2001 (13% moderate-severe pain market). Ketorolac (Toradol), introduced in 1990, achieved $281 million peak U.S. sales in 1994 before its market share was eroded by generic competition and concerns about its safety (see below). As the only orally active nonnarcotic analgesics indicated for moderate-severe pain, tramadol and ketorolac together account for 15% of the $4.9 billion market for drugs to treat moderate-severe pain.

The major concern with narcotics, which constitute the largest segment of the U.S. market for treatment of moderate-to-severe pain, is the potential for addiction and loss of activity (tolerance) with continued use. These concerns cause many physicians to withhold, underdose, or shorten the course of therapy with narcotics. As a result, pain is not alleviated, patients

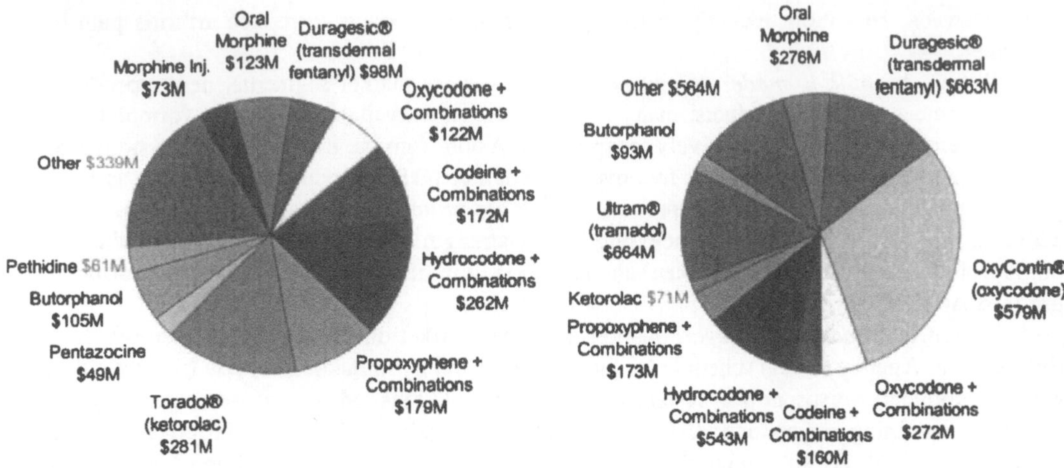

Figure 3 Analgesics for moderate-severe pain, U.S. market. (From IMS Health 1994, 2001 Retail and Provider Perspective, used with permission.)

request more medication, and the physician is faced with the decision of whether he/she is supporting ''drug-seeking behavior'' or treating a seriously ill patient. In many instances, this leads to an even more conservative use of narcotics with future treatments. This scenario helps to explain the rapid acceptance of higher-potency nonnarcotic products like ketorolac, bromfenac, and tramadol, which are currently expanding the market potential for higher-potency analgesics.

1. Ketorolac

Ketorolac is the only NSAID available for use in the United States as both an injectable and an oral analgesic. Following a 2-year Food and Drug Administration (FDA) priority review, ketorolac was approved in an intramuscular (i.m.) injectable formulation in November 1989, and launched in May 1990. The oral formulation was approved in December 1991. Ketorolac

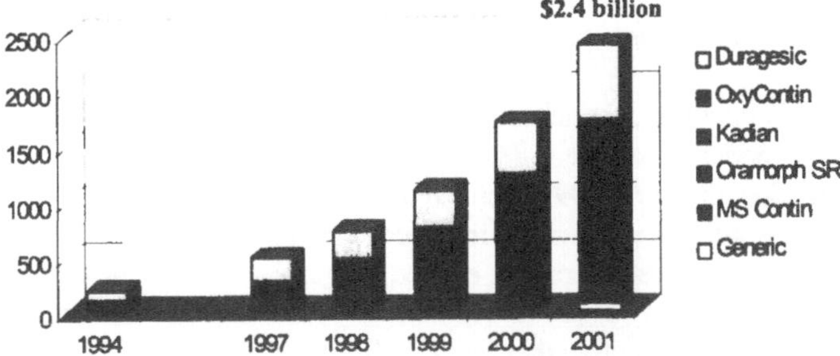

Figure 4 Sustained-release narcotic analgesics: U.S. sales. Sustained-release narcotic analgesic sales have been increasing at a compound annualized growth rate of 42% since 1994 when only two products (MS Contin, Duragesic) dominated the U.S. market. (From IMS Health 1994–2001 Retail and Provider Perspective, used with permission.)

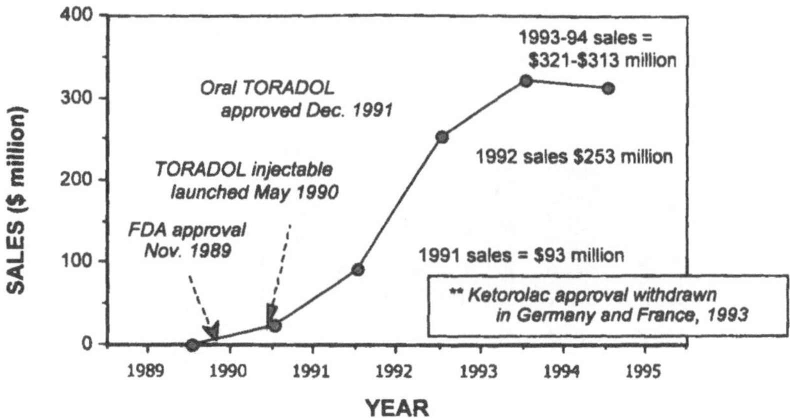

Figure 5 Ketorolac (Toradol) worldwide sales. (From Syntex Corporation, Annual Reports, 1990–1994; Roche Laboratories, 1995.) Ketorolac is now a generic product. For comparison, U.S. annual sales for the year 2001 were $2.2 million for Toradol and $71 million for generic ketorolac. (From IMS Health 2001 Retail and Provider Perspective, used with permission.)

sales data may serve to illustrate the potential market value of a newly introduced higher-potency analgesic.

Ketorolac is generally regarded as being as effective as low doses of morphine for the treatment of postoperative pain. It is limited to short-term pain management (no more than 5 days) owing to the increased frequency and severity of adverse reactions associated with longer-term treatment. After 4 years on the market, Toradol reached total worldwide sales of $321 million. This declined modestly in 1994 following withdrawal of the drug from Germany and France over concerns about ketorolac-induced deaths from bleeding and renal toxicity in older patients. Following expiration of ketorolac's patent in 1995, total U.S. sales have declined 75% from their 1994 peak; the volume of prescription doses has declined only modestly.

Ketorolac's early success may reflect its higher-efficacy analgesic profile, combined with "user frustration" with other compounds on the market and an eagerness to seek newer treatments that overcome limitations of currently available products.

2. Butorphanol

Another example of the intense interest in newer nonnarcotic analgesic products comes from the introduction of an intranasal formulation of butorphanol (Stadol NS) in 1992. Stadol injection was introduced for postoperative pain in 1978. Stadol was not introduced in an oral formulation owing to limited oral bioavailability. The newer nasal spray formulation, which has between 61 and 69% of the bioavailability of an intravenous (i.v.) dose, is promoted primarily for migraine; its rapid acceptance over the injectable formulation is shown in Figure 6. Over 80% of Stadol prescription doses and sales revenue currently comes from the intranasal formulation; the combined products achieved estimated 2001 U.S. sales of $93 million (Fig. 1). These data indicate the importance of the more "user-friendly" nasal spray versus parenteral dosing as well as renewed promotional activity on a then 14-year-old product. However, concerns about the growing abuse liability of the nasal formulation prompted the manufacturer to move butorphanol to Schedule IV of the Controlled Substances Act in 1997.

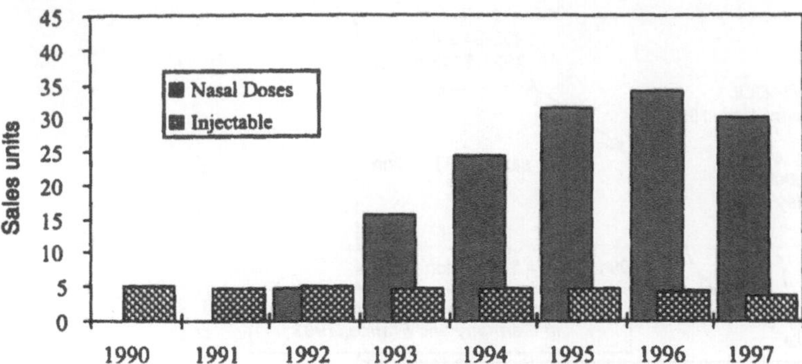

Figure 6 Butorphanol (Stadol) unit sales (U.S.). Estimated individual patient doses per year, 1990–1997. The nasal spray formulation of butorphanol tartrate increased total unit volume 6–7× higher than the injectable (i.m., s.c.) formulation of butorphanol tratrate; 1997 sales were $109 million for the nasal spray formulation and $22 million for the injectable formulation. Butorphanol is now a generic product. For comparison, U.S. annual sales for the year 2001 were $78 million for Stadol NS and $15 million for all sources of injectable butorphanol tartrate. (From IMS Health 2001 Retail and Provider Perspective, used with permission.)

3. Tramadol

As shown in Figure 7, tramadol (Ultram, originated in 1977 as Tramal by Grünenthal in Germany) has become the most successful nonnarcotic product in the market for moderate-severe pain in the United States.

Tramadol is a potent nonnarcotic analgesic that is indicated for the treatment of moderate-severe acute or chronic pain. Tramadol analgesia is mediated by both opioid (mu) and nonopioid (inhibition of monoamine reuptake) mechanisms. It is a mixture of two enantiomers, both of which are required for full analgesic activity. The (+)-enantiomer inhibits serotonin reuptake and has weak affinity for opioid receptors, whereas the (−)-enantiomer inhibits norepinephrine reuptake. Each enantiomer independently produces centrally mediated analgesia and the combi-

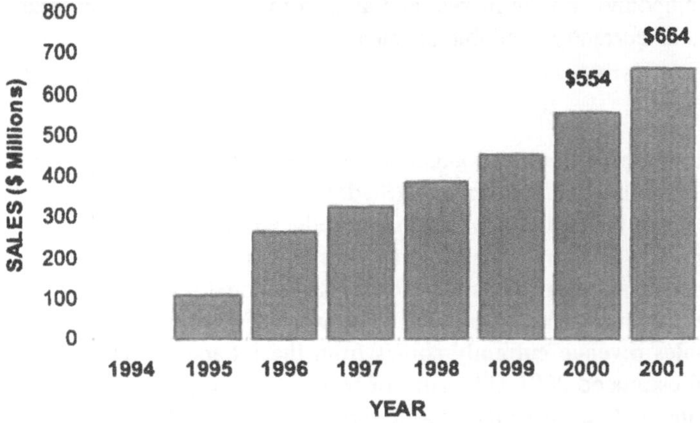

Figure 7 Tramadol (Ultran) U.S. sales. Tramadol sales have been increasing at a compound annualized growth rate of 35% since Ultram was introduced to the U.S. market in 1995. Generic versions of tramadol are expected to be introduced to the U.S. market in 2002. (From IMS Health 1995–2001 Retail and Provider Perspective, used with permission.)

nation of enantiomers (i.e., racemic tramadol) produces an analgesia greater than the additive effect of each enantiomer alone. Tramadol is not scheduled as a drug of abuse in the United States, but concerns about its possible abuse liability have led to increased surveillance. A warning against its use in opioid-dependent patients was added to its label indications in 1996.

Tramadol was developed for the U.S. market by Johnson & Johnson (Ortho-McNeil). A U.S. NDA was filed in late 1993 and the product was launched in April 1995. In 1997, it accounted for 16% of the $2.0 billion U.S. market for drugs used to treat moderate-severe pain. Despite increased sales growth to $664 million in 2001, its market share has declined to 13%, in part due to explosive growth of OxyContin, and it may fall further in 2002 due to the expected introduction of generic formulations. A newer tramadol-plus-acetaminophen formulation (Ultracet) was introduced in late 2001 and sustained-release formulations are expected to follow soon.

B. Growth of the Mild-Moderate Pain Market

Nonnarcotic analgesics, including acetaminophen and NSAIDs, such as ibuprofen, are widely used to treat mild-to-moderate pain. NSAIDs are thought to produce analgesia by inhibiting activity of cyclooxygenase enzymes (COX-1 and COX-2), thereby reducing inflammation at the site of injury or disease. Recent advances in NSAID analgesia have focused on reducing adverse gastrointestinal (GI) side effects. The introduction of two selective COX-2 inhibitors in 1999 transformed the overall market for anti-inflammatory–antiarthritic and other mild-moderate pain products from relative stagnation to increasing at a rate of 34% per year between 1999 and 2001. As shown in Figure 8, Celebrex and Vioxx have led the pack with a compound annualized growth rate of 75% since 1999. Aspirin, acetaminophen, and other NSAIDs have all had declining market value since 1994 (Table 1).

C. Growth of the Special-Purpose Analgesic Market

As indicated in Table 1, the U.S. market for antimigraine drugs has expanded more than any other individual segment during the past 7 years to approximately $1.7 billion in 2001. This has occurred largely through the 1995 introduction of sumitriptan (Imitrex), a selective 5-HT_{1d} receptor agonist, which was followed by the introduction of three 5-$HT_{1d/1b}$ agonist drugs in 1997–1998 (zolmitriptan, Zomig; naratriptan, Amerge; rizatriptan, Maxalt). One additional

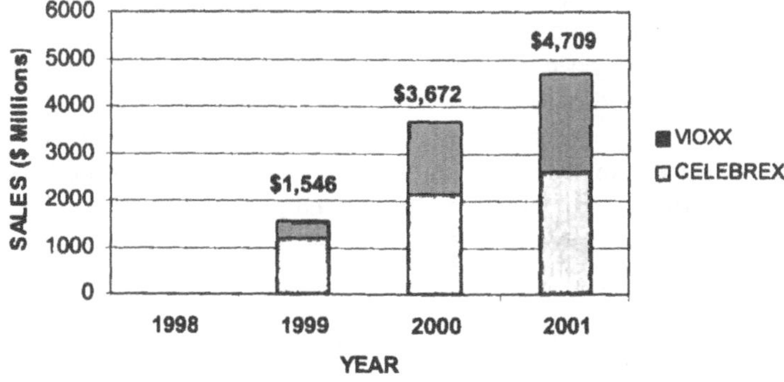

Figure 8 COX-2 inhibitors U.S. sales. COX-2 sales have been increasing at a compound annualized growth rate of 75% since Celebrex and Vioxx were introduced to the U.S. market in 1999. (From IMS Health 1999–2001 Retail and Provider Perspective, used with permission.)

Table 2 New Opioid-related Analgesics and Narcotic Antagonists in the U.S. Market (1990–2001)

Compound	Originator	Year introduced
Fentanyl patch, Duragesic	Janssen	1991
Butorphanol intranasal, Stadol NS	Bristol-Myers Squibb	1992
Levomethadyl acetate, Orlaam[a]	Roxane	1993
Fentanyl oral, Oralet	Anesta/Abbott	1994
Naltrexone, ReVia (opioid antagonist)	DuPont Merck	1995
Nalmefene, Revex (opioid antagonist)	Ohmeda	1995
Tramadol, Ultram	J&J/Ortho-McNeil	1995
Oxycodone (contr. rel.), Oxycontin	Purdue Pharma	1996
Morphine (contr. rel.), Kadian	Zeneca	1996
Remifentanil, Ultiva[b]	Glaxo Wellcome	1996
Hydrocodone + ibuprofen, Vicoprofen	Knoll	1997
Fentanyl, Actiq	Anesta/Abbott	1999
Tramadol + acetaminophen, Ultracet	J&J/Ortho-McNeil	2000

[a] Ultra-long-acting methadone analog; use restricted to opioid dependence.
[b] Ultra-short-acting mu agonist analgesic-anesthetic (esterase-metabolized opioid).

5-$HT_{1d/1b}$ agonist was introduced in 2001 (almotriptan, Axert) and a fifth compound was approved in 2001 and is expected to be introduced in 2002 (frovatriptan, Frova). This market segment is expected to continue to grow sharply with the introduction of several additional serotonin-subtype-selective drugs that are likely to be introduced within the next 1–2 years (see below).

Other special-purpose products that are currently expanding this category include two intra-articular viscosupplementation products indicated for pain associated with osteoarthritis (Synvisc, with 2001 sales of $180 million; Hyalgan with 2001 sales of $65 million), pentosan polysulfate, a macromolecular carbohydrate derivative for pain and discomfort associated with interstitial cystitis (Elmiron, 2001 sales of $49 million), and a new lidocaine dermal patch indicated for relief of pain associated with postherpetic neuralgia (Lidoderm, 2001 sales of $47 million).

Four compounds approved for use in depression (paroxetine, Paxil; nefazodone, Serzone) or epilepsy (lamotrigine, Lamictal; gabapentin, Neurontin) may have adjunctive usefulness in the treatment of postherpetic neuralgia, diabetic neuropathy, or other chronic pain conditions. None have been approved for use as an analgesic in humans, but clinical studies (of paroxetine, nefazodone, gabapentin) and preclinical studies (of lamotrigine) suggest that additional clinical evaluation may be warranted to further develop the analgesic profile of these and related compounds. None of these have been included in the estimation of the U.S. analgesic market (Table 1), but it is widely believed that gabapentin off-label use in treating chronic pain may be valued in excess of $1 billion annual sales in the United States.

III. RECENTLY APPROVED ANALGESICS (IN THE UNITED STATES)

Since 1990, 39 new analgesic or narcotic antagonist products have been approved by the FDA and launched for use in the United States, with 23 of these appearing since 1997 (Tables 2–

Table 3 New Anti-inflammatory Analgesics and Antiarthritic Drugs in the U.S. Market (1990–2001)

Compound	Originator	Year introduced
Ketorolac, Toradol[a]	Roche/Syntex	1990
Naproxen (controlled rel.), Naprelan[a]	Wyeth-Ayerst	1996
Bromfenac sodium, Duract[a,b]	Wyeth-Ayerst	1997 (X)
Diclofenac + misoprostel, Arthrotec[c]	Searle	1997
Leflunomide, Arava[d]	Aventis	1998
Etanercept, Enbrel[e]	Immunex/Wyeth-Ayerst	1998
Infliximab, Remicade[e]	Centocor	1999
Celecoxib, Celebrex[f]	Searle/Pfizer	1999
Rofecoxib, Vioxx[f]	Merck	1999
Meloxican, Mobic[g]	Boehringer Ingelheim	2000
Anakinra, Kineret[h]	Amgen	2001
Valdecoxib, Bextra[f]	Pharmacia-Searle/Pfizer	2002[i]

[a] COX-1 NSAID anti-inflammatory/analgesic.
[b] Bromfenac was withdrawn in 1998 due to hepatic toxicity and deaths.
[c] COX-1 NSAID anti-inflammatory/analgesic with PGE_1 analog for gastric mucosal protection.
[d] Disease-modifying antiarthritic drug (DMARD).
[e] TNFα antagonist.
[f] COX-2 antagonist.
[g] COX-2/COX-1 antagonist.
[h] IL-1 receptor antagonist.
[i] FDA approval November 2001; full launch in April 2002.
(X) Product withdrawn.

4). Of the 39 total new products, 26 are new chemical entities. The other 13 are new formulations of older, already approved products or reintroductions of older products with new uses (naltrexone, an opioid antagonist now indicated for treatment of both opioid dependence and alcoholism, and Duraclon clonidine, indicated for epidural use as an adjunct to narcotic analgesics in advanced cancer pain). It is interesting to note that many new products are special-use products indicated for migraine (six products), metastatic bone pain (two products), viscosupplementation for osteoarthritis (two products), interstitial cystitis, and as an adjunct to the use of opioids in chronic cancer pain (one product each), rather than general-use products such as opioids and NSAIDS that still dominate the market.

Three products approved during the past 5 years are combinations of older, approved drugs that are reported to have enhanced efficacy compared to either product used alone (hydrocodone plus ibuprofen, Vicoprofen; tramadol plus acetaminophen, Ultracet) or that are intended to have a greater GI safety profile than the active analgesic used alone (diclofenac plus misoprostel, Arthrotec).

Among the newer single-entity products not already discussed in other sections, four new disease-modifying products for treating rheumatoid arthritis and other inflammatory diseases (leflunomide, Arava; etanercept, Enbrel; infliximab, Remicade; anakinra, Kineret) offer significant new treatment options that may transform the management of severe inflammatory diseases. Because these do not have primary indications as analgesic drugs, they are not included in the analgesic market values presented in previous tables.

Table 4 New Antimigraine and Special-use Analgesics in the U.S. Market (1990–2001)

Compound	Originator	Year introduced
Strontium-89 chloride, Metastron[a]	Amersham	1993
Sumitriptan, Imitrex[b]	Glaxo Wellcome	1995
Pentosan polysulfate, Elmiron[c]	Ivax/Baker Norton	1996
Ropivacaine, Naropin[d]	Astra	1996
Clonidine epidural, Duraclon[e]	Roxane	1997
Samarium 153-EDTMP, Quadramet[f]	DuPont Merck	1997
Hyaluronate, Hyalgan[g]	Sanofi	1997
Hylan, Synvisc[g]	Wyeth-Ayerst	1997
Zolmitriptan, Zomig[b]	Zeneca	1997
Naratriptan, Amerge[b]	Glaxo Wellcome	1998
Rizatriptan, Maxalt[b]	Merck	1998
Lidocaine patch, Lidoderm[h]	Endo/Hind	1999
Almotriptan, Axert[b]	Pharmacia/Almirall	2001
Frovatriptan, Frova[b]	Elan/Vernalis	2002[i]

[a] Radionuclide for metastatic bone pain.
[b] 5-HT_{1d} or mixed $5\text{-HT}_{1b/1d}$ agonist for migraine pain.
[c] Pain and discomfort associated with interstitial cystitis.
[d] Long-acting spinal/epidural/local anesthetic-analgesic.
[e] Analgesic adjunct in advanced cancer pain.
[f] Radionuclide for metastatic bone pain; phase IV studies for refractory rheumatoid arthritis.
[g] Intra-articular viscosupplementation for osteoarthritis.
[h] Dermal patch approved for relief of pain associated with postherpetic neuralgia.
[i] FDA approval August 2001; launch expected in 2002.

IV. DEFICIENCIES OF CURRENT THERAPIES

Although morphine and other narcotic analgesics are considered the most effective analgesics, many patients who use them do not obtain complete pain relief, and they are ineffective for other patients. Narcotic analgesics also produce a wide range of adverse side effects that may include opioid bowel dysfunction, sedation, nausea, vomiting, decreased respiratory function, addiction, and death. In addition, owing to their potential for abuse, narcotic analgesics are strictly regulated by the DEA under the Controlled Substances Act, which imposes strict registration, record-keeping, and reporting requirements, security controls, and restrictions on narcotic analgesic prescriptions.

Although NSAIDs are generally effective for mild or moderate pain, many patients are unable to tolerate NSAIDs because of GI side effects. Traditional NSAIDs can produce significant adverse effects on the stomach and GI tract, including GI ulcers and bleeding. In addition, prolonged use can cause liver and kidney failure. COX-2 inhibitors appear to produce fewer GI ulcers than NSAIDs but may be less effective for acute pain. For most patients with moderate-to-severe pain, NSAIDs and COX-2 inhibitors do not produce complete pain relief.

A summary of significant unmet medical needs that are driving the discovery of newer analgesic compounds is shown in Table 5.

The evaluation of new drugs with new mechanisms of action to treat chronic pain, especially rheumatoid and osteoarthritis, neuropathic pain, and cancer pain, is one of the most intense

Table 5 Significant Unmet Medical Needs

Moderate-severe pain analgesics with significantly reduced side effects, reduced addiction potential, and not cross-tolerant to morphine for cancer/chronic pain
Mild-moderate pain analgesics with reduced side effects and improved analgesic profiles
Neuropathic pain
Visceral pain
Drugs with novel mechanisms of action and/or designed to treat specific disease states will be increasingly important in the future.

areas of development for new analgesics today. New 1× or 2×/day formulations of narcotic analgesics or NSAIDs with longer durations of action or improved side effect profiles have already made a significant impact in the marketplace; others are on the way. Without regard to mechanism of action, several criteria that I have used to identify new drugs for treating chronic pain are presented in Table 6.

Table 6 Idealized Criteria for New Analgesic Therapy in Chronic Pain

Analgesic properties
Moderate-strong analgesic activity (ibuprofen or codeine combinations)
Delayed onset of action is acceptable for treating chronic pain; fast onset of action is required for treating acute or breakthrough pain
No or low analgesic tolerance profile
Not cross-tolerant to morphine
Side effect profile compatible with chronic use
Nonsedating
No respiratory depression
Minimal GI, cardiovascular, renal effects
No or minimal physical drug dependence
Minimal mood-altering activity (non-drug-seeking)
Not immunosuppressant
Pharmaceutics considerations
Acceptable bioavailability for oral use preferred; alternatives = nasal, rectal, transdermal, or injectable use
Half-life and duration of action consistent with chronic use: 1–2×/day dosing
No drug accumulation with chronic use
Nontoxic metabolite(s)
Known and acceptable drug interactions; compatible use with opioids, NSAIDs, acetaminophen
Acceptable for use in elderly population
Mechanism of action considerations
Nonopioid mechanisms of action may be preferred
Agonists at non-mu opioid receptors may have advantages
Indirect opioid agonists/peptide releasers, opioid potentiators, and opioid tolerance inhibitors may be useful
Drugs with novel or "unknown" mechanisms of action deserve high attention
Analgesics that also treat the emotional/psychological aspects of chronic pain, stress, or depression would be welcome

To evaluate general themes in analgesic drug discovery and to compare the profiles of new drugs and formulations that are or have been in development during the past 20+ years, I started a database several years ago that now has over 1800 products that have been identified as in various stages of preclinical discovery through clinical development and commercial launch in the United States and elsewhere throughout the world (see Appendix II: "21-Year Survey of Analgesics in Development for Treatment of Acute or Chronic Pain"). This database covers compounds mentioned in the scientific literature, company communications, or trade sources worldwide (Pharmaprojects, Scrip, etc.). Additional compounds were added from current literature or corporate press releases to create a comprehensive survey of analgesics in development for treatment of acute or chronic pain. Some compounds in this list may not have a specific indication for the treatment of pain, but pain has been mentioned among investigational uses in the Pharmaprojects database or in the open literature.

Using this database, I have identified six basic themes in analgesic drug discovery, which are covered in the following section.

V. THEMES IN ANALGESIC DISCOVERY

A. Theme 1: Narcotic Combination Products

Increased analgesic potency, and/or
Increased analgesic efficacy, and/or
Reduced side effect profile, and/or
Reduced tolerance/dependence potential

Oral narcotic-acetaminophen or narcotic-aspirin combination analgesics represent the largest category of drugs currently available in the United States for treating acute or chronic pain. All currently marketed analgesic combination products for moderate-to-severe pain are mixtures of codeine, hydrocodone, oxycodone, or propoxyphene with aspirin, acetaminophen, or ibuprofen (see Appendix I: "Currently Marketed Analgesics"). Because of the inclusion of a narcotic analgesic in these combined-dose formulations, all currently marketed combination analgesics are controlled substances under classifications C-II, C-III, or C-IV in the United States. Oxycodone combinations (Percodan, Percocet, Roxicet, Tylox) have the more restrictive C-II designation since oxycodone is generally regarded as being a more potent analgesic (hence, greater abuse liability) than codeine, hydrocodone, or propoxyphene combination products.

As previously indicated in Table 2, Vicoprofen (hydrocodone plus ibuprofen) became the first ibuprofen-containing combination opioid analgesic on the U.S. market in 1997. Ibuprofen is widely regarded as having a higher level of analgesic and anti-inflammatory activity than aspirin or acetaminophen; hence it is hoped that ibuprofen combination analgesics will have a greater efficacy than aspirin or acetaminophen combination analgesics. An oxycodone-plus-ibuprofen analgesic was filed for FDA approval at the end of 2001 (Table 7). Interestingly, there is no codeine-plus-ibuprofen analgesic available in the United States owing to the difficulty of showing greater analgesic activity in a codeine-ibuprofen combination product than obtained with ibuprofen alone.

At least six new analgesic combination products containing dextromethorphan have been reported to be in development by Algos Pharmaceutical Corp. (now merged with Endo Pharmaceuticals) under the hypothesis that dextromethorphan, a weak NMDA antagonist that has been the active ingredient in many OTC cough syrups for many years, may potentiate the analgesic activity, reduce the side effect profile, and reduce the tolerance potential of opioid or NSAID analgesics. The first of these products, MorphiDex, received a nonapprovable letter from the

Table 7 Selected Analgesic Combinations in Worldwide Clinical Development (1998–2001)

Composition	Sponsor	Status
Oxycodone + ibuprofen	Forest Labs	NDA filed
MorphiDex (morphine + dextromethorphan)	Endo (Algos)	Phase III
Acetaminophen + dextromethorphan[a]	Algos/McNeil	Phase III
MT 100 (naproxen + metoclopramide)	Pozen	Phase III
HydrocoDex (hydrocodone + dextromethorphan)	Endo (Algos)	Phase II
Ibuprofen + dextromethorphan[a]	Algos/McNeil	Phase II
Methadone + dextromethorphan	Endo (Algos)	Phase II
PTI-501 (morphine + naloxone; injectable)	Pain Therapeutics	Phase II
PTI-555 (morphine + naltrexone)	Pain Therapeutics	Phase II
PTI-601 (tramadol + naltrexone)	Pain Therapeutics	Phase II
PTI-701 (hydrocodone + naltrexone)	Pain Therapeutics	Phase II
PTI-801 (oxycodone + naltrexone)	Pain Therapeutics	Phase II
MT 400 (triptan + NSAID, unspecified)	Pozen	Phase II
Colykade (opioid + CCK_B antagonist)	Panos/ML Therap.	Phase II
Devacade (opioid + CCK_A antagonist)	Panos/ML Therap.	Phase II
OxycoDex (oxycodone + dextromethorphan)	Endo (Algos)	Phase I
Alvimopan + opioid analgesic	Adolor	Phase I

[a] Development status unclear following Algos merger with Endo Pharmaceuticals (July 2000).
Source: Pharmaprojects, Scrip, company reports updated to February 2002 (see Appendix II).

FDA in August 1999, and is reportedly back in phase III clinical trials to obtain additional efficacy and long-term safety data needed for drug approval.

Other combination analgesics follow similar mechanistic themes. Pozen is developing several combination products for faster onset of action and possibly greater efficacy in the treatment of migraine. Pain Therapeutics is developing narcotic analgesic combination products with ultralow doses of naloxone or naltrexone with the objective of obtaining enhanced potency and/or reduced tolerance potential. Panos is developing narcotic analgesic combination products with CCK_A or CCK_B antagonists with similar goals. Adolor is developing a narcotic analgesic combination product with alvimopan, an investigational peripherally restricted μ opioid antagonist designed to block opioid receptors throughout the GI tract, with the goal of developing a GI side-effect-free opioid analgesic.

B. Theme 2: Central Opioid Receptor Analgesics

Opioid-active partial mu agonist
Morphine metabolite (M6G)
Mu-delta opioid analgesic
Kappa agonist analgesic
Controlled-release drug delivery systems

Newer single-entity products and drug delivery strategies in clinical development may provide additional opportunities to provide pain control using different mechanisms of action than currently available medications. Table 8 lists some of the more advanced and/or more novel centrally acting opioid analgesic drugs that are in clinical development.

Not surprisingly, the majority of these products are sustained-release preparations of older narcotic analgesic drugs with oral or parenteral timed-delivery ranging from 1× per day to 3

Table 8 Selected Central Opioid Analgesics in Worldwide Clinical Development (1998–2001)

Compound	Mechanism of action	Sponsor	Status
Morphine	Morphelan 24-hr	Elan	NDA filed
Hydromorphone	OROS delivery	J&J/Alza	NDA filed
Propiram	Partial mu agonist	Shire/Roberts	Phase III
Fentanyl	E-trans delivery	J&J/Alza	Phase III
Sufentanil	DUROS 3-month delivery	Durect	Phase III
Morphine	DepoFoam delivery	Skye Pharma	Phase III
Oxymorphone	TIMERx delivery	Endo	Phase III
Tramadol	24-hr extended release	Biovail	Phase III
Morphine	AERx delivery (lung)	Aradigm	Phase II
Morphine	Intranasal delivery	Nastech	Phase II
M6G[a]	Morphine metabolite	CeNeS/ML Labs	Phase II
TRK-820	Kappa agonist	Toray/Daiichi	Phase II
DPI-3290	Mu-delta agonist	Ardent/Organon Teknika	Phase II
Fentanyl	7-day transdermal	Purdue/3M	Phase I

[a] Morphine-6-gluconate (morphine active metabolite).
Source: Pharmaprojects, Scrip, company reports updated to February 2002 (see Appendix II).

months of continuous drug delivery for the management of chronic pain. Other products are being developed with transdermal, nasal, or pulmonary drug delivery mechanisms.

Only three novel products have been identified in this group: M6G, a mu agonist morphine metabolite; DPI 3290, a mu-delta agonist analgesic; and TRK 820, a kappa agonist analgesic. Each is reported to be in phase II clinical trials.

C. Theme 3: Peripheral Opioid Receptor Analgesics

Peripheral mu agonist
Peripheral kappa agonist

Five novel single-entity products are in phase I or phase II development that are reported to be peripherally restricted mu, mu-delta, or kappa agonist analgesics. These compounds are intended to produce morphine-like analgesic effects without the central-nervous-system side effects associated with older narcotic analgesics. Some proof-of-concept results reported in company press

Table 9 Selected Peripheral Opioid Analgesics in Worldwide Clinical Development (1998–2001)

Compound	Mechanism of action	Sponsor	Status
Asimadoline	Kappa agonist[a,b]	Merck KGaA (Germany)	Phase II
Loperamide	Mu agonist[a,c]	Adolor	Phase II
Frakefamide	Mu-delta agonist[a]	AstraZeneca/Shire	Phase II
ADL 10-0101	Kappa agonist[a]	Adolor	Phase II
ADL 10-0116	Kappa agonist[a]	Adolor	Phase I

[a] Peripherally acting.
[b] Asimadoline clinical trials are for IBS (negative phase II postoperative pain trials).
[c] Loperamide (ADL 2-1294) clinical trials are for topical-dermal and ophthalmic indications.
Source: Pharmaprojects, Scrip, company reports updated to February 2002 (see Appendix II).

releases support this hypothesis, but some clinical tests have been negative. Larger double-blind clinical trials are still required to validate this hypothesis.

D. Theme 4: Anti-inflammatory Analgesics

COX-2 inhibitors
COX-LO inhibitors
COX–nitric-oxide-releasing compounds
Disease-modifying compounds

At least three second-generation COX-2 antagonists are either in phase III clinical development or in drug registration. Etoricoxib has been approved by the FDA and is expected to be introduced in 2002. Parecoxib, which received a nonapprovable letter from the FDA in 2001, is back in phase III development. It may become the first injectable COX-2 antagonist to reach the U.S. market with an indication for postoperative pain. If approved, it would join ketorolac as the only injectable NSAIDs approved for postoperative pain. Several other orally active COX-2 antagonists or mixed COX/5-lipoxygenase (5-LO) antagonists are in advanced clinical development in the United States and other parts of the world.

Other anti-inflammatory–antiarthritic approaches in earlier clinical testing include additional cytokine antagonists, a C5a complement inhibitor, and several NSAID-NO compounds that are modified to release nitric oxide locally at stomach and intestinal mucosa for cytoprotective activity.

E. Theme 5: Antimigraine Compounds

5-HT_{1d}, 5-HT_{1b} "triptan-like" compounds
Botulinum toxin
Glycine site antagonist

Following the recent release of several new antimigraine drugs, at least six additional serotonin 5-HT_{1d} or $5\text{-HT}_{1d/1b}$ receptor agonist compounds are in advanced clinical testing (Table 11).

Table 10 Selected Anti-inflammatory Analgesics in Worldwide Clinical Development (1998–2001)

Compound	Mechanism of action	Sponsor	Status
Etoricoxib	COX-2 inhibitor	Merck	Registered
Parecoxib	COX-2 inhibitor (i.v.)	Pharmacia	Phase III
JTE-522	COX-2 inhibitor	Japan Tobacco/J&J	Phase III
ML-3000	COX/5-LO inhibitor	Merckle/Forest	Phase III
Pelubiprofen	NSAID, T-cell stimulant	Sankyo	Phase III
Pexelizumab[a]	C5a complement inhibitor	Alexion/P&G	Phase III
CBF-BS2	G-6P-DH inhibitor	KS Biomedix	Phase II
HP-228	Cytokine antagonist	Lion Biosciences	Phase II
NCX-4016[b]	NO-aspirin	NicOx	Phase I

[a] Pexelizumab (5G1.1-SC) phase III trials for reduction of inflammation and bleeding following coronary bypass surgery; additional trials reported underway for joint destruction in rheumatoid arthritis.
[b] NCX-4016 phase II for restenosis; phase I indication for pain.
Source: Pharmaprojects, Scrip, company reports updated to February 2002 (see Appendix II).

Table 11 Selected Antimigraine Drugs in Worldwide Clinical Development (1998–2001)

Compound	Mechanism of action	Sponsor	Status
Eletriptan	5-HT_{1d} partial agonist	Pfizer	NDA filed[a]
Flunarizine	Calcium channel antagonist	Johnson & Johnson	Phase III[a]
MT 300	D.H.E. formulation[b]	Pozen	Phase III
BIBN-4096	CGRP antagonist[c]	Boehringer Ingelheim	Phase II
Tonabersat	(Unidentified)	GlaxoSmithKline	Phase II
(S)-fluoxetine	5-HT uptake inhibitor	Sepracor	Phase II
PNU-142633	5-HT_{1d} agonist	Pharmacia	Phase II
MT 500	5-HT_{1b} antagonist	Pozen/Roche	Phase I[d]
ALX-0646	5-HT_{1b} agonist	NPS/Forest	Phase I
Donitriptan	5-$HT_{1b/1d}$ agonist	bioMerieux-Pierre Fabre	Phase I
Cannabis	Cannabinoid	GW Pharmaceuticals	Phase I[e]

[a] Launched in Europe.
[b] D.H.E. = dihydroergotamine.
[c] CGRP = calcitonin gene-related peptide.
[d] Migraine prophylaxis.
[e] High THC cannabis; phase III development for cancer pain; phase I for migraine.
NOTE: See also MT 100 and MT 400 analgesic combinations for migraine (Table 7).
Source: Pharmaprojects, Scrip, company reports updated to February 2002 (see Appendix II).

Other novel approaches for migraine include a calcium channel antagonist, a new faster-onset formulation of dihydroergotamine, a CGRP antagonist, and a high-potency, purified formulation of tetrahydrocannabinol (cannabis).

F. Theme 6: Novel Mechanism of Action

Ion channel blocking drugs
Cannabinoid analgesics
Muscarinic/nicotinic/alpha-2 agonist drugs
Special-use products

Analgesics with novel or unknown mechanisms of action deserve greater attention for evaluation in chronic pain situations since they may offer the potential for greater efficacy for intractable neuropathic pain or visceral pain. It makes little sense, barring advances in site-specific drug delivery, to believe that the tenth new opioid mu agonist or the twenty-first NSAID will have any greater activity in areas with unmet medical need than products that have been on the market for the past 10–20 years. It is encouraging to see that many smaller biopharmaceutical companies have taken a lead in developing drugs with novel mechanisms of action.

Drugs with novel mechanisms of action that are in clinical development include a neuron-selective calcium channel antagonist (ziconotide) intended for intrathecal delivery in patients with intractable cancer pain, a compound working through a novel neuronal-selective nicotinic cholinergic approach (ABT-594), a high-potency cannabinoid preparation for chronic pain (cannabis) and a nonpsychoactive cannabinoid (CT-3) for acute or chronic pain, an NMDA ion channel antagonist (CNS-5161) that may be active in neuropathic or chronic pain, a nitric-oxide-releasing NSAID and a nitric-oxide-releasing derivative of acetaminophen that may have greater safety than the parent compounds from which they are derived, high-strength topical capsaicin for the management of neuropathic pain, and a compound with mixed vascular cell adhesion (VCAM) and monocyte chemoattractant protein antagonist activity (AGIX-4207). A summary

Table 12 Selected Novel-mechanism-of-action Analgesics, Anti-inflammatory Drugs, and Antiarthritic Drugs in Worldwide Clinical Development (1998–2001)

Compound	Mechanism of action	Sponsor	Status
Dexmedetomidine	Alpha-2 agonist	Abbott	Launched[a]
Ziconotide	Ca^{2+} channel antagonist	Elan	Prelaunch[b]
Cannabis	Cannabinoid	GW Pharmaceuticals	Phase III[c]
ABT-594	Nicotinic $\alpha4\beta2$ agonist	Abbott	Phase II
CNS-5161	NMDA ion channel antagonist	CeNeS	Phase II
HCT 3012	NO-naproxen[d]	NicOx/AstraZeneca	Phase II
Transdolor	Capsaicin topical	NeurogesX	Phase II
CT-3	Cannabinoid derivative[e]	Atlantic Technology	Phase I
AGIX-4207	VCAM-1/MCP-1 antagonist	AtheroBenics	Phase I
NCX 701	NO-acetaminophen[d]	NicOx	Phase I

[a] Dexmedetomidine (i.v.) approved for sedation; investigational intrathecal delivery in cancer pain.
[b] Ziconotide is FDA "approvable" for intrathecal delivery in cancer pain; launch date unknown.
[c] High THC cannabis; phase III development for cancer pain; phase I for migraine.
[d] Nitric-oxide-releasing derivative.
[e] Nonpsychoactive cannabinoid.
Source: Pharmaprojects, Scrip, company reports updated to February 2002 (see Appendix II).

of the development status of these compounds is presented in Table 12. Other compounds with novel mechanisms of action are presented in Appendix II.

Novel preclinical approaches that are or have been under investigation for acute or chronic pain include adenosine antagonists, bradykinin antagonists, CCK agonists and antagonists, dopaminergics, glutamate release inhibitors, IL-1 antagonists, NO synthase inhibitors, prostaglandin receptor antagonists, and NK-1 or NK-2 substance P antagonists. A selection of these compounds and their current status is also presented in Appendix II.

It is natural to expect that drugs with novel mechanisms of action may be riskier to develop than new formulations or simple derivatives of older marketed products. Indeed, only two of 10 novel compounds in clinical development that I mentioned in a paper in 1998 (7) appear to remain in clinical development today. However, for those that succeed, the medical importance and the return on investment may be exceptionally favorable, as with tramadol (Fig. 7) and COX-2 inhibitors (Fig. 8).

VI. RECENTLY DISCONTINUED DRUGS AND EXPERIMENTAL COMPOUNDS

Some novel mechanisms of action have not yielded useful drugs to date despite multiple entries into clinical trials (e.g., enkephalinase inhibitors). Many drugs have been dropped from clinical evaluation due to lack of effectiveness, unresolved safety concerns, lack of competitive advantages over other more advanced drugs in the marketplace, or because of periodic changes in the direction of research programs in both large and small pharmaceutical companies. Among the newer drugs that have been dropped recently or suspended from clinical development are several NSAID-like anti-inflammatory-antiarthritic drugs (bromfenac, GI-245402, parcetasal), a COX-2 inhibitor (D-1367), two 5-HT_{1d} antagonists (alniditan, BMS-181885) and a 5-HT_{1f} antagonist (LY-334370) for migraine, a serotonin neuromodulator (UP-26-91), a GABA modulator (pregabalin), a bradykinin antagonist (Bradycor), two NK-1 antagonists (lanepitant, GR-

Table 13 Recently Discontinued Drugs and Experimental Compounds in Clinical Development (1997–2001)

Compound	Mechanism of action	Sponsor	Status[a]
Bromfenac	NSAID	Wyeth-Ayerst	Marketed
Parcetasal	PGSI	Medea Research	NDA filed
Pregabalin[b]	GABA modulator	Pfizer	Phase III
LY-334370	5-HT_{1f} agonist	Lilly/Synaptic	Phase III
Bay 12-9566	Stromelysin/MMP inhib.	Bayer	Phase III
Alniditan	5-HT_{1d} antagonist	Johnson & Johnson	Phase II
Ganaxolone[c]	Epalon neurosteroid	Purdue/CoCensys	Phase II
UP-26-91	5-HT neuromodulator	UPSA/BMS	Phase II
Sameridine	Spinal anesthetic	AstraZeneca	Phase II
GR-205171	NK-1 antagonist	Glaxo Wellcome	Phase II
Moxilubant	LTB4 antagonist	Novartis (Ciba Geigy)	Phase II
LY-297802	Muscarinic M1 agonist	Lilly/Novo Nordisk	Phase II
Lanepitant	NK-1 antagonist	Lilly	Phase II
CereCRIB	Encapsulated bovine adrenochromaffin cells; release of catecholamines, enkephalins, and other analgesic peptides	CytoTherapeutics	Phase II
BMS-181885	5-HT_{1d} antagonist	Bristol-Myers Squibb	Phase I
D-1367	COX-2 inhibitor	Celltech	Phase I
GI-245402	MMP-TNF inhibitor	Glaxo Wellcome	Phase I
GR-79236	Adenosine A1 agonist	Glaxo Wellcome	Phase I
D-5410	MMP/TNF inhibitor	Celltech	Phase I

[a] Status when discontinued.
[b] Pregabalin phase III neuropathic pain trials discontinued owing to positive mouse carcinogenicity data; phase III epilepsy trials continuing.
[c] Ganaxolone continues in phase II trials for epilepsy (negative phase II migraine trials).
Source: Pharmaprojects, Scrip, company reports updated to February 2002 (see Appendix II).

205171), and an anesthetic-analgesic (sameridine). A summary of the development status of these compounds is presented in Table 13. Other compounds are presented in Appendix II.

VII. CONCLUSIONS

Opioid-related analgesics, opioid combination drugs, and sustained-release oral opioid formulations represent the greatest number of products on the market and in clinical development for the treatment of moderate-severe acute and chronic pain.

Non-mu opioid analgesics (e.g., kappa or delta agonists) and/or peripherally acting opioid analgesics have promising preclinical profiles but have yet to demonstrate clinical usefulness in wide-scale clinical trials.

Drugs such as NMDA antagonists, CCK antagonists, or ultra-low-dose opioid antagonists, each of which may potentiate opioid effectiveness while preventing analgesic tolerance development, may have significant impact if preclinical studies are verified in wide-scale clinical trials now underway.

NSAID COX-1 inhibitors continue to represent the mainstay treatment for mild-moderate acute and chronic pain and inflammation, but the risk of GI ulceration and bleeding is a major limitation. Newer COX-2 inhibitors, mixed COX/5-LO inhibitors, or nitric-oxide-releasing NSAIDs hold considerable promise for providing potent anti-inflammatory and antiarthritic effects with less GI ulceration.

Selected cytokine antagonists have demonstrated their importance in treating inflammation and arthritic disease by reducing the pathology of the disease and reducing pain and disability. MMP inhibitors and other mechanism-specific antagonists of the inflammatory cascade may provide additional methods to control or reduce the biological basis for pain and disability in some inflammatory and arthritic diseases.

Neuron-selective ion channel antagonists, excitatory amino acid antagonists, and regulators of GABA or glutamate release hold significant promise in treating neuropathic and other forms of chronic pain. However, their efficacy remains to be established in clinical trials against both inflammatory and noninflammatory pain.

5-HT/NE uptake inhibitors, antidepressants, and subtype-selective serotonin agonists have demonstrated usefulness in treating acute and chronic pain or as analgesic adjuncts. Newer antimigraine drugs with mixed $5\text{-HT}_{1d/1b}$ agonist activity promise greater efficacy, faster onset, and fewer side effects in migraine treatment.

Somatostatin and calcitonin analogs may have selected usefulness in chronic pain situations, but currently available peptides are not orally active and may require advanced dosing techniques (intranasal, intrathecal) to be effective.

Recently approved special-use analgesics include an ultra-short-acting fentanyl analog for use in anesthesia or for short painful procedures, oral transmucosal fentanyl for breakthrough cancer pain, rhenium or samarium radionuclides for treating metastatic bone cancer pain, epidural clonidine as an adjunct in intractable cancer pain, pentosan polysulfate for pain associated with interstitial cystitis, and the lidocaine patch for postherpetic neuralgia. These newer special-use drugs may increase the effectiveness of or reduce the need for more traditional analgesic therapy.

Other classes of analgesics with novel or unknown mechanisms of action deserve greater attention for evaluation for chronic pain. There is a strong and growing need for improved analgesic therapies; the market potential for newer improved drugs is strong.

REFERENCES

1. World Health Organization. Cancer Pain Relief and Palliative Care. Report of a WHO Expert Committee, Technical Report Series, No. 804. Geneva: World Health Organization, 1990.
2. World Health Organization. Cancer Pain Relief, 2nd ed, with a guide to opioid availability. Geneva: World Health Organization, 1996.
3. World Health Organization. Cancer Pain Relief and Palliative Care in Children. Geneva: World Health Organization, 1998.
4. Carr DB, Jacox AK, Chapman CR, et al. Acute Pain Management: Operative or Medical Procedures and Trauma Clinical Practice Guideline No. 1. AHCPR Publication No. 92-0032. Rockville, MD: Agency for Health Care Policy and Research, U.S. Department of Health and Human Services, Public Health Service, February 1992.
5. Jacox A, Carr DB, Payne R, et al. Management of Cancer Pain. Clinical Practice Guideline No. 9. AHCPR Publication No. 94-0592. Rockville, MD: Agency for Health Care Policy and Research, U.S. Department of Health and Human Services, Public Health Service, March 1994.
6. Goudas L, Carr DB, Bloch R, Galk E, Ioannidis JPA, Terrin N, Gialeli-Goudas M, Chew P, Lau J. Management of Cancer Pain. File Inventory, Evidence Report/Technology Assessment Number 35. AHRQ Publication No. 02-E002. Rockville, MD: Agency for Healthcare Research and Quality, October 2001. http://www.ahrq.gov/clinic/capaininv.htm.

7. Schmidt WK. Overview of current and investigational drugs for the treatment of chronic pain. National Managed Health Care Congress (NMHCC). 2nd Annual Conference on Therapeutic Developments in Chronic Pain, Annapolis, MD, May 18, 1998.
8. Schmidt WK. Pharmacological approaches to the treatment of chronic pain: current and investigational drugs. IBC International Business Communications Conference on Advances in Therapeutic Development for Chronic Pain, San Diego, CA, February 24–25, 1994.
9. Schmidt WK. Survey of current and investigational drugs for the treatment of acute and chronic pain. Global Business Research Ltd. Conference on Pain Control, New Concepts and Therapeutic Applications, Princeton, NJ, October 3–5, 1994.
10. Schmidt WK. Survey of current and investigational drugs for the treatment of acute and chronic pain. American Pain Society, November 9, 1995.
11. Schmidt WK. An overview of current and investigational drugs for the treatment of chronic pain. National Managed Health Care Congress (NMHCC) Conference on Therapeutic Developments in Chronic Pain, Washington, DC, June 26, 1997.
12. Schmidt WK. Drug development for analgesia. Conference on Contemporary Issues and Challenges for Today's Pain Practitioner, Eastern Pain Association Scientific Meeting 2000, New York, December 8, 2000.

Data regarding drugs in clinical development are supported by references obtained in the open literature or from generally accessible trade sources (e.g. Scrip World Pharmaceutical News, Pharmaprojects, PR Newswire, Business Wire, AP News, Reuters). Pharmaprojects source data (©2002, PJB Publications, Surrey, UK) are used with permission.

All market value estimates are derived from IMS Health Retail Provider Perspective (IMS Health 1994–2002) unless otherwise noted and are used with permission.

31

Novel Mu, Delta, and Kappa Agonists

Potential for Development of Novel Analgesic Agents

Frank Porreca
University of Arizona Health Sciences Center, Tucson, Arizona, U.S.A.

Victor J. Hruby
University of Arizona, Tucson, Arizona, U.S.A.

I. INTRODUCTION

Current opioid analgesics such as morphine are known to exert their specific pharmacological effects through the mu (μ) opioid receptor. Although powerful and effective pain killers, opioid μ-agonists have many undesirable side effects including analgesic tolerance, respiratory depression, constipation, and abuse liability, that limit their utilization for long-term treatment of severe pain without hospitalization. Thus, efforts to discover new modalities for control of pain by the discovery of novel opioid analgesics that have high selectivity for other, more recently discovered, opioid receptors [delta (δ) and kappa (κ) receptors], or that have unique biological activity profiles, are receiving increasingly urgent attention. In this chapter, we will briefly profile some of the most promising agonist leads in this area, including compounds with mixed activity at opioid δ and μ receptors and extremely high selectivity for opioid κ receptors. Such compounds include δ agonist–μ agonists and μ agonist–δ antagonists that appear to have promise as ligands with unique biological activity profiles and may offer approaches to limit the development of tolerance. Because of page limitations, not all lead compounds will be covered, but we will provide selected examples of each class of promising lead compounds and provide the reader with the various structures that appear to be promising in the development of new modalities of bioactivity. There is still much to learn about the biological potential of these various classes of compounds, especially as very few of them have been used in human medicine in a controlled clinical setting. Nonetheless, it is hoped that this brief review will stimulate others to do a more detailed examination of the problem and lead to the development of new ligands for the opioid receptors.

II. δ-OPIOID AGONIST LIGANDS

The realization that there were different opioid receptor types came originally from pharmacological evidence (1–4), but it was only recently that structurally distinct opioid receptors were isolated and their primary structure determined (5). Thus far, three different opioid receptors, referred to as mu (μ), delta (δ), and kappa (κ) have been cloned and stably transfected into cell lines. Although there is much pharmacological evidence for distinct subtypes of these receptors (e.g., 6), thus far no subtypes have been structurally identified. However, development of ligands that have specific affinity for δ, κ, and μ compounds have continued, especially for the former two, because there is much evidence that δ and κ ligands have different biological activity profiles, especially for side effects.

A. Development of Selective δ Type and Subtype Agonist Ligands

Although DADLE (Tables 1 and 2) has often been viewed and used as a δ-opioid receptor ligand, in fact, it has virtually no binding affinity selectivity and only modest selectivity in the mouse vas deferens (MVD) δ versus guinea pig ileum (GPI) (μ) bioassay systems. The first major successes in obtaining δ-selective ligands came from modification of enkephalin sequences either in linear ligands such as [DSer(*O*ᵗBu)^2,Thr(*O*ᵗBu)^6]leucine enkephalin (7) or in cyclic, conformationally constrained, analogues such as c-[DPen^2, DPen^5]enkephalin (DPDPE) (8). The latter compound has found extensive use by most investigators as the prototypical δ-opioid receptor selective ligand because of its high stability against chemical and enzymatic degradation (9,10), its conformation restriction by cyclization which allowed the determination of solution (11) and crystal (12) structures, and its lack of toxicity in studies in vivo (13).

Table 1 Binding Affinities of Selective Agonists for the δ-Receptor

	Binding affinities-EC_{50} or *Ki* (nM)			
Compound	δ	μ	μ/δ	Ref.
1 *H*-Tyr-c[DPen-Gly-Phe-DPen]OH (DPDPE)	1.2	720	600	18
2 *H*-Tyr-DAla-Gly-Phe-DLeu-OH (DADLE)	3.3	10.3	3.1	14,15
3 *H*-Tyr-DSer(OᵗBu)-Gly-Phe-Leu-Thr(Oᵗ/Bu) (BUBU)	4.7	475	100	7
4 *H*-Tyr-DAla-Gly-(2*R*,3*S*)∇EPhe-Leu	13	3200	250	17
5 *H*-Tyr-c[DPen-Gly-Phe(*p*Cl)-DPen]-OH	1.6	980	570	19,20
6 *H*-Tyr-c[DPen-Gly-Phe(*p*F)-DPen]-OH	2.5	620	250	20
7 *H*-Tyr-c[DPen-Gly-Phe-LCys]-OH	0.90	180	200	13,21
8 *H*-Tyr-c[DPen-Gly-(2*S*,3*S*)β-MePhe-DPen]-OH	38	69,000	1,800	22
9 *H*-Tyr-[DPen-Gly-Phe-LCys]-Phe-OH	1.4	280	200	24
10 *H*-Tyr-c[DPen-Gly-Phe(*p*Cl)-LCys]-Phe-OH	0.27	260	960	24
11 *H*-Tyr-c[DPen-Gly-Phe-LCys]-Trp-OH	0.12	300	2,500	—
12 *H*-Tyr-c[DPen-Gly-Phe(*p*-Br)-LPen]-Phe-OH	0.20	4,200	21,000	25
13 [(2*S*,3*R*)TMT^1]-DPDPE	5.0	4,300	850	26
14 Deltorphin I	0.31	205	660	27
15 Deltorphin II	0.71	2,400	3,400	27
16 *H*-Tyr-c[DPen-Phe-Asp-Pen]-Nle-Gly-NH_2	3.7	26,000	7,000	29
17 *H*-Tyr-D-Met-Phe-His-Leu-nBuG-Asp-NH_2	0.04	820	20,000	30
18 *H*-Tyr-DAla-(*R*)Atc-Asp-Ile-Ile-Gly-NH_2	4.0	4,500	1,100	31
19 *H*-Tyr-DAla-(*R*)Atc-Glu-Ile-Ile-Gly-NH_2	0.51	730	1,400	31
20 Tan-67	1.1	2,300	2,100	32
21 SNC-80	1.1	2,500	2,300	33,35
22 SL 3111	8.4	17,000	2,000	34
23 *H*-Tyr-c[DPen-Gly-Phe(*p*F)-LPen]-Phe-OH	0.43	1,600	3,800	25
24 *H*-Tyr-Tic-NH-CH_2-CH(Ph)-CO_2Et(I)	0.57	890	1,600	36

Table 2 Bioassay Potencies of Selective Agonists for the δ-Receptor

Compound	Potencies—EC_{50} or *K*i (nM)			Ref.
	MVD	GPI	μ/δ	
1 *H*-Tyr-c[DPen-Gly-Phe-DPen]-OH(DPDPE)	3.9	11,300	2,900	8,18
2 *H*-Tyr-DAla-Gly-Phe-DLeu-OH(DADLE)	0.27	24	90	14,15
3 *H*-Tyr-D-Ser(*O*'Bu)-Gly-Phe-Leu-Thr(*O*'Bu) (BUBU)	0.60	2,800	4,700	7
4 *H*-Tyr-DAla-Gly-(2*R*,3*S*)∇EPhe-Leu	34	64	1.9	16,17
5 *H*-Tyr-c[DPen-Gly-Phe-Phe(*p*Cl)-DPen]-OH	0.89	4,800	5,400	19,20
6 *H*-Tyr-c[DPen-Gly-Phe(*p*F)-DPen]-OH	0.84	5,000	6,000	20
7 *H*-Tyr-c[DPen-Gly-Phe-LCys]-OH	0.32	210	660	13,21
8 *H*-Tyr-c[DPen-Gly-(2*S*,3*S*)β-MePhe-DPen]-OH	39	59,000	1,500	22
9 *H*-Tyr-c[DPen-Gly-Phe-LCys]-Phe-OH	0.016	83	2,700	24
11 *H*-Tyr-c[DPen-Gly-Phe-LCys]-Trp-OH	0.042	114	670	—
12 *H*-Tyr-c[DPen-Gly-Phe(*p*-Br)-LPen]-Phe-OH	0.18	3400	19,000	25
13 [(2*S*,3*R*)-TMT[1]]DPDPE	1.8	O at 60μM	>45,000	26
14 Deltorphin I	0.15	3,150	21,000	27
15 Deltorphin II	0.71	2,400	3,500	27
16 *H*-Tyr-c[DPen-Phe-Asp-LPen]-Nle-Gly-NH_2	6.3	68,000	11,000	29
17 *H*-Tyr-DMet-Phe-His-Leu-*N*BuG-Asp-NH_2	0.56	580	1,000	30
18 *H*-Tyr-D-Ala-(*R*)Atc-Asp-Ile-Ile-Gly-NH_2	0.07	6,600	92,000	31
19 DAla-(*R*)Atc-Glu-Ile-Ile-Gly-NH_2	0.09	19,000	22,000	31
20 Tan-67	50	26,000	520	32
21 SNC-80	2.7	5,500	2,000	33,35
22 SL 3111	85	39,000	460	34
23 *H*-Tyr-c[DPen-Gly-Phe(*p*F)-LPen]-Phe-OH	0.016	740	45,000	25
24 *H*-Tyr-Tic-NH-CH_2-CH(Ph)-CO_2Et(I)	1.28	ND	ND	36

Although DPDPE has been a very useful tool for examining agonist activity at δ-opioid receptors, recent pharmacological studies, and studies using μ-receptor knockout animals, have suggested that there is a μ-component to the bioactivity of DPDPE in vivo (Yamamura HI, Hruby YJ., Porreca F, unpublished observations). This lack of complete selectivity actually was realized earlier, and thus several laboratories have continued to search for more selective δ-opioid receptor ligands both in binding affinities and in in vitro and in vivo bioassays. A number of highly potent and receptor-selective agonist ligands for the δ-receptor have been identified in several laboratories (see Tables 1 and 2). Of the earlier δ-opioid receptor-selective agonists ligands, the cyclic conformationally constrained analogue c[DPen[2], DPen[5]]enkephalin (**1**; DPDPE) has been most widely used as the prototypical delta ligand owing to its good potency and high selectivity both in binding assays (see Table 1) and bioassays (see Table 2), and its remarkable stability in vitro and in vivo to proteolytic degradation. The linear peptides DADLE (**2**; see Tables 1 and 2) (14,15), BUBU (**3**) (7), and **4** (16,17) have been used quite often as well, but they suffer from lack of selectivity in either binding (**2**,**3**) or bioassay (**2**,**4**) studies. Radiolabeled DPDPE often has been used in binding studies, although because of its slow on and off rates (18), these studies have suffered as some investigators have not studied their cold ligands at equilibrium with radiolabeled DPDPE. A better ligand for binding studies is [Phe(pCl)[4]]DPDPE (**5**; see Tables 1 and 2) because it has much faster on and off rates than DPDPE (19), is slightly more potent, and has equal or more selective bioactivities than DPDPE. A potentially even better ligand would be [Phe(pF)[4]]DPDPE (**6**; see Tables 1 and 2) (20), but it has not been radiolabeled. c[DPen[2],LCys[5]]enkephalin (**7**; DPLCE) (13,21), although slightly more potent than DPDPE (see Tables 1 and 2) is somewhat less selective than DPDPE and not suitable for most in vitro and in vivo studies of δ-receptor-mediated bioactivities.

A very interesting compound is the topographically constrained analogue of DPDPE, [(2*S*,3*S*)β-MePhe[4]]DPDPE (**8**; see Tables 1 and 2) (22). Its selectivity is good, but it suffers from reduced affinity and potency relative to DPDPE. Nonetheless, it has become a useful ligand for examining effects of side chain conformation on binding and transduction at δ-opioid receptors (23).

[Phe[6]]DPLCE (**9**; see Tables 1 and 2) and especially the Phe(p-Cl)[4] analogue **10** (see Table 1) (24) were potent and δ-opioid receptor-selective in binding assays (see Table 1). Compound **9** (see Table 2) was highly potent and selective in the in vitro bioassays for the δ-receptor with an EC_{50} value of 16 pmol in the MVD assay. To our knowledge, this is the most potent ligand known in the MVD assay (see also **23**;Table 2). The Trp[6]-analogue **11** (see Tables 1 and 2) has very high-binding affinities and δ-opioid receptor selectivities (see Table 1) as well, and maintains high potency and δ-opioid receptor selectivity in the MVD assay (see Table 2). Much higher binding selectivity is seen for the [Phe(pBr)[4],Phe[6]]DPLPE analogue (**12**; see Table 1) with a δ-opioid receptor-binding selectivity of over 20,000 (see Table 1), making it perhaps the most selective δ-agonist ligand yet observed in binding affinity assays. Interestingly, both **12** and, especially, the Phe(pF)[4] analogue **23** (see Table 2) were found to have extraordinary selectivities for the MVD (δ) versus GPI (μ)-receptors [well over four orders of magnitude; (25)].

The highly conformationally and topographically constrained cyclic enkephalin analogue **13**, [(2*S*,3*R*)TMT[1]]DPDPE (TMT = β methyl-2′, 6′-dimethyltyrosine) (26), has an exceptional biological activity and binding affinity profile. Although its binding affinity and δ-opioid receptor selectivity in binding assays (see Table 1) is similar to that of DPDPE, the compound has no agonist activity at the GPI (μ)-receptor (see Table 2) up to 60 μM, the highest concentration that could be measured under standard assay conditions. Currently, this unique ligand for the δ-opioid receptor is under investigation as the first example of a δ-opioid receptor-specific agonist.

An important discovery more than a decade ago provided the first examples of highly δ opioid-selective ligand found in nature (frog skins) (27–28) with both deltorphin I (*H*-Tyr-D-Ala-Phe-Asp-Val-Val-Gly-NH_2; **14**; Tables 1 and 2), deltorphin II (*H*-Tyr-D-Ala-Phe-Glu-Val-Val-Gly-NH_2; **15**; (see Tables 1 and 2), and dermenkephalin. Subsequently, cyclic (**16**) and linear (**17–19**) analogues of these and other deltorphins have been synthesized. Some of them have excellent receptor-binding affinity selectivities (see Table 1) and selectivities in the MVD versus GPI biological assays (see Table 2); and they show no evidence of μ-receptor activity in pharmacological studies and in μ-receptor knockout mice (Yamamura HI, Hruby VJ, Porreca F, unpublished observations). Interestingly, the most selective analogue for binding affinity (**17**; see Table 1) is highly selective (see Table 2) in the bioassays. Several of these analogues clearly are worthy of further study (and also the cyclic analogue **16** for its conformation) for their biological activities in vivo to obtain a more complete picture of their antinociceptive activities. Very recently, structure–activity relations of deltorphins have been comprehensively reviewed by Lazarus et al. (37).

After many years of effort, a few nonpeptide ligands with reasonable potencies and good selectivities for δ-opioid receptors have been developed (**20,21,22**; see Tables 1 and 2; structures are shown in Fig. 1) (32–34). Based on data presented in the literature thus far, they seem to have quite different structure–activity relations. TAN-67 (32) and BW 373U86 were initially derived from screening programs in industry and were obtained as a result of subsequent improvements to initial leads by standard medicinal chemistry approaches. Subsequently, Rice and colleagues (33) developed SNC 80, the methylether of (−)BW 373U86, as a highly selective, nonpeptidic δ-agonist. SL-3111 was designed as a nonpeptide peptidomimetic based on the structure, conformation, and topographical relations of pharmacophore elements from, among

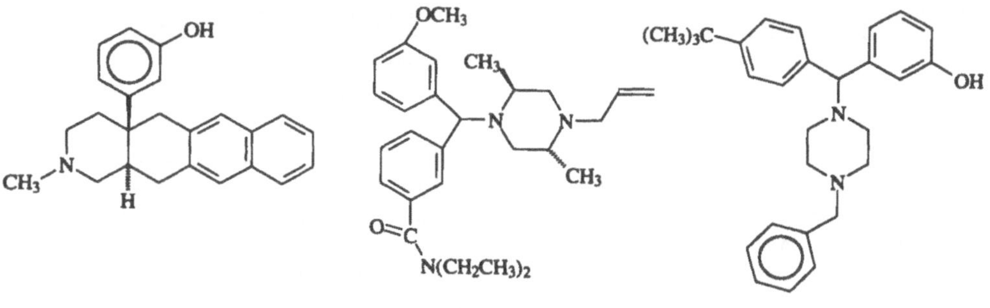

Tan-67 SNC-80 SL-3111

Figure 1 Structures of selective nonpeptide and opioid receptor-selective ligands.

other compounds, [(2*S*,3*R*) TMT[1]]DPDPE (34), and currently this compound is under further investigation.

Some aspects of the pharmacology of SNC 80 are worthy of mention. Specifically, (1) SNC 80 shows a δ (vs. μ) selectivity ratio of 2300 in radioligand-binding assays in brain tissue; (2) SNC 80 shows a GPI/MVD ratio (i.e., δ selectivity) of 2400; (3) the concentration–effect curve of SNC 80 in the MVD is displaced 270-fold to the right by ICI 174,864 (δ-antagonist) and 1.6-fold to the right by CTAP (μ-antagonist); (4) SNC 80 produces antinociception (tail-flick and hot-plate tests) following intracranial–ventricular (i.c.v.) or intrathecal (i.th.) administration to mice, although with somewhat lower potency compared with DPDPE (selective δ-ligand); (5) SNC 80 produces maximal antinociception following subcutaneous or intraperitoneal (i.p.) administration to mice with potency approximately threefold lower than systemic morphine; (6) the antinociceptive actions of i.p. SNC 80 in mice are antagonized by i.c.v. naloxone or i.c.v. ICI 174,864 (δ-antagonist), but not by pretreatment with β-funaltrexamine (μ-antagonist), suggesting that the observed antinociception is mediated (at least in large part) by supraspinal δ- (but not μ)-receptors (35). These data suggest that appropriate agonists at the opioid δ-receptor can mediate antinociception following systemic administration. Although the pharmacology of compounds such as SNC 80 and SL3111 is limited, it is clear that such compounds show promise, although improvements in efficacy and in vivo potency will be needed.

B. Development of Peptide Ligands with Mixed Activity at μ- and δ-Opioid Receptors

The discovery of the enkephalins in the late 1970s and the subsequent discovery of other endogenous peptides that interact with opioid receptors, as well as the discovery of multiple opioid receptors, led to efforts initially to obtain μ-opioid receptor peptide ligands with high selectivity and agonist potency at μ-opioid receptors. Two of the earliest successes were DAMGO (**25**) and PLO17 (**26**) (Tables 3 and 4). Both of these modified peptides showed good μ-receptor selectivity in binding assays (see Table 3), but only modest selectivity in the classic GPI (μ) and MVD (δ) bioassays for opioids (see Table 4). Subsequently, even more potent and μ-opioid receptor-selective ligands such as **27** and **28** (see Table 4) were developed. These and other μ-selective agonist ligands were studied for their in vivo antinociception properties, and although some had high in vivo potency, they usually have the same undesirable side effects as morphine and other μ-selective ligands.

Table 3 Binding Affinities of Compounds with Mixed μ–δ Receptor Binding

Compound	Binding affinity (nM)			
	μ	δ	δ–μ	Ref.
25 *H*-Tyr-DAla-Gly-*N*MePhe-NHCH$_2$OH(DAMGO)	3.9	700	180	38
26 *H*-Tyr-Pro-*N*MePhe-DPro-NH$_2$(PLO17)	5.5	10,000	1,800	39
27 *H*-Tyr-D-Met(*O*)-Gly-*N*MePhe-ol	0.29	1,250	4,300	41
28 *H*-Tyr-DArg-Phe-Lys-NH$_2$	1.7	19,000	11,000	42
29 (*H*-Tyr-DAla-Gly-Phe-NH)$_2$ (Biphalin)	1.4	2.6	1.8	43–45
30 (*H*-Tyr-DAla-Gly-Phe(*pF*)-NH-)$_2$	0.64	0.31	0.5	46
31 *H*-Tyr-c[DCys-Gly-Phe-DCys]-Ser(β-DGlc)-Gly-NH$_2$	53	26	0.5	47
32 *H*-Tyr-c[DOrn-Phe-D-Pro-Gly-]	0.88	13.2	15	48
33 *H*-Tyr-c[DOrn-Trp-DPro-Gly-]	2.1	10.	5	49
34 *H*-DMT-c[DOrn-Nal(2′)-DPro-Gly]	0.46	0.46	1	49,50
35 *H*-DMT-Tic-NH-(CH$_2$)$_3$-Ph	0.40	0.087	0.22	50
36 *H*-Tyr-(1*R*,2*S*)-Ahh^2-Gly-Phe-Leu-OH	0.25	0.010	0.04	51

Serious work on developing μ-selective peptide or peptidomimetic agonist ligands with high potency and selectivity for the μ-opioid receptor has been absent for the last 10–15 years. However, various pharmacological experiments during this period led to the hypothesis that ligands that interacted as agonists or mixed agonists–antagonists at both the μ- and δ-opioid receptors might have very useful properties for the treatment of pain without undesirable side effects on respiration, gut transit, and addiction. Studies of Takemori and colleagues suggested that occupation of opioid δ-receptors by either naltrindole or 5′-naltrindole isothiocyanate prevented the development of tolerance to morphine-induced antinociception as well as the development of physical dependence (or the expression of abstinence) to morphine in mice (53,54). These findings and those of our laboratory have been confirmed in the rat using osmotic minipump infusion of BW 373U86 (55); BW 373U86 prevented the development of the motor signs of morphine abstinence (jumping, wet-dog shakes, head shakes, forelimb tremors, digging, and teeth chattering) in a dose-related fashion, suggesting that occupation of the opioid δ-receptor can prevent the development of tolerance and dependence to morphine (see also 56,57).

Table 4 Bioassay Potencies of Compounds with Mixed μ–δ Bioactivity

Compound	Bioassay (nM)			
	MVD	GPI	δ–μ	Ref.
25 *H*-Tyr-DAla-Gly-*N*MePhe-NH$_2$(DAMGO)	33	4.5	7.3	40
26 *H*-Tyr-Pro-*N*MePhe-DPro-NH$_2$(PLO17)	240	34	7.1	40
27 *H*-Tyr-DMet(*O*)-Gly-*N*MePhe-ol	—	0.0025	—	41
28 *H*-Tyr-DArg-Pro-Lys-NH$_2$(DALDA)	800	3.2	250	42
29 (*H*-Tyr-DAla-Gly-Phe-NH)$_2$ (Biphalin)	27	8.8	3.4	43–45
30 (*H*-Tyr-DAla-Gly-Phe(*pF*)-NH)$_2$	1.3	2.1	0.62	46
31 *H*-Tyr-c[DCys-Gly-Phe-DCys]-Ser(β-Gluc)-GlyNH$_2$	13	60	0.20	47
32 *H*-Tyr-c[DOrn-Phe-DPro-Gly-]	4.9	2.1	2.2	48
33 *H*-Tyr-c[DOrn-Trp-DPro-Gly-]	16	28	0.64	48
34 *H*-DMT-c[DOrn-Nal(2′)-DPro-Gly-]	2.1	7.9	0.27	49,50
35 *H*-DMT-Tic-NH-(CH$_2$)$_3$Phe	1.7	100	0.017	49

This idea was also given considerable support when it was discovered (43) that biphalin (**29**; see Tables 3 and 4) (44,45) with nearly equivalent 1- to 3-nM–binding affinities and 10- to 30-nM–MVD and GPI (μ) bioassay potencies, nonetheless was as potent as, or more potent than, etorphine, which had been thought to be the most potent opioid ligand known in antinociception assays. This nearly 1000-fold enhancement in analgesic efficacy of biphalin relative to its binding and bioassay potency was remarkable and the mechanism for this is still unknown. Furthermore, this compound was bioactive as an analgesic when given peripherally with a potency equal to morphine. Its binding affinity (see Table 3) and biological potency (see Table 4) could be significantly enhanced at both the μ- and the δ-opioid receptors by substitution of the Phe^4 and $Phe^{4\prime}$ with *p*-fluoro substitution on the aromatic ring (**30**). These compounds currently are being developed for human clinical trials.

Another novel approach that has led to enkephalin analogues with surprisingly potent analgesic activities is illustrated by the cyclic glycopeptide analogue **31** (see Tables 3 and 4). Although this cyclic peptide has only modest affinity for the μ- and δ-opioid receptors (see Table 3) and modest potency in the MVD and GPI bioassays (see Table 4), compound **31** has potent analgesic activities and apparently crosses the blood–brain barrier quite effectively, as analgesia can be observed following peripheral administration.

A very interesting new class of mixed μ/δ ligands are the β-casomorphin analogues **32–34**, and the 2-position constrained enkephalin analogues **35** and **36** (see Tables 3 and 4). These ligands bind with high affinity to μ- and δ-opioid receptors and have potent mixed μ-agonist activity and δ-antagonist activity in the GPI and MVD bioassays, respectively. Recently, Schiller et al. (52) have pointed out the small changes in structure that can affect agonist versus antagonist activities (52). Pharmacological evidence suggests that these compounds may have excellent analgesic properties with a low potential for addiction. This exciting new development suggests another new modality for treatment of pain, which thus far has not been examined in humans, but that deserves careful scrutiny.

III. LIGANDS WITH HIGH AFFINITY AND GOOD SELECTIVITY FOR κ-OPIOID RECEPTORS

It has been suggested for some time that development of κ-opioid ligands for treatment of certain pain states may have distinct advantages over μ-opioid ligands because of their low addiction potential and lack of effects on gut motility. However, nonpeptide agonists selective for the κ-receptor have a major drawback in that they cause dysphoria in animals and humans; therefore, there is an adversive reaction to taking such compounds. However, it is suggested that dynorphin-related peptides may not suffer from such effects; hence, efforts have been made to obtain analogues that are more selective for the κ-opioid receptor than the naturally occurring dynorphins. Table 5 gives some of the potent or selective dynorphins that have been reported to date.

One of the earliest compounds that was shown to be more potent in κ-receptor–binding affinity and also more selective by nearly an order of magnitude over the dynorphins is **37** (see Table 5). The D-Pro in position 10 (**37**; see Table 5) of dynorphin A surprisingly imparts these properties on dynorphin A. Interestingly, cyclization through a $DPen^5$ Cys^{11} substitution (**38**; see Table 5) led to a analogue with similar κ- versus δ-opioid receptor selectivity to **37**, whereas cyclization of dynorphin A(1–13) by a Cys^8, $DCys^{13}$ substitution (**39**; see Table 5) leads to an analogue with affinity identical to that of the κ-receptor for [D-Pro^{10}]dynorphin A(1–11) analogue **37**.

An interesting finding was the observation that the tyrosine in position 1 of dynorphin could be substituted by a $pBrPhe^1$- (**40**; see Table 5) or even a simple Phe^1- (**41**; see Table 5)

Table 5 Binding Affinities of Compounds with Agonist Selectivity for the κ-Receptor

	Binding affinities EC_{50} or *Ki* (nM)			Selectivities		
Compound	μ	δ	κ	μ/κ	δ/κ	Ref.
37 [D-Pro[10]]DynA-(1–11)	2.0	7.5	0.032	63	230	58
38 c[DPen[5], Cys[11]]DynA-(1–11)	1.3	86	0.52	2.4	170	59
39 c[Cys[8],DCys[13]]DynA-(1–13)	0.38	1.9	0.035	11	55	59
40 [*p*BrPhe[1],D-Ala[8]]DynA-(1–11)	47	1100	1.8	26	610	60
41 [Phe[1],DPro[10]]DynA-(1–11)	120.	390	2.4	50	160	60
42 [DAla[3]]DynA-(1–11)	200	1000	0.76	350	1300	61
43 [*N*-BnTyr[1],D-Pro[10]]DynA-(1–11)	31	180	0.029	1100	6,100	62,63
44 [*N*-PrTyr[1],DAla[3]]DynA-(1–11)	1400	3900	5.2	270	750	64
45 *N*-MeTyr-Gly-Gly-Phe-Leu-Arg-NMeArg-DLeu-OH	4.5	27	1.9	2.4	14	65

and still retain high nanomolar affinity for the δ-opioid receptor, and fair-to-excellent κ- versus μ-opioid receptor selectivity.

Replacement of the Gly[3] by D-Ala[3] (**42**; see Table 5) led to an analogue with subnamolar affinity for the κ-opioid receptor and an excellent selectivity for the κ-receptor versus the δ- and μ-receptor. This compound also has considerably greater stability against proteolytic degradation than dynorphin A. Interestingly, substitution of the D-Pro[10] analogue with *N*-alkyl substitutients in the Tyr position led to potent and exceptionally selective κ-ligands, such as **43** (see Table 5), similar substitutions of the D-Ala[3] analogues led to analogues such as **44** (see Table 5) which had somewhat reduced affinity for the κ-receptor and slightly reduced selectivity for the κ- versus μ- and κ- versus δ-opioid receptors. Investigation of the conformational and structural origins of these different affinities and selectivities for κ-opioid receptors should provide new insights into the structural and conformation features critical to molecular recognition and receptor transduction of ligands at κ-opioid receptors and their potential use in the treatment of pain. The [*N*-MeTyr[1], *N*-MeArg[7], DLeu[8]]dynorphin A-(1–8) analogue **45** (see Table 5) deserves comment because although it has only modest selectivity for the κ-opioid receptor, it has nanomolar binding at all three opioid receptors and is systemically active in producing analgesia (57), suggesting it is quite stable to proteolytic breakdown in vivo and possibly crosses the blood–brain barrier or readily enters the CSF.

An additional important strategy is the development of opioid κ-ligands that do not penetrate the blood–brain barrier and thus produce their analgesic actions in the periphery. Recently, an all D-amino acid tetrapeptide motif has been discovered, using a combinatorial library of 6.25 million tetrapeptides, which demonstrates outstanding selectivity for κ- rather than μ- or δ-opioid receptors (66). One compound from this series, DPhe-DPhe-DNle-DArg-NH_2 (FE 200041; Table 6) shows high affinity (i.e., 1 nM or lower) and selectivity (i.e., > 30,000-fold)

Table 6 Values at the Cloned Human κ (hKOR), μ (hMOR), and δ (hDOR) Opioid Receptors

Compounds	hKOR (nM)	hMOR (nM)	hDOR (nM)
FE 200041	0.146	4570	>10,000
(−)U50,488	1.120	2400	7100
Enadoline (CI-977)	0.160	320	707

Table 7 Antinociceptive A_{50} Values of FE 200041 in Assays of Mouse and Rat Antinociception and Effects on the Rotarod

Antinociceptive tests	FE 200041 (A_{50})
Mouse acetic acid writhing	0.030 mg/kg, i.v.
Mouse acetic acid writhing	3.0 mg/kg, p.o.
Rat acetic acid writhing	0.094 mg/kg, s.c.
Rat 2% formalin flinch	(Phase-I) 0.396 and (phase-II) 0.551 mg/kg, i.v.
Mouse hot-water (52°C) tail-flick	13.48 mg/kg, i.v.
Rat hot-water (52°C) tail-flick	>10.00 mg/kg, s.c.
Mouse rotarod	5.04 mg/kg, i.v.

at opioid κ-receptors (66; Vanderah TW, et al., unpublished results). FE 200041 was shown to be an agonist by the inhibition of forskolin-stimulated adenylate cyclase using R1G1 thymoma cell line membranes (67). Additionally, this tetrapeptide produces strong antinociception following systemic administration in assays emphasizing peripheral sites of action, such as the mouse acetic acid writhing test, but does not show antinociceptive effects in assays requiring penetration to the brain (see Table 7). FE 200041 does not produce inhibition of gastrointestinal transit, suggesting that it may be a useful molecule for the production of peripheral antinociception without either dysphoria or constipation.

Fedotozine is another molecule with κ-opioid properties. This compound is a lipophilic κ-agonist, with structural features similar to U50,488 (**47**; see Table 6), and was designed as an analgesic that would remain in the periphery after oral administration for the indication of irritable bowel syndrome and dyspepsia. However, the compound was discontinued after demonstrating low affinity and selectivity for its targeted κ-receptor in the gastrointestinal tract of dogs (68). Finally, another purported peripheral κ-agonist, asimadoline, was evaluated by E. Merck for the treatment of rheumatic pain and osteoarthritis. Asimadoline possesses a biophysical profile similar to several peripherally selective antihistamines. It has a characteristic distribution of lipophilic and hydrophilic structural elements that may result in active transport out of the CNS by membrane pumps in the brain capillary endothelium (69). However, asimadoline was discontinued in clinical trials owing to the CNS side effects of dysphoria (69,70), suggesting significant penetration of this molecule to the brain, at least at doses that produce significant analgesia.

The studies described in the foregoing indicate that further work on addiction, dysphoria, gut motility, respiration, and other potential in vivo side effects with the highly selective peptide κ-ligands are needed. However, these recent findings also suggest that highly selective and peripherally acting κ-agonist ligands may have considerable potential as analgesic agents and that the discovery of such molecules with outstanding selectivity for the κ-receptor may offer a novel approach to the control of pain without significant side effect liability.

ACKNOWLEDGMENT

The studies reported from our laboratories were supported by grants from the U.S. Public Health Service, National Institute of Drug Abuse. The opinions expressed are those of the authors and do not necessarily reflect those of the U.S. Public Health Service.

REFERENCES

1. Martin WR, Eades JA, Thompson JA, Huppler RA, Gilbert PE. The effects of morphine and nalorphine-like drugs in the nondependent chronic spinal dog. J Pharm Exp Ther 1976; 197:517–532.
2. Iwamoto ET, Martin WR. Multiple opioid receptors. Med Res Rev 1981; 1:411–440.
3. Lord JAH, Waterfield AA, Hughes J, Kosterlitz HW. Endogenous opioid peptides; multiple agonists and receptors. Nature 1977; 267:495–499.
4. Chavkin C, James IF, Goldstein A. Dynorphin is a specific endogenous ligand for the κ opioid receptor. Science 1982; 215:413–415.
5. Moitto K, Magendzo K, Evans CJ. Molecular characterization of opioid receptors [review]. In: Tseng LF, ed. The Pharmacology of Opioid Peptides. New Jersey: Harwood Academic Press, 1995:57–71.
6. Porreca F, Bilsky EJ, Lai J. Pharmacological characterization of opioid δ and *k* receptors. In: Tseng LF, ed. The Pharmacology of Opioid Peptides. New Jersey: Harwood Academic Press, 1995:219–248.
7. Gacel G, Dange V, Breuzē P, Delay–Goyet P, Roques BP. Development of conformationally constrained linear peptides exhibiting a high affinity and pronounced selectivity for δ-opioid receptors. J Med Chem 1988; 31:1891–1897.
8. Mosberg HI, Hurst R, Hruby VJ, Gee K, Yamamura HI, Galligan JJ, Burks TJ. Bis-penicillamine enkephalins possess highly improved specificity toward delta opioid receptors. Proc Natl Acad Sci USA 1983; 80:5871–5874.
9. Weber SJ, Greene DL, Hruby VJ, Yamamura HI, Porreca F, Davis TP. Whole body and brain distribution of [^3H]cyclic[D-Pen^2,D-Pen^5] enkephalin after intraperitoneal, intravenous, oral and subcutaneous administration. J Pharmacol Exp Ther 1992; 263:1308–1316.
10. Greene DL, Hau VS, Abbruscato TJ, Bartosz H, Misicka A, Lipkowski AW, Hom S, Gillespie TJ, Hruby VJ, Davis TP. Enkephalin analog prodrugs: assessment of in vitro conversion, enzyme cleavage characterization and blood–brain permeability. J Pharmacol Exp Ther 1996; 277:1366–1375.
11. Hruby VJ, Kao L–F, Pettitt BM, Karplus M. The conformational properties of the delta opioid peptide [D-Pen^2, D-Pen^5] enkephalin in aqueous solution determined by NMR and energy minimization calculations. J Am Chem Soc 1988; 110:3351–3359.
12. Flippen–Anderson JL, Hruby VJ, Collins N, George C, Cudney B. X-ray structure of [D-Pen^2, δD-Pen^5]enkephalin, a highly potent, delta opioid receptor selective compound: comparisons with proposed solution conformations. J Am Chem Soc 1994; 116:7523–7531.
13. Rapaka RS, Porreca, F. Development of delta opioid peptides as non-addicting analgesics. Pharm Res 1991; 8:1–8.
14. Sakaguchi Y, Shimohigashi Y, Waki M, Kato T, Costa T, Herz A. Synthesis and activity of a series of morphiceptin analogs containing phenylalanine homologs in position 4. In: Shiba T, Sakakibara S, eds. Peptide Chemistry 1987: Proceedings Japanese Peptide Symposium, Osaka: Protein Research Foundation, 1988:577–580.
15. Rigaudy P, Garbay–Jaureguiberry C, Jacquemin–Sablon A, LePecq JB, Roques BP, Synthesis and binding properties to DNA and to opioid receptors of enkephalin–ellipticinum conjugates. Int J Pept Protein Res 1987; 30:347–355.
16. Kimura H, Stammer CH, Shimohigashi Y, Ren-Lin C, Stewart J. The synthesis, bioactivity and enzyme stability of D-Ala^2, Δ^EPhe^4, Leu^5-enkephalins. Biochem Biophys Res Commun 1983; 115: 112–115.
17. Shimohigashi Y, Costa T, Pfeiffer A, Herz A, Kimura H, Stammer CH. Δ^EPhe-enkephalin analogs: delta receptors in rat brain are different from those in mouse vas deferens. FEBS Lett 1987; 222: 71–74.
18. Akiyama K, Gee KW, Mosberg HI, Hruby VJ, Yamamura HI. Characterization of [^3H][2-D-penicillamine,5-D-penicillamine]-enkephalin binding to delta opiate receptors in the rat brain and neuroblastoma–glioma hybrid cell line (NG 108–15). Proc Natl Acad Sci USA 1985; 82:2543–2547.
19. Vaughn LK, Knapp RJ, Tóth G, Wan YP, Hruby VJ, Yamamura HI. A high affinity, highly selective

ligand for the delta opioid receptor:[^3H]-[D-Pen^2,pCI-Phe^4, D-Pen^5]-enkephalin. Life Sci 1989; 45: 1001–1008.

20. Tóth G, Kramer TH, Knapp R, Lui GK, Davis P, Burks TF, Yamamura HI, Hruby VJ. [D-Pen^{2}D-Pen^5] enkephalin (DPDPE) analogues with increased affinity and selectivity for delta opioid receptors. J Med Chem 1990; 33:249–253.
21. Mosberg HI, Hurst R, Hruby VJ, Galligan JJ, Burks TF, Gee K, Yamamura HI. Conformationally constrained cyclic enkephalin analogs with pronounced delta opioid receptor agonist selectivity. Life Sci 1983; 32:2565–2569.
22. Hruby VJ, Toth G, Gehrig CA, Kao C–F, Knapp R, Liu GK, Yamamura HI, Kramer TH, Davis P, Burks TF. Topographically designed analogues of [D-Pen^{2}D-Pen^5] enkephalin. J Med Chem 1991; 34:1823–1830.
23. Hruby VJ, Li G, Haskell–Luevano C, Shenderovich MD. Design of peptides, proteins, and peptidomimetics in chi space. Biopolymers (Pept Sci) 1997; 43:219–266.
24. Bartosz–Bechowski H, Davis P, Zalewska T, Slaninova J, Porreca F, Yamamura HI, Hruby VJ. Cyclic enkephalins analogues with exceptional potency at peripheral delta opioid receptors. J Med Chem 1994; 37:146–150.
25. Hruby VJ, Bartosz–Bechowski H, Davis P, Slaninova J, Zalewska T, Stropova D, Porreca F, Yamamura HI. Cyclic enkephalin analogues with exceptional potency and selectivity for δ-opioid receptors. J Med Chem 1997; 40:3957–3962.
26. Qian X, Shenderovich MD, Kövér KE, Davis P, Horváth R, Zalewska T, Yamamura HI, Porreca F, Hruby VJ. Probing the stereochemical requirements for receptor recognition of δ opioid agonists through topographic modifications in position 1. J Am Chem Soc 1996; 118:7280–7290.
27. Erspamer V, Melchiori P, Falconieri–Erspamer G, Negri L, Corsi R, Baraa D, Simmaco M, Kriel G. Deltorphins: a family of naturally occurring peptides with high affinity and selectivity for δ opioid binding sites. Proc Natl Acad Sci USA 1989; 86:5188–5192.
28. Sagan S, Amiche M, Delfour A, Moz A, Camus A, Nicolas P. Molecular determinants of receptor affinity and selectivity of the natural Δ-opioid agonist, dermenkephalin. J Biol Chem 1989; 264: 17100–17106.
29. Misicka A, Lipkowski AW, Horvath P, Davis P, Yamamura HI, Porreca F, Hruby VJ. Design of cyclic deltorphins and dermenkephalins with a disulfide bridge leads to analogues with high selectivity for delta opioid receptors. J Med Chem 1994; 37:141–145.
30. Sasaki Y, Chiba T. Novel deltorphin analogues with potent δ agonist δ antagonist or mixed μ antagonist/δ agonist properties. J Med Chem 1995; 38:3995–3999.
31. Toth G, Darula Z, Péter A, Fülöp F, Tourwē D, Jaspers H, Verheyden P, Böcskey Z, Töth Z, Borsodi A. Conformationally constrained deltorphin analogs with 2-aminotetralin-2-carboxylic acid in position 3. J Med Chem 1997; 40:990–995.
32. Suzuki T, Tsuji M, Mori T, Misawa M, Endoh T, Nigase H. Effects of a highly selective nonpeptide δ opioid receptor agonist Tan-67 on morphine-induced antinociception in mice. Life Sci 1995; 57: 155–168.
33. Calderon SN, Rothman RB, Porreca F, Flippen–Anderson JL, McNutt RW, Xu H, Smith LE, Bilsky EJ, Davis P, Rice KC. Probes for narcotic receptor mediated phenomina. 19. Synthesis of (+)-4-[(αR)$_3$-α((2S5R)-4-allyl-25-dimethyl-1-piperazinyl)-3-methoxybenzyl]-N_1N-diethylbenzamide (SNC80) A highly selective nonpeptide δ opioid receptor agonist. J Med Chem 1994; 37:2125–2128.
34. Liao S, Alfaro–Lopez J, Shenderovich MD, Hosohata K, Lin J, Li X, Stropova D, Davis P, Jernigan KA, Porreca F, Yamamura HI, Hruby VJ. De novo design, synthesis, and biological activities of high-affinity, and selective non-peptide agonists of the delta-opioid receptor. J Med Chem 1998; 41: 4767–4776.
35. Bilsky EJ, Calderon SN, Wang T, Bernstein RN, Davis P, Hruby VJ, McNutt RW, Rothman RB, Rice KC, Porreca F. SNC 80, a selective, non-peptidic and systemically active opioid delta agonist. J Pharmacol Exp Ther 1995; 273:359–366.
36. Schiller PW, Weltrowska G, Berezowska I, Lemieux C, Chung NN, Carpenter KA, Wilkes BC. A new class of dipeptide derivatives that are potent and selective δ opioid agonists. In: Tam J, Hodges

R, eds. Peptides: Chemistry, Structure, Biology, Proceedings 15th American Peptide Symposium 1999:514–516.

37. Lazarus LH, Bryant SD, Cooper PS, Salvadori S. What peptides these deltorphins be. Prog Neurobiol 1999; 57:377–420.
38. Gacel G, Zajac JM, Delay-Goyet P, Daugé V, Roques PB. Investigation of structural parameters involved in the μ and δ opioid receptor discrimination of linear enkephalin-related peptides. J Med Chem 1988; 31:377–383.
39. Chang KJ, Wei ET, Killian A, Chang JK. Potent morphiceptin analogs: structure activity relationships and morphine-like activities. J Pharmacol Exp Ther 1983; 227:403–408.
40. Aldrich JV. Analgesics. In: Wolff ME, ed. Burger's Medicinal Chemistry and Drug Discovery. New York: John Wiley & Sons, 1996:321–441.
41. Kiso Y, Yamaguchi M, Akita T, Moritoki H, Takei M, Nakamura H. Super-active enkephalin analogues. Naturwissenschaften 1981; 68:210–212.

41a. Quiron R, Kiso Y, Pert CB. Syndyphalin DS-25: a highly selective ligand for μ opioid receptors. FEBS Lett 1982; 141:203–206.

42. Schiller PW, Nguyen TMD, Chung NN, Lemieux C. Dermorphin analogues carrying an increased positive net charge in their "message" domain display extremely high μ opioid receptor selectivity. J Med Chem 1989; 32:698–703.
43. Horan PJ, Mattia A, Bilsky EJ, Weber SJ, Davis TP, Yamamura HI, Malatynska E, Applyard SM, Slaninová J, Misicka A, Lipkowski AW, Hruby VJ, Porreca F. Antinociceptive profile of biphalin, a dimeric enkephalin analog. J Pharmacol Exp Ther 1993; 265:1446–1454.
44. Misicka A, Lipkowski AW, Horvath R, Davis P, Porreca F, Yamamura HI, Hruby VJ. Structure–activity relationships of analogues of highly potent opioid peptide, biphalin. Regul Pept 1994; S131–S132.
45. Lipkowski AW, Konecka AM, Sroczynska I. Double enkephalins-synthesis, activity on guinea-pig ileum, and analgesic effect. Peptides 1982; 3:697–700.
46. Misicka A, Lipkowski AW, Horvath R, Davis P, Porreca F, Yamamura HI, Hruby VJ. Structure–activity relationships of biphalin. The synthesis and biological activities of new analogues with modifications in positions 3 and 4. Life Sci 1997; 60:1263–1269.
47. Polt R, Porreca F, Szabo LZ, Bilsky EJ, Davis P, Abbruscato TJ, Davis TP, Horvath R, Yamamura HI, Hruby VJ. Glycopeptide enkephalin analogues produce analgesia in mice: evidence for penetration of the blood–brain barrier. Proc Natl Acad Sci USA 1994; 91:7114–7118.
48. Schmidt R, Vogel D, Mrestani–Klaus C, Brandt W, Neubert K, Chung NN, Lemieux C, Schiller PW. Cyclic β-casomorphin analogues with mixed μ agonist/δ antagonist properties: synthesis, pharmacological characterization and conformational aspects. J Med Chem 1994; 37:1136–1144.
49. Schiller PW, Weltrowska G, Schmidt R, Nguyen TM–D, Berezowsk I, Lemieux C, Chung NN, Carpenter KA, Wilkes BC. Four different types of opioid peptides with mixed μ agonist/δ antagonist properties. Analgesia 1995; 1:703–706.
50. Schiller PW, Schmidt R, Weltrowska G, Berezowska I, Nguyen TM–D, Dupuis S, Chung NN, Lemieux C, Wilkes BC, Carpernter KA. Conformationally constrained opioid peptide analogues with novel activity profiles. Lett Pept Sci 1998; 5:209–214.
51. Horikawa M, Shiferi Y, Yumoto N, Yoshikawa S, Nakajima T, Ohfume Y. Synthesis of potent leu-enkephalin analogs possessing β-hydroxy-α, α-disubstituted-α-amino acid and their characterization to opioid receptors. Bioorg Med Chem Letts 1998; 8:2027–2032.
52. Schiller PW, Wetrowska G, Schmidt R, Berezowska I, Nguyen TMD, Lemieux C, Chung NN, Carpenter KA, Wilkes BC. Subtleties of structure–agonist versus antagonist relationships of opioid peptides and peptidomimetics. J Rec Sign Transduction Res 1999; 19:573–588.
53. Abdelhamid EE, Sultana M, Portoghese PS, Takemori AE. Selective blockage of delta opioid receptors prevents the development of morphine tolerance and dependence in mice. J Pharmacol Exp Ther 1991; 258:299–303.
54. Miyamoto Y, Portoghese PS, Takemori AE. Involvement of delta 2 opioid receptors in the development of morphine dependence in mice. J Pharmacol Exp Ther 264:11415, 1993.
55. Lee PH, McNutt RW, Chang KJ. A nonpeptidic delta opioid receptor agonist, BW373U86, attenuates

the development and expression of morphine abstinence precipitated by naloxone in rat. J Pharmacol Exp Ther 1993; 267:8837.

56. Fundytus ME, Schiller PW, Shapiro M, Weltrowska G, Coderre TJ. Attenuation of morphine tolerance and dependence with the highly selective delta-opioid receptor antagonist TIPP[psi]. Eur J Pharmacol 1995; 286:105–108.

57. Schmidt R, Wilkes BC, Chung NN, Lemieux C, Schiller PW. Effect of aromatic amino acid substitutions in the 3-position of cyclic beta-casomorphin analogues on mu-opioid agonist/delta-opioid antagonist properties. Int J Pept Protein Res 1996; 48:411–419.

58. Gairin JE, Gouarderes C, Mazarguil H, Alvinerie P, Cross J. [D-Pro10]dynorphin-(1–11) is a highly potent and selective ligand for κ opioid receptors. Eur J Pharm 1984; 106:457–458.

59. Kawasaki AM, Knapp RJ, Kramer TH, Walton A, Wire WS, Hashimoto S, Yamamura HI, Porreca F, Burks TH, Hruby VJ. Design and synthesis of highly potent and selective cyclic dynorphin A analogs. II. New analogs. J Med Chem 1993; 36:750–757.

60. Kawasaki AM, Knapp RJ, Walton A, Wire WS, Zalewska T, Yamamura HI, Porreca F, Burks TK, Hruby VJ. Synthesis, opioid binding affinities, and potencies of dynorphin A analogues substituted in the 1,6,7,8 and 10 positions. Int J Pept Protein Res 1993; 42:411–419.

61. Lung FD–T, Meyer JP, Li G, Lou BS, Stropova D, Davis P, Yamamura HI, Porreca F, Hruby VJ. Highly kappa receptor selective dynorphin A analogues with modifications in position 3 of dynorphin A (1–11)-NH_2. J Med Chem 1995; 38:585–586.

62. Choi H, Murray TF, DeLander GE, Caldwell V, Aldrich JV. N-Terminal alkylated derivatives of [D-Pro^{10}]dynorphin A-(1–11) are highly selective for κ-opioid receptor. J Med Chem 1992; 35:4638–4639.

63. Soderstrom K, Choi H, Berman FW, Aldrich JV, Murray TF. N-Alkylated derivatives of [D-Pro^{10}]dynorphin A(1–11) are high affinity-partial agonists at the cloned rat κ-opioid receptor. Eur J Pharmacol 1997; 338:191–197.

64. Meyer J–P, Lung FD, Davis P, DeLeon I, Gillespie T, Davis TP, Porreca F, Yamamura HI, Hruby VJ. Synthesis and biological activities of enzymatically stable and highly selective Dyn A-(1–11)-NH_2 analogs. In: Kaumaya PTP, Hodges RS, eds. Peptides: Chemistry, Structure and Biology. Proceedings of the 14th American Peptide Symposium, Mayflower Scientific, Kingswinford, England, 1996:625–626.

65. Nazazawa T, Furuya Y, Kaneko T, Yamatsu K, Yoshino H, Tachibana S. Analgesia produced by E-2078, a systemically active dynorphin analog in mice. J Pharmacol Exp Ther 1990; 252:1247–1254.

66. Houghten RA, Ny P, Bidlack JM, Dooley CT. kappa Tetrapeptide ligands induce peripheral analgesia, Soc Neurosci Abstr 1998:495.9.

67. Dooley CT, Ny P, Bidlack JM, Houghten RA. Selective ligands for the μ, δ and κ opioid receptors identified from a single mixture based tetrapeptide positional scanning combinatorial library. J Biol Chem 1998; 273:18848–18856.

68. Pascaud X, Honde C, Gallou LE, Chanoine B, Roman F, Bueno F, Junien JL. Effects of fedotozine on gastrointestinal activity in dogs: mechanisms of action and related pharmacokinetics. J Pharm Pharmacol 1990; 42:546–552.

69. Seelig A, Gottschlich R, Devant R. A method to determine the ability of drugs to diffuse through the blood–brain barrier. Proc Natl Acad Sci USA 1994; 91:68–72.

70. Barber A, Bartoszyk GD, Bender HM, Gottschlich R, Greiner HE, Harting J, Mauler F, Minck K–O, Murray RD, Simon M, Seyfried CA. A pharmacological profile of the novel, peripherally-selective κ-opioid receptor agonist, EMD 61753. Br J Pharmacol 1994; 113:1317–1327.

32

Delta-Receptor, Nonpeptide Agonists

The Development of Safe, Strong Analgesics with a Novel Mechanism of Action

Hugh O. Pettit and Kwen-Jen Chang
Ardent Pharmaceuticals, Inc., Durham, North Carolina, U.S.A.

I. INTRODUCTION

Patients are prescribed mu (μ) opiate receptor agonists to manage moderate to severe symptoms of pain. Other than μ-agonists, such as fentanyl and morphine, no other types of drugs can be used to adequately treat patients with severe pain (1–3). However, physicians do know that μ-agonist treatment will also produce significant side effects that, in some cases, are life-threatening (1–3). The major drawback to the use of μ-analgesics is a substantial adverse side effect profile that includes respiratory depression (RD), nausea, emesis, constipation, and addiction (1,4,5). Physicians actually limit the amount of drug that is prescribed to compensate for these adverse effects (1,5). Consequently, patients do not receive adequate relief from severe symptoms of pain (1,2,6).

The ultimate goal of researchers in the analgesic field has been to develop an analgesic with a minimal side effect profile that can be used to treat severe pain. Despite decades of research this goal remains unmet. New analgesics have been discovered, but these drugs are roughly as efficacious as aspirin and cannot be used to manage severe pain. New treatments for severe pain are generally either analogues of known μ-agonists with a modified duration of action, or simply common μ-agonists with different formulations (e.g., transdermal patches). The amount of drug patients receive is still limited by side effects produced by these "new and improved" drugs. A strong analgesic with minimal side effects is strongly needed.

II. δ-RECEPTOR ANALGESICS

The development of delta (δ) opiate receptor analgesics has made significant progress following the discovery of BW373U86 [(±)-4-((α*R**)-α-((2*S**,5*R**)-4-allyl-2,5-dimethyl-1-piperazinyl)-3-hydroxybenzyl)-*N*,*N*-diethylbenzamide], the first nonpeptide δ-agonist (7). BW373U86 does produce analgesic effects (8); however, the effects are mild (e.g., aspirin-like) and probably cannot be used to treat severe pain. Similar effects have been observed with other nonpeptide δ-agonists, such as the methylated form of (+)BW373U86, SNC-80 (9,10).

One major drawback to δ-receptor agonists is that some nonpeptide δ-agonists produce a single, brief seizure episode (11). It is important to note that δ-agonist-induced seizures are not severe. The seizure-like activity is very brief, with a duration of less than 30 s, and no permanent or long-term effects have been observed. The mechanism of action of the seizure activity is logically the δ-receptor; however, research does indicate a neuromodulatory role between δ- and μ-opiate receptor mechanisms. In mice, seizure activity produced by BW373U86 can be dose-dependently blocked by administration of the δ-antagonist naltrindole (12), the benzodiazepine, midazolam (11,12), and by the μ-agonist, fentanyl (12). Apparently, central mechanisms mediate the effect, as central administration of some δ-peptides does produce seizure-like activity (13). Interestingly, however, some δ-peptide agonists do not produce seizures (13), suggesting that the development of a potent δ-agonist that does not produce seizures is possible.

A complex interaction between δ- and μ-opiate receptors does take place (12). Additive analgesic effects are produced by combining the μ-agonist (fentanyl) with the δ-agonist BW373U86. In contrast, BW373U86 seizure activity is dose-dependently blocked by fentanyl administration, and muscle rigidity induced by fentanyl is attenuated by BW373U86 (12). New research has examined the effects of a δ-agonist on other unwanted side effects of μ-agonists. Deaths resulting from μ-specific agonists are primarily caused by RD, the most serious and dangerous side effect of μ-agonists (1,5). Therefore, a series of experiments were conducted to determine if the administration of a δ-agonist could affect the RD caused by μ-agonist analgesics.

In these studies, male Sprague–Dawley rats (275–375 g) were first anesthetized with pentobarbital (Nembutal; 5 mg/kg i.p.). A stainless steel guide cannula was implanted into the right lateral ventricle and fixed with instant glue (Eastman 910 adhesive). Stereotaxic coordinates were AP (from bregma) = −0.8 mm and L (from the sagital sinus) = 1.2 mm. Following a 3-day-recovery period, subjects were anesthetized with 3% halothane to allow cannulation of the femoral artery and vein with PE50 tubing. After a 60-min anesthesia and surgery recovery period, in a plastic restraining device, alfentanil was infused through the venous line and blood samples were collected with use of the arterial line. For intracranial–ventricular (i.c.v.) administration, injections were accomplished by the insertion of a 30-g cannula (7.5 mm in length) into the guide cannula and (60 min later) by the infusion of drugs over a 30-s period in a volume of 10–20 μL. Arterial blood was withdrawn into a syringe prewetted with heparin and analyzed with a blood gas analyzer for determinations of P_{CO_2}, P_{O_2}, and pH (Instrumentation Laboratory, Model 1306 PH/Gas Analyzer). Antinociception was also assessed right after blood collection time points, by placing a radiant lamp heat source beneath the tail to record tail-flick response latencies. The intensity of the lamp was adjusted so that all rats had a mean latency response of 4 s before drug treatment. An automatic 10-s cutoff time allowed multiple tests without excessive tissue injury.

Figure 1 depicts the effects of the δ-agonist peptides, DPDPE ([D-pen^2-D-pen^5]-enkephalin, 14) and deltorphin II (15–17) on RD produced by a continuous intravenous (i.v.) infusion of the μ-analgesic, alfentanil. Following infusion into the lateral ventricles of rats, both peptides significantly attenuated alfentanil-induced RD in a dose-dependent manner (see Fig. 1, top panel). Alfentanil-induced analgesia, however, was not affected by either deltorphin II or DPDPE administration (see Fig. 1, bottom panel). The effects of the nonpeptide δ-agonist (+)BW373U86, on alfentanil-induced RD are presented in Fig. 2. Similar to the effects observed with DPDPE and deltorphin II, a substantial inhibition of the RD induced by alfentanil was produced by systemic (e.g., i.v.) (+)BW373U86 administration, with no observed effect on analgesia (see Fig. 2). More detailed findings are reported elsewhere (18). Similar results have also been obtained with another nonpeptide δ-agonist, SNC 80, and all effects can be attenuated

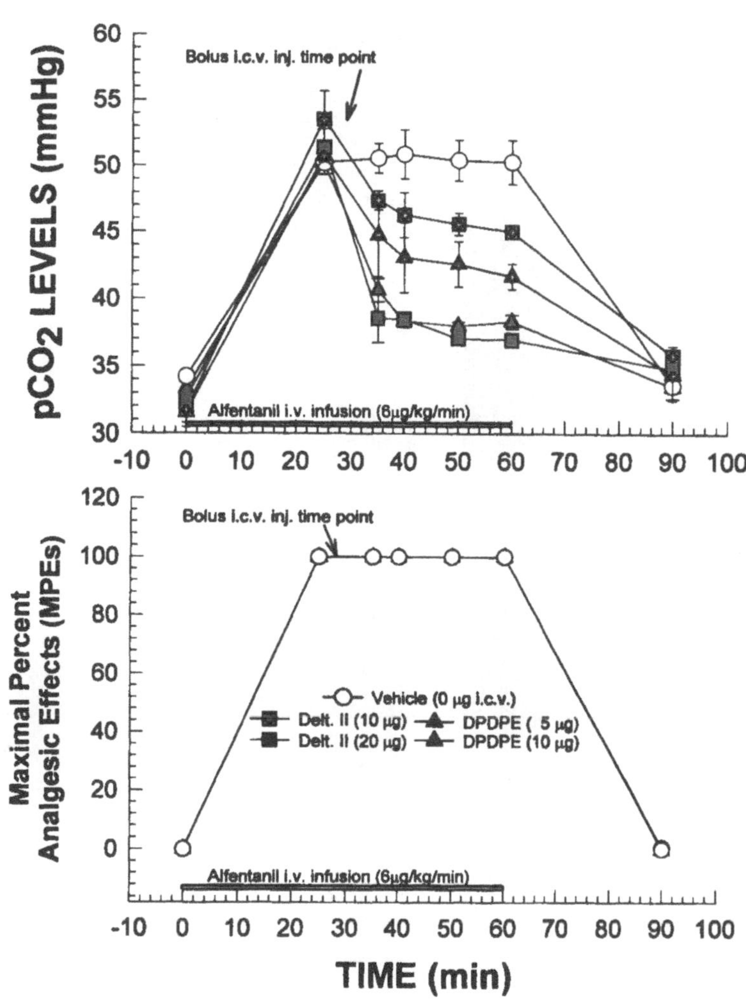

Figure 1 The effects of deltorphin II (Delt. II) and DPDPE on respiratory depression and antinociception induced by a constant infusion of alfentanil: The period of alfentanil infusion is indicated by the solid bar. Deltorphin II or DPDPE were infused into the lateral ventricle of rats approximately 30 min into the alfentanil infusion. Immediately following the infusion of each peptide, significant decreases were observed in Pco_2 levels (top panel). Results demonstrate that the respiratory depressive effects of alfentanil can be attenuated by δ-selective peptides. Antinociceptive effects of alfentanil (bottom panel) were not affected by either deltorphin II or DPDPE. Note that when the alfentanil infusion was discontinued, at the 60-min time point, Pco_2 and analgesic effects returned to control values. All values are presented as the mean ± SEM.

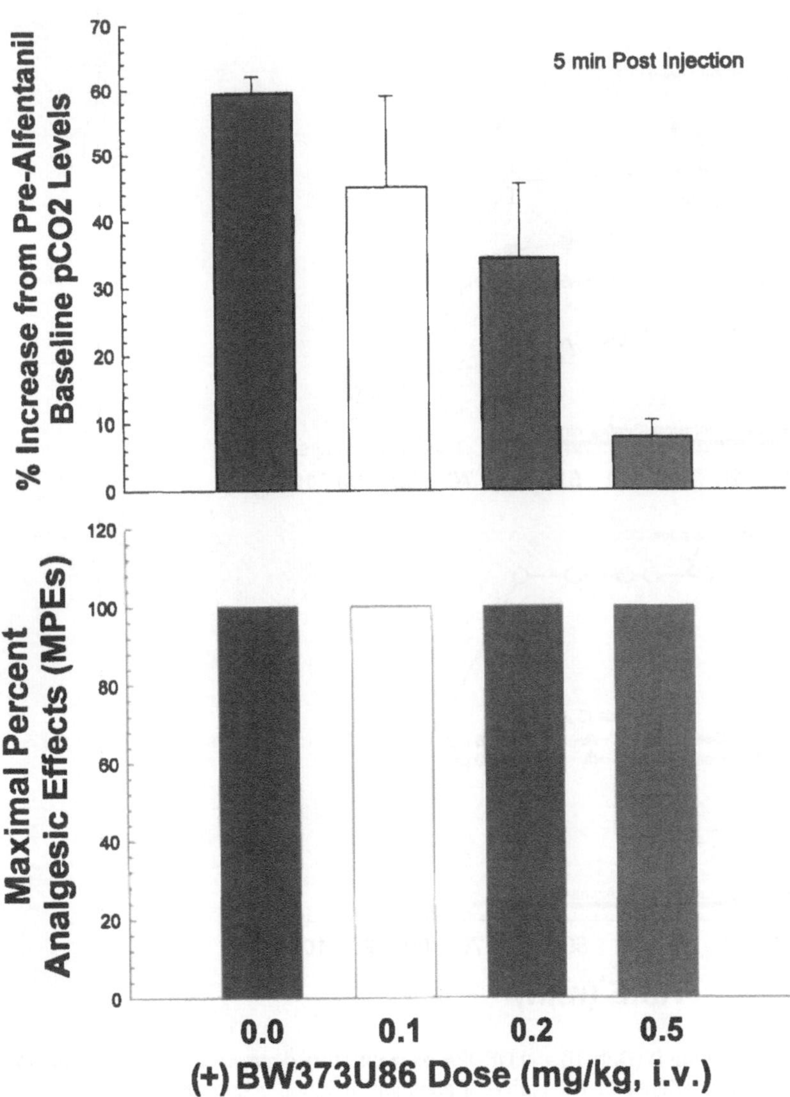

Figure 2 The effect of (+)BW373U86 on respiratory depression and antinociception induced by a continuous infusion of alfentanil: Similar to results presented in Fig. 1, the intravenous administration of the nonpeptide δ-agonist, (+)BW373U86, significantly reduced, in a dose-dependent manner, the respiratory depression produced by alfentanil. Antinociceptive effects of alfentanil were not affected by (+)BW373U86 administration. Significant attenuating effects of (+)BW373U86 were observed throughout the entire alfentanil-infusion period; however, data are presented from only the 5-min period after (+)BW373U86 administration to highlight the dose-dependent results. All values are presented as the mean ± SEM.

with use of a δ-antagonist (results not shown). Overall, these results indicate that δ-agonists can selectively inhibit the RD produced by a strong μ-analgesic compound.

III. DEVELOPMENT OF SYNERGISTIC δ- AND μ-RECEPTOR ANALGESICS

The foregoing findings that (1) μ-compounds can attenuate δ-receptor–induced seizure activity, (2) δ-compounds can attenuate μ-receptor–induced muscle rigidity, and (3) δ-compounds can attenuate μ-receptor–induced RD, all suggest that a compound with appropriately mixed δ–μ activity could serve a strong analgesic with a significantly reduced side effect profile. The benzhydrylpiperazine DPI3290 [3-((α-*R*)-α-((2*S*,5*R*)-4-allyl-2,5-dimethyl-1-piperazinyl)-3-hydroxybenzyl)-*N*-(3-fluorophenyl)-*N*-methylbenzamide] has recently been developed as a strong analgesic with minimal RD effects (19).

DPI3290 is a potent opioid agonist with mixed δ-, μ-, and κ-receptor activity. The activity of DPI3290 is greatest at δ, with moderate μ and more minimal activity at κ-opioid receptor subtypes. The mixed activity serves to produce strong analgesic effects through μ-receptor activation with an antagonism of μ-related side effects by, primarily, δ-receptor actions. Effects at κ-receptors are thought, theoretically, to counteract the euphoric effect produced by μ-receptor activation.

Strong analgesic effects are produced by DPI3290 in mice, rats, dogs, and monkeys after systemic administration. Its analgesic potency is about ten times greater than morphine and about one-tenth the potency of fentanyl. A therapeutic index (e.g., the ratio of the ED_{50} dose that produces RD effects over the ED_{50} dose for analgesia) produces a measure of the separation between the beneficial effects of analgesia and the adverse side effect of RD. Morphine and fentanyl have a therapeutic index of about 2–4, indicating a poor separation between analgesia and RD. The therapeutic index of DPI3290 is greater than 25. The results reveal that DPI3290 can produce strong analgesic effects with a significantly reduced ability to produce RD.

In a variety of nonhuman species, DPI3290 has a significantly better safety profile than the strong analgesics used in the clinic today. DPI3290 is currently undergoing stringent safety and efficacy testing in phase I human clinical trials as a strong analgesic to be used in postoperative surgical applications. The effort to develop a potent analgesic with significantly reduced levels of side effects has been exhaustive. Recent discoveries now reveal that the clinical management of severe pain may finally be possible with the use of δ-pharmaceuticals.

REFERENCES

1. Inturrisi CE. Opiate analgesic therapy in cancer pain. In: Forley KM, ed. Advances in Pain Research and Therapy. New York: Raven Press, 1990:133–154.
2. Clotz MA, Nahata MC. Clinical uses of fentanyl, sufentanil, and alfentanil. Clin Pharm 1991; 10: 581–593.
3. Holder KA, Dougherty TB, Chiang JS. Postoperative pain management. Cancer Bull 1995; 47:43–51.
4. Chang K–J. Opioid receptors: multiplicity and sequelae of ligand–receptor interactions. In: Conn M, ed. The Receptors. New York: Academic Press, 1984:1–81.
5. Reisine T, Pasternak G. In: Molinoff PB, Ruddon RW, eds. The Pharmacological Basis of Therapeutics. 9th ed. New York: Macmillan, 1993:521–555.
6. McGilliard KL, Takemori AE. Antagonism by naloxone of narcotic-induced respiratory depression and analgesia. J Pharmacol Exp Ther 1978; 207:494–503.

7. Chang K–J, Rigdon GC, Howard JL, McNutt RW. A novel, potent and selective nonpeptidic delta opioid receptor agonist BW373U86. J Pharmacol Exp Ther 1993; 267:852–857.
8. Wild KD, McCormick J, Bilsky EJ, Vanderah T, McNutt RW, Chang K–J, Porreca F. Antinociceptive action of BW373U86 in the mouse. J Pharmacol Exp Ther 1993; 267:858–865.
9. Calderon SN, Rothman RB, Porreca F, Flippen–Anderson JL, McNutt RW, Xu H, Smith LE, Bilsky EJ, Davis P, Rice KC. Probes for narcotic receptor mediated phenomena. 191. Synthesis of (+)-4-[(αR)-α((2S,5R)-4-allyl-2,5-dimethyl-1-piperazinyl)-3-methoxybenzyl]-*N*,*N*-diethylbenzamide (SNC 80): a highly selective, nonpeptide delta opioid receptor agonist. J Med Chem 1994; 37:2125–2128.
10. Bilsky EJ, Calderon SN, Wang T, Bernstein RN, Davis P, Hruby VJ, McNutt RW, Rothman RB, Rice KC, Porreca F. SNC 80, A selective, nonpeptidic and systemically active opioid delta agonist. J Pharmacol Exp Ther 1995; 273:359–366.
11. Comer SD, Hoenicke EM, Sable, AI, McNutt RW, Chang K–J, De Costa BR, Mosberg HI, Woods, JH. Convulsive effects of systemic administration of the delta opioid agonist BW373U86 in mice. J Pharmacol Exp Ther 1993; 267:888–895.
12. O'Neill, SJ, Collins MA, Pettit HO, McNutt RW, Chang K–J. Antagonistic modulation between the delta opioid agonist BW373U86 and the mu opioid agonist fentanyl in mice. J Pharmacol Exp Ther 1997; 282:271–277.
13. Tortella FC, Robles L, Mosberg HI, Holaday JW. Electroencephalographic assessment of the role of delta receptors in opioid peptide-induced seizures. Neuropeptides 1984; 5:213–216.
14. Mosberg HI, Hurst R, Hruby VJ, Gee K, Yamamura HI, Galligan JJ, Burks TF. Bis-penicillamine enkephalins possess highly improved specificity toward delta opioid receptors. Proc Natl Acad Sci USA 1983; 80:5871–5874.
15. Kreil G, Barra D, Simmaco M, Erspamer V, Falconierei–Erspamer G, Negri L, Severini C, Corsi R, Melchiorri P. Deltorphin, a novel amphibian skin peptide with high selectivity and affinity for δ opioid receptors. Eur J Pharmacol 1989; 162:123–128.
16. Erspamer V, Melchiorri P, Falconieri–Erspamer G, Negri L, Corsi R, Severini C, Barra D, Simmaco M, Kriel G. Deltorphins: a family of naturally occurring peptides with high affinity and selectivity for δ opioid binding sites. Proc Natl Acad Sci USA 1989; 86:5188–5192.
17. Jiang Q, Mosberg HI, Porreca F. Antinociceptive effects of [D-Ala^2]deltorphin II, a highly selective δ agonist in vivo. Life Sci 1990; 47:PL-43–PL-47.
18. Su Y–F, McNutt RW, Chang K–J. delta-Opioid ligands reverse alfentanil-induced respiratory depression but not antinociception. J Pharmacol Exp Ther 1998; 287:815–823.
19. Pettit HO, Su Y–F, O'Neill SJ, Bishop MJ, McNutt RW, Chang K–J. DPI3290: a δ/μ agonist with strong analgesia and minimal respiratory depression. (submitted)

33

Peripheral Opioid Analgesia

Neuroimmune Interactions and Therapeutic Implications

Halina Machelska and Christoph Stein
Free University Berlin, Berlin, Germany

I. INTRODUCTION

Recent research has shown that effective inhibition of pain by endogenous mechanisms is not exclusively generated within the central nervous system (CNS). Such intrinsic pain control can also occur in the periphery, mediated by an interaction between immune cells and peripheral sensory nerve endings. This neuroimmune link has emerged during studies concerning the peripheral antinociceptive actions of locally applied exogenous opioid receptor agonists. A prerequisite for the manifestation of such peripheral effects seems to be inflammation, accompanied by hyperalgesia of the tissue from which the nociceptive impulses arise. Opioid receptors are present on peripheral sensory nerves and are up-regulated during the development of inflammation. Their endogenous ligands, opioid peptides, are synthesized in circulating immune cells, which under pathological conditions, migrate preferentially to injured sites. Under environmental stressful stimuli or in response to releasing agents (e.g., corticotropin-releasing factor, cytokines) these immunocytes can secrete opioids to activate peripheral opioid receptors and to produce analgesia by inhibiting either the excitability of these nerves or the release of excitatory, proinflammatory neuropeptides. Suppression of the immune system abolishes these effects. This chapter will present the discoveries that led to this concept and therapeutic implications resulting therefrom.

II. PERIPHERAL OPIOID RECEPTORS

Anatomical (1–5) and molecular (6) studies have shown that all three opioid receptors, mu (μ), delta (δ), and kappa (κ), are expressed within sensory neurons. They have been found on cell bodies in the dorsal root ganglia (3,6) and on central (7) and peripheral terminals of primary afferent neurons in animals (1,2,5) and in humans (4). Pharmacological experiments indicate that the characteristics of these receptors are very similar to those in the brain (2). In vivo experiments have shown that the peripheral antinociceptive effects of μ-, δ-, and κ-selective agonists were abolished by pretreament with capsaicin, a selective neurotoxin of primary afferent neurons (8).

A. Peripheral Opioid Receptors in Inflammation

Opioid receptors are synthesized in the dorsal root ganglia (3,6). Axonal transport is responsible for delivering macromolecules from the cell body to nerve terminals. After the induction of peripheral inflammation, the axonal transport of opioid receptors in fibers of the sciatic nerve is greatly enhanced (2). Subsequently, the density of opioid receptors on cutaneous nerve fibers in the inflamed tissue increases and this increase is abolished by ligating the sciatic nerve (2). These findings indicate that inflammation enhances the peripherally directed axonal transport of opioid receptors, which leads to an increase in their number (up-regulation) on peripheral nerve terminals.

In addition, preexistent, but possibly inactive, neuronal opioid receptors may undergo changes owing to the specific milieu (e.g., low pH) of inflamed tissue, and thus be rendered active. Indeed, low pH increases opioid agonist efficacy in vitro by altering the interaction of opioid receptors with G proteins in neuronal membranes. Furthermore, inflammation entails a disruption of the perineurium (a normally rather impermeable barrier sheath encasing peripheral nerve fibers) and increases the number of peripheral sensory nerve terminals in inflamed tissue, a phenomenon known as "sprouting" (9).

Activation of these receptors results in potent peripherally mediated analgesia which is greatly enhanced in inflammation either of subcutaneous tissue, viscera, or joints (10). Central effects can be excluded by using compounds that do not cross the blood–brain barrier (11) or by the local application of small, systemically inactive doses of agents (10). Rigorous criteria, such as reversibility by standard opioid antagonists (e.g., naloxone), dose-dependency, and stereospecificity, have been applied to demonstrate the opioid receptor-specificity of these peripheral effects. The comparison of agonists with differing affinities for the three types of opioid receptors (μ, δ and κ) has shown that ligands with a preference for μ-receptors are generally most potent, but δ- and κ-ligands are active as well. Considering the different characteristics of the various inflammatory models, it is conceivable that, depending on the nature and stage of the inflammatory reaction, different types of local opioid receptors become active. Thus, depending on the particular circumstances, all three receptor types can be present and functionally active in peripheral tissues (10).

Apart from primary afferent neurons, it has been suggested that opioid receptors are also located on sympathetic postganglionic neuron (SPN) terminals and that they may contribute to peripheral opioid antinociception in bradykinin hyperalgesia (12). However, there are reports arguing against the involvement of sympathetic neurons in this model, and studies attempting the direct demonstration of opioid receptor mRNA in sympathetic ganglia have produced negative results (8). Moreover, recent studies using chemical sympathectomy with 6-hydroxydopamine have shown that peripheral antinociception mediated by μ-, δ-, and κ-opioid receptors is independent of SPN in Freund's adjuvant inflammation (8).

Finally, opioid-binding sites and the expression of opioid receptor transcripts have been conclusively demonstrated in immune cells (2,13). Opioid-mediated modulation of the proliferation of these cells and several of their functions (e.g., chemotaxis, superoxide and cytokine production, mast cell degranulation) has been reported (14,15). These immunomodulatory actions can be stimulatory as well as inhibitory (15,16) and have been ascribed to the activation of opioid receptors (13). However, the significance of those effects relative to nociception has not yet been investigated.

III. PERIPHERAL ENDOGENOUS OPIOID PEPTIDES

Opioid peptides are the natural ligands at opioid receptors. Three families of these peptides are well characterized in the central nervous and neuroendocrine systems. Each family derives from a distinct gene and precursor protein, namely proopiomelanocortin (POMC), proenkephalin (PENK), and prodynorphin (PDYN). Appropriate processing yields their respective major representative opioid peptides β-endorphin (β-END), enkephalin (ENK), and dynorphin (DYN). Each peptide exhibits different affinities and selectivities for the three opioid receptor types: μ (β-END, ENK), δ (ENK, β-END), and κ (DYN) (17). Recently, two additional endogenous opioid peptides have been isolated from bovine brain: endomorphin-1 and endomorphin-2 (18), although their precursors are not yet known. Both peptides are considered μ-receptor ligands having the highest specificity and affinity for these receptors of any endogenous substance so far described (18).

A. Immune Cells

During evolution, POMC-derived peptides are well conserved (19). Their presence and production were first reported in human lymphocytes by Blalock and Smith (20). Since then, POMC-related opioid peptides have been found in immune cells of many vertebrates and nonvertebrates (15,19,20). To determine whether these immune-competent cells actually synthesize POMC, rather than simply absorbing related peptides from plasma, mRNA-encoding POMC was sought for and demonstrated in many of these studies (15,19). In spite of the initial notion that only truncated forms of POMC mRNA are present in immune cells (15,21), recently, full-length POMC mRNA identical in sequence with that isolated from the pituitary gland has been demonstrated in rat mononuclear leukocytes. This POMC transcript is spliced in the same way as the pituitary transcript and, consequently, contains the sequence for the signal peptide. The 31-kDa–POMC protein was also proteolytically processed in a way consistent with the pituitary gland (22).

PENK-derived opioid peptides have also been detected in human and rodent immune cells (23). On in vitro stimulation or under pathological conditions, these cells express enhanced levels of PENK mRNA, probably as a result of the induction of transcription factors (e.g., NF-κB) and the subsequent activation of the preproenkephalin promoter. In subpopulations of these cells, this mRNA is highly homologous to brain PENK mRNA, abundant, and apparently translated, because immunoreactive ENK is present or is released (23). The appropriate enzymes necessary for posttranslational processing of both POMC and PENK have also been identified in immune cells (24).

Thus, a growing body of evidence indicates that both POMC- and PENK-derived opioid peptides are produced by immune cells. These immune-derived opioid peptides apparently play a substantial role in modulation of inflammatory pain (25). Persistent inflammation is a pathophysiological in vivo stimulus for the immune system and represents a condition that is closer to the clinical setting than some of the early in vitro studies. In a rat model of unilateral localized paw inflammation, mRNAs encoding POMC and PENK and their respective opioid peptide products, β-END and ENK are found predominantly within inflamed tissue (26). Histomorphological (1) and double-staining procedures (26,27) have identified the opioid-containing cells as T and B lymphocytes as well as monocytes and macrophages. Small amounts of DYN are also detectable by immunocytochemistry (28). Recent studies investigating the production, release, and antinociceptive effects of lymphocyte-derived β-END in relation to cell trafficking have suggested that β-END-producing lymphocytes home to inflamed tissue where they secrete the opioid to inhibit pain. Afterward, they travel to the regional lymph nodes, depeleted of the peptide (27). This migratory pattern is reminiscent of memory-type T cells. The trafficking of those cells is not random, but-they are specifically directed to sites of antigenic or microbial invasion (e.g., inflammatory lesions of the skin) (29). Consistent with this notion, β-END was indeed found mostly in memory-type T cells (27). These findings suggest that local signals not only stimulate the synthesis of opioid peptides in different types of resident inflammatory cells, but also attract opioid-containing cells from the circulation to the site of tissue injury to reduce pain.

The mechanisms underlying the migration of opioid-containing immunocytes to inflamed tissue are beginning to be unraveled. Extensive studies of the last 10 years revealed that extravasation of immune cells is a multistep process involving the sequential activation of various adhesion molecules located on immune cells and vascular endothelium. Initially, the circulating leukocytes are captured and roll on the endothelial cells of vessels, a process mediated by selectins present on leukocytes (L-selectin) and endothelial cells (P- and E-selectins). The rolling leukocytes can then be activated by chemoattractants, which leads to up-regulation and increased avidity of integrins. These mediate the firm adhesion of leukocytes to endothelial cells via immunoglobulin ligands. Finally, the leukocytes transmigrate through the endothelial wall and are directed to the sites of inflammation. Interruption of the leukocyte–endothelial cell cascade (e.g., by monoclonal antibodies against adhesion molecules or by blocking agents such as polysaccharides) can block immune cell extravasation (29). Recently, it has been shown that such treatment can also influence endogenous pain control in inflammation. Pretreatment of rats with a selectin blocker (fucoidin) (30) results in a blockade of the infiltration of END-containing immunocytes, a consequent decrease of the END content in the inflamed tissue and, thus, abolishes endogenous opioid analgesia (31). These findings indicate that the immune system uses mechanisms of cell migration not only to fight pathogens, but also to control pain within injured tissue. Thus, pain may be exacerbated by measures inhibiting the immigration of opioid-producing cells or, conversely, analgesia may be conveyed by adhesive interactions that recruit those cells to injured tissue.

B. Other Sources

The classic loci for opioids in the periphery are the adrenals and the pituitary glands, but these have been excluded as sources for opioid ligands at peripheral receptors (32). PENK mRNA and its peptides as well as DYN have been found in sensory ganglia (33,34); DYN is also found in peripheral terminals of sensory nerves (28). Also β-END and endomorphin-2 have been detected in cultured human and rat spinal ganglion neurons (35,36). However, direct functional evidence on the role of nociceptor-derived opioid peptides in peripheral nociceptive transmission is still lacking.

IV. INTERACTION OF IMMUNE-DERIVED OPIOIDS AND PERIPHERAL OPIOID RECEPTORS

Endogenous opioid peptides are released by different kinds of stress. Following cold water swim, nociceptive thresholds increase selectively in inflamed tissue, and this effect is blocked by peripherally acting opioid antagonists (1,32,37). Moreover, this effect is abolished by antibodies against opioid peptides and by immunosuppression (1,26,37). Together, these findings suggest that peripheral opioid receptors can mediate local antinociception following their activation by opioids released from immune cells during stress. Recent studies have supported this notion by the direct demonstration of opioid peptide release within subcutaneous tissue following a noxious thermal stimulus (38).

The exact mechanisms and stimuli triggering the opioid secretion within inflamed tissue are being investigated. Corticotropin-releasing factor (CRF) is a major physiological secretagogue for opioid peptides in the pituitary. Its releasing effects are potentiated by interleukin-1β (IL-1), and IL-1 (and other cytokines) can stimulate β-END release directly. Receptors for each of these agents are present on immune cells and up-regulated within inflamed tissue (39). In vivo, the local application of small, systemically inactive doses of CRF, IL-1, and other cytokines produces potent antinociceptive effects in inflamed, but not in noninflamed tissue (39,40). These effects are reversible by immunosuppression, by passive immunization with antibodies against opioid peptides, and by opioid antagonists. Furthermore, short-term incubation with CRF or IL-1 can release β-END in immune cell suspensions prepared from lymph nodes in vitro (27,41). This release is specific to CRF and IL-1 receptors, it is calcium-dependent and mimicked by elevated extracellular concentrations of potassium. This is consistent with a regulated pathway of release from secretory vesicles, as in neurons and endocrine cells (27). In summary, these findings indicate that CRF and cytokines can cause secretion of opioids from immune cells, which subsequently activate opioid receptors on sensory nerves to inhibit nociception. The most important endogenous secretagogue appears to be locally produced CRF, because endogenous analgesia in inflamed tissue is abolished when the synthesis of CRF in inflamed tissue is inhibited by antisense oligodeoxynucleotides or when antagonists and antibodies against CRF are administered locally (41).

Opioids produce antinociception by several mechanisms. They increase potassium and decrease calcium currents in the soma of dorsal root ganglion sensory neurons through interactions with G proteins (G_i, or G_o; or both). Recently, the inhibition of a tetrodotoxin-resistant sodium current by a μ-opioid agonist was also described. Provided that these events are similar throughout the neuron, they may underly the following observations. Opioids attenuate the excitability of the peripheral nociceptive terminal and the propagation of action potentials. Similar to their effects at the soma and at central terminals, opioids inhibit the (calcium-dependent) release of excitatory proinflammatory compounds (e.g., substance P) from peripheral sensory nerve endings. In addition, morphine inhibits the antidromic vasodilation evoked by stimulation of C fibers. These mechanisms may also account for opioid anti-inflammatory and antiarthritic actions (9).

V. CLINICAL IMPLICATIONS

Opioid receptors are present on peripheral terminals of nerve fibers in human synovia (4). That intra-articular naloxone antagonizes the analgesia of locally applied morphine indicates that these receptors are capable of mediating analgesia in humans (42). In search for the endogenous ligands, inflamed synovial tissue from patients undergoing arthroscopic knee surgery was examined. Opioid peptides (mainly β-END and ENK) were found in synovial lining cells and in immune cells, such as lymphocytes, macrophages, and mast cells (4). The interaction of synovial opioids with peripheral opioid receptors was examined in patients undergoing knee surgery. Blocking of intra-articular opioid receptors by the local administration of the antagonist naloxone resulted in significantly increased postoperative pain. This pain-enhancing effect was demonstrated by subjective measures as well as by increased supplemental analgesic requirements (43). Taken together, these findings suggest that in a stressful (e.g., postoperative) situation, opioids are tonically released from inflamed tissue and activate peripheral opioid receptors to attenuate clinical pain.

Importantly, these endogenous opioids do not interfere with exogenous morphine (i.e., intra-articular morphine is an equally potent analgesic in patients with and without opioid-producing inflammatory synovial cells) (4). This suggests that, in contrast to the rapid development of tolerance in the CNS, the immune cell-derived opioids do not produce cross-tolerance to morphine at peripheral opioid receptors. This finding is at variance with some animal experiments that have used exogenous agonists to produce tolerance at peripheral opioid receptors (4). Importantly, however, in these studies normal animals without inflammation were pretreated with repeated opioid injections to induce tolerance. Because the number, affinity, and coupling efficacy of opioid receptors appear to be markedly enhanced under inflammatory conditions (2,9), these studies do not permit conclusions about tolerance in the clinical situation. Indeed, earlier studies have suggested that tolerance to peripheral opioid antinociception does not occur when the opioid pretreatment is performed in presence of brief, transient inflammatory stimuli (44). These considerations raise questions whether tolerance development is different at central versus peripheral opioid receptors and in inflamed versus noninflamed tissue. Clarification of these issues is important for the treatment of chronic pain in arthritis and other inflammatory conditions with peripherally acting opioids.

VI. CONCLUSIONS

The nervous and immune systems communicate with each other through the cytokines expressed in the nervous system and neuropeptides expressed in immune cells. Interactions of immune-derived opioid peptides and opioid receptors located in peripheral inflamed tissue lead to engogenous analgesia (20,21,25,45). Thus, it appears that, in addition to their immunological functions, immunocytes are involved in intrinsic pain inhibition. This provides new insights into pain associated with a compromised immune system, as in the aquired immunodeficiency syndrome or in cancer. Furthermore, the activation of opioid production and release from immune cells may be a novel approach to the development of peripherally acting analgesics. As such drugs would be targeted toward events in peripheral injured tissue, these analgesics should lack unwanted central side effects typically associated with opioids.

Melzack and Wall originally proposed that activation of the first central transmission cells in the dorsal horn marks the beginning of the sequence of intrinsic antinociceptive activities that occur when the body sustains damage (46). Evidently this is only one possible mechanism. Intrinsic pain inhibition can be achieved even earlier through the attenuation of afferent sensory nerve activity at the peripheral endings by immune-derived opioid peptides. Thus, the selection and filtering of incoming information is not restricted to the brain and spinal cord, but already occurs in the periphery through an interaction of the immune and sensory nervous systems.

REFERENCES

1. Stein C, Hassan AHS, Przewlocki R, Gramsch C, Peter K, Herz A. Opioids from immunocytes interact with receptors on sensory nerves to inhibit nociception in inflammation. Proc Natl Acad Sci USA 1990; 87:5935–5939.
2. Hassan AHS, Ableitner A, Stein C, Herz A. Inflammation of the rat paw enhances axonal transport of opioid receptors in the sciatic nerve and increases their density in the inflamed tissue. Neuroscience 1993; 55:185–195.
3. Ji R–R, Zhang Q, Law P–Y, Low HH, Elde R, Hökfelt T. Expression of μ-, δ-, and κ-opioid receptor-like immunoreactivities in rat dorsal root ganglia after carrageenan-induced inflammation. J Neurosci 1995; 15:8156–8166.

4. Stein C, Pflüger M, Yassouridis A, Hoelzl J, Lehrberger K, Welte C, Hassan AH. No tolerance to peripheral morphine analgesia in presence of opioid expression in inflamed synovia. J Clin Invest 1996; 98:793–799.
5. Coggeshall RE, Zhou S, Carlton SM. Opioid receptors on peripheral sensory axons. Brain Res 1997; 764:126–132.
6. Mansour A, Fox CA, Akil H, Watson SJ. Opioid-receptor mRNA expression in the rat CNS: anatomical and functional implications. Trends Neurosci 1995; 18:22–29.
7. LaMotte C, Pert CB, Snyder SH. Opiate receptor binding in primate spinal cord: distribution and changes after dorsal root section. Brain Res 1976; 112:407–412.
8. Zhou L, Zhang Q, Stein C, Schäfer M. Contribution of opioid receptors on primary afferent versus sympathetic neurons to peripheral opioid analgesia. J Pharmacol Exp Ther 1998; 261:1–7.
9. Stein C, Schäfer M, Cabot PJ, Carter L, Zhang Q, Zhou L, Gasior M. Peripheral opioid analgesia. Pain Rev 1997; 4:171–185.
10. Stein C. Peripheral mechanisms of opioid analgesia. Anesth Analg 1993; 76:182–191.
11. Barber A, Gottschlich R. Central and peripheral nervous system. Novel developments with selective, non-peptidic kappa-opioid receptor agonists. Exp Opin Invest Drugs 1997; 6:1351–1368.
12. Taiwo YO, Levine JD. Kappa- and delta-opioids block sympathetically dependent hyperalgesia. J Neurosci 1991; 11:928–932.
13. Sharp BM, Roy S, Bidlack JM. Evidence for opioid receptors on cells involved in host defense and the immune system. J Neuroimmunol 1998; 83:45–56.
14. Bryant HU, Holaday JW. Opioids in immunologic processes. In: Herz A, ed. Opioids II. Berlin: Springer-Verlag, 1993:551–570.
15. Panerai AE, Sacerdote P. β-Endorphin in the immune system: a role at last? Immunol Today 1997; 18:317–319.
16. Heijnen CJ, Kavelaars A, Ballieux RE. Beta-endorphin: cytokine and neuropeptide. Immunol Rev 1991; 119:41–63.
17. Höllt V. Opioid peptide processing and receptor selectivity. Annu Rev Pharmacol Toxicol 1986; 26: 59–77.
18. Zadina JE, Hackler L, Ge L–J, Kastin AJ. A potent and selective endogenous agonist for the μ-opiate receptor. Nature 1997; 386:499–502.
19. Ottaviani E, Franchini A, Franceschi C. Pro-opiomelanocortin-derived peptides, cytokines, and nitric oxide in immune responses and stress: an evolutionary approach. Int Rev Cytol 1997; 170:79–141.
20. Blalock JE. The syntax of immune–neuroendocrine communication. Immunol Today 1994; 15:504–511.
21. Sharp B, Yaksh T. Pain killers of the immune system. T lymphocyte produce opioid immunopeptides that control pain at sites of inflammation. Nat Med 1997; 3:831–832.
22. Lyons PD, Blalock JE. Pro-opioimelanocortin gene expression and protein processing in rat mononuclear leukocytes. J Neuroimmunol 1997; 78:47–56.
23. Weisinger G. The transcriptional regulation of the preproenkephalin gene. Biochem J 1995; 307: 617–629.
24. Vindrola O, Mayer AMS, Citera G, Spitzer JA, Espinoza LR. Prohormone convertases PC2 and PC3 in rat neutrophils and macrophages. Neuropeptides 1994; 27:235–244.
25. Stein C. Mechanisms of disease: the control of pain in peripheral tissue by opioids. N Engl J Med 1995; 332:1685–1690.
26. Przewlocki R, Hassan AHS, Lason W, Epplen C, Herz A, Stein C. Gene expression and localization of opioid peptides in immune cells of inflamed tissue. Functional role in antinociception. Neuroscience 1992; 48:491–500.
27. Cabot PJ, Carter L, Gaiddon C, Zhang Q, Schäfer M, Loeffler JP, Stein C. Immune cell-derived β-endorphin: production, release and control of inflammatory pain in rats. J Clin Invest 1997; 100: 142–148.
28. Hassan AHS, Przewlocki R, Herz A, Stein C. Dynorphin, a preferential ligand for kappa-opioid receptors, is present in nerve fibers and immune cells within inflamed tissue of the rat. Neurosci Lett 1992; 140:85–88.

29. Butcher EC, Picker LJ. Lymphocyte homing homeostasis. Science 1996; 272:60–66.
30. Ley K, Linnemann G, Meinen M, Stoolman LM, Gaehtgens P. Fucoidin, but not polyphosphomannan PPME, inhibits leukocyte rolling in venules of the rat mesentery. Blood 1993; 81:177–185.
31. Machelska H, Cabot PJ, Mousa SA, Zhang Q, Stein C. Pain control in inflammation governed by selectins. Nat Med 1998; 4:1425–1428.
32. Parsons CG, Czlonkowski A, Stein C, Herz A. Peripheral opioid receptors mediating antinociception in inflammation. Activation by endogenous opioids and role of the pituitary–adrenal axis. Pain 1990; 41:81–93.
33. Pohl M, Ballet S, Collin E, Mauborgne A, Bourgoin S, Benoliel JJ, Hamon M, Cesselin F. Enkephalinergic and dynorphinergic neurons in the spinal cord and dorsal root ganglia of the polyarthritic rat—in vivo release and cDNA hybridization studies. Brain Res 1997; 749:18–28.
34. Przewlocki R, Gramsch C, Pasi A, Herz A. Characterization and localization of immunoreactive dynorphin, alpha-neoendorphin, met-enkephalin and substance P in human spinal cord. Brain Res 1983; 280:95–103.
35. Kim JH, Kim SU, Kito S. Immunocytochemical demonstration of beta-endorphin and beta-lipotropin in cultured human spinal ganglion neurons. Brain Res 1984; 304:192–196.
36. Martin–Schild S, Zadina JE, Geral AA, Vigh S, Kastin AJ. Localization of endomorphin-2-like immunoreactivity in the rat medulla and spinal cord. Peptides 1997; 18:1641–1649.
37. Stein C, Gramsch C, Herz A. Intrinsic mechanisms of antinociception in inflammation. Local opioid receptors and β-endorphin. J Neurosci 1990; 10:1292–1298.
38. Yonehara N, Takiuchi S, Imai Y, Inoki R. Opioid peptide release evoked by noxious stimulation of the hind instep of rats. Regul Pept 1993; 48:365–372.
39. Schafer M, Mousa SA, Stein C. Corticotropin-releasing factor in antinociception and inflammation. Eur J Pharmacol 1997; 323:1–10.
40. Schäfer M, Carter L, Stein C. Interleukin-1β and corticotropin-releasing-factor inhibit pain by releasing opioids from immune cells in inflamed tissue. Proc Natl Acad Sci USA 1994; 91:4219–4223.
41. Schäfer M, Mousa SA, Zhang Q, Carter L, Stein C. Expression of corticotropin-releasing factor in inflamed tissue is required for intrinsic peripheral opioid analgesia. Proc Natl Acad Sci USA 1996; 93:6096–6100.
42. Stein C, Comisel K, Haimerl E, Yassouridis A, Lehrberger K, Herz A, Peter K. Analgesic effect of intraarticular morphine after arthroscopic knee surgery. N Engl J Med 1991; 325:1123–1126.
43. Stein C, Hassan AHS, Lehrberger K, Giefing J, Yassouridis A. Local analgesic effect of endogenous opioid peptides. Lancet 1993; 342:321–324.
44. Ferreira SH, Lorenzetti BB, Rae GA. Is methylnalorphinium the prototype of an ideal peripheral analgesic. Eur J Pharmacol 1984; 99:23–29.
45. Jessop DS. β-Endorphin in the immune system—mediator of pain and stress? Lancet 1998; 351: 1828–1829.
46. Melzack R, Wall PD. Pain mechanisms: a new theory. Science 1965; 150:971–973.

34

Profile of ADL 2-1294, an Opioid Antihyperalgesic Agent with Selectivity for Peripheral Mu-Opiate Receptors

Diane L. DeHaven-Hudkins
Adolor Corporation, Malvern, Pennsylvania, U.S.A.

I. INTRODUCTION

Research conducted over the past 10 years has demonstrated that opiates can produce antinociception by peripheral as well as central mechanisms. Antinociception resulting from stimulation of peripheral opiate receptors has been reported in situations where chemical, thermal, or mechanical insult has resulted in hyperalgesia. Preclinical studies in rodents and clinical studies in humans have shown that potent antinociception results from injection of opiates directly into inflamed tissue at doses that are systemically inactive (1,2). Local actions of opiates are mediated through the μ, δ, and κ receptors (3–5), are stereoselective (3,4), reversible with antagonist treatment (4,5), and exhibit greater potency and efficacy compared with local (6) or systemic (7) administration of nonsteroidal anti-inflammatory agents (NSAIDs).

In humans, local administration of μ-opioid agonists to inflamed tissues produces antinociception at doses well below those that result in systemic effects. This has been demonstrated with intra-articular (i.art.) administration of morphine to patients following arthroscopic surgery (8–12) or to patients suffering from osteoarthritis (13). Local injection of morphine at the site of an experimental second-degree burn injury (14), or direct application of a solution of 0.05% morphine to the abraded corneas of patients following intraocular surgery resulted in significant analgesia (15). Similarly, infiltration of 1 mg morphine into a dental surgery site (16) or 10 μg of fentanyl into the periodontal ligaments of patients with inflamed tooth pulp (17) provided peripherally mediated pain relief. The efficacy of topically applied morphine in alleviating back pain has also been reported (18). Importantly, in some of the clinical studies, a prolonged duration of action, naloxone reversibility, and a lack of systemic side effects have been observed, confirming that opiate receptors in the periphery of humans respond to local administration of opioid agonists. The efficacy observed following local administration of morphine in clinical situations where pain has resulted from diverse inflammatory insults suggests that the specific type of stimulus that produces pain is not as critical as the presence of inflammation to observe peripheral antinociception. This observation concurs with animal data that suggest that inflammation is necessary for the complete expression of opioid receptors in the periphery (19–23). Inflammation is thought to open the perineurial sheath, which allows a drug to gain access to preexistent opioid receptors present on the peripheral nerve terminal (23,24). Populations of

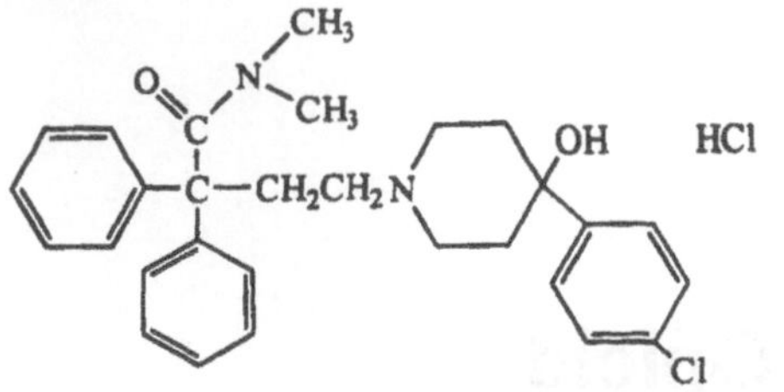

Figure 1 Structure of ADL 2-1294 (loperamide hydrochloride).

cutaneous sensory afferents responsive to local application of DAMGO and lacking the protective perineurial sheath have also been described (25). Collectively, the data support the notion that opiates play a prominent role in mediating antinociception locally at the level of the primary afferent nerve terminal, and that peripheral antinociception can be dissociated from the centrally mediated analgesia produced by certain opiate agonists.

The ideal characteristics of an opioid agonist with selectivity for receptors in the periphery are as follows:

Potency superior to morphine and full efficacy following local administration
Lack of penetration through the blood–brain barrier
Lack of efficacy in central measures of analgesia

Such a compound would be best described as an *antihyperalgesic* agent, because it reduces pain responses to baseline levels without producing analgesia by central mechanisms and without compromising normal function. ADL 2-1294 (loperamide hydrochloride; Fig. 1) is a compound that exhibits the profile of an antihyperalgesic therapeutic agent (26).

II. IN VITRO PROFILE OF ADL 2-1294

The mechanism of action of ADL 2-1294 is consistent with agonist activity at the μ-opioid receptor, as it inhibited binding to the receptor with nanomolar potency, was a full agonist as evidenced by stimulation of [^{35}S]GTPγS binding and inhibition of cAMP accumulation, and its effects were naloxone-reversible (27). Using membranes prepared from the cloned human opioid receptor expressed in Chinese hamster ovary (CHO) cells, the selectivity of ADL 2-1294 for the μ-subtype was 15-fold greater than that for the δ-subtype, and 350-fold greater than that for the κ-opioid receptor, as determined by competition with the binding of [^{3}H]diprenorphine (Table 1). The mean EC_{50} value of ADL 2-1294 to stimulate the binding of [^{35}S]GTPγS was

Table 1 The In Vitro Profile of ADL 2-1294 and Morphine at Cloned Human Opioid Receptors

	K_i(nM)			Receptor selectivity		μ Receptor EC_{50}(nM)	
Compound	μ	δ	κ	μ/δ	μ/κ	GTPγS	cAMP
ADL 2-1294	3.3 ± 1.6 (3)	48 ± 6 (4)	1156 ± 124 (3)	15	350	19 ± 1.1 (7)	27 ± 6 (3)
Morphine	19.3 ± 4.3 (4)	171 ± 55 (4)	273 ± 56 (3)	9	14	115 ± 1.4 (7)	ND

Data are the mean ± S.E.M., with the number of determinations shown in parentheses. ND, not determined.

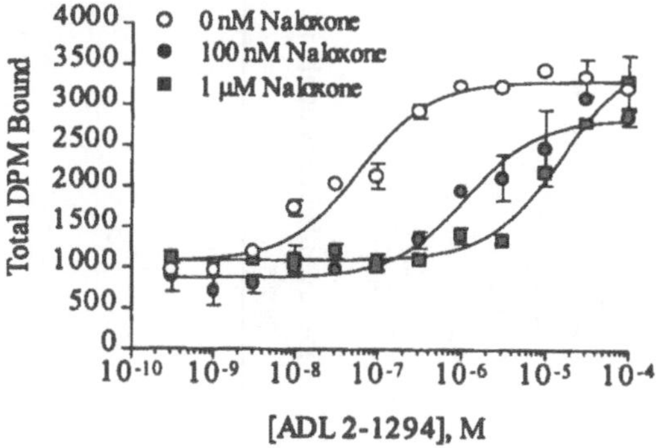

Figure 2 Stimulation of [^{35}S]GTPγS binding by ADL 2-1294 and its antagonism by naloxone: Data are the mean ± SEM of two independent experiments. Each experiment was performed as an individual 12-point dose–response curve in singlicate.

19 nM, compared with a mean EC_{50} value of 115 nM for morphine (see Table 1), and the maximum stimulation by ADL 2-1294 was threefold, compared with the twofold stimulation produced by morphine. Naloxone was a competitive inhibitor of the stimulation of [^{35}S]GTPγS binding produced by ADL 2-1294 (Fig. 2), in which increasing concentrations of naloxone caused a parallel shift to the right of the dose–response curve for ADL 2-1294, without decreasing the maximal stimulation. ADL 2-1294 also inhibited forskolin-stimulated cAMP accumulation in CHO cells in a concentration-dependent manner, with a mean IC_{50} value of 27 nM and maximal inhibition of 54 ± 6%. The effects of loperamide in isolated tissue preparations were consistent with the mechanism of action being μ-agonism (27).

III. EFFICACY IN MODELS OF INFLAMMATORY PAIN FOLLOWING LOCAL INJECTION OF ADL 2-1294

ADL 2-1294 is a potent and fully efficacious antihyperalgesic agent when administered locally under conditions of inflammatory pain (Table 2). The first evaluation of the local antihyperalgesic effects of ADL 2-1294 used the knee joint compression model in the rat, in which robust hyperalgesia to μ- or κ-agonists can be measured by the change in blood pressure that results from the sympathetic response to the painful stimulus of compression of the inflamed knee joint (5). Figure 3 demonstrates that following intra-articular injection of ADL 2-1294 (0.3 mg), the pain response evoked by knee joint compression was reduced to a level comparable with that induced by morphine at a dose tenfold lower than that of morphine (28,29). The antihyperalgesia produced by ADL 2-1294 was naloxone-reversible and, in contrast to that produced by morphine, did not result in catalepsy. Furthermore, morphine, but not ADL 2-1294, produced analgesia following i.m. or contralateral joint injection, demonstrating that ADL 2-1294 exerts its effects locally and lacks systemic bioavailability.

Formalin-induced flinching behavior can be inhibited by opiates that are injected centrally (30,31), systemically (31,32), or locally (7,33). Opiate agonists with peripheral selectivity inhibit flinching only during the late phase (34,35), where, unlike in the early phase, the presence of inflammation is prominent. This was the case for ADL 2-1294 (27,29), which demonstrated an A_{50} value of 6 (1.6–21) μg intrapaw against late-phase formalin-induced flinching and failed to inhibit early-phase flinching at doses up to 300 μg intrapaw (see Table 2). Its potency was

Table 2 Pharmacology of ADL 2-1294 in Models of Inflammatory Pain

Assay	Species	Route[a]	Antinociceptive effect: ADL 2-1294	Antinociceptive effect: Morphine	Ref.
Kaolin/carrageenan-induced hyperalgesia	Rat	i.art.	Maximal antinociception at 0.3 mg	Maximal antinociception at 3 mg	27, 29
Formalin-induced flinching, late phase	Rat	i.paw	A_{50} = 6 μg	A_{50} = 72 μg	27, 29
Formalin-induced flinching, early phase	Rat	i.paw	No effect up to 300 μg	A_{50} = 180 μg	27, 29
FCA-induced hyperalgesia	Rat	i.pl.	ED_{50} = 21 μg	ED_{50} = 14 μg	27, 29
FCA-induced hyperalgesia	Rat	Topical	Dose-dependent antihyperalgesia at 3 and 10%	Not determined	Adolor Corporation, unpublished data
Tape–stripping-induced hyperalgesia	Rat	i.paw	ED_{50} = 71 μg	ED_{50} = 293 μg	27, 29
Erythema-induced hyperalgesia	Rat	Topical	Dose-dependent antihyperalgesia at 1.67 and 5%	Not determined	42
First- and second-degree–burn-induced hyperalgesia	Rat	i.pl.	Dose-dependent antihyperalgesia at 100 and 120 μg	Not determined	39–41
Compound 48/80-induced itch	Mouse	s.c.	I_{50} = 1.3 mg/kg	I_{50} = 0.38 mg/kg	DeHaven-Hudkins et al., in press

[a] i.art., intra-articular; i.paw, intrapaw; Lipl., intraplantar; s.c., subcutaneous.

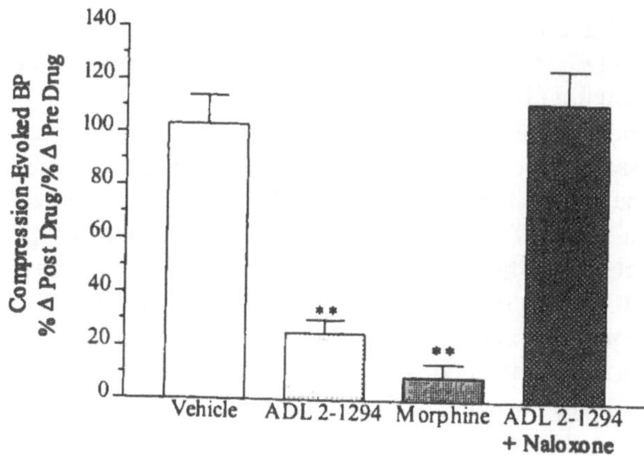

Figure 3 Effect of intra-articular (i.art.) ADL 2-1294 or morphine on blood pressure (BP) changes evoked by compression of the inflamed knee joint: ADL 2-1294 (0.3 mg) or morphine (3 mg) was injected i.art. at 3 h following the induction of inflammation (n = 4/group). Naloxone was injected i.p. at a dose of 1 mg/kg (n = 4). ** = Significantly different from vehicle; Dunnett's test, $p < 0.01$.

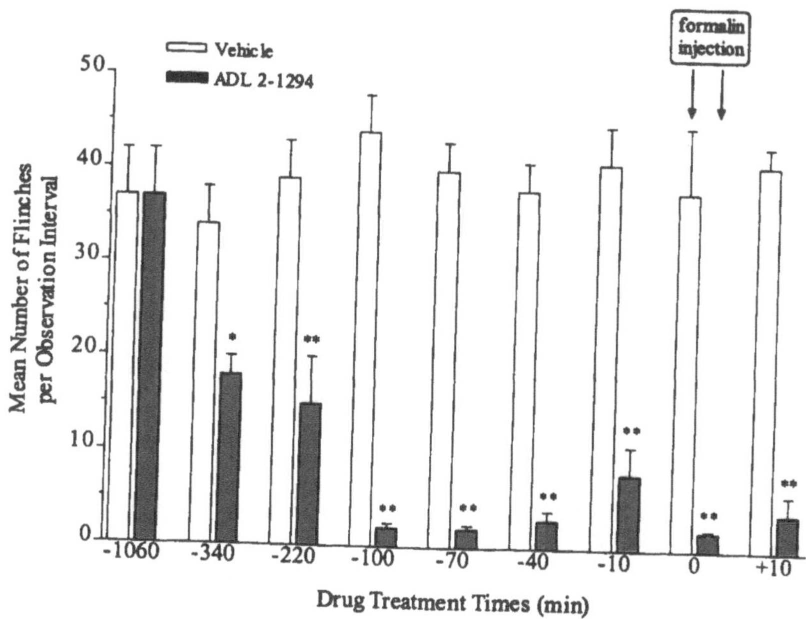

Figure 4 Time course of the antagonism by ADL 2-1294 of late-phase formalin-induced flinching: ADL 2-1294 at a dose of 100 μg or vehicle (n = 8–11/group) was injected i.paw at various times before or after the injection of 50 μL of 5% formalin. The number of flinches occurring during the 20- to 35-min interval following the injection of formalin was counted. Data are the mean ± SEM of the average number of flinches per 5-min observation interval. Significantly different from vehicle, Bonferroni's multiple comparison test: * = $p < 0.05$; ** = $p < 0.01$.

12-fold greater than that of morphine (see Table 2). The antihyperalgesia produced by ADL 2-1294 was prolonged and its onset was rapid (Fig. 4), as evidenced by maximal antihyperalgesia when it was administered 10 min after formalin (10 min before observation).

Additional evidence for the local and peripheral selectivity of the antihyperalgesia produced by ADL 2-1294 in the formalin assay was obtained by examining late-phase flinching behavior following injection of drug into the contralateral paw (27,29). If ADL 2-1294 possessed central or systemic analgesic activity as a result of intrapaw injection, antinociception would be observed when ADL 2-1294 was injected into the paw opposite the paw that was injected with formalin. ADL 2-1294 at a dose of 100 μg intrapaw exhibited antihyperalgesia when injected ipsilateral to formalin, but failed to produce antinociception when injected into the paw contralateral to formalin (27,29). These data support the notion that ADL 2-1294 is a peripherally selective compound that acts locally without any anesthetic effects and without producing centrally mediated analgesia following systemic absorption.

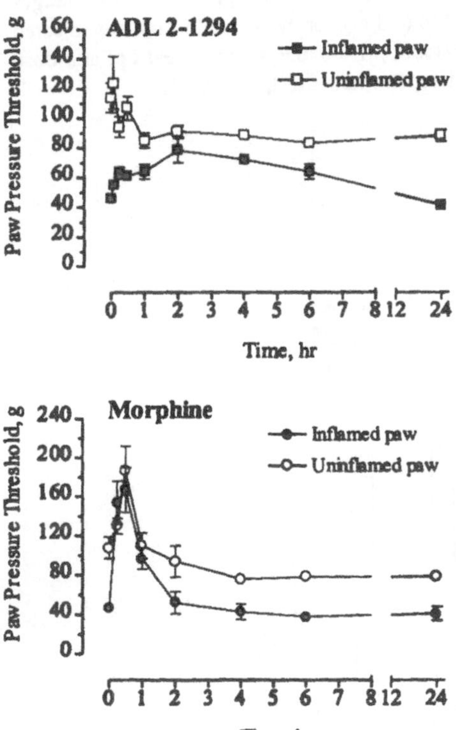

Figure 5 Time course of the antagonism by ADL 2-1294 or morphine of FCA-induced hyperalgesia: FCA was injected i.pl. and hyperalgesia was allowed to develop for 24 h. ADL 2-1294 at a dose of 100 μg (n = 11–13) or morphine at a dose of 300 μg (n = 8–13) was then injected i.pl. into the inflamed paw (t = 0). The paw pressure threshold (PPT) in grams was read in each paw before drug injection and at various times up to 24 h following treatment. Each point is the mean ± SEM PPT in grams at the respective time points. The PPT values for ADL 2-1294 in the inflamed paw were significantly different from baseline at 15 min ($p < 0.01$), 30 min ($p < 0.05$), and at 1, 2, 4, and 6 h (all $p < 0.01$; Dunnett's test). Following morphine treatment, the PPT values in the inflamed paw were significantly different from baseline at 15 min, 30 min, and 1 h ($p < 0.01$; Dunnett's test). Morphine also produced significant antinociception in the uninflamed paw at 30 min ($p < 0.01$; Dunnett's test).

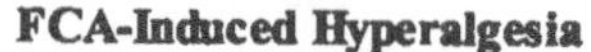

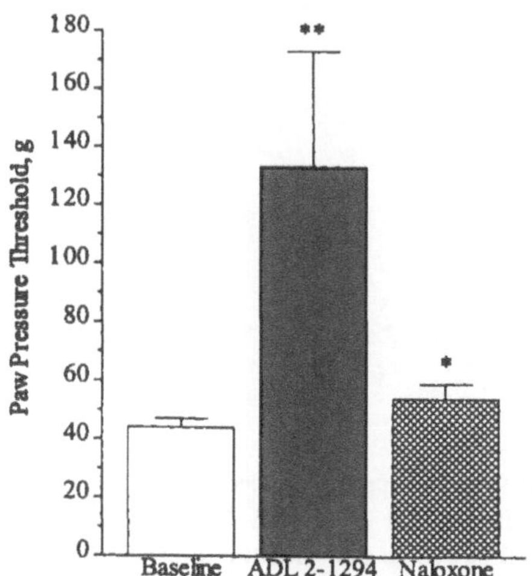

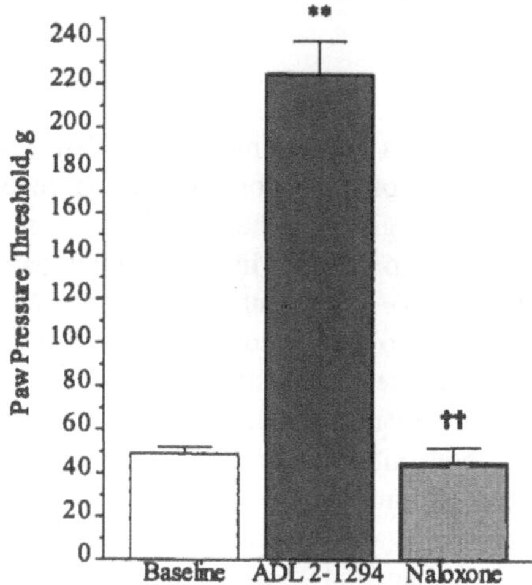

Figure 6 Antagonism by naloxone of the antihyperalgesia produced by local injection of ADL 2-1294: FCA-induced hyperalgesia: naloxone (10 mg/kg s.c.) was injected 15 min before the i.pl. administration of 300 μg of ADL 2-1294. PPTs were read at 2 h following ADL 2-1294. Values are the mean ± SEM PPT in grams (n = 5–11). The PPT values in the inflamed paw of rats treated with ADL 2-1294 were significantly different from baseline values ($p < 0.01$, Tukey), and PPT values for naloxone-pretreated rats were significantly different from rats treated with ADL 2-1294 alone ($p < 0.05$, Tukey). Tape–stripping-induced hyperalgesia: naloxone (10 mg/kg s.c.) was injected 15 min before the i.pl. administration of 300 μg of ADL 2-1294. PPTs were read at 15 min after ADL 2-1294. Values are the mean ± SEM PPT in grams (n = 6–14). The PPT values in the inflamed paw of rats treated with ADL 2-1294 were significantly different from baseline values (** = $p < 0.0001$, Tukey), and PPT values for naloxone-pretreated rats were significantly different from rats treated with ADL 2-1294 alone (* = $p < 0.05$; †† = $p < 0.001$, Tukey).

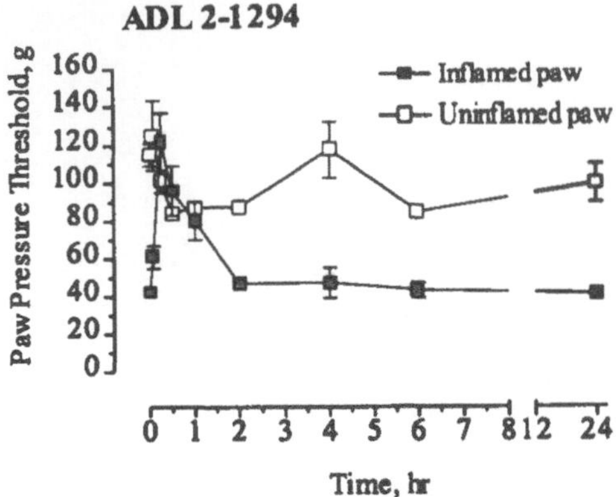

Figure 7 Time course of the antagonism by ADL 2-1294 of tape–stripping-induced hyperalgesia: Tape stripping was performed, and hyperalgesia was allowed to develop for 24 h. ADL 2-1294 at a dose of 100 μg (n = 15–17) was injected i.paw into the tape-stripped paw. The paw pressure threshold (PPT) in grams was read in each paw before drug injection and at various times following treatment up to 24 h postdrug. Each point is the mean ± SEM PPT in grams at the respective time points. The PPT values in the inflamed paw were significantly different from baseline at 15 min, 30 min, and 1 h following treatment ($p < 0.01$; Dunnett's test).

Freund's complete adjuvant (FCA)-induced hyperalgesia is another model of inflammatory pain that is sensitive to the effects of local administration of μ-, δ-, or κ-opioid agonists into inflamed tissue (4,36,37). A dose of 100 μg of ADL 2-1294, given by the intraplantar route, produced a significant and dose-dependent attenuation of the hyperalgesia in the inflamed paw (27,29), lasting from 5 min to 6 h after a single injection (Fig. 5). Treatment with ADL 2-1294 elevated the paw pressure threshold (PPT) in the inflamed paw to a level comparable with that of an untreated and uninflamed paw, without producing further elevations that would be indicative of systemic or CNS effects. In contrast, morphine, which can produce analgesia by both systemic and CNS mechanisms, elevated PPT values in both inflamed and uninflamed paws (see Fig. 5). The antihyperalgesia produced by intraplantar administration of ADL 2-1294 was dose-dependent, with an ED_{50}, defined as the dose that produced a 50% increase over baseline, of 21 μg. ADL 2-1294 was equipotent to morphine when evaluated at 15 min postinjection, its peak time of analgesia (see Table 2). The antihyperalgesia produced by intraplantar injection of 300 μg of ADL 2-1294 into the inflamed paw was completely antagonized by pretreatment with naloxone at a subcutaneous dose of 10 mg/kg, given 15 min before ADL 2-1294 (Fig. 6).

Tape–stripping-induced hyperalgesia is a model of inflammatory pain developed in our laboratory (6) that uses repetitive application and removal of Scotch tape to the dorsal surface of the rat paw to produce an abrasion injury by removal of the stratum corneum layer of the epidermis. The hyperalgesia that results from the tape-stripping procedure was ameliorated by local injection of μ-agonists or by nonselective κ-agonists that have nanomolar affinity for the μ-receptor, but not by agonists selective for the δ- or κ-subtypes (6). These data suggest that following local administration of opioid agonists, the tape-stripping model of hyperalgesia is selective for μ-agonists. ADL 2-1294 exhibits peripheral antihyperalgesia in this model (27,29) with a potency fourfold greater than the μ-agonists DAMGO (ED_{50} = 269 μg) or morphine (ED_{50} = 293 μg) when injected into the dorsal surface of the rat hindpaw (6). Antihyperalgesia was observed in the inflamed paw at 15 min, 30 min, and 1 h following injection (Fig. 7).

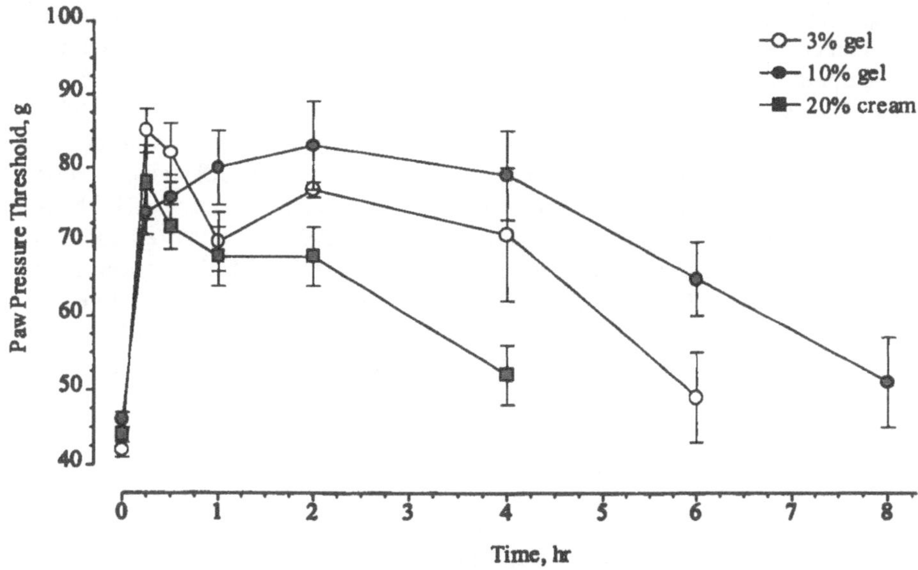

Figure 8 Time course of the antihyperalgesia produced by topical formulations of ADL 2-1294 against FCA-induced hyperalgesia: FCA was injected i.pl. and hyperalgesia was allowed to develop for 24 h. Baseline PPT measurements were taken ($t = 0$), and then approximately 100 mg of each formulation was applied to the inflamed paw. The paw pressure threshold (PPT) in grams was read in each paw before topical application of formulation and at various times up to 8 h following treatment. Each point is the mean ± SEM PPT in grams at the respective time points. The PPT values for the 20% cream in the inflamed paw were significantly different from baseline at 15 min, 30 min, 1 h, and 2 h (all $p < 0.01$). The PPT values for the 3% gel in the inflamed paw were significantly different from baseline at 15 min, 30 min, 1 h, 2 h, and 4 h (all $p < 0.01$), and for the 10% gel at 15 min, 30 min, 1 h, 2 h, 4 h, and 6 h (all $p < 0.01$; Dunnett's test).

Treatment with ADL 2-1294 elevated the PPT value in the inflamed paw to a level comparable with that of an untreated and uninflamed paw, without producing further elevations in the inflamed paw or drug effects in the uninflamed paw, which would be indicative of systemic or CNS effects. In contrast, morphine, which can produce analgesia by both systemic and CNS mechanisms, elevated PPT values in both inflamed and uninflamed paws. The antihyperalgesia produced by ADL 2-1294 against tape–stripping-induced hyperalgesia at 15 min after intrapaw injection was antagonized by naloxone (see Fig. 6).

The hyperalgesia that occurs in response to a first- or second-degree burn injury (38) is also ameliorated by local injection of ADL 2-1294 to Sprague–Dawley rats (39–41). Injection of 100 or 120 μg of ADL 2-1294 significantly attenuated withdrawal latencies to a thermal stimulus, with a time to peak effect of 30 min and duration of less than 60 min (39,40). An increase in latency in the contralateral foot is not observed following drug injection into the injured foot (39).

IV. EFFICACY IN MODELS OF INFLAMMATORY PAIN FOLLOWING TOPICAL APPLICATION

The efficacy of ADL 2-1294 administered by the topical route has been demonstrated with application of both cream and gel formulations. Following topical application of ADL 2-1294 cream in strengths of 1.67 and 5%, dose-dependent antihyperalgesia to a heat stimulus was observed against an erythema injury induced by a thermal burn (42). The antihyperalgesia produced by topical application of ADL 2-1294 cream was reversed by naloxone.

Our laboratory has evaluated a variety of topical formulations for efficacy in the FCA-induced hyperalgesia model as a means to determine the optimal drug concentrations and combinations of excipients that result in maximal efficacy with rapid onset and prolonged duration. In this model, inflammation in the rat paw was induced by intraplantar injection of FCA. At 24 h following FCA injection, baseline paw pressure threshold readings were taken and then approximately 100 mg of a formulation containing either 20% ADL 2-1294 in a cream base, or ADL 2-1294 in strengths of 3 or 10% in a gel base, was applied to the dorsal and ventral surfaces of the inflamed paw. Application of a cream formulation containing 20% ADL 2-1294 or a gel formulation in strengths of 3 or 10% ADL 2-1294 resulted in significant antihyperalgesia (Fig. 8). With the 20% cream, antihyperalgesia was present from 15 min to 2 h after application. The gel formulation substantially improved the duration of the antihyperalgesia compared with the 20% cream. The 3% gel produced significant antihyperalgesia that lasted from 15 min to 4 h. Increasing the concentration of ADL 2-1294 to 10% in the same gel formulation resulted in antihyperalgesia that was present from 15 min up to 6 h after application. This time course was similar to that which occurs following intraplantar injection (see Fig. 5). At no time did PPT values increase in the uninflamed paw, suggesting a lack of systemic bioavailability of ADL 2-1294 following topical application in these formulations.

V. EFFICACY OF ADL 2-1294 IN A RODENT MODEL OF PRURITUS

Kuriyashi et al. (43) have described a model of scratching behavior in the mouse in which injection of the pruritogenic agent compound 48/80 into the nape of the neck resulted in robust scratching of the injected site. An investigation of the pharmacology of opiate compounds in this model has shown that κ-, μ-, or δ-agonists produced a dose-dependent inhibition of scratching, whereas the opiate antagonist naloxone itself was without effect (44). ADL 2-1294 also produced a dose-dependent inhibition of scratching behavior when injected into the same site as compound 48/80, with an ED_{50} value of 1.3 (0.61–1.9) mg/kg (DeHaven-Hudkins et al., in press). Local administration of ADL 2-1294 may therefore have potential usefulness as an agent for the treatment of skin disorders in which itching is one of the primary hallmarks of discomfort.

VI. LACK OF ANALGESIA FOLLOWING SYSTEMIC ADMINISTRATION

Loperamide has consistently failed to show evidence of activity in assays that measure acute pain or centrally mediated analgesia. When loperamide was administered intravenously to either mice or rats, analgesia was not observed until doses that approached the LD_{50} were given (45, 46). Following oral administration in rats, loperamide failed to exhibit analgesia in the tail-withdrawal test at doses up to 160 mg/kg (47), in the tail-pinch test at doses up to 80 mg/kg, and in the Randall–Selitto test at doses up to 16 mg/kg (48). Similarly, loperamide was a weak analgesic in the mouse hot-plate test with an oral ED_{50} of 42 mg/kg (48), and exhibited efficacy only at high doses in the tail-withdrawal test in the mouse following subcutaneous or oral administration (45). In mice, morphine-like side effects were not observed with loperamide at subcutaneous doses of 80 mg/kg or 20 mg/kg intraperitoneal, which were nearly equivalent to the subcutaneous LD_{50} values of 75 mg/kg and 28 mg/kg intraperitoneal (49). The only reported behavioral effect was the occurrence of clonic seizures in mice treated subcutaneously with 80 mg/kg (49).

VII. PHARMACOKINETICS OF ADL 2-1294

Pharmacokinetic data with loperamide have demonstrated that it fails to cross the blood–brain barrier (50,51), at least in part because it is a substrate for the drug-transporting *p*-glycoproteins (MDR) in brain and, therefore, is actively "pumped out" of the brain (51). Classic pharmacokinetic studies performed in the 1970s found that following oral dosing of 1.25 mg/kg to rats, most of the drug was localized to the stomach and intestines, with extremely low levels (<0.022 μg/g wet weight) in the brain (50). With intravenous injection of 5 mg/kg of [^{3}H]loperamide in mice, most of the radioactivity was found in the lung, liver, and kidney, with levels in brain of <1 μg/g (46). Recently, Schinkel and co-workers (51) have reported that mice lacking the *mdr* transporter gene exhibited a 14-fold increase in the levels of loperamide in brain and exhibited opiate-like behaviors after an oral dose of 1 mg/kg (51). Owing to the highly lipophilic nature of loperamide, its pharmacokinetic profile is such that it remains localized at the site of application when administered orally (or locally by injection), and in intravenous administration, high levels are found in the lung, the first tissue at which the compound reaches a large surface area of lipid membranes.

VIII. SAFETY AND EFFICACY OF ADL 2-1294 AS AN ANTIHYPERALGESIC AGENT IN HUMANS

The safety profile of loperamide following oral administration has established that it is well tolerated by this route (52). Clinical studies have demonstrated that it does not possess abuse potential (53) or dependence liability (54) when administered orally. The compound is an unscheduled drug in the United States that is available over-the-counter in certain antidiarrheal preparations. Safety studies by the topical route of administration have shown that doses of 0.06–377 mg of a cream containing 5% ADL 2-1294 applied to body surface areas up to 8% were well tolerated (Adolor Corporation, unpublished data). Measurement of plasma concentrations of drug from the topical safety studies demonstrated that the levels were well below the 2–10 ng/mL reported after oral administration of 18–54 mg of drug (55). Topically applied ADL 2-1294 has demonstrated efficacy in an experimental human model of burn pain and in pain resulting from injury to the eye (Adolor Corporation, unpublished data).

IX. SUMMARY

The unique pharmacokinetic properties that make loperamide an effective antidiarrheal agent are the same properties that make it an ideal antihyperalgesic agent for local administration. Following local administration, ADL 2-1294 produces antihyperalgesia by its accessibility to the peripheral opioid receptor. It is not distributed systemically, as demonstrated by the lack of effect when it is injected into the contralateral knee in the compression model or into the contralateral paw in the formalin and burn models, and by its lack of effect on uninflamed paw pressure thresholds in the FCA- and tape-stripping-induced hyperalgesia assays. ADL 2-1294 demonstrated antihyperalgesia in numerous animal models of inflammatory pain. In the studies where dose–response relations were determined, ADL 2-1294 exhibited potency and efficacy equal to or better than those of morphine following local administration. ADL 2-1294 produced antihyperalgesia by local effects, whereas the effects of morphine were mediated by local, systemic, and CNS actions. The activity of ADL 2-1294 in an animal model of itch suggests new therapeutic indications for this topical antihyperalgesic agent. Since ADL 2-1294 does not cross the blood–brain barrier or produce its effects systemically, it appears to be a superior drug of choice for treatment of inflammatory pain when administration of drug directly at the site of injury is possible. ADL 2-1294 has potential therapeutic usefulness as a peripherally selective opiate antihyperalgesic agent that lacks many of the side effects associated with opiate administration.

ACKNOWLEDGMENTS

I thank Bob DeHaven, Jeff Daubert, and Joel Cassel for performing the in vitro experiments with ADL 2-1294, and Dr. Erik Mansson for the cloning and expression of the opioid receptors. The technical support of Luz Cortes Burgos, Susan Gottshall, Sue Long, Mike Koblish, and Dr. Patrick Little for the in vivo studies is gratefully acknowledged. Lastly, I thank our collaborators Dr. Jerry Collins, Dr. Alan Cowan, and Dr. Tony Yaksh for sharing their data and for their insightful comments.

REFERENCES

1. Hargreaves K, Joris JL. The peripheral analgesic effects of opioids. APS J 1993; 2:51–59.
2. Stein C. The control of pain in peripheral tissue by opioids. N Engl J Med 1995; 332:1685–1690.
3. Joris JL, Dubner R, Hargreaves KM. Opioid analgesia at peripheral sites: a target for opioids released during stress and inflammation? Anesth Analg 1987; 66:1277–1281.
4. Stein C, Millan MJ, Shippenberg TS, Peter K, Herz A. Peripheral opioid receptors mediating antinociception in inflammation. Evidence for involvement of mu, delta, and kappa receptors. J Pharmacol Exp Ther 1989; 248:1269–1275.
5. Nagasaka H, Awad H, Yaksh TL. Peripheral and spinal actions of opioids in the blockade of the autonomic response evoked by compression of the inflamed knee joint. Anesthesiology 1996; 85: 808–816.
6. Cortes Burgos L, DeHaven-Hudkins DL. Tape stripping-induced hyperalgesia as a model for the evaluation of analgesic agents. Soc Neurosci Abstr 1996; 22:1315.
7. Wheeler–Aceto H. Characterization of nociception and edema after formalin-induced tissue injury in the rat: pharmacological analysis of opioid activity. PhD dissertation, Temple University, Philadelphia, PA, 1994.
8. Stein C, Comisel K, Haimerl E, Yassouridis A, Lehrberger K, Herz A, Peter K. Analgesic effect of intraarticular morphine after arthroscopic knee surgery. N Engl J Med 1991; 325:1123–1126.
9. Stein C, Hassan AHS, Lehrberger K, Giefing J, Yassouridis A. Local analgesic effect of endogenous opioid peptides. Lancet 1993; 342:321–324.
10. Reuben SS, Connelly NR. Postarthroscopic meniscus repair analgesia with intraarticular ketorolac or morphine. Anesth Analg 1996; 82:1036–1039.
11. Kalso E, Tramer MR, Carroll D, McQuay HJ, Moore RA. Pain relief from intra-articular morphine after knee surgery: a qualitative systematic review. Pain 1997; 71:127–134.
12. Whitford A, Healy M, Joshi GP, McCarroll SM, O'Brien TM. The effect of tourniquet release time on the analgesic efficacy of intraarticular morphine after arthroscopic knee surgery. Anesth Analg 1997; 84:791–793.
13. Likar R, Schafer M, Paulak F, Sittl R, Pipam W, Schalk H, Geissler D, Bernatzky G. Intraarticular morphine analgesia in chronic pain patients with osteoarthritis. Anesth Analg 1997; 84:1313–1317.

14. Moiniche S, Dahl JB, Kehlet H. Peripheral antinociceptive effects of morphine after burn injury. Acta Anaesthesiol Scand 1993; 37:710–712.
15. Peyman GA, Rahimy MH, Fernandes ML. Effects of morphine on corneal sensitivity and epithelial wound healing: implications for topical ophthalmic analgesia. Br J Ophthalmol 1994; 78:138–141.
16. Likar R, Sittl R, Gragger K, Pipam W, Blatnig H, Breschan C, Schalk HV, Stein C, Schafer M. Peripheral morphine analgesia in dental surgery. Pain 1998; 76:145–150.
17. Uhle RA, Reader A, Nist R, Weaver J, Meck M, Meyers WJ. Peripheral opioid analgesia in teeth with symptomatic inflamed pulps. Anesth Prog 1997; 44:90–95.
18. Tennant F, Moll D, DePaulo V. Topical morphine for peripheral pain. Lancet 1993; 342:1047–1048.
19. Przewlocki R, Hassan AHS, Lason W, Epplen C, Herz A, Stein C. Gene expression and localization of opioid peptides in immune cells of inflamed tissue: functional role in antinociception. Neuroscience 1992; 48:491–500.
20. Hassan AHS, Ableitner A, Stein C, Herz A. Inflammation of the rat paw enhances axonal transport of opioid receptors in the sciatic nerve and increases their density in the inflamed tissue. Neuroscience 1993; 55:185–195.
21. Schafer M, Carter L, Stein C. Interleukin 1β and corticotropin-releasing factor inhibit pain by releasing opioids from immune cells in inflamed tissue. Proc Natl Acad Sci USA 1994; 91:4219–4223.
22. Cabot PJ, Carter L, Gaiddon C, Zhang Q, Schafer M, Loeffler JP, Stein C. Immune cell-derived β-endorphin: production, release, and control of inflammatory pain in rats. J Clin Invest 1997; 100: 142–148.
23. Zhou L, Zhang Q, Stein C, Schafer M. Contribution of opioid receptors on primary afferent versus sympathetic neurons to peripheral opioid analgesia. J Pharmacol Exp Ther 1998; 286:1000–1006.
24. Antonijevic I, Mousa SA, Schafer M, Stein C. Perineurial defect and peripheral opioid analgesia in inflammation. J Neurosci 1995; 15:165–172.
25. Coggeshall RE, Zhou S, Carlton SM. Opioid receptors on peripheral sensory axons. Brain Res 1997; 764:126–132.
26. Adolor Corporation. U.S. Patent 5,849,761, December 15, 1998.
27. DeHaven–Hudkins DL, Cortes Burgos L, Cassel JA, Daubert JD, DeHaven RN, Mansson E, Nagasaka H, Yu G, Yaksh T. Loperamide (ADL 2-1294), an opioid antihyperalgesic agent with peripheral selectivity. J Pharmacol Exp Ther 1999; 289:494–502.
28. Giagnoni G, Casiraghi R, Senini L, Revel D, Parolaro D, Sala M, Gori E. Loperamide: evidence of interaction with μ and δ opioid receptors. Life Sci 1983; 33(suppl 1):315–318.
29. DeHaven–Hudkins DL, Cortes Burgos L, Nagasaka H, Yaksh T. ADL 2-1294, a peripherally selective opiate analgesic. Soc Neurosci Abstr 1996; 22:1362.
30. Calcagnetti DJ, Helmstetter FJ, Fanselow M. Analgesia produced by centrally administered DAGO, DPDPE and U50488H in the formalin test. Eur J Pharmacol 1988; 153:117–122.
31. Murray CW, Cowan A. Tonic pain perception in the mouse: differential modulation by three receptor-selective opioid agonists. J Pharmacol Exp Ther 1991; 257:335–341.
32. Wheeler–Aceto H, Cowan A. Standardization of the rat paw formalin test for the evaluation of analgesics. Psychopharmacology 1981; 104:35–44.
33. Hong Y, Abbott FV. Peripheral opioid modulation of pain and inflammation in the formalin test. Eur J Pharmacol 1995; 277:21–28.
34. Oluyomi AO, Hart SL, Smith TW. Differential antinociceptive effects of morphine and methylmorphine in the formalin test. Pain 1992; 49:415–418.
35. Rogers H, Birch PJ, Harrison SM, Palmer E, Manchee GR, Judd DB, Naylor A, Scopes DIC, Hayes AG. GR94839, a κ-opioid agonist with limited access to the central nervous system, has antinociceptive activity. Br J Pharmacol 1992; 106:783–789.
36. Stein C, Millan MJ, Yassouridis A, Herz A. Antinociceptive effects of μ- and κ-agonists in inflammation are enhanced by a peripheral opioid receptor-specific mechanism. Eur J Pharmacol 1988; 155: 255–264.
37. Stein C, Millan MJ, Shippenberg TS, Herz A. Peripheral effect of fentanyl upon nociception in inflamed tissue of the rat. Neurosci Lett 1988; 84:225–228.
38. Collins JG, LaMotte CC, Franco K, Shimada SG, Iwase Y. A model of hyperalgesia induced by

thermal injury in the rat. 17th Annual Scientific Meeting, American Pain Society, San Diego, CA, Nov 5–8, 1998:abstr 604.
39. Collins JG, Shimada SG, Krocheski K. Profound analgesia produced in rats by a mu opiate agonist with peripheral selectivity. Anesth Analg 1998; 86:S266.
40. Collins JG, Shimada SG. Effects of a peripherally limited mu opiate agonist (ADL 2-1294) on hyperalgesia resulting from thermal injury. 17th Annual Scientific Meeting, American Pain Society, San Diego, CA, Nov 5–8, 1998:abstr 733.
41. Iwase Y, Franco K, Shimada S, Collins JG. The response of rats from different vendors to the opioid agonist, ADL 2-1294. 17th Annual Scientific Meeting, American Pain Society, San Diego, CA, Nov 5–8, 1998:abstr 732.
42. Nozaki–Taguchi N, Yaksh TL. Characterization of the antihyperalgesic action of a novel peripheral mu-opioid receptor agonist—loperamide. Anesthesiology 1999; 90:225–234.
43. Kuraishi Y, Nagasawa T, Hayashi K, Satoh M. Scratching behavior induced by pruritogenic but not algesiogenic agents in mice. Eur J Pharmacol 1995; 275:229–233.
44. Kehner GB, Cowan A. Studies on the antipruritic potential of agonists at mu, kappa and delta opioid receptors. NIDA Res Monogr 1997; 178:88.
45. Hurwitz A, Sztern MI, Looney GA, Ben–Zvi Z. Loperamide effects on hepatobiliary function, intestinal transit and analgesia in mice. Life Sci 1994; 54:1687–1698.
46. Wuster M, Herz A. Opiate agonist action of antidiarrheal agents in vitro and in vivo—findings in support for selective action. Naunyn Schmiedebergs Arch Pharmacol 1978; 301:187–194.
47. Niemegeers CJE, Lenaerts FM, Janssen PAJ. Loperamide (R 18 553), a novel type of antidiarrheal agent. Part 1: In vivo oral pharmacology and acute toxicity. Comparison with morphine, codeine, diphenoxylate, and difenoxine. Arzneimittelforschung Drug Res 1974; 24:1633–1636.
48. Bianchi C, Goi A. On the antidiarrhoeal and analgesic properties of diphenoxylate, difenoxine and loperamide in mice and rats. Arzneimittelforschung Drug Res 1977; 27:1040–1043.
49. Niemegeers CJE, Lenaerts FM, Janssen PAJ. Loperamide (R 18 553), a novel type of antidiarrheal agent. Part 2. In vivo parenteral pharmacology and acute toxicity in mice. Comparison with morphine, codeine and diphenoxylate. Arzneimittelforschung Drug Res 1974; 24:1636–1641.
50. Heykants J, Michiels M, Knaeps A, Brugmans J. Loperamide (R 18 553), a novel type of antidiarrheal agent. Arzneimittelforschung Drug Res 1974; 24:1649–1653.
51. Schinkel AH, Wagenaar E, Mol CAAM, van Deemter L. *p*-Glycoprotein in the blood–brain barrier of mice influences the brain penetration and pharmacological activity of many drugs. J Clin Invest 1996; 97:2517–2524.
52. Ericsson CD, Johnson PC. Safety and efficacy of loperamide. Am J Med 1990; 88(suppl 6A):10S–14S.
53. Jaffe JH, Kanzler M, Green J. Abuse potential of loperamide. Clin Pharmacol Ther 1980; 28:812–819.
54. Korey A, Zilm DH, Sellers EM. Dependence liability of two antidiarrheals, nufenoxole and loperamide. Clin Pharmacol Ther 1980; 27:659–664.
55. Weintraub HS, Killinger JM, Keykants J, Kanzler M, Jaffe JH. Studies on the elimination rate of loperamide in man after administration of increasing oral doses of loperamide. Curr Ther Res 1977; 21:867–876.

35
Controlled-Release Opioids

Allan J. Miller and Kevin J. Smith
Napp Pharmaceuticals Ltd., Cambridge, England

I. INTRODUCTION

This chapter reviews a range of controlled-release opioid preparations available for oral, rectal, and transdermal administration in a wide variety of pain states (Table 1). MS Contin® tablets, the first marketed controlled-release opioid, have been in clinical use for almost two decades. Others have only more recently been developed or become available. Compared with short-acting, immediate-release opioids that typically are administered every 4–6 h, controlled-release opioids have the advantage of a prolonged dosing interval. For oral or rectal preparations, a once- or twice-daily–dosing regimen is common. For transdermal products, dosing intervals can range from 2 up to 7 days. Some preparations such as OxyContin® tablets do not require patients to be stabilized on an immediate-release opioid. Analgesic therapy can be initiated directly with the controlled-release product. The prolonged dosing interval provides greater global acceptability, sustained pain relief, minimal intrusion into patients' lives, improved compliance, and an opportunity for a full, uninterrupted night's sleep (1,2).

II. CONTROLLED-RELEASE MORPHINE

A. MS Contin Tablets

The development of MS Contin tablets* as the first controlled-release opioid preparation, introduced in the United Kingdom in 1981, represented a significant advance in the management of pain. This formulation uses the Contin® system, a patented delivery system, that controls the rate of active drug release within the gastrointestinal tract.

1. Pharmacokinetic Studies

Figure 1 shows the mean plasma morphine concentration–time profile at steady state in cancer patients after administration of MS Contin tablets.

This manuscript was submitted to editors in 1999.

* This product is marketed in 42 countries under a variety of trade names (see Table 1); for the convenience of the reader of this chapter, the product designation used in the cited publications has been changed to MS Contin.

Table 1 Controlled-Release Opioids

Single entity opioids	Trade name	Strengths	Other trade names
Oral q12h			
Codeine tablet q12h	Codeine Contin	50, 100, 150, 200 mg	
Dihydrocodeine tablet q12h	DHC Continus	60, 90, 120 mg	Codidol, Codicontin, Dicodin, Didor, Dolcontin
Hydromorphone capsule q12h	Palladone-SR	2, 4, 8, 16, 24 mg	Opidol depot, Opidol Depot, Opidol depotkapslar, Opidol Retard-Kapseln, Hydal retard, Palladon, Palladone Contin, Palladone LP, Palladone CR, Hydromorphone Continus, Hydromorph Contin, Hydromorphone CR
Morphine capsule q12h	Skenan LP Capsules	10, 30, 60, 100, 200 mg	Zomorph, M-Eslon, Duralgin, Capros
Morphine suspension q12h	MS Contin	20, 30, 60, 100, 200 mg	MST Continus, Moscontin, Mundidol retard, Contalgin, Dolcontin, MST, MCR
Morphine tablet q12h	MS Contin	5, 10, 15, 30, 60, 100, 200 mg	MST Continus, Moscontin, Mundidol retard, Substidol retard, Contalgin, Dolcontin, Morficontin, Morcontin Continus, MST Noceptin, Loseptin
	Oramorph SR (UK)	15, 30, 60, 100 mg	SRM-Rhotard
	Oramorph SR (US)	15, 30, 60, 100 mg	
Oxycodone tablet q12h	OxyContin	5, 10, 20, 40, 80 mg; 160 mg in development	Oxygesic
Oral q12–24h			
Morphine capsule q12–24h	Kadian	20, 50, 100 mg	Kapanol, Morcap SR
Oral q24h			
Hydromorphone capsule q24h	Palladone XL	12, 16, 24, 32 mg	
Morphine capsule q24h	MXL Capsules	30, 60, 90, 120, 150, 200 mg	Morphine OD, MXL Contin, MST Continus, Emexel Continus, Emexel, Exelgesic, MS-Mondiem, Mundidol Uno retard, Substitol retard, Contalgin Uno, Dolcontin Unotard, Sevre-Long, MS Mono, MST Uno, MST Mono, Uni MST, MCR Uno
Rectal q12–24h			
Morphine suppository q12–24h	MS Contin	30, 60, 100, 200, 300 mg	MST Continus, Mundidol retard, Exelgesic CR
Transdermal			
Fentanyl transdermal system q3d	Duragesic	25, 50, 75, 100 μg/h	Durogesic

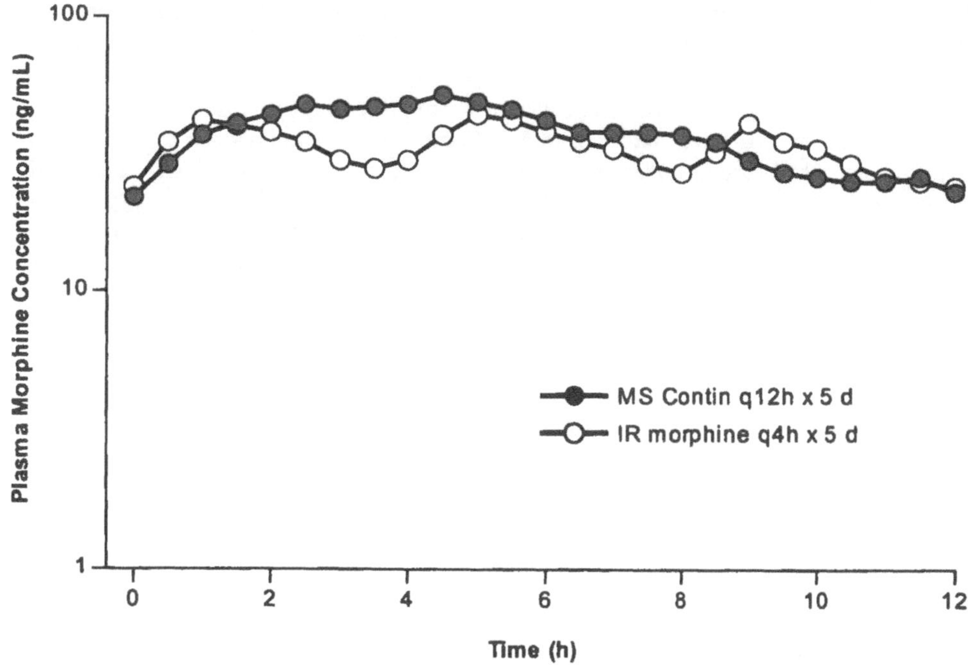

Figure 1 Mean steady-state plasma morphine concentrations following administration of MS Contin tablets administered every 12 h, or oral morphine solution administered every 4 h in cancer patients. The mean total daily morphine dose was 183.9 ± 140.0 mg. (From Ref. 3.)

For all controlled-release preparations it is essential to ensure that the pharmacokinetic properties are reasonably well maintained in the presence of food so that dosing can proceed independent of dietary status. Two studies have confirmed that the rate and extent of morphine absorption, and the other pharmacokinetic characteristics studied, were unaffected when MS Contin tablets were administered together with a high-fat meal (4,5).

The bioequivalence and dose proportionality of MS Contin tablets have been demonstrated across a range of dosage strengths in healthy volunteers (1,6). In a more recent study in naltrexone-blocked volunteers, the 200-mg tablet was bioequivalent to two 100-mg tablets (7). This feature, combined with the recognized linearity in the pharmacokinetics of morphine (8,9), facilitates the titration of individual patients to optimum pain control.

2. Clinical Studies

More than 100 studies have documented the efficacy and safety of MS Contin tablets; the majority of these studies were conducted in a cancer pain population, or they used postoperative pain models. Kaiko et al. (1) reviewed the results of nine U.S. multicenter, sequential crossover, dose titration studies of MS Contin tablets. The studies demonstrated the prolonged analgesic efficacy of this preparation in the treatment of patients with moderate to severe cancer pain. Approximately 93% of patients achieved satisfactory to excellent analgesia on a 12-h regimen when appropriate dose titration was allowed. In global evaluations by patients and investigators, MS Contin tablets provided a significant improvement in both effectiveness and safety over immediate-release morphine and prestudy analgesics. Because these studies were unblinded, it is likely that the results were influenced by the patients' evaluation of the long and convenient duration of action of MS Contin tablets.

More recently, Warfield (10) reviewed the results of ten published, randomized, double-blind, repeated-dose, comparative studies with MS Contin tablets administered every 12 h to cancer pain patients. MS Contin tablets were uniformly effective; 98% of patients completed a treatment course of 12-h therapy. All studies showed consistent pain control with mean pain scores, converted to a common 10-point scale, ranging from 1.1 to 2.9. There was little need for rescue medication. Side effects were generally minimal. In the seven trials in which immediate-release morphine was the comparative agent, MS Contin tablets administered every 12 h were equally as effective as immediate-release morphine given every 4 h in the same total daily doses.

In an open-label study, MS Contin was also effective in patients with severe, chronic acquired immune deficiency syndrome (AIDS) pain (11). Pain intensity decreased by 50–65% (from severe to mild–moderate or mild). For patients with neuropathic pain, there was an approximately 50% reduction in overall mean pain. Side effects were limited or manageable in most patients.

B. MS Contin Suspension

The development of the first controlled-release suspension in the Contin system may be of particular benefit to patients with early dysphagia.

A pharmacokinetic study in healthy volunteers showed the equivalence of MS Contin suspension and MS Contin tablets (12). The controlled-release properties and availability of morphine were maintained when MS Contin suspension was administered together with a high-fat meal (13).

Two clinical studies have confirmed the clinical equivalence of the MS Contin tablet and suspension preparations (Napp Pharmaceuticals, unpublished data).

C. MS Contin Suppositories

Clinical practice guidelines on cancer pain management from several national organizations recommend the rectal route of opioid administration as an alternative to the oral route before more invasive routes of administration are considered (14,15).

A single-dose, bioavailability study in healthy subjects given a rectal enema the evening before dosing demonstrated that the mean systemic availability of morphine was approximately 40% higher with the suppositories than with an equivalent dose of MS Contin tablets administered orally (16). These findings are consistent with a partial avoidance of hepatic first-pass metabolism following rectal administration. In a subsequent steady-state, crossover study in cancer patients, oral tablets and suppositories administered every 12 h were equivalent in the extent of morphine absorption (17). In both studies, the peak plasma concentration (C_{max}) associated with the suppository was approximately 70% that of the oral reference.

MS Contin suppositories provide a level of pain control comparable with that achieved following oral administration of MS Contin tablets when given every 12 h in a 1:1 dosage ratio (18). Although recommended for 12-h dosing, a double-blind, crossover study in patients with cancer pain showed that the pharmacokinetics of MS Contin suppositories support 24-h administration (19).

D. Kapanol® and Kadian® Capsules

1. Pharmacokinetic Studies

Kapanol, an oral sustained-release morphine preparation, is available for once- or twice-daily administration. Single-dose pharmacokinetic studies showed that the rate of morphine absorption from Kapanol was markedly reduced compared with MS Contin (20). Dose-proportional pharmacokinetic responses of morphine and its 3- and 6-glucuronide metabolites was confirmed across the range of capsule strengths.

In vitro studies with Kapanol have shown a doubling of the dissolution rate of morphine in simulated intestinal fluid (physiological alkaline pH) compared with that in simulated gastric fluid (acidic pH) (21). These findings suggest that drugs or pathological conditions that influence gastrointestinal pH may change the absorption rate of Kapanol.

Food intake has an effect on the absorption of Kapanol. Kaiko (22) demonstrated that plasma morphine concentrations were significantly lower 5–10 h after dosing with Kapanol after a high-fat meal than under fasted conditions. These results are consistent with those of an earlier study that demonstrated a food-related delay in the absorption of morphine from Kapanol (20).

A steady-state study compared Kapanol capsules administered every 12 h with MS Contin tablets every 12 h and morphine solution every 4 h in cancer patients (23). The mean profile associated with Kapanol was particularly smooth; fluctuations were markedly smaller than those associated with the other two preparations. Another steady-state study compared once-daily administration of Kapanol capsules with MS Contin tablets every 12 h in patients with moderate to severe cancer pain (24). The mean profile associated with once-daily administration of Kapanol showed a much greater degree of fluctuation (compared with 12-h administration) which was similar to that observed with MS Contin tablets 12 h (Fig. 2).

A single-dose pharmacokinetic study demonstrated that Kapanol capsules (3 × 20 mg) and MXL capsule 60 mg had similar bioavailability when both preparations were administered in a fasting state (see later) (26).

2. Clinical Studies

MS Contin was significantly more effective than Kapanol in all measures of peak and total analgesic effects in a single-dose, double-blind, parallel-group comparative study in postorthopedic surgery patients (27). Despite the use of the same dosage for each product, the results showed a difference in efficacy that has usually been associated with an approximate twofold difference in morphine dosage.

Although the pharmacokinetic and pharmacodynamic profiles of Kapanol differ from those of MS Contin tablets, two randomized, double-blind studies have shown no differences in efficacy or safety between the two products at steady state (24,28). Because patients in both studies were typically titrated with immediate-release morphine to a pain level that was less than moderate, the ability to detect differences between the two preparations was reduced. The controlled conditions for comparison also do not reflect the true degree of pain in the population of cancer and other patients who are routinely treated with oral morphine; these patients typically have moderate to severe pain when therapy with MS Contin tablets or Kapanol is initiated. The

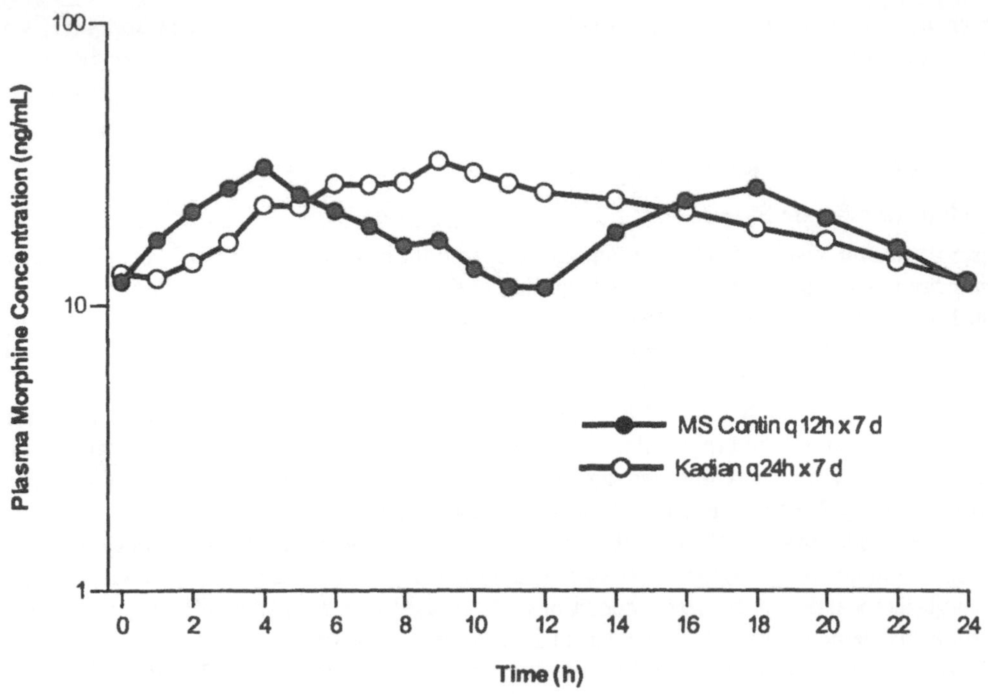

Figure 2 Mean steady-state plasma morphine concentrations after administration of Kadian every 24 h or MS Contin every 12 h in patients with cancer pain. Plasma concentrations normalized to a 100-mg dose q24h. (From Ref. 25.)

combination of "no difference" results and the lack of an internal measure of analgesic assay sensitivity fail to provide for a definitive conclusion of equivalence (29–31).

E. Oramorph® SR Tablets (United Kingdom and United States)

Oramorph SR tablets, sustained-release oral morphine tablets, marketed in the United Kingdom have a different delivery system, different pharmacokinetics, and different bioavailability from those marketed under the same brand name in the United States (32–34). These differences are of some concern for patients in whom one product may be substituted for another without their physicians appreciating the significant differences in pharmacokinetics, and perhaps therapeutic effects, between them.

1. Pharmacokinetic Studies

Oramorph SR Tablets (United Kingdom). A comparative study of MS Contin and Oramorph SR™ in healthy volunteers demonstrated that the mean plasma profiles were bioequivalent in the fasting state, but the peak plasma morphine concentration from Oramorph SR increased significantly in the presence of food (5). A later study of identical design confirmed the equivalence of the preparations in extent of absorption, but the fasting C_{max} associated with

Oramorph SR was greater than that of MS Contin. In the presence of food, there was no difference in C_{max} values between preparations (32).

Oramorph SR Tablets (United States). In a single-dose pharmacokinetic study, the peak plasma concentration and overall bioavailability of Oramorph SR were lower than that observed with MS Contin (35). Differing pharmacokinetic responses were also observed in relation to food intake. In single-dose studies, food consumption did not significantly affect the rate or extent of morphine absorption after dosing with MS Contin (4); however, Oramorph SR showed higher bioavailability in the presence of food (36).

In a repeated-dose pharmacokinetic study, food had no clinically significant effect on the oral bioavailability of Oramorph SR (37). In contrast to the single-dose studies, however, this study was not an appropriately rigorous test of the fasted state.

Because the two preparations are not bioequivalent, Oramorph SR and MS Contin are not considered therapeutically equivalent in clinical use (38).

2. Clinical Studies: Oramorph SR Tablets (United States)

The lack of therapeutic equivalence has been demonstrated in a single-dose, randomized, double-blind, parallel-group study comparing the relative potency of Oramorph SR and MS Contin in patients with postoperative pain (39). Estimates of relative potency from two measures (sum of pain intensity difference and total pain relief) showed that MS Contin was nearly twice as potent as Oramorph SR. MS Contin provided greater peak, total, and duration of analgesia, without a higher incidence of adverse events.

Cooper et al. (40) also compared the analgesic efficacy of MS Contin with Oramorph SR in patients with postorthopedic surgery pain. At the same total dosage, MS Contin provided more rapid and greater peak analgesia with fewer adverse effects than Oramorph SR.

In an open-label, comparative efficacy study of the two preparations in patients with advanced cancer, MS Contin tablets were considered preferable because of the smaller tablet size and longer duration of analgesic effect (41).

F. MXL™ Capsules

Introduced in Germany in 1995, MXL capsules, a multiparticulate morphine formulation, were the first once-a-day opioid analgesic.

1. Pharmacokinetic Studies

The selection of a preferred plasma profile for MXL capsules was based on experience gained with MS Contin tablets. The benefit of an early onset, combined with the need for a prolonged duration of action, indicated that an early peak concentration (relative to the proposed 24-h interval) was desirable. The mean profile in healthy volunteers administered a single dose of MXL capsules is illustrated in Fig. 3. Important features of this profile include an early peak concentration from the MXL capsule, which matches that of a single MS Contin tablet, and plasma concentrations that are maintained over a 24-h period (42). The profiles of the two glucuronide metabolites parallel those of the parent compound (43). In the presence of a high-fat breakfast, the profile shows a greater degree of retardation with a maintained bioavailability of morphine.

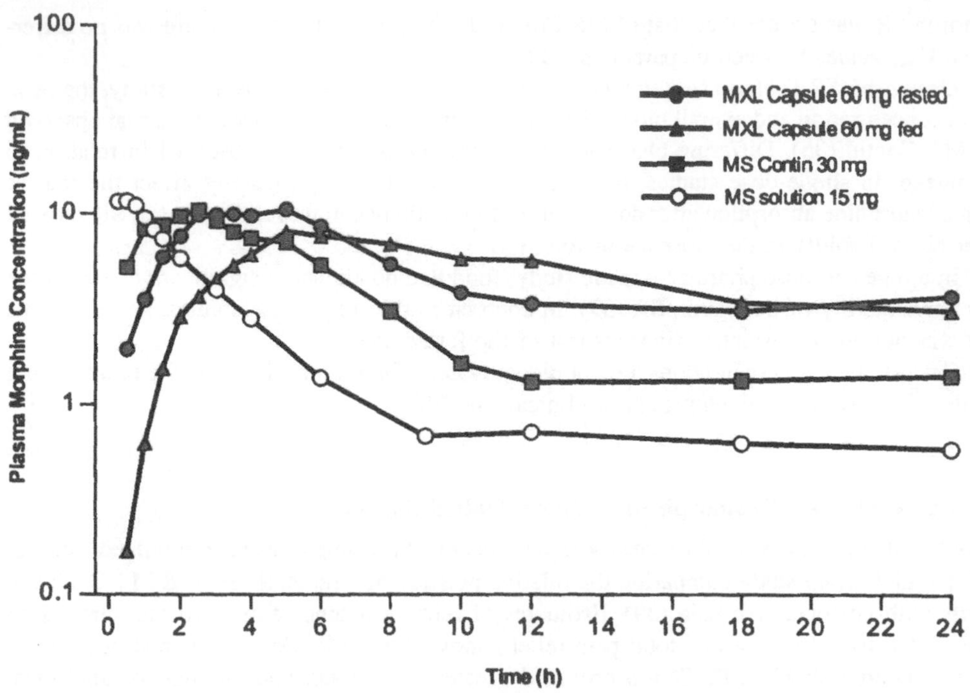

Figure 3 Mean plasma morphine concentrations following administration of a single MXL capsule (fasted or fed), MS Contin tablet, or immediate-release solution in healthy volunteers. (From Napp Pharmaceuticals, unpublished data.)

2. Clinical Studies

MXL capsules administered once daily provide efficacy and tolerability that is equivalent to MS Contin tablets administered every 12 h or immediate-release morphine administered every 4 h. Figure 4 illustrates the distribution of morning pain scores before administration of MXL. The majority of patients were reporting no pain at all; pain scores were equivalent between the two treatments. These data were collected against a background of equivalent use of rescue medication (44).

III. CONTROLLED-RELEASE HYDROMORPHONE

Hydromorphone is a semisynthetic congener of morphine, differing structurally from morphine by the substitution of an oxygen for the 6-hydroxyl group and by the hydrogenation of the 7–8 double bond of the morphine molecule (Fig. 5). Hydromorphone is a μ-selective full opioid agonist with a potency five to ten times greater than that of morphine. In some patients, hydromorphone produces a different response from morphine in terms of pain relief and side effect intensity (45,46), although the reason for this difference is not fully understood. In the United States and Canada, hydromorphone was the strong opioid of choice until morphine became commercially available as the first controlled-release strong opioid formulation.

Morphine is metabolized to a 6-glucuronide which may contribute significantly to the

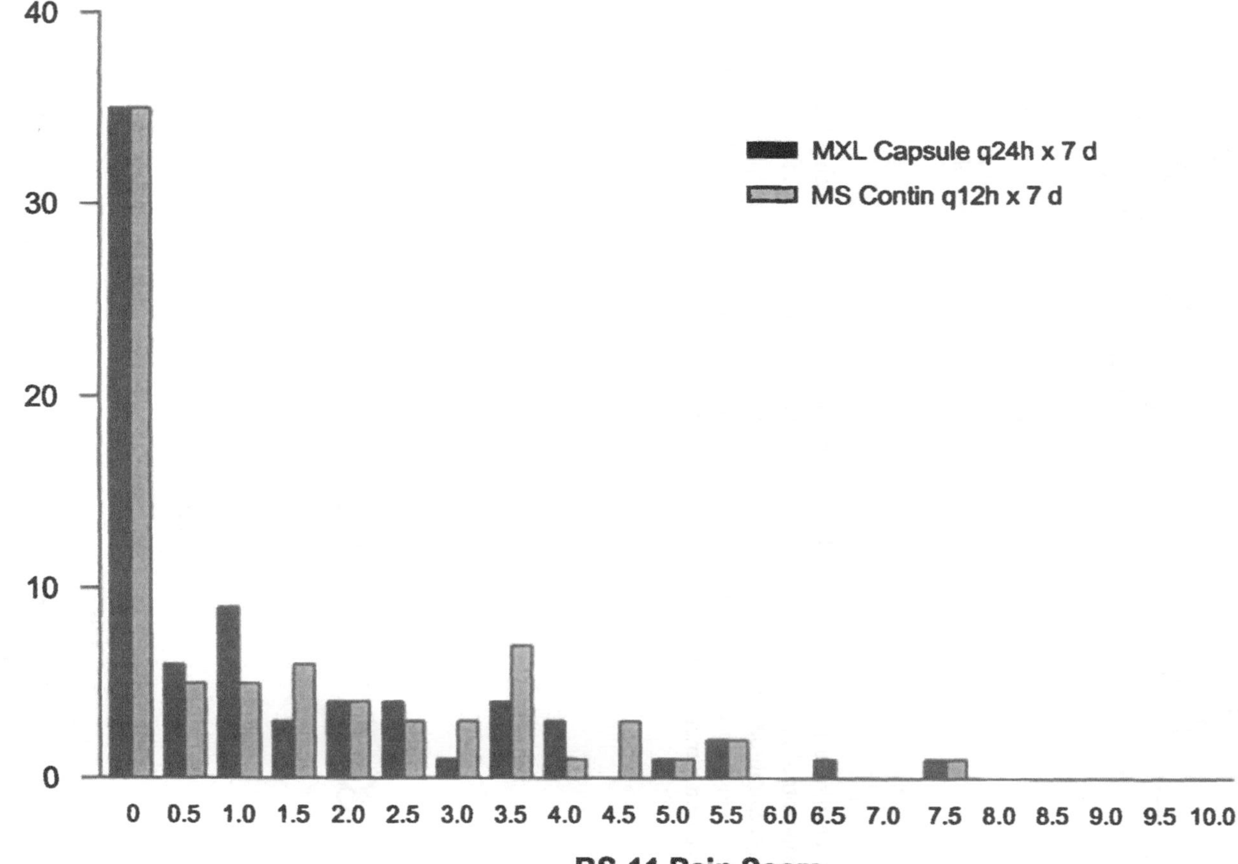

Figure 4 Morning (predose) pain scores following once-daily administration of MXL Capsules or twice-daily administration of MS Contin tablets in patients with cancer pain. The majority of patients received 60 mg of morphine per day. Scores represent the means from the last 3 days of each treatment period. 0 = no pain to 10 = worst pain imaginable. (From Napp Pharmaceuticals, unpublished data.)

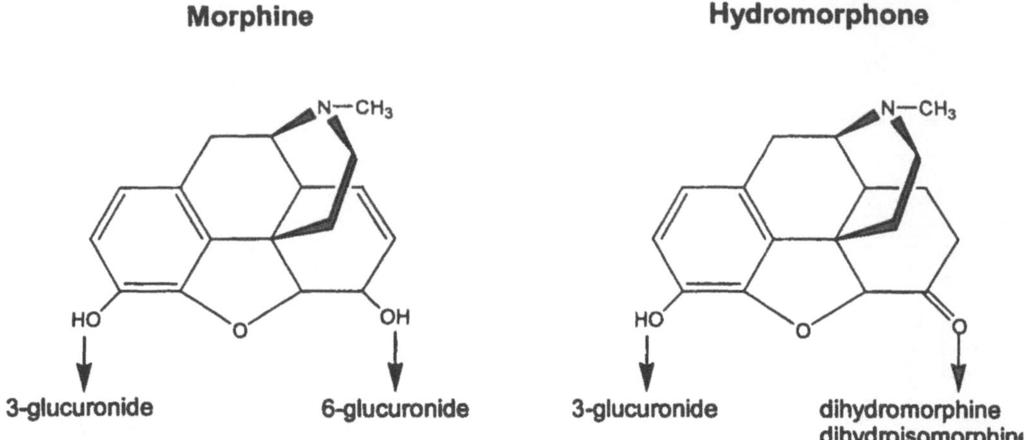

Figure 5 Principal metabolic pathways of morphine and hydromorphone.

overall response. Indeed, it has been suggested that the absence of a clear relationship between plasma morphine concentration and analgesic response may be due to the presence of morphine-6-glucuronide in concentrations severalfold greater than those of the parent compound. Hydromorphone does not form such an active metabolite, but it remains to be established whether this feature is reflected in a more predictable pharmacokinetic–pharmacodynamic relationship.

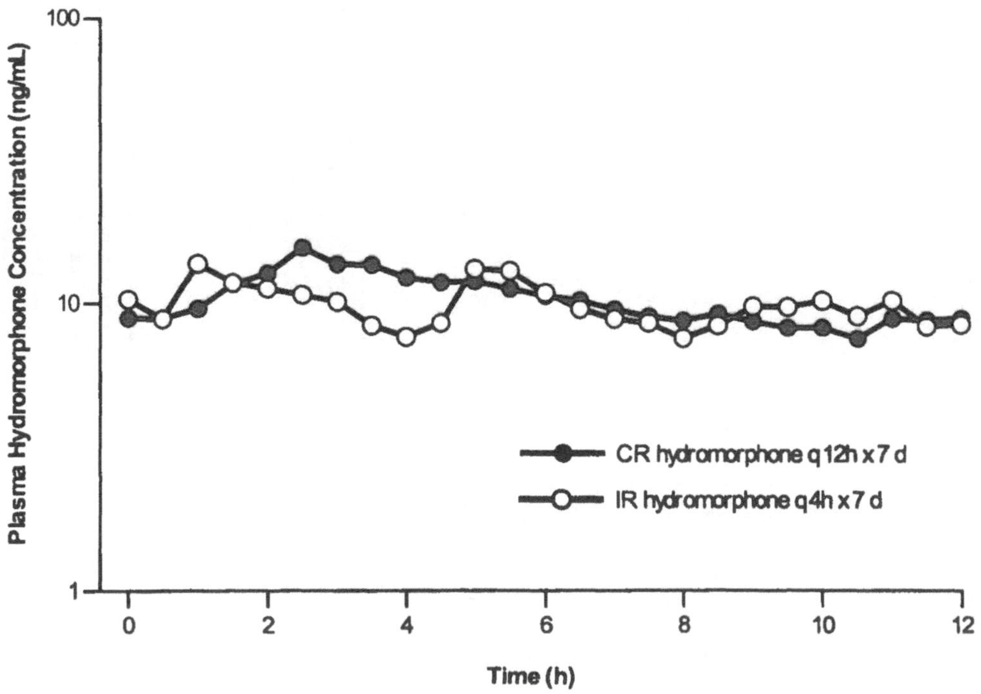

Figure 6 Mean steady-state plasma hydromorphone concentrations following every 12-h administration of Palladone-SR capsules or every 4-h administration of immediate-release hydromorphone to patients with cancer pain. The mean daily hydromorphone dose was 48 ± 11 mg. (From Ref. 48.)

A. Palladone-MXL™ Capsules

Palladone-SR capsules is a controlled-release hydromorphone product developed for every 12-h dosing. A single-dose study in healthy volunteers (47) and a steady-state study in cancer patients (48) have confirmed the controlled-release characteristics of Palladone-SR capsules. The mean plasma profiles obtained with Palladone-SR and immediate-release hydromorphone in the steady-state study are compared in Fig. 6. There was a linear relationship between plasma hydromorphone concentrations and dose, indicating a dose-proportional bioavailability for both controlled- and immediate-release preparations.

In a clinical study, Palladone-SR capsules were equally as effective as immediate-release hydromorphone administered every 4 h in terms of pain scores and the use of rescue medication. Tolerability, as determined by nausea and sedation scores and the frequency and severity of other side effects, was also similar between the two treatments (49).

B. Palladone-XL™ Capsules

A second controlled-release hydromorphone product Palladone XL has been developed to provide consistent plasma hydromorphone concentrations over a 24-h period. Palladone XL is characterized by a biphasic plasma concentration–time curve with the concentration maintained at a plateau for over 24 h (Fig. 7). The biphasic absorption is apparent from both an early and a late peak in the plasma hydromorphone profile utilizing the ATC™ delivery system. The rationale is to provide an initially prompt onset of analgesia as well as a second peak analgesic effect that ensures 24 h duration (Purdue Pharma, unpublished data).

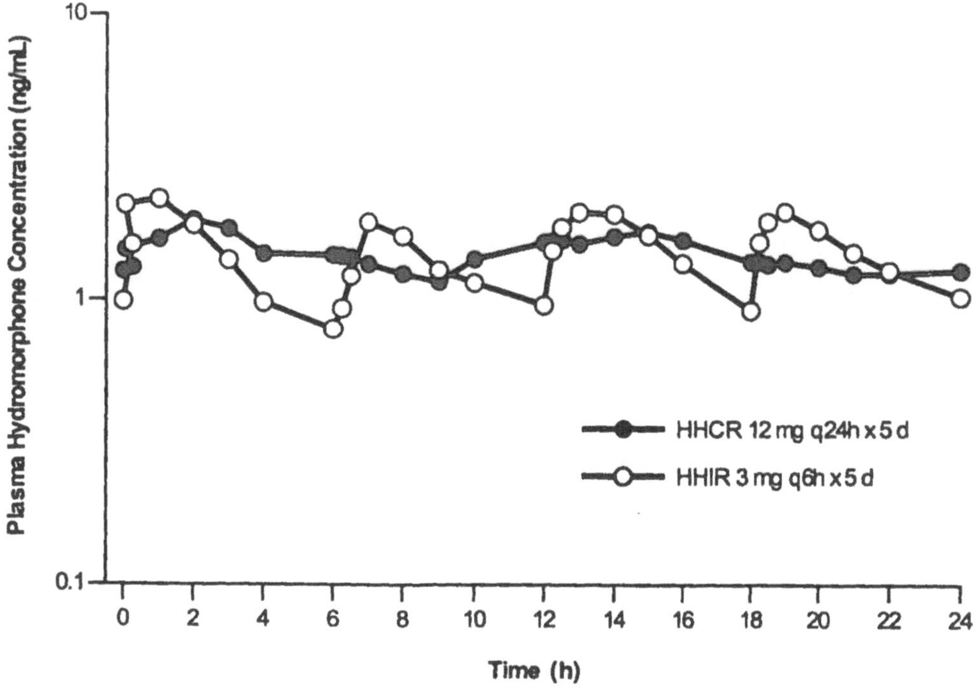

Figure 7 Mean steady-state plasma hydromorphone concentrations following administration of Palladone XL (HHCR) every 24-h or immediate-release hydromorphone (HHIR) every 6 h in normal volunteers. (From Purdue Pharma, unpublished data.)

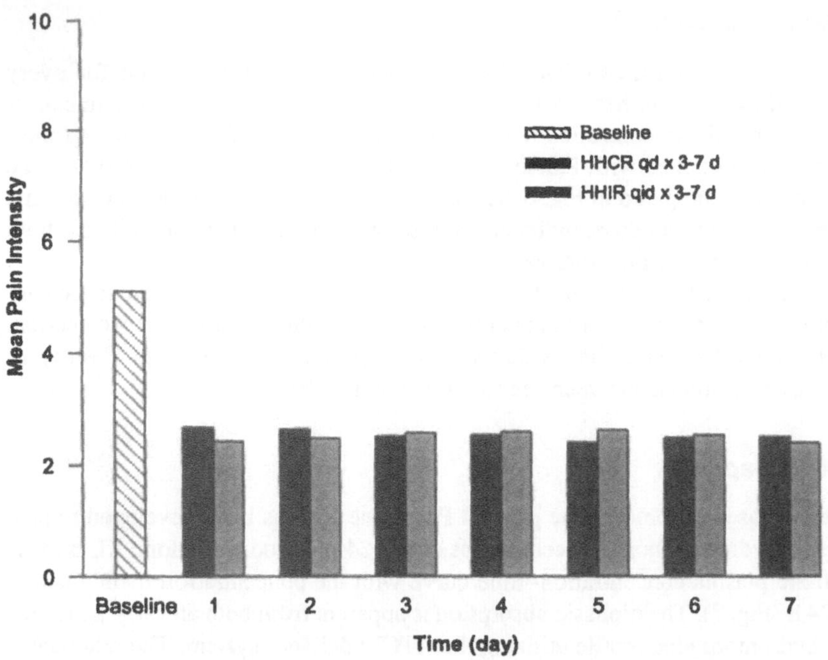

Figure 8 Mean of average pain intensity by day in patients treated with Palladone XL (HHCR) once daily or immediate-release hydromorphone (HHIR) four times daily for 3–7 days. The total daily hydromorphone dose ranged from 12 to 84 mg. 0, no pain to 10, worst pain imaginable. (From Purdue Pharma, unpublished data.)

At steady state in normal volunteers, Palladone XL is equally as bioavailable as immediate-release hydromorphone (Dilaudid™). Fluctuation is approximately one-third that of the immediate-release product. Steady-state pharmacokinetics of Palladone XL evaluated in a diverse patient population showed dose proportionality across the 12- to 84-mg–dose range.

There is no significant food effect. When the capsule contents are sprinkled over applesauce, hydromorphone absorption is equivalent to that observed with the intact capsule.

Palladone XL once-daily was comparable in efficacy to immediate-release hydromorphone four times daily in two randomized, double-blind, two-way crossover studies of identical design (Purdue Pharma, unpublished data). Of patients randomized to treatment, 75–83% had chronic cancer pain. The 24-h duration of effect of Palladone XL was shown by stable pain intensity and low rescue use over the 3- to 7-day–dosing period (Fig. 8). When assessed at four intervals over the course of the day, pain control was not significantly different by time of day over the 24 h dosing interval with Palladone XL treatment (Fig. 9). Trough plasma hydromorphone concentrations were also higher with the controlled-release product. The safety profiles of both controlled- and immediate-release products were comparable.

IV. CONTROLLED-RELEASE OXYCODONE

A. OxyContin Tablets

Oxycodone is a semisynthetic derivative of thebaine. It is a full opioid agonist that has been in clinical use for over 80 years. In contrast to morphine which interacts primarily with μ-opioid

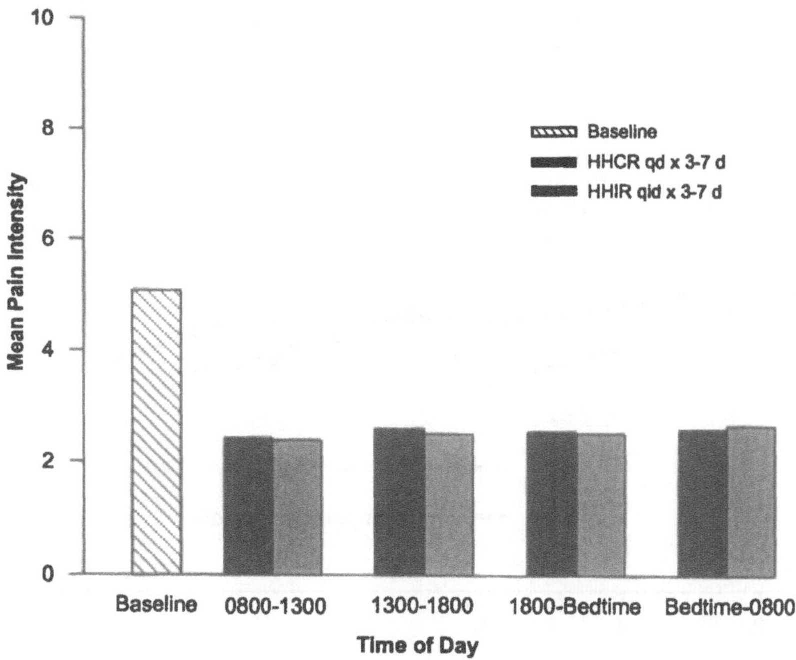

Figure 9 Mean of average pain intensity by time of day in patients treated with Palladone XL (HHCR) once daily or immediate-release hydromorphone (HHIR) four times daily for the mean of the last 2 days before the final day. The total daily hydromorphone dose ranged from 12 to 84 mg. 0 = no pain to 10 = worst pain imaginable. (From Purdue Pharma, unpublished data.)

receptors, there is evidence that oxycodone has particular activity at κ-opioid receptors (50). When given orally, oxycodone is twice as potent as morphine (51,52).

1. Pharmacokinetic Studies

OxyContin tablets have been developed using a second-generation Contin delivery system called AcroContin™. The properties of the AcroContin matrix impart an initial rapid absorption of oxycodone, followed by a more prolonged absorption of the drug substance (53). Onset of action occurs within 1 h in most patients. A more protracted phase follows so that effective plasma oxycodone concentrations are assured over a 12-h–dosing interval.

Because oxycodone is not subject to an extensive first-pass metabolism following oral administration like most other opioids, its oral bioavailability ranges between 60 and 87%. The higher oral bioavailability of oxycodone compared with that for morphine is associated with a significant reduction in interpatient variability in both the rate and extent of absorption (54). Steady-state plasma concentrations are achieved within 24–36 h (55).

Oxycodone® is extensively metabolized and eliminated primarily in the urine as unconjugated (principally noroxycodone and oxymorphone) and conjugated metabolites. Noroxycodone is considered to have weak analgesic activity and, at best, probably plays no role in clinical analgesic activity after oxycodone administration. Although known to have pharmacological activity, oxymorphone is not clinically significant after oxycodone administration: the pharmacodynamic effects of oxycodone were not substantially altered when quinidine pretreatment was

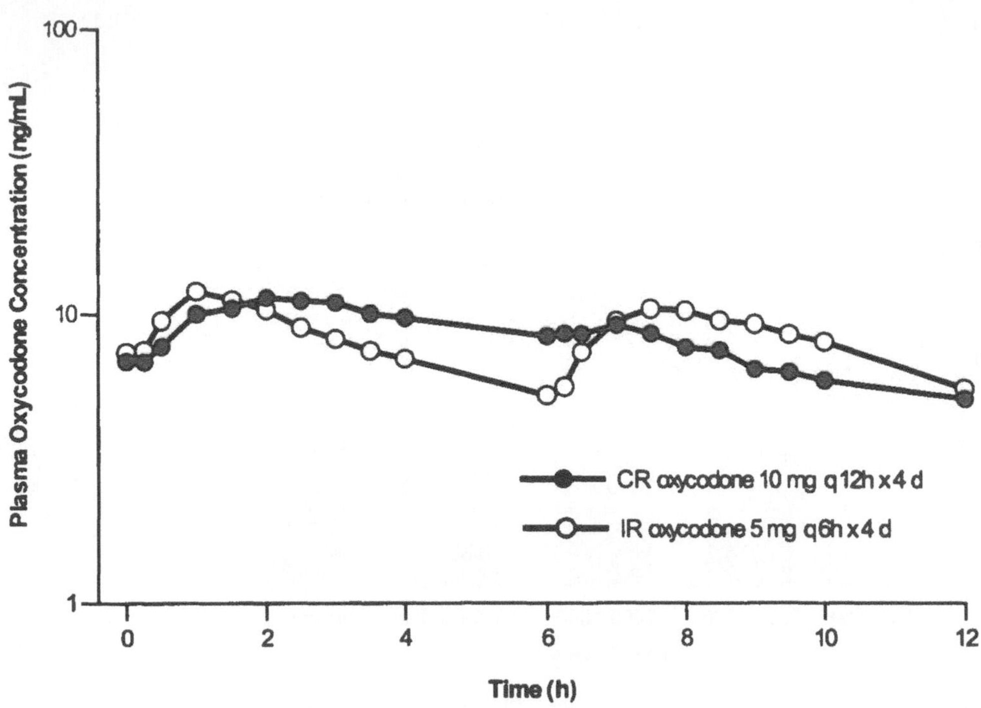

Figure 10 Mean steady-state plasma oxycodone concentrations following twice-daily administration of OxyContin tablets or 6-hourly administration of immediate-release oxycodone in healthy volunteers. (From Ref. 55.)

used to block the formation of oxymorphone (56). The parent compound appears to be solely responsible for the analgesic response (57).

Single-dose and steady-state studies in healthy volunteers have confirmed the controlled-release properties of OxyContin tablets. The mean steady-state plasma profile obtained with OxyContin administered every 12 h compared with that for immediate-release oxycodone given every 6 h is shown in Fig. 10. The two dosage regimens were equivalent in terms of AUC, C_{max}, C_{min}, and fluctuation (55). A number of dose–proportionality/bioequivalence studies have confirmed the equivalence of the available tablet strengths across a broad dosage range (58–60) (Fig. 11). A high-fat meal had no effect on the plasma profile of a single 40-mg dose; AUC and C_{max} values were equivalent under fed and fasted conditions (61).

Pharmacokinetic studies of OxyContin tablets in special patient groups have revealed increased AUCs in the elderly (15%), patients with renal impairment (60%), and patients with hepatic impairment (90%) compared with healthy volunteers (63). The differences are considered less than those observed for morphine or its 6-glucuronide metabolite in these special patient populations. Female volunteers also exhibited plasma concentrations that averaged 25% greater than those recorded in males (57). As with other opioids, careful titration of oxycodone is advised in these special patient groups.

2. Clinical Studies

The efficacy and tolerability of controlled-release oxycodone has been investigated in a variety of pain syndromes, including cancer pain (64–74); Purdue Pharma, unpublished data), osteoar-

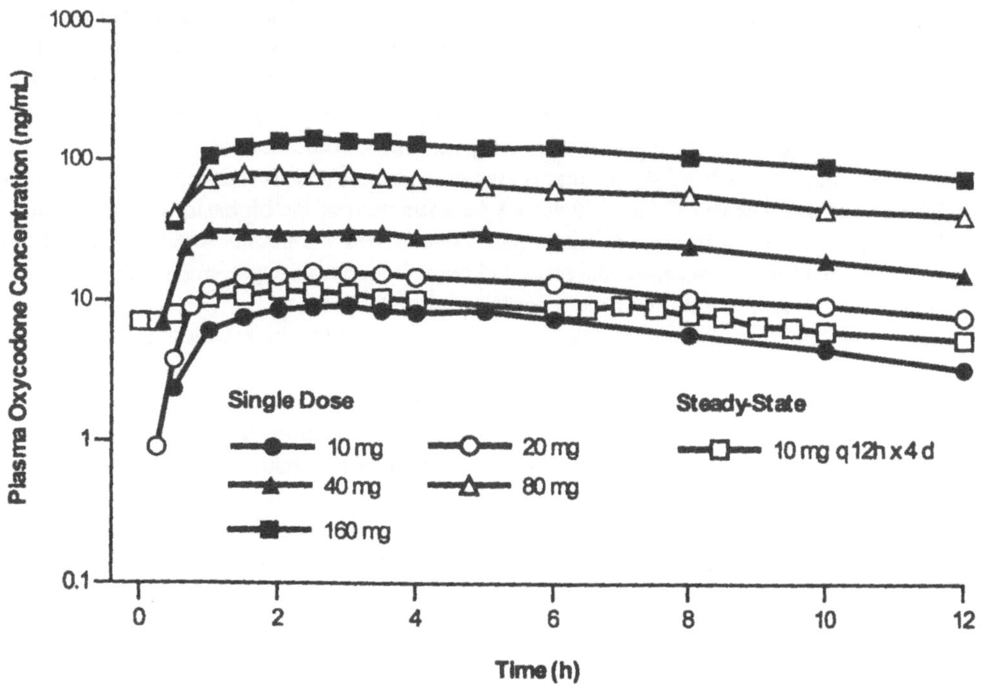

Figure 11 Mean plasma oxycodone concentrations following single or repeated oral doses of OxyContin tablets. (From Ref. 62 and Purdue Pharma, unpublished data.)

thritis (75–77), chronic low-back pain (78), postherpetic neuralgia (79), and postoperative pain (51,52,80–83).

Controlled-release oxycodone provided a rational alternative to controlled-release morphine in the management of moderate to severe cancer pain in three randomized, double-blind trials (64,68,70). Both drugs were equally effective in relieving pain and shared similar adverse event profiles. In one study (70), small differences were observed in side effects that could be significant for individual patients: controlled-release oxycodone-treated patients had no hallucinations (compared with 4% of patients reporting hallucinations in the controlled-release morphine-treated group) and significantly less itching. Heiskanen and Kalso (64) also showed more vomiting with morphine, but more constipation with oxycodone.

Controlled-release oxycodone also provided efficacy comparable with controlled-release hydromorphone in a randomized, double-blind, crossover study in patients with chronic cancer pain (65). There were no significant differences in pain intensity, rescue use, sedation, or nausea scores, or patient preference between the two drugs. Two patients treated with controlled-release hydromorphone experienced hallucinations. No hallucinations were reported in patients given controlled-release oxycodone.

These data, together with data from other studies with immediate-release oxycodone (84,85), indicate a clear trend toward a lower incidence of central nervous system (CNS) excitatory effects, especially hallucinations, with oxycodone compared with other opioids such as morphine. Cramond et al. (86) have proposed an underlying mechanism for this observation: the oxycodone metabolite oxymorphone-3-glucuronide (OM3G) was markedly less potent than its structural analogue morphine-3-glucuronide (M3G) in eliciting CNS excitatory behavioral effects following supraspinal administration in rats.

Although the benefits of the use of controlled-release oxycodone in cancer pain are well documented, the advantages in postoperative pain management are often less fully appreciated. In a double-blind, randomized, placebo-controlled trial, Narcessian et al. (82) showed that rehabilitation hospital length of stay and therapeutic requirements following discharge were significantly reduced in total-knee arthroplasty patients given OxyContin tablets.

Several clinical trials have shown that patients can be titrated to stable pain control with controlled-release oxycodone (87,88), which may be a function of the biphasic-release formulation (53). Once established in clinical trials, pain control was maintained over the long-term without development of tolerance to analgesia, although interestingly, patients became tolerant to typical opioid adverse events (with the exception of constipation).

Clinicians regard controlled-release oxycodone as similar in efficacy and safety to controlled-release morphine and oxycodone has accepted use in both malignant and nonmalignant chronic pain therapy (89). The use of controlled-release oxycodone in osteoarthritis results in improved analgesia with trends toward improvements in function. Successful treatment of chronic low back pain (78) and, perhaps surprisingly, neuropathic pain (74,79) have also been established in clinical trials.

Long-term trials in nonmalignant pain have shown that the risk of addiction or abuse with opioids is low if appropriate patients are selected for treatment (90). Experience with controlled-release oxycodone in clinical trials supports this observation.

V. CONTROLLED-RELEASE DIHYDROCODEINE

A. DHC Continus® Tablets

Dihydrocodeine has been used for many years as an effective analgesic therapy for moderately severe pain. The compound is considered a step 2 analgesic in the three-step ladder developed by the World Health Organization (WHO) for the use of analgesics in cancer pain (91). Although DHC Continus tablets were developed primarily to treat moderately severe pain in cancer patients before stronger opioids were required, the preparation lends itself to other categories of disease associated with pain (e.g., chronic rheumatoid arthritis, chronic osteoarthritis, chronic back pain, and ankylosing spondylitis) when nonsteroidal anti-inflammatory drugs (NSAIDs) and mild analgesics fail to control pain. DHC Continus tablets are also indicated for postoperative pain.

A steady-state study in healthy volunteers has confirmed that DHC Continus tablets administered every 12 h provide a fluctuation comparable with that of conventional dihydrocodeine given every 8 h. A clinical study showed the efficacy of DHC Continus tablets in moderate to severe pain of osteoarthritis (Napp Pharmaceuticals, unpublished data).

VI. CONTROLLED-RELEASE CODEINE

A. Codeine Contin® Tablets

Codeine Contin tablets provided an equivalent bioavailability of codeine and a significantly prolonged time to maximum plasma concentration when compared with immediate-release tablets and liquid formulations in single-dose studies (Purdue Pharma, unpublished data) and steady-state studies (92). In addition the three strengths of 100, 200, and 300 mg demonstrate dose-proportional bioavailability. A dose–response relationship for Codeine Contin has been established in the range of 200–600 mg/day in patients with cancer pain (93). The response to the combination of acetaminophen plus codeine (600/60 mg) given four times a day was approximately equivalent to 150 mg of controlled-release codeine given twice a day.

In a placebo-controlled, double-blind, crossover study, Codeine Contin tablets provided significant reductions in pain intensity and in the use of rescue acetaminophen plus codeine in patients with chronic cancer pain (94). Using a similar study design, the efficacy of 12-h Codeine Contin tablets was also confirmed in chronic nonmalignant pain (95).

VII. TRANSDERMAL FENTANYL

A. Duragesic® Transdermal System

Fentanyl is a synthetic phenylpiperidine opioid analgesic and primarily a μ-receptor agonist that has been used in anesthesia and intensive care since the 1960s (96). Following systemic administration, the duration of action is 30–60 min, and is mainly influenced by its distribution to other tissues. Fentanyl is metabolized in the liver to inactive metabolites (primarily norfentanyl). The terminal half-life-ranges from 2 to 7 h. Parenteral fentanyl is 75–100 times more potent than intravenous morphine (97). Its low molecular weight and relatively high lipophilicity render the molecule an excellent candidate for transdermal delivery.

1. Pharmacokinetics

Studies with transdermal (TTS) fentanyl applied over samples of cadaver skin of the same individual have shown that the transdermal absorption of fentanyl is essentially the same from the chest, abdomen, and thigh (98). The skin permeability constant of fentanyl is reported as 60- to 120-fold lower than the regional blood supply to a chest skin area. As a result, the permeation of fentanyl through the skin is a much slower process than is permitted by the local blood supply under normal physiological conditions (99). Bioavailability studies have shown that 92% of the dose delivered by TTS fentanyl reached the systemic circulation as unchanged fentanyl (100), confirming that metabolism during transdermal penetration can be neglected.

Multiple patches provide an opportunity to meet higher dosage requirements, although the absence of an immediate-release oral dosage form for breakthrough pain is a limiting factor in the use of fentanyl.

Because of the absorption process, fentanyl concentrations are hardly measurable until 2 h after application, and it takes 8- to 16-h latency until full clinical fentanyl effects are observed after the first TTS. Consequently, if effective fentanyl blood concentrations are required in the immediate postoperative period, TTS fentanyl should be applied 12–18 h before surgery (99). Each application is recommended for 72-h duration, and patients reach steady-state plasma concentrations within 12–24 h after the second application. An illustration of mean and group minimum and maximum plasma fentanyl concentrations achieved following five successive applications is presented in Fig. 12. Following TTS removal, serum fentanyl concentrations decline gradually, with an apparent half-life of 16 h (97). The slow decay is not a function of low clearance, but a slow washout from the cutaneous reservoir.

2. Clinical Studies

Zech et al. (96) reviewed the use of transdermal fentanyl in cancer pain management. In most of the trials reported the TTS was changed every 72 h, but the authors reported a 48-h change

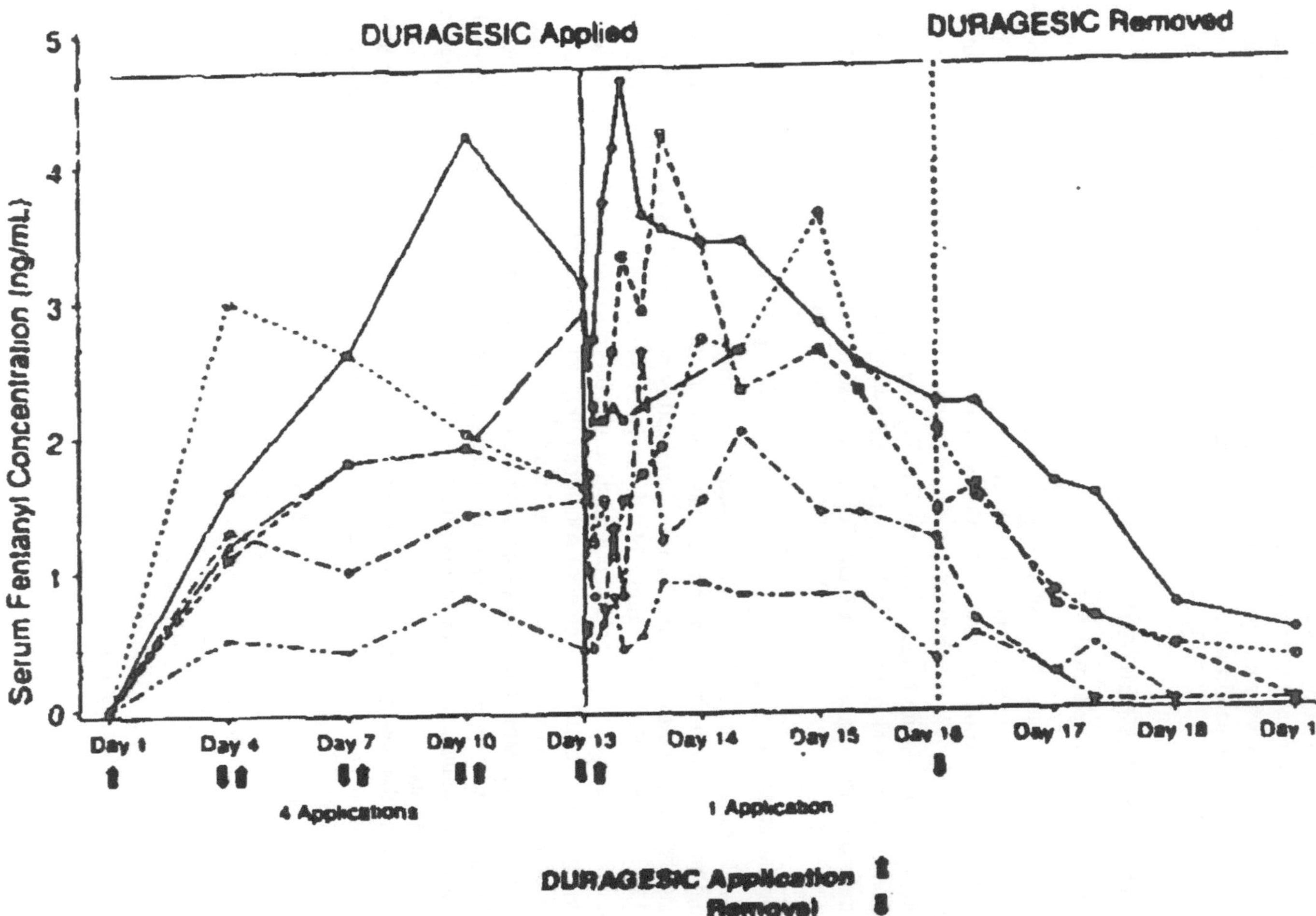

Figure 12 Serum fentanyl concentrations following five successive applications of Duragesic™ 100 µg/h. (From Ref. 101.)

in a substantial number of patients. More recently, TTS fentanyl appeared to be equally as effective as oral sustained-release morphine in cancer pain patients; however, the study design precluded a definitive conclusion for efficacy because it was an open-label study and because it lacked an internal measure of assay sensitivity (102). Fentanyl was associated with greater sleep disturbance and shorter sleep duration than morphine, but a lower incidence of constipation and daytime drowsiness. Quality of life assessments showed no difference between treatments.

Transdermal fentanyl has also been effective in the treatment of low-back pain (103), although its use in postoperative pain is limited by safety issues and by the slow onset of action.

VIII. DISCUSSION

There is still a desire among some clinical pharmacologists for a controlled-release opioid preparation with a flat plasma profile mimicking a constant intravenous infusion. The thinking behind this concept is the old one of a therapeutic window; however, it has not been proven with opioids in the treatment of pain. Each individual's pain is different and requires different doses and plasma concentrations for optimum relief of pain. Each patient has to be individually titrated to pain control and each dose increment has to be followed by an incremental increase of pain relief to establish opioid sensitivity and to successfully titrate to pain relief. For each compound, there is no universally applicable therapeutic window.

Although an early t_{max} after the first dose provides greater and longer duration pain relief compared with products with flatter profiles (27,39), there is a need for opioids other than morphine in the treatment of severe pain. Opioid substitution with, for example, hydromorphone has in many open trials and case reports provided increased analgesia and better tolerance in the 20% of cancer pain patients who do not respond to morphine. Controlled trials designed to confirm these studies are now ongoing in morphine-intolerant or insensitive patients.

There is increasing acceptance that patients with severe pain from chronic nonmalignant conditions have less than optimum pain management when treated with combination analgesics and NSAIDs alone. The majority of these patients are still in severe pain and will continue to remain so. The fear of addiction, abuse, tolerance, and untimely death often prevents both doctors, patients, and caregivers from prescribing and accepting morphine. Oxycodone has been studied in controlled trials in osteoarthritis, rheumatoid arthritis, and acute and chronic back pain. In all of these conditions, oxycodone has provided significant pain relief. Oxycodone also has the potential advantages of rapid onset and prolonged duration of pain relief, more predictable kinetic and clinical responses, and the absence of active metabolites.

The ongoing search for new treatments continues. Although the use of some newly developed drugs may well become established, the strong opioids will remain the bedrock of treatment.

REFERENCES

1. Kaiko RF, Grandy RP, Oshlack B, Pav J, Horodniak J, Thomas G, Ingber E, Goldenheim PD. The United States experience with oral controlled-release morphine (MS Contin tablets). Parts I and II. Review of nine dose titration studies and clinical pharmacology of 15-mg, 30-mg, 60-mg and 100-mg tablet strengths in normal subjects. Cancer 1989; 63:2348–2354.

2. Kaiko RF. The use of controlled-release opioids. In: Parris WCV, ed. Cancer Pain Management: Principles and Practice. Boston: Butterworth-Heinemann, 1997:69–90.
3. Thirlwell MP, Sloan PA, Maroun JA, Boos GJ, Besner J–G, Stewart JH, Mount BM. Pharmacokinetics and clinical efficacy of oral morphine solution and controlled-release morphine tablets in cancer patients. Cancer 1989; 63:2275–2283.
4. Kaiko RF, Lazarus H, Cronin C, Grandy RP, Thomas GB, Goldenheim PD. Controlled-release morphine bioavailability (MS Contin tablets) in the presence and absence of food. Hospice J 1990; 6:17–30.
5. Houston AC, Yeang Y. The influence of food on the pharmacokinetics of morphine from two controlled release preparations. Br J Clin Res 1991; 2:201–209.
6. Smith KJ, Miller AJ, McKellar J, Court M. Morphine at gramme doses: kinetics, dynamics and clinical need. Postgrad Med J 1991; 67(suppl 2):S55–S59.
7. Kaiko RF, Grandy RP, Reder RF, Goldenheim PD, Sackler RS. A bioequivalence study of oral controlled-release morphine using naltrexone blockade. J Clin Pharmacol 1995; 35:499–504.
8. Säwe J. Morphine and its 3- and 6-glucuronides in plasma and urine during chronic oral administration in cancer patients. In: Foley KM, Inturrisi CE, eds. Advances in Pain Research and Therapy. Vol 8. New York: Raven Press, 1986:45–55.
9. McQuay HJ, Carroll D, Faura CC, Gavaghan DJ, Hand CW, Moore RA. Oral morphine in cancer pain: influences on morphine and metabolite concentration. Clin Pharmacol Ther 1990; 48:236–244.
10. Warfield CA. Controlled-release morphine tablets in patients with chronic cancer pain: a narrative review of controlled clinical trials. Cancer 1998; 82:2299–2306.
11. Kaplan R, Conant M, Cundiff D, Maciewicz R, Ries K, Slagle S, Slywka J, Buckley B. Sustained-release morphine sulfate in the management of pain associated with acquired immune deficiency syndrome. J Pain Sympt Manage 1996; 12:150–160.
12. Smith KJ, Leslie ST, Miller AJ, Sinclair KA, Smith AT. The pharmacokinetics of morphine from MST Continus suspension. 5th Congress of the European Association for Palliative Care. London, Sept 10–13, 1997:S37; abstr P-041.
13. Smith KJ, McKellar J, Sinclair KA, Smith AT, Yeang YY. The influence of food on the pharmacokinetics of morphine from MST Continus suspension. 7th World Congress on Pain. Paris, Aug 22–27, 1993:382; abstr 1004.
14. Jacox A, Carr DB, Payne R, Berde CB, Brietbart W, Cain JM, Chapman CR, Cleeland CS, Ferrell BR, Finley RS, Hester NO, Hill CS Jr, Leak WD, Lipman AG, Logan CL, McGarvey CL, Miaskowski CA, Mulder DS, Paice JA, Shapiro BS, Silberstein EB, Smith RS, Stover J, Tsou CV, Vecchiarelli L, Weissman DE. Management of Cancer Pain. Clinical Practice Guideline No. 9. Rockville, Md: Agency for Health Care Policy and Research, U. S. Department of Health and Human Services, Public Health Service, March 1994. AHCPR Publication No. 94-0592.
15. Practice guidelines for cancer pain management: a report by the American Society of Anesthesiologists Task Force on Pain Management, Cancer Pain Section. Anesthesiology 1996; 84:1243–1257.
16. Babul N, Darke AC, Anslow JA, Krishnamurthy TN. Pharmacokinetics of two novel rectal controlled-release morphine formulations. J Pain Sympt Manage 1992; 7:400–405.
17. Darke A, Moulin D, Provencher L, Laberge F, Harsanyi Z, Babul N. Efficacy, safety and pharmacokinetics of controlled release morphine suppositories and tablets in cancer pain. Clin Pharmacol Ther 1995; 57:165; abstr PII-6.
18. Babul N, Provencher L, Laberge F, Harsanyi Z, Moulin D. Comparative efficacy and safety of controlled-release morphine suppositories and tablets in cancer pain. J Clin Pharmacol 1998; 38: 74–81.
19. Bruera E, Belzile M, Pituskin E, Ford I, Harsanyi Z, Darke A. Efficacy and safety of morphine sulfate controlled-release suppositories (MS-CRS) administered once daily and twice daily for severe cancer pain. J Palliat Care 1998; 14:117.
20. Maccarrone C, West RJ, Broomhead AF, Hodsman GP. Single dose pharmacokinetics of Kapanol, a new oral sustained-release morphine formulation. Drug Invest 1994; 7:262–274.
21. Kaiko R, Weingarten B, Comack I, Rotshteyn Y, Oshlack B. Influence of pH and food on dissolution

and plasma morphine with sustained-release morphine (Kapanol/Kadian). 8th World Congress on Pain, Vancouver, BC, Aug 17–22, 1996:287; abstr 229.

22. Kaiko RF. The effect of food intake on the pharmacokinetics of sustained-release morphine sulfate capsules. Clin Ther 1997; 19:296–303.
23. Gourlay GK, Plummer JL, Cherry DA, Onley MM. A comparison of Kapanol (a new sustained-release morphine formulation), MST Continus, and morphine solution in cancer patients: pharmacokinetic aspects of morphine and morphine metabolites. In: Gebhart GF, Hammond DL, Jensen TS, eds. Progress in Pain Research and Management. Vol 2. Proceedings of the 7th World Congress on Pain. Seattle: IASP Press, 1994:631–643.
24. Gourlay GK, Cherry DA, Onley MM, Tordoff SG, Conn DA, Hood GM, Plummer JL. Pharmacokinetics and pharmacodynamics of twenty-four-hourly Kapanol compared to twelve-hourly MS Contin in the treatment of severe cancer pain. Pain 1997; 69:295–302.
25. Faulding Laboratories. Kadian. In: Physicians' Desk Reference. 53rd ed. Montvale, NJ: Medical Economics, 1999:995–999.
26. Broomhead A, West R, Eglinton L, Jones M, Bubner R, Sienko D, Knox, K. Comparative single-dose pharmacokinetics of sustained-release and modified-release morphine sulfate capsules under fed and fasting conditions. Clin Drug Invest 1997; 13:162–170.
27. Brown CR, Moodie JE, Bisley–Phillips EJ. Analgesic pharmacodynamics of oral morphine sulfate controlled-release tablets (MS Contin, M) and sustained-release capsules (Kadian/Kapanol, K). 15th Annual Scientific Meeting of the American Pain Society, Washington, DC, Nov 14–17, 1996:A-67; abstr 676.
28. Kerr RO. Clinical experience with 12–24 hourly Kapanol. GlaxoWellcome Symposium, Pain Control—Current Practice and New Developments. Amsterdam, Oct 28, 1995.
29. Modell W, Houde RW. Factors influencing clinical evaluation of drugs. JAMA 1958; 167:2190–2199.
30. Cooper SA. Commentary. Single-dose analgesic studies: the upside and downside of assay sensitivity. In: Max MB, Portenoy RK, Laska EM, eds. Advances in Pain Research and Therapy. Vol 18. New York: Raven Press, 1991:117–124.
31. US Food and Drug Administration. Guideline for the Clinical Evaluation of Analgesic Drugs. Rockville, MD: US Department of Health and Human Services, 1992.
32. Drake J, Kirkpatrick CT, Aliyar CA, Crawford FE, Gibson P, Horth CE. Effect of food on the comparative pharmacokinetics of modified-release morphine tablet formulations: Oramorph SR and MST Continus. Br J Clin Pharmacol 1996; 41:417–420.
33. Miller AJ, Smith KJ. Effect of food on the comparative pharmacokinetics of modified-release morphine tablet formulations, Oramorph SR and MST Continus. Br J Clin Pharmacol 1996; 42: 645.
34. Drake J, Horth CE, Crawford FE. Effect of food on the comparative pharmacokinetics of modified-release morphine tablet formulations, Oramorph SR and MST Continus: a reply. Br J Clin Pharmacol 1996; 42:646–647.
35. Hunt TL, Kaiko RF. Comparison of the pharmacokinetic profiles of two oral controlled-release morphine formulations in healthy young adults. Clin Ther 1991; 13:482–488.
36. Kaiko R, Grandy R, Thomas G, Goldenheim P. A single-dose study of the effect of food ingestion and timing of dose administration on the pharmacokinetic profile of 30-mg sustained-release morphine sulfate tablets. Curr Ther Res 1990; 47:869–878.
37. Bass J, Shepard KV, Lee JW, Hulse J. An evaluation of the effect of food on the oral bioavailability of sustained-release morphine sulfate tablets (Oramorph SR) after multiple doses. J Clin Pharmacol 1992; 32:1003–1007.
38. Approved Drug Products with Therapeutic Equivalence Evaluations. 19th ed. Rockville, MD: U.S. Dept of Health and Human Services, Food and Drug Administration, 1999:3-235–3-236.
39. Bloomfield SS, Cissell GB, Mitchel J, Barden TP, Kaiko RF, Fitzmartin RD, Grandy RP, Komorowski J, Goldenheim PD. Analgesic efficacy and potency of two oral controlled-release morphine preparations. Clin Pharmacol Ther 1993; 53:469–478.
40. Cooper SA, Fitzmartin R, Slywka J, Buckley BJ, Kaiko R, Goldenheim PD, Mooar P, Witte JF,

Hersh EV. Analgesic efficacy and safety of two oral controlled-release morphine preparations in orthopedic postoperative pain. Adv Ther 1994; 11:213–227.
41. Sherman LM. The use of sustained-release morphine in a hospice setting. Pharmatherapeutica 1987; 5:99–102.
42. Smith KJ, Miller AJ, Sinclair KA, Smith AT. A novel once-daily morphine preparation: pharmacokinetic development. 8th World Congress on Pain, Vancouver, BC, Aug 17–22, 1996:284–285; abstr 221.
43. Smith KJ, Leslie ST, Miller AJ, Sinclair KA, Smith AT. MXL capsules: pharmacokinetics of glucuronide metabolites. 5th Congress of the European Association for Palliative Care. London, Sept 10–13, 1997:S38; abstr P-042.
44. O'Brien T, Mortimer PG, McDonald CJ, Miller AJ. A randomized crossover study comparing the efficacy and tolerability of a novel once-daily morphine preparation (MXL capsules) with MST Continus tablets in cancer patients with severe pain. Palliat Med 1997; 11:475–482.
45. Portenoy RK, Foley KN, Inturrisi CE. The nature of opioid responsiveness and its implications for neuropathic pain: new hypotheses derived from studies of opioid infusions. Pain 1990; 43:273–286.
46. Galer BS, Coyle N, Pasternak GW, Portenoy RK. Individual variability in the response to different opioids: report of five cases. Pain 1992; 49:87–91.
47. Smith KJ, Leslie ST, Miller AJ, Sinclair KA, Smith AT. The pharmacokinetics of hydromorphone from Palladone SR capsules. 5th Congress of the European Association for Palliative Care. London Sept 10–13, 1997:S85; abstr P-256.
48. Hagen N, Thirwell MP, Dhaliwal HS, Babul N, Harsanyi Z, Darke AC. Steady-state pharmacokinetics of hydromorphone and hydromorphone-3-glucuronide in cancer patients after immediate and controlled-release hydromorphone. J Clin Pharmacol 1995; 35:37–44.
49. Hays H, Hagen N, Thirlwell M, Dhaliwal H, Babul N, Harsanyi Z, Darke AC. Comparative clinical efficacy and safety of immediate release and controlled release hydromorphone for chronic severe cancer pain. Cancer 1994; 74:1808–1816.
50. Ross FB, Smith MT. The intrinsic antinociceptive effects of oxycodone appear to be κ-opioid receptor mediated. Pain 1997; 73:151–157.
51. Kaiko R, Lacouture P, Hopf K, Brown J, Goldenheim PD. Analgesic onset and potency of oral controlled-release (CR) oxycodone and CR morphine. Clin Pharmacol Ther 1996; 59:130; abstr PI-4.
52. Curtis GB, Johnson GH, Clark P, Taylor R, Brown J, O'Callaghan R, Shi M, Lacouture PG. Relative potency of controlled-release oxycodone and controlled-release morphine in a postoperative pain model. Eur J Clin Pharmacol 1999; 55:425–429.
53. Mandema JW, Kaiko RF, Oshlack B, Reder RF, Stanski DR. Characterization and validation of a pharmacokinetic model for controlled-release oxycodone. Br J Clin Pharmacol 1996; 42:747–756.
54. Colucci RD, Swanton RE, Thomas GB, Kaiko RF. Retrospective analysis of relative variability of controlled-release oxycodone and morphine absorption in normal volunteers. J Clin Pharmacol 1998; 38:875; abstr 596.
55. Reder RF, Oshlack B, Miotto JB, Benziger DP, Kaiko RF. Steady-state bioavailability of controlled-release oxycodone in normal subjects. Clin Ther 1996; 18:95–105.
56. Heiskanen T, Olkkola KT, Kalso E. Effect of blocking CYP2D6 on the pharmacokinetics and pharmacodynamics of oxycodone. Clin Pharmacol Ther 1998; 64:603–611.
57. Kaiko RF, Benziger DP, Fitzmartin RD, Burke BE, Reder RF, Goldenheim PD. Pharmacokinetics–pharmacodynamic relationships of controlled-release oxycodone. Clin Pharmacol Ther 1996; 59:52–61.
58. Benziger DP, Levy SA, Fitzmartin RD, Reder RF. Dose proportionality of 10, 20, and 40 mg controlled-release oxycodone hydrochloride tablets (OxyContin). Pharmacotherapy 1995; 15:391; abstr 188.
59. Benziger DP, Miotto J, Grandy RP, Thomas GB, Swanton RE, Fitzmartin R. A pharmacokinetic/pharmacodynamic study of controlled-release oxycodone. J Pain Sympt Manage 1997; 13:75–82.
60. Kaiko R, Lockhart E, Grandy R, Reder R. Bioequivalency of an 80 mg controlled release oxycodone

(OxyContin) tablet compared to two 40 mg CR oxycodone tablets. 5th Congress of the European Association for Palliative Care. London, Sept 10–13, 1997:S33; abstr P-019.

61. Benziger DP, Kaiko RF, Miotto JB, Fitzmartin RD, Reder RF, Chasin M. Differential effects of food on the bioavailability of controlled-release oxycodone tablets and immediate-release oxycodone solution. J Pharm Sci 1996; 85:407–410.
62. Purdue Pharma L.P. OxyContin. In: Physicians' Desk Reference. 53rd ed. Montvale, NJ: Medical Economics, 1999:2569–2574.
63. Benziger DP, Cheng C, Miotto J, Grandy R. Comparative pharmacokinetics of controlled-release oxycodone (OxyContin) in special populations. 8th World Congress on Pain. Vancouver, BC, Aug 17–22, 1996:285; abstr 223.
64. Heiskanen T, Kalso E. Controlled-release oxycodone and morphine in cancer-related pain. Pain 1997; 73:37–45.
65. Hagen NA, Babul N. Comparative clinical efficacy and safety of a novel controlled-release oxycodone formulation and controlled-release hydromorphone in the treatment of cancer pain. Cancer 1997; 79:1428–1437.
66. Stambaugh JE, Reder RF, Stambaugh M, Davis M. Double-blind, randomized, two-period crossover efficacy and pharmacokinetic comparison of immediate-release oxycodone (IR) and controlled-release oxycodone (CR) in cancer patients with pain. Clin Pharmacol Ther 1997; 61:197; abstr PIII-13.
67. Allende-Perez SR, Iwan T, Shi M, Lockhart E. Treatment of cancer pain with q12h oral controlled-release oxycodone OxyContin (CR Oxy). 17th International Cancer Congress. Rio de Janeiro, Aug 23–28, 1998:156; abstr 664.
68. Bruera E, Belzile M, Pituskin E, Fainsinger R, Darke A, Harsanyi Z, Babul N, Ford I. Randomized, double-blind, cross-over trial comparing safety and efficacy of oral controlled-release oxycodone with controlled-release morphine in patients with cancer pain. J Clin Oncol 1998; 16:3222–3229.
69. Kaplan R, Parris WC-V, Citron ML, Zhukovsky DR, Reder RF, Buckley BJ, Kaiko RF. Comparison of controlled-release and immediate-release oxycodone tablets in patients with cancer pain. J Clin Oncol 1998; 16:3230–3237.
70. Mucci–LoRusso P, Berman BS, Silberstein PT, Citron ML, Bressler L, Weinstein SM, Kaiko RF, Buckley BJ, Reder RF. Controlled-release oxycodone compared with controlled-release morphine in the treatment of cancer pain: a randomized, double-blind, parallel-group study. Eur J Pain 1998; 2:239–249.
71. Parris WC–V, Johnson BW Jr, Croghan MK, Moore MR, Khojasteh A, Reder RF, Kaiko RF, Buckley BJ. The use of controlled-release oxycodone for the treatment of chronic cancer pain: a randomized, double-blind study. J Pain Sympt Manage 1998; 16:205–211.
72. Citron ML, Kaplan R, Parris WC–V, Croghan MK, Herbst LH, Rosenbluth RJ, Reder RF, Slagle NS, Buckley BJ, Kaiko RF. Long-term administration of controlled-release oxycodone tablets for the treatment of cancer pain. Cancer Invest 1998; 16:562–571.
73. Reder RF, Buckley B. Open-label clinical use study of controlled-release (CR) oxycodone tablets (OxyContin) administered orally every 12 hours for the management of pain. 17th Annual Scientific Meeting of the American Pain Society. San Diego, CA, Nov 5–8, 1998:129; abstr 723.
74. Buckley B, Reder RF. Controlled-release (CR) oxycodone tablets (OxyContin) administered orally every 12 hours: patients with neuropathic pain. 17th Annual Scientific Meeting of the American Pain Society. San Diego, CA, Nov 5–8, 1998:130; abstr 725.
75. Roth S, Burch F, Fleischmann R, Dietz F, Rutstein J, Iwan T, Kaiko R, Lacouture P. The effect of controlled-release (CR) oxycodone on pain intensity and activities in patients with pain secondary to osteoarthritis. 14th Annual Scientific Meeting of the American Pain Society. Los Angeles, CA, Nov 9–12, 1995:A-147; abstr 95884.
76. Roth S, Iwan T, Hou Y, Fitzmartin R, Kaiko R, Lacouture PG. Long term opioid administration: stable doses and pain control with reduction in side effects overtime. 8th World Congress on Pain. Vancouver, BC, Aug 17–22, 1996:53; abstr 168.
77. Caldwell JR, Hale ME, Boyd RE, Hague JM, Iwan T, Shi M, Lacouture PG. Treatment of osteoar-

thritis pain with controlled release oxycodone or fixed combination oxycodone plus acetaminophen added to nonsteroidal antiinflammatory drugs: a double blind, randomized, multicenter, placebo controlled trial. J Rheumatol 1999; 26:862–869.
78. Fleischmann R, Iwan T, Kaiko R, Lacouture PG. Chronic low back pain (LBP) treatment with controlled-release (CR) and immediate-release (IR) oxycodone. 8th World Congress on Pain. Vancouver, BC, Aug 17–22, 1996:493; abstr 184.
79. Watson CPN, Babul N. Efficacy of oxycodone in neuropathic pain: a randomized trial in postherpetic neuralgia. Neurology 1998; 50:1837–1841.
80. Sunshine A, Olson NZ, Colon A, Rivera J, Kaiko RF, Fitzmartin RD, Reder RF, Goldenheim PD. Analgesic efficacy of controlled release oxycodone in postoperative pain. J Clin Pharmacol 1996; 36:595–603.
81. Ginsberg B, Sinatra R, Crews J, Hord A, Adler L, Lockhart E. Conversion from IV PCA morphine to oral controlled release oxycodone (OxyContin) for post-operative pain management. Anesth Analg 1998; 86:S271.
82. Narcessian E, Cheville A, Chen A. OxyContin following unilateral total knee arthroplasty: a double-blind randomized controlled trial. 17th Annual Scientific Meeting of the American Pain Society. San Diego, CA, Nov 5–8, 1998:127; abstr 719.
83. Reuben SS, Connelly NR, Maciolek H. Postoperative analgesia with controlled-release oxycodone for outpatient anterior cruciate ligament surgery. Anesth Analg 1999; 88:1286–1291.
84. Kalso E, Vainio A. Morphine and oxycodone hydrochloride in the management of cancer pain. Clin Pharmacol Ther 1990; 47:639–646.
85. Maddocks I, Somogyi A, Abbott F, Hayball P, Parker D. Attenuation of morphine-induced delirium in palliative care by substitution with infusion of oxycodone. J Pain Sympt Manage 1996; 12:182–189.
86. Cramond TR, Ross FB, Smith MT. Oxymorphone-3-glucuronide has no intrinsic antinociceptive effects in a manner analogous to morphine-3-glucuronide. 8th World Congress on Pain. Vancouver, BC, Aug 17–22, 1996:395–396; abstr 226.
87. Salzman RT, Roberts MS, Wild J, Fabian C, Reder RF, Goldenheim PD. Can a controlled-release oral dose form of oxycodone be used as readily as an immediate-release form for the purpose of titrating to stable pain control? J Pain Sympt Manage 1999; 18:271–279.
88. Reder R, Lacouture P, Kaiko R, Fitzmartin R, Goldenheim P. Ease of titration to stable pain control in chronic pain patients with controlled-release oral oxycodone (OxyContin) tablets. 8th World Congress on Pain. Vancouver, BC, Aug 17–22, 1996:53–54; abstr 171.
89. Reder RF, Fitzmartin RD. Physician survey of attitudes about controlled-release oxycodone (OXYCR). 14th Annual Scientific Meeting of the American Pain Society. Los Angeles, CA, Nov 9–12, 1995:A-144; abstr 95878.
90. McQuay HJ. Opioids in chronic pain. Br J Anaesth 1989; 63:213–226.
91. Cancer Pain Relief. Geneva: World Health Organization, 1986.
92. Band CJ, Band PR, Deschamps M, Besner J–G, Coldman AJ. Human pharmacokinetic study of immediate-release (codeine phosphate) and sustained-release (codeine Contin) codeine. J Clin Pharmacol 1994; 34:938–943.
93. Chary S, Goughnour BR, Moulin DE, Thorpe WR, Harsanyi Z, Darke AC. The dose–response relationship of controlled-release codeine (Codeine Contin) in chronic cancer pain. J Pain Symptom Manage 1994; 9:363–371.
94. Dhaliwal HS, Sloan P, Arkinstall WW, Thirlwell MP, Babul N, Harsanyi Z, Darke AC. Randomized evaluation of controlled-release codeine and placebo in chronic cancer pain. J Pain Symptom Manage 1995; 10:612–623.
95. Arkinstall W, Sandler A, Goughnour B, Babul N, Harsanyi Z, Darke AC. Efficacy of controlled-release codeine in chronic non-malignant pain: a randomized, placebo-controlled clinical trial. Pain 1995; 62:169–178.
96. Zech DFJ, Lehmann KA, Grond S. Transdermal (TTS) fentanyl in cancer pain management. Prog Palliat Care 1994; 2:37–42.
97. Gourlay GK, Mather LE. Postoperative pain management with TTS fentanyl: pharmacokinetics and

pharmacodynamics. In: Lehmann KA, Zech D, eds. Transdermal Fentanyl. Heidelberg: Springer, 1991:119–140.

98. Roy SD, Flynn GL. Transdermal delivery of narcotic analgesics: pH, anatomical and subject influences of cutaneous permeability of fentanyl and sufentanil. Pharm Res 1990; 7:842–847.
99. Lehmann KA, Zech D. Transdermal fentanyl: clinical pharmacology. J Pain Sympt Manage 1992; 7:S8–16.
100. Varvel JR, Shafer SL, Hwang SS, Coen PA, Stanski DR. Absorption characteristics of transdermally administered fentanyl. Anesthesiology 1989; 70:928–934.
101. Janssen Pharmaceutica, Inc. Duragesic. In: Physicians' Desk Reference. 53rd ed. Montvale, NJ: Medical Economics, 1998:1297–1301.
102. Ahmedzai S, Brooks D. Transdermal fentanyl versus sustained-release oral morphine in cancer pain: preference, efficacy and quality of life. The TTS-Fentanyl Comparative Trial Group. J Pain Sympt Manage 1997; 13:254–261.
103. Simpson RK Jr, Edmondson EA, Constant CF, Collier C. Transdermal fentanyl as treatment for chronic low back pain. J Pain Sympt Manage 1997; 14:218–224.

36

NMDA-Receptor Antagonists as Enhancers of Analgesic Activity

The MorphiDex™ Morphine–Dextromethorphan Combination

Frank S. Caruso
Caruso Pharmaceutical Consultation Services, Cape May, New Jersey, U.S.A.

Donald D. Price
University of Florida, Gainesville, Florida, U.S.A.

David J. Mayer*
Medical College of Virginia, Richmond, Virginia, U.S.A. (retired)

Jianren Mao
MGH Pain Center, Massachusetts General Hospital, and Harvard Medical School, Boston, Massachusetts, U.S.A.

Eileen M. Shalhoub
Johnson & Johnson Pharmaceutical Research and Development, Titusville, New Jersey, U.S.A.

Ronald Goldblum
Elan Pharmaceuticals, San Diego, California, U.S.A.

I. OVERVIEW OF *N*-METHYL-D-ASPARTATE (NMDA) RECEPTOR MECHANISMS OF PAIN

Dorsal neurons are the origin of ascending pathways subserving "normal" pain and pathophysiological pain. Impulses in primary nociceptive afferents evoke brief high-intensity excitation followed by a lower-intensity, prolonged impulse discharge in dorsal horn nociceptive neurons (1). Furthermore, continuous input over C polymodal nociceptive afferents, but not other types of nociceptive afferents, additionally evokes temporal summation by activation of NMDA-receptors (2,3). These mechanisms are considered to provide part of the basis for centrally mediated hyperalgesia that occurs in persistent pain states, such as inflammatory pain that follows tissue injury. This hyperalgesia is a normal consequence of injury and subsides with healing of the injured tissue. Generally, similar central mechanisms of hyperalgesia also occur with nerve injury (4,5). Temporal summation of C-afferent-evoked responses of dorsal horn nocicep-

* Retired.

tive neurons is likely to be mediated by the release of glutamate–aspartate and their activation of NMDA-receptors, leading to prolonged depolarizations (3,6).

Studies using in vitro preparations have shown that NMDA-receptor antagonists powerfully block prolonged depolarizations evoked in dorsal horn neurons (3,6) and block the temporal summation evoked by electrical stimulation of C afferents, without reducing the responses of these same neurons to A fiber stimulation (1–3,6). Temporal summation of C afferent-evoked responses in dorsal horn neurons reflects some of the mechanisms underlying centrally mediated hyperalgesias that occur after nerve injury or after inflammation (1–6). Both phenomena involve the same NMDA-receptor mechanism and at least some of the same intracellular consequences of NMDA-receptor activation. Temporal summation has long been considered a central neural mechanism that has a critical role in pathophysiological pain.

The direct participation of temporal summation of C-fiber-mediated responses of dorsal horn nociceptive neurons in normal pain is shown in human psychophysical experiments on the "second-pain" response. Both second-pain and C-afferent-evoked impulse discharges of dorsal horn nociceptive neurons progressively increase in magnitude if the stimulus that activates the C nociceptive afferents occurs at a frequency greater than once every 3 s (1,6,7). If the same NMDA-receptor mechanism underlies both electrophysiological and psychophysical expressions of slow temporal summation, then both phenomena should be antagonized by NMDA-receptor antagonists. In a direct test of this hypothesis, oral doses of dextromethorphan (DM), an NMDA-receptor antagonist, and vehicle control were given on a double-blind basis to healthy human subjects who rated intensities of first and second pain in response to repeated brief stimuli (7). DM doses of 30 and 45 mg, but not 15 mg, were effective in attenuating temporal summation of second pain, a psychophysical correlate of temporal summation of C-afferent-mediated responses of dorsal horn nociceptive neurons, termed windup. These results further confirm temporal summation of second pain as a psychophysical correlate of windup by providing evidence that DM selectively reduces temporal summation of second pain, as has been shown for windup.

Windup is now considered to be related to central mechanisms of hyperalgesia (1,4,6). Similar to what occurs following tissue injury, tonic input from nociceptive C afferents is thought to lead to central sensitization of dorsal horn neurons by means of a windup mechanism (1,4,6). Moreover, slow temporal summation, electrophysiological and behavioral indices of hyperalgesia can be blocked by NMDA-receptor antagonists, and windup itself can be enhanced by tissue injury-evoked hyperalgesia (2,3). To a certain extent, windup has come to serve as a predictive model for pharmacological and other manipulations that may be used to modulate central mechanisms of hyperalgesia (1–4).

II. NMDA-RECEPTOR MECHANISMS OF HYPERALGESIA AND NARCOTIC TOLERANCE–DEPENDENCE

Within the last few years, several studies have directly or indirectly indicated that narcotic tolerance and narcotic-induced hyperalgesia involve some of the same NMDA-receptor mechanisms that occur during inflammatory and neuropathic pain (6,8). Of relevant interest is that NMDA-receptor activation plays a critically important role in tolerance to the analgesic effects of narcotics, dependence on narcotics, and narcotic-induced thermal hyperalgesia (6). The prevention of analgesic tolerance and hyperalgesia by NMDA-receptor antagonists suggests a role for excitatory amino acids in these phenomena. The site of the NMDA-receptor action is likely within the spinal cord dorsal horn (1,6). Taken together, data on neurogenic and inflammatory thermal hyperalgesia and morphine tolerance–dependence suggest that central activation of

NMDA-receptors is strategically involved in both thermal hyperalgesia and in the development of narcotic tolerance and dependence.

Thermal hyperalgesia associated with narcotic tolerance can also be potently reversed by intrathecal treatment with dizocilpine (MK 801; a prototype NMDA-receptor antagonist), indicating that NMDA-receptors are critical for the expression of thermal hyperalgesia in morphine-tolerant rats (8). Thermal hyperalgesia develops in association with the development of morphine tolerance and dependence, and NMDA-receptor antagonists potently prevent both the development of morphine tolerance and thermal hyperalgesia. Therefore, it is very likely that the development of morphine tolerance or dependence and the associated thermal hyperalgesia may involve a common NMDA-receptor mechanism.

Protein kinase C (PKC) also is involved in the development of morphine tolerance and dependence in rats. Spinal cord levels of membrane-bound PKC (the translocated form of PKC) increase significantly, specifically within the superficial laminae of the dorsal horn (laminae I-II), following the development of morphine tolerance and dependence, and GM1 ganglioside potently attenuates both the increase in membrane-bound PKC and the development of tolerance to the analgesic effect of morphine (9). In addition, the GM1 ganglioside also effectively prevents the development of thermal hyperalgesia associated with the development of morphine tolerance and dependence (9). Similarly, behavioral studies have indicated that nitric oxide (NO) is involved in thermal hyperalgesia induced by peripheral nerve injury or intrathecal NMDA administration. NO is involved in the development of morphine tolerance and dependence (6). Taken together, these data indicate that intracellular PKC and NO may mediate neurogenic and inflammatory thermal hyperalgesia and the development of narcotic tolerance and dependence, both of which are associated with NMDA-receptor activation. Thus, converging lines of evidence strongly suggest that NMDA-receptor–mediated intracellular PKC and NO changes may be associated with thermal hyperalgesia that occurs following the development of narcotic tolerance and dependence, as well as with hyperalgesia following nerve injury.

Several lines of research from different laboratories have demonstrated that postsynaptic opioid mu (μ)-receptor occupation by an exogenous ligand, such as morphine, may initiate the activation of PKC (6). Activation of PKC then increases the sensitivity of the NMDA-receptor by the same mechanisms that occur during persistent pain states. At the same time, activated PKC may uncouple the G protein associated with the opioid μ-receptor or modulate the μ-activated potassium channel. In either case, the net result is reduced responsiveness of the μ-receptor to an exogenous opioid and, hence, the development of tolerance. The two major components of this mechanism are a positive-feedback loop, wherein the NMDA-receptor becomes progressively sensitized as a result of repeated opioid administration, and a negative-feedback loop, wherein activation of PKC reduces the sensitivity of the μ-receptor.

The model makes the following predictions: (1) hyperalgesia should be associated with opioid tolerance, and this hyperalgesia should be blocked by an NMDA-receptor antagonist; (2) opioid tolerance should be blocked by an NMDA-receptor antagonist to some extent; (3) a preexisting hyperalgesic state, such as that brought about by chronic constrictive nerve injury, should be associated with increased resistance to the analgesic effects of morphine (i.e., "tolerance"). Laboratory results support these predictions and have several clinical implications (6). There is experimental support for the long-held impressions that patients with neuropathic pain are resistant to opioid analgesics and that hyperalgesia and tolerance develop in some patients who have taken narcotic analgesics for extended periods. These problems may be prevented by the coadministration of nontoxic NMDA-receptor antagonists with opioids. Combining NMDA-receptor antagonists with opioid, and even nonopioid analgesics, may be a way of increasing their analgesic potency, in addition to preventing tolerance and dependence. Nonclinical animal studies demonstrate the practicality of the combined administration of nontoxic NMDA-receptor antagonists with various types of analgesic drugs.

III. USE OF DEXTROMETHORPHAN TO ENHANCE MORPHINE SULFATE ANALGESIA AND PREVENT MORPHINE SULFATE TOLERANCE

Several key points were demonstrated in a study specifically designed to evaluate the practical feasibility of the combined oral administration of morphine sulfate (MS) and dextromethorphan (DM), an NMDA-receptor antagonist. DM prevented the development of tolerance to the antinociceptive effects of MS (15, 24, or 32 mg/kg) (10) and attenuated signs of naloxone-precipitated physical dependence on morphine in rats. A range of ratios of MS to DM (2:1, 1:1, and 1:2) was effective. An important feature of this DM-mediated prevention of the development of morphine tolerance is that selective ratios of MS to DM and not absolute DM amount seemed effective. The results indicate a therapeutic window for potential clinical utility of this MS–DM-combination treatment regimen. Finally, DM increased the antinociceptive effects of MS even with a single administration of an MS–DM (1:1) combination. These results indicate that oral treatment that combines DM with opioid analgesics may be a powerful approach for simultaneously preventing opioid tolerance and dependence and enhancing analgesia in humans.

A critical feature of this study was the demonstration that DM increased the antinociceptive effects of low doses of MS. This result is similar to that obtained using 48-h delivery of MS and DM through a subcutaneous osmotic pump (11). Although the highest DM dose (64 mg/kg) alone used in the experiments produced some antinociception by itself, no changes in baseline tail-flick latencies were observed in rats receiving lower doses (30 or 15 mg/kg) of DM alone. These results, taken together, indicate that greater antinociception resulting from MS–DM combinations is not simply an additive effect of MS and DM. Clinically, this would mean that DM not only might be able to prevent morphine tolerance when coadministered with MS, but also could enhance morphine analgesia, thereby possibly reducing the dose of opioid analgesics required for pain relief. DM potently facilitates morphine analgesia, at least in part by preventing or reversing tolerance (6). Oral DM also facilitates analgesia produced by other opioid analgesics (Mao J, Price DD, Caruso FJ, Mayer DJ, unpublished observations), suggesting the possibility of other combination analgesic products.

IV. OVERVIEW OF MORPHIDEX CLINICAL STUDIES

Based on the pooled results of two dose-response studies over the 2:1 to 1:2 MS–DM range (60:30, 60:60, and 60:120 mg), the 1:1 ratio was chosen for clinical development as providing the best enhancement of analgesia with the least exposure to DM (Fig. 1). The clinical program evaluating the safety and efficacy of MorphiDex capsules, a 1:1 ratio combination product of morphine sulfate, USP (MS) and dextromethorphan hydrobromide, USP (DM), is summarized in the following.

A. Controlled, Single-Dose, Postsurgical Pain Studies

The clinical program to date included six single-dose, double-blind, placebo-controlled studies in patients with moderate-to-severe postsurgical pain which compared treatment with MorphiDex capsules, morphine alone, or dextromethorphan alone.

Categorical scales were used to evaluate pain relief (0, none; 1, a little; 2, some; 3, a lot;

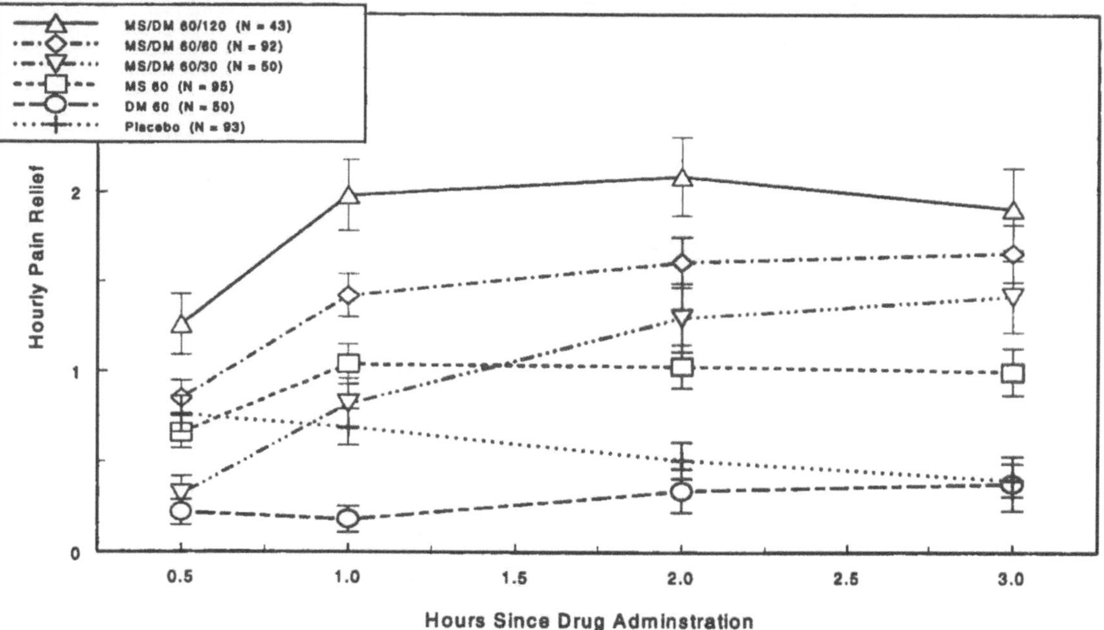

Figure 1 Pain relief over time for single doses of MS/DM 2:1, 1:1, and 1:2 ratios, MS, DM, and placebo; pool of two dental postsurgical pain studies: MS, morphine sulfate, USP; DM, dextromethorphan hydrobromide, USP; N, number of subjects; dosages are in milligrams.

4, complete) and pain intensity (0, none; 1, mild; 2, moderate; 3, severe). Pain intensity was also evaluated on a 100-mm visual–analog scale (VAS) from none to worst pain. The primary efficacy variables total pain relief (TOTPAR) sum of pain intensity differences (SPID), and VAS SPID (where measured) were calculated as area under the curve (AUC) over the entire postdose observation interval. Additional primary efficacy measures included time to meaningful pain relief (timed by means of a stopwatch), percentage of patients who achieved meaningful pain relief, time to remedication, and percentage of patients who remedicated. Safety was evaluated by the patient-reported incidence of adverse experiences.

1. Dental Postsurgical Pain

Although morphine is not customarily used in dental postoperative pain, this clinical model of analgesia has become a satisfactory predictor of the pain relief qualities of many types of opioid and nonopioid analgesics.

Efficacy data were pooled for three single-dose, double-blind, parallel-group studies that evaluated MorphiDex 60:60 mg (144 patients), MS 60 mg (146 patients), DM 60 mg (100 patients), and placebo (145 patients) in patients with moderate-to-severe pain following the surgical extraction of one or more impacted third molars. Evaluations were made over a 6- or 8-h interval after treatment. The percentage of possible total pain relief achieved (% TOTPAR; Fig. 2) and the percentage of possible sum of the pain intensity difference (% SPID) were significantly greater for MorphiDex 60:60 mg than for MS 60 mg ($p = 0.006$ and 0.003, respectively). The time to onset of meaningful relief was significantly shorter (better) for MorphiDex 60:60 mg than for MS 60 mg, whereas the time to use of rescue medication was significantly longer (better) ($p = 0.04$ and 0.02, respectively). The duration of action of MorphiDex 60:60

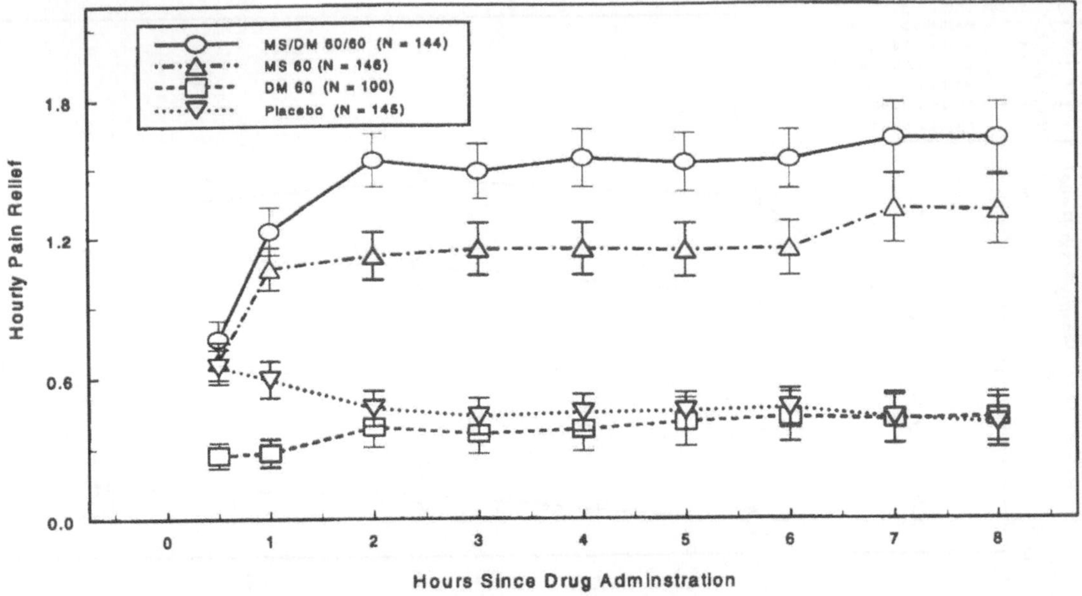

Figure 2 Pain relief over time for single doses of MorphiDex (MS/DM 1:1 ratio), MS, DM, and placebo; pool of three dental postsurgical pain studies: MS, morphine sulfate, USP; DM, dextromethorphan hydrobromide, USP; N, number of subjects; dosages are in milligrams.

mg was at least 8 h. MorphiDex 60:60 mg was rated significantly more highly by patients than MS 60 mg ($p = 0.007$). Both MS-containing treatments were significantly better than DM 60 mg or placebo for each of these measures, and DM 60 mg never differed significantly from placebo. The enhancement of MS analgesia was demonstrated with a dose of DM that had no analgesic effect when administered alone (10).

A study in 24 healthy men showed no pharmacokinetic interaction when MS and DM were given together in MorphiDex 1:1 ratio capsules. Thus, the enhancement of morphine's analgesic effect by the addition of DM is not due to an influence of DM on the metabolism of morphine (12).

2. Orthopedic Postsurgical Pain

In a pool of two similar orthopedic postsurgical pain studies, evaluable patients took MorphiDex 60:60 mg (86 patients), MS 60 mg (83 patients), DM 60 mg (45 patients), or placebo (87 patients). Both studies included patients with moderate to severe pain following orthopedic surgery involving osteotomy. Evaluations were made over an 8-h interval after treatment. Efficacy variables included categorical TOTPAR and SPID, VAS SPID, time to onset of meaningful relief, time to use of rescue medication, an overall rating, and a pain relief satisfaction rating.

The numerical order of best to worst efficacy variable values was MorphiDex 60:60 mg > MS 60 mg > DM 60 mg > placebo for every variable. MorphiDex 60:60 mg was significantly superior to MS 60 mg for TOTPAR (Fig. 3) and pain relief satisfaction rating, and to DM 60 mg and placebo for all the foregoing variables. The duration of action of MorphiDex 60:60 mg was at least 8 h. MS 60 mg was significantly better than DM 60 mg for SPID, VAS SPID, time

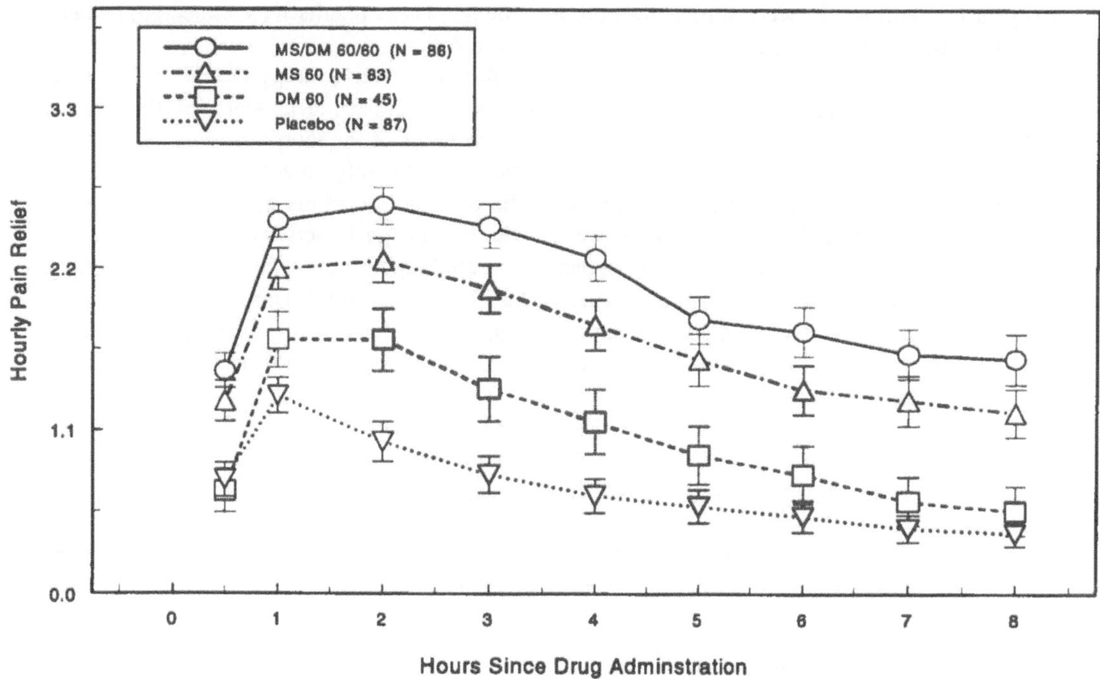

Figure 3 Pain relief over time for single doses of MorphiDex (MS/DM 1:1 ratio), MS, DM, and placebo; pool of two orthopedic postsurgical pain studies: MS, morphine sulfate, USP; DM, dextromethorphan hydrobromide, USP; N, number of subjects; dosages are in milligrams.

to onset of meaningful relief, and overall evaluation. DM 60 mg was usually significantly more effective than placebo (12).

A subset of 75 patients in one of these studies last took prestudy analgesic more than 4 h before study medication. For this subset, MorphiDex 30:30 mg (18 patients) provided pain relief equivalent to that for MS 60 mg (19 patients) with a significantly faster onset of meaningful pain relief ($p = 0.05$).

MorphiDex 60:60 mg (17 patients) was approximately twice as effective as MS 60 mg alone for TOTPAR ($p = 0.001$), SPID ($p = 0.04$), and VAS SPID ($p = 0.06$) with a significantly greater percentage of patients showing meaningful relief ($p = 0.003$) and a significantly shorter time to meaningful relief ($p < 0.001$).

Higher levels of residual nonstudy opioids for patients in the pooled studies most likely account for the low study sensitivity to the difference between MorphiDex 60:60 mg and MS 60 mg administered alone, and the apparent analgesic efficacy of DM 60 mg administered alone.

B. Double-Blind, Multiple-Dose Studies in Patients with Cancer or Other Chronic Pain

1. Two-Week per Treatment Crossover Study

The 77 patients who received both double-blind treatments, MorphiDex 15:15 mg and MS 30 mg, in this 4-week crossover study were included in the efficacy analyses. During the double-blind period, average daily pain, pain at dosing, daily satisfaction with pain relief, and global drug assessment scores were similar for both treatments. These results were expected, because patients titrated their dose to achieve satisfactory pain relief.

The study had 90% power to detect a 0.5 difference in the average number of capsules taken per day. The average number of capsules taken per day did not differ significantly between treatments; however, each MorphiDex capsule contained half of the morphine dose of each MS capsule. Thus, the average daily morphine dose was significantly lower ($p < 0.001$) during MorphiDex treatment (80.3 mg) compared with the average morphine daily dose during MS treatment (161.5 mg). These results demonstrate that the analgesic activity of MorphiDex 15: 15 mg is equivalent to that of MS 30 mg in patients treated repetitively with oral opioid therapy. DM 15 mg enhances the analgesic properties of MS 15 mg in MorphiDex.

The average number of doses per day was significantly lower ($p = 0.04$) for MorphiDex (3.58 doses) than for MS (3.73 doses). Additionally, the average time between doses ($p = 0.05$) and the average time from the last dose of the day to the first dose of the next day (overnight interval; $p = 0.01$) were both significantly longer for MorphiDex (6.99 and 9.83 h, respectively) than for MS (6.42 and 8.90 h, respectively). These results demonstrate that DM 15 mg enhances the duration of the analgesic effect of MS 15 mg and may provide a more convenient dosing schedule (13).

With no washout period between treatments, the study had limited ability to detect any differences between treatments in the patient incidences of adverse events.

2. Four-Week, Parallel Group Study

In the 4-week parallel group study, patients titrated their dose of MS 30 mg or MorphiDex 30:30 mg capsules to achieve satisfactory pain relief. Those who met entry criteria and completed at least 3 weeks of treatment were evaluable for efficacy. For all measures except patients' global assessment of effectiveness of study medication, results were analyzed by mean change from baseline for each of the 4 weeks of the double-blind period. Data for patients' global assessment of study medication were collected and analyzed for weeks 2 and 4.

MorphiDex capsules (92 patients) provided pain control equal to that of MS alone (93 patients), but with a significantly lower morphine daily dose during week 4 ($p = 0.044$), and with a comparable side effect profile. Patients in each group rated their double-blind treatment as better, no different, or worse compared with their run-in morphine medication. Double-blind MorphiDex was statistically significantly better than double-blind MS for this comparative global rating ($p = 0.026$). Daily morphine dose escalation over 4 weeks occurred with MS (16 mg) as compared with little increase for MorphiDex (1.6 mg). The increases differed significantly between the treatments ($p = 0.025$) (13), suggesting a reduction in tolerance to morphine analgesia.

C. Open-Label, Multiple-Dose Study of Conversion from Other Opioids to Morphidex Treatment in Patients with Cancer or Other Chronic Pain

A 2-week, open-label study in patients with moderate to severe cancer or other chronic pain was conducted to gain experience in converting patients' medication from other opioids to MorphiDex. The 457 patients who did not take prohibited medications on 5 or more days and who completed at least 10 days of study drug treatment were included in the efficacy analyses.

After a first MorphiDex dose containing one-half their morphine-equivalent prestudy dose, patients could titrate their dose to achieve satisfactory pain control. During week 2 of MorphiDex treatment, patients took significantly less morphine (78.7% of their prestudy morphine-equivalent daily dose; $p = 0.0001$), and rated MorphiDex significantly better than they had rated their prestudy opioid at baseline ($p = 0.001$). The mean number of MorphiDex doses per day was 3.6. Half of the patients took a median of 1, 2, or 3 doses per day, whereas an additional 27% most commonly took 4 doses daily (14).

In a 26-week extension of this study, 96.6% of patient treatment days were managed with no rescue medication. The MorphiDex side effect profile was similar to that expected with morphine treatment. MorphiDex capsules were generally well tolerated during long-term treatment, as shown by clinical laboratory evaluations, vital signs, and neurological examinations.

D. Abuse Liability

An initial study in postopioid-abusing subjects showed no difference in addiction liability or naloxone-induced withdrawal between subjects who received oral MS 60 mg alone or with up to 120 mg of DM.

In a second study, which was a balanced Latin square four-way crossover, 20 postopioid-abusing subjects were randomized to receive double-blind, single oral doses to evaluate MS/DM 180:180 mg, MS 180 mg, DM 180 mg, and placebo. Subjects were evaluated over a 6-h interval after treatment. There was no indication of the potentiation of any subjective, behavioral, or physiological effect of morphine when coadministered with dextromethorphan. In contrast, morphine antagonized the dysphoric and pressor effects of dextromethorphan. The potentiation of morphine analgesia by dextromethorphan observed in other studies thus seems selective in that it does not extend to the euphorigenic and subjective effects of morphine that are indicative of abuse potential. There is no evidence that MS/DM 180:180 mg has any greater abuse liability than MS 180 mg (15).

E. Respiratory Depression

A double-blind, single-dose, crossover study compared the respiratory depressant effects of oral MorphiDex 60:60 mg, MS 60 mg, DM 60 mg, and placebo over 6 h in 16 healthy subjects. There was a similar degree of respiratory depression for MorphiDex 60:60 mg and MS 60 mg, with only a slightly longer duration after MorphiDex treatment (15).

V. SUMMARY AND CONCLUSION

Six double-blind, placebo-controlled, single-dose clinical trials of MorphiDex capsules in patients with moderate to severe postsurgical pain demonstrated a significantly faster onset of meaningful pain relief and enhanced analgesia compared with the same dose of morphine alone, and at least an 8-h duration of effect. MorphiDex side effects were comparable with side effects for the same dose of morphine.

Multiple dose studies comparing MorphiDex treatment with MS alone in patients with cancer and other chronic pain showed that patients taking MorphiDex capsules require significantly less morphine to achieve satisfactory pain control. Additionally, patients took fewer doses per day during MorphiDex treatment, suggesting a longer duration of action compared with morphine alone.

Generally, long-term MorphiDex treatment provided comprehensive pain control. Most patients required no other opioid analgesic for breakthrough pain. Patients with cancer or other chronic pain were significantly more satisfied with MorphiDex than with their previous opioid medications.

A clinical pharmacokinetic interaction study showed no clinically relevant differences in the metabolism of morphine and dextromethorphan when they are coadministered. Therefore, enhancement of morphine analgesia is likely due to a separate mechanism, possibly antagonism of the NMDA receptor.

There was no indication of increased abuse liability or naloxone-induced withdrawal effects of morphine with concurrent dextromethorphan administration. Respiratory depressant effects and adverse events owing to morphine were not enhanced during MorphiDex treatment.

In conclusion, clinical studies showed that MorphiDex capsules provide an alternative to currently available opioids and may provide more effective pain control with a convenient-dosing regimen.

REFERENCES

1. Price DD, Mao J, Mayer DJ. Central neural mechanisms of normal and abnormal pain states. In: Fields HL, Liebeskind JC, eds. Pharmacological Approaches to the Treatment of Pain: New Concepts and Critical Issues, Progress in Pain Research and Management. Vol. 1. Seattle: IASP Press, 1994: 61–84.
2. Dickenson AH, Sullivan AF. Differential effects of excitatory amino acid antagonists on dorsal horn nociceptive neurons in the rat. Brain Res 1990; 506:31–39.
3. Woolf CJ, Thompson SWN. The induction and maintenance of central sensitization is dependent on *N*-methyl-D-aspartic acid receptor activation; implications for the treatment of post-injury pain hypersensitivity states. Pain 1991; 44:293–299.
4. Dubner R. Neuronal plasticity and pain following peripheral tissue inflammation or nerve injury. In: Bond M, Charlton E, Woolf CJ, eds. Proceedings of 5th World Congress on Pain. Pain Research and Clinical Management. Vol. 5. Amsterdam: Elsevier, 1991:263–276.
5. Ren K, Hylden JL, Williams GM, Ruda MA, Dubner R. The effects of a non-competitive NMDA-receptor antagonist, MK-801, on behavioral hyperalgesia and dorsal horn neuronal activity in rats with unilateral inflammation. Pain 1992; 50:331–344.
6. Mao J, Price DD, Mayer DJ. Mechanisms of hyperalgesia and morphine tolerance: a current view of their possible interactions. Pain 1995; 62:259–274.
7. Price DD, Mao J, Frenk H, Mayer DJ. The *N*-methyl-D-aspartate receptor antagonist dextromethorphan selectively reduces temporal summation of second pain in man. Pain 1994; 59:165–174.
8. Mao J, Price DD, Mayer DJ. Thermal hyperalgesia in association with the development of morphine tolerance and dependence in rats: prevention and reversal by excitatory amino acid antagonists. J Neurosci 1994; 14:2301–2312.
9. Mayer DJ, Mao J, Price DD. The development of morphine tolerance and dependence is associated with translocation of protein kinase C. Pain 1995; 61:365–374.
10. Mao J, Price DD, Caruso F, Mayer DJ. Oral administration of dextromethorphan prevents the development of morphine tolerance and dependence in rats. Pain 1996; 67:361–368.
11. Manning B, Mao J, Frenk H, Price DD, Mayer DJ. Continuous co-administration of dextromethorphan or MK-801 with morphine: attenuation of morphine dependence and naloxone reversible attenuation or morphine tolerance. Pain 1996; 67:79–88.
12. Caruso FS. MorphiDex pharmacokinetic studies and single-dose efficacy analgesic studies in patients with postoperative pain. J Pain Sympt Manage 2000; 19:S31–S36.
13. Katz NP. MorphiDex (MS:DM) double-blind, multiple-dose studies in chronic pain patients. J Pain Sympt Manage 2000; 19:S37–S41.
14. Chevlen E. Morphine with dextromethorphan: conversion from other opioid analgesics. J Pain Sympt Manage 2000; 19:S42–S49.
15. Jasinskl DR. Abuse potential of morphine/dextromethorphan combinations. J Pain Sympt Manage 2000; 19:S26–S30.

37
CCK Antagonist Potentiation of Opioid Analgesia

Leslie L. Iversen
University of Oxford, Oxford, England

I. INTRODUCTION

Cholecystokinin (CCK) is one of the most abundant of the neuropeptides that are present in small neurons in many regions of the brain and spinal cord (1,2). Several of these (e.g., spinal cord dorsal horn and brain stem) correspond to areas containing high levels of endogenous opioids, and there has been a growing awareness of functional interactions between the CCK and opioid systems. CCK and the opioids tend to have opposite effects on food intake, motor behavior, and responsiveness to painful stimuli (3), leading to the suggestion that the CCK system may represent an "antiopioid" or "antianalgesic" mechanism. The discovery of nonpeptide drugs that act as CCK antagonists (4–6) offers a new series of tools with which to investigate the interactions of the CCK and opioid systems, and it becomes apparent that under some conditions CCK antagonists can enhance the analgesic effects of both exogenous and endogenous opioids. This brief review will give a summary of these findings; for more detailed reviews see elsewhere (7–9).

II. CCK ANTAGONISTS ENHANCE OPIOID ANALGESIA

The first reports of the ability of CCK to reduce analgesic responses to either exogenously administered or endogenously released opioids (10,11) were soon followed by studies showing that CCK antagonist drugs had the opposite effect (12–14). The CCK antagonists not only enhanced opioid responses, they also appeared able to reverse existing morphine tolerance (12–13). The enhancement of analgesic responses to morphine or opioid peptides and reversal of tolerance have been reported in a number of different acute pain models (rat and mouse tail-flick, hot-plate, paw-pressure, primate tail-withdrawal, dental dolorimetry), and these results have been reviewed in detail elsewhere (7–9). CCK antagonists also strongly potentiated analgesic responses (mouse hot-plate, rat tail-flick) to the enkephalinase inhibitors RB 101 and RB 211 (15,16), and they were able to convert "nonresponders" to "responders" in a rat electroacupuncture model (17).

The CCK antagonists, however, do not potentiate opiate responses in all experimental pain models. In the formalin test in mice the CCK antagonist PD-134,308 was reported to enhance the analgesic effects of morphine in the late phase of the test, but not in the initial phase

(18). In the rat model of inflammatory pain induced by intraplantar injection of carrageenin, CCK antagonists were either ineffective in enhancing the antinociceptive effects of morphine (19), or effective only at a particular time after carrageenin injection and in those animals with the most severe hyperalgesic response (20). The effects of the CCK antagonists may also be "state-dependent" and are seen most prominently in animals that have not been acclimatized to the laboratory environment or accustomed to handling (21), suggesting that the CCK system may be activated by fearful stimuli. This may possibly explain why the effectiveness of CCK antagonists in enhancing opiate responses was diminished after repeated administration of proglumide or lorgumide (22).

Perhaps the most impressive results are those obtained with CCK antagonists in animal models of neuropathic pain. Xu et al. (23) reported that intrathecal injections of morphine alone were ineffective in preventing the self-mutilating behavior that develops after sciatic nerve section in the rat. The CCK antagonist CI 988 (given s.c.) was also ineffective when given alone, but when morphine and CI 988 were coadministered self-mutilation behavior was significantly inhibited. Nichols et al. (24) also found that the CCK antagonist L-365,260, although ineffective when given alone in a rat nerve ligation model of neuropathic pain, restored morphine analgesia when coadministered with the opiate. CI 988 was also able to restore normal morphine inhibitory responses in a flexor reflex test in the rat, when the effectiveness of morphine had been reduced after sciatic nerve section (25). In some studies of neuropathic pain, involving peripheral nerve ligation of 5-weeks duration (26) or spinal cord injury (27), CCK antagonists have been reported to be effective in reversing hyperalgesia when given alone without any accompanying opiate drug.

The great majority of published studies have utilized CCK antagonists that exhibit selectivity for the CCK-2 subtype receptor, although some earlier studies obtained positive results with the CCK-1–selective compound devazepide. However, it is likely that, at least in rodent studies, these results can be attributed to the ability of devazepide at higher doses to act also at CCK-2 sites (8) as CCK-1 receptors are not present in rodent spinal cord or brain. In humans and monkeys, however, the situation is more complicated as the CCK-1 receptor is the predominant subtype in spinal cord and brain stem, while the CCK-2 receptor is predominant in the rest of the brain (28). Another so far unexplained feature of the CCK antagonist–opiate interaction is that most studies have revealed an inverted U-shaped dose–response curve when increasing doses of CCK antagonist were administered, with high doses no longer being effective (7,8).

III. MECHANISMS UNDERLYING CCK–OPIATE INTERACTIONS

Although a number of regions of CNS contain both CCK and endorphin- or enkephalin-containing neurons, the most obvious target site for an interaction between the two systems is the primary afferent neuron. Ghilardi et al. (29) showed that CCK receptor-binding sites could be visualized autoradiographically on a substantial proportion of primary sensory neurons in rat, rabbit, and monkey trigeminal and dorsal root ganglia (DRG). Even in the monkey, in which spinal cord and brain stem contains largely CCK-1 receptors, the sensory neurons expressed predominantly the CCK-2 receptor subtype. Liu et al. (30) showed by patch-clamp recording from isolated rat DRG cells that CCK could reverse the inhibition of calcium current produced by activation of the μ-opioid receptor. As this inhibition is thought to play a key role in mediating the effects of opioids in inhibiting the release of primary afferent neurotransmitters and neuropeptides, the effect of CCK at this site may be to dampen or block opioid actions. Zhou et al. (31), furthermore, showed that systemic morphine caused a marked increase in the release of endogenous CCK in the perfusate of rat spinal cord. They suggested that the opioid-induced release of CCK may represent a self-limiting process for opioid effects at the spinal cord level. As opioid receptors (and presumably CCK-2 receptors) are present on the peripheral terminals of primary afferent neurons as well as on their central processes, one might expect that CCK–opiate interactions could occur at such peripheral sites. Schäfer et al. (32) have indeed reported that injection of CCK locally into the inflamed rat paw attenuated the local analgesic effects of μ-opioid agonists.

Changes in the expression of the peptide CCK and its receptor (CCK-2) on primary afferent neurons may play a key role in the alterations in pain sensitivity and opiate responsiveness that occur in chronic pain conditions. In animal models of neuropathic pain involving peripheral nerve section, Hökfelt and colleagues have shown that there are marked increases in the expression of both CCK-1 and CCK-2 receptors in primary afferent neurons, with many DRG cells that normally do not express either the peptide or the receptor becoming positive (23,33,34). The time course of these changes parallels the slow development of hyperalgesia in the animals, and it was suggested that the up-regulation of the CCK system in response to nerve injury might explain the opioid-insensitivity of the accompanying pain. On the other hand, in inflammatory pain models there is no such up-regulation of the peptide CCK or its receptor, but instead, a heightened sensitivity to opiates accompanied by a diminished release of CCK (9,19).

The primary afferent neuron, however, may be only one of several sites at which the CCK and opioid systems interact. Han and his colleagues in Beijing (35–37) have implicated CCK-containing neurons in rat ventral tegmentum, nucleus accumbens, and amygdala in such interactions. Very small doses of CCK (0.1–0.5 ng) injected bilaterally into rat nucleus accumbens antagonized the analgesic effects of systemically administered morphine (35), whereas CCK-containing neurons in ventral tegmentum were activated by peripheral noxious stimuli (36) and the CCK content of neurons in the amygdala was increased in morphine-tolerant animals (37).

IV. EFFECTS OF CCK ANTAGONISTS ON OPIATE TOLERANCE AND DEPENDENCE

Several studies have reported that CCK antagonists can reverse morphine tolerance or prevent its development. In animals already tolerant to morphine, a single low dose of CCK antagonist restored analgesic responsiveness to morphine (12,38), or coadministration of a CCK antagonist with morphine prevented the development of tolerance (7,8,13,39,40). However, coadministration of a CCK antagonist with morphine did not prevent the subsequent withdrawal signs seen after challenge with the opiate receptor antagonist naloxone (7,8,39). The mechanisms underlying the effects of CCK antagonists on opiate tolerance remain unclear. One possibility is that the development of such tolerance is due to an increase in activity of the endogenous CCK system in the spinal cord after long exposure to opiates, but no experimental evidence is available to support this hypothesis.

The subjective effects of CCK antagonists do not resemble those of opiates. CCK antagonists failed to antagonize morphine in rats trained to recognize morphine as a discriminative stimulus (41,42), and did not alter the pattern of heroin self-administration in heroin-dependent animals (42). Rats could not be trained to recognize the CCK-2 antagonist L-365,260 as a discriminative stimulus (41), suggesting that it produces little subjective effect in normal animals—perhaps because there is little tonic activity in the endogenous CCK systems. This would also explain why CCK antagonists have no significant effects on basal levels of pain sensitivity, and why human subjects were unable to distinguish L-365,260 from placebo in clinical trials (43). The lack of interaction of CCK antagonists with morphine in drug-discrimination studies and the inability of CCK antagonists to alter physical dependence and withdrawal suggest that the mechanisms involved in mediating the analgesic and rewarding effects of opiates are different. This was also suggested by previous studies that showed that although tolerance develops to the analgesic effects of morphine, this is not true for the discriminative properties of the drug(44).

The question of whether tolerance develops to the opiate-enhancing effects of CCK antagonists on prolonged treatment is not easy to answer. One study showed that the opiate-enhancing effects of intrathecally administered proglumide was absent 1 week after a single dose of proglumide or after daily injections of proglumide for a week. Similar results were reported for lorglumide (22). On the other hand, several studies with the newer generation of more potent CCK antagonists have failed to observe any diminution in the opiate-enhancing effects of these drugs after prolonged treatment (8,13,39,40). Long-term administration of a CCK antagonist (once or twice a day for 5 days) in combination with the enkephalinase inhibitor RB101 also showed only a weak degree of tolerance, with no alteration in peak antinociceptive responses, but a small reduction in their duration (45).

V. CLINICAL STUDIES

There has not yet been any definitive test of the CCK antagonists as adjuncts to opiate analgesics in the clinic. An early study of the effects of proglumide in healthy volunteers (using a skin thermal stimulation model) showed an enhancement of opiate analgesia (46), but a subsequent study with proglumide in 80 postoperative patients suffering moderate to severe pain failed to show any effect on morphine analgesia, using a patient-controlled analgesia model (47). Proglumide, however, is a first-generation CCK antagonist, with only weak affinity for the CCK receptor, and it could be argued that postoperative pain—with a considerable inflammatory pain element—is not the most likely to respond to CCK antagonists. Clinical trials with one of the more potent CCK antagonists in a more suitable clinical context are needed before the usefulness of the concept can be properly evaluated.

REFERENCES

1. Reeve JR, Eysselein V, Solomon TE, Go VLW, eds. Cholecystokinin. Ann NY Acad Sci 1994; 713.
2. Crawley JN, Corwin RL. Biological actions of cholecystokinin. Peptides 1994; 15:731–755.
3. Iversen SD. CCK and opioid analgesia. In: Dourish CT, Cooper SJ, Iversen SD, Iversen LL, eds. Multiple Cholecystokinin Receptors in the CNS. Oxford: Oxford University Press, 1992:433–438.
4. Freidinger RM. Synthesis of non-peptide CCK antagonists. In: Dourish CT, Cooper SJ, Iversen SD, Iversen LL, eds. Multiple Cholecystokinin Receptors in the CNS. Oxford: Oxford University Press 1992:8–27.
5. Rasmussen K. Therapeutic potential of cholecystokinin-B antagonists. Exp Opin Invest Drugs 1995; 4:313–322.
6. Wettstein JG, Bueno L, Junien JL. CCK antagonists: pharmacology and therapeutic interest. Pharmac Ther 1994; 62:267–282.
7. Baber NS, Dourish CT, Hill DR. The role of caerulein and CCK antagonists in nociception. Pain 1989; 39:307–328.
8. Dourish CT. The role of CCK_A and CCK_B receptors in mediating the inhibitor effect of CCK on opioid analgesia. In: Dourish CT, Cooper SJ, Iversen SD, Iversen LL, eds. Multiple Cholecystokinin Receptors in the CNS. Oxford: Oxford University Press, 1992:455–479.
9. Stanfa L, Dickenson A, Xu XJ, Wiesenfeld-Hallin Z. Cholecystokinin and morphine analgesia: variations on a theme. Trends Pharmacol Sci 1994; 15:65–66.

10. Faris PL, Komisaruk BR, Watkins LR, Mayer DJ. Evidence for the neuropeptide cholecystokinin as an antagonist of opiate analgesia. Science 1983; 219:310–312.
11. Kellstein DE, Mayer DJ. CCK and opioid analgesia. In: Dourish CT, Cooper SJ, Iversen SD, Iversen LL, eds. Multiple Cholecystokinin Receptors in the CNS. Oxford: Oxford University Press, 1992: 439–454.
12. Watkins LR, Kinscheck IB, Mayer DJ. Potentiation of opiate analgesia and apparent reversal of morphine tolerance by proglumide. Science 1984; 224:395–396.
13. Dourish CT, Hawley D, Iversen SD. Enhancement of morphine analgesia and prevention of morphine tolerance in the rat by the cholecystokinin antagonist L-364,718. Eur J Pharmacol 1988; 147:469–472.
14. Wiesenfeld–Hallin Z, Xu XJ, Horwell DC, Hökfelt T. PD 134308, a selective antagonist of cholecystokinin type B receptor, enhances the analgesic effect of morphine and synergistically interacts with intrathecal galanin to depress spinal nociceptive reflexes. Proc Natl Acad Sci USA 1990; 87:7105–7109.
15. Maldonado R, Derrien M, Noble F, Roques BP. Association of the peptidase inhibitor RB 101 and a CCK antagonist strongly enhances antinociceptive responses. Neuroreport 1993; 4:947–950.
16. Valverde O, Maldonado R, Fournie–Zaluski MC, Roques BP. Cholecystokinin B antagonists strongly potentiate antinociception mediated by endogenous enkephalins. J Pharmacol Exp Ther 1994; 270: 77–88.
17. Han JS. The role of CCK in electro-acupuncture analgesia and electro-acupuncture tolerance. In: Dourish CT, Cooper SJ, Iversen SD, Iversen LL, eds. Multiple Cholecystokinin Receptors in the CNS. Oxford: Oxford University Press, 1992:480–502.
18. Noble F, Blommaert A, Fournie–Zaluski MC, Roques BP. A selective CCK_B receptor antagonist potentiates μ-, but not δ-opioid receptor mediated antinociception in the formalin test. Eur J Pharmacol 1995; 273:145–151.
19. Stanfa LC, Dickenson AH. Cholecystokinin as a factor in the enhanced potency of spinal morphine following carrageenin inflammation. Br J Pharmacol 1993; 108:967–973.
20. Perrot S, Idänpään–Heikkilä JJ, Guilbaud G, Kayser V. The enhancement of morphine antinociception by a CCK_B receptor antagonist in the rat depends on the phase of inflammation and the intensity of carrageenin-induced hyperalgesia. Pain 1998; 74:269–274.
21. Lavigne GJ, Millington WR, Mueller GP. The CCK_A and CCK_B receptor antagonists devazepide and L-365,260 enhance morphine antinociception only in non-acclimated rats exposed to a novel environment. Neuropeptides 1992; 21:119–129.
22. Kellstein DE, Mayer DJ. Chronic administration of cholecystokinin antagonists reverses the enhancement of spinal morphine analgesia induced by acute pretreatment. Brain Res 1990; 516:263–270.
23. Xu XJ, Puke MJC, Verge VMK, Wiesenfeld–Hallin Z, Hughes J, Hökfelt T. Up-regulation of cholecystokinin in primary sensory neurons is associated with morphine insensitivity in experimental neuropathic pain in the rat. Neurosci Lett 1993; 152:129–132.
24. Nichols ML, Bian D, Ossipv MH, Lai J, Porreca F. Regulation of morphine antiallodynic efficacy by cholecystokinin in a model of neuropathic pain in rats. J Pharmacol Exp Ther 1995; 275:1339–1345.
25. Xu XJ, Hökfelt T, Hughes J, Wiesenfeld–Hallin Z. The CCK_B antagonist CI988 enhances the reflex-depressive effect of morphine in axotomized rats. Neuroreport 1994; 5:718–720.
26. Yamamoto T, Nozaki–Taguchi N. Role of cholecystokinin-B receptor in the maintenance of thermal hyperalgesia induced by unilateral constriction injury to the sciatic nerve in the rat. Neurosci Lett 1995; 202:89–92.
27. Xu XJ, Hao JX, Seiger A, Hughes J, Hökfelt T, Wiesenfeld–Hallin Z. Chronic pain-related behaviors in spinally injured rats: evidence for functional alterations of the endogenous cholecystokinin and opioid systems. Pain 1994; 56:271–277.
28. Hill DR, Shaw TM, Woodruff GN. Binding sites for ^{125}I-cholecystokinin in primate spinal cord are of the CCK-A subclass. Neurosci Lett 1988; 89:133–139.
29. Ghilardi JR, Allen CJ, Vigna SR, McVey DC, Mantyh PW. Trigeminal and dorsal root ganglion neurons express CCK receptor binding sites in the rat, rabbit and monkey: possible site of opiate–CCK analgesic interactions. J Neurosci 1992; 12:4854–4866.

30. Liu NJ, Xu T, Li CQ, Yu YX, Kang HG, Han JS. Cholecystokinin octapeptide reverses μ-opioid-receptor–mediated inhibition of calcium current in rat dorsal root ganglion neurons. J Pharmacol Exp Ther 1995; 275:1293–1299.
31. Zhou Y, Sun YH, Zhang ZW, Han JS. Increased release of immunoreactive cholecystokinin octapeptide by morphine and potentiation of μ-opioid analgesia by CCK_B receptor antagonist L-365,260 in rat spinal cord. Eur J Pharmacol 1993; 234:147–154.
32. Schäfer M, Zhou L, Stein C. Cholecystokinin inhibits peripheral opioid analgesia in inflamed tissue. Neuroscience 1998; 82:603–611.
33. Verge VMK, Wiesenfeld–Hallin Z, Hökfelt T. Cholecystokinin in mammalian primary sensory neurons and spinal cord: in situ hybridization studies in rat and monkey. Eur J Neurosci 1993; 5:240–250.
34. Zhang X, Dagerlind A, Elde RP, Castel MN, Broberger C, Wiesenfeld–Hallin Z, Hökfelt T. Marked increase in cholecystokinin B receptor messenger RNA levels in rat dorsal root ganglia after peripheral axotomy. Neuroscience 1993; 57:227–233.
35. Pu SF, Zhuang HX, Han JS. Cholecystokinin octapeptide (CCK-8) antagonizes morphine analgesia in nucleus accumbens of the rat via the CCK-B receptor. Brain Res 1994; 657:159–164.
36. Ma QP, Zhou Y, Han JS. Noxious stimulation accelerated the expression of c-*fos* protooncogene in cholecystokininergic and dopaminergic neurons in the ventral tegmental area. Peptides 1993; 14: 561–566.
37. Pu S, Zhuang H, Lu Z, Wu X, Han JS. Cholecystokinin gene expression in rat amygdaloid neurons: normal distribution and effect of morphine tolerance. Mol Brain Res 1994; 21:183–189.
38. Hoffmann O, Wiesenfeld–Hallin Z. The CCK-B receptor antagonist CI988 reverses tolerance to morphine in rats. Neuroreport 1994; 5:2565–2568.
39. Xu XJ, Wiesenfeld–Hallin Z, Hughes J, Horwell DC, Hökfelt T. CI988, a selective antagonist of $cholecystokinin_B$ receptors, prevents morphine tolerance in the rat. Br J Pharmacol 1992; 105:591–596.
40. Idänpään–Heikkilä JJ, Guilbaud G, Kayser V. Prevention of tolerance to the antinociceptive effects of systemic morphine by a selective cholecystokinin-B receptor antagonist in a rat model of peripheral neuropathy. J Pharmacol Exp Ther 1997; 282:1366–1372.
41. Jackson A, Tattersall D, Bentley G, Rycroft W, Bourson A, Hargreaves R, Tricklebank M, Iversen S. An investigation into the discriminative stimulus and reinforcing properties of the CCK_B-receptor antagonist L-365,260 in rats. Neuropeptides 1994; 26:343–353.
42. Higgins GA, Joharchi N, Wang Y, Corrigall WA, Sellers EM. The CCK receptor antagonist devazepide does not modify opioid self-administration or drug discrimination: comparison with the dopamine antagonist haloperidol. Brain Res 1994; 640:246–254.
43. Kramer MS, Cutler NR, Ballenger JC, Patterson WM, Mendels J, Chenault A, Shrivastava R, Matzura–Wolfe D, Lines C, Reines S. A placebo controlled trial of L-365,260, a CCK_B antagonist, in panic disorder. Biol Psychiatry 1995; 37:462–466.
44. Colpaert FC, Niemegeers CJE, Janssen PAJ. Studies on the regulation of sensitivity to the narcotic cue. Neuropharmacology 1978; 17:705–713.
45. Valverde O, Blommaert AGS, Fournie–Zaluski MC, Roques BP, Maldonado R. Weak tolerance to the antinociceptive effect induced by the association of a peptidase inhibitor and a CCK_B receptor antagonist. Eur J Pharmacol 1995; 286:79–93.
46. Price DD, von der Gruen A, Miller J, Rafii A, Price C. Potentiation of systemic morphine analgesia in humans by proglumide, a cholecystokinin antagonist. Anesth Analg 1985; 64:801–806.
47. Lehmann KA, Schlüsener M, Arabatis P. Failure of proglumide, a cholecystokinin antagonist, to potentiate clinical morphine analgesia. Anesth Analg 1989; 68:31–36.

38
Profile of NSAID + Opioid Combination Analgesics

Abraham Sunshine
Analgesic Development Ltd. and NYU School of Medicine, New York, New York, U.S.A.

In the management of acute pain and cancer pain, stepped levels of treatment intensity are recommended. The initial treatment is usually a nonopioid analgesic, such as aspirin, salicylate salt, acetaminophen, or a nonsteroidal anti-inflammatory drug (NSAID) (1). If this treatment, at the recommended doses is inadequate, simply increasing the dose will not result in a proportional increase in analgesia (2). Furthermore, the risk of adverse effects increases with these higher doses. Therefore, the addition of a low-dose opioid is recommended (1). The combination can be given as two individual doses or in a combination tablet or capsule. Oral narcotic–acetaminophen or narcotic–aspirin combinations represent a large category of drugs currently available in the United States for treating acute and chronic pain. Their popularity is due to the ease of prescribing the combination product, the minimization of abuse of the opioid alone, and the considerable marketing effort for the combinations. The currently marketed analgesic combinations for pain in the United States are mixtures of either codeine, hydrocodone, oxycodone, or propoxyphene with aspirin, acetaminophen, or ibuprofen. Ibuprofen at 200 mg has an analgesic efficacy equal to or greater than aspirin or acetaminophen 650 mg. Ibuprofen at 400 mg is widely considered to have a higher level of analgesic activity than aspirin or acetaminophen at 650 mg (3,4). Hence, it is reasonable that a 400-mg ibuprofen combination with a low-dose opioid would undoubtedly have greater efficacy than a combination of 650 mg of aspirin or acetaminophen with the same amount of the opioid.

For approval to market a combination product, the policy of the U.S. Federal Drug Administration (FDA) requires a clinical trial in which the efficacy of the combination is significantly better than both of the individual ingredients, and that the marketed NSAID alone is significantly better than placebo. The reader is referred to the analgesic guidelines for a fuller discussion of the FDA requirements (5). This seemingly easy, simple requirement has not been satisfied in many clinical trials. Statistical issues are presented in a recent publication (6). The failure to fulfill the combination policy of the FDA is a result of many different factors. It requires experienced investigators and expertly conducted clinical trials to demonstrate differences between the active products of the combination. It is far less challenging to show differences between placebo and an active compound. Other factors that influence the success of the trial are variability in the absorption of the oral analgesic. This can be influenced by the fasting or fed state, depending on the compound. Furthermore, the formulation of the new combination may change the rate and extent of absorption of each component of the combination in comparison with the individual ingredients alone (5,7).

Some clinical models do not readily detect the opioid or the addition of an opioid to a NSAID. For example, to demonstrate the analgesic efficacy of codeine 30 mg in comparison with placebo, or its contribution to an analgesic combination, is an extremely difficult task, particularly when it is studied in the dental extraction pain model. Codeine 60 mg can be demonstrated to be effective (Fig. 1) (8). However this dose is in excess of the dose of codeine frequently used in combination. Failed clinical trials are rarely reported in the literature and thus the difficulty in meeting the combination guidelines with ibuprofen and codeine may not be appreciated. In one failed study the authors suggest the upside sensitivity of the model may be a factor (9). In another study the authors did not demonstrate the superiority of the combinations on the first-dose administration, but did on the sixth dose (10). To date there is no codeine plus ibuprofen combination that is approved for use in the United States.

The first successful NSAID–opioid NDA approved was for Vicoprofen, a combination product manufactured by Knoll Pharmaceutical containing 200 mg of ibuprofen and 7.5 mg of hydrocodone (7). Two clinical trials submitted to the FDA demonstrated substantial evidence for the contribution of hydrocodone to the analgesic effect of ibuprofen (7). One of these studies was conducted at a dose level of 200 mg ibuprofen and 7.5 mg of hydrocodone (Fig. 2; Table 1). A recent publication describes in further detail the foregoing study (11). The combination was significantly superior to placebo and significantly superior to either hydrocodone or ibuprofen alone for most parameters. Hydrocodone 7.5 mg was not significantly different from placebo. The second study was conducted at a dose of 400 mg of ibuprofen and 15 mg of hydrocodone, (Fig. 3; Table 2) (12). The combination was significantly different from ibuprofen and placebo. Hydrocodone alone was not included in the study. Another study at this dosage level confirmed

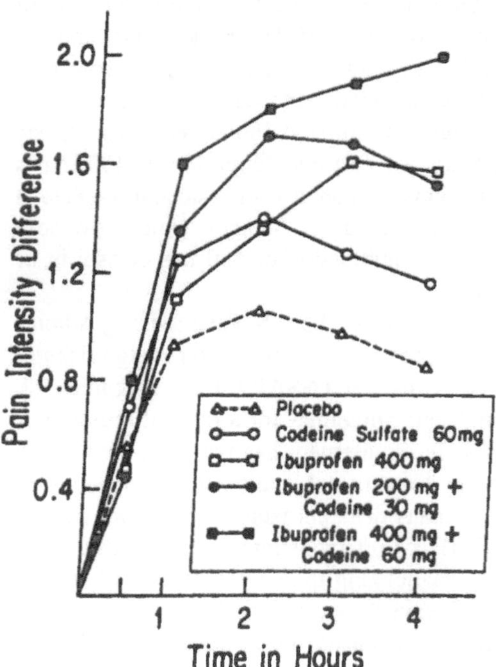

Figure 1 Time–effect curve: mean PID. Scores are calculated by subtracting the pain intensity score from the pain intensity at 0 h. Patient responses were scored on a four-point scale as; 0 = no pain, 1 = slight pain, 2 = moderate pain, and 3 = severe pain. (From Ref. 8.)

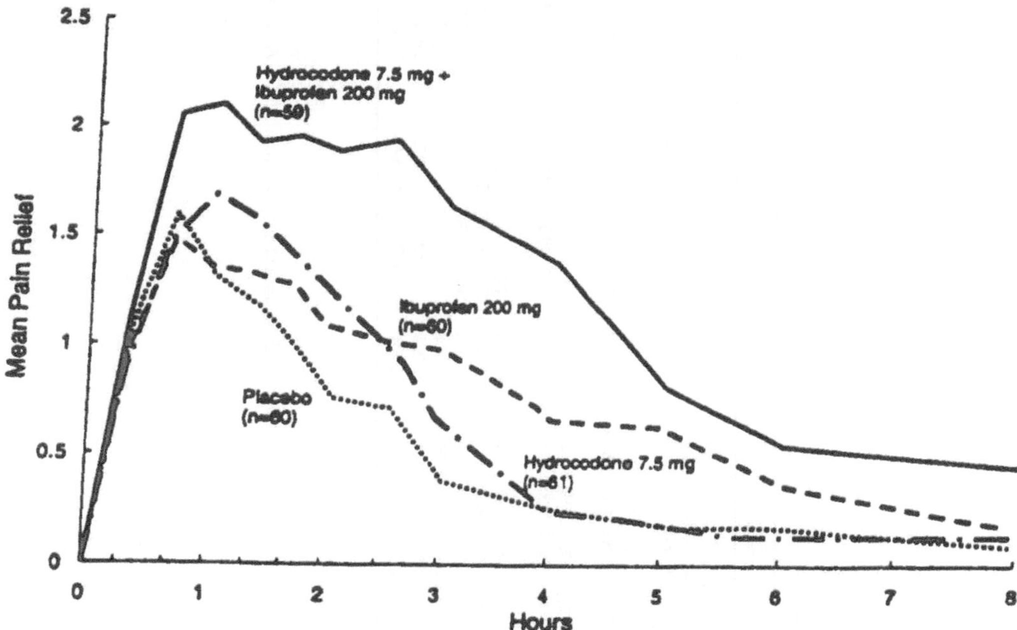

Figure 2 Time–effect curves for 7.5-mg hydrocodone, 200-mg ibuprofen, the combination of 7.5-mg hydrocodone with 200-mg ibuprofen and placebo: Mean pain relief scores are plotted. (From Ref. 11.)

the superiority of the combination to each component and placebo. Hydrocodone 15 mg was not significantly different from placebo in thc third study (Fig. 4) (11).

The Summary Basis of Approval available on the Internet at the FDA's homepage gives further insight into the NDA approval process and the findings of the FDA (7). In single-dose studies, not discussed in the foregoing, a significant dose–response was not demonstrated between the one- and two-tablet–dose regimens, although mean differences were in the anticipated direction. The efficacy data from the 30-day study compared one and two tablets of Vicoprofen and acetaminophen with codeine 600 mg/60 mg. Overall the highest dose of Vicoprofen was significantly better than the other two treatments. The low-dose Vicoprofen was numerically, but not statistically, better than APAP/codeine. The high-dose (two tablets) was studied in only 230 patients and fell short of the 300 patients required by the FDA for 30-day administration. Therefore, the flexibility in dosage that is available with Vicodin, hydrocodone/acetaminophen 5 mg/500 mg, 7.5 mg/750 mg, and 10 mg/660 mg is not available with Vicoprofen (13).

When an NSAID (ibuprofen) combination is preferred the only one approved in the United States at this time is ibuprofen with hydrocodone (Vicoprofen). In clinical practice it would seem reasonable to initially administer the Vicoprofen with an additional 200 mg of ibuprofen to obtain the maximum benefit of the ibuprofen analgesia. If additional analgesia is required, and if the patient tolerated a single tablet of Vicoprofen, the clinician could carefully consider giving two Vicoprofen tablets at one time. This would provide 400 mg of ibuprofen and 15 mg of hydrocodone. However, the approved dosage is not to exceed five tablets in 24 h (13). Other NSAID combinations are under development, including ibuprofen with oxycodone (see Chap. 30).

In summary, opioid–NSAID combination analgesics are indicated in the management of pain and form an intermediate step on the WHO ladder.

Table 1 Means (Standard Deviations), Sample Sizes, and Fisher's Protected LSD Comparisons

Treatment	Assessment time point (in hours from dosing)												
	0.33	0.5	0.67	1	1.33	1.67	2	2.5	3	4	5	6	8
Vicoprofen 200/7.5 mg (*n* = 59)[e]	0.42 (0.65)	0.68 (0.62)	0.93 (0.76)	1.00 (0.85)	0.95 (0.94)	0.93 (0.96)	0.92 (0.93)	0.95 (0.95)	0.81 (0.94)	0.64 (0.87)	0.34 (0.71)	0.22 (0.59)	0.19 (0.57)
	[59][a] A[d]	[59] A	[59] A	[59] A	[41] A	[34] A	[33] A	[32] A	[32] A	[26] A	[22] A	[14] A	[8] A
Ibuprofen 200 mg (*n* = 60)	0.37 (0.64)	0.47 (0.59)	0.57 (0.65)	0.60 (0.85)	0.67 (0.80)	0.62 (0.83)	0.48 (0.79)	0.47 (0.79)	0.47 (0.79)	0.33 (0.77)	0.28 (0.72)	0.18 (0.57)	0.00 (0.18)
	[60] A	[60] A	[60] B	[60] A	[33] A	[28] A	[25] B	[21] B	[19] B	[18] B	[11] A	[11] A	[5] B
Hydrocodone 7.5 mg (*n* = 61)	0.31 (0.59)	0.44 (0.60)	0.57 (0.76)	0.80 (0.87)	0.74 (0.83)	0.70 (0.82)	0.59 (0.84)	0.48 (0.83)	0.31 (0.67)	0.07 (0.48)	0.07 (0.31)	0.03 (0.18)	0.02 (0.13)
	[61] A	[61] A	[61] B	[61] A	[38] A	[34] A	[30] B	[24] B	[21] B	[13] C	[5] B	[3] A	[1] B
Placebo (*n* = 60)	0.48 (0.65)	0.60 (0.69)	0.72 (0.85)	0.67 (0.93)	0.62 (0.88)	0.55 (0.85)	0.42 (0.81)	0.37 (0.74)	0.22 (0.56)	0.15 (0.48)	0.13 (0.47)	0.12 (0.45)	0.07 (0.36)
	[60] A	[60] A	[60] AB	[60] A	[32] A	[26] A	[23] B	[15] B	[14] B	[9] BC	[6] AB	[4] A	[3] AB
Treatment p-value[b]	0.468	0.125	0.029	0.066	0.166	0.091	0.008	<0.001	<0.001	<0.001	0.032	0.143	0.020
Trt*Baseline p-value[c]	0.216	0.155	0.222	0.049	0.073	0.074	0.049	0.052	0.304	0.068	0.522	0.700	0.655
RMS Error[b]	0.629	0.623	0.757	0.870	0.861	0.868	0.848	0.833	0.753	0.671	0.574	0.475	0.355

[a] Represents the number of subjects evaluating efficacy at that time point (i.e., number of active subjects).

[b] Model: PID = μ + Trt(i)+ baseline(i) + error

[c] Model: PID = μ + Trt(i) + baseline(j) + Trt*Baseline(ij) + error

[d] Protected LSD based on model LSMEANS. Same letters indicate nonsignificant treatment differences. Different letters indicate the overall treatment p-value from ANOVA < = 0.05.

[e] Represents the number of subjects analyzed for efficacy based on extrapolated data.

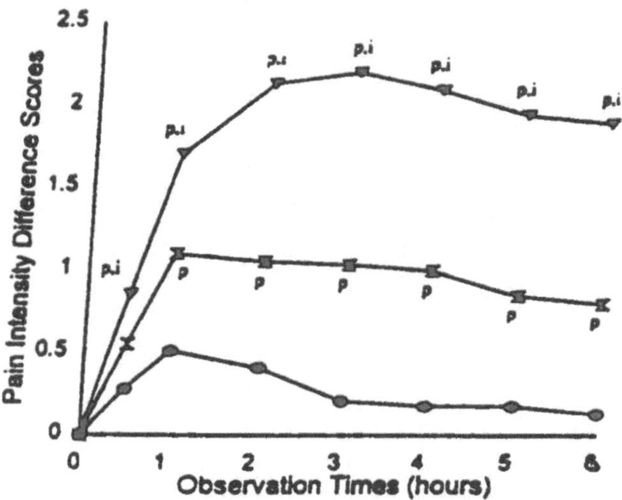

Figure 3 Time–effect curve for mean pain intensity difference: Statistically significant treatment differences: p, significantly superior to placebo; i, significantly superior to 400 mg of ibuprofen based on Fisher's protected least-significant difference test, p ≤ 0.05., placebo; ●, ibuprofen 400 mg; ⧗, hydrocodone 15 mg with ibuprofen 400 mg; ▼. (From Ref. 12.)

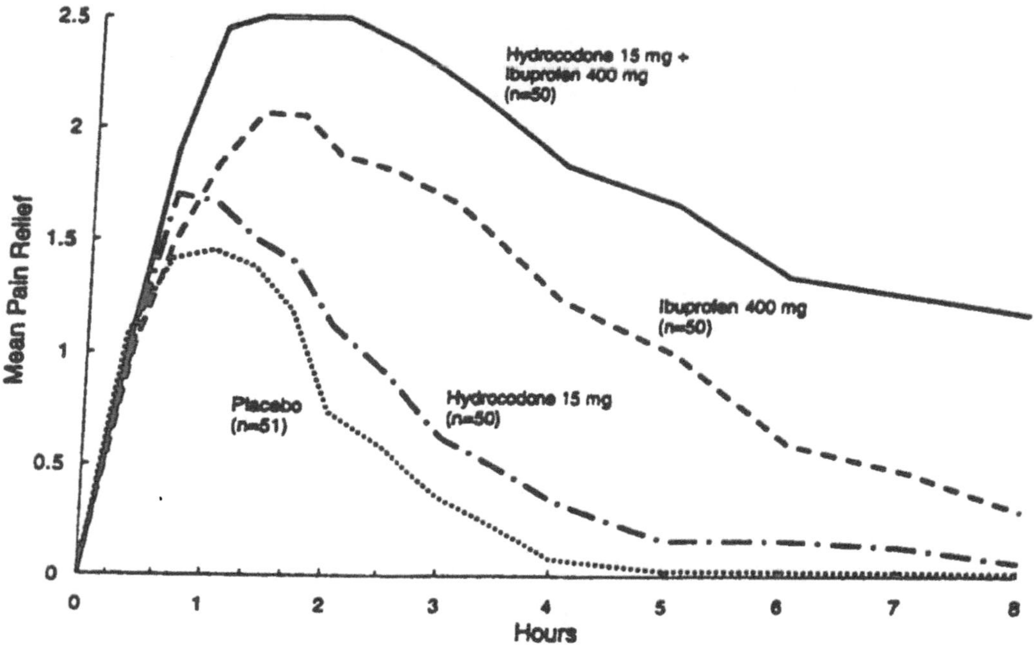

Figure 4 Time–effect curves for 15 mg of hydrocodone, 400 mg of ibuprofen, the combination of 15 mg of hydrocodone with 400 mg of ibuprofen, and placebo: Mean pain relief scores are plotted. (From Ref. 11.)

Table 2 Means (Standard Deviations), Sample Sizes, and Fisher's Protected LSD Comparisons

Treatment	Assessment time point (in hours from dosing)													
	0.5		1		2		3		4		5		6	
Vicoprofen 400/15 mg (n = 40)[e]	0.85	(0.70)	1.70	(0.72)	2.13	(0.69)	2.20	(0.61)	2.10	(0.63)	1.95	(0.64)	1.90	(0.67)
	[40][a]	A[d]	[40]	A	[40]	A	[40]	A	[40]	A	[40]	A	[40]	A
Ibuprofen 400 mg (n = 40)	0.55	(0.60)	1.10	(0.74)	1.05	(0.88)	1.00	(0.85)	1.00	(0.78)	0.85	(0.74)	0.80	(0.69)
	[40]	B	[40]	B	[39]	B	[34]	B	[30]	B	[30]	B	[30]	B
Placebo (n = 39)	0.28	(0.56)	0.41	(0.79)	0.38	(0.63)	0.18	(0.56)	0.18	(0.51)	0.18	(0.51)	0.18	(0.41)
	[39]	B	[39]	C	[25]	C	[20]	C	[12]	C	[7]	C	[7]	C
Treatment P-value[b]	<0.001		<0.001		<0.001		<0.001		<0.001		<0.001		<0.001	
Trt*baseline P-value[c]	0.914		0.332		0.205		0.343		0.198		0.105		0.071	
RMS error[b]	0.614		0.693		0.693		0.646		0.626		0.601		0.557	

[a] Represents the number of subjects evaluating efficacy at that time point (i.e., number of active subjects).

[b] Model: PID = μ + Trt(i) + baseline(j) + error.

[c] Model: PID = μ + Trt(i) + baseline(j) + Trt*baseline(ij) + error.

[d] Protected LSD based on model LSMEANS. Same letters indicate nonsignificant treatment differences. Different letters indicate the overall treatment p-value from ANOVA < = 0.05.

[e] Represents the number of subjects analyzed for efficacy based on extrapolated data.

REFERENCES

1. Max MB, Payne R, Edwards WT, Sunshine A, Inturrisi CE. Principles of Analgesic Use in the Treatment of Acute Pain and Cancer Pain. 4th ed. Glenview, IL; American Pain Society, 1999.
2. Laska EM, Sunshine A, Wanderling JA, Meisner MJ. Quantitative differences in aspirin analgesia in three models of clinical pain. J Clin Pharmacol 1982; 22:531–542.
3. Cooper SA. Five studies on ibuprofen for postsurgical dental pain. In:Proceedings of a Symposium—Motrin (Ibuprofen) Past, Present and Future. Am J Med 1984; 77:70–77.
4. Sunshine A, Olson NZ. Nonnarcotic analgesics. In: Wall PD, Melzack R, eds. Textbook of Pain, 3rd ed. New York: Churchill Livingstone; 1994:923–942.
5. U.S. Food and Drug Administration. Guideline for the Clinical Evaluation of Analgesic Drugs. Rockville, MD. Revised 1992; Docket No. 91D-04525.
6. Laska E, Meisner M, Tang D–I. Classification of the effectiveness of combination treatments. Statist Med 1997; 16:2211–2228.
7. New Drug Approval Package for Vicoprofen. Supplied over the Internet by CDER Freedom of Electronic Information Office, April 28, 1998; (http://www.fda.gov/cder/foi/nda/index.htm).
8. Sunshine A, Roure C, Olson NZ, Laska E, Zorilla C, Rivera J. Analgesic efficacy of two ibuprofen–codeine combinations for the treatment of post-episiotomy and post-operative pain. Clin Pharmacol Ther 1987; 42:374–380.
9. Cooper SA, Engel J, Ladov M, Precheur H, Rosenheck A, Rauch D. Analgesic efficacy of an ibuprofen–codeine combination. Pharmacotherapy 1982; 2:162–167.
10. Quiding H, Grimstad J, Rusten K, Stubhaug A, Bremnes J, Breivik H. Ibuprofen plus codeine, ibuprofen, and placebo in a single and multidose cross-over comparison for coxarthrosis pain. Pain 1992; 50:303–307.
11. Wideman GL, Keffer M, Morris E, Doyle RT, Jiang JG, Beaver WT. Analgesic efficacy of a combination of hydrocodone with ibuprofen in postoperative pain. Clin Pharmacol Ther 1999; 65:66–76.
12. Sunshine A, Olson NZ, O'Neill E, Ramos I, Doyle RT. Analgesic efficacy of a hydrocodone with ibuprofen combination compared with ibuprofen alone for the treatment of acute postoperative pain. J Clin Pharmacol 1997; 37:908–915.
13. Physician's Desk Reference. 53 ed. Montvale, NJ: Medical Economics Company, 1999;1489.

39
NSAIDs and COX-2 Inhibitors

Alan Naylor
GlaxoSmithKline, Harlow, Essex, England

I. HISTORICAL INTRODUCTION

Nonsteroidal anti-inflammatory drugs in the form of salicylates have been used for centuries for the control of pain and inflammation. Acetylsalicylic acid, aspirin, was the first of this class to be synthesized by Felix Hoffman in 1899 and thus became generally available for medical use. Since the profile of activity of this class was clearly different from the glucocorticoids, they were named "nonsteroidal anti-inflammatory drugs" (NSAIDs).

In 1971, the pioneering work of Vane (1) demonstrated that aspirin inhibited the formation of prostaglandins via inhibition of the cyclooxygenase (COX) enzyme. COX is the enzyme responsible for the conversion of arachidonic acid, released from membrane phospholipids by the action of phopholipase, into the endoperoxide Prostaglandin G_2 via the cyclooxygenase reaction, and subsequently via a hydroperoxidase-mediated conversion to Prostaglandin H_2, the precursor to the wide range of prostanoids known today (Fig. 1). The bifunctional enzyme responsible for the conversion of arachidonic acid to PGH_2 is colloquially referred to as "cyclo-oxygenase (COX)" although it is more correctly named "prostaglandin H_2 synthase (PGHS)."

II. PHYSIOLOGICAL AND PATHOLOGICAL EFFECTS OF PROSTAGLANDINS

Prostaglandins are produced ubiquitously and have diverse biological functions, being involved in both physiological and pathological functions (Table 1). For example, prostacylin and PGE_2 are known to be cytoprotective in the gastrointestinal tract and are also responsible for maintaining normal renal function. Prostaglandins are also involved in a host of inflammatory and nociceptive pathologies and are released by a variety of cells involved in the inflammatory process.

Prostaglandins produce the characteristic symptoms of inflammation by several mechanisms. Prostaglandin-mediated vasodilatation of small blood vessels is responsible for the redness, heat, and edema associated with typical inflammatory responses. Prostaglandins also sensitize peripheral nociceptors that are responsible for transmitting painful stimuli to the central nervous system. There is also an increasing amount of evidence that prostaglandins may be directly involved in nociceptive processing in the central nervous system (2).

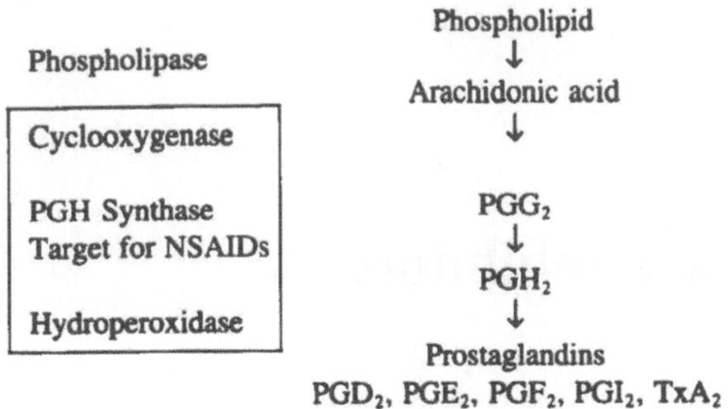

Figure 1 Biosynthesis of prostaglandins: target for NSAID drugs.

III. NONSTEROIDAL ANTI-INFLAMMATORY DRUGS (NSAIDs)

Hoffman could not have imagined that aspirin would become the forerunner of a large family of nonsteroidal anti-inflammatory drugs (NSAIDs), which, by virtue of their ability to inhibit cyclooxygenase, have become the mainstay of treatment of inflammatory disease such as rheumatoid arthritis, osteoarthritis, and a range of musculoskeletal disorders, e.g., back pain. Such is the widespread use of this class of agent that they accounted for 54% of the prescription analgesic market in 1996.

NSAIDs can be categorized broadly into carboxylic acids, which include the anthranilic acids and arylacetic acids, enolic acids, and nonacidic compounds (Table 2).

Despite providing first-line therapy for inflammatory pain for many years, NSAIDs are associated with a significant side-effect liability. The most pronounced of these is gastrointestinal toxicity in the form of gastric erosions and, in extreme cases, overt ulceration and bleeding. It has been estimated that, in the United Kingdom alone, over 1500 deaths and 15,000 hospital admissions per year are associated with NSAID-induced gastrotoxicity. The gastric toxicity of these agents is believed to result from inhibition of cytoprotective prostaglandins, e.g., prostacyclin and prostaglandin E_2, which regulate gastric blood flow and mucus secretion. A detailed study on the relative propensity of NSAIDs to cause gastrointestinal damage has been reported by Langman et al. (3), who employed epidemiological data to rank them in order of toxicity (Table 3).

In addition to detectable gastrointestinal damage, the use of NSAIDs is often associated with adverse symptomatic events such as dyspepsia, diarrhea, and gastric pain. It is these symptomatic effects that often result in the physician switching to an alternative NSAID on the basis of poor tolerability to a specific agent.

Table 1 Physiological and Pathological Roles of Prostaglandins

Physiological functions	Pathological functions
Vascular smooth muscle—control of blood flow	Vasodilatation—heat, edema, vascular permeability
Platelet aggregation	Inflammation
Renal blood flow—salt balance	Sensitization of peripheral nerve fibres
Gastric blood flow—mucus secretion	Stimulation of tissue damage
Uterine muscle tone—ovulation	Cell proliferation—tumor cells
Bronchial smooth muscle tone	Brain—fever, inflammation
Brain spinal cord—neuronal transmission?	

Table 2 Classification of NSAIDs

Arylacetic acids		Salicylic/anthranilic acids	
Representative examples		Representative examples	
Diclofenac 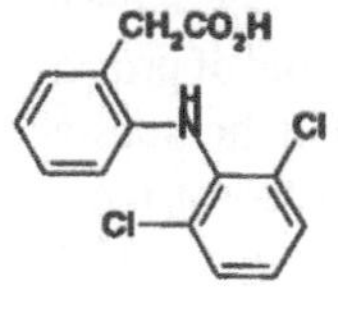	Indomethacin 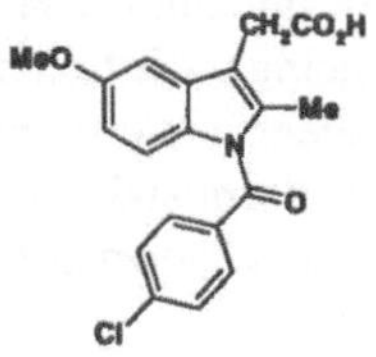	Acetylsalicylic acid (aspirin) 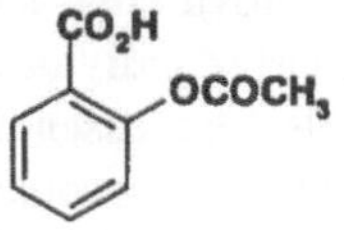	Meclofenamic acid 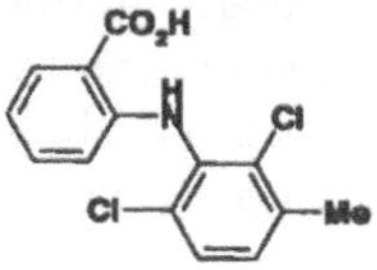
Others in class		Others in class	
Fenclofenac	Tolmetin	Diflunisal	Flufenamic acid
Alclofenac	Etodolac		Mefenamic acid
	Sulindac		
Nabumetone (prodrug of 6-methoxy-naphthyl acetic acid)			
Arylpropionic acids		**Enolic acids/pyrazolones**	
Representative examples		Representative examples	
Ibuprofen 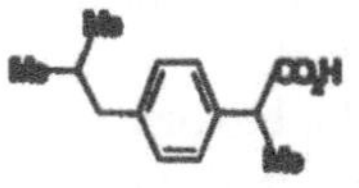	Naproxen 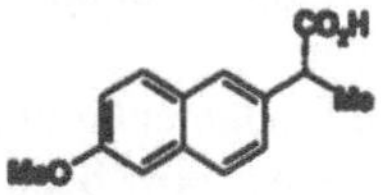	Piroxicam 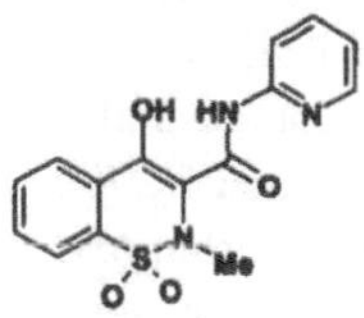	Phenylbutazone 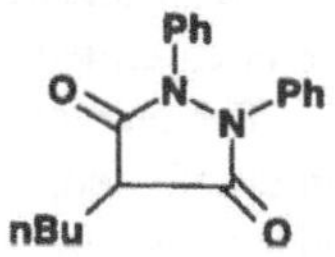
Others in class		Others in class	
Fenoprofen	Oxaprozin	Isoxicam	Azapropazone
Ketoprofen	Tiaprofenic acid	Tenoxicam	
Flurbiprofen			

Table 3 Relative Gastrointestinal Safety of NSAIDs

NSAID	Odds ratio (95% confidence interval) for acute GI bleeding (3)
None	4.5 (3.6–5.6)
Ibuprofen	2.0 (1.4–2.8)
Diclofenac	4.2 (2.6–6.8)
Naproxen	9.1 (5.5–15.1)
Indomethacin	11.3 (6.3–20.3)
Piroxicam	13.7 (7.1–26.3)
Ketoprofen	23.7 (7.6–74.2)
Azapropazone	31.5 (10.3–96.9)

Various strategies have been employed to overcome or counteract the gastrointestinal toxicity of NSAIDs (4). The use of high doses of H_2-receptor antagonists, proton-pump inhibitors, and sucralfate has produced varying degrees of success. Misoprostol, a prostaglandin E_1 analog, has also been shown to significantly reduce serious gastrointestinal side-effects but its use is associated with other significant side effects.

To a much lesser degree, NSAIDs have also been associated with serious renal toxicities, particularly in patients with cardiovascular morbidities or impaired renal function. Thus, elderly patients represent the main cohort of individuals experiencing these toxicities. The role of prostaglandins in the kidney is complex, but essentially these agents are present to maintain homeostasis. In particular, prostaglandins are produced to offset hormonally induced vasoconstriction such as occurs in hypertension, and it is the inhibition of vasodilatory prostaglandins by NSAIDs that results in nephritis.

The discovery of two distinct isoforms of cyclooxygenase, COX-1 and COX-2, has been a major advance in identifying a strategy for separating the beneficial effects of NSAIDs from their associated toxicities.

IV. ISOFORMS OF CYCLOOXYGENASE

For many years only a single isoform of COX or Prostaglandin-H_2 synthase (PGHS) was known. This isoform was first purified from sheep seminal vesicles as described by Lands et al. in 1976 (5). It has now been shown that at least two isoforms of the enzyme exist, which, although identical in biochemical function, have very different pathophysiological roles. These isoforms have been called COX-1 and COX-2.

The enzyme isolated by Lands et al., on which the fundamental prostaglandin biology has been elucidated, is currently termed COX-1. This enzyme has now been well characterized and cDNA clones have been obtained from many species. The mRNA for COX-1 encodes a protein of 599–602 amino acids, depending on species, which exhibits approximately 90% identity between mammalian species. COX-1 has been found to be constitutively expressed and widely distributed throughout most mammalian tissue, particularly stomach, intestine, kidney, and platelets, and is regarded as a "housekeeping" enzyme responsible for maintaining homeostasis.

More recently a second isoform of the enzyme, COX-2, has been characterized from several species, including humans. In contrast to COX-1, COX-2 is not widely expressed under normal physiological conditions but is up-regulated in cells such as synoviocytes, fibroblasts, monocytes, and macrophages under the influence of proinflammatory mediators, e.g., TNF and IL-1 (6–8). The COX-2 gene was originally identified in several studies on the regulation of gene expression in response to mitogen challenge in chick embryo fibroblasts (9) and in Swiss 3T3 cells, in which the mRNA, found to be induced by phorbol-ester and originally called TIS10 was ultimately associated with that of murine COX-2 (10). The induction of the COX-2 gene by mitogens was found to be inhibited by glucocorticoids such as dexamethasone (10,11) whereas expression of COX-1 was insensitive to the presence of dexamethasone.

Across species, the cDNA for COX-2 possesses approximately 60% homology with that of COX-1. Interestingly, the mRNA for COX-1 is ca. 2.8 kb whereas that for COX-2 is ca. 4.5 kb and, in contrast with COX-1, contains several Shaw-Kamen instability sequences (AUUA) in the 3′-untranslated region typical of immediate early-response genes. Furthermore, the promoter region of the COX-2 gene contains a number of potential binding sites for transcription factors such as NF-kB, CCAAT/enhancer-binding protein (C/EBP), also referred to as the nuclear factor for IL-6 or NF-IL6, and the cyclic-AMP-responsive-binding protein (CREBP). These transcription factors are known to be stimulated by proinflammatory cytokines (Fig. 2).

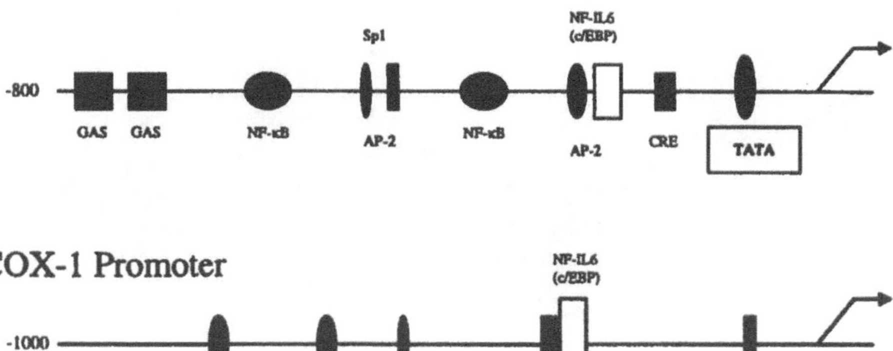

Figure 2 Comparison of promoter regions of COX-2 and COX-1.

Both COX-1 and COX-2 are membrane-bound, heme-containing, homodimeric glycoproteins of approximately 71 kda mass. Both isoforms are found in the endoplasmic reticulum and, particularly COX-2, in the nuclear envelope of the cell. Both proteins also contain linked cyclooxygenase and peroxidase activities, and the kinetics of formation of PGH_2 is identical in both isoforms, consistent with the finding that the amino acid sequence around the active site channel is highly conserved.

A summary comparison of the protein and gene structures of the two isoforms is shown in Figure 3.

A recent X-ray crystallographic study of human COX-2 by Luong et al. (12) has shown the structure to be similar to that of sheep COX-1, the structure of which had previously been elucidated by Picot et al. (13). The enzyme consists of three separate protein domains (Fig. 4). An N-terminal beta sheet EGF-like domain, so named as a result of its structural similarity to that of Epidermal Growth Factor (EGF), is believed to be responsible for maintaining the structural integrity of the dimer. Contiguous to the EGF-like domain is a helical amphipathic region

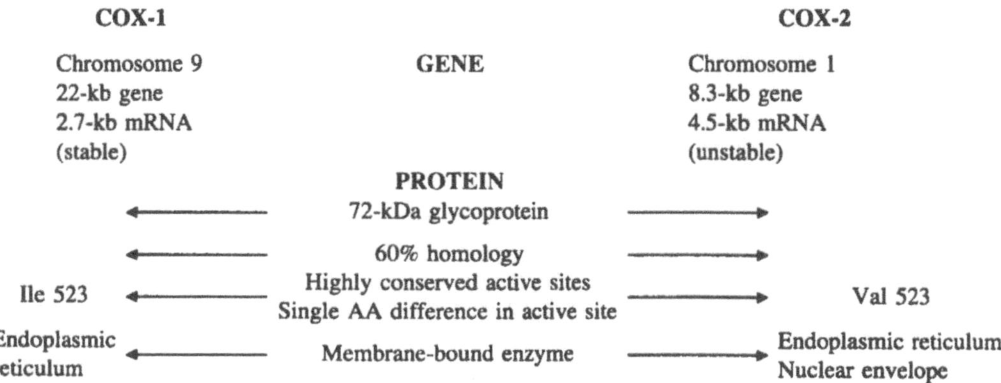

Figure 3 Comparison of protein and gene structures for COX-1 and COX-2.

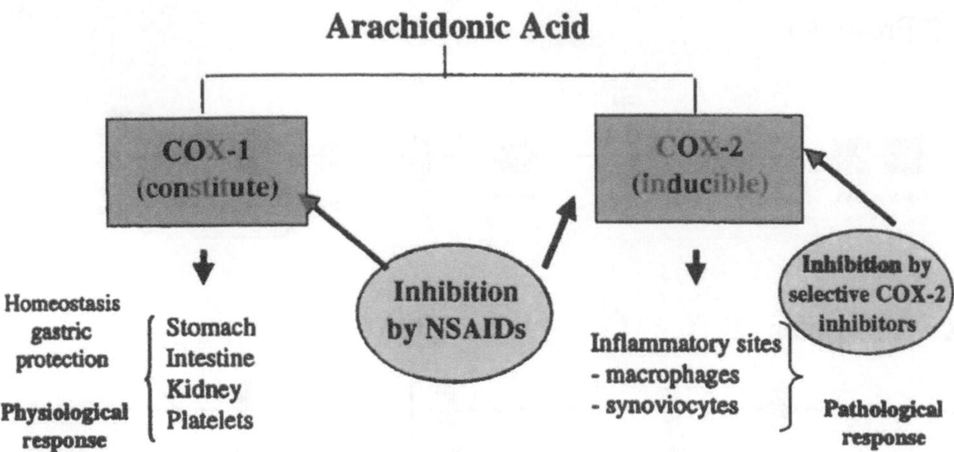

Figure 4 The "COX-2 Hypothesis."

that is responsible for "anchoring" the enzyme into the cell membrane. The enzymes are monotopic, i.e., they do not cross the lipid bilayer, but are simply anchored into the cell membrane. This lipophilic domain provides a channel from the cell membrane to the active catalytic site of the enzyme containing the cyclooxygenase and peroxidase functionalities. This region has been shown to be the site at which a variety of NSAIDs bind.

The overall amino acid sequence identity between human COX-1 and COX-2 is 63%; however, the only difference between the two isoforms in the active site is a region that occurs at residue 523 in which the isoleucine residue in COX-1 is replaced by a valine residue in COX-2. This single difference has been shown to have a significant effect on the overall size and shape of the binding site (12) and may be the basis for the selectivity of at least some of the recently identified classes of selective COX-2 inhibitors to be discussed later.

V. THE "COX-2 HYPOTHESIS" AS THE BASIS FOR A SAFER CLASS OF NSAID

The identification of the inducible isoform COX-2 led to the hypothesis that selective inhibitors of COX-2 might provide effective analgesic and anti-inflammatory agents that would be devoid of the gastrointestinal (GI) toxicity associated with the nonselective inhibitors, i.e., the NSAIDs. The basis of the hypothesis, which is summarized in Figure 4, is that selective COX-2 inhibitors would only inhibit the inducible form of the enzyme, up-regulated at sites of inflammation, but would not inhibit the production of prostanoids via COX-1, which are involved in maintaining homeostasis and protection of the gastric mucosa.

Early support for this hypothesis was provided by Seibert's group at Searle, which compared the potencies of indomethacin and an early selective COX-2 inhibitor, SC 58125, at inhibiting prostanoid production in the inflamed mouse paw and GI tract and correlated this data with the COX-2 selectivity observed in vitro (14). Although both agents were shown to be potent analgesics, the COX-2 inhibitor produced was significantly less ulcerogenic than indomethacin (Table 4).

The pioneering work of the Searle group provided a rational explanation for the safety profile of the structurally related analgesic/antiinflammatory agent DuP 697 (Fig. 6), which had been investigated by the DuPont group some years earlier (15). Similarly, the sulfonamide

Table 4 Preclinical Validation of the "Cox-2 Hypothesis"

Inhibitor	COX-2 selectivity[a]	ED_{50}(mg/kg) PG inflamm. (COX-2)	PG GI (COX-1)	Analgesia	GI toxicity
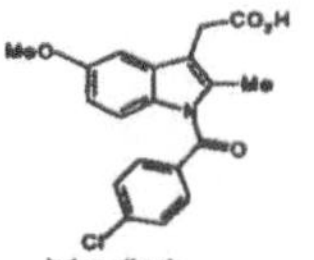 Indomethacin	3	0.4	0.4	2.0	8.0
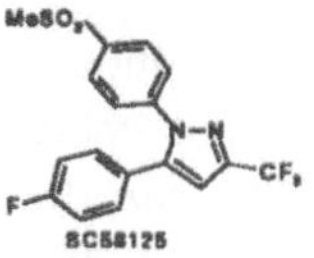 SC58125	>200	0.1	>10	10	>600

[a] Mouse recombinant enzyme essays.
Source: Adapted from Seibert et al. (14).

derivatives nimesulide and flosulide (Fig. 7), which had previously been evaluated clinically, were also shown to have selectivity for the COX-2 isoform (16).

Subsequent to the initial validation of the hypothesis, there has been an explosion of interest in this class of agent by the pharmaceutical industry and many new COX-2 inhibitors have emerged over the past few years. The main classes of COX-2 inhibitors and key examples are summarized in the following section.

VI. CLASSES OF SELECTIVE COX-2 INHIBITORS

The intensive search for selective inhibitors of COX-2 has focused largely on three main structural classes of compounds, tricyclic inhibitors based on DuP 697 and SC 58125, methanesulfonamide derivatives derived from nimesulide and flosulide and structurally modified NSAIDs. The key compounds in each category are summarized below. More comprehensive discussions on the various structural modifications can be found in reviews by Carter (17), Kalgutkar (18), and Talley (19), and de Leval (20) since a comprehensive coverage of the structural classes is beyond the scope of this chapter.

VII. TRICYCLIC INHIBITORS

Interest in this class has obviously been stimulated by the early work of Searle, which has produced the majority of agents in this field. The generic structure of this class can be represented as shown in Figure 5, which illustrates a cyclic template that can be heterocyclic, carbocyclic, or even a double bond, substituted by a phenyl ring, bearing either a sulfone or sulfonamido substituent in the para position (R1). Juxtaposed is a side chain (R2), which is normally a substituted aryl or heteroaryl moiety but can be replaced by an alkoxy, aryloxy, or cycloalkyl derivative.

Prototype molecules of this structural class are DuP 697 and SC 58125. A wide variety of structural modifications to this template have been made, culminating in the introduction of Celebrex (celecoxib), from Searle (now Pfizer/Pharmacia), and Vioxx (rofecoxib), from Merck. Both agents are potent, highly selective inhibitors of COX-2. Celebrex is reported to have an IC_{50} of 40nM against recombinant human COX-2 and a selectivity ratio of 375, whereas Vioxx

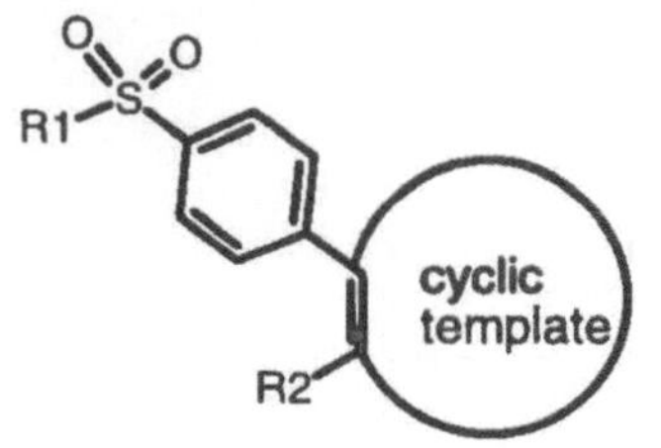

Figure 5 Generalized structure of the tricyclic class of inhibitors.

is claimed to have an IC_{50} of 18nM and a selectivity ratio of 800. However, caution should be exercised in interpreting inhibitory data from different laboratories even when comparable preparations are being employed. Many factors can influence the data obtained from enzyme preparations such as species, incubation time, and enzyme source, e.g., cell, microsome, and purified and human blood (21). Furthermore, the kinetics of inhibition are very complex with time dependency being a factor particularly when measuring COX-2 potency. The latter phenomenon will be discussed later.

Pfizer and Merck are currently engaged in launching backup molecules to their first-generation inhibitors, both of which fall into the tricyclic category. Arcoxia (etoricoxib), from Merck, is claimed to demonstrate superior selectivity for COX-2 compared with the previous agents. In human whole blood the compound shows greater than 100-fold selectivity compared with 35-fold and 7.6-fold for Vioxx and Celebrex respectively. Against recombinant human COX-2 the compound is reported to have an IC_{50} of 79nM and greater than 600-fold selectivity over COX-1 (22). Arcoxia was launched in the United Kingdom in 2002 although it has not yet been approved in the United States following Merck's withdrawal of the NDA.

Pfizer/Pharmacia has recently launched Bextra (valdecoxib) as a follow-up to Celebrex. Bextra is reported to have an IC_{50} of 5nM against recombinant human COX-2 and 28,000-fold selectivity over COX-1. In common with other COX-2 inhibitors, the selectivity measured in whole blood is much lower than against recombinant enzyme, and for Bextra is 28-fold, with an IC_{50} of 890nM (23). Bextra was launched in the United States in April 2002 and was approved in Europe in July 2002. Pfizer/Pharmacia has also launched Dynastat, a water-soluble pro-drug of Bextra as the first injectable COX-2 inhibitor for the treatment of acute pain. Approval in Europe was obtained in November 2001, however the FDA has requested additional data before granting approval in the United States. A detailed description of the pharmacokinetic and pharmacodynamic profile has been published (24). Since a number of pharmaceutical companies are active in pursuing compounds of this general structural class it is anticipated that more agents of this type will be introduced into clinical usae in the future and a review of the latest disclosures has recently been published (20).

Clinical data on the available COX-2 inhibitors will be discussed later.

VIII. METHANESULPHONAMIDE INHIBITORS

Following the discovery that NS-398 (Fig. 7) showed significant selectivity at inhibiting the COX-2 isoform (25), two related compounds, nimesulide and flosulide, were also reinvestigated and found to be COX-2 selective (26,27). Both agents have been used clinically as analgesic/anti-inflammatory agents although flosulide (28) has since been discontinued. Several related structures have subsequently been synthesized. In particular, replacement of the ether oxygen of flosulide by a sulfur atom provided the Merck compound L745337 (27) that was used in early "hypothesis-proving" studies.

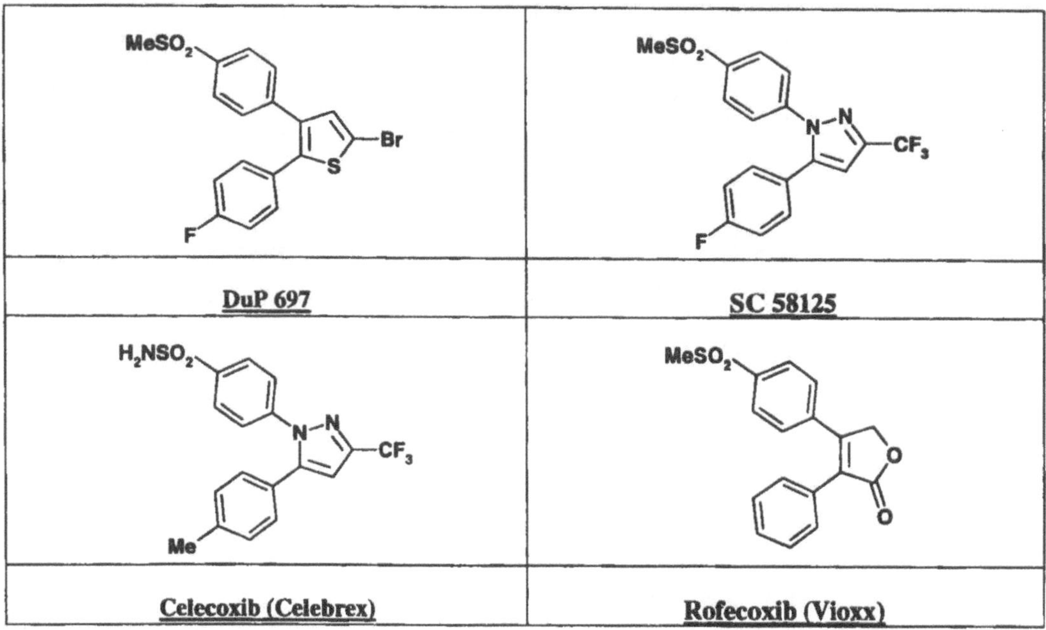

Figure 6 Key tricyclic inhibitors.

IX. MODIFICATION OF NSAIDs

Several groups have explored the strategy of modifying known NSAID molecules to introduce COX-2 selectivity, largely based on the premise that the NSAID-binding pocket in COX-2 is larger than that in COX-1. Thus the group at Merck has modified the structure of indomethacin to produce L-761,066, which shows high selectivity for COX-2 (29,30) (Fig. 8). The Abbott group has also modified indomethacin in a different manner to identify the thiazole (Fig. 8, panel "1") (31). Several patents have appeared recently claiming additional analogs of indomethacin exhibiting COX-2 selectivity (20). Modification of zomepirac by the Roche group has resulted in the selective analog (Fig. 8, panel "2") (32).

Relatively simple modifications to known NSAIDs have been successful in introducing selectivity, as exemplified by meta-substituted analogs of diclofenac such as (Fig. 8, panel "3"),

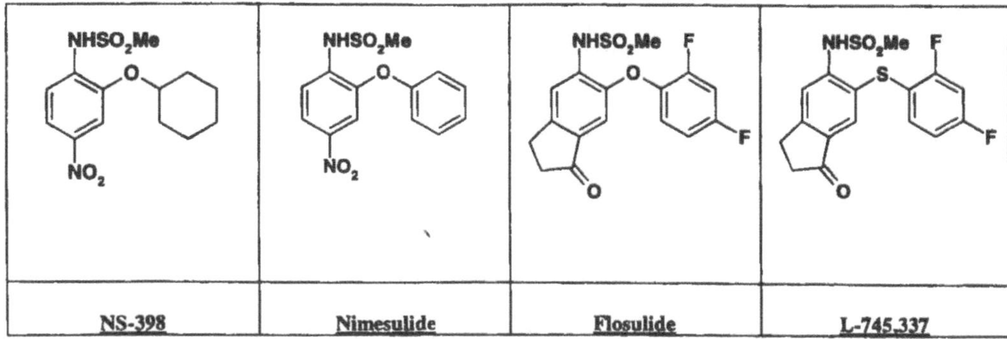

Figure 7 Key methanesulphonamide inhibitors.

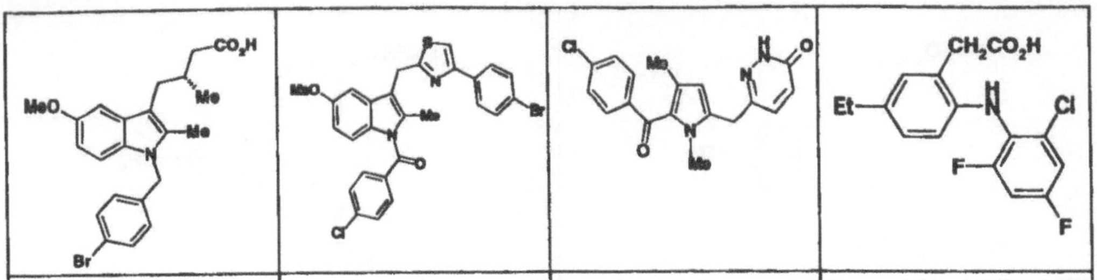

L-761,066	(1)	(2)	(3)

Figure 8 Modification of NSAIDs to selective COX-2 inhibitors.

being investigated by Novartis (33). Several other NSAIDs have also recently been modified to provide selective COX-2 inhibitors (18).

X. MECHANISM OF INHIBITION

A. Structural Basis

The protein structure of COX-2 and differences between COX-2 and COX-1 have been discussed earlier. Arg120 has been shown to be very important for arachidonate and NSAID binding to the active site since site-directed mutagenesis of the arginine residue to either glutamine or glutamate diminishes the binding of arachidonate and the inhibitory activity of NSAIDs (34). However, a recent publication has shown that the interaction with Arg120 is via a hydrogen-bonding network rather than an ionic interaction and that this interaction is much less important in COX-2 than COX-1 (35). It is also believed that the methanesulfonamide class of inhibitors also interact via hydrogen bonding of the methanesulfonamide moiety with Arg120 in a similar fashion to the carboxylic acid–containing inhibitors.

An explanation for the COX-2 selectivity of the tricyclic class of inhibitor has been provided by cocrystallisation of inhibitors with the enzyme (36). X-ray crystallographic examination reveals that the sulfone/sulfonamide moieties bind to Arg513, which is located in a side pocket that is accessible only in COX-2. This results from the presence of Val523 at the entrance to the side pocket in COX-2, which is replaced by the bulkier isoleucine residue in COX-1. The overall size of the binding site of COX-2 is significantly larger in COX-2. Furthermore, there is greater conformational flexibility at the apex of the active site, with Ile384 having Phe503 as a neighbor in COX-1 as opposed to leucine in COX-2 (37).

A cartoon summary explaining the rationale is given in Figure 9.

B. Enzyme Kinetics

Many of the highly selective COX-2 inhibitors exhibit time-dependent inhibition of COX-2 while weakly inhibiting COX-1 in a time-independent fashion (Fig. 10). Thus maximum inhibition of COX-2 will develop over a period of time and the selectivity at earlier time points will be lower than at longer time points, at which point some inhibitors appear to be pseudo-irreversible at COX-2 (38). This phenomenon is probably a contributory factor to the variability in data obtained from different groups.

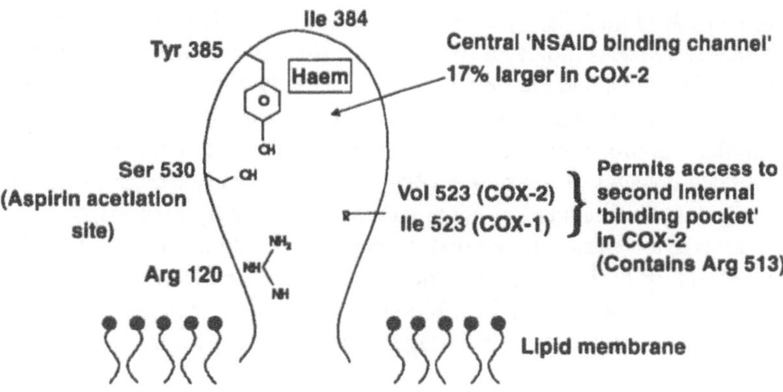

Figure 9 Mechanism of selective inhibition.

XI. CLINICAL EXPERIENCE WITH COX-2 INHIBITORS

The first clinically available selective COX-2 inhibitors were Celebrex (celecoxib) from Searle (now Pfizer/Pharmacia) and Vioxx (rofecoxib) from Merck-Frosst (Fig. 6). Celebrex, which is claimed to have 375-fold selectivity for human COX-2 over COX-1, was originally approved by the FDA for the treatment of signs and symptoms of osteoarthritis (OA) and rheumatoid arthritis (RA) in adults at recommended doses of 100 mg twice daily or 200 mg once daily for the treatment of OA, and 100–200 mg twice daily for the treatment of RA. Celebrex was not initially approved for the treatment of acute pain. Data presented from an early single-dose dental pain study indicated that the efficacy of 200 mg Celebrex was similar to 650 mg aspirin but inferior to 550 mg naproxen sodium (39). Furthermore, in a multiple-dose trial in postorthopedic surgery pain, the data were inconsistent. Recently, however, the drug has gained FDA approval for the treatment of acute pain and primary dysmenorrhea in adults.

Early endoscopic studies in a total of 4500 arthritic patients taking doses between 50 and 400 mg twice daily for periods ranging from 12 to 24 weeks have clearly demonstrated that the compound has a much lower ulcerogenic potential than NSAIDs and this safety profile has now been confirmed over 3 years of extensive clinical usage.

COX-2

$$E + I \underset{}{\overset{K_i}{\rightleftharpoons}} EI \underset{K_{off}}{\overset{K_{on}}{\rightleftharpoons}} EI^*$$

- Initial phase competitive/reversible (EI)
- later-phase-"tight binding"(EI*) pseudo-irreversible
- IC_{50} values sensitive to preincubation period

COX-1

$$E + I \underset{}{\overset{K_i}{\rightleftharpoons}} EI$$

- Reversible inhibiton (EI)
- IC_{50} values independent of preincubation period

Figure 10. Enzyme kinetics of inhibition.

Vioxx was approved in the United States in May 1999 and in the United Kingdom in June 1999. In the United States, Vioxx is indicated for the relief of signs and symptoms of OA, the management of acute pain in adults, and the treatment of primary dysmenorrhea. An indication for the treatment of RA was not sought at that time, although approval has recently been granted. In the United Kingdom, approval has been granted for symptomatic relief in the treatment of OA. The recommended dosages of Vioxx are 12.5–25 mg once daily for the treatment of OA and 50 mg once daily for the treatment of acute pain and primary dysmenorrhea.

Initial endoscopic studies again demonstrated that the compound, administered at both 25 mg and 50 mg daily for periods up to 24 weeks, produced a much lower ulceration rate than ibuprofen at 2400 mg daily. Furthermore, occult fecal blood loss associated with the same dose regimes over a 4-week period was studied using ^{51}Cr-tagged red blood cells and shown to be no greater than that in the placebo group.

Despite the impressive gastrointestinal (GI) safety data, the labeling of both agents carries the same GI safety warnings associated with standard NSAIDs. Both Pfizer/Pharmacia and Merck have conducted long-term outcome studies to evaluate the GI safety more thoroughly, particularly with respect to the incidence of serious upper-GI events such as perforations and bleeds. The VIGOR (Vioxx Gastrointestinal Outcome Research) study was conducted in 8076 patients and excluded patients taking low-dose aspirin, whereas the CLASS (Celebrex Long-term Arthritis Safety Study) study admitted those patients taking low dose aspirin. These trials showed that patients who were not taking aspirin had significantly fewer symptomatic and complicated ulcers than patients taking nonselective NSAIDs; however, a significant risk reduction was not demonstrated in those patients in the CLASS study who were taking low-dose aspirin. The results from the VIGOR study however showed an increased relative risk of developing thrombotic cardiovascular events with Vioxx treatment compared with naproxen. In the CLASS study there was no significant difference in the cardiovascular event rates between Celebrex and NSAIDs. The apparent increased cardiovascular risk of Vioxx compared to naproxen is consistent with the absence of an anti-platelet effect being associated with selective COX-2 inhibition. The apparent differences between Vioxx and Celebrex with respect to cardiovascular risk factors may be attributable to differences in study design, in particular the study entrance criteria with respect to patients taking low-dose aspirin; however, further studies are required to confirm whether this is the only explanation or whether other factors are involved (40).

As a result of these studies Pfizer/Pharmacia's Celebrex label has been modified to state that the cardiovascular risk is equivalent to traditional NSAIDs; however, no change to the gastrointestinal safety warning was introduced. In contrast labeling changes for Merck's Vioxx included statements that Vioxx had demonstrated a clear gastrointestinal safety advantage over NSAIDs, but also included information referring to the apparent increased risk of cardiovascular thrombotic events.

Clinical experience with the recent COX-2 inhibitors, Arcoxia and Bextra, is limited; however, Merck has recently reported that Arcoxia has performed significantly better than naproxen in a clinical trial in patients with ankylosing spondylitis, in terms of pain control and global assessment. Recent reports of skin hypersensitivity with Pfizer/Pharmacia's Bextra have caused some concern and is under review by the FDA.

XII. OTHER POTENTIAL INDICATIONS OF COX-2 INHIBITORS

A. Colon Cancer

Epidemiological data have indicated that chronic NSAID usage results in a reduction in the incidence of colon cancer (41,42). More recently, animal experiments in the *min* mouse model of adenamatous polyposis have shown COX-2 inhibitors to reduce the number of polyps (43). The susceptibility of these mice to the growth of polyps is due to a defect in the *Apc* gene that is similar to that associated with the occurrence of adenomatous polyposis in humans, a condition that can progress to colonic cancer.

The FDA has recently granted approval for the use of Celebrex as an adjunct to the treatment of adenamatous colorectal polyps in cases of familial adenomatous polyposis.

The full potential of these agents for the treatment of colon cancer remains to be established; however, considerable animal data now illustrates that COX-2 expression may contribute to tumorigenesis (44). Furthermore, increased COX-2 expression has been reported in a range of other human cancers including breast (45), lung (46), prostate (47), and skin (48) cancer.

B. Alzheimer's Disease

There have been several epidemiological studies that suggest the use of NSAIDs delays onset or slows the progression of Alzheimer's disease (AD) (49–52). Further evidence for this potential has been provided by a small clinical trial using indomethacin, which demonstrated a slowing of disease progression relative to placebo over a 6-month period (53). In addition, neuronal COX-2 expression has been shown to be elevated in the AD brain (54).

Despite this, the precise mechanism is currently not clear. In vitro COX-2 inhibitors reduce prostaglandin production from activated microglial cells, suggesting an anti-inflammatory mechanism may be important, although Pasinetti has speculated that COX-2 induction may be related to oxidative stress and the formation of neurotoxic prostanoid derivatives (55).

Although initial short-term studies on the effectiveness of COX-2 inhibitors in the treatment of AD have been disappointing both Celebrex and Vioxx are undergoing long-term prevention trials and the outcome of these studies is eagerly awaited.

C. Preterm Labor

Indomethacin has been known for several years to delay the onset of preterm labor; however, this agent is not widely used owing to its adverse effects on closure of the ductus arteriosus. More recently, Bennet has employed the COX-2 selective inhibitor nimesulide to successfully delay labor in a "high-risk" case and demonstrated no adverse effects on fetal renal or ductal blood flow (56).

Merck has recently demonstrated the efficacy of Vioxx for this condition in a Phase III study in 118 patients who were at 22–34 weeks of gestation.

XIII. POTENTIAL ADVERSE EFFECTS OF COX-2 INHIBITORS

Since NSAIDs inhibit COX-2 as well as COX-1, there are unlikely to be many adverse events associated with the use of COX-2 inhibitors that would be unlikely to occur with NSAIDs at equi-efficacious doses. There is some evidence from the recent large outcome studies that the absence of the COX-1 inhibitory activity may lead to an increased susceptibility to cardiovascular events through further clarification is still required. Furthermore, should the increased therapeutic window for these agents encourage the use of much higher doses than recommended, particularly for highly specific second-generation COX-2 inhibitors, it is possible that unanticipated adverse events could occur. It is becoming clear that COX-2 inhibitors will not provide any advantage over NSAIDs with respect to renal side-effects. Similarly, there is still no clear evidence on the effects of selective COX-2 inhibitors on asthmatic individuals having aspirin sensitivity.

It has been reported that COX-2 expression can be induced in the vascular endothelium by platelet microparticles (57) and that PGI_2 production was reduced by COX-2 inhibitors. This induction of COX-2 occurs via a mechanism that is independent of TXA_2 activation and thus the effects of selective COX-2 inhibition on the homeostatic mechanism of endothelial activation remain to be established.

Data from studies in experimental models of colitis in rats have shown that inhibition of COX-2 causes exacerbation of the condition resulting in perforation of the bowel (58). On a similar theme, the COX-2 knockout mouse has been shown to have increased susceptibility to dextran sodium sulfate–induced colonic inflammation (59). These effects have been attributed to impairment of the healing and repair process by inhibition of prostaglandin production. However, from the considerable clinical safety data available on Vioxx and Celebrex, there is no evidence to date that these effects translate to humans.

XIV. FUTURE PERSPECTIVES

It is arguable that the introduction of COX-2 inhibitors represents the most significant breakthrough in the treatment of inflammatory pain and inflammation since the wider usage of aspirin was made possible by Hoffman over 100 years ago. It will be interesting to observe how the clinical use and market for COX-2 inhibitors develops over the next 10 years. The discovery of NSAIDs heralded the introduction of a plethora of agents of this class, and in view of the ongoing activity in this field, it is likely that many more COX-2 inhibitors will be available in the future.

What will second-generation inhibitors offer? It is likely that future compounds will possess extremely high selectivity for the COX-2 isoform, which should enable much higher doses to be used than has previously been possible with NSAIDs. Whether this is likely to bring added clinical benefit with respect to pain and inflammation over NSAIDs remains to be determined. However, the possibility of safely increasing the dose may facilitate the discovery and exploitation of other potential applications, some of which, such as cancer, are only just emerging. Clearly, neither of the currently available agents has a fully comprehensive package of indications, as mentioned earlier, and future compounds are likely to address these shortcomings. Furthermore, complete removal of the NSAID GI warning label has still not been achieved and is a key objective of those engaged in this field.

The individual patient response to a given NSAID has been found to be quite variable and clinicians will often switch the treatment two or three times before finding an NSAID that is both reasonably well tolerated and providing effective pain relief. The precise reasons for this are not entirely clear but interpatient variability related to pharmacokinetic parameters is likely to be a contributory factor (60). The attainment of a consistent patient response will still be a challenge for the new COX-2 inhibitors for which dose-proportional exposure is lost at doses only slightly higher than the recommended clinical doses. (See Prescribing information on Celebrex and Vioxx).

Alternative approaches to the modulation of prostanoid-induced hyperalgesia and inflammation are also being pursued, particularly with regard to the identification of selective antagonists for the G-protein-coupled 7-trans membrane domain receptors. Receptors of the EP and IP classes are inducible prostaglandin synthetases are receiving close attention currently, and it will be informative to determine how the analgesic, anti-inflammatory, and safety profiles of such agents compare with those of the COX-2 inhibitors.

REFERENCES

1. Vane JR. Nature New Biol 1971; 231:232–235.
2. (a) Yaksh TL, Svesson C. In: Vane JR, Botting RM, eds. Therapeutic Roles of Selective COX-2 Inhibitors. Willliam Harvey Press, 2001:168–190. (b) Hoffman C. Curr Med Chem 2000; 7(11): 1113–1120.
3. Langman MJS, Morgan L, Worral A. Br Med J 1985; 290:347–349.
4. Donnelly MT, Hawkey CJ. Aliment Pharmacol Ther 1997; 11:227–236.
5. Hemler M, Lands WEM, Smith WL. J Biol Chem 1976; 251:5575–5579.
6. Raz A, et al. J Biol Chem 1988; 253:3022–3028.
7. Fu J, Masferrer J, et al. J Clin Invest 1990; 86:1375–1379.
8. Masferrer JL, et al. Proc Natl Acad Sci USA 1992; 89:3917–3921.
9. Xie W, Chipman D, Robertson R, Erikson R, Simmons D. Proc Natl Acad Sci USA 1991; 88:2692.
10. Kujubu DA, et al. J Biol Chem 1991; 266:12866–12872.
11. O'Banion MK, et al. J Biol Chem 1991; 266:23261–23267.
12. Luong C, et al. Nature Struct Biol 1996; 3:927–933.
13. Picot D, et al. Nature 1994; 367:243–249.
14. Seibert K, et al. Proc Natl Acad Sci USA 1994; 91:12013–12017.
15. Gans K, et al. J Pharm Exp Ther 1989; 254:180.
16. Pairet M, van Ryn J, Mauz A, Schierok H, Diederen W, Turck D. Selective cyclooxygenase-2 inhibitors: pharmacology, clinical effects and therapeutic potential. Dordecht: Kluwer Academic Publishers, 1998, 27–46.
17. Carter JS. Exp Opin Ther Patents 1997; 8:21–29.
18. Kalgutkar AS. Exp Opin Ther Patents 1999; 9:831–849.
19. Talley JJ. In: King FD, Oxford AW, eds. Progress in Medicinal Chemistry. Elsevier Science. 1999; 36:201–233.
20. De Leval X, et al. Expert Opin Ther Patients 2002; 12(7):969–989.
21. Warner DW, Pairet M, van Ryn J. In: Vane JR, Bottin RM, eds. Therapeutic Roles of Selective COX-2 Inhibitors. William Harvey Press, 2001:76–94.
22. Riendeau D, et al. J Pharm Expt Ther 2001; 296(2):558–566.
23. Talley JT, et al. J Med Chem 2000; 43:775–777.
24. Cheer SM, Goa KL. Drugs 2001; 61–1133.
25. Masferrer JL, et al. Proc Natl Acad Sci USA 1994; 91:3228–3232.
26. Rabasseda X. Drugs Today 1996; 365–384.
27. Li CS, et al. J Med Chem 1995; 38:4897–4905.
28. Weisenberg-Bottcher I, et al. Agents Actions 1989; 26:240–242.
29. Black WC, et al. Bioorg Med Chem Lett 1996; 6:725–730.
30. Leblanc Y, et al. Bioorg Med Chem Lett 1996; 6:731–736.
31. Abbott Labs WO 9839330, 1998.
32. Barnett JW, et al. Eur Pat Appl EP 714895, 1996.
33. Novartis, Pat Appl WO 9911605, 1999.
34. Bhattacharyya DK, et al. J Biol Chem 1996; 271:2179–2184.
35. Rieke JC, et al. J Biol Chem 1999; 274:17109–17114.
36. Kurumbail RG, et al. Nature 1996; 384:644–648.
37. Luong C, et al. Nature Struct Biol 1996; 3:927–933.
38. Oulett M, Percival MD. Biochem J 1995; 305:247–251.
39. Hubbard RC, et al. J Invest Med 1996; 44:293A.
40. Hochberg MC. Clinical and Exptl Rheumatol 2001; 19(6 Suppl 25):S15–S22.
41. Kune GA, Kune S, Watso LF. Cancer Res 1988; 48:4399–4404.
42. Peleg II, Maiboch HT, Brown SH, Wilcox CM. Arch Intern Med 1994; 154:394–399.
43. Oshima M, Dinchuk JE, Kargman SL, Oshima H, Hancock B, Kwong E, Trzaskos JM, Evans JF, Taketo MM. Cell 1996; 87:803–809.
44. Sheng H, Kirkland SC, Isakson P, Coffey RJ, Morrow J, Beachamp RD, DuBois RN. J Clin Invest 1997; 99:2254–2259.

45. Hwang D, Scollard D, Byrene J, Levine E. J Nat Cancer Inst 1998; 90:455–460.
46. Wolff H, Saukkonen K, Anttila S, Karjalainen A, Vainio H, Ristimaki A. Cancer Res 1998; 58: 4997–5001.
47. Gupta S, Srivastava M, Ahmed N, Bostwick DG, Mukhtar H. Prostate 2000; 42:73–78.
48. Bucman S, Gresham A, Hale P, Hruza G, Anast J, Maferrer J, Pentland AP. Carcinogenesis 1998; 19:723–729.
49. Breitner JC, Welsh KA, Helms MJ, Gaskell PC, Gau BA, Roses AD, Pericak-Vance MA, Saunders AM. Neurobiol Aging 1995; 16:523–530.
50. McGeer PL, Schulzer M, McGeer EG. Neurology 1996; 47:425–432.
51. Rich JB, Rasmusson DX, Folstein MF, Carson KA, Kawas C, Brandt J. Neurology 1995; 45:51–55.
52. McGeer EG, McGeer PL. Curr Pharm Des 1999; 5:821–836.
53. Rogers J, Kirby LC, Hempelman SR, Berry DL, McGeer PL, Kaszniak AW, Zalinski J, Cofield M, Mansukhani L, Willson P, et al. Neurology 1993; 43:1609–1611.
54. Pasinetti GM, Aisen PS. Neuroscience 1998; 87:319–324.
55. Pasinetti GM. J Neurosci 1998; 54:1–6.
56. Sawdy R, Slater D, Fisk N, Edmonds DK, Bennett P. Lancet 1997; 350:265–266.
57. Barry OP, Pratico D, Lawson JA, Fitzgerald GA. J Clin Invest 1997; 99:2118–2127.
58. Reuter BK, Asfaha S, Buret A, Sharkey KA, Wallace JL. J Clin Invest 1996; 98:2076–2085.
59. Morteau O, Morham SG, Sellon R, Dieleman LA, Langenbach R, Smithies O, Sartor RB. J Clin Invest 2000; 105:469–478.
60. Brune K. Agents Actions 1985; (Suppl):1759–1763.

40
COX-2–Specific Inhibitors
Celecoxib and Second-Generation Agents

William G. Bensen
St. Joseph's Hospital, McMaster University, Hamilton, Ontario, Canada

I. INTRODUCTION

Nonsteroidal anti-inflammatory drugs (NSAIDs) reduce pain and inflammation by inhibiting cyclooxygenase (COX), the enzyme that initiates the biotransformation of arachidonic acid to the prostanoids (1). As discussed in Chapter 39, a second isoform of COX (COX-2), which is induced by cytokines and suppressed by glucocorticoids, was discovered in 1989 in the laboratory of Dr. Philip Needleman (2). Subsequent studies revealed that the isoform COX-1 is constitutively expressed in virtually all tissues, where it initiates the production of prostaglandins involved in physiological "housekeeping" functions, such as gastrointestinal protection and hemostasis (3). In contrast, in most tissues, COX-2 is an inducible enzyme that produces prostaglandins that produce pain and inflammation in response to tissue injury (4). With the discovery that COX exists as these two, distinct isoforms came the awareness that NSAIDs inhibit both COX-1 and COX-2 and, therefore, produce therapeutic anti-inflammatory and analgesic effects, as well as adverse effects on gastrointestinal (GI) mucosa, platelet aggregation, and renal function (5–7).

The ability to characterize the molecular structures of the NSAID-binding sites of COX-1 and COX-2 permitted the development of a novel class of agents, the COX-2–specific inhibitors. The COX-2 molecule contains an NSAID-binding site that is larger than the analogous binding site of COX-1. COX-2–specific agents are able to bind to the larger COX-2-binding site, but not to the smaller binding site found on COX-1, whereas conventional NSAIDs are able to bind to either COX isoform (8). It has been hypothesized that, by sparing the constitutive activity of COX-1, COX-2–specific inhibitors may relieve pain and inflammation with less risk of gastrointestinal or hemostasis complications than is associated with NSAID therapy (9,10). Celecoxib (Celebrex), the first COX-2–specific inhibitor to become commercially available, was approved for the relief of the signs and symptoms of osteoarthritis and rheumatoid arthritis by the U. S. Food and Drug Administration (FDA) in December 1998. A second, rofecoxib (Vioxx), was released in 1999, and two second-generation COX-2–specific inhibitors, valdecoxib and parecoxib, are currently being evaluated in phase III clinical trials.

II. COX-2 SPECIFICITY

A. Biological Versus Clinical Definitions

In any discussion of COX-2 inhibition, it is necessary to distinguish clearly between agents that are relatively COX-2–selective, and agents that are COX-2–specific. Several NSAIDs possess some degree of selectivity for COX-2, but at dosages used clinically, still produce profound inhibition of COX-1 (11). In contrast, COX-2–specific inhibitors are agents that produce little or no inhibition of COX-1 at dosages that are used clinically (12). Many in vitro and ex vivo systems have been developed to characterize the effects of anti-inflammatory drugs on COX-1 and COX-2; however, for an agent to be considered clinically COX-2–specific, it is necessary to demonstrate analgesic and anti-inflammatory efficacy with little or no risk of gastrointestinal toxicity or COX-1–mediated platelet inhibition (12). The hypothesis that COX-2–specific inhibition should reduce pain and inflammation with little gastrointestinal toxicity or antiplatelet effect has been confirmed in both animal models and in clinical studies.

B. Preclinical Findings

Masferrer and colleagues (10) examined the anti-inflammatory, analgesic, and gastrointestinal effects of the specific COX-2 inhibitor NS-938, in comparison with indomethacin, in rats. An inflammatory site was prepared by subcutaneous introduction of air into the intracapsular area of the back (the rate "air pouch" model of inflammation). Injection of carrageenan into this air pouch produces a rapid inflammatory response, including induction of COX-2 messenger ribonucleic acid (mRNA) and protein with an associated increase in inflammatory prostaglandins. Oral administration of indomethacin 1 h before carrageenan injection significantly reduced prostaglandin production both at the site of inflammation and in the stomach, whereas the COX-2–specific inhibitor NS-398 inhibited prostaglandin production only at the site of inflammation. Gastric lesions were evident in animals that had been treated with indomethacin, although no gastric lesions were observed with NS-398 administration, even when administered at 100 times the anti-inflammatory dosage.

Seibert and colleagues (9) compared the analgesic and anti-inflammatory effects of indomethacin and the COX-2–specific inhibitor SC-58125. Tissue injury was produced by injecting a 1% carrageenan solution into the hindpaw of male rats. This results in significant paw edema (a measure of inflammation) and hyperalgesia (as measured by a reduced latency of removal of the carrageenan-injected paw from a heat source). Paw edema and hyperalgesia following injection of carrageenan were reduced by oral administration of both indomethacin and SC-58125. However, whereas oral administration of indomethacin damaged the gastric mucosa and caused intestinal ulcers, even very high dosages of SC-58125 (as much as 30–60 times the ED_{50} for edema) did not.

Using a similar paw edema model, Zhang and colleagues (13) reported that oral administration of SC-58635 (celecoxib) 3 h after carrageenan injection reduced paw edema and hyperalgesia in a dose-dependent manner, and was similar in effectiveness to the nonspecific NSAID ketorolac. Gastrointestinal toxicity was not reported in this study.

These findings provided an initial confirmation of the hypothesis that COX-2–specific inhibition reduces pain and inflammation with less risk of gastrointestinal toxicity than nonselective COX inhibition. The results of these preclinical studies have been confirmed in clinical trials of the COX-2–specific inhibitor celecoxib.

III. CELECOXIB CLINICAL STUDIES: RELIEVING ARTHRITIS PAIN AND INFLAMMATION

The primary goals for managing arthritis are to relieve joint pain, reduce joint inflammation, and minimize disability caused by restricted joint movement. NSAIDs, which have analgesic and anti-inflammatory properties, are currently one component of the standard of care in relieving these signs and symptoms of arthritis, although NSAID therapy is associated with a substantial risk of gastrointestinal toxicity (5).

COX-2–specific inhibitors, such as celecoxib, offer an alternative therapy for the relief of arthritis pain and inflammation. Extensive clinical trials, conducted in over 6000 patients with either osteoarthritis or rheumatoid arthritis, have established that celecoxib possesses anti-inflammatory and analgesic activities comparable with those of commonly prescribed NSAIDs, but with a significant reduction in the incidence of endoscopically determined gastrointestinal injury.

A. Osteoarthritis

In a pilot efficacy study, 293 patients with osteoarthritis of the knee were randomly assigned in a double-blind fashion to 2 weeks of treatment with celecoxib (40, 100, or 200 mg b.i.d.) or placebo (14). Before initiation of treatment, arthritis "flare" was induced by withdrawing anti-inflammatory drugs. Evaluations of clinical response included physician and patient global assessments of arthritis, the Osteoarthritis Severity Index, patient's evaluation of arthritis pain on a visual analog scale, and classification of functional capacity. Assessments were conducted at baseline and after 1 and 2 weeks of therapy.

Patient assessments of osteoarthritis pain by the visual analog scale and the patient global assessments after 1 and 2 weeks of celecoxib treatment or placebo are shown in Fig. 1. In the visual analog scale, all improvements (i.e., decreases from baseline) in mean patient ratings of pain were significantly greater with celecoxib than placebo ($p \leq 0.048$), except for the 40-mg–b.i.d. celecoxib dosage at week 2 ($p = 0.083$). In the patient global osteoarthritis assessment, all improvements from baseline (i.e., decreases in mean scores) between celecoxib and placebo were statistically significant ($p \leq 0.011$) except for the 100-mg–b.i.d. celecoxib dosage at week 2.

These efficacy findings have been confirmed in a recent phase III clinical trial of 1004 patients with osteoarthritis of the knee in a flare state. The results of this trial, which have at present appeared only in abstract form, were presented at the 1998 meeting of the American College of Rheumatology in San Diego, California (15). Patients with osteoarthritis of the knee in a flare state were randomly assigned to receive celecoxib (50, 100, or 200 mg b.i.d.), naproxen (500 mg b.i.d.), or placebo for up to 12 weeks. Celecoxib dosages of 100 and 200 mg b.i.d. provided significant reduction in patient and physician assessments of arthritis severity. These reductions were comparable with that observed with naproxen 500 mg b.i.d., and significantly better than placebo. Celecoxib 50 m.g. b.i.d. was significantly superior to placebo, although this dosage was not as effective as the 100- to 200-mg dosages. Celecoxib appeared well tolerated in this study; the incidence of adverse events and withdrawals due to adverse events with celecoxib were comparable with those observed with placebo, and the incidence of adverse events with celecoxib was not dose-related.

B. Rheumatoid Arthritis

This pilot study enrolled 330 patients with rheumatoid arthritis who were then randomly allocated in a double-blind manner to 4 weeks of treatment with celecoxib (40, 200, or 400 mg

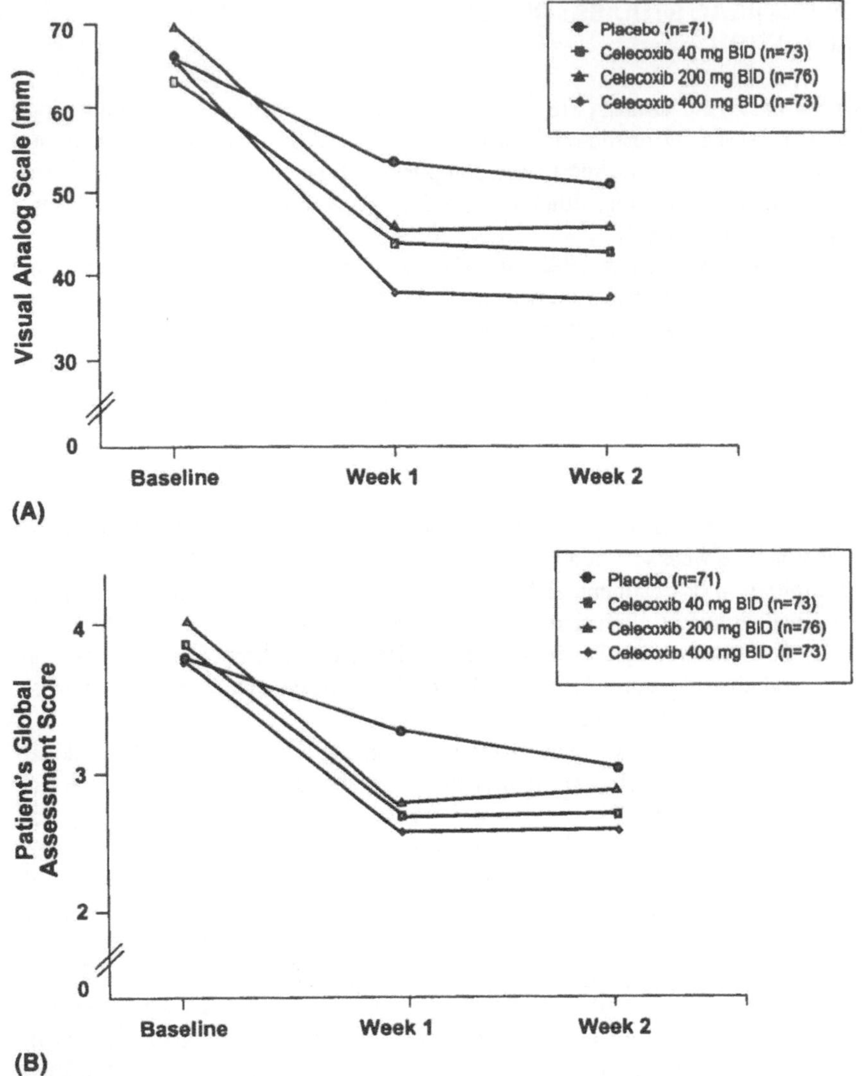

Figure 1 Pilot efficacy trial in osteoarthritis of the knee in a flare state: (A) mean values for patient assessments of osteoarthritis pain by visual analog scale (scale range: 0–100 mm); (B) mean values (scale range: 0–5) for patient global assessments. (From Ref. 15.)

b.i.d.) or placebo (14). Before randomization, an arthritis flare state was induced by withdrawing other anti-inflammatory medications. Evaluations included the patient and physician global assessments of arthritis, patient visual analog scale assessment of pain, and classification of functional capacity, as well as an evaluation of joint swelling, joint tenderness or pain, and duration of morning stiffness. Arthritis assessments were carried out after 1, 2, and 4 weeks of therapy.

In the global assessments, improvement in the mean change from baseline scores at weeks 1, 2, and 4 for celecoxib at dosages of 200 and 400 mg b.i.d. were statistically significantly ($p \leq 0.001$) superior to the assessments with placebo. At the same time, the scores for celecoxib 40 mg indicated a significant improvement compared with placebo only at week 1 ($p \leq 0.001$). Similarly, the reduction in mean values for the number of tender or painful joints was statistically significant ($p \leq 0.005$) for celecoxib at dosages of 200 and 400 mg b.i.d. compared with placebo at weeks 1, 2, and 4, whereas the mean change from baseline for the 40-mg–b.i.d. dosage was not statistically discernible from placebo at any time point. Patient global assessments and the number of tender or painful joints, which are representative of the overall trial results, are shown in Fig. 2.

These data demonstrate that at doses of 200 and 400 mg b.i.d., celecoxib is significantly more effective than placebo in ameliorating the signs and symptoms of rheumatoid arthritis. The 40-mg–b.i.d. dosage appears to be less effective, which is consistent with the observation that similar numbers of patients withdrew for lack of efficacy in the celecoxib 40-mg–b.i.d. group (17%) and the placebo group (18%). In contrast, withdrawals attributable to lack of efficacy were observed in only 4 and 6% of the 200- and 400-mg–b.i.d. groups, respectively.

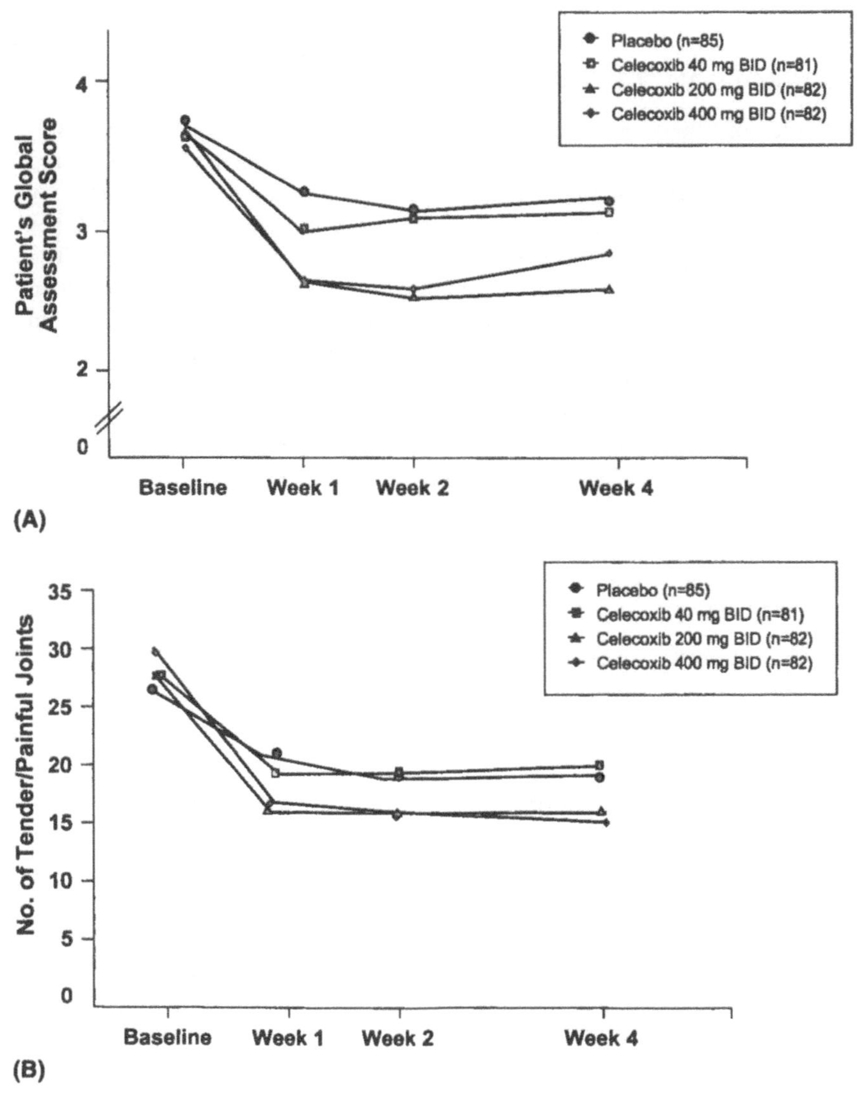

Figure 2 Pilot efficacy trial in rheumatoid arthritis in a flare state: (A) mean values for patient global assessments; (B) number of tender or painful joints. (From Ref. 15.)

The efficacy of the 200-mg–b.i.d. celecoxib dosage in the symptomatic relief of rheumatoid arthritis was corroborated in a recent phase III study presented at the annual meeting of the American College of Rheumatology in San Diego, CA. Patients with rheumatoid arthritis in a flare state ($N = 1149$) were randomly assigned to receive celecoxib (100-, 200-, or 400-mg b.i.d.), naproxen (500-mg b.i.d.), or placebo for 12 weeks (16). As measured by patient and physician global evaluations of arthritis severity, all dosages of celecoxib provided relief from arthritis symptoms that was superior to placebo and comparable with that observed with naproxen. In a second trial, conducted in Europe, 655 patients with a diagnosis of rheumatoid arthritis for at least 6 months were randomly assigned to receive either celecoxib (200-mg b.i.d.) or diclofenac SR (75-mg b.i.d.) for 24 weeks (17). Several measures of arthritis severity, including global assessments of function by the patient and the physician, and the total number of swollen or painful joints, improved during treatment to a comparable degree in both treatment groups.

C. Gastrointestinal and Platelet Effects

In the foregoing pilot study of patients with RA (13), the effects of two celecoxib dosages (100- or 200-mg b.i.d.) and naproxen (500-mg b.i.d.) on gastrointestinal erosions and ulcers were examined in a separate group of healthy subjects. Gastrointestinal ulceration, as determined by upper GI endoscopy, was not present in any placebo- or celecoxib-treated subject ($n = 32$ per group). In contrast, 6 subjects (19%) who received naproxen exhibited one or more ulcers. The combined incidence of gastric erosions or ulcers varied between 9 and 13% for subjects who received celecoxib or placebo, compared with 72% of subjects who received naproxen. For both ulcers and combined erosions and ulcers, the incidence with naproxen was significantly greater than the incidence with placebo or either celecoxib dosage ($p \leq 0.11$).

The same investigators compared the effects of celecoxib and aspirin on collagen-induced platelet aggregation. Six healthy male subjects received celecoxib (400-mg b.i.d.) for 6 days, followed by a 7-day drug-free washout period, and a single dose of aspirin on day 14. Platelet aggregation was evaluated at baseline and 2, 4, and 12 h after the last dose of celecoxib, and then again before aspirin administration and 2 and 4 h after aspirin administration. Collagen-induced platelet aggregation was unchanged by administration of celecoxib at all evaluated time points. In contrast, platelet aggregation 2 h after aspirin administration was reduced to about 25% of its predose level.

IV. SECOND-GENERATION COX-2–SPECIFIC INHIBITORS

A group of "second-generation" COX-2–specific inhibitors, such as valdecoxib and parecoxib, possess even an even greater degree of specificity for the COX-2 isoforms than celecoxib. The effectiveness of these compounds for the management of pain is currently undergoing evaluation in clinical trials. It is hypothesized that these agents should produce a strong analgesic effect, perhaps comparable with that of a mild opioid, but with less risk of side effects, particularly sedation and dependence liability.

V. CONCLUSIONS

The discovery of COX-2–specific inhibitors that appear to relieve pain and inflammation with less risk of toxicity than nonspecific COX-1/COX-2 inhibitors represents a major advance in anti-inflammatory and analgesic therapy.

Celecoxib appears to be both safe and effective for the treatment of the signs and symptoms of osteoarthritis and rheumatoid arthritis. In clinical trials, celecoxib was associated with a markedly lower rate of gastroduodenal injury than seen typically with NSAIDs, and also appears to possess little or no antiplatelet effect. Incidences of most adverse events, including gastrointestinal bleeding, and withdrawal rates because of adverse events with celecoxib were similar to placebo. Its COX-2–specific inhibitory properties thus introduce the possibility of effective relief of arthritic and other types of pain and inflammation with less risk of the COX-1–dependent toxicity observed with NSAIDs.

REFERENCES

1. Abramson SR, Weissman G. The mechanisms of action of nonsteroidal anti-inflammatory drugs. Arthritis Rheum 1989; 32:1–9.
2. Masferrer JL, Seibert K, Zweifel BS, Needleman P. Endogenous glucocorticoids regulate an inducible cyclooxygenase enzyme. Proc Natl Acad Sci USA 1992; 89:3917–3921.
3. Campbell WB, Halushka PV. Lipid-derived autacoids. In: Goodman and Gilman's The Phamacological Basis of Therapeutics. 9th ed. New York: McGraw-Hill, 1996:601–616.
4. Griswold DE, Adams JL. Constitutive cyclooxygenase (COX-1) and inducible cyclooxygenase (COX-2): rationale for selective inhibition and progress to date. Med Res Rev 1996; 16:181–206.
5. Allison MC, Howatson AG, Torrance CJ, Lee FD, Russell R. Gastrointestinal damage associated with the use of nonsteroidal antiinflammatory drugs. N Engl J Med 1992; 327:749–754.
6. Schafer AI. Effects of nonsteroidal antiinflammatory drugs on platelet function and systemic hemostasis. J Clin Pharmacol 1995; 35:209–2189.
7. Palmer BF. Renal complications associated with use of nonsteroidal anti-inflammatory agents. J Invest Med 1995; 43:516–533.
8. Kurumbail RG, Stevens AM, Gierse JK, McDonald JJ, Stegeman RA, Pak JY, Gildehaus D, Miyashiro JM, Penning TD, Seibert K, Isakson PC, Stallings WC. Structural basis for selective inhibition of cyclooxygenase-2 by anti-inflammatory agents. Nature 1996; 384:644–648.
9. Seibert K, Zhang Y, Leahy K, Hauser S, Masferrer J, Perkins W, Lee L, Isakson P. Pharmacological and biochemical demonstration of the role of cyclooxygenase in inflammation and pain. Proc Natl Acad Sci USA 1994; 91:12013–12017.
10. Masferrer J, Zweifel B, Manning PT, Hauser SD, Leahy KM, Smith WG, Isakson PC, Seibert K. Selective inhibition of inducible cyclooxygenase 2 in vivo is anti-inflammatory and non-ulcerogenic. Proc Natl Acad Sci USA 1994; 91:3228–3232.
11. Simons LS. Nonsteroidal antiinflammatory drugs and their effects: the importance of COX "selectivity." J Clin Rheumatol 1996; 3:135–140.
12. Lipsky LPE, Abramson SB, Crofford L, Dubois RN, Simon LS, van de Putte LBA. The classification of cyclooxygenase inhibitors. J Rheumatol 1998; 25:2298–2303.
13. Zhang Y, Shaffer A, Portanova J, Seibert K, Isakson PC. Inhibition of cyclooxygenase-2 rapidly reverses inflammatory hyperalgesia and prostaglandin E_2 production. J Pharmacol Exp Ther 1997; 283:1069–1075.
14. Simon LS, Lanza FL, Lipsky PE, Hubbard RC, Talwalker S, Schwartz BD, Isakson PC, Geis GS. Preliminary study of the safety and efficacy of SC-58635, a novel cyclooxygenase 2 inhibitor: efficacy and safety in two placebo-controlled trials in osteoarthritis and rheumatoid arthritis, and studies of gastrointestinal and platelet effects. Arthritis Rheum 1998; 41:1591–1602.
15. Hubbard RC, Geis GS, Woods EM, Yu S, Zhao W. Efficacy, tolerability, and safety of celecoxib, a specific COX-2 inhibitor, in osteoarthritis. Arthritis Rheum 1998; 41(suppl 9):S196; abstr 982.
16. Geis GS, Hubbard R, Callison D, Yu S, Zhao W. Safety and efficacy of celecoxib, a specific COX-2 inhibitor, in patients with rheumatoid arthritis. Arthritis Rheum 1998; 41(suppl 9):S364; abstr 1990.
17. Geis GS, Stead H, Morant SV, Naudin R, Hubbard HC. Efficacy and safety of celecoxib, a specific COX-2 inhibitor, in patients with rheumatoid arthritis. Arthritis Rheum 1998; 41(suppl 9):S316; abstr 1699.

41

NK_1 Receptor Antagonists

Potential Analgesics?

Raymond G. Hill
Merck Sharp & Dohme, Harlow, Essex, England

I. INTRODUCTION

Substance P is one of the most abundant peptides in mammalian primary afferent fibers and has long been thought to have a specific role in pain perception (1). It is clearly not the only substance involved in this, and the nociceptive transmission process from primary afferent neurons into the central nervous system (CNS) is complex. Within the dorsal horn of the spinal cord, many different afferent sensory neurons synapse onto secondary neurons within the dorsal horn of the spinal cord that provide the secondary nociceptive relay. Additionally, even within individual nerve terminals, there are multiple transmitter systems. The likelihood is, therefore, that numerous transmitter substances are released from the terminals of primary afferent neurons within the spinal cord's dorsal horn in response to a single noxious peripheral stimulus. Accordingly, it is necessary to ask whether blocking the effects of just one of these substances would be likely to give an analgesic effect. Blocking the effects of glutamate, the ubiquitous sensory transmitter, would most likely give clinical analgesia because, as far as we know, every primary afferent neuron releases glutamate along with the other transmitters it contains (1). Additionally, it is already known that the blockade of the *N*-methyl-D-aspartate (NMDA) subset of glutamate receptors in humans with agents such as ketamine will produce analgesia (2,3). We also know from these studies in humans that there is an extremely high probability of unacceptable side effects by blocking the effects of glutamate at all NMDA receptors. Use of a pharmacological antagonist to block the effects of a single peptide neuromodulator, such as substance P, which is found in just a proportion of unmyelinated primary afferent neurons, increases the probability that there will be fewer side effects than with blockade of the effects of glutamate. This is because the presence of substance P in only a proportion of sensory fibers ensures there is not a complete block of neurotransmission. But for the same reason, there is likely to be an unpredictable analgesic efficacy with a maximum effect smaller than could be produced with NMDA receptor blockade and probably smaller than that which would be seen with an opioid drug, such as morphine, that has multiple sites of action (4). The compromise is thus between unwanted side effects and the presence or absence of effective analgesia. The key questions related to therapeutic efficacy are now being asked in clinical studies with potent antagonists of the effects of substance P that have recently been discovered (5–7).

II. SUBSTANCE P AND NOCICEPTION

Tachykinin has been adopted as the generic name for the family of peptides to which substance P belongs. There are three main mammalian tachykinin peptides: substance P itself, neurokinin (NK) A, and neurokinin B, although, as a whole, in the animal kingdom there are many other peptides that are structurally and functionally similar (8). This chapter will deal with substance P and the NK_1 receptor, at which we believe substance P is the preferential agonist.

Substance P and neurokinin A come from the same protein precursor molecule, preprotachykinin; hence, it is not surprising that they are found in the same sensory neurons. Although we believe neurokinin A is the preferred ligand for the NK_2 receptor, it is important to remember that it is also a prime ligand for the NK_1 receptor and, as in the dorsal horn of the spinal cord where there are few if any NK_2 receptors, but abundant NK_1 sites, it probably acts together with substance P at the NK_1 receptor (9,10). NK_2 and NK_3 receptors may well be of great interest in the future but, at present, we know far more about the NK_1 receptor.

Before the advent of effective substance P or NK_1 receptor antagonists, there were already several reasons for believing substance P was involved in nociception. In addition to the aforementioned presence of substance P in primary afferents, NK_1 receptors were identified in the dorsal horn of the spinal cord, initially by autoradiography (9) and, more recently, by elegant immunocytochemistry, using a specific antibody to the NK_1 receptor (11,12) on the target nociceptive secondary neurons. Neurochemically, substance P is released only after intense, constant peripheral stimuli such as demonstrated in experiments done by Duggan et al. (13) using the immunomicroprobe technique. In dorsal root ganglion (DRG) cells, preprotachykinin message is up-regulated after peripheral tissue damage (14), and within the dorsal horn of the spinal cord, an up-regulation of NK_1 receptors is seen after peripheral tissue inflammation or damage (15).

By using substance P itself, or close analogues that are more metabolically stable, intrathecal injection can be shown to produce hyperalgesia to a variety of noxious stimuli (16). In the dorsal horn, both nociceptive and low-threshold neurons are readily excited by substance P (17,18). It is necessary, however, to relate these effects to a feasible physiology that would confirm that substance P is important in nociception.

A. Substance P Receptor Antagonists

Although some pharmacological antagonists were available more than 10 years ago, these were synthetic peptides, rather than the small heterocycles we have today. These first generation compounds were simple analogues of substance P, with D-amino acids substituted in critical positions of the sequence to reduce the agonist efficacy and make them into antagonists (19). At least that was the theory, and although useable antagonism was seen on some isolated tissues (19,20) within the central nervous system, these compounds had direct effects that obscured any antagonism of the effects of substance P. In experiments on isolated spinal cord, for example, ventral root depolarizations produced by substance P were seen to be potentiated, rather than blocked, when the peptide antagonist [D-Pro^2, D-Trp^{7,9}]-substance P was added. When a higher concentration of the antagonist was added alone, it produced a direct depolarization (20). When a microionophoretic technique was used to directly apply this agent to dorsal horn neurons, the neuronal excitation produced by substance P was blocked only by concentrations of the putative antagonist that also reduced the excitation of the same neuron produced by glutamate (20). When injected intrathecally, these first-generation peptide antagonists caused permanent locomotor paralysis (21) and histologically identifiable motoneuron degeneration (22). This effect is not a consequence of NK_1 receptor blockade and has not been seen with modern NK_1 receptor antagonists (20–22; also, see later discussion).

There were no suitably selective and potent NK_1 antagonists for detailed studies on nociceptive physiology until 1990, when scientists from Pfizer published the first paper describing a potent, novel, nonpeptide antagonist of the effects of substance P at the human NK_1 receptor (23). Within 5 years of the publication of the structure of this molecule, there was an assortment of clinical candidates ready for evaluation from several different companies (5–7). The combination of molecular pharmacology, with site-directed mutagenesis to determine which amino acid residues were involved in the binding of agonists and antagonists, and targeted medicinal chemistry allowed confident description of a pharmacophore for the NK_1 receptor (5,6,24,25). In the cloned human NK_1 receptor, it was possible to identify critical residues, that were important for the occurrence of binding to produce antagonism and that were different from the residues at which agonism occurred (24,25).

B. Substance P Receptor Antagonists and Nociception

With these new, nonpeptide antagonists as tools, it is possible to gain additional evidence that the NK_1 receptor may be involved in nociception. NK_1 receptor antagonists block the windup and facilitation of a spinal nociceptive reflex with little effect on the baseline reflex (26,27). Also, they can block the activation of dorsal horn neurons by adequate noxious stimuli (28) or after inflammatory facilitation (29). After initial studies using a rat-selective NK_1 receptor antagonist, RP-76580 (26), it appeared that spinal reflex studies in the rabbit were more useful for human clinical candidate evaluation because rabbits have an NK_1 receptor with a pharmacological profile closely resembling that of the human receptor (30). In general, the facilitation, the windup, and the afterdischarge following noxious stimuli are reduced by NK_1 receptor antagonists in all species yet tested, but the baseline reflex is less sensitive (26). NMDA receptor antagonists can reduce all of the components of this reflex, as can opiates (31). Coadministration of morphine and the NK_1 receptor antagonist gives an additive interaction against nociceptive flexor reflexes. This may be therapeutically important because the emetic effects of morphine are blocked by NK_1 receptor antagonists (32).

Many behavioral studies have been published on the putative antinociceptive effects of NK_1 receptor antagonists. It is necessary to critically examine these studies and to ask if appropriate controls have been performed using the inactive enantiomers of the compounds in question. In particular, it is important to evaluate whether effects such as nonspecific ion channel blockade had been eliminated (33,34). If these criteria are applied strictly, there are then few studies that provide unequivocal evidence of antinociceptive effects. Most workers would now agree that NK_1 antagonists do not have selective antinociceptive effects in the classic tail-flick, hot-plate, and paw-pressure tests in which opioids work very well, but in which few other classes of agents are effective (34). If inflammation is used to produce hyperalgesia or to directly evoke a behavioral response, as in the formalin test (34–37), antinociceptive effects can be demonstrated with NK_1 receptor antagonists. In the gerbil, a small animal with NK_1 receptors that have a pharmacological profiles similar to those in humans, Rupniak and her colleagues have developed a variant of the formalin test in which formalin is used as a baseline inflammatory stimulus to produce thermal hyperalgesia. The brain penetrant NK_1 antagonist CP-99,994 gave a dose-related depression of this hyperalgesia (35). This response could be separated from that seen with the less active enantiomer. Giving NK_1 antagonists intrathecally appears to facilitate the production of an enantioselective effect (36). Rupniak et al. (38), using a brain-penetrant NK_1 receptor antagonist L-733,060 that has a long duration of action, achieved an impressive separation of specific from nonspecific effects by being able to preserve a central effect at a time when peripheral drug concentrations were quite low (38). L-733,060, and its less active enantiomer, L-733,061 have a 300-fold difference in their affinity for the human NK_1 receptor. In the gerbil, using a simple assay of foot-tapping produced by intracerebroventricular injection of the stable NK_1 agonist, GR 73632 (38,39), it was possible to block the effect of the agonist by increasing doses of L-733,060 (ED_{50} = 250 mg/kg) but 10 mg/kg of L-733,061 was inactive. In this foot-tapping test, it was possible to measure the central duration of action of ED_{90} doses (about 1 mg/kilogram) of L-733,060 or CP-99,994 by pretreating the animals and then challenging them with intracerebral ventricular (icv) NK_1 agonists at different times after pretreatment. L733,060 maintained blockade of the NK_1 receptor for up to 4 h after treatment, whereas the effects of CP-99,994 diminished after 2 h. This is a pharmacological half-life difference, because in the gerbil, the plasma half-lifes of these two compounds are similar at about 90 min (39). By using a 3-h pretreatment before injecting formalin, Rupniak et al. (38) showed that the second phase of the formalin response was attenuated by L-733,060 (ED_{50} = 170 mg/kg) with a clear dose–response relation and with plasma levels that one would expect to give cerebrospinal fluid (CSF) levels that are adequate for 95% occupancy of the NK_1 receptor. Carefully controlled studies such as these suggest that NK_1 antagonists might be worthy of clinical evaluation as analgesics. Published work in the last couple of years has included several studies using tests that are claimed to be more relevant to acute and chronic pain states in humans. For example, in rats when hyperalgesia and allodynia were produced as a consequence of chronic constriction injury of one sciatic nerve, effective antinociception was produced by RP 67580 (40) and GR 205171 (41). In a similar paradigm in guinea pigs, SDZ-NKT-343, LY-303,870, and RPR-100,893 all had antihyperalgesic properties (42). In an incisional model of postoperative pain, PD 154,075 prevented the development of thermal and mechanical hypersensitivity (43), and CI-1021 blocked the mechanical hypersensitivity produced in rats with streptazocin-induced diabetes.

III. NEURONAL PLASTICITY IN SUBSTANCE P SYSTEMS

The reasons for believing that substance P, acting at NK_1 receptors, might be important in nociception are progressively becoming stronger. Following an inflammatory stimulus, a tactile hypersensitivity develops that can be measured behaviorally, and single dorsal horn neurons respond more intensely to a peripheral stimulus. This effect is long-lasting, and although it is maximal in the first day, it is only after about 5 days that the responses to a peripheral stimulus return to their normal magnitude. At the time this increased responsiveness to mechanical stimuli is seen, the number of neurons staining for substance P in the dorsal root ganglia increases on the ipsilateral side and, also, to a somewhat lesser extent, on the contralateral side, and the amount of mRNA for preprotachykinin also increases (45). This seems to be due to a change in the particular population of fibers that drive the dorsal horn neurons after the inflammation is established. In the presence of inflammation, even gentle stimuli at Aβ strength will evoke an after discharge in dorsal horn neurons and an enhanced behavioral response. However, in the rat, the selective NK_1 antagonist RP-67580 blocks these effects, suggesting that substance P is the key transmitter substance involved. Immunocytochemistry of ganglia taken from these animals shows that the increases in substance P in the presence of inflammation is partly seen in neurons that also stain with an antibody for the β-subunit of cholera toxin, a specific marker for myelinated fibers. In other words, neurons that give rise to myelinated axons and that normally do not make substance P seem to become capable of manufacturing substance P after a prolonged inflammatory stimulus (45). The authors of the paper call this a phylogenetic switch.

It may be that our assumptions about which fibers release substance P (and possibly other peptides) needs to be reviewed. This study is further evidence of plasticity in the systems mediating nociception.

IV. CLINICAL STUDIES WITH SUBSTANCE P RECEPTOR ANTAGONISTS

There is now abundant evidence that substance P is part of the nociceptive process in mammals, so it is surprising that pain studies with an NK_1 antagonist have so far been equivocal in humans. There is a single report in the literature (46) showing that CP-99,994 has analgesic properties against dental postsurgical pain in humans, but other, similar studies have shown that L-754,030 is not effective against dental pain (47). This latter compound is clearly capable of blocking central NK_1 receptors in humans, since it is an effective and long-acting antiemetic (48). Lanepitant has been ineffective against osteoarthritis pain (49) and acute migraine headache (50). L-758,298 (51) and GR-205,171 have also failed in trials against acute migraine.

The inability of the animal data to predict efficacy in humans, is probably not due to the limited range of tests in which the NK_1 receptor antagonists work, because even severe paradigms are capable of showing efficacy. For example, following chronic constriction injury of the sciatic nerve in the rat, which is a relatively intractable test with similarities to neuropathic pain in humans, NK_1 antagonists can have antinociceptive effects (41).

V. CONCLUSIONS

We clearly do not yet know all the answers, and clinical studies with NK_1 antagonists in pain are continuing. It seems that NK_1 receptor activation is not important in acute-phase pain, such as the direct nociceptive process which is probably involved in assays such as the hot-plate test. But evidence is abundant that it is important in persistent inflammatory pain in animals, if not in humans. One possible explanation for the mismatch between clinical and preclinical data is that a large component of persistent pain in humans may be due to CNS reprograming and that, at this stage, the NK_1 receptor may no longer be important, although its activation may have been involved earlier in the process leading to a maintained pain state. There is much circumstantial evidence for involvement of substance P in nociception in humans, for example, spinal CSF levels of substance P are elevated in patients with osteoarthritis (53), and in a group of subjects with congenital insensitivity to pain, CSF substance P was decreased (54). The story of clinical pain and substance P is not yet over, and it is clear from other clinical investigations that pharmacological blockade of the NK_1 receptor is likely to be important therapeutically. Although there is published evidence for useful antiemetic (48) and antidepressant (55) effects in humans, the full scope of the clinical usefulness of NK_1 antagonist compounds remains to be established.

REFERENCES

1. Salt TE, Hill RG. Neurotransmitter candidates of somatosensory primary afferent fibers. Neuroscience 1983; 10:1083–1103.
2. Warnke T, Stubhaug A, Jorum E. Ketamine, an NMDA receptor antagonist, suppresses spatial and temporal properties of burn induced hyperalgesia in man: a double blind cross over comparison with morphine and placebo. Pain 1997; 72:99–106.

3. Stubhaug A, Breivik H, Eide PK, Kreunen M, Foss A. Mapping of punctate hyperalgesia around a surgical incision demonstrates that ketamine is a powerful suppressor of central sensitisation to pain following surgery. Acta Anaesth Scand 1997; 41:1124–1132.
4. Hill RG, Morris R, Pepper CM. Electrophysiological studies on the actions of opioids, with particular reference to the production of analgesia. In: Hughes J, Collier HOJ, Rance MJ, Tyers MB, eds. Opioids Past, Present and Future. London: Taylor & Francis, 1983;61–78.
5. Mills SG. Recent advances in neurokinin receptor antagonists. Annu Rep Med Chem 1997; 32:51–60.
6. Giardina GAM, Raveglia LF, Grugni M. Lead generation and lead optimization processes in the discovery of selective nonpeptide neurokinin receptor antagonists. Drugs Future 1997; 22:1235–1257.
7. Longmore J, Hill RG, Hargreaves RJ. Neurokinin-receptor antagonists: pharmacological tools and therapeutic drugs. Can J Physiol Pharmacol 1997; 75:612–621.
8. Iversen LL. History of tachykinin receptors. In: Buck SH, ed. The Tachykinin Receptors. Totowa, NJ: Humana Press, 1994;23–27.
9. Yashpal K, Dam TV, Quirion R. Quantitative autoradiographic distribution of multiple neurokinin binding sites in rat spinal cord. Brain Res 1990; 506:259–266.
10. Humpel C, Saria A. Characterisation of neurokinin binding sites in rat brain membranes using highly selective ligands. Neuropeptides 1993; 25:65–71.
11. Bleazard L, Hill RG, Morris R. The correlation between the distribution of the NK_1 receptor and the action of tachykinin agonists in the dorsal horn of the rat indicates that substance P does not have a functional role on substantia gelatinosa (lamina II) neurons. J Neurosci 1994; 14:7655–7664.
12. Mantyh PW, DeMaster E, Malhotra E, Ghilardi JR, Rogers SD, Mantyh CR, Liu H, Basbaum AI, Vigna SR, Maggio JE, Simone DA. Receptor endocytosis and dendrite reshaping in spinal neurons after somatosensory stimulation. Science 1995; 268:1629–1632.
13. Duggan AW, Weihe E. Central transmission of impulses in nociceptors: events in the superficial dorsal horn. In: Basbaum AI, Besson JM, eds. Towards a New Pharmacotherapy of Pain: Beyond Morphine. Chichester: John Wiley, 1991;35–67.
14. Marchand JE, Wurm WH, Kato T, Kream RM. Altered tachykinin expression by dorsal root ganglion neurons in a rat model of neuropathic pain. Pain 1994; 58:219–231.
15. Abbadie C, Brown JL, Mantyh PW, Basbaum AI. Spinal cord substance P receptor immunoreactivity increases in both inflammatory and nerve injury models of persistent pain. Neuroscience 1996; 70: 201–209.
16. Cridland RA, Henry JL. Comparison of the effects of substance P, neurokinin A, physaelamin and eledoisin in facilitating a nociceptive reflex in the rat. Brain Res 1986; 381:93–99.
17. Salt TE, Morris R, Hill RG. Distribution of substance P-responsive and nociceptive neurons in relation to substance P—immunoreactivity within caudal trigeminal nucleus of the rat. Brain Res 1983; 273:217–228.
18. Dougherty PM, Willis WD. Enhancement of spinothalamic neuron responses to chemical and mechanical stimuli following combined microiontophoretic application of *N*-methyl-D-aspartic acid and substance P. Pain 1991; 47:85–93.
19. Engberg G, Svensson TH, Rosell S, Folkers K. A synthetic peptide as an antagonist of substance P. Nature 1981; 293:222–223.
20. Salt TE, DeVries GJ, Rodriguez RE, Cahusac PMB, Morris R, Hill RG. Evaluation of (D-Pro^2, D-Trp^{7,9})–substance P as an antagonist of substance P responses in the rat central nervous system. Neurosci Lett 1982; 30:291–295.
21. Rodriguez RE, Salt TE, Cahusac PMB, Hill RG. The behavioral effects of intrathecally administered [D-Pro^2, D-Trp^{7,9}]–substance P, an analogue with presumed antagonist actions in the rat. Neuropharmacology 1983; 22:173–176.
22. Hokfelt T, Vincent S, Hellsten L, Rosell S, Folkers K, Markey K, Goldstein M, Cuello C. Immunohistochemical evidence for a neurotoxic action of [D-Pro^2, D-Trp^{7,9}]–substance P, an analogue with substance P antagonistic activity. Acta Physiol Scand 1981; 113:571–573.
23. Snider RM, Constantine JW, Lowe JA, Longo KP, Lebel WS, Woody HA, Drozda SE, Desai MC,

Vinick FJ, Spencer RW, Hess HJ. A potent nonpeptide antagonist of the substance P (NK_1) receptor. Science 1991; 251:435–439.

24. Fong TM, Yu H, Strader CD. Molecular basis for the species selectivity of the neurokinin-1 receptor antagonists CP-96,345 and RP 67580. J Biol Chem 1992; 267:25668–25671.
25. Longmore JL, Swain CJ, Hill RG. Neurokinin receptors. Drug News Perspect 1995; 8:5–23.
26. Laird JMA, Hargreaves RJ, Hill RG. Effect of RP 67580, a non-peptide neurokinin-1 receptor antagonist, on facilitation of a nociceptive spinal flexion reflex in the rat. Br J Pharmacol 1993; 109:713–718.
27. Xu XJ, Dalsgaard CJ, Wiesenfeld–Hallin Z. Intrathecal CP-96,345 blocks reflex facilitation induced in rats by substance P and C-fibre conditioning stimulation. Eur J Pharmacol 1992; 216:337–344.
28. Radhakrishnan V, Henry JL. Novel substance P antagonist, CP-96,345, blocks responses of cat spinal dorsal horn neurons to noxious cutaneous stimulation and to substance P. Neurosci Lett 1991; 132: 39–43.
29. Rees H, Sluka KA, Urban L, Walpole CJ, Willis WD. The effects of SDZ NKT 343, a potent NK_1 receptor antagonist, on cutaneous responses of primate spinothalamic tract neurones sensitized by intradermal capsaicin injection. Exp Brain Res 1998; 121:355–358.
30. Boyce S, Laird JMA, Tattersall FD, Rupniak NMJ, Hargreaves RJ, Hill RG. Antinociceptive effects of NK_1 receptor antagonists: comparison of behavioral and electrophysiological tests. Proceedings 7th World Congress on Pain, 1993; Abstr 641.
31. Xu XJ, Dalsgaard CJ, Wiesenfeld–Hallin Z. Spinal substance P and *N*-methyl-D-aspartate receptors are co-activated in the induction of central sensitisation of the nociceptive flexor reflex. Neuroscience 1992; 51:641–648.
32. Gardner CJ, Twissel DJ, Dale TJ, Gale JD, Jordan CC, Kilpatrick GJ, Bountra C, Ward P. The broad spectrum anti-emetic activity of the novel nonpeptide tachykinin NK_1 receptor antagonist GR 203040. Br J Pharmacol 1995; 116:3158–3163.
33. Rupniak, NMJ, Boyce S, Williams AR, Cook G, Longmore JL, Seabrook GS, Caesar M, Iversen SD, Hill RG. Antinociceptive activity of NK_1 receptor antagonists: non-specific effects of racemic RP 67580. Br J Pharmacol 1993; 110:1607–1613.
34. Hill RG. Tachykinin receptors and nociception. In: Buck S, ed. The Tachykinin Receptors. Humana Press: New York, 1994;471–498.
35. Rupniak NMJ, Webb JK, Williams AR, Carlson E, Boyce S, Hill RG. Antinociceptive activity of the tachykinin NK_1 receptor antagonist CP-99,994 in conscious gerbils. Br J Pharmacol 1995; 116: 1937–1943.
36. Yamamoto T, Yaksh TL. Stereospecific effects of a non-peptidic NK_1 selective antagonist CP-96,345: antinociception in the absence of motor dysfunction. Life Sci 1991; 49:1955–1963.
37. Ma Q–P, Woolf CJ. Tachykinin NK_1 receptor antagonist RP 67580 attenuates progressive hypersensitivity of flexor reflex during experimental inflammation in rats. Eur J Pharmacol 1997; 322:165–171.
38. Rupniak NMJ, Carlson E, Boyce S, Webb JK, Hill RG. Enantioselective inhibition of the formalin paw late phase by the NK_1 receptor antagonist L-733,060 in gerbils. Pain 1996; 67:189–195.
39. Rupniak NMJ, Tattersall FD, Williams AR, Rycroft W, Carlson EJ, Cascieri MA, Sadowski S, Ber E, Hale JJ, Mills SG, Macoss M, Seward E, Huscroft I, Swain CJ, Hill RG, Hargreaves RJ. In vitro and in vivo predictors of the anti-emetic activity of tachykinin NK_1 receptor antagonists. Eur J Pharmacol 1997; 326:201–209.
40. Coudore–Civiale M–A, Courteix C, Eschalier A, Fialip J. Effect of tachykinin receptor antagonists in experimental neuropathic pain. Eur J Pharmacol 1998; 361:175–184.
41. Cumberbatch MJ, Wyatt A, Boyce S, Hill RG, Rupniak NMJ. Reversal of behavioral and electrophysiological correlates of experimental peripheral neuropathy by the NK_1 receptor antagonist GR 205171 in rats. Neuropharmacology 1998; 37:1535–1543.
42. Campbell EA, Gentry CT, Patel S, Panesar MS, Walpole CSJ, Urban L. Selective neurokinin-1 receptor antagonists are anti-hyperalgesic in a model of neuropathic pain in the guinea pig. Neuroscience 1998; 87:527–532.
43. Gonzalez MI, Field MJ, Holloman EF, Hughes J, Oles RJ, Singh L. Evaluation of PD 154075, a

tachykinin NK_1 receptor antagonist, in a rat model of postoperative pain. Eur J Pharmacol 1998; 344:115–120.

44. Field MJ, McLeary S, Boden P, Suman–Chauhan N, Hughes J, Singh L. Involvement of the central tachykinin NK_1 receptor during maintenance of mechanical hypersensitivity induced by diabetes in the rat. J Pharmacol Exp Ther 1998; 285:1226–1232.
45. Neumann S, Doubell TP, Leslie T, Woolf CJ. Inflammatory pain hypersensitivity mediated by phenotypic switch in myelinated primary sensory neurons. Nature 1996; 384:360–364.
46. Dionne RA, Max MB, Gordon SM, Parada S, Sang C, Gracely RH, Sethna NF, MacLean DB. The substance P receptor antagonist CP-99,994 reduces acute postoperative pain. Clin Pharmacol Ther 1998; 64:562–568.
47. Reinhardt RR, Laub JB, Fricke JR, Polis AB, Gertz BJ. Comparison of a neurokinin-1 antagonist, L-745,030, to placebo, acetaminophen and ibuprofen in the dental pain model. Clin Pharmacol Ther 1998; 63:168.
48. Navari RM, Reinhardt RR, Gralla RJ, Kris MG, Hesketh PJ, Khojasteh A, Kindler H, Grote TH, Pendergrass K, Grunberg SM, Carides AD, Gertz BJ. Reduction of cisplatin-induced emesis by a selective neurokinin-1 receptor antagonist. N Engl J Med 1999; 340:190–195.
49. Goldstein DJ, Wang O, Todd LE. Lanepitant in osteoarthritis pain. Clin Pharmacol Ther 1998; 63: 143.
50. Goldstein DJ, Wang O, Saper JR, Stolz R, Silberstein SD, Mathew NT. Ineffectiveness of neurokinin-1 antagonist in acute migraine: a crossover study. Cephalalgia 1997; 17:785–790.
51. Norman B, Panebianco D, Block GA. A placebo-controlled, in-clinic study to explore the preliminary safety and efficacy of intravenous L-758,298 (a prodrug of the NK_1 receptor antagonist L-745,030) in the acute treatment of migraine. Cephalalgia 1998; 18:38.
52. Connor HE, Bertin L, Gillies S, Beattie DT, Ward P. Clinical evaluation of a novel, potent, CNS penetrating NK_1 receptor antagonist in the acute treatment of migraine. Cephalalgia 1998; 18:23.
53. Lindh C, Liu Z, Lyrenas S, Ordeberg G, Nyberg F. Elevated cerebrospinal fluid substance P-like immunoreactivity in patients with painful osteoarthritis, but not in patients with rhizopathic pain from a herniated lumbar disc. Scand J Rheumatol 1997; 26:468–472.
54. Nagamitsu S, Matsuishi T, Ohnishi A, Kato H, Decreased CSF levels of substance P in patients with congenital sensory neuropathy with anhidrosis. Neurology 1997; 48:1133.
55. Kramer MS, Cutler N, Feighner J, et al. Distinct mechanism for antidepressant activity by blockade of central substance P receptors. Science 1998; 281:1640–1645.

42
Vanilloids

Allan I. Basbaum and David J. Julius
University of California, San Francisco, San Francisco, California, U.S.A.

Wendye R. Robbins
NeurogesX, Inc., San Carlos, and Stanford University, Stanford, California, U.S.A.

I. INTRODUCTION

Traditional views of the "pain" pathway describe a primary afferent nociceptor that contacts a spinothalamic tract neuron. The latter projects to thalamocortical neurons that transmit the "pain" message to the cortex. Recent studies, of course, have emphasized the heterogeneity of these central circuits. Of particular importance is the evidence that there are multiple classes of primary afferent nociceptor with cell bodies in the trigeminal and dorsal root ganglion (DRG) and that subpopulations of nociceptors express molecules that are unique and, in fact, are not found in other parts of the nervous system (1). Among the many molecules that have a very specific association with the primary afferent nociceptor are the tetrodotoxin resistant Na channel (TTX-R), transient receptor potential channels (TRP), and the $P2X_3$ subtype of purinergic receptor.

One of the first molecules to be specifically associated with the nociceptor was the vanilloid/capsaicin receptor. Sensitivity to vanilloid compounds in many respects is the defining feature of the primary afferent nociceptor. The term vanilloid refers to a group of substances related structurally and pharmacologically to capsaicin, the pungent ingredient of chili peppers. Because the vanilloid receptor is selectively expressed in the primary afferent nociceptor (see below), it likely represents a target for the development of novel analgesic drugs.

II. CAPSAICIN AND SENSORY NEURONS

Capsaicin first attracted scientific interest because of its ability to produce a selective activation and sensitization of nociceptive sensory neurons, including both C- and Aδ-fibers, without affecting other types of sensory neuron (2–4). Based on the distribution of the capsaicin receptor (see below) and on the physiological responses of single cells in vitro, it is clear capsaicin acts on both the peptide-containing population of primary afferent nociceptors, which synthesize substance P and calcitonin gene-related peptide (CGRP), and also on the non-peptide containing population, which is characterized by its binding of the lectin IB4 (5–7).

Because of the widespread distribution of nociceptive C-fibers (in somatic and visceral tissue), and because of their involvement in peripheral effector mechanisms (as well as in sensory transmission), it follows that the physiological effects of capsaicin in the whole animal are numerous. The main ones are:

Immediate pain (familiar to anyone who has eaten a hot curry, or experienced sore fingers and eyes after cutting up chili peppers);

A variety of autonomic effects resulting from peripheral release of substance P and CGRP, which induces profound vasodilatation, while release of substance P promotes vascular leakage and protein extravasation. The latter are prominent components of the neurogenic inflammatory response, namely rubor (redness), calor (heat) and tumor (swelling) (8);

In neonatal animals (studied mainly in rats), capsaicin in high doses causes permanent ablation of the two major subpopulations of nociceptive primary afferent neurons. In adult animals, degeneration of C-fiber axons and terminals occurs, but irreversible loss of cell bodies is limited (3);

An antinociceptive effect of varying duration, associated with desensitization of nociceptive afferent fibers following the initial excitation;

A more prolonged antinociceptive effect secondary to the neurodegenerative effect of capsaicin on the peripheral terminals of C fibers. The cellular mechanisms underlying the neurodegenerative consequences of capsaicin likely involve both necrotic and apoptotic (i.e., programmed) cell death; and

A fall in body temperature (9). This is a reflex response generated by thermosensitive neurons in the hypothalamus following capsaicin activation of primary afferent fibers.

III. MEMBRANE EFFECTS OF VANILLOIDS

The principal action of capsaicin and other vanilloids on the sensory neuron membrane is to produce a non-selective increase in cation permeability, associated with the opening of a distinct type of cation channel (10). The inward current responsible for depolarization and excitation of the neurons is carried mainly by sodium ions, but the channel is also permeable to divalent cations, including calcium. Thus activation by capsaicin causes calcium entry (11). The well-defined cellular specificity and pattern of membrane response to capsaicin and related compounds suggested that a specific vanilloid receptor must be expressed by sensory neurons, and this idea gained support with the discoveries of capsazepine, a selective competitive antagonist (12), and of resiniferatoxin (RTX) [see Ref. (13) for references], a naturally-occurring vanilloid of high potency, which allowed receptor labelling to be carried out. The latter showed properties and a distribution pattern that corresponded closely with the pharmacological findings. Final proof came with the successful cloning and expression of the receptor (14), an advance that is providing important new insights into the biophysical properties of vanilloid receptors and the into the mechanisms through which nociceptors detect noxious stimuli. Characterization of the receptor has also opened up new avenues for the development of drugs that specifically target the nociceptor.

IV. PROPERTIES OF THE CLONED VANILLOID RECEPTOR, VR1

The vanilloid receptor (VR1) consists of 838 amino acids, and possesses 6 membrane-spanning domains (TM1-6) with a long intracellular N-terminal tail and a pore-forming loop region between TM5 and TM6 corresponding to that seen in many transmembrane ion channels. Although the overall topology of the receptor resembles that proposed for numerous other ion channels (such as voltage-gated potassium channels), VR1 displays greatest similarity to the family of TRP channels, the founding member of which was identified as an essential component of the fly phototransduction pathway. Subsequent studies have demonstrated that many members of the TRP channel family, including VR1, participate in one or more aspect of sensory transduction (see below). The mammalian TRP channel family is now recognized to be quite large and it continues to expand (15). According to the new TRP channel nomenclature, VR1 is also called TRPV1.

When the TRPV1 clone is introduced into frog oocytes or non-neuronal mammalian cells in culture (which normally do not express this channel), the channel that is produced is largely identical to native vanilloid/capsaicin receptors, with regard to their biophysical and pharmacological properties. Importantly, although studies performed prior to the cloning of the receptor described two subtypes of vanilloid receptor (C-type and R-type, based on their differential responses to capsaicin and resiniferatoxin, respectively (16)), the properties of both the C and R subtype can be recapitulated by expression of TRPV1. This suggests that the C and R subtypes reflect a differential action of capsaicin and resiniferatoxin on the same receptor, i.e. the difference lies in the way in which these molecules interact at the same receptor.

A. Distribution of TRPV1

TRPV1 expression in the spinal cord and brainstem of rat, studied by antibody labelling (5, 7), corresponds to the distribution of nociceptive afferent nerve terminals including both the peptidergic group (of which 85% are TRPV1-positive) and the non-peptidergic IB4 lectin-expressing group (of which 60–80% are TRPV1-positive). Expression of TRPV1 mRNA is more intense, and in some studies largely confined to a subpopulation of sensory neuron cell bodies, including those of the nodose ganglion as well as somatic sensory ganglia (7, 17). Recent studies, however, have provided evidence for a broader distribution of the receptor, but clearly at much lower levels, based on in situ hybridization analysis (18). Whether those levels are physiologically relevant remains to be determined. Capsaicin has also been reported to activate mast cells and glioma cells (19, 20), but whether this is due a direct action via TRPV1 has yet to be firmly established. Finally, there is an interesting report demonstrating TRPV1 message and protein in epithelial cells of the bladder wall (21). Interestingly, the latter cells are unusual in that they express other receptors typically associated with primary afferent neurons, such as the PTX_3 subtype of ATP-sensitive purinergic receptor.

B. The Vanilloid Receptor Is a Detector of Noxious Heat

When expressed in heterologous systems (frog oocytes or transfected mammalian cells), TRPV1 shows a remarkable characteristic of heat sensitivity (7, 14). Thus, increases in ambient temperature promote robust channel opening, even in TRPV1-containing membrane patches that have been excised from the cell surface. The thermal responsiveness of the channel is characterized by two salient properties: the temperature threshold under normal conditions is ~43°C, similar to the psychophysical response threshold in humans and primates; and the cooperativity of channel opening is extremely steep ($Q_{10} > 20$), suggesting that heat sensitivity is, indeed, a specialized and specific functional property of the channel. These and other findings support the idea that TRPV1 is a molecular thermometer whose thermal response properties underlie heat sensitivity in some sensory nerve fibers.

Several studies (22, 23) have shown that a subpopulation of sensory neurons responds to stimulation with noxious heat, showing a reversible inward (i.e., depolarizing) membrane current associated with the opening of non-selective cation channels, with a temperature threshold corresponding to that of nociceptors. In one population, whose temperature threshold averages 46°C, heat-sensitivity is invariably accompanied by capsaicin-sensitivity, consistent with the hypothesis that TRPV1 represents the membrane transducer; these cells likely correspond to heat-sensitive unmyelinated C-fibers and myelinated Type II Aδ fibers (24). A second population, with a higher temperature threshold (52°C) consists of capsaicin-insensitive cells, and probably corresponds to Type I Aδ fibers. A likely candidate for this high-threshold heat sensor is TRPV2 (or VRL-1), a close molecular cousin of TRPV1 whose functional properties and cellular distribution match that of high-threshold heat-evoked currents observed in cultured sensory neurons and nerve fibers (25, 26).

V. TRPV1: POLYMODAL SIGNAL DETECTOR

The existence of a specific membrane receptor for vanilloids, and its coupling to ion channels, raises the obvious question of whether there are endogenous ligands that regulate nociceptor excitability by acting on TRPV1. One candidate is acidic protons because extracellular protons are able to mimic (27) and potentiate (28, 29) the effects of vanilloids on isolated sensory neurons. Like the actions of capsaicin, these effects are blocked by the non-specific channel blocking drug, ruthenium red. In some studies, the competitive capsaicin antagonist, capsazepine, has also been found to block proton-induced effects (30), suggesting that protons could represent a physiological ligand for the capsaicin receptor. It must be remembered that other proton-activated channels that are not vanilloid-sensitive are known to occur in sensory neurons (31), but at least one major component (the sustained phase) of the proton response fits the criteria of a TRPV1-mediated current. Indeed, the cloned TRPV1 receptor also shows the property of sensitivity to acidic solutions in which acidification below pH 6.0 leads to channel opening (at room temperature) or causes increased sensitivity to vanilloids and heat with more moderate changes in extracellular pH. Thus the TRPV1-associated ion channel is directly modulated by several distinct stimuli, namely vanilloids, heat, and protons; since all three can act on excised membrane patches, it is likely that sensitivity to these chemical and thermal stimuli is an integral property of the TRPV1 protein and does not depend on cellular signal transduction pathways.

Capsaicin bears structural homology to a number of bioactive lipids, especially those of the ethanolamide variety, suggesting that TRPV1 is activated by endogenous ligands of this type. Indeed, recent studies have demonstrated that the endogenous cannabinoid receptor agonist, anandamide, can also activate native or cloned vanilloid receptors (32, 33). Further evidence for pharmacological cross-over between cannabinoid and vanilloid receptors comes from the observation that the synthetic cannabinoid re-uptake blocker, AM404, is also a TRPV1 agonist (34). Responses of TRPV1 to anandamide and AM404 are specific in that they are inhibited by the vanilloid antagonist, capsazepine (but not by cannabinoid-receptor antagonists), and a variety of other cannabinoid-receptor agonists (endogenous and synthetic) have no effect on TRPV1. Moreover, structure-function studies of cloned TRPV1 show that residues involved in capsaicin activation are also important for anandamide recognition (35). These observations suggest that anandamide or other structurally related lipids function as activators or modulators of TRPV1 in vivo (i.e., endovanilloids). These molecules may be released by macrophages, neutrophils, or endothelial cells during inflammation and contribute to thermal hyperalgesia by lowering thermal thresholds for channel activation.

Protons and lipids may contribute to thermal hypersensitivity because they bind to TRPV1 directly and function as allosteric modulators of the channel complex (1). However, a variety of other factors that bind to their own receptors on sensory neurons are also known to augment responses to heat or capsaicin. Presumably, these agents, such as bradykinin (23) and nerve growth factor (NGF) (36), alter TRPV1 function indirectly through second messenger signalling cascades. Recent studies of native and cloned vanilloid receptors support this idea and suggest that activation of phospholipase C is a key step in this regulatory pathway. Candidate downstream mechanisms include the hydrolysis of membrane lipids, such as phosphatidylinositol bisphosphate, that exert a tonic inhibitory effect on TRPV1 (37), and/or phosphorylation of the channel by protein kinase C (38–40).

A. Function of TRPV1: Studies of Mice in Which the Gene Has Been Deleted

As predicted from the properties of TRPV1, deletion of the gene in mice resulted in complete loss of the response to vanilloids, including capsaicin and resiniferatoxin (41, 42). For example, single cells from dorsal root ganglion no longer show activation by capsaicin and the neurogenic inflammatory response to capsaicin is abrogated. Further, the hypothermic response to capsaicin is lost, and mutant mice will drink water spiked with capsaicin (a wild-type mouse will not). Consistent with the physiological properties of the channel, mutant mice also showed significantly altered thermal pain sensitivity. Interestingly however, the mice showed normal response to temperatures around

45°C, namely near the threshold for the channel. The greatest deficits were observed at higher temperatures (>50°C). This seemingly paradoxical result can be best explained from an analysis of the effects of gene deletion on the physiological properties of nociceptors studied in a skin-attached ex vivo preparation. As expected, the number of C fibers that responded to noxious temperatures (>45°C) was significantly reduced compared to control, and those that responded showed a reduced maximal discharge at the highest temperatures.

Although only 17% of C fibers responded to noxious thermal stimuli in the mutant (compared to 54% in wild-type mice), their threshold for responding was equivalent to the wild type. We assume that the preservation of normal responsiveness near the threshold of TRPV1 reflects the residual activity of these thermal nociceptors in the mutant mice. A full complement of nociceptors is not required to maintain acute pain responsiveness around 45°C, however, at higher temperatures, there is reduced responding because this behavior results from the summated activity of many C fibers (and in the mutant mice, there are many fewer).

In addition to showing deficits in acute pain responsiveness, we found that there was a very significant decrease in thermal sensitization in the setting of tissue injury produced by injection of complete Freund's adjuvant into the hindpaw of the mouse. Furthermore, the thermal sensitization produced by defined components of the inflammatory milieu, notably bradykinin and NGF, was also attenuated in the TRPV1 mutant mice (37). These results are consistent with studies concerning bradykinin and NGF regulation of the receptor, and raise the important possibility that drugs that target TRPV1 may prove useful for pain associated with tissue injury. Although thermal sensitization is not a major clinical problem, it is of interest to examine the possibility that the extreme pain that characterizes injury to viscera may reflect a contribution of TRPV1 expressed by these normally (silent) nociceptors (43). Conceivably in the setting of significant inflammation, the thermal threshold of visceral afferents drops close to body temperature.

B. Clinical Applications

Clinically, vanilloids (notably capsaicinoids) have been used for medicinal, dietary, and other purposes for centuries (43,44). More recently, the potential utility of capsaicinoids for specific clinical conditions has been emphasized. To some extent the attractiveness of these drugs reflects the discrete localization of the vanilloid receptors, which should limit their side-effect profile. Autonomic, motor, enteric, and most central neurons are likely to be insensitive. Empirically, compounds with activity at the vanilloid receptor have potential utility against a number of unmyelinated afferent fiber disorders including those of the gut, bladder, and peripheral nervous system.

Gut Cytoprotection

The gastrointestinal tract is richly supplied by afferent fibers originating from the dorsal root ganglia. These fibers travel with the sympathetic (splanchnic, colonic, and hypogastric) and sacral parasympathetic (pelvic) nerves. Vagal afferents originating from the nodose ganglia also supply the GI tract down to the transverse colon and capsaicin-sensitive afferent neurons are important contributors to gastric defense mechanisms. Endogenous ligands for vanilloid receptors in the gut probably include lipoxygenase and other inflammatory mediators. Presence of these ligands at localized sites of inflammation and activation of capsaicin-sensitive fibers produces warning (visceral) pain symptoms (45).

Rat studies involving administration of intragastric capsaicin have shown that stimulation of capsaicin-sensitive afferents produce synergistic protective effects, including enhancement of motility (46), arteriolar dilatation (47–49), alteration of secretions (50), and mucosal sparing (51, 52). In 1996, Kang showed (in rats) that intragastric administration of capsaicin is superior to cimetidine in promoting the healing of chemically induced gastric ulcer (53). These authors reported that capsaicin increased gastric mucosal blood flow (measured by laser Doppler) while cimetidine had the opposite effect. Food containing capsaicinoids and other vanilloid agonists may offer gut protection by initiating the same protective actions.

Bladder

Among other types of receptors, the bladder is richly innervated by capsaicin-sensitive afferent fibers. These fibers detect distension and the presence of irritant chemicals inside the vesicle. In turn, they trigger reflex bladder contraction. As noted above, it was recently reported that the TRPV1 receptor is also expressed by non-neural uro-epithelial cells (54). Although it was previously thought that these cells only serve a barrier function, they are responsive to mechanical and chemical stimuli, and release nitric oxide and ATP. Whether there are other natural ligands of these uro-epithelial cells remains to be determined, as does the consequence of TRPV1 agonist induced activation of these putative barrier cells.

Afferent signalling by activated sensory afferents stimulates micturation. In less mature animals, the impulse is a reflex mediated between local (bladder) C-fibers and the spinal cord. In humans, the C-fiber–spinal cord reflex is overridden as the conscious brain learns to assert control of micturation in response to pressure signals. After complete spinal cord transection, bladder pressure signaling is lost and arreflexia results (neurogenic bladder). In time, the immature C-fiber–spinal cord reflex route reemerges and the bladder may empty spontaneously (55). In diverse disorders such as benign prostatic hyperplasia (BPH), interstitial cystitis, urinary tract infection (UTI), and others, it is believed that ongoing stimulation of the C-fiber–spinal cord reflex may stimulate sensations of need for urinary frequency. Additionally, patients often report sensations of "burning," another indication that capsaicin-sensitive afferent fiber activation is occurring in these disorders.

Bladder instilled resiniferatoxin (RTX) is theorized to dampen the signaling that initiates the micturation reflex allowing the bladder to reach a higher filling capacity before requiring emptying. Indeed, intra-vesicle RTX was shown in animal models to block frequent urination (56). This ultrapotent TRPV1 agonist is now in phase II trials for the treatment of pain and urinary frequency associated with interstitial cystitis.

Vanilloids for the Treatment of Pain

Pain is generally described as a noxious sensation that stimulates a protective response from the organism. Most pains are acute, and resolve when the painful stimulus is removed. However, some pain syndromes may become chronic, persisting despite optimization or healing of the affected area. There is evidence that the barrage from capsaicin-sensitive afferent fibers contributes to the persistence of many syndromes of chronic pain, including diverse disorders such as post-herpetic neuralgia, peripheral neuropathy, mucositis, enteritis, cystitis, pancreatitis, arthritis, and bony fractures.

When placed adjacent to innervated human epidermis, capsaicin-induced desensitization of nociceptors produces localized cutaneous effects, including vasodilatation and changes in thermal and mechanical sensations (57, 58). The Kennedy group was the first to demonstrate the mechanism of action of topically administered capsaicin. In their 1999 study, normal volunteers underwent daily application of low dose (0.075%) topical capsaicin for 3 weeks followed by serial biopsies and quantitative sensory testing. The authors noted that there was a reduced presence of capsaicin sensitive fibers in the epidermis (with lesser effect on fibers deep to the dermal-epidermal junction) after initial week exposure (59). However, six weeks after cessation of capsaicin exposure, repeat biopsies showed that epidermal nerve fibers had significantly regenerated.

As noted above, there is a profound loss of function of nociceptors after topical administration of capsaicin. This may result from transient desensitization or from frank destruction of the peripheral terminals of TRPV1 expressing nociceptors. In the 1980s, several groups initiated clinical studies with low dose capsaicin containing formulations for the treatment of pain associated with post-herpetic neuralgia, diabetic neuropathy, and osteoarthritis. However, reports of equivocal analgesia and poor compliance associated with the low dose formulations deterred ongoing interest (60–63).

In 1994, the use of significantly higher doses of topical capsaicinoids (>5%) for the treatment of neuropathic pain was explored. After a modestly positive result in one patient with HIV-associated neuropathy, we explored various methods of optimizing the formulation of topical capsaicin for use in patients with intractable pain. In a subsequent uncontrolled pilot study of ten patients with intractable neuropathies, we showed (WR) that topical exposure to high dose nonivamide cream after regional anesthesia produced relief of chronic pain in several subjects for prolonged amounts of time (64). Since that time, several groups have demonstrated in controlled studies that exposure to high dose capsaicinoids can produce analgesia for prolonged intervals.

VI. CONCLUDING REMARKS

It has taken about 50 years from the time that the unusual pharmacological properties of capsaicin–notably its selective excitatory and neurotoxic effects on nociceptive afferent neurons–were first described, to reach the point of recognizing the vanilloid receptor as a distinct molecular entity, forming a ligand-gated ion channel with the specific property of thermosensitivity, and probably playing a major role in nociceptive transduction. The cloning and expression of TRPV1 has already led to the development of novel ligands for the receptor, which hopefully will have even greater selectivity and clinical value. Many questions remain to be explored. For example: what are the physiological ligands for the vanilloid receptor, and under what conditions are they released? Are there subtypes of TRPV1 and, if so, what are their distributions and functional properties? What is the nature and function of non-neuronal vanilloid receptors? How is vanilloid receptor expression regulated, and does it alter in pathological conditions? Finally, and perhaps most importantly, to what extent does the vanilloid receptor constitute a useful target for the development of novel analgesic drugs?

REFERENCES

1. Julius D, Basbaum AI. Nature 2001; 413: 203–210.
2. Holzer P. Pharmacol Rev 1991; 43:143–201.
3. Jancso G, Kiraly E, Jancso-Gabor A. Nature 1977; 270:741–743.
4. Szolcsanyi J. In: Wood J, ed. Capsaicin in the Study of Pain. London: Academic Press, 1993:1–26.
5. Guo A, et al. Eur J Neurosci 1999; 11:946–958.
6. Snider WD, McMahon SB. Neuron 1998; 20:629–632.
7. Tominaga M, et al. Neuron 1998; 21:531–543.
8. Levine J, Taiwo Y. In: Wall PD, Melzack R, eds. Textbook of Pain. Edinburgh: Churchill Livingstone, 1994:45–56.
9. Jancso-Gabor A, et al. J Physiol 1970; 206:495–507.
10. Bevan S, Szolcsanyi J. Trends Pharmacol Sci 1990; 11:330–333.
11. Wood JN, et al. J Neurosci 1988; 8:3208–3220.
12. Bevan S, et al. Br J Pharmacol 1992; 107:544–552.
13. Szallasi A, Blumberg PM. Pharmacol Rev 1999; 51:159–212.
14. Caterina MJ, et al. Nature 1977; 389:816–824.
15. Montell C, et al. Mol Cell 2002; 9:229–231.
16. Szallasi A, et al. Mol Pharmacol 1999; 56:581–587.
17. Michael GJ, Priestley JV. J Neurosci 1999; 19:1844–1854.
18. Mezey E, et al. Proc Natl Acad Sci USA 2000; 97:3655–3660.
19. Biro T, et al. Blood 1998; 91:1332–1340.
20. Biro T, et al. Brain Res Mol Brain Res 1998; 56:89–98.
21. Birder LA, et al. Nat Neurosci 2002; 5:856–860.
22. Nagy I, Rang HP. J Physiol Proceedings of the Physiological Society 1998; 37P.
23. Cesare P, McNaughton P. Proc Natl Acad Sci USA 1996; 93:15435–15439.
24. Raja SN, Meyer RA, Raingkamp M, Campbell JN, eds. Peripheral neural mechanisms of nociception New York: Churchill-Livingstone, 1999.
25. Caterina MJ, et al. Nature 1999; 398:436–441.
26. Ahluwalia J, Rang H, Nagy I. Eur J Neurosci 2002; 16:1483–1489.

27. Bevan S, Yeats J. J Physiol 1991; 433:145–161.
28. Kress M, et al. Neurosci Lett 1996; 211:5–8.
29. Petersen M, LaMotte RH. Pain 1993; 54:37–42.
30. Bevan S, Geppetti P. Protons: Trends Neurosci 1994; 17:509–512.
31. Waldmann R, et al. Ann NY Acad Sci 1999; 868:67–76.
32. Zygmunt PM, et al. Nature 1999; 400:452–457.
33. Smart D, et al. Br J Pharmacol 2000; 129:227–230.
34. Zygmunt PM, et al. Eur J Pharmacol 2000; 396:39–42.
35. Jordt SE, Julius D. Cell 2002; 108:421–430.
36. Shu X-Q, Mendell LM. Proc Natl Acad Sci USA 1999; 96:7693–7696.
37. Chuang HH, et al. Nature 2001; 411:957–962.
38. Cesare P, et al. Neuron 1999; 23:617–62.
39. Premkumar LS, Ahern GP. Nature 2000; 408:985–990.
40. Tominaga M, et al. Proc Natl Acad Sci USA 2001; 98:6951–6956.
41. Davis JB, et al. Nature 2000; 405:183–187.
42. Schmidt R, et al. J Neurosci 1995; 15:333–341.
43. Hogyes A. Arch Exp Pathol Pharmak 1878; 9:117.
44. Fusco BM, Giacovazzo M. Am J Physiol Gastrointest Liver Physiol 2000; 278:G834–G838.
46. Takeuchi K, et al. Jpn J Pharmacol 1991; 55:147–155.
47. Kang JY, et al. Gut 1998; 42:344–350.
48. Matsumoto Y, et al. Am J Physiol Gastrointest Liver Physiol 2001; 280:G897–G903.
49. Lippe IT, et al. Br J Pharmacol 1989; 96:91–100.
50. Takeuchi K, et al. Gastroenterology 1991; 101:951–961.
51. Yeoh KG, et al. Dig Dis Sci 1995; 40:580–583.
52. Uchida M, et al. Jpn J Pharmacol 1991; 55:279–282.
53. Kang JY, et al. Gut 1996; 38:832–836.
54. Birder LA, et al. Proc Natl Acad Sci USA 2001; 98:13396–13401.
55. de Groat WC. Urology 1997;50(6A Suppl):36–52.
56. Craft RM, et al. Pain 1993; 55:205–215.
57. Szolcsanyi J. J Physiol (Paris) 1977; 73:251–259.
58. Carpenter SE, Lynn B. Br J Pharmacol 1981; 73:755–758.
59. Nolano M, et al. Pain 1999; 81:135–145.
60. Capsaicin Study Group. Diabetes Care 1992; 15:159–165.
61. Bernstein JE, et al. J Am Acad Dermatol 1987; 17:93–96.
62. Rains C, Bryson HM. Drugs Aging 1995; 7:317–328.
63. Watson CPN, et al. Pain 1988; 33:333–340.
64. Robbins WR, et al. Anesth Analg 1998; 86:579–583.

43
The Development of Bradykinin Antagonists as Therapeutic Agents

Martin N. Perkins
AstraZeneca R&D Montreal, Montreal, Quebec, Canada

I. INTRODUCTION

There is considerable evidence to suggest that kinins play a major role in the initiation and maintenance of inflammatory conditions. A detailed review of the production and pharmacology of kinins is beyond the scope of this chapter, but it is worth stressing that kinin production is one of the first responses of the body to trauma or inflammation and continues for as long as such stimuli are present. Kinins are formed rapidly from their precursor molecules: bradykinin (Bk) being cleaved from high molecular weight kininogen (HMWK) in plasma, and kallidin being formed from low molecular weight kininogen (LMWK) (1). They are, therefore, ideally placed to play a role both in the initiation and maintenance of inflammatory processes and the accompanying pain. Surprisingly, for such ubiquitous mediators of inflammation, no kinin receptor antagonist has been successfully taken to the clinic, primarily owing to the difficulty in synthesizing an orally active kinin receptor antagonist. In the last decade this has changed with, initially, the synthesis of antagonists based on substitutions of the peptide structure of Bk and, more recently, the development of small-molecule nonpeptide antagonists.

Even so, there are very few kinin antagonists currently in the clinical stages of development, and none at all known to be in clinical trials for pain, although this indication is included in most patent applications. This reflects both the relatively recent timescale in which kinin antagonists have been developed, as well as the necessity to consider indications for which topical or intravenous administration is a viable option owing to the peptidic nature of the first generation of kinin receptor antagonists. This chapter will cover both those antagonists that have been taken through the initial stages of development, but subsequently abandoned, as well as those still in development. It will also attempt to put these novel potential therapeutic agents in the context of what is known about kinin involvement in pathophysiological processes. This chapter will not attempt to review the vast body of preclinical, experimental literature supporting a role for kinins in many diverse conditions, but will focus on studies relating directly to the clinical conditions for which kinin antagonists have been considered as therapeutic agents. The equally important issue of possible side effects of such drugs will also be addressed.

A. Kinin Receptors

Kinins act on two distinct receptors, the B_1 and B_2 receptor (2), which are both typical G protein-coupled receptors (3,4), although there is, surprisingly in view of the similarity of their preferred ligands, little homology between the two receptors (5). The preferred ligands for the B_2 receptor are Bk and kallidin, and those for the B_1 receptor are the only active metabolites of Bk and kallidin, namely, des-Arg^9Bk and des-Arg^{10}kallidin.

Although there are two receptors, only antagonists for the B_2 receptor that have been taken into development as therapeutic agents. This partly reflects that it is only recently that the B_1 receptor has been implicated in pathophysiological processes. Consequently, the development of orally active B_1 receptor antagonists is less advanced than those targeted toward the B_2 receptor.

II. POTENTIAL THERAPEUTIC AREAS FOR KININ ANTAGONISTS

A. Inflammation

Kinins are proinflammatory, producing vasodilation, plasma extravasation, and edema, as well as the release of other inflammatory mediators. Vasodilation is caused, primarily, by the release of nitric oxide and prostacyclin from endothelial cells, leading to relaxation of arterial smooth muscle and an increase in blood flow. Edema is a consequence of an increase in the permeability of endothelial cells as well as intracapillary pressure from kinin-induced venoconstriction concomitant with arteriovasodilation. Kinins also act on immunocompetent cells that can release further inflammatory mediators (e.g., prostaglandins and cytokines). Kinin antagonists have been anti-inflammatory in animal models, providing the preclinical basis for considering kinin antagonists as therapeutic agents in asthma, allergic rhinitis, pancreatitis, and septic shock. In addition, there are animal studies suggesting that kinins may contribute to the sequelae following a cerebral infarct: kinin production being activated by ischemia and resulting in cerebral edema.

B. Kinins and Inflammatory Pain

Kinins are clearly involved in the initiation and maintenance of inflammatory pain, both directly, at the level of the nociceptor itself, and indirectly by actions on other tissues involved in inflammation per se. The result is both activation and sensitization of nociceptors, the latter leading to a reduced threshold to noxious stimulation that probably contributes to the "tenderness" associated with inflammatory conditions in humans.

Although both B_1 and B_2 receptors are involved in nociception, most evidence supports a role for the B_2 receptor in activating and sensitizing the nociceptor. Activation leads to a depolarization of the sensory neuron, primarily mediated by an increase in sodium ion conductance, activation of phospholipase C, and stimulation of protein kinase C (6,7). Bk increases neuronal activity in nociceptive fibers in vitro and in vivo (7–9) as well as causing pain in animals (10–12) and humans (13,14) and also sensitizes nociceptors, lowering their threshold to noxious stimuli (15–17). There are many studies in animals suggesting kinins contribute to the initiation and maintenance of inflammatory pain and both B_2 and B_1 receptors are involved in this process. The clinical conditions that have been considered are arthritic pain as well as acute "inflammatory" pain such as postsurgical pain.

C. Peptide Antagonists at Kinin Receptors

The first generation of kinin receptors antagonists were based on substitutions to the structure of Bk. A few of these were subsequently taken into the early phases of clinical development, but this therapeutic approach has been largely discontinued for two main reasons: First, being peptidic in nature they lacked oral bioavailability which limits the indications for which they could be considered. The relatively short half-life of such compounds caused by enzymatic breakdown was also an issue with the first generation of such antagonists. The second reason for largely abandoning this approach has been the recent development of potent nonpeptide antagonists of the kinin B_2 receptor with oral availability. Despite that peptidic antagonists will probably never succeed as therapeutic agents, they have had, and continue to have, great value in providing potent, specific pharmacological tools to explore the role of kinins in both physiological and pathophysiological animal models.

As yet, there are no nonpeptide B_1 receptor antagonists known to be in clinical development, although this is an area where there is increasing interest within the pharmaceutical industry.

1. NPC-567 (Scios Nova)

NPC-567 (D-Arg^0[Hyp^3-D-Phe^7]Bk was one of the first kinin B_2 receptor antagonists to be taken into development as a potential drug. It is a peptide antagonist with good potency and selectivity for the B_2 kinin receptor and shows efficacy in animal models of inflammatory pain as well as being an anti-inflammatory agent by itself, inhibiting carrageenan-induced hyperalgesia and edema in rats (18,19,20). In mice, local administration of NPC-567 as well as the related peptide antagonist NPC 349 (D-Arg^0[Hyp^3-Thi^{5,8}-D-Phe^7]Bk) inhibited both the initial and delayed phases of formalin-induced nocifensor responses (21). Both antagonists inhibited Bk-induced increases in discharge rate of canine testicular polymodal afferents (22) and NPC-567 reduced capsaicin-induced edema in mice (23).

A possible role in asthma or allergic rhinitis was suggested by a series of studies in sheep allergic to *Ascaris suum* antigen, in which NPC-567 attenuated the delayed increase in lung resistance to allergen (24–26). However, in humans NPC-567 failed to attenuate the response to intranasal Bk (27) and did not alleviate the symptoms of experimental rhinovirus cold (28). NPC-567 entered phase I/II clinical trials for asthma in 1989, but development has been discontinued. The most likely reason for the absence of efficacy in humans is metabolic instability; NPC-567 is subject to degradation by peptidases.

More recently, Scios Nova developed a series of pseudopeptide kinin antagonists such as NPC-18688 and NPC-18521 (29). There has been little published work on this series of antagonists but NPC-18688 has been demonstrated to inhibit formalin-induced nocifensor responses and edema in mice (30). NPC-18521 reduces Bk- and carrageenan-induced edema in rats as well as formalin and capsaicin-induced licking in mice and rats and abdominal writhing in mice (31). However, NPC-18521 was also observed to cause edema and hyperalgesia by itself, a response not related to kinin receptor activation, but probably secondary to mast cell degranulation (31). Both of these antagonists are believed to be in development for the indications of inflammatory diseases and endotoxic shock, but their current status is unclear.

2. Icatibant (Hoe 140; Hoechst)

Hock et al. (32) discovered one of the most potent peptide antagonist at the B_2 receptor known to date, Hoe 140, now known as icatibant (D-Arg-[Hyp^3, Thi^5, D-Tic^7, Oic^8]Bk). Icatibant has high potency at the B_2 kinin receptor in several species as well as humans, with pA_2 values varying between 7 and 9 (32,33). Icatibant has also inhibited Bk-evoked responses in vivo (34,35). More importantly, it marked a milestone in the development of Bk antagonists in that it was metabolically stable; substitution with the unnatural amino acids D-Tic and Oic rendered it resistant to peptidase degradation (36). The combination of potency and metabolic stability ensured that it rapidly became the gold standard reference B_2 kinin receptor antagonist in preclinical studies aimed at elucidating the role of kinins in vitro and in vivo. It is fair to say that the discovery of, first, NPC-567 and then icatibant, revitalized the kinin field providing for the first time potent, selective pharmacological tools.

Icatibant administered locally or systemically reduces Bk-induced plasma extravazation and edema in vivo in animal studies (33–35) and reduces carrageenan or noxious heat-evoked edema (37). Icatibant has also alleviated the hyperalgesia associated with inflammatory stimuli in several studies (21,38,39), supporting a role for a B_2 kinin receptor antagonist in inflammatory pain.

Although the numerous studies with icatibant in animal models have provided strong evidence for kinin B_2 receptor involvement in many conditions when there is an underlying inflammatory component, the lack of oral activity of this peptidic antagonist clearly severely limited its therapeutic potential. However, in spite of this, icatibant, given as an aerosol, was taken into development with clinical trials in patients with seasonal allergic rhinitis, house dust mite rhinitis, and asthma. The results were mixed, with no significant efficacy in alleviating the symptoms of allergic rhinitis and asthma, but a positive effect against house dust mite allergic rhinitis (40). Clinical development of icatibant has now been discontinued.

4. Deltibank (CP-0127; Cortech)

A novel approach to developing a kinin B_2 antagonist was adopted by Cortech with a series of bissuccinimidoalkane peptide dimers. CP-0127 (bissuccimidohexane (L-Cys^6)-1), later named deltibant, is a dimer of matching peptide B_2 antagonists (D-Arg^0-Arg^1-Pro^2-Hyp^3-Gly^4-Phe^5-Cys^6-D-Phe^7-Leu^8-Arg^9), with a bissuccinimidoalkane moeity cross-linking the substituted cysteine amino acid residues (41). CP-0127 is a potent, competitive antagonist at the B_2 kinin receptor with pA_2 values of 7.7 and 8.5 in the guinea pig ileum and rat uterus smooth muscle bioassay, respectively (41). It is active in vivo, inhibiting Bk-induced hypotension and plasma extravazation in rabbits and rats (42–44). CP-0127 was also able to increase survival time after endotoxic shock in rabbits and rats (43,44), a finding that supported clinical trials for the indications of sepsis and inflammatory response syndrome (SIRS). These trials were halted, however, due to unexpected increases in mortality in rodent toxicology studies, although these findings were, subsequently, not reproduced. Subsequently, CP-0127, was developed for the indication of traumatic head injury, but this was discontinued in 1997 owing to lack of efficacy in phase II trials. More recently, Cortech has extended the concept of these peptide dimers with heterogeneous dimers, combining activity at different receptors. B-9340 has both B_1 and B_2 kinin receptor antagonist activity, and dimers with kinin receptor antagonist activity coupled with μ-opioid receptor agonism (e.g., CP-0719) have been synthesized. Although these approaches are interesting, none of these compounds are currently in clinical development, and it is likely that they will be limited by a lack of oral activity.

D. Nonpeptide Antagonists at Kinin Receptors

1. WIN 64338 (Sterling Winthrop)

The first functional nonpeptide kinin antagonist was, actually, developed almost a decade ago by Sterling Winthrop (45). WIN 64338, ([[4-[[2-[[bis(cyclohexylamino)methylene]amino]-3-(2-naphthyl)-1-oxopropyl]amino]phyenyl]methyl]tributylphosphonium chloride monohydrochloride) inhibits Bk binding to the human B_2 receptor (K_i-64 nM) and antagonizes Bk-induced responses with pA_2 values between 7 and 8 (45). WIN 64338 also inhibits Bk-induced activation of trigeminal nerve terminals in the rabbit and guinea pig (46). Interestingly, one report suggested

WIN 64338 preferentially inhibited a B_1 receptor-mediated cGMP response in bovine endothelial cells (47), suggesting its kinin receptor specificity may be tissue- or species-dependent. Further development was, however, discontinued relatively quickly. Further Bk antagonists based on a model of this compound together with a cyclic peptide antagonist are reportedly being explored by Roche Bioscience.

2. FR173657 (Fujisawa)

FR173657 ((*E*)-3-(6-acetamido-3-pyridyl)-*N*-[*N*-[2,4-dichloro-3-[(2-methyl-8-quinolinyl)oxymethyl]phenyl]-*N*-methylaminocarbonylmethyl]acrylamide) is a recent, potent, nonpeptide kinin B_2 receptor antagonist which, together with a closely related derivative, FR184280, is being taken into clinical development for the indications of pain and inflammation. FR173657 is a potent, competitive antagonist, inhibiting binding of Bk to the human B_2 kinin receptor with a K_i value of 3 nM (48), with no affinity for the human B_1 kinin receptor and no effect on histamine or acetylcholine-induced contractions of smooth muscle (48,49). FR173657 inhibits Bk-induced responses in vivo, abolishing Bk-induced hypotension, plasma extravazation and bronchoconstriction when given intravenously or subcutaneously in the rat (50). FR173657 also inhibits Bk-induced bronchoconstriction in guinea pigs with an ED_{50} of 0.075 mg/kg (48). FR173657 prevents visceral plasma extravazation induced by Bk in the rat, with complete inhibition at 30 nmol/kg s.c., although Bk-induced paw edema was reduced only by a maximum of approximately 50% at 3 μmol/kg (50). FR173657 is orally active, although its potency in the rat varied between studies. Asano et al. (48) reported an ED_{50} of 6.8 mg/kg p.o. in inhibiting carrageenan-induced paw edema in the rat, whereas Majima et al. (51) reported a 50–77% inhibition of carrageenan-induced pleural plasma extravasation with 30 mg/kg. FR173657 virtually abolished Bk-induced behavioral nocifensor responses in the rat when given both orally and subcutaneously and reduced thermal hyperalgesia when given subcutaneously (52). It is virtually equipotent i.v. with the most potent peptide B_2 kinin receptor antagonist, icatibant, in inhibiting carrageenan-induced pleurisy in rats, with a duration of action in excess of 4 h (51). More recently, oral administration of FR173657 has reduced allergic skin reactions in guinea pigs, suggesting a potential for a kinin antagonist in human allergic diseases (53).

There appears to be species differences relative to oral bioavailability of FR173657 with a figure of 44% reported for the guinea pig, but only 7% in the rat (48). In view of the relatively low value in the rat, determination of oral bioavailability in the primate or human is clearly important. Other nonpeptide antagonists belonging to this class (e.g., FR167344, FR165649) also have potent kinin B_2 antagonists and are active orally, but there are still no reported studies relating to potential antinociceptive actions of these antagonists (49,54).

E. Other Nonpeptide Kinin B_2 Receptor Antagonists

In addition to the nonpeptide kinin B_2 antagonists described in the foregoing, there are several others in early preclinical stages of development about which little is known.

For example, Fournier recently developed a nonpeptide antagonist, LF-16-0335 (1-[[3-(2,4-dimethylquiniolin-8-yl)oxymethyl]-2,4-dichloro-phenyl]sulfonyl]-2(*S*)-[[4-[4-(amino-iminomethyl)phenyl-carbonyl]piperazin-1-y]carbonyl]pyrrolidine), which is a potent, competitive kinin B_2 receptor antagonist with K_i values ranging from 0.84 to 2.34 nM at the human B_2 receptor LF-16-0335 antagonised Bk-induced inositolphosphate production in a cell line with a pA_2 of 8.3 (55). There are, as yet, no reported studies on its activity in vivo, although a related compound, LF-16-0687, has reduced brain edema in rats. Another recent B_2 receptor antagonist has been presented by Menarini (MEN-11270) which has activity in vitro comparable with that of Hoe 140 and greater than FR-173657; however, further information on this compound is not yet available.

This is clearly an area in which there is much activity within the pharmaceutical industry and it is known that several other pharmaceutical companies have active preclinical programs aimed toward this potential therapeutic target.

F. Kinin B_1 Antagonists

There have been fewer kinin B_1 receptor antagonists developed, which partly reflects that historically it was the B_2 kinin receptor that was thought to mediate most of the effects of kinins. However, it is now increasingly recognized that the B_1 receptor plays an important role in inflammatory conditions, particularly in the maintenance of the hyperalgesia accompanying persistent inflammation. As with the kinin B_2 receptor, peptide antagonists for the B_1 receptor have been known for some years, but these exhibit the same weaknesses as the early B_2 receptor antagonists: namely, lack of oral availability. However, there has been a preliminary report of potent nonpeptide B_1 receptor antagonists from Pharmacopeia. Two of these, PS-322835 and PS-020990, inhibit binding of the B_1 agonist, desArg^{10}kallidin in a human cell line with K_i values in the low nanomolar range and are functional antagonists of Bk-induced phosphatidylinositol turnover and calcium mobilization in the same cell line. The structures of these antagonists, however, are not yet known.

III. SIDE EFFECTS OF KININ RECEPTOR ANTAGONISTS

The side effect profile of kinin antagonists will, as with all therapeutic agents, fall into two areas: nonspecific- and mechanism-based side effects. Nonspecific side effects are, by nature, idiosyncratic to the compound or compound class and are difficult to predict. The only kinin antagonists to have been taken into a clinical trial and, therefore, been assessed for tolerability in humans, are peptide-based antagonists such as deltibant (Cortech) and icatibant (Hoechst), and in both cases, tolerability was reported to be acceptable in humans.

Of more importance for the use of kinin antagonists as therapeutic agents is the possibility of mechanism-based side effects. As kinins are produced in any significant amount only in response to trauma or an inflammatory episode, it has been believed that there is little or no physiological role for kinins. This appears to be true, for in the many studies characterizing kinin antagonists there have been no reports of significant effects on the basal functioning of physiological systems, such as the cardiovascular, respiratory, and renal systems. The first generation of peptide kinin antagonists, such as [Thi^{5,8}-D-Phe^7]Bk, have been reported to possess partial agonist activity in some models in vitro and have been reported to cause edema in rats, which was blocked by antihistamines (56). Histamine release has been demonstrated in vitro but this did not appear to be a kinin receptor-mediated phenomenon and may be related to the presence of positive charges on these molecules (57). Edema and hyperalgesia in mice and rats has also been reported for pseudopeptide antagonists such as NPC 18521, also apparently due to mast cell degranulation (31). NPC 567 and a similar peptide antagonist (NPC 349) have also caused pain, wheal, and flare in humans after intracutaneous injection, an effect partially reduced by antihistamines (13), suggesting a similar mechanism in humans. As similar responses in animals were reduced by antihistamines, but not by icatibant, it is unlikely these are due to an action on kinin receptors per se, but are probably a nonspecific effect peculiar to peptidergic structures. No such effects have yet been reported for the nonpeptide kinin antagonists.

One area of potential concern, however, is the use of kinin antagonists as therapeutic agents if there is a concomitant risk of cardiac ischemia. Bk is released during cardiac ischemia (58) and has markedly reduced the severity of ischemia-induced arrhythmias in dogs (59). Subsequently, a series of reports from this laboratory provided strong evidence that Bk serves a cardioprotective role following cardiac ischemia (60). In particular, the B_2 receptor antagonist, Hoe 140, prevented the protective effect of "ischemic preconditioning" in dogs (61), suggesting that in cases of cardiac insufficiency a kinin antagonist may be detrimental. It is not clear, however, whether this effect is species-dependent, as Hoe 140 failed to prevent the protective effect of ischemic preconditioning in rats (62).

In addition, kinin B_2 receptor antagonists may be detrimental when coadministered with angiotensin-converting enzyme (ACE) inhibitors. ACE inhibitors can reduce the ventricular hypertrophy that develops in hypertension and one study has shown that Hoe-140 prevents the beneficial effect of ramipril, an ACE inhibitor (63). Hoe 140 also abolished the reduction in infarct size seen after administration of an angiotensin II type I receptor antagonist, although not affecting the size of the infarct by itself (64). These findings suggest that any future development of kinin antagonists may need to include studies to determine whether they have any potential to exacerbate the effect of cardiovascular stress on the heart.

IV. SUMMARY AND FUTURE DIRECTIONS

It is clear from the animal studies that there is every reason to expect kinin B_2 receptor antagonists to have therapeutic potential as analgesics in humans in conditions of inflammatory pain. However, it is also true that there is no study in humans demonstrating such efficacy, nor are there any clinical trials reported to be ongoing for pain, although most patent applications cite this as a potential indication. This probably reflects the fact that only very recently have orally active nonpeptide antagonists been developed, and it is reasonable to assume it will not be long before this concept is tested in the clinic. In view of the large number of potential indications for a kinin antagonist, it is, perhaps, fair to say that kinin antagonists are therapeutic agents in search of an indication.

Farther into the future, however, it is likely that kinin B_1 receptor antagonists will be developed and evaluated for efficacy in chronic inflammatory pain. It will be interesting to see in the next few years whether kinin receptor antagonists prove to be a truly novel treatment for one of the most common pain conditions in humans.

REFERENCES

1. Bhoola KD, Figueroa CD, Worthy K. Bioregulation of kinins: kallikreins, kininogens, and kininases. Pharmacol Rev 1992; 44:1–80.
2. Hall JM. Bradykinin receptors: pharmacological properties and biological roles. Pharmacol Ther 1992; 56:131–190.
3. McEarchern AE, Shelton ER, Bhakta S, et al. Expression cloning of a rat B_2 bradykinin receptor. Proc Nat Acad Sci USA 1991; 88:7724–7728.
4. Hess JF, Borkowski JA, Young GS, Strader CD, Ransom RW. Cloning and pharmacological characterization of a human bradykinin (BK-2) receptor. Biochem Biophys Res Commun 1992; 184:260–268.
5. Menke JG, Borkowski JA, Bierilo K, et al. Expression cloning of a human B_1 bradykinin receptor. J Biol Chem 1994; 269:21583–21586.

6. Burgess GM, Mullaney I, McNeil M, Coote PR, Minhas A, Wood JN. Activation of guanylate cyclase by bradykinin in rat sensory neurones is mediated by calcium influx: possible role of the increase in cyclic GMP. J Neurochem 1989; 53:1212–1218.
7. Dray A, Patel IA, Perkins MN, Rueff A. Bradykinin-induced activation of nociceptors: receptor and mechanistic studies on the neonatal rat spinal cord–tail preparation in vitro. Br J Pharmacol 1992; 107:1129–1134.
8. Mizumura K, Minagawa M, Tsuji Y, Kumasawa T. The effects of bradykinin agonists and antagonists on visceral polymodal receptor activities. Pain 1990; 40:221–227.
9. Sengupta JN, Gebhart GF. Characterization of mechanosensitive pelvic nerve afferent fibres innervating the colon of the rat. J Neurophysiol 1994; 71:2046–2070.
10. Ferreira SH, Lorenzetti BB, Cunha FQ, Poole S. Bradykinin release of TNF-alpha plays a key role in the development of inflammatory hyperalgesia. Agents Actions Suppl 1993; 38:7–9.
11. Khasar SG, Green PG, Levine JD. Comparison of intradermal and subcutaneous hyperalgesic effects of inflammatory mediators in the rat. Neurosci Lett 1993; 153:215–218.
12. Davis AJ, Kelly D, Perkins MN. The induction of des-Arg^9-bradykinin-mediated hyperalgesia in the rat by inflammatory stimuli. Braz J Med Biol Res 1994; 27:1793–1802.
13. Kingden–Milles D, Klement W. Pain and inflammation evoked in the human skin by bradykinin receptor antagonists. Eur J Pharmacol 1992; 218:183–185.
14. Whalley ET, Clegg S, Stewart JM, Vavrek RJ. The effect of kinin agonists and antagonists on the pain response of the human blister base. Arch Pharmacol 1987; 336:652–655.
15. Birrell GJ, McQueen DS, Iggo A, Grubb BD. Prostanoid-induced potentiation of the excitatory and sensitizing effects of bradykinin on articular mechanoniceptors in the rat ankle joint. Neuroscience 1993; 54:536–544.
16. Rueff A, Dray A. Sensitization of peripheral afferent fibres in the in vitro neonatal rat spinal cord–tail by bradykinin and prostaglandins. Neuroscience 1993; 54:527–535.
17. Khan AA, Raja SN, Manning DC, Campbell JN, Meyer RA. The effects of bradykinin and sequence-related analogs on the response properties of cutaneous nociceptors in monkeys. Somatosens Motor Res 1991; 9:97–106.
18. Steranka LR, Manning D, DeHass CJ, et al. Bradykinin as a pain mediator: receptors are localized to sensory neurons, and antagonists have analgesic actions. Proc Nat Acad Sci USA 1988; 85:3245–3249.
19. Costello AH, Hargreaves KM. Suppression of carrageenan-induced hyperalgesia, hyperthermia and edema by a bradykinin antagonist. Eur J Pharmacol 1989; 171:259–263.
20. Burch RM, DeHaas C. A bradykinin antagonist inhibits carrageenan edema in rats. Naunyn-Schmiedebergs Arch Pharmacol 1990; 342:2–93.
21. Correa CR, Calixto JB. Evidence for participation of B_1 and B_2 kinin receptors in formalin-induced nociceptive response in the mouse. Br J Pharmacol 1993; 110:193–198.
22. Kumazawa T, Mizumura M, Minagawa M, Tsuji Y. Sensitizing effect of bradykinin on the heat responses of the visceral nociceptor. J Neurophysiol 1991; 66:1819–1824.
23. Mantione CR, Rodriguez R. A bradykinin $(BK)_1$ receptor antagonist blocks capsaicin-induced ear edema in mice. Br J Pharmacol 1990; 99:516–518.
24. Abraham WM. The potential role of bradykinin antagonist in the treatment of asthma. Agents Actions Suppl 1992; 38:439–449.
25. Soler M, Sielczak M, Abraham WM. A bradykinin-antagonist blocks antigen-induced airway hyper-responsiveness and inflammation in sheep. Pulmon Pharmacol 1990; 3:9–15.
26. Abraham WM, Ahmed A, Cortes A, et al. Airway effects of inhaled bradykinin, substance P, and neurokinin A in sheep. J Allergy Clin Immunol 1991; 87:557–564.
27. Pongracic JA, Naclerio RM, Reynolds CJ, Proud D. A competitive kinin receptor antagonist, [DArg^0, Hyp^3, DPhe^7]-bradykinin, does not affect the response to nasal provocation with bradykinin. Br J Clin Pharmacol 1991; 31:287–290.
28. Higgins PG, Barrow GI, Tyrell DA. A study of the efficacy of the bradykinin antagonist, NPC 567, in rhinovirus infections in human volunteers. Antiviral Res 1990; 14:339–344.
29. Mavunkel BJ, Lu Z, Goehring RR, et al. Synthesis and characterization of pseudopeptide bradykinin

B_2 receptor antagonists containing the 1,3,8-triazaspiro[4,5]decan-4-one ring system. J Med Chem 1996; 39:3169–3173.
30. Correa CR, Kyle DJ, Chakraverty S, Calixto JB. Antinociceptive profile of pseudopeptide B_2 bradykinin receptor antagonist NPC 18688 in mice. Br J Pharmacol 1996; 117:552–558.
31. DeCampos ROP, Alves RV, Kyle DJ, Chakravarty S, Mavunkel BJ, Calixto JB. Antioedematogenic and antinociceptive actions of NPC 18521, a novel bradykinin B_2 receptor antagonist. Eur J Pharmacol 1996; 316:227–286.
32. Hock FJ, Wirth K, Albus U, et al. Hoe-140 a new potent long acting bradykinin antagonist: in vitro studies. Br J Pharmacol 1991; 102:769–773.
33. Lembeck F, Griesbacher T, Eckhardt M, Henke S, Briepohl G, Knolle J. New long-acting, potent bradykinin antagonists. Br J Pharmacol 1991; 102:297–304.
34. Griesbacher T, Lembeck F. Effect of bradykinin antagonists on bradykinin-induced plasma extravasation, venoconstriction, prostaglandin E_2 release, nociceptor stimulation and contraction of the iris sphincter in the rabbit. Br J Pharmacol 1997; 92:333–340.
35. Wirth K, Hock FJ, Albus U, et al. Hoe 140 a new potent and long acting bradykinin-antagonist: in vivo studies. Br J Pharmacol 1991; 102:774–777.
36. Bond AP, Breipohl G, Worthy K, Campion G, Dieppe PA, Bhoola KD. Metabolism and characterisation of kinins and Hoe 140 (kinin antagonist) in the synovial fluid of patients with inflammatory joint diseases. Agents Actions Suppl 1992; 38:582–589.
37. Wirth KJ, Alpermann HG, Satoh R, Inazu M. The bradykinin antagonist Hoe 140 inhibits carrageenan—and thermically induced paw edema in rats. Agents Actions Suppl 1992; 38:428–431.
38. Perkins MN, Campbell E, Dray A. Antinoniceptive activity of the bradykinin B_1 and B_2 receptor antagonist, desArg^9(Leu^8)-Bk and HOE 140, in two models of persistent hyperalgesia in the rat. Pain 1993; 53:191–197.
39. Dray A, Perkins MN. Bradykinin and inflammatory pain. Trends Neurosci 1993; 16:99–104.
40. Austin CE, Foreman JC, Scadding GK. Reduction by Hoe 140, the B_2 kinin receptor antagonist, of antigen-induced nasal blockage. Br J Pharmacol 1994; 111:969–971.
41. Cheronis JC, Whalley ET, Nguyen KT, et al. A new class of bradykinin antagonists: synthesis and in vitro activity of bissuccinimidoalkane peptide dimers. J Med Chem 1992; 35:1563–1572.
42. Breil I, Koch T, Goldberg S, Neuhof H, van Ackern K. Influence of B_2 receptor antagonists on bradykinin-induced vasodilation and edema formation in isolated rabbit hindlimbs. Inflamm Res 1995; 44:212–216.
43. Christopher TA, Ma XL, Gauthier TW, Lefer AM. Beneficial actions of CO-0127, a novel bradykinin receptor antagonist, in murine traumatic shock. Am J Physiol 1994; 266:867–873.
44. Whalley ET, Solomon JA, Modafferi DM, Bonham KA, Cheronis JC. CP-0127, a novel potent bradykinin antagonist, increases survival in rat and rabbit models of endotoxin shock. Agents Actions Suppl 1992; 38:413–420.
45. Sawutz DG, Salvino JM, Dolle RE, et al. The nonpeptide WIN 64388 is a bradykinin B_2 receptor antagonist. Proc Natl Acad Sci USA 1994; 91:4693–4697.
46. Hall JM, Figin M, Butt SK, Geppetti P. Inhibition of bradykinin-evoked trigeminal nerve stimulation by the non-peptide bradykinin B_2 receptor antagonist WIN 64338 in vivo and in vitro. Br J Pharmacol 1995; 116:164–168.
47. Wirth KJ, Scholkens BA, Wiener G. The bradykinin B_2 receptor antagonist WIN 64338 inhibits the effect of des-Arg^9-bradykinin in endothelial cells. Eur J Pharmacol 1994; 288:R1–R2.
48. Asano M, Inamura N, Hator C, et al. The identification of an orally active, nonpeptide bradykinin B_2 receptor antagonist, FR173657. Br J Pharmacol 1997; 120:617–624.
49. Inamura N, Asano M, Kayakiri H, Hatori C, Oku T, Nakahara K. Characterization of FR173657, a novel nonpeptide B_2 antagonist: in vitro and in vivo studies. Can J Physiol Pharmacol 1997; 75: 622–628.
50. Griesbacher T, Legat FJ. Effects of FR173657, a non-peptide B_2 antagonist, on kinin-induced hypotension, visceral and peripheral edema formation and bronchoconstriction. Br J Pharmacol 1997; 120:933–939.
51. Majima M, Kawashima N, Hiroshi I, Katori M. Effects of an orally active nonpeptide bradykinin

B_2 receptor antagonist, FR173657, on plasma exudation in rat carrageenin-induced pleurisy. Br J Pharmacol 1997; 121:723–730.

52. Griesbacher T, Amann R, Sametz W, Diethart S, Juan H. The nonpeptide B_2 receptor antagonist FR173657: inhibition of effects of bradykinin related to its role in nociception. Br J Pharmacol 1998; 124:1328–1334.
53. Mori T, Inamura T. Inhibition of guinea-pig skin allergic reactions by nonpeptide bradykinin B_2 receptor antagonist FR173657. Int Arch Allergy Immunol 1998; 116:278–283.
54. Asano M, Hatori C, Sawai H, et al. Pharmacological characterization of a nonpeptide bradykinin B_2 receptor antagonist, FR165649, and agonist, FR190997. Br J Pharmacol 1998; 124:441–446.
55. Pruneau D, Luccarini J–M, Fouchet C, et al. LF 16-0335, a novel potent and selective nonpeptide antagonist of the human bradykinin B_2 receptor. Br J Pharmacol 1998; 125:365–372.
56. Wang J–P, Hsu M–F, Ouyang C, Teng C–M. Edematous response caused by [Thi^5,8-D-Phe^7]bradykinin, a B_2 receptor antagonist, is due to mast cell degranulation. Eur J Pharmacol 1989; 161:143–149.
57. Devillier P, Drapeau G, Renoux M, Regoli D. Role of the N-terminal arginine in the histamine-releasing activity of substance P, bradykinin and related peptides. Eur J Pharmacol 1989; 168:53–60.
58. Ahmad M, Zeitlin IJ, Parratt JR, Kolar F. Kinin release from normally perfused and ischaemic isolated rat hearts: effect of strain. Immunopharmacology 1996; 33:297–298.
59. Vegh A, Szekeres L, Parratt JR. Local intracoronary infusions of bradykinin profoundly reduce the severity of ischaemia-induced arrythmias in anaesthetised dogs. Br J Pharmacol 1991; 104:294–295.
60. Parratt JR, Vegh A, Papp JG. Bradykinin as an endogenous myocardial protective substance with particular reference to ischemic preconditioning—a brief review of the evidence. Can J Physiol Pharmacol 1995; 73:837–842.
61. Vegh A, Papp JG, Parratt J. Attenuation of the antiarryhthmic effect of ischaemic preconditioning by blockade of bradykinin B_2 receptors. Br J Pharmacol 1994; 113:1167–1172.
62. Bouchard J–F, Chouinard J, Lamontagne D. Role of kinins in the endothelial protective effect of ischemic preconditioning. Br J Pharmacol 1998; 123:413–420.
63. Linz W, Scholkens BA. A specific B_2-bradykinin receptor antagonist HOE 140 abolishes the antihypertrophic effect of ramipril. Br J Pharmacol 1992; 105:771–772.
64. Jalowy A, Rainer S, Hilmar D, Behrends MHG, Facc F. Infarct size reduction by AT1-receptor blockade through a signal cascade of AT2-receptor activation, bradykinin and prostaglandins in pigs. J Am Coll Cardiol 1998; 32:1787–1796.

44

The Treatment of Neuropathic Pain

Anticonvulsants, Antidepressants, Na Channel Blockers, NMDA Receptor Blockers, and Capsaicin

David Bowsher
Pain Research Institute, Liverpool, England

I. INTRODUCTION AND HISTORY

Neuropathic pains have been described piecemeal: Only recently has it been recognized that they all possess certain common features that distinguish them from nociceptive pains. Chief among these is that they are not elicited by nociceptor stimulation, from which it follows that their transmission brainward does not employ the same synapses and pathways as nociceptive pains elicited by nociceptor stimulation, with all the pharmacological implications that this carries. Most neuropathic–type pains reveal a partial sensory deficit, particularly for nonnoxious temperature and sharpness, in the painful area; and when true allodynia (pain elicited by a discrete nonnoxious stimulus) occurs, it is pathognomonic of neuropathic pain. Trigeminal neuralgia (tic douloureux) is the odd man out among neuropathic pains in that there is no overt sensory deficit, although one can be detected instrumentally (1,2), and allodynia is the main if not only feature of which the patient complains. Long periods of remission are also not a feature of other neuropathic pain conditions. Other neuropathic pains encompass conditions as diverse as central poststroke pain (''thalamic syndrome''), syringomyelia, postherpetic neuralgia (PHN), painful diabetic neuropathy, and (posttraumatic) complex regional pain syndromes. Also, there are many mixed nociceptive–neuropathic pains, not only in malignant disease, but also in conditions such as herniated intervertebral disk and postamputation (phantom) limb pain.

In 1853, Trousseau (3) described trigeminal neuralgia as being ''epileptiform.'' The first reports of anticonvulsant therapy (phenytoin) were published 90 years later by Bergouignan (4). In 1962, Blom (5) introduced carbamazepine for the treatment of trigeminal neuralgia, and this has remained the standard therapy ever since. It must, however, be recognized that the vast majority of trigeminal neuralgia patients so treated eventually escape from drug control and require interventional treatment, of which microvascular decompression appears to be the treatment of choice (6,7), apparently because a mechanical factor (compression of the juxtapontine root by a blood vessel) appears to be responsible in almost all cases (8). Long-term carbamazepine therapy for trigeminal neuralgia produces some degree of cognitive impairment in virtually all patients, and other side effects in many. This has led to trials of other anticonvulsants, such as baclofen (9), a γ-aminobutyric acid ($GABA_B$) agonist, and lamotrigine (10), an atypical sodium channel blocker, with antiglutamate activity (11), with some degree of success.

Because trigeminal neuralgia was the first form of neuropathic pain for which a virtually specific treatment was discovered, an unfortunate tendency was established (and still persists) to treat any neuropathic pain (but particularly if its designation includes the word "neuralgia") with carbamazepine. Trigeminal (and glossopharyngeal) neuralgia is unique in that its leading feature is allodynia, whereas ongoing background pain is either absent or of little import in comparison with triggered shooting pains (allodynia). Kugelberg and Lindblom (12) showed that tactile allodynia in trigeminal neuralgia is subserved by Aβ-primary afferents, whereas Nurmikko et al. (13) were able to demonstrate that tactile allodynia in postherpetic neuralgia is due to activity evoked in rapidly adapting (dynamic) low-threshold (Aβ) mechanoreceptors. The implication of GABAergic mechanisms has been experimentally demonstrated (14). Although allodynia is present in 100% of cases of trigeminal neuralgia, it is exhibited by more than 90% of patients with PHN. Most patients with complex regional pain syndromes (causalgia and reflex sympathetic dystrophy) and about half of patients with central poststroke pain (CPSP), formerly known as "thalamic syndrome," and spinal cord damage (syringomyelia and spinal cord injury) have allodynia, but it is relatively uncommon in painful diabetic neuropathy, one of the most frequently occurring neuropathic pain conditions.

In all forms of neuropathic pain, except most cases of trigeminal neuralgia, there is a background pain, often burning or burning/freezing in nature, which can be pathophysiologically differentiated from allodynia in animals (15) and humans (16). Similar to allodynia, this pain is abolished by local anesthesia, but returns as soon as Aβ-function returns and before Aδ- and C-function return (13). It has been observed, particularly in CPSP (17), but also in PHN, that in many instances there is no pain when the patient is perfectly immobile. Thus neuropathic pain may be attributed to a changed central state ("sensitization"; 18) in which pain is maintained or triggered by low-intensity peripheral input, perhaps altered (19). However, peripheral neurectomy or neurotomy, although it may abolish allodynia, frequently produces anesthesia dolorosa, a severe neuropathic pain that is frequently worse than the pain for which the lesion was carried out. Anesthesia dolorosa can also be produced by section of the central nociceptive pathway, the anterolateral white funiculus of the spinal cord.

A further observation, which has some bearing on treatment, should be recorded. This is that most subjects who acquire shingles, or who undergo cerebral infarction involving the ventroposterior thalamic nucleus, or who have diabetic neuropathy, do not suffer from neuropathic pain. Moreover, some patients with neuropathic pain undergo spontaneous recovery. These observations suggest that the development of pain may depend on the level, or concentration, of certain receptors within the central nervous system (CNS) (20). What these receptors are, or might be, is still unknown, but subtypes of noradrenaline (norepinephrine), GABA, glutamate, *N*-methyl-D-aspartate (NMDA), and adenosine receptors, all have been implicated [see Canavero and Bonicalzi (21) for the role of GABA and glutamate in central pain].

Finally, the dynamic nature of the pathophysiology is illustrated by the response to treatment. Both PHN (22,23) and CPSP (24) respond to a far greater extent if treated early with antidepressants than if treatment is initiated at a later stage.

II. TREATMENT OF NEUROPATHIC PAIN

A. Anticonvulsants

The use of anticonvulsants, particularly carbamazepine (an atypical tricyclic), for the treatment of trigeminal neuralgia has already been mentioned. There has been a tendency to use anticonvulsants, particularly carbamazepine or valproate (valproic acid) (25) in other neuropathic conditions, especially when the shooting or stabbing pains of allodynia are a prominent feature. There is unhappily little objective evidence that any positive result has been achieved by their use. Thus, Leijon and Boivie (26), in a double-blind, crossover, placebo-controlled trial of 15 patients with CPSP found that although 5 patients reported some pain relief with carbamazepine, the effect did not reach statistical significance in comparison with placebo. A systematic review (27) confirmed these effects on CPSP, and interestingly found that anticonvulsants had some effectiveness (number needed to treat = 2.5) in diabetic neuropathy, in which allodynia is rare; there appeared to be no significant effect in postherpetic neuralgia, in agreement with Bowsher (28).

The atypical anticonvulsant lamotrigine—its use in trigeminal neuralgia is referred to in the foregoing—has also been reported to have been successfully used in cases of central pain (29).

Many communications at the Eighth World Congress on Pain (1996), and some subsequent publications, reported the apparent success of another anticonvulsant, gabapentin in various neuropathic pains (30). There is a published report on its use in reflex sympathetic dystrophy (31); and very recently, a multicenter trial (32,33) has confirmed that gabapentin is superior to placebo in the treatment of painful diabetic neuropathy and postherpetic neuralgia (97). Unfortunately, it has not yet been tested against amitriptyline (see Sec. II.B), compared with which it is expected to have fewer side effects. Another GABA analogue, vigabatrin, in open trials has had little effect, thus stressing the differential importance of receptor subtypes. The benzodiazepine antidepressant lorazepam, which depresses activity in the reticular formation as well as having a GABAergic effect, is not effective in the treatment of neuropathic pain (34).

B. Antidepressants

The first recorded use of a tricyclic antidepressant (amitriptyline) for neuropathic pain (postherpetic neuralgia) was by Woodforde et al. in 1965 (35), in the belief that depression formed a major part of the illness. Demonstration of true therapeutic effect independent of depression was achieved in a double-blind, placebo-controlled, crossover trial (36). Other effective tricyclic [nortriptyline, desipramine (37)] and tetracyclic antidepressants [maprotiline (38)], similar to amitriptyline, are reuptake inhibitors of either norepinephrine and serotonin (5-HT), or principally of norepinephrine only; their effectiveness in the treatment of postherpetic neuralgia has been reviewed (39). Ardid and Guilbaud (40) were able to demonstrate, in an animal model of mononeuropathy, that the adrenergic action of these compounds is the effective component of their therapeutic action. Their effectiveness in central neuropathic pain has also been objectively demonstrated (24,26).

Imipramine, which is also a combined tricyclic norepinephrine and 5-HT reuptake inhibitor, has long been the most commonly used drug for the treatment of painful diabetic neuropathy (41). However, most clinicians concur that amitriptyline and drugs with a very similar pharmacological profile are the most effective in the treatment of neuropathic pain (42), including diabetic neuropathy (43). The dose of oral amitriptyline and related drugs usually prescribed for neuropathic pain rises gradually to 75 mg/day (50 mg in the elderly or infirm), and rises above this only if inadequate beneficial effects are seen at full dose (44), if 75 mg is ineffective. These doses are lower than those used in the treatment of depression. Nevertheless, they frequently produce undesirable side effects, sometimes necessitating the abandonment of treatment (e.g., 5 out of 37 in a recent publication) (43); how many patients fail to comply fully with antidepressant treatment because of side effects is unknown, but the proportion is undoubtedly high. Dry mouth is the most common side effect, and can be alleviated by the concomitant use of artificial saliva or chewing gum (45). Nevertheless, a metanalysis concludes that "antidepressants are effective in relieving neuropathic pain" (46).

That early treatment with antidepressants is more effective than late, logically led to a trial of preemptive treatment of elderly patients with acute shingles (not PHN, defined as a neuropathic pain persisting or recurring at the site of acute shingles 3 months or more after rash appearance) with low-dose amitriptyline. The probability of pain still being present 6 months after acute shingles compared with a placebo-treated group was 0.015 (47). Although this is of obvious value to an at-risk group (50% of patients with shingles at age 60 and 75% at age 70 develop PHN) (48), it is more difficult to assess risk in other groups. However, a high proportion of diabetics develop painful neuropathy (49), and might perhaps benefit from preemptive treatment if risk factors can be more closely identified.

Although they have fewer undesirable side effects and, therefore, are much used in the treatment of depression, the more recently developed specific serotonin-reuptake inhibitors (SSRIs) seem to have little effect on neuropathic diabetic pain (fluoxetine; 50) in comparison with tricyclics, although a single report suggests that paroxetine has some effect on the pain of diabetic neuropathy (51).

There are as yet no published controlled trials of the even newer specific adrenergic-reuptake inhibitors (reboxetine and viloxazine); but they are eagerly awaited.

There is one published report (28) and considerable anecdotal evidence that the addition of the sympathomimetic dextroamphetamine (5 mg b.i.d.), which stimulates both α- and β-adrenoceptors, to an adrenergically active antidepressant enhances the activity of the latter, and may produce an effect when an antidepressant alone has failed to do so.

C. Sodium Channel Blockers

This class of drug was developed for its antiarrhythmic properties; but it also has an effect on nerve conduction. This was the rationale for the introduction of flecainide and tocainide (52) for the treatment of trigeminal neuralgia. These drugs were also tried in other forms of neuropathic pain. They were, however, soon abandoned because of their high toxicity. Mexiletine was introduced for the treatment of diabetic neuropathy (53), and has subsequently been validated (54). It has also been used successfully to treat painful traumatic mononeuropathy (55) and, experimentally, it has relieved allodynia-like symptoms in rats (56). It has proved particularly useful as an adjunct to amitriptyline in the treatment of recalcitrant CPSP (24). In my own experience, it is more effective when started at a high dose (400 mg, followed by 200 mg every 6-h by mouth) to monitored hospitalized patients than when it is given in increasing doses to ambulant patients. Its effects in PHN have been considerably less marked.

Lidocaine (lignocaine) is a local anesthetic that blocks sodium channels. Boas et al. (57) reported its analgesic effect when given systemically (i.v.) in conditions with neuropathic pain. Its duration of action is short, but it frequently alleviates the pain to a considerable extent, and it has been stated that intravenous infusions at intervals may have a long-term effect on some neuropathic pains. Wallace et al. (58) showed that a plasma lidocaine concentration of 1.5 μg/mL, or more, induced significant alleviation of pain in peripheral neuropathy following intravenous infusion. Five percent lidocaine has recently been reintroduced in the form of patches (59) for the treatment of PHN; blood level measurements of 0.1 μg/mL indicated that there was no significant systemic absorption, suggesting a purely local effect. The most recent observations on 32 patients (98) show a highly significant therapeutic effect.

D. *N*-Methyl-D-Aspartate Receptor Antagonists

As stated in the introduction, neuropathic pain involves an element of central sensitization, and NMDA receptor-mediated processes have been shown to be concerned in such sensitization (60).

Experimental work (61) suggests that lidocaine acts to block NMDA-mediated transmission in the spinal cord in addition to its local anesthetic action. Two NMDA receptor antagonists are available to clinicians; one of them, dextromethorphan (62) has rather low NMDA receptor antagonist activity. The other substance, the general anesthetic ketamine, has much more pronounced activity, and it has been successfully used to alleviate various neuropathic pain syndromes (63–65), including PHN (66) and phantom limb pain (68). In accordance with the dynamic pathophysiological nature of neuropathic pain, ketamine is less effective in long-standing neuropathic pain and more effective in such pain of shorter duration (69). Unwanted side effects have been troublesome with this drug, and great efforts are being made to find an NMDA receptor antagonist with fewer side effects; meanwhile, the use of oral ketamine (70) and improvements in infusion techniques (71) are to some extent allaying the problem; Takahashi et al. (72) have obtained successful long-term pain relief following low-dose (25 $\mu g/kg\ h^{-1}$) epidural infusion for 10 days.

The opioid drug methadone, unlike other opioids, is an NMDA receptor antagonist (73,74), and also functions as a norepinephrine-reuptake inhibitor (75). It has been successfully used in neuropathic pains occurring in cancer patients (76–78). Clinical experience of this drug in nonmalignant neuropathic pain has yet to be published; it seems likely to be promising.

Very recently, another NMDA receptor antagonist, amantadine, has been successfully used in a single intravenous bolus dose in three cases of neuropathic pain of peripheral origin (79,80).

E. Adenosine

A naturally occurring substance that has antiarrhythmic activity because it blocks Ca^{2+} channels is adenosine. It also inhibits neurally mediated norepinephrine release. Adenosine receptors are found in the substantia gelatinosa (81). Its duration of action is measured in seconds because it is very rapidly eliminated. Intramuscular injection of adenosine monophosphate (AMP) has been reported to prevent PHN in 17 out of 32 patients with acute herpes zoster (82). Relief of neuropathic pain has been reported following continuous intravenous infusion of adenosine (83). Intrathecal adenosine (500 or 1000 μg) has recently been shown to reduce neuropathic pain and allodynia for a median of 24 hours after injection in 12 of 14 patients (84). Adenosine has been recently reviewed by Sollevi (85). There may be some future for an artificial adenosine receptor agonist.

F. Topical Agents

Since it has long been known that painful peripheral neuropathies cease to be painful following local anesthesia (for as long as large fibers remain inactivated), it is not surprising that in earlier times much therapeutic effort was directed at the painful peripheral locus. Mention has already been made of lidocaine patches (59,60). Even in recent years, in addition to local anesthetic creams (86,87), attention has been given to aspirin-in-chloroform lotion (88), topical NSAIDs, and vinca alkaloids (89), as well as to herbal remedies, such as *Hypericum* extract (possibly the most promising). Topical NSAIDs have been ineffective (90), as has aspirin-in-chloroform (91).

However, neuropathic pain depends on an altered central state as well as peripheral input, so it is not surprising that most topical "remedies," with the possible exception of lidocaine patches, have turned out to be "flashes in the pan." One topical application, however—capsaicin—deserves more serious consideration.

Capsaicin acts on nonmyelinated peripheral afferent fibers to deplete substance P (92) and other transmitter peptides; the net effect of this is first to stimulate and then to destroy C fibers

(93). On the (probably erroneous) assumption that the pain of peripheral neuropathies is due to activation of primary afferent C fibers, topical capsaicin was introduced as a therapy. A degree of success has been claimed. However, a review of trials (94) suggests that relief is obtained by one in four patients with painful diabetic neuropathy (95), but that there is no significant benefit in postherpetic neuralgia or painful distal polyneuropathy (96). Many patients abandoned trials because of the severe initial burning induced by capsaicin.

When used for pain arising from skin (97) or subcutaneous soft tissues, the action of capsaicin is very rapid, some alleviation usually being seen within 48 h. By contrast, when it is effective in neuropathic pain, it is usually 6–8 weeks before any significant effect is seen. This leads one to speculate on the possibility that the capsaicin effect in such cases is not due to primary afferent C-fiber inactivation, but to transsynaptic effects within the spinal dorsal horn. Be that as it may, topical capsaicin has a place in the treatment of refractory PHN because it is sometimes effective in long-standing cases in whom systemic medication has produced no benefit.

III. CONCLUSION

There is usually no difficulty in diagnosing trigeminal neuralgia, which should be treated with anticonvulsants in the first instance (with careful monitoring of side effects, particularly cognitive impairment), and subsequently passed on for interventional treatment, probably microvascular decompression.

The clinician should be able to diagnose other forms of neuropathic pain because of the differential sensory deficit (distinguishable with a warm finger and a cold spoon) and by allodynia (to be distinguished from hyperpathia) if present. Whether central or "peripheral," the first line of treatment probably should still be amitriptyline or a related tricyclic (the action of which is greatly enhanced in the case of PHN by antiviral treatment of herpes zoster (98)). Failure to respond indicates additional adrenergic or Na channel blocking (mexiletine) therapy in the first instance, followed by trials of drugs acting on GABA (gabapentin) systems—drugs such as gabapentin, now known not to act on GABA receptors but on a subunit of voltage-sensitive Ca2+ channels (99)—and NMDA receptors (ketamine, ?methadone). Topical lidocaine patches can be useful in peripheral neuropathies, and in the case of long-standing recalcitrant PHN, topical capsaicin may sometimes be helpful.

REFERENCES

1. Nurmikko TJ. Altered cutaneous sensation in trigeminal neuralgia. Arch Neurol 1991; 48:523–527.
2. Bowsher D, Miles J, Haggett C, Eldridge P. Trigeminal neuralgia: a quantitative sensory perception threshold study in patients who had had no previous invasive procedures. J Neurosurg 1997; 86: 190–192.
3. Trousseau A. De la névralgie épileptiforme. Arch Gén Méd 1853; 57:33–44.
4. Bergouignan M. Cures heureuses de névralgies faciales essentielles par le diphenyl-hydantoinate de soude. Rev Laryngol Otol Rhinol 1942; 63:34–41.
5. Blom S. Trigeminal neuralgia. Its treatment with a new anticonvulsant drug (G32883). Lancet 1962; 1:839–840.
6. Janetta PJ. Microsurgical approach to the trigeminal nerve for tic douloureux. Prog Neurol Surg 1976; 7:180–200.
7. Barker FG, Janetta PJ, Bissonette DJ, et al. The long-term outcome of microvascular decompression for trigeminal neuralgia. N Engl J Med 1996; 334:1077–1083.

8. Meaney JFM, Miles JB, Nixon TE, et al. Vascular contact with the fifth cranial nerve at the pons in patients with trigeminal neuralgia: detection with 3D FISP imaging. AJR Am J Roentgenol 1994; 163:1447–1452.
9. Fromm GH, Terrence CF, Chattha AS. Baclofen in the treatment of trigeminal neuralgia: double-blind study and long-term follow-up. Ann Neurol 1984; 15:240–244.
10. Zakrzewska JM, Chaudry Z, Nurmikko TJ, Patton DW, Mullens EL. Lamotrigine (Lamictal) in refractory trigeminal neuralgia: results from a double-blind placebo controlled crossover trial. Pain 1997; 73:223–230.
11. Leach MJ, Lees G, Riddall DR. Lamotrigine: mechanisms of action. In: Levy RH, Mattson RH, Meldrum BS, eds. Antiepileptic Drugs. 4th ed. New York: Raven Press, 1995:861–869.
12. Kugelberg E, Lindblom U. The mechanism of the pain in trigeminal neuralgia. J Neurol Neurosurg Psychiatry 1959; 22:36–43.
13. Nurmikko T, Wells C, Bowsher D. Pain and allodynia in postherpetic neuralgia: role of somatic and sympathetic systems. Acta Neurol Scand 1991; 84:146–152.
14. Cui J–G, Linderoth B, Meyerson BA. Effects of spinal cord stimulation on touch-evoked allodynia involve GABA-ergic mechanisms. An experimental study in the mononeuropathic rat. Pain 1996; 66:287–296.
15. Jett M–F, McGuirk J, Waligora D, Hunter JC. The effects of mexiletine, desipramine and fluoxetine in rat models involving central sensitisation. Pain 1997; 69:161–169.
16. Mailis A, Amani N, Umana M, Basur R, Roe S. Effect of intravenous sodium amytal on cutaneous sensory abnormalities, spontaneous pain, and algometric pain pressure thresholds in neuropathic pain patients: a placebo-controlled study. II. Pain 1997; 70:69–82.
17. Bowsher D. Central pain: clinical and physiological characteristics. J Neurol Neurosurg Psychiatry 1996; 61:62–69.
18. Woolf CJ. Evidence for a central component of post-injury pain hypersensitivity. Nature 1983; 306: 686–688.
19. Baron R, Haendler G, Schulte H. Afferent large fiber polyneuropathy predicts the development of postherpetic neuralgia. Pain 1997; 73:231–238.
20. Bowsher D. Central pain. Pain Rev 1995; 2:175–186.
21. Canavero S, Bonicalzi V. The neurochemistry of central pain: evidence from clinical studies, hypothesis, and therapeutic implications. Pain 1998; 74:109–114.
22. Bhala BB, Ramamoorthy C, Bowsher D, Yelnoorker KN. Shingles and postherpetic neuralgia. Clin J Pain 1988; 4:169–174.
23. Bowsher D. Acute shingles and postherpetic neuralgia: effects of acyclovir and outcome of treatment with amitriptyline. Br J Gen Prac 1992; 42:244–246.
24. Bowsher D. The management of central post-stroke pain. Postgrad Med J 1995; 71:598–604.
25. Raftery H. The management of postherpetic pain using sodium valproate and amitriptyline. Irish Med J 1975; 72:399–401.
26. Leijon G, Boivie J. Central post-stroke pain—a controlled trial of amitriptyline and carbamazepine. Pain 1989; 36:27–36.
27. McQuay H, Carroll D, Jadad AR, Wiffen P, Moore A. Anticonvulsant drugs for the management of pain: a systematic review. Br Med J 1995; 31:1047–1052.
28. Bowsher D. Postherpetic neuralgia and its treatment: a retrospective survey of 191 patients. J Pain Sympt Manage 1996; 12:290–299.
29. Canavero S, Bonicalzi V. Lamotrigine control of central pain. Pain 1996; 68:179–181.
30. Rosner H, Rubin L, Kestenbaum A. Gabapentin adjunctive therapy in neuropathic pain states. Clin J Pain 1996; 12:56–58.
31. Mellick GA, Mellick LB. Reflex sympathetic dystrophy treated with gabapentin. Arch Phys Med Rehabil 1997; 78:98–105.
32. Backjona M, Hes MS, LaMoreaux LK, Graofalo EA, Koto EM, US Study Group 210. Gabapentin (GBP, Neurontin) reduces pain in diabetics with painful peripheral neuropathy: results of a double-blind, placebo-controlled trial (945–210) [Abstract]. American Pain Society Meeting, New Orleans, Oct 1997.

33. Backonja M, Beydoun A, Edwards KR, Schwartz SL, Fonseca V, Hes M, LaMoreaux L, Garofalo E. Gabapentin for the symptomatic treatment of painful neuropathy in patients with diabetes mellitus: a randomized controlled trial. JAMA 1998; 280:1831–1836.
33a. Rowbotham M, Harden N, Stacey B, Bernstein P, Magnus-Miller L, for the Gabapentin Postherpetic Neuralgia Study Group. Gabapentin for the treatment of postherpetic neuralgia: a randomized controlled trial. JAMA 1998; 280:1837–1842.
34. Max MB, Schafer SC, Culnane M, Smoller B, Dubner R, Gracely RH. Amitriptyline but not lorazepam relieves postherpetic neuralgia. Neurology 1988; 38:1427–1432.
35. Woodforde JM, Dwyer B, McEwen BW, et al. The treatment of postherpetic neuralgia. Med J Aust 1965; 2:869–872.
36. Watson CP, Evans RJ, Reed K, Merskey H, Goldsmith L, Warsh J. Amitriptyline versus placebo in postherpetic neuralgia. Neurology 1982; 32:671–673.
37. Kishore-Kumar R, Max MB, Schafer SC, Gaughan AM, Smoller B, Gracely RH, Dubner R. Desipramine relieves postherpetic neuralgia. Clin Pharmacol Ther 1990; 47:305–312.
38. Watson CPN, Chipman M, Reed K, Evans RJ, Birkett N. Amitriptyline versus maprotiline in postherpetic neuralgia: a randomized double-blind crossover trial. Pain 1992; 48:29–36.
39. Max MB. Treatment of post-herpetic neuralgia: antidepressants. Ann Neurol 1994; 35:50–53.
40. Ardid D, Guilbaud G. Antinociceptive effects of acute and "chronic" injections of tricyclic antidepressant drugs in a new model of mononeuropathy in rats. Pain 1992; 49:279–287.
41. Kvinesdal B, Molin J, Fröland A, Gram LF. Imipramine treatment of painful diabetic neuropathy. JAMA 1984; 251:1727–1730.
42. Richeimer SH, Bajwa ZH, Kahraman SS, Ransil BJ, Warfield CA. Utilization patterns of tricyclic antidepressants in a multidisciplinary pain clinic: a survey. Clin J Pain 1997; 13:324–329.
43. Vrethem M, Boivie J, Arnqvist H, Holmgren H, Lindström T, Thorell LH. A comparison of amitriptyline and maprotiline in the treatment of polyneuropathy in diabetics and non-diabetics. Clin J Pain 1997; 13:313–323.
44. Bowsher D. The management of postherpetic neuralgia. Postgrad Med J 1997; 73:623–629.
45. Bowsher D. Post-herpetic neuralgia in older patients. Incidence and optimal treatment. Drugs Aging 1994; 5:411–418.
46. McQuay HJ, Tramèr M, Nye BA, Carroll D, Wiffen PJ, Moore RA. A systematic review of antidepressants in neuropathic pain. Pain 1996; 68:217–227.
47. Bowsher D. The effects of pre-emptive treatment of postherpetic neuralgia with amitriptyline: a randomized double-blind placebo-controlled trial. J Pain Sympt Manage 1997; 13:327–331.
48. DeMoragas JM, Kierland RR. The outcome of patients with herpes zoster. Arch Dermatol 1957; 75: 193–196.
49. Benbow SJ, Cossins L, MacFarlane IA. Painful diabetic neuropathy. Diabetic Med 1999; 16:632–644.
50. Max M, Lynch SA, Muir J, et al. Effects of desipramine, amitriptyline, and fluoxetine on pain in diabetic neuropathy. N Engl J Med 1992; 326:1250–1256.
51. Sindrup SH, Gram LF, Brosen K, Eshøj O, Mogensen EF. The selective serotonin reuptake inhibitor paroxetine is effective in the treatment of diabetic neuropathy symptoms. Pain 1990; 42:135–144.
52. Lindstrom P, Lindblom U. The analgesic effect of tocainide in trigeminal neuralgia. Pain 1987; 28: 45–50.
53. Dejgard A, Petersen P, Kastrup J. Mexiletine for treatment of chronic painful diabetic neuropathy. Lancet 1988; 1:9–11.
54. Oskarsson P, Ljunggren JG, Lins PE. Efficacy and safety of mexiletine in the treatment of painful diabetic neuropathy. The Mexiletine Study Group. Diabetes Care 1997; 20:1594–1597.
55. Chabal C, Jacobson L, Mariano A, Chaney E, Britell CW. The use of oral mexiletine for the treatment of pain after peripheral nerve injury. Anesthesiology 1992; 76:513–517.
56. Xu X–J, Hao J–X, Seiger A, Staffan A, Lindblom U, Wiesenfeld–Hallin Z. Systemic mexiletine relieves chronic allodynia-like symptoms in rats with ischemic spinal cord injury. Anesth Analg 1992; 74:649–652.

57. Boas RA, Covino BG, Shanharian A. Analgesic response to i.v. lignocaine. Br J Anaesth 1982; 54: 501–505.
58. Wallace MS, Dyck JB, Rossi SS, Yaksh TL. Computer-controlled lidocaine infusion for the evaluation of neuropathic pain after peripheral nerve injury. Pain 1996; 66:69–77.
59. Rowbotham MC, Davies PS, Verkempinck C, Galer BS. Lidocaine patch: a double-blind controlled study of a new treatment method for post-herpetic neuralgia. Pain 1996; 65:39–44.
60. Galer BS, Rowbotham MC, Perander J, Friedman E. Topical lidocaine patch relieves postherpetic neuralgia more effectively than a vehicle topical patch: results of an enriched enrollment study. Pain 1999; 80:533–538.
61. Woolf CJ, Thompson SW. The induction and maintenance of central sensitization is dependent on *N*-methyl-D-aspartic acid receptor activation: implications for the treatment of post-injury pain hypersensitivity states. Pain 1991; 44:293–299.
62. Nagy I, Woolf CJ. Lignocaine selectively reduces C fibre-evoked neuronal activity in rat spinal cord in vitro by decreasing *N*-methyl-D-aspartate and neurokinin receptor-mediated post-synaptic depolarizations; implications for the development of novel centrally acting analgesics. Pain 1996; 64:59–70.
63. Price DD, Mao J, Frenk H, Mayer DJ. The *N*-methyl-D-aspartate receptor antagonist dextromethorphan selectively reduces temporal summation of second pain in man. Pain 1994; 59:165–174.
64. Backjona M, Arndt G, Gombar KA, Check B, Zimmermann M. Response of chronic neuropathic pain syndromes to ketamine: a preliminary study. Pain 1994; 56:51–57.
65. Felsby S, Nielsen J, Arendt–Nielsen L, Jensen TS. NMDA receptor blockade in chronic neuropathic pain: a comparison of ketamine and magnesium chloride. Pain 1995; 64:283–291.
66. Max MB, Byas–Smith MG, Gracely RH, Bennett GJ. Intravenous infusion of the NMDA antagonist, ketamine, in chronic posttraumatic pain with allodynia: a double-blind comparison to alfentanil and placebo. Clin Neuropharmacol 1995; 18:360–368.
67. Eide PK, Jørum E, Stubhaug A, Bremnes J, Breivik H. Relief of post-herpetic neuralgia with the *N*-methyl-D-aspartic acid receptor antagonist ketamine: a double-blind, cross-over comparison with morphine and placebo. Pain 1994; 58:347–354.
68. Stannard CF, Porter GE. Ketamine hydrochloride in the treatment of phantom limb pain. Pain 1993; 54:227–230.
69. Mathisen LC, Skjelbred P, Skoglund LA, Øye I. Effect of ketamine, an NMDA receptor inhibitor, in acute and chronic orofacial pain. Pain 1995; 61:215–220.
70. Luczak J, Dickenson AH, Kotlinska–Lemieszek A. The role of ketamine, an NMDA receptor antagonist, in the management of pain. Progr Palliat Care 1995; 3:127–134.
71. Eide PK, Stubhaug A, Øye I, Breivik H. Continuous subcutaneous administration of the *N*-methyl-D-aspartic acid (NMDA) receptor antagonist ketamine in the treatment of post-herpetic neuralgia. Pain 1995; 61:221–228.
72. Takahashi H, Miyazaki M, Nanbu T, Yanagida H, Morita S. The NMDA-receptor antagonist ketamine abolishes neuropathic pain after epidural administration in a clinical case. Pain 1998; 75:391–394.
73. Ebert B, Andersen S, Krosgaard–Larsen P. Ketobemidone, methadone and pethidine are non-competitive *N*-methyl D-aspartate (NMDA) antagonists in the rat cortex and spinal cord. Neurosci Lett 1995; 187:165–168.
74. Gorman Al, Elliott KJ, Inturrisi CE. The D- and L-isomers of methadone bind to the non-competitive site on the NMDA receptor in rat forebrain and spinal cord. Neurosci Lett 1997; 223:5–8.
75. Codd EE, Shank RP, Schupsky JJ, Raffa RB. Serotonin and norepinephrine uptake inhibiting activity of centrally acting analgesics: structural determinants and role in antinociception. J Pharmacol Exp Ther 1995; 274:1263–1270.
76. Morley JS, Makin MK. Comments on Ripamonti et al. Pain 1997; 70:109–115. Pain 1997; 73:114 [Letter].
77. Morley JS, Makin MK. The use of methadone in cancer pain poorly responsive to other opioids. Pain Rev 1998; 5:51–58.
78. Makin MK, O'Donnell V, Skinner JM, Ellershaw JE. Methadone in the management of cancer related neuropathic pain. Pain Clin 1998; 10:275–279.

79. Eisenberg E, Pud D. Can patients with chronic neuropathic pain be cured by acute administration of the NMDA receptor antagonist amantadine? Pain 1998; 74:337–340.
80. Pud D, Eisenberg E, Spitzer A, Adler R, Fried G, Yarnitsky D. The NMDA receptor antagonist amantadine reduces surgical neuropathic pain in cancer patients: a double-blind, randomized, placebo controlled trial. Pain 1998; 75:349–354.
81. Choca JL, Green RD, Proudfit HK. Adenosine A_1 and A_2 receptors in the substantia gelatinosa are located predominantly on intrinsic neurones: an autoradiographic study. J Pharmacol Exp Ther 1988; 247:757–764.
82. Sklar SH, Blue WT, Alexander EJ, et al. Herpes zoster, the treatment and prevention of neuralgia by adenosine monophosphate. JAMA 1985; 253:1427–1430.
83. Sollevi A, Belfrage M, Lundeberg T, Segerdahl M, Hansson P. Systemic adenosine infusion: a new treatment modality to alleviate neuropathic pain. Pain 1995; 61:155–158.
84. Belfrage M, Segerdahl M, Arner S, Sollevi A. The safety and efficacy of intrathecal adenosine in patients with chronic neuropathic pain. Anesth Analg 1999; 89:136–142.
85. Sollevi A. Adenosine for pain control. Acta Anaesthesiol Scand Suppl 1997; 110:135–136.
86. Rowbotham MC, Fields HL. Topical lidocaine reduces pain in post-herpetic neuralgia. Pain 1989; 38:297–301.
87. Collins PD. EMLA cream and herpetic neuralgia. Med J Aust 1991; 155:206–207.
88. King RB. Concerning the management of pain associated with herpes zoster and of postherpetic neuralgia. Pain 1988; 33:73–78.
89. Csillik B, Knyihar–Csillik E, Szucs A. Treatment of chronic pain syndromes with iontophoresis of vinca alkaloids to the skin of patients. Neuroscience 1982; 31:87–90.
90. McQuay H, Carroll D, Moxon A, Glynn CJ, Moore RA. Benzydamine cream for the treatment of post-herpetic neuralgia: minimum duration of treatment periods in a crossover trial. Pain 1990; 40: 131–135.
91. Bowsher D, Gill H. Aspirin-in-chloroform for the topical treatment of postherpetic neuralgia: a double-blind trial. J Pain Soc 1991; 9:16–17.
92. Carpenter SE, Lynn B. Vascular and sensory responses human skin to mild injury after topical treatment with capsaicin. Br J Pharmacol 1981; 73:755–758.
93. Lynn B. Capsaicin: actions on nociceptive C-fibres and therapeutic potential. Pain 1990; 41:61–69.
94. McQuay H, Moore A. Capaicin. In: An Evidence-Based Resource for Pain Relief. Oxford: Oxford University Press, 1998:249–250.
95. Capsaicin Study Group. Treatment of painful diabetic neuropathy with topical capsaicin. A multicenter, double-blind, vehicle-controlled study. Arch Intern Med 1991; 151:2225–2229.
96. Low PA, Opfer–Gehrking, TL, Dyck PJ, Litchy WJ, O'Brien PC. Double-blind, placebo controlled study of the application of capsaicin cream in chronic distal painful polyneuropathy. Pain 1995; 62: 163–168.
97. Beydoun A, Dyke DBS, Morrow TJ, Casey KL. Topical capsaicin attenuates heat pain and Aδ fiber-mediated laser-evoked potentials. Pain 1996; 65:189–196.
98. Bowsher D. The effects of acyclovir therapy for herpes zoster on treatment outcome in postherpetic neuralgia: a randomised study. Eur J Pain 1994; 15:9–12.
99. Taylor CP, Gee NS, Sutz, Koesis JD, Welty DF, Brown JP, Dooley DJ, Boden P, Singh L. A summary of mechanistic hypotheses of gabapentin pharmacology. Epilepsy Res 1998; 29:233–249.

45

N-Methyl-D-Aspartate (NMDA) Receptors as a Target for Pain Therapy

Boris A. Chizh
Grünenthal GmbH Research Centre, Aachen, Germany

P. Max Headley
School of Medical Sciences, University of Bristol, Bristol, England

I. INTRODUCTION

With L-glutamate being the major excitatory neurotransmitter in the central nervous system (CNS), glutamate receptors have inescapably been the focus of interest as central targets for analgesia. The longer history and better understanding of the function and role of receptors for *N*-methyl-D-aspartate (NMDA) are explained by early discoveries of selective agonists and antagonists in pioneering studies by Watkins and colleagues (for review see Ref. 1). The initial expectations of a quick route for NMDA antagonists into the pain clinic were followed by a tide of disappointment resulting from a palette of specific side effects. In this chapter we describe some current approaches to the development of new analgesics based on recent advances in the understanding of the NMDA receptor complex. Given the very large literature on this topic, it has not been possible for us within the scope of this short review to embrace all aspects or to cite more than a small selection of the relevant references; reviews are cited where possible.

II. PROPERTIES OF NMDA RECEPTORS AND THEIR ROLE IN THE PATHOPHYSIOLOGY OF NOCICEPTION

NMDA receptors are a functionally and structurally defined class of glutamate receptor (Fig. 1). There is plentiful evidence for the involvement of these receptors in nociception and pain (2–5). Glutamate is present in primary nociceptive afferents and may be released, together with some neuropeptides, after peripheral noxious stimulation (6). Under normal physiological conditions, however, fast synaptic transmission in the dorsal horn of the spinal cord is mostly mediated by non-NMDA glutamate receptors (7,8); hence, NMDA receptors have a limited role in the short-duration physiological nociception that underlies daily experience of painful stimuli (9, 10). Several unique physiological properties of the NMDA receptor–channel complex mean that it is better suited for mediating longer term modulation and synaptic plasticity over a time-scale of seconds or more, rather than synaptic transmission over a time-scale of milliseconds

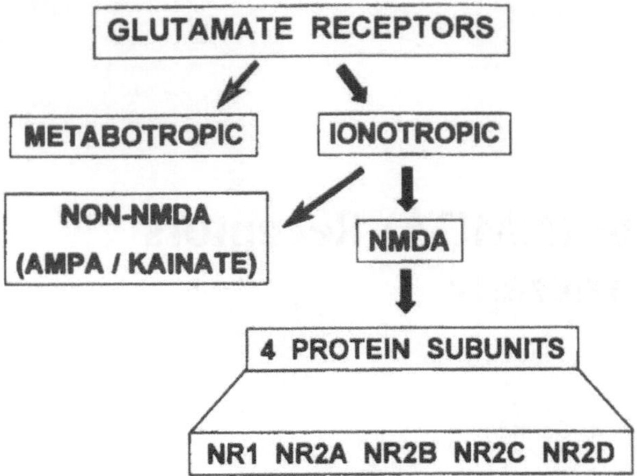

Figure 1 A classification of glutamate receptors: Glutamate can act on metabotropic receptors, which activate intracellular messenger systems, and on ionotropic receptors, which directly gate ion channels. These receptors are classified by glutamate analogues known as AMPA, kainate, and NMDA. NMDA receptors consist of four or five protein subunits. These ''heteromeric'' assemblies are made up of obligatory NR1 unit(s) and one (or two) types of the four currently recognized NR2 subunits (NR2A–2D). The different subunits are differentially distributed in the CNS and different combinations influence receptor properties (see text).

(Fig. 2). These properties include the relatively slow time course of channel openings, the high permeability of channels for calcium, the block of NMDA channels at resting membrane potentials by extracellular Mg^{2+}, with the result that the channels conduct appreciable current only when the membrane has been depolarized by other mechanisms (voltage dependence), and the presence of several modulatory sites on the receptor complex. For nociceptive transmission, NMDA receptor-mediated plasticity is thought to manifest itself initially as hyperalgesia and allodynia and, subsequently, as pain chronification.

The role of NMDA receptors in pain chronification mechanisms is often modeled by their role in the process of windup (4). Synchronous activation of unmyelinated afferent fibers results in the release of glutamate that causes subsynaptic depolarization sufficient to relieve the magnesium block of the resting NMDA receptor channel. With repeated stimulation, the slow NMDA receptor-mediated components of the depolarizations sum over a time scale of seconds, resulting in a progressive increase of the spiking response of dorsal horn neurons (11). NMDA antagonists can block this cumulative depolarization and windup in vitro (12, but see Ref. 13) and in vivo, both in experimental animals (14,15) and in humans (16). This process may follow tissue damage, inflammation, nerve injury, or other events known to trigger ongoing activity in nociceptors. Where prolonged, the NMDA receptor-mediated calcium influx into the postsynaptic cell may lead to a cascade of intracellular events, resulting in long-term pronociceptive plasticity.

Simple depolarization is not the only factor determining the NMDA receptor contribution to nociceptive processing. This follows from the observation that in the spinal cord in a postsurgical situation, NMDA receptors mediate low levels of tonic ongoing activity, but not the superimposed and much more vigorous phasic nociceptive responses (10) that must reflect greater membrane depolarization; this argues that, under these conditions, voltage-dependence is not a primary mechanism underlying NMDA receptor involvement in nociceptive processing. Two types of mechanism are plausible to explain this unexpected observation.

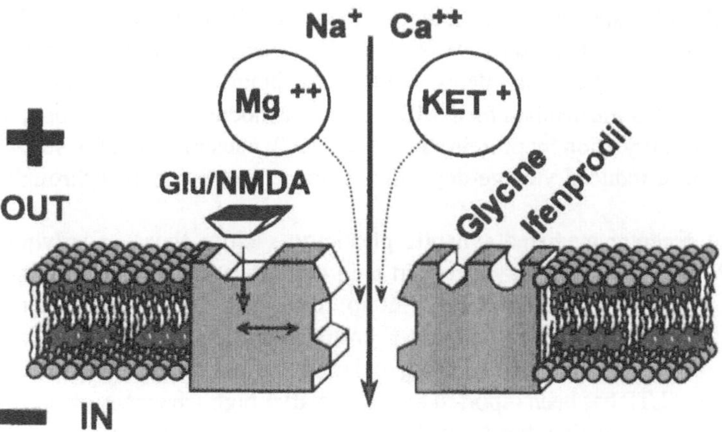

Figure 2 Simplified diagram of the NMDA receptor channel complex showing the sites discussed in this chapter. The strong voltage gradient across the membrane (equivalent to over 20,000 V/mm) drives positively charged ions into the channel, but only when it has been opened following binding of L-glutamate to its recognition site. Sodium ions carry most of the charge across the membrane and thereby mediate the transient depolarization that underlies excitatory synaptic events. A particular feature of the NMDA channel is its permeability to calcium, which can trigger longer-lasting intracellular biochemical events. Magnesium ions in the extracellular medium are also driven into the channel, but cannot penetrate; therefore, they block the channel. The degree of block depends on the voltage gradient driving the magnesium ions into the channel; this means that when the cell has been depolarized (as by activation of other glutamate receptors) the magnesium block will be relieved and more current will flow through NMDA channels. Dissociative anesthetics, such as ketamine, also block the channel, but unlike magnesium they bind in the channel for longer periods (variably between compounds), thereby blocking subsequent synaptic activation and acting as effective NMDA antagonists. Glycine is an obligatory "coagonist" at its recognition site (glycine$_B$) and prevents the very rapid desensitization that otherwise reduces effective channel function; antagonists at this site can therefore increase desensitization; thus, they form a functionally different group of NMDA antagonists. The ifenprodil-binding (polyamine) site is restricted to some subunit combinations (and thus some brain regions) and is another site at which NMDA antagonists can act. There are yet more sites on the NMDA complex that are not discussed in this chapter.

NMDA receptors, similar to other ionotropic glutamate receptors, are composed of several protein subunits (see Fig. 1) that can be assembled heteromerically in various combinations. The functional properties of native NMDA receptors, such as magnesium sensitivity and modulation by glycine or polyamines, are associated with different subunit composition of the heteromeric assemblies (17). Spinal cord neurons from immature rats possess NMDA receptors with low magnesium sensitivity and, as a result, low–voltage-dependence (18), properties evidently associated with the inclusion of NR2C or NR2D subunits. The mRNA for these subunits is present, together with NR1 subunit mRNA, in adult rat spinal cord (19). It is, therefore, likely that the spinal cord possesses NMDA receptors that show less–voltage-dependence than is generally expected, which may alter our views on how NMDA receptors are involved in nociception.

An alternative (but not mutually exclusive) mechanism involves neuropeptides, several of which modulate NMDA receptor-mediated synaptic events. The tachykinins, substance P and neurokinin A, are colocalized, and presumably coreleased, with glutamate from the terminals of nociceptive primary afferents (20), and they positively modulate NMDA receptor-mediated responses (21,22). Thyrotropin-releasing hormone (TRH) is another neuropeptide present in the spinal cord that can selectively facilitate NMDA receptor-mediated activity (23). Neuropeptide release that follows intense noxious stimulation (24) is, therefore, likely to enhance NMDA receptor-mediated activity under conditions of intense nociceptive inputs, such as following surgical trauma (10,25). A suggested mechanism for NMDA receptor modulation by neuropeptides is calcium-dependent phosphorylation by protein kinase C (PKC), causing a relief of magnesium block (26) and, in turn, a reduced voltage-dependence and enhanced current through the NMDA channel.

Other forms of NMDA receptor-mediated synaptic plasticity, such as those underlying long-term potentiation (LTP) (27), may also play a role in pain chronification. LTP is a long-lasting phenomenon (hours, as opposed to minutes for windup) associated with an increase in synaptic efficacy after high-frequency activation of input neurons. In the hippocampus, where LTP is best characterized, it is believed to underlie learning and memory formation. In the spinal cord, NMDA receptor-dependent LTP has been reported to develop after high-frequency primary afferent stimulation (28,29). The observation that NMDA antagonists block the process of LTP in the hippocampus and cerebral cortex provides a ready explanation for some of the side effects that many NMDA antagonists cause in humans. There are, however, various strategies that may result in the development of NMDA antagonists that differentiate between spinal cord and forebrain mechanisms (see later).

III. CLASSES OF NMDA ANTAGONISTS

There are several sites on the NMDA receptor complex at which NMDA antagonists can act. The most obvious is the NMDA recognition site itself (1,30). The disadvantage of targeting this site has been that the available antagonists are glutamate analogues that are polarized and, therefore, show poor CNS penetration (Table 1). Moreover, this has seemed a rather blunderbuss approach that would affect all NMDA receptor function and thereby cause unacceptable side effects. However, the precise recognition site is likely to vary with subunit composition, and since subunits are differentially distributed in the CNS (31), antagonists that could target receptors with particular subunit composition would have regionally limited sites of action, allowing specific functions to be targeted and limiting side effects. Such antagonists have yet to be developed.

Ketamine was already in clinical use as a dissociative anesthetic when it was found to act in vivo as an NMDA antagonist of moderate selectivity (30,32); low doses of ketamine are relatively selective at blocking NMDA receptors, whereas at higher doses this compound interacts with muscarinic, adrenergic, and dopaminergic mechanisms (33,34). Subsequently, its mechanism of action as an NMDA antagonist was determined to be by blocking the ion channel, a mechanism referred to as uncompetitive block. Other clinically available NMDA antagonists (dextromethorphan, memantine, and amantadine) and many other compounds act by this mechanism (see Table 1).

There has recently been much interest in two modulatory sites on the NMDA receptor complex. The best characterized is that for glycine (35) (see Fig. 2). Endogenous glycine limits desensitization of NMDA receptors; consequently, $glycine_B$ antagonists increase the rate of desensitization to glutamate, thus inhibiting NMDA receptor-mediated synaptic responses (see Sec. IV).

Another modulatory site is the "polyamine" site (see Fig. 2). This site has been linked to the inclusion of the NR2B subunit in receptors (89) and, in consequence, occurs in anatomically restricted sites in the CNS. Antagonists have now been developed that interact with this site and that modulate NMDA receptor-mediated processes rather selectively (see the following).

Table 1 Examples of NMDA Antagonists of Various Classes[a]

Regulatory site	Compound	Effectiveness in pain
PCP-sensitive channel site	MK-801	Frequently used in preclinical studies, highly selective and potent NMDA antagonist. Antinociceptive or antihyperalgesic in a variety of models of subacute and chronic pain. Not used in humans because of high psychotomimetic activity.
	Ketamine	Most frequently used NMDA antagonist in the clinic, active in a variety of pain states, including posttraumatic, postoperative, and neuropathic pain (see text). Clinical use for analgesia is frequently limited by side effects.
	Dextromethorphan	Weak NMDA antagonist. Effective as analgesic in some, but not in other clinical studies (see text).
	Memantine	Antinociceptive or antihyperalgesic in a variety of preclinical pain models (100,101); clinical analgesic effectiveness has not been reported.
	Amantadine	Weak NMDA antagonist, effective as analgesic in some recent clinical trials (see text).
Glutamate (NMDA) recognition site	D-AP5	Highly selective and potent NMDA antagonist. Frequently used in preclinical in vitro studies. Poor penetration into the CNS.
	CPP	Selective and potent NMDA antagonist. Poor penetration into the CNS; somewhat better with CPP-ene.
	CGS19755 (Selfotel)	Selective and potent NMDA antagonist. Development stopped because of side effect in humans.
Glycine_B allosteric site	HA-966	Partial agonist, antinociceptive in some chronic pain models.
	5,7-Dichlorokynurenate	Potent and selective glycine_B antagonist in vitro. Poor penetration into the CNS.
	L-701,324	Selective glycine_B antagonist with reasonable penetration into the CNS. Antinociceptive or antihyperalgesic in inflammatory pain models (79).
	ACEA-1021	Glycine_B/AMPA antagonist with reasonable penetration into the CNS. Antinociceptive or antihyperalgesic in chronic pain models. Well tolerated in humans (86).
	Mrz2/576	Selective glycine_B antagonist, good CNS permeability (87). Antinociceptive in acute inflammatory and chronic pain models (80).
Ifenprodil-sensitive allosteric site	Ifenprodil	Limited selectivity for NMDA receptors. Antinociceptive in some preclinical pain models, including acute pain tests (94).
	CP-101,606	Selective NR2B antagonist. Antinociceptive in inflammatory pain models (95).
	Ro 25-6981	Selective NR2B antagonist (98). No published reports on antinociceptive activity.

[a] Members of all classes have been tested in animal models of acute and neuropathic pain. In humans, only ketamine, dextromethorphan, and amantadine have so far been subjected to controlled trials that have been published.

NMDA antagonists acting at these sites are currently available (see Table 1), and several have been tested in pain states in man (see Sec. IV.C).

IV. THE USE OF NMDA ANTAGONISTS AS ANALGESICS

These different classes of NMDA antagonist have been tested in a variety of animal pain models, and some of them have made their way into clinical trials. As a result we now have, or very soon will have, substantial information on the pharmacological profiles of different groups of antagonists, their different side effect profiles, and to some extent their effectiveness in different pain states.

A. Antinociceptive Profile of NMDA Antagonists in Preclinical Tests

Given the theoretical considerations just outlined, it comes as little surprise that NMDA antagonists are largely ineffective in acute pain models, such as tail-flick (37,38). On the other hand, there is a plethora of reports that NMDA antagonists are effective in a variety of subacute or chronic pain models (2,3). The palette of pain models in which NMDA antagonists are antinociceptive includes windup, acute and chronic inflammation, peripheral and central neuropathy, and postoperative situations. Importantly, NMDA antagonists are not only effective in preventing the development of pronociceptive changes, but may also reduce hyperalgesia, even when the changes have already developed (39). The ability to block the development of hyperalgesia in preclinical models suggests that NMDA antagonists might be effective as preemptive analgesic agents under clinical conditions. The antinociceptive profile is generally very similar for all classes of compound tested to date, but the side effect profile can vary considerably.

B. Interaction with Opioid Analgesics in Preclinical Studies

There are two potentially important interactions between NMDA antagonists and opioid analgesics: synergism in analgesia, and inhibition of opioid tolerance and dependence.

Some preclinical studies report a synergistic interaction between opioids and NMDA antagonists. Interestingly, this synergism is found in acute pain models, in which NMDA antagonists are normally rather inactive (37); for example, competitive and uncompetitive NMDA antagonists potentiate morphine antinociception in the hot-plate test and tail-flick tests (40,41).

In a number of studies and in several species, competitive, channel-blocking, and glycine$_B$ site NMDA antagonists have reduced the development of tolerance to the analgesic effect of opioids (42–44). Similarly, competitive and channel-blocking NMDA antagonists may be able to reverse established tolerance to morphine (42).

The mechanisms of the synergistic interaction with opioids and of attenuation of opioid tolerance by NMDA antagonists are not entirely clear. It has been shown that μ-opioid receptor activation can positively modulate the NMDA receptor in trigeminal neurons (45), a mechanism involving protein kinase C (PKC)-mediated phosphorylation of the receptor causing a decrease in magnesium sensitivity (46). Consistent with this, the development of morphine tolerance has been associated with an increase in concentration of a specific PKC isoform (PKC$_\gamma$) in superficial laminae of spinal dorsal horn; this effect was prevented by MK-801 (dizocilpine) (42). It is notable that PKC$_\gamma$ seems to play an important role in pain chronification, in particular in the development of neuropathic pain (36). Under neuropathic conditions animals may show reduced opioid sensitivity (42) and opioids are relatively ineffective in treating neuropathic pain in the clinic (47).

C. Clinical Experience with NMDA Antagonists

Paradoxically, those few NMDA antagonists that are now clinically available made their way into human use before their mechanism of action was understood to be by NMDA antagonism. Most of the information on the analgesic effectiveness of NMDA antagonists has been accumulated with ketamine, but there are some data with other channel-blocking antagonists, including dextromethorphan and amantadine. There is one case report using a competitive antagonist, but still no reports with glycine site or polyamine site antagonists.

At subanesthetic doses, the effects of ketamine on sensation appear to be rather selectively antihyperalgesic. Thus, in a placebo-controlled human study, a low intravenous dose of ketamine (0.5 mg/kg) reduced both pain rating and withdrawal reflex to repeated electrical stimuli, but not to single stimuli (48).

In randomized placebo-controlled studies, intra- and postoperative intravenous infusions of ketamine prevented postoperative secondary mechanical hyperalgesia and allodynia (5). In agreement with the idea of the importance of NMDA receptors in triggering pronociceptive plasticity in the CNS (see foregoing), ketamine has been tried for preemptive analgesia and was more effective when given before than after the operation (49,50). Interestingly, there are reports on effectiveness of low-dose infusion of ketamine in posttraumatic pain (51).

Another important field of application of ketamine is for neuropathic pain. Several studies report a relief of both spontaneous and evoked pain by prolonged treatment with ketamine of patients with neuropathic pain syndromes of either peripheral or central origin (52–54). In double-blind studies, ketamine produced significant (vs. placebo) relief of spontaneous pain, aloodynia, and windup-like pain in patients with postherpetic neuralgia (55) or with phantom pain (56).

Some groups report effectiveness of ketamine in neuropathic pain after chronic subcutaneous infusion (57) or oral administration (58–60). This effect could, at least in part, be mediated by the main metabolite of ketamine, norketamine, which has a somewhat lower affinity for the channel site of the NMDA receptor (61). These administration regimens are likely to avoid sudden peaks in plasma concentration, and this seems to minimize the psychotomimetic actions that are a frequent side effect of ketamine and the major problem limiting its use as an analgesic (see Sec. V).

Dextromethorphan was first introduced as an antitussive agent, and only more than 35 years later was it found to have the properties of an open-channel NMDA blocker (for review see Ref. 62). Dextromethorphan selectively reduced temporal summation of second pain (16). However, in double-blind, randomized, controlled crossover trials, it was largely ineffective in neuropathic pain at doses causing no adverse effects (63). It was also ineffective in human capsaicin-induced ongoing pain and mechanical hypersensitivity (64), but showed some effectiveness when tested at much higher doses (65).

Amantadine has recently been assessed in clinical trials and has been reported to be effective in neuropathic pain with a reduced side effect profile (66).

V. DRAWBACKS AND PROBLEMS ASSOCIATED WITH THE USE OF NMDA ANTAGONISTS

The tendency to have dysphoric and psychotomimetic effects is the major problem limiting the clinical use of ketamine and dextromethorphan for the treatment of pain. These effects have been reported for a variety of NMDA antagonists used in humans, the most typical example being phencyclidine (PCP; ''angel dust''). The mechanisms of this effect are not yet fully understood, but are likely to result from block of NMDA receptor-mediated control over dopamine and serotonin systems (33,67) that influence conscious perception. In animals, stereotypic behavior is thought to predict possible psychotomimetic actions in humans; the compounds that are known to cause pronounced psychotomimetic effects in humans (e.g., PCP, MK-801, ketamine) are all able to evoke stereotypic behavior (68).

These neurotransmitter changes plus associated activation of glutamatergic transmission (67) could be a mechanism of the NMDA antagonist-induced, area-specific neurotoxicity, which is seen as vacuolarization and necrosis of neurons in the retrosplenial cortex and cingulate area (69). Increased glucose metabolism seen specifically in these brain areas is another implication of the enhanced neuronal activity after NMDA antagonist administration (70).

Other side effects seen in pain patients include memory deficits, ataxia, dizziness, and sedation.

VI. CURRENT APPROACHES TO THE DEVELOPMENT OF NMDA ANTAGONISTS AS ANALGESICS

Regulation of NMDA receptor function can be achieved though diverse binding sites, such as the glutamate recognition site, the glycine$_B$ site, the polyamine site, and sites within the ion channel (see Fig. 2). The block at these different sites causes distinct pharmacological effects. Three mechanisms are currently recognized to contribute to these differences. First, the channel blockers may have different voltage dependencies and kinetics of their interaction with the channel. Second, glycine$_B$ antagonists can act rather variably to restore receptor desensitization. Third, antagonists of all classes may have different subtype selectivity (i.e., for receptors with different subunit composition) (see Ref. 17 for a review).

A. Fast Kinetics Channel Blockers

Channel block can occur only when the channel has been opened following activation of the NMDA recognition site (open channel block) (30,71). The result is that current will pass during the initial period that corresponds to fast synaptic transmission, but the prolonged currents that correspond to more pathological processes will be blocked preferentially. Those agents that have high affinity remain bound in the channel for prolonged periods and thereby block all phases of subsequent synaptic responses; this applies to ketamine. In contrast those channel blockers that leave the channel again before the next synaptic event, rather than staying bound in the channel for prolonged periods, will repeatedly permit the early phase of synaptic transmission to proceed (68,72). Adamantane derivatives including memantine are noncompetitive antagonists, with lower affinity and more rapid kinetics (i.e., they leave the channel rapidly) and so have theoretical advantages in this respect (73).

An additional consideration is the variable relief of channel block when the cell is strongly excited (voltage-dependence of block). When the voltage gradient across the membrane is reduced, low-affinity blockers can escape from the channel (see Fig. 2); high-affinity blockers will remain strongly bound. Strong depolarizations can be expected during physiological synaptic excitation, which will therefore be spared by low-affinity, but not high-affinity, channel blockers. In contrast much pathological activation is likely to involve prolonged, but smaller, depolarizations insufficient to dislodge the blockers (73).

These mechanisms in combination are thought to be relevant for chronic pain situations. NMDA receptors mediate tonic activity of spinal dorsal horn neurons, presumably associated with continuous neurotransmitter release caused by peripheral injury (10,25). The windup model of pronociceptive plasticity in the spinal cord involves summation of slow synaptic components that may mimic the situation during a continuous barrage of nociceptive impulses during inflammation, or from ectopic sites after nerve injury (4,74). Importantly, the fast kinetics channel blocker, memantine, reduced windup more than short-term physiological responses to noxious pinch stimuli, whereas the slower blockers ketamine and MK-801 did not differentiate between these two types of responses (75).

The proposed inverse correlation between the affinity to the PCP site and frequency of side effects seems, to some extent, to hold true for those few channel blockers that have been used in humans. Thus, the low-to-medium affinity ligands memantine and dextromethorphan have a long history of a safe use as an antiparkinsonian and antitussive drug, respectively (although memantine has been reported to produce typical psychotomimetic effects in some groups of patients) (68,76).

A further possible reason for differences between channel blockers would be differential interaction with receptor subtypes. NR2A and NR2B subunits are found extensively in the forebrain, so that compounds that have less effect on these units might have advantages. Most current channel blockers show little or no selectivity between subtypes; however, MK-801 shows preference for NR2A and NR2B subtypes (17,77) and has strong psychotomimetic potential, whereas dextromethorphan shows some selectivity for NR2C subunits (78) and shows less psychotomimetic potential.

B. Glycine$_B$ Antagonists

The accumulated animal data with this class of NMDA antagonists are most encouraging. They are antinociceptive in models of inflammatory (79,80) and neuropathic pain (81). As with other classes of NMDA antagonists, glycine$_B$ antagonists have been reported to block the development of morphine tolerance (44). On the other hand, PCP-like stereotypic behavior, neuronal vacuolarization, and increase in brain glucose utilization have not been seen with glycine$_B$ antagonists (35,82,83). Interestingly, and in contrast to other classes of NMDA antagonist, glycine$_B$ antagonists have been reported to have antipsychotic activity in some animal models (84), and to antagonize the behavioral effects of some psychostimulants, including NMDA channel blockers such as PCP and MK-801 (85). Other side effects typical for NMDA antagonists, such as sedation, also seem to be minimal with glycine$_B$ antagonists (79,83).

The beneficial profile of this class of NMDA antagonists in preclinical studies has triggered the further development of several glycine$_B$ compounds. The clinical evaluation of such antagonists has been hampered until recently by the lack of compounds with acceptable pharmacokinetic or physicochemical properties (mostly the permeability of the blood–brain barrier and solubility). Preliminary reports with some compounds that have entered phase I studies as potential neuroprotective agents (e.g., ACEA 1021) indicate a lack of PCP-like psychotomimetic effects at plasma concentrations higher than those that are effective in animal studies (86).

There are various possible explanations for the lower side effect profile of glycine$_B$ antagonists. One is that they interact preferentially with NR2C–subunit-containing receptors (17), which appear to be expressed in spinal cord and cerebellum more than forebrain (18,31); these antagonists may therefore cause antinociception and ataxia, but have less psychotomimetic potential.

Another explanation relates to the desensitization caused by glycine$_B$ antagonists (see foregoing), which implies a preferential reduction of prolonged (pathological) activation of NMDA receptor, as compared with transient (physiological) events (82). Interestingly, low-to-medium affinity glycine$_B$ antagonists seem to affect the peak NMDA current relatively less (87) and, therefore, might be better than high-affinity antagonists in terms of separation between slow and fast components of NMDA–receptor-mediated events.

C. Ifenprodil-like Compounds

Ifenprodil and structurally related compounds (see Table 1) act at a distinct site that may be associated with the polyamine site (88,89). They block the NMDA receptor in a noncompetitive, activity-dependent, voltage-independent manner (90). They have a high selectivity for NR1/NR2B over NR1/NR2A receptor subtypes (17,91), and some evidence also indicates selectivity over receptors containing NR2C or NR2D subunits (92,93). Therefore, it is of considerable interest that ifenprodil and a derivative, CP-101,606, have been antinociceptive in a variety of pain models, including carrageenan- and capsaicin-induced hyperalgesia, phenylquinone writhing, and hot-plate tests (94,95). Notably, both ifenprodil (96) and CP101,606 (95,97) have fewer behavioral side effects typical for NMDA antagonists (stereotypic behavior, hyperlocomotion, and motor impairment).

The reasons for the apparent selectivity of this antinociceptive effect is not entirely clear. There is an apparent inconsistency between the lack of side effects at antinociceptive doses on the one hand and, on the other hand, the high levels of binding of ifenprodil-like compounds in forebrain (93,98), the high selectivity of this group towards NR2B-containing receptors, and the predominant forebrain localization of these receptors (31,99). An action as an NMDA antagonist is also hard to reconcile with the report that ifenprodil-induced antinociception was fully antagonized by naloxone (94).

VII. CONCLUSIONS AND PERSPECTIVES

Although some of the clinically available NMDA antagonists are effective in different clinical pain states, several serious side effects limit their use. Current strategies for developing safer compounds are aimed at selectively inhibiting pathological NMDA receptor activation without affecting normal physiological processes; these strategies depend on both different kinetics of the block and subtype selectivity. Several approaches look promising; they include development of fast kinetics channel blockers and of antagonists of the glycine site at the NMDA receptor. Recent encouraging preclinical results with ifenprodil-like compounds make this approach potentially important, although there are still theoretical questions to be clarified. Other approaches to minimizing the specific side effects exploit interactions between the NMDA receptor and other systems (e.g., opioids and tachykinins). Although there is preclinical evidence that a combination of NMDA antagonists and opioid agonists or neurokinin antagonists will be synergistic in analgesia, thus reducing the risk of specific side effects, the success depends on the availability of well-tolerated compounds for critical proof-of-principle studies in humans.

REFERENCES

1. Watkins JC, Evans RH. Excitatory amino acid transmitters. Annu Rev Pharmacol Toxicol 1981; 21:165–204.
2. Meller ST, Gebhart GF. Nitric oxide (NO) and nociceptive processing in the spinal cord. Pain 1993; 52:127–136.

3. Woolf CJ, Chong M–S. Pre-emptive analgesia—treating post operative pain by preventing the establishment of central sensitization. Anesth Analg 1993; 77:362–379.
4. Dickenson AH. A cure for wind up: NMDA receptor antagonists as potential analgesics. Trends Pharmacol Sci 1990; 11:307–309.
5. Stubhaug A, Breivik H, Eide PK, Kreunen M, Foss A. Ketamine reduces postoperative hyperalgesia. In: Jensen TS, Turner JA, Wiesenfeld–Hallin Z, eds. Proceedings of the 8th World Congress on Pain. Seattle: IASP Press, 1997:333–342.
6. Headley PM, Grillner S. Excitatory amino acids and synaptic transmission: the evidence for a physiological function. Trends Pharmacol Sci 1990; 11:205–211.
7. Yoshimura M, Jessel T. Amino acid-mediated EPSPs at primary afferent synapses with substantia gelatinosa neurones in the rat spinal cord. J Physiol 1990; 430:315–335.
8. King AE, LopezGarcia JA. Excitatory amino acid receptor-mediated neurotransmission from cutaneous afferents in rat dorsal horn in vitro. J Physiol 1993; 472:443–457.
9. Headley PM, Parsons CG, West DC. The role of *N*-methylaspartate receptors in mediating responses of rat and cat spinal neurones to defined sensory stimuli. J Physiol 1987; 385:169–188.
10. Chizh BA, Cumberbatch MJ, Herrero JF, Stirk GC, Headley PM. Stimulus intensity, cell excitation and the *N*-methyl-D-aspartate receptor component of sensory responses in the rat spinal cord in vivo. Neuroscience 1997; 80:251–265.
11. Mendell LM. Physiological properties of unmyelinated fiber projections to the spinal cord. Exp Neurol 1966; 16:316–332.
12. Thompson SWN, King AE, Woolf CJ. Activity-dependent changes in rat ventral horn neurons in vitro; summation of prolonged afferent evoked postsynaptic depolarizations produce a D-2-amino-5-phosphonovaleric acid sensitive windup. Eur J Neurosci 1990; 2:638–649.
13. Baranauskas G, Nistri A. NMDA receptor-independent mechanisms responsible for the rate of rise of cumulative depolarization evoked by trains of dorsal root stimuli on rat spinal motoneurones. Brain Res 1996; 738:329–332.
14. Davies SN, Lodge D. Evidence for involvement of *N*-methylaspartate receptors in "wind-up" of class 2 neurones in the dorsal horn of the rat. Brain Res 1987; 424:402–406.
15. Dickenson AH, Sullivan AF. Evidence for a role of the NMDA receptor in the frequency-dependent potentiation of deep rat dorsal horn nociceptive neurones following C-fibre stimulation. Neuropharmacology 1987; 26:1235–1238.
16. Price DD, Mao J, Frenk H, Mayer DJ. The *N*-methyl-D-aspartate receptor antagonist dextromethorphan selectively reduces temporal summation of second pain in man. Pain 1994; 59:165–174.
17. Sucher NJ, Awobuluyi M, Choi YB, Lipton SA. NMDA receptors: from genes to channels. Trends Pharmacol Sci 1996; 17:348–355.
18. Momiyama A, Feldmeyer D, Cull–Candy SG. Identification of a native low-conductance NMDA channel with reduced sensitivity to Mg^{2+} in rat central neurones. J Physiol 1996; 494:479–492.
19. Tölle TR, Berthele A, Zieglgänsberger W, Seeburg PH, Wisden W. The differential expression of 16 NMDA and non-NMDA receptor subunits in the rat spinal cord and in periaqueductal gray. J Neurosci 1993; 13:5009–5028.
20. DeBiasi S, Rustioni A. Glutamate and substance P coexist in primary afferent terminals in the superficial laminae of spinal cord. Proc Natl Acad Sci USA 1988; 85:7820–7824.
21. Dougherty PM, Palecek J, Zorn S, Willis WD. Combined application of excitatory amino acids and substance P produces long-lasting changes in responses of primate spinothalamic tract neurons. Brain Res Rev 1993; 18:227–246.
22. Rusin KI, Bleakman D, Chard PS, Randic M, Miller RJ. Tachykinins potentiate *N*-methyl-D-aspartate responses in acutely isolated neurons from the dorsal horn. J Neurochem 1993; 60:952–960.
23. Chizh BA, Headley PM. Thyrotropin-releasing hormone facilitates spinal nociceptive responses by potentiating NMDA receptor-mediated transmission. Eur J Pharmacol 1996; 300:183–189.
24. Duggan AW, Riley RC, Mark MA, Macmillan SJA, Schaible HG. Afferent volley patterns and the spinal release of immunoreactive substance P in the dorsal horn of the anaesthetized spinal cat. Neuroscience 1995; 65:849–858.

25. Hartell NA, Headley PM. NMDA-receptor contribution to spinal nociceptive reflexes: influence of stimulus parameters and of preparatory surgery. Neuropharmacology 1996; 35:1567–1572.
26. Raymond LA, Blackstone CD, Huganir RL. Phosphorylation of amino acid neurotransmitter receptors in synaptic plasticity. Trends Neurosci 1993; 16:147–153.
27. Bliss TVP, Collingridge GL. A synaptic model of memory: long-term potentiation in the hippocampus. Nature 1993; 361:31–39.
28. Pockett S. Long-term potentiation and depression in the intermediate gray matter of rat spinal cord in vitro. Neuroscience 1995; 67:791–798.
29. Liu XG, Sandkühler J. Long-term potentiation of C-fiber-evoked potentials in the rat spinal dorsal horn is prevented by spinal *N*-methyl-D-aspartic acid receptor blockage. Neurosci Lett 1995; 191: 43–46.
30. Lodge D, Collingridge GL, eds. The Pharmacology of Excitatory Amino Acids. Amsterdam: Elsevier, 1990.
31. Monyer H, Burnashev N, Laurie DJ, Sakmann B, Seeburg PH. Developmental and regional expression in the rat brain and functional properties of four NMDA receptors. Neuron 1994; 12:529–540.
32. Anis NA, Berry SC, Burton NR, Lodge D. The dissociative anaesthetics, ketamine and phencyclidine, selectively reduce excitation of central mammalian neurones by *N*-methyl-aspartate. Br J Pharmacol 1983; 79:565–575.
33. White PF, Way WL, Trevor AJ. Ketamine—its pharmacology and therapeutic uses. Anesthesiology 1982; 56:119–136.
34. Johnson KM, Jones SM. Neuropharmacology of phencyclidine: basic mechanisms and therapeutic potential. Annu Rev Pharmacol Toxicol 1990; 30:707–750.
35. Kemp JA, Leeson PD. The glycine site of the NMDA receptor—five years on. Trends Pharmacol Sci 1993; 14:20–25.
36. Malmberg AB, Chen C, Tonegawa S, Basbaum AI. Preserved acute pain and reduced neuropathic pain in mice lacking PKCgamma. Science 1998; 278:279–283.
37. Advokat C, Rutherford D. Selective antinociceptive effect of excitatory amino acid antagonists in intact and acute spinal rats. Pharmacol Biochem Behav 1995; 51:855–860.
38. Lutfy K, Cai SX, Woodward RM, Weber E. Antinociceptive effects of NMDA and non-NMDA receptor antagonists in the tail flick test in mice. Pain 1997; 70:31–40.
39. Woolf CJ, Thompson SWN. The induction and maintenance of central sensitization is dependent on *N*-methyl-D-aspartic acid receptor activation; implications for the treatment of post-injury pain hypersensitivity states. Pain 1991; 44:293–299.
40. Dambisya YM, Lee TL. Antinociceptive effects of ketamine–opioid combinations in the mouse tail flick test. Methods Find Exp Clin Pharmacol 1995; 16:179–184.
41. Wiesenfeld–Hallin Z. Combined opioid–NMDA antagonist therapies. What advantage do they offer for the control of pain syndromes? Drugs 1998; 55:1–4.
42. Mao J, Price DD, Mayer DJ. Mechanisms of hyperalgesia and morphine tolerance: a current view of their possible interactions. Pain 1995; 62:259–274.
43. Gonzalez P, Cabello P, Germany A, Norris B, Contreras E. Decrease of tolerance to, and physical dependence on, morphine by glutamate receptor antagonists. Eur J Pharmacol 1997; 332:257–262.
44. Lufty K, Shen K–Z, Kwon IS, Cai SX, Woodward RM, Keana JFW, Weber E. Blockade of morphine tolerance by ACEA-1328, a novel NMDA receptor/glycine site antagonist. Eur J Pharmacol 1995; 273:187–189.
45. Chen L, Huang L–YM. Sustained potentiation of NMDA receptor-mediated glutamate responses through activation of protein kinase C by a mu-opioid. Neuron 1991; 7:319–326.
46. Chen L, Huang L–YM. Protein kinase C reduces Mg^{2+} block of NMDA-receptor channels as a mechanism of modulation. Nature 1992; 356:521–523.
47. Arnér S, Meyerson B. Opioids in neuropathic pain. Pain Digest 1993; 3:15–22.
48. Arendt–Nielsen L, Petersen–Felix S, Fisher M, Bak P, Bjerring P, Zbinden AM. The effect of *N*-methyl-D-aspartate antagonist (ketamine) on single and repeated nociceptive stimuli: a placebo-controlled experimental human study. Anesth Analg 1995; 81:63–68.
49. Barbieri M, Colnaghi E, Tommasino C, Zangrillo A, Galli L, Torri G. Efficacy of the NMDA

antagonist ketamine in preemptive analgesia. In: Jensen TS, Turner JA, Wiesenfeld–Hallin Z, eds. Proceedings of the 8th World Congress on Pain. Seattle: IASP Press, 1997:343–349.
50. Fu ES, Miguel R, Scharf JE. Preemptive ketamine decreases postoperative narcotic requirements in patients undergoing abdominal surgery. Anesth Analg 1997; 84:1086–1090.
51. Gurnani A, Sharma PK, Rautela RS, Bhattacharya A. Analgesia for acute musculoskeletal trauma: low-dose subcutaneous infusion of ketamine. Anaesth Intensive Care 1996; 24:32–36.
52. Felsby S, Nielsen J, Arendt–Nielsen L, Jensen TS. NMDA receptor blockade in chronic neuropathic pain: a comparison of ketamine and magnesium chloride. Pain 1996; 64:283–291.
53. Backonja M, Arndt G, Gombar KA, Check B, Zimmerman M. Response of chronic neuropathic pain syndromes to ketamine: a preliminary study. Pain 1994; 56:51–57.
54. Stannard CF, Porter GE. Ketamine hydrochloride in the treatment of phantom limb pain. Pain 1993; 54:227–230.
55. Eide PK, Jørum E, Stubhaug A, Bremnes J, Breivik H. Relief of post-herpetic neuralgia with the *N*-methyl-D-aspartic acid receptor antagonist ketamine: a double-blind, cross-over comparison with morphine and placebo. Pain 1994; 58:347–354.
56. Nikolajsen L, Hansen CL, Nielsen J, Keller J, Arendt–Nielsen L, Jensen TS. The effect of ketamine on phantom pain: a central neuropathic disorder maintained by peripheral input. Pain 1996; 67:69–77.
57. Eide PK, Stubhaug A, Øye I, Breivik H. Continuous subcutaneous administration of the *N*-methyl-D-aspartatic acid (NMDA) receptor antagonist ketamine in the treatment of post-herpetic neuralgia. Pain 1995; 61:221–228.
58. Hoffmann V, Coppejans H, Vercauteren M, Adriaensen H. Successful treatment of postherpetic neuralgia with oral ketamine. Clin J Pain 1994; 10:240–242.
59. Broadley KE, Kurowska A, Tookman A. Ketamine injection used orally. Palliat Med 1996; 10: 247–250.
60. Nikolajsen L, Hansen PO, Jensen TS. Oral ketamine therapy in the treatment of postamputation stump pain. Acta Anaesthesiol Scand 1997; 41:427–429.
61. Ebert B, Mikkelsen S, Thorkildsen C, Borgbjerg FM. Norketamine, the main metabolite of ketamine, is a non-competitive NMDA receptor antagonist in the rat cortex and spinal cord. Eur J Pharmacol 1997; 333:99–104.
62. Tortella FC, Pellicano M, Bowery NG. Dextromethorphan and neuromodulation: old drug coughs up new activities. Trends Pharmacol Sci 1989; 10:501–507.
63. McQuay HJ, Carroll D, Jadad AR, Glynn CJ, Jack T, Moore RA, Wiffen PJ. Dextromethorphan for the treatment of neuropathic pain: a double-blind randomised controlled crossover trial with integral n-of-1 design. Pain 1994; 59:127–133.
64. Kinnman E, Nygards EB, Hansson P. Effects of dextromethorphan in clinical doses on capsaicin-induced ongoing pain and mechanical hypersensitivity. J Pain Symptom Manage 1997; 14:195–201.
65. Nelson KA, Park KM, Robinovitz E, Tsigos C, Max MB. High-dose oral dextromethorphan versus placebo in painful diabetic neuropathy and postherpetic neuralgia. Neurology 1997; 48:1212–1218.
66. Pud D, Eisenberg E, Spitzer A, Adler R, Fried G, Yarnitsky D. The NMDA receptor antagonist amantadine reduces surgical neuropathic pain in cancer patients: a double blind, randomized, placebo controlled trial. Pain 1998; 75:349–354.
67. Moghaddam B, Adams B, Verma A, Daly D. Activation of glutamatergic neurotransmission by ketamine: a novel step in the pathway from NMDA receptor blockade to dopaminergic and cognitive disruptions associated with the prefrontal cortex. J Neurosci 1997; 17:2921–2927.
68. Rogawski MA. Therapeutic potential of excitatory amino acid antagonists: channel blockers and 2,3-benzodiazepines. Trends Pharmacol Sci 1993; 14:325–331.
69. Olney JW, Labruyere J, Wang G, Wozniak DF, Price MT, Sesma MA. NMDA antagonist neurotoxicity: mechanism and prevention. Science 1991; 254:1515–1518.
70. Hargreaves RJ, Rigby M, Smith D, Hill RG, Iversen LL. Competitive as well as uncompetitive *N*-methyl-D-aspartate receptor antagonists affect cortical neuronal morphology and cerebral glucose metabolism. Neurochem Res 1993; 18:1263–1269.

71. MacDonald JF, Miljkovic Z, Pennefather. Use-dependent block of excitatory amino acid currents in cultured neurons by ketamine. J Neurophysiol. 1987; 58:251–266.
72. Chen H–SV, Pellegrini JW, Aggarwal SK, Lei SZ, Warach S, Jensen FE, Lipton SA. Open-channel block of *N*-methyl-D-aspartate (NMDA) responses by memantine: therapeutic advantage against NMDA receptor-mediated neurotoxicity. J Neurosci 1992; 12:4427–4436.
73. Parsons CG, Grüner R, Rozental J, Millar J, Lodge D. Patch clamp studies on the kinetics and selectivity of *N*-methyl-D-aspartate receptor antagonism by memantine (1-amino-3,5-dimethyladamantan). Neuropharmacology 1993; 32:1337–1350.
74. Ren K. Wind-up and the NMDA receptor: from animal studies to humans. Pain 1994; 59:157–158.
75. Jones MW, McClean M, Parsons CG, Headley PM. The in vivo relevance of the varied channel-blocking properties of uncompetitive NMDA antagonists: tests on spinal neurones. Neuropharmacology 2001; (in press).
76. Kornhuber J, Weller M. Psychotogenicity and *N*-methyl-D-aspartate receptor antagonism: implications for neuroprotective pharmacotherapy. Biol Psychiatry 1997; 41:135–144.
77. Bresink I, Benke TA, Collett VJ, Seal AJ, Parsons CG, Henley JM, Collingridge GL. Effects of memantine on recombinant rat NMDA receptors expressed in HEK 293 cells. Br J Pharmacol 1996; 119:195–204.
78. Monaghan DT, Larsen H. NR1 and NR2 subunit contributions to *N*-methyl-D-aspartate receptor channel blocker pharmacology. J Pharmacol Exp Ther 1997; 280:614–620.
79. Laird JMA, Mason GS, Webb J, Hill RG, Hargreaves RJ. Effects of a partial agonist and a full antagonist acting at the glycine site of the NMDA receptor on inflammation-induced mechanical hyperalgesia in rats. Br J Pharmacol 1996; 117:1487–1492.
80. McClean M, Headley PM, Parsons CG. The glycine$_B$ antagonist, Mrz 2/576, is antinociceptive in behavioural tests. Soc Neurosci Abstr 1997; 23:367.12.
81. Mao J, Price DD, Hayes RL, Lu J, Mayer DJ. Differential roles of NMDA and non-NMDA receptor activation in induction and maintenance of thermal hyperalgesia in rats with painful peripheral mononeuropathy. Brain Res 1992; 598:271–278.
82. Danysz W, Parsons CG, Bresink I, Quack G. Glutamate in CNS disorders. Drug News Perspect 1995; 8:261–277.
83. Kretschmer BD, Kratzer U, Breithecker K, Koch M. ACEA 1021, a glycine site antagonist with minor psychotomimetic and amnestic effects in rats. Eur J Pharmacol 1997; 331:109–116.
84. Bristow LJ, Landon L, Saywell KL, Tricklebank MD. The glycine/NMDA receptor antagonist, L-701,324 reverses isolation-induced deficits in prepulse inhibition in the rat. Psychopharmacology 1995; 118:230–232.
85. Bristow LJ, Hutson PH, Thorn L, Tricklebank MD. The glycine/NMDA receptor antagonist, R-(+)-HA-966, blocks activation of the mesolimbic dopaminergic system induced by phencyclidine and dizocilpine (MK-801) in rodents. Br J Pharmacol 1993; 108:1156–1163.
86. Kulagowski JJ. Glycine-site NMDA receptor antagonists: an update. Exp Opin Ther Patents 1996; 6:1069–1079.
87. Parsons CG, Danysz W, Quack G, Hartmann S, Lorenz B, Wollenburg C, Baran L, Przegalinski E, Kostowski W, Krzascik P, Chizh BA, Headley PM. Novel systemically active antagonists of the glycine site of the *N*-methyl-D-aspartate receptor: electrophysiological, biochemical and behavioral characterization. J Pharmacol Exp Ther 1997; 283:1264–1275.
88. Kashiwagi K, Fukuchi J, Chao J, Igarashi K, Williams K. An aspartate residue in the extracellular loop of the *N*-methyl-D-aspartate receptor controls sensitivity to spermine and protons. Mol Pharmacol 1996; 49:1131–1141.
89. Gallagher MJ, Huang H, Pritchett DB, Lynch DR. Interactions between ifenprodil and the NR2B subunit of the *N*-methyl-D-aspartate receptor. J Biol Chem 1996; 271:9603–9611.
90. Kew JN, Trube G, Kemp JA. A novel mechanism of activity-dependent NMDA receptor antagonism describes the effect of ifenprodil in rat cultured cortical neurones. J Physiol 1996; 497:761–772.
91. Williams K. Ifenprodil discriminates subtypes of the *N*-methyl-D-aspartate receptor: selectivity and mechanism at recombinant heteromeric receptors. Mol Pharmacol 1993; 44:851–859.

92. Williams K. Pharmacological properties of recombinant *N*-methyl-D-aspartate (NMDA) receptors containing the epsilon4 (NR2D) subunit. Neurosci Lett 1995; 184:181–184.
93. Menniti F, Chenard B, Collins M, Ducat M, Shalaby I, White F. CP-101,606, a potent neuroprotectant selective for forebrain neurons. Eur J Pharmacol 1997; 331:117–126.
94. Bernardi M, Bertolini A, Szczawinska K, Genedani S. Blockade of the polyamine site of NMDA receptors produces antinociception and enhances the effect of morphine in mice. Eur J Pharmacol 1996; 298:51–55.
95. Taniguchi K, Shinjo K, Mizutani M, Shimada K, Ishikawa T, Menniti F, S S, Nagahisa A. Antinociceptive activity of CP-101,606, an NMDA receptor NR2B subunit antagonist. Br J Pharmacol 1997; 122:809–812.
96. Jackson A, Sanger DJ. Is the discriminative stimulus produced by phencyclidine due to an interaction with *N*-methyl-D-aspartate receptors? Psychopharmacology 1988; 96:87–92.
97. Tsuchida E, Rice M, Bullock R. The neuroprotective effect of the forebrain-selective NMDA antagonist CP101,606 upon focal ischemic brain damage caused by acute subdural hematoma in the rat. J Neurotrauma 1997; 14:409–417.
98. Mutel V, Buchy D, Klingelschmidt A, Messer J, Bleuel Z, Kemp JA, Richards JG. In vitro binding properties in rat brain of [^{3}H]Ro 25-6981, a potent and selective antagonist of NMDA receptors containing NR2B subunits. J Neurochem 1998; 70:2147–2155.
99. Hollmann M, Heinemann S. Cloned glutamate receptors. Annu Rev Neurosci 1994; 17:31–108.
100. Eisenberg E, Vos BP, Strassman AM. The NMDA antagonist memantine blocks pain behavior in a rat model of formalin-induced facial pain. Pain 1993; 54:301–307.
101. Eisenberg E, LaCross S, Strassman AM. The effects of the clinically tested NMDA receptor antagonist memantine on carrageenan-induced thermal hyperalgesia. Eur J Pharmacol 1994; 255:123–129.

46

Profile of Ketamine, CPP, Dextromethorphan, and Memantine

Jeff Gelblum
Mt. Sinai Medical Center, Miami, Florida, U.S.A.

I. INTRODUCTION

Disturbances of nervous system monoamine activity are thought to play a role in various psychiatric and neurological disorders of depression, anxiety, panic, phobia pain, and seizure. In particular, glutamate and serotonin (5-HT) play a significant role in the maintenance of neuronal functioning in two important ways. These monoamine neurotransmitters can alter postsynaptic flux, resulting in excessive depolarizations. This would be termed an *ionotropic effect.* These neurotransmitters can also affect the secondary-messenger system, resulting in the production of transcription factors that can cause or block neuronal gene expression (Wong et al., 1995). Glutamate and serotonin act on specific receptors located throughout the nervous system and other organ systems, including heart, gut, and blood cells. Drugs that alter the receptor binding of glutamate and serotonin may play a significant role in the management of acute and chronic pain syndromes, which are often accompanied by prominent behavioral features of panic, anxiety, depression, and sleep disturbance. This chapter will explore the role of the antiglutamate effects of ketamine, memantine, dextromethorphan, and CPP as well as the serotonergic effects of mCPP. Modulation of these two monoamine pathways may be useful in helping to dampen neuronal hyperexcitability, a desirable goal in the treatment of many neurological ills.

II. GLUTAMATE

The ability of certain amino acids such as glutamate to excite cortical neurons was first observed in the late 1950s. By the early 1980s glutamate was established as a central nervous system (CNS) neurotransmitter (Rothman and Olney, 1988). Other excitatory chemicals, including aspartate and homocysteate, may also act as neurotransmitters. Glutamate fibers give rise to major pathways throughout the brain cortex, thalamus, cochlea, olfactory bulb, and retina (Karschin et al., 1988). In the peripheral nervous system large myelinated primary somatosensory fibers utilize glutamate. The regulation of corticothalamic glutamate neurotransmission may explain sensory gating problems in schizophrenia (Hargreaves and Cain, 1992). Disruption of hippocampal glutamate may contribute to Alzheimer's dementia (Butleman, 1989). Glutamate-induced excitation has been shown to destroy CNS neurons by local and systemic application. This usually occurs by uncontrolled flux of calcium ions into neurons as well as uncontrolled activation of nitric oxide synthase, the enzyme responsible for buildup of nitric oxide. Physiologically, intraneuronal formation of nitric oxide may function as a retrograde second messenger serving to potentiate synaptic transmission required for memory formation (Dawson and Dawson, 1991).

Excessive glutamate activity is also implicated in ischemic brain injury, seizures, and such neurodegenerative disorders as amyotrophic lateral sclerosis (ALS) and Huntington's chorea. In the latter disease, the symptom severity correlates well with cerebrospinal fluid (CSF) glutamate concentrations (Meldrum and Garthwaite, 1990).

Glutamate exerts its excitational effects by way of distinct receptor-binding sites, enabling various ionotropic and second-messenger effects. The principal ionotropic receptors are the *N*-methyl-D-aspartate (NMDA), α-amino-3-hydroxy-5-methyl-4-isoxazole propionic acid (AMPA), and kainate receptors. The naming of these receptors is based on their respective activations by these synthetic glutamate derivatives. These channels are voltage-dependent and govern the influx of calcium and sodium. When bound by glutamate, the NMDA channel gives rise to a sodium and channel flux resulting in prolonged postsynaptic neuronal depolarization, sometimes up to 500 ms in duration. At rest, physiological concentrations of magnesium will block this channel. A depolarizing voltage, however, will abolish this blockade. In contrast, AMPA and kainate channel activations result in brief depolarizations of just a few milliseconds duration. Their subunit compositions determine permeability to sodium alone or sodium in combination with calcium. These channels are not physiologically blocked by magnesium (Sagratella, 1995).

Multiple subunits of the NMDA receptor have been demonstrated (Narkai, 1998). Further evaluation of these NMDA receptor subunits may be useful in the development of new pharmacological agents.

A. Glutamate-Mediated Pain

A single brief noxious stimulus applied to the limb will result first in a pricking pain conveyed by the afferent high-frequency, brief-latency, myelinated Aδ fibers. However, a moment later, the afferent long-latency unmyelinated C fibers will convey a burning, throbbing, aching pain. The same second-order nociceptive neuron will receive both of these impulses in sequence. Repetition of the brief noxious stimulus at less than 3-s intervals will result in magnification of the secondary burning component conveyed by the C fibers. This is termed temporal summation or "windup."

Temporal summation is recorded from dorsal horn nociceptive neurons stimulated by C-fiber afferents. In particular, neurons from dorsal horn laminae I and V will then transmit impulses to the spinothalamic tract. There, further magnification may occur. Dorsal horn temporal summation is dependent on glutamate activation of the NMDA receptor (Davies and Lodge, 1987). This results in a prolonged depolarization. This prolonged depolarization causes a phenomenon of long-term potentiation that activates the nitric oxide synthase cascade. Here, nitric oxide plays a role in the amplification and coding of the windup response. Since the 1950s slow, temporal summation has been recognized to play a critical role in the pathophysiology of chronic neurogenic pain (Noorderbos, 1959). More recently, this concept has incorporated nitric oxide-mediated dorsal horn long-term potentiation.

Numerous studies have demonstrated the role of the glutamate NMDA receptor in the evolution of prolonged dorsal horn depolarization. Microinstallation of glutamate results in depolarization of the cells as has been documented by patch-clamp studies (Urban and Randic, 1984). In vivo animal studies have shown NMDA receptor antagonists to block prolonged depolarization and temporal summation of electrically stimulated C afferent fibers without abolishing

Aδ activation. Other studies have shown NMDA blockade to inhibit nociceptive neuron excitability induced by formalin, Freund's adjuvant, carrageenan, and wide-dynamic–range neuron receptor field expansion (Murray et al., 1991). Inflammatory electrical stimulus and mustard oil chemical nerve stimuli can be attenuated by NMDA antagonism (Price et al., 1994). Thus, in vitro and in vivo studies implicate the glutamate NMDA receptors in spinal cord dorsal horn as a common intermediate in the maintenance and amplification of neurogenic and perhaps nociceptive pain.

In addition to modulating neuronal behavior, the NMDA receptor plays a crucial role in neuronal development. During embryogenesis, nerve cell migration, dendrite spine formation, and embryonic synapse formation are guided by NMDA receptors. Postnatally, ocular dominance columns in the visual cortex as well as spatial representation in the somatosensory parietal cortex rely on NMDA-induced long-term potentiation (Hotter and Wasterlain, 1990). These activities can be blocked by NMDA antagonists, which could theoretically limit their clinical application in the prenatal and pediatric settings.

III. KETAMINE

Ketamine functions as a noncompetitive NMDA blocker (Anis et al., 1983). At high doses it causes dissociative anesthesia, whereby subjects are awake but dissociated from the environment. This anesthetic effect may be due to inhibition of the NMDA activity in the hippocampus, which is responsible for registration of new memories. There, the initiation of long-term potentiation occurs whereby an NMDA channel calcium influx triggers the nitric oxide second-messenger system. However, in lower doses, ketamine may induce a psychotic state similar to schizophrenia. This is also seen with another NMDA blocker, the hallucinogen phencyclidine hydrochloride (PCP). The ability of such NMDA blockers as ketamine and PCP to induce a transient schizophrenic state suggests that disorders of this particular channel may play a pathogenic role in this disease. Conversely, glycine, an amino acid potentiator of the NMDA channel may ameliorate some psychotic features of schizophrenia. Immunohistochemical findings suggest increased proliferation of NMDA and non-NMDA receptor density in specific regions of the schizophrenic brain (Kornhuber et al., 1989). Schizophrenic patients and those with schizophrenic predispositions appear to be particularly sensitive to the disorganizing effects of ketamine and may show profound behavioral abnormality for several weeks, after even a single low dose.

Aside from anesthetic applications, ketamine has been used as an analgesic, and sedative drug for many years. In the intravenous dose of 0.125–0.35 mg/kg, ketamine relieves phantom limb pain (Stannard, 1993). This effect is not reversed by naloxone, suggesting a mechanism of action completely independent from the opiates. Other studies at 0.075 mg/kg have shown analgesic effects in patients suffering from postherpetic neuralgia pain who failed low-dose morphine (Eide, 1994). This is in keeping with clinical studies showing that opiates are often less effective in relieving neurogenic pain than nociceptive pain. The effectiveness of ketamine in relieving truncal and limb postherpetic neuralgia pain suggests a role of NMDA receptors at the spinal cord level, particularly the dorsal horn, as well as supraspinal thalamic regions. Present data indicate that NMDA receptors are responsible for the maintenance of allodynic pain, as may be reflected by dorsal horn nociceptive neuronal windup. A possible explanation is that excited hypersensitized dorsal horn pain cells respond to activity from low-threshold afferent Aβ fibers. An NMDA antagonist will reverse this hyperexcitability. In animals, dorsal horn windup is inhibited by low-dose ketamine, whereas it is enhanced by low-dose morphine (Van-Pragg, 1990). This further differentiates the analgesic role of NMDA blockade versus opiate agonism. Moreover, NMDA blockade does not alter tactile or thermal sensory threshold.

Thus, an NMDA antagonist such as ketamine may reduce allodynia by reduction of dorsal horn neuronal excitability. After-sensation pain and radiant pain may be further inhibited by ketamine as would be implicated by additional attenuation of afferent Aβ-fiber pathways.

IV. MEMANTINE

Memantine was first introduced in 1964 as an antiviral drug against type A2 influenza. Memantine is a derivative of amantadine, a drug presently used in the treatment of Parkinson's and flu syndromes. Its primary effect is as a short-duration noncompetitive inhibitor of the open NMDA channel, thereby preventing prolonged neuronal influx of sodium and calcium (Bormann, 1989). Also it decreases monoamine oxydase (MAO) activity in the liver, brain, and kidney, thereby possibly retarding degradation of such CNS amines as serotonin (5-HT), norepinephrine, and dopamine (Wesemann et al., 1982). Increases in brain dopamine would theoretically have a beneficial effect in the treatment of Parkinson's disease. The use of an NMDA antagonist such as memantine in the treatment of Parkinson's disease lies not only in possible dopamine potentiation by MAO inhibition, but also in behavioral activation, as has been shown in rodents with suppressed glutamatergic transmission. This behavioral activation by memantine occurs in rodent brain even in the absence of dopamine (Carlsson and Carlsson, 1989). Human data, however, are limited in confirming a primary disturbance of limbic or cortical glutamatergic function in parkinsonian conditions, exclusive of dopamine. Significant inhibition of cerebral glutamatergic function may contribute to the pathophysiology of hallucinosis and schizophrenia, as has been previously discussed. This could theoretically limit the tolerable-dosing ranges in parkinsonian patients.

In addition to antiparkinsonian effects, memantine has been studied in epilepsy. Patch-clamp and animal investigations of epilepsy-prone rats have shown memantine to inhibit seizure-causing prolonged depolarizations by NMDA channel calcium influx (Parsons and Gruner, 1993). Neurotoxicity studies have demonstrated the ability of memantine to protect neonatal rat forebrain from ischemic injury caused by bilateral carotid occlusion. This occurred at dosages of 10–20 mg/kg. The memantine-treated rat stroke model demonstrated 30% reduction of infarct size, compared with sham-occluded, placebo-matched controls (Sefel Nasir et al., 1990). Other neuroprotective models have shown protection of retinal, cortical neuronal, and cortical glial cells against endogenous glutamate agonism in an environment of elevated extracellular calcium and decreased magnesium. These effects were seen at relatively low memantine concentrations of 6–12 μM. An NMDA–receptor-mediated neurotoxicity is thought to comprise a final common pathway in multiple neurological disease processes. Alzheimer's dementia studies have shown memantine tolerability and possible benefit at low doses (Cortelmeyer and Erbier, 1992). More recently, possibly owing to memantine's historic antiviral spectrum of activity, AIDS dementia studies are underway. Here, memantine may help to deactivate HIV protein coat injury of the neuronal cell (Lipton and Gendelman, 1995). This aspect of AIDS-related neuronal injury resembles the mechanism of neuronal damage in stroke, trauma, epilepsy, neuropathic pain, and several neurogenic diseases. HIV-infected monocytes produce low molecular weight neurotoxins that activate the neuron's NMDA receptor directly as well as indirectly by interfering with glial cells' glutamate reuptake. Thus, CNS glutamate concentrations are elevated against a background of increased neuronal NMDA receptor sensitivity. The L-type calcium channel blocker nimodipine may also play a similar role in dampening–diminishing glutamate's injury to HIV-infected nerve cells (Dreyer et al., 1990). The role of memantine as an adjunct to antiretroviral therapy in AIDS dementia is especially promising because of its history of safe use in patients with other diseases as well as its blockade of only open NMDA ion channels for a short time.

Analgesic studies of low-dose memantine have shown promise particularly in the settings of painful diabetic neuropathy and postherpetic neuralgia, presumably owing to this agent's ability to inhibit dorsal horn C–fiber-mediated windup. In a recent study, nocturnal neuropathic pain was significantly ameliorated. Prior studies have shown memantine's inhibition of carrageenan-induced thermal paw pain as well as formalin-induced facial pain in rats. This may suggest an additional mechanism of action relying on tissue-induced injury, as could be evoked in nociceptive impulses (Eisenberg et al.; 1994). Most likely both neurogenic and nociceptive stimulus inhibition may incorporate common pathways at the dorsal horn.

V. DEXTROMETHORPHAN

Dextromethorphan is presently available as an antitussive in many over-the-counter preparations. Its noncompetitive NMDA-blocking effects have been documented since the late 1980s. Single human oral dosages of 30 mg attenuate the secondary temporal summation pain of electroshock, but not the first pain. This is in keeping with the functioning of dorsal horn NMDA activation. Other human studies using noxious thermal (burn) stimuli in moderate dosages (60–120 mg/day) resulted in similar reduction of secondary, but not primary hyperalgesia (Ilkjaer et al., 1997). Clinical trials have specifically tested dextromethorphan at varying dosages in the treatment of painful diabetic neuropathy and postherpetic neuralgia. Dextromethorphan at mean doses of 381 mg/day decreased neuropathic pain by 24%, whereas no effect was seen in postherpetic neuralgia. Expectedly, high-dose side effects of sedation and ataxia caused subject dropout (Nelson et al., 1997). Other anecdotal reports at varying dextromethorphan dosages suggest equivocal analgesic benefit. Other reports have shown high-dose dextromethorphan to be useful as a preinduction analgesic in the treatment of postamputation stump pain.

VI. CPP

3-(2-Carboxypiperazine-4-yl)-1-phosphonic acid (CPP) is a competitive NMDA blocker. It exhibits anticonvulsant activity in many animal models of epilepsy. One of its derivatives, cPPene, has demonstrated similar effect. Typical animal models used to evaluate antiepileptic drugs include those agents' ability to protect against electroconvulsive shock, induced seizures, and seizures caused by such proconvulsant chemicals as pentalene-tetrazol and mercaptopropionic acid. Typically, genetically epilepsy-prone Sprague–Dawley rats are obtained. These animals are then exposed to the ictal stimuli noted.

The noncompetitive NMDA antagonists ketamine, memantine, and dextromethorphan have demonstrated anticonvulsant and analgesic benefits. This is due to their ability to dampen glutamate-induced neuronal hyperexcitability of brain and spinal cord areas. Dizocilpine (MK-801) has been evaluated in neuroprotective stroke models. This characteristic may arise from inhibition of ischemia-induced excessive calcium influx, as is commonly associated with neuronal death of stroke and other neurodegenerative processes. Unfortunately, hallucinatory side effects similar to those seen with PCP, another noncompetitive NMDA antagonist, have limited its clinical applicability.

Similarly, the competitive NMDA receptor antagonist CPP and its derivatives possess anticonvulsant benefit in the epilepsy-prone rat. Moreover, several excitatory behavioral effects of increased locomotion, head weaving, circling, and ataxia are not seen here as are commonly encountered with the noncompetitive NMDA antagonists (DeSarro and DeSarro, 1993). Additionally these agents offer longer-lasting anticonvulsant activity, as well as a higher therapeutic index. Anticonvulsant therapeutic index is defined as toxic dosage required for impaired performance in 50% of the animals (TD_{50}) divided by effective dosage in preventing 50% of sound-induced clonic (ED_{50}) seizure. Whether the increased therapeutic index of CPP yields better tolerability and efficacy in human subjects remains to be seen.

The role of competitive versus noncompetitive NMDA blockers in the analgesic setting is not well established. Thus far, most of the clinical trials exploring the role of NMDA blockade in the management of painful neuropathy and postherpetic neuralgia have relied on the noncompetitive NMDA antagonists. Certainly, the role of such competitive antagonists as CPP may prove beneficial in helping to dampen glutamate-dependent dorsal horn windup, as is known to occur in these patients. This windup is the basis of pathological pain transmission at the spinal level and should not interfere with normal sensory processing, in that CPP-treated patients demonstrated no impairment of warm and cold, skin pinch, proprioception, tendon reflexes, coordination, or motor performance (Gordh et al., 1995).

VII. mCPP

meta-Chlorophenylpiperazine (mCPP) is a nonselective 5-HT receptor agonist–antagonist that is used extensively in the evaluation of psychiatric and pain disorders to assess central serotonergic functioning. It is the major hepatic metabolite of trazodone, a triazolopyridine derivative presently marketed as an antidepressant (Desyrel) (Klaasen et al., 1998). Trazodone has a somewhat complex pharmacology. Through the mCPP metabolite, it acts as an agonist at 5-HT_{1A}, 5-HT_{1B}, 5-HT_{1C}, and 5-HT_{1D} postsynaptic receptor sites. Trazodone is an antagonist at the 5-HT_2 postsynaptic site. mCPP has minor antagonism at this 5-HT_2 site (Kennett et al., 1994). The major antidepressant action of trazodone is probably through its antagonism at the 5-HT_2 site, as this would cause an inhibition of a postsynaptic phosphatidylinositol second-messenger system. Furthermore, blocking this particular receptor site may shift synaptic serotonin over to 5-HT_{1A} receptors. This may result in the antidepressant effect. Significant 5-HT_2 receptor blockade also results in a down-regulation of the postsynaptic 5-HT_2 receptor density, which would ameliorate many negative components of depression.

The 5-HT_2 receptor is predominantly blocked by trazodone, and it is also blocked by other antidepressants, mianserine and nefazodone (Serzone) (Cyr, 1996). It is less effectively blocked by mCPP. Excessive 5-HT_2 receptor activation and subsequent amplification of the phosphatidylinositol second-messenger system is believed to account for many of the negative behavioral problems accompanying depression, including anxiety, temperature changes, sleep irregularities, hallucinations, psychosis, and panic. The 5-HT_2 receptor and its A and C subtypes may mediate the hallucinatory effects of LSD. Thus, blocking this receptors action would have important consequences in the control of the multiple negative behavioral components of depression as well as chronic pain (Nelson, 1994).

mCPP agonism at 5-HT_{1A}, 5-HT_{1B}, 5-HT_{1C}, and 5-HT_{1D} sites should theoretically elicit several beneficial behavioral and analgesic effects (Saxena, 1995). Stimulation of 5-HT_{1A} receptors should mediate antidepressant, antiobsessive compulsive, antipanic, and antibulimic properties. Stimulation of 5-HT_{1B} and 5-HT_{1D} receptors should elicit antimigrainous effects, similar in action to the triptan class of medications that utilize these receptors specifically to reverse cranial vessel inflammation and dilation.

Binding at the 5-HT_{1A}, 5-HT_{1B}, and 5-HT_{1D} receptors activates an alternative second-messenger system. Here a GTP-binding protein, Gs, is activated, stimulating adenylate cyclase which produces more postsynaptic intraneuronal cAMP. Incidentally, 5-HT_{1A} and 5-HT_3 binding also results in an ionotropic effect of increased postsynaptic potassium influx (Stam et al., 1992).

These effects are in contradistinction to the phosphatidylinositol system activated by 5-HT_2 receptor binding. 5-HT_{1C} site-binding may also elicit increased postsynaptic phosphatidylinositol synthesis, similar in action to 5-HT_2 receptor activation. Indeed, the binding of mCPP specifically to the 5-HT_{1C} site may theoretically account for some negative behavioral consequences of anxiety commonly encountered with this agent (Glennon, 1990).

In animal studies, low-dose trazodone (0.05–1 mg/kg) is primarily a 5-HT_2 antagonist. However, at higher dosages (6–8 mg/kg) 5-HT_1 agonist activity occurs primarily through the mCPP metabolite (Eison et al., 1990). Thus, in animal and human studies, mCPP has played a useful role in evaluating the clinical effects of 5-HT_1 activation in various psychiatric and pain disorders. Some clinical data indicate that modulation of the serotonergic system can alter symptoms of excessive obsessive–compulsive disorder. Orally administered mCPP in obsessive–compulsive subjects demonstrated an exacerbation of symptoms with worsened anxiety, dysphoria, and depression. However, after 4 months of coadministered clomipramine, mCPP no longer exacerbated OCD symptoms suggesting that clomipramine is able to down-regulate postsynaptic serotonin receptors, such as would be activated by the mCPP pharmacological probe (Kahn and Wetzler, 1991). Inconsistent studies on the efficacy of various tricyclics and selective serotonin-reuptake inhibitors (SSRI) medications in the treatment of OCD suggest that this complex disorder is caused not only by various perturbations of the serotonin system, but may also involve the adrenergic system. Nevertheless, mCPP continues to play a role in understanding the various psychiatric clinical manifestations of 5-HT_{1C} activation. Peripherally administered mCPP will cause anorexia in a decerebrate rat (Kaplan, 1998). This effect is active at caudal brain stem areas. Clinical studies using mCPP in cocaine addicts have shown diminished hostility as a direct consequence of this serotonin agonism (Handelsman, 1998).

Migraine pain studies have incorporated mCPP to address serotonin receptor hyperresponsiveness in these individuals. In humans, a bolus dose of mCPP will cause migraine pain in susceptible individuals as well as alcohol craving in abstinent alcoholics. However, chronic treatment with antidepressant serotinin-reuptake inhibitors suppressed these responses to mCPP, most likely owing to down-regulation of postsynaptic 5-HT_{1C} and 5-HT_2 receptors (Leone, 1998). Thus, serotonin-reuptake inhibitors may play a unique role in down-regulating postsynaptic receptors, resulting in an analgesic benefit that is independent of opiate mechanisms. Coadministration of the selective serotonin-reuptake inhibitor fluvoxamine significantly potentiated analgesia at the κ-3 opioid and to a lesser extent at the μ, δ, and κ-1 opiate receptors in the mouse (Schreiber, 1996). Moreover, nefazodone demonstrated analgesic benefit in mice exposed to hot-plate burn stimuli (Pick, 1992). This effect was independent of opiates. Thus, pain models exploring the role of 5-HT_1 and 5-HT_2 receptor activation through mCPP administration may be useful in explaining behavioral symptoms of panic associated with anxiety and pain, as well as serve as an avenue for further drug development. Indeed, potent blockade at the sites by chemically altered mCPP derivatives could be of significant use in anxiolytic and analgesic settings.

VIII. CONCLUSION

Neurogenic and other pain mechanisms that utilize the NMDA glutamate receptor are found at spinal, supraspinal, and cortical regions. Sustained neuronal firing can be inhibited by NMDA glutamate blockade. These depolarizations may account for various components of neurogenic and possibly nociceptive pain, including allodynia, windup, aftersensation, and radiant pain found in such clinical conditions as diabetic neuropathy and postherpetic neuralgia. These two conditions are the usual settings whereby clinical trials are underway.

Such glutamate-blocking agents as ketamine, memantine, dextromethorphan and CPP alleviate this pain mechanism in human and animal models. Their analgesic benefit is distinctive and perhaps superior to opiates, particularly in neurogenic pain models (Herman, 1995). Indeed, they may serve to lessen dependency on opiate analgesic strategies as well as ameliorate the opiate withdrawal process. Similarly, down-regulation of anxiolytic and nociceptive postsynaptic serotonergic receptors by mCPP may offer a useful adjuvant analgesic role. Thus, these diverse classes of drugs have multiple clinical applications in pain, psychiatry, epilepsy, and neurodegenerative settings, in that disturbances of NMDA and serotonin receptors have been identified at various regions of the nervous system in patients with these disorders.

Moreover, new pharmacological research may identify more NMDA and serotonin receptor subtypes that may possess different functional and pharmacokinetic profiles offering new treatments of improved efficacy and tolerability. These may be used in tandem with selective nitric oxide synthase inhibitors as well as glutamate-depleting and blocking anticonvulsants to limit the nervous system's "learning" of pain in response to peripheral injuries of traumatic, metabolic, infectious, or drug-induced etiologies.

REFERENCES

Anis NA, Berry SC, Burton NR, Lodge D. The dissociative anesthetics ketamine and phencyclidine selectively reduce excitation of central mammalion neurons by methyl-aspartate. Br J Pharmacol 1983; 71:565–875.

Bormann J. Memantine is a potent blocker of NMDA receptor channels. Eur J Pharmacol 1989; 166:591.

Butelman ER. A novel NMDA antagonist, MK 801, impairs performance in a hippocampal dependant spatial learning task. Pharmacol Biochem Behav 1989; 34:13–16.

Carlsson M, Carlsson A. The NMDA antagonist MK-801 causes marked locomotor stimulation in monoamine-depleted mice. J Neurol Transm 1989; 75:221–226.

Cortelmeyer R, Erbler H. Memantine in the treatment of mild to moderate dementia syndrome. A double-blind placebo controlled study. Arzneimittelforschung 1992; 42:904–913.

Cyr M. Nefazodone: its place among antidepressants. Ann Pharmacother 1996; 30:1006–1012.

Davies SN, Lodge D. Evidence for involvement of NMDA receptors in "wind up" of class 2 neurons in the dorsal horn of the rat. Brain Res 1987; 424:402–406.

Dawson VL, Dawson TM. Nitric oxide mediates glutamate neurotoxicity in primary cortical cultures. Proc Natl Acad Sci 1991; 88:6368–6371.

Desarro GB, DeSarro A. Anti-convulsant properties of noncompetitive antagonists of the NMDA receptor in genetically epilepsy-prone rats: comparison with cPPene. Neuropharmacology 1993; 32:51–58.

Dreyer EB, Kaiser PK, Offermann JT, Lipton SA. HIV-1 coat protein neurotoxicity prevented by calcium channel antagonists. Science 1990; 248:364–367.

Eide PK, Jorum E, Stubhaug A. Relief of post herpetic neuralgia with the NMDA receptor antagonist ketamine: a double-blind, cross over comparison with morphine and placebo. Pain 1994; 58:347–354.

Eisenberg E, LaCross S, Strassman A. The effects of the clinically tested NMDA receptor antagonist memantine on the carrageenan-induced thermal hyperalgesia in rats. Eur J Pharmacol 1994; 225: 123–129.

Eison AS, Eison MS, Torrente JR. Nefazodone: pre-clinical pharmacology of a new antidepressant. Psychopharm Bull 1990; 26:311.

Glennon NA. Serotonin receptors: clinical implications. Neurosci Biobehav Rev 1990; 14:35–47.

Gordh T, Karlsten N, Kristensen J. Intervention with spinal NMDA, adrenosine and NO systems for pain modulation. Ann Med 1995; 27:229–234.

Gortemeyer R, Erbles H. Memantine in the treatment of mild to moderate dementia syndrome. A double-blind placebo controlled study. Arzneimittelforschung 1992; 42:904–913.

Handelsman L. Hostility is associated with a heightened prolactin response to MCPP in abstinent cocaine addicts. Psychiatry Res 1998; 80:1–12.

Hargreaves EL, Cain DP. Hyperactivity, hyper-reactivity, and sensorimotor deficits induced by low doses of NMDA non-competitive channel blocker MK801. Behav Brain Res 1992; 47:23.

Herman BH. The effects of NMDA receptor antagonists and nitric oxide synthase inhibitors on opioid tolerance and withdrawal. Neuropsychopharmacology 1995; 13:269–293.

Hottor H, Wasterlain CG. Excitatory amino acids in the developing brain: ontogeny, plasticity, and excitotoxicity. Pediatr Neurol 1990; 6:219.

Ilkjaer S, Dirks J, Brennum J. Effect of systemic NMDA receptor antagonist (dextromethorphan) on primary and secondary hyperalgesia in humans. Br J Anaesth 1997; 79:600–605.

Kahn NS, Wetzler S. mCPP as a probe of serotonin function. Biol Psychiatry 1991; 30:1139–1166.

Kaplan JM. Serotonin receptors in the caudal brainstem are necessary and sufficient for the anorectic effect of peripherally administered mCPP. Psychopharmacology (Berl) 1998; 137:43–49.

Karschin A, Aizenman E, Lipton SA. The interaction of agonists and non-competitive antagonists at the excitatory amino acid receptors in rat, retinal ganglion cells in vitro. J Neuroscience 1988; 8:28895–2906.

Kennett GA, Lightower S, deBrasi V. Effect of chronic administration of selective 5-HT and noradrenaline uptake inhibitors on a putative index of $5HT_{2C}/_{2B}$ receptor function. Neuropharmacology 1994; 22: 1581–1588.

Klaasen T, Ho KL, Westenberg HG. Serotonin syndrome after challenge with the 5-HT agonist metachorophenylpiperazine. Psychiatry Res 1998; 79:207–212.

Kornhuber J, Mack-Burkhardt F, Riederer P, Hebenstreit GF, Reynolds CP, Andrews HB, Beckman H. [^{3}H]MK-801 binding sites in post-mortem brain regions of schizophrenic patients. J Neurol Transm 1989; 77:231–236.

Leone M. 5-HT1a receptor hypersensitivity in migraine is suggested by the mCPP test. Neuroreport 1998; 9:2605–2608.

Lipton S, Gendelman H. Dementia associated with the acquired immunodeficiency syndrome. N Engl J Med 1995; ■:934–940.

Meldrum B, Garthwaite J. Excitatory amino acid neuro-1 toxicity and neurodegenerative disease. Trends Pharmacol Sci 1990; 11:167–172.

Murray CW, Cowan A, Larson AA. Nesokinin and NMDA antagonists (but not a kainic acid antagonist) are anti-nociceptive in the mouse formalin model. Pain 1991; 44:179–185.

Narkai M. The pharmacology of native NMDA receptor subtypes: different receptors control the release of different striatal and spinal transmitters. Prog Neuropsychopharmacol Biol Psychiatry 1998; 22: 35–64.

Nelson EC. An open-label study of nefazodone in the treatment of depression with and without comorbid obsessive compulsive disorder. Ann Clin Psychiatry 1994; 6:249–153.

Nelson KA, Park KM, Rabinovitz E. High dose oral dextromethorphan versus placebo in painful diabetic neuropathy and post-herpetic neuralgia. Neurology 1997; 48:1212–1218.

Noordenbos W. Pain. Amsterdam: Elsevier 1959.

Parsons C, Gruner R. Patch clamp studies on the kinetics and selectivity of NMDA receptor antagonism by memantine. Neuropharmacology 1993; 32:1337–1350.

Pick CG. Potentiation of opioid analgesia by the anti-depressant nefazodone. Eur J Pharmacol 1992; 211: 375–381.

Price D, Mao J, Flaerk H, Mayer D. The NMDA receptor antagonist dextromethrophan selectively reduced temporal summation of second pain in man. Pain 1994; 59:165–174.

Rothman SM, Olney JW. Excitotoxicity and the NMDA receptor. Trends Neurosci 1987; 10:299–302.

Sagratella S. NMDA antagonists: anti-epileptic-neuroprotective drugs with diversified neuro-pharmacological profiles. Pharmacol Res 1995; 32:1–13.

Saxena PN. Serotonin receptors: sub-types, functional responses and therapeutic relevance. Pharmacol Ther 1995; 66:339–369.

Schreiber S. The antinocicepetive effect of fluvoxamine. Eur Neuropsychopharmacol 1996; 6:2810–284.

Sef el Nasir M, Peruche B, et al. Neuroprotective effect of memantine demonstrated in vivo and in vitro. Eur J Pharmacol 1990; 185:19–24.

Stam NJ, Van Huizen F, Van Alebee K. Geromic organization, coding sequence and functional expression of human 5-HT_2 and 5-HT_{1a} receptor genes. Eur J Pharmacol 1992; 227:153–162.

Stannard CF, Porter GE. Ketamine hydrochloride in the treatment of phantom limb pain. Pain 1993; 54: 227–230.

Urban L, Randic M. Slow excitatory transmission in rat dorsal horn: possible mediation by peptides. Brain Res 1984; 290:336–341.

Van Pragg H. The role of glutamate in opiate descending inhibition of nociceptive spinal reflexes. Brain Res 1990; 524:101–105.

Wesemann W, Ekenna O. Efficacy of 1-aminoadamantanes on the MAO activity in brain, liver, and kidney of the rat. Arzneimittelforschung 1982; 32:1241–1243.

Wong CS, Cherng CH, Ho ST. Clinical applications of excitatory amino acid antagonists in pain management. Acta Anaesthesiol Scand 1995; 33:227–232.

47

GV 196771A, a New Glycine Site Antagonist of the NMDA Receptor with Potent Antihyperalgesic Activity

M. Quartaroli, C. Carignani, G. Dal Forno, M. Mugnaini, A. Ugolini, R. Arban, L. Bettelini, D. G. Trist, E. Ratti, R. Di Fabio, and M. Corsi
GlaxoSmithKline S.p.A., Verona, Italy

I. INTRODUCTION

Central sensitization is a condition of enhanced excitability of spinal cord neurons that contributes to the exaggerated pain sensation (hyperalgesia) associated with prolonged tissue or nerve injury. *N*-Methyl-D-aspartate (NMDA) receptors are thought to play a key role in central sensitization. We have tested this hypothesis by characterizing in vitro and in vivo a novel antagonist of the NMDA receptor acting on its glycine site, GV 196771A [*E*-4,6-dichloro-3-(2-oxo-1-phenylpyrrolidin-3-ylidenemethyl)-1*H*-indole-2-carboxylic acid sodium salt]. GV 196771A exhibits an elevated affinity for the NMDA glycine-binding site in rat cerebral cortex membranes ($pK_i = 7.56$). Moreover, GV 196771A competitively and potently antagonizes the activation of NMDA receptors produced by glycine in the presence of NMDA in primary cultures of cortical, spinal, and hippocampal neurons ($pK_B = 7.46$, 8.04, and 7.86, respectively). In isolated baby rat spinal cords, 10 μM GV 196771A depressed windup, an electrical correlate of central sensitization.

The antihyperalgesic properties of GV 196771A were studied in a model of chronic constriction injury (CCI) of the rat sciatic nerve and in the mice formalin test. In the CCI model, GV 196771A (3 mg/kg twice a day p.o.) administered before and then for 10 days after nerve ligature blocked the development of thermal hyperalgesia. Moreover, GV 196771A (1–10 mg/kg, p.o.) reversed the hyperalgesia when tested after the establishment of the CCI-induced hyperalgesia. In the formalin test, GV 196771A (0.1–10 mg/kg p.o.) dose-dependently reduced the duration of the licking time of the late phase. These observations strengthen the view that NMDA receptors play a key role in the events underlying plastic phenomena, including hyperalgesia. Importantly, antagonists of the NMDA glycine site receptor could offer a novel mechanism in the approach to pain control.

Glutamate is the dominant excitatory neurotransmitter of the mammalian central nervous system (CNS). Almost all types of central neurons can be excited by glutamate acting on a variety of ligand-gated ion channels or G protein-coupled (metabotropic) receptors (1–3). Glutamatergic transmission is critically involved in many important events of the CNS, such as synaptic plasticity in the developing and adult brain, as well as neuronal survival and death (4–9).

The glutamate-gated ion channel receptors have been classified in three main categories: those sensitive to the agonist *N*-methyl-D-aspartate (NMDA receptors), those sensitive to the agonist kainate (kainate receptors) and those sensitive to the agonist α-amino-3-hydroxy-5-methylisoxazole-4-propionate (AMPA receptors) (10). Molecular cloning studies have revealed that NMDA receptors are heteromultimeric protein complexes, composed of at least two subunits, $NMDAR_1$ (NR_1) and $NMDAR_2$ (NR_2) (11–13).

Whereas NR_1 exists in several variants generated by alternative splicing from a single gene, four distinct genes are responsible for the expression of NR_{2A}, NR_{2B}, NR_{2C}, and NR_{2D} (1). The NMDA receptor is blocked by external physiological Mg^{2+} at resting membrane potential. Depolarization removes this block, allowing entry of Ca^{2+} that in turn can activate a variety of signal transduction pathways (14,15). As a consequence of this mechanism, NMDA receptors can function as detectors of temporally coincident synaptic inputs to the same neuron. Such a cascade of events is thought to be at the basis of the long-term potentiation (LTP) of synaptic inputs to CA_1 pyramidal neurons in the hippocampus, an event responsible for certain forms of learning (16). However, the crucial role of NMDA-based detectors of coincident activity is not restricted to hippocampal synaptic plasticity. Indeed, evidence is present to support the crucial role of the NMDA receptors in other forms of neuronal plasticity induced by prolonged electrical activity. Peripheral tissue injury or inflammation induces a state of sensory hypersensitivity that manifests itself as allodynia (decreased pain threshold) and hyperalgesia (an increased response to noxious stimuli). This pain hypersensitivity results from both an increase in transduction sensitivity of primary afferent receptors and an increase in the excitability of spinal cord neurons (17). Several lines of investigation have shown the involvement of the glutamatergic system in the development and maintenance of pain hypersensitivity. Iontophoretic applications of glutamate produce a facilitation of responses to low- and high-intensity of mechanical stimulation of the skin (18), whereas an increase in glutamate release has been observed in rat spinal cord after injection of an irritant agent or nerve injury (19,20). Moreover, it appears that the dorsal horn neuronal plasticity and hyperexcitability following tissue injury involves the effect of excitatory amino acids on NMDA receptors. In fact, NMDA antagonists have been shown to suppress formalin-induced pain behavior (21), hyperalgesia induced by chronic constriction injury to the rat sciatic nerve (22,23) and peripheral inflammation (24).

The NMDA receptor is unique because opening of the channel requires the simultaneous binding of glutamate and glycine (25,26). Therefore, the NMDA receptor blockade can also be obtained through the antagonism of the glycine site, which may represent a centerpiece for a novel strategy to explore in vivo the role of NMDA receptors (23,24,27,28). Therefore, to further study the role of NMDA receptors in chronic pain, we have employed a novel, potent and selective antagonist of the glycine site, GV 196771A (*E*-4,6-dichloro-3-(2-oxo-1-phenylpyrrolidin-3-ylidenemethyl)-1*H*-indole-2-carboxylic acid sodium salt) (Fig. 1).

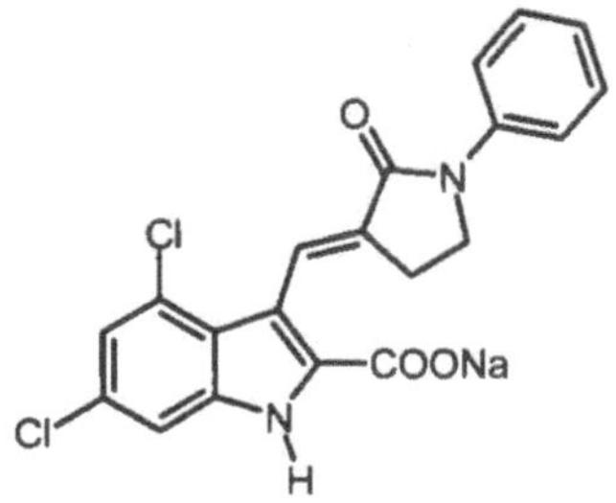

Figure 1 Chemical structure of GV 196771A.

II. MATERIALS AND METHODS

A. Binding Studies

1. Animals and Tissue Preparation

Male Sprague–Dawley rats (200–250 g) were used. Animals were supplied by Charles River (Lecco, Italy) and were allowed food and water until used. Immediately after sacrifice, brains were removed and used for the preparation of cerebral cortex synaptic membranes to be employed in radioligand-binding studies.

The protocols used for the preparation of membranes for [^{3}H]glycine-binding experiments were as described by Mugnaini et al. (29), whereas for [^{3}H]AMPA or [^{3}H]kainic acid experiments were as described by Giberti et al. (30).

For [^{3}H]TCP-binding experiments, extensively washed membranes were prepared, as described by Foster and Wong (31), with some additional modifications to further reduce the presence of endogenous amino acids, as follows: Briefly, the cerebral cortex tissue was homogenized with a Polytron PT-MR 3000. (Littau, Switzerland) in 9 volumes (v/original wet weight) of 0.32-M sucrose and centrifuged at 1000 *g* for 10 min. The supernatant was centrifuged again at 10,000 *g* for 10 min, and the upper "buffy coat" of the resulting pellet was collected and frozen in liquid N_2 for approximately 30 s. After thawing at room temperature and resuspension in 20 volumes of MilliQ water (MilliQ ultra-pure water system; Millipore, France) the suspension was sonicated for 30 s (model 300 sonic dismembrator; Fisher, Milano, Italy) and centrifuged at 50,000 *g* for 20 min. The last three steps were repeated three more times, with the addition of an incubation at 25°C for 20 min before the last centrifugation. The final pellet was resuspended in 10 volumes of MilliQ water and dialyzed (D0655 dialysis tubing; Sigma, St. Louis, MO) against 5 L of Tris/HCl 5 mM (pH 7.7) for 72 h, with the dialysis buffer refreshed every day. Finally, membranes were centrifuged at 50,000 *g* for 20 min and the pellet was resuspended in 3 volumes of MilliQ water, aliquoted, frozen in liquid N_2 and conserved at −80°C until the day of the experiment. Only laboratory glassware previously treated at high temperature (250°C) for more than 4 h or treated with 1 M HCl and then extensively washed with fresh MilliQ water was used throughout the preparation procedure.

[^{3}H]Glycine-Binding Assay. Displacement experiments with [^{3}H]glycine were performed, as described by Mugnaini et al. (29). GV196771A was dissolved in DMSO at 5 mM and tested at seven concentrations in duplicate (0.1 nM–100 μM) in five separate experiments.

Antagonism of the Glycine-Induced [^{3}H]TCP Binding Enhancement. [^{3}H]TCP (1-[1-(2-thienyl)cyclohexyl] piperidine)-binding experiments were performed as follows: To minimize glycine contamination all steps were performed in laboratory glassware previously treated at high-temperature (250°C) for more than 4 h or treated with 1 M HCl and then extensively washed with fresh MilliQ water. Briefly, on the day of the experiment, rat cerebral cortex membranes were homogenized in 20 volumes of 5 mM of Tris/HCl (pH 7.7) and centrifuged at 48,000 *g* for 15 min. Pellets were then given four cycles of washing, each cycle consisting of resuspending the membranes in 20 volumes of buffer, incubating at 25°C for 20 min and centrifuging at 48,000 *g* for 15 min. Glycine concentration–response curves (CRC) at enhancing [^{3}H]TCP binding were obtained in the presence of increasing concentration of GV 196771A and 1 μM glutamic acid. Final pellets were resuspended in 30 volumes of buffer, and [^{3}H]TCP binding was performed in a final volume of 1000 μL containing: 180 μL of buffer, 100 μL of buffer with 1 μM glutamic acid (final concentration), 20 μL of buffer containing increasing concentrations of glycine (from 0.1 nM–100 μM final concentration, including intermediate concentrations), 100 μL of buffer with 10 time, the final desired concentration of GV 196771A, 100 μL of buffer with the radioligand ([^{3}H]TCP at a final concentration of 2.5 nM) and 500 μL of final membrane suspension. The reaction was allowed to proceed for 2 h at 30°C and then stopped by filtration through fiberglass filters (GF/C, Whatman International; Maidstone, UK) on a Brandel M48R cell harvester (Brandel, Gaithersburg, MD), followed by rapid washing of the filters two times with 3 mL ice-cold buffer. Filters were collected in polyethylene vials (Biovials; Beckman) to which 3.5 mL of scintillation fluid (Filter Count, Packard Instruments) were added. The vials were capped, shaken, and counted in a Packard TRI-CARB 1900 CA liquid scintillation analyzer. CRC to glycine in the absence (control) or presence of antagonist (0.3, 1, and 3 μM GV 196771A) were simultaneously obtained in the same experiment with each incubation performed in triplicate.

[^{3}H]AMPA and [^{3}H]Kainic Acid-Binding Assay. Displacement experiments with [^{3}H]AMPA were performed essentially as previously described (30). [^{3}H]Kainic acid-displacement experiments were performed as follows: Membranes for [^{3}H]kainic acid-binding assay were incubated (60 min, 4°C) in tris/acetate 50 mM (pH 7.10) with 2 nM radioligand. The reaction was stopped by dilution with ice-cold buffer solution and filtration, as indicated for the [^{3}H]TCP-binding assay.

GV 196771A was dissolved in DMSO at 5 mM and tested at five concentrations in duplicate (10 nM–100μM); glutamic acid, at six concentrations in duplicate (1 nM–100 μM), was the reference compound tested as a positive control.

2. Data Analysis for Binding Experiments

Data of [^{3}H]glycine and [^{3}H]kainic acid displacement experiments were analyzed using the nonlinear curve-fitting program LIGAND (32) to determine the inhibition constants of displacer ligands (K_i); the required K_D values of the radioligands were set to 177 nM and 2.19 nM, as previously determined in saturation studies with [^{3}H]glycine and [^{3}H]kainic acid, respectively (data not shown). Given the ability of [^{3}H]AMPA to label two populations of binding sites in the conditions employed in this study (30), and the consequent complexity of estimation of K_i values, data of [^{3}H]AMPA displacement experiments were analyzed using ALLFIT (33), and only the concentration of displacer ligands inhibiting 50% of [^{3}H]AMPA-specific binding (IC_{50}) were estimated. K_i and IC_{50} values have been expressed as pK_i ($-\log K_i$) and pIC_{50} ($-\log IC_{50}$) ±SEM. In [^{3}H]TCP-binding experiments, CRCs to glycine in the presence of increasing concentrations of GV 196771A were simultaneously fitted to Eq. (1)

$$[^3\text{H}]\text{TCP binding} = \frac{[A]^n R_{max}}{[A]^n + ([\text{EC}_{50}](1 + [B]^m/K)^n} \tag{1}$$

Glycine-induced [^{3}H]TCP binding, is equal to total [^{3}H]TCP binding minus basal binding, where $[A]$ is the concentration of agonist; R_{max} is the maximal glycine-induced [^{3}H]TCP binding; EC_{50} is the agonist concentration capable of producing 50% of maximal response; n is the Hill slope factor of the glycine concentration–response curves; $[B]$ is the concentration of antagonist; m is the "Schild plot" slope parameter (34); and K is a parameter that measures the potency of the antagonist and corresponds to the apparent equilibrium dissociation constant of the antagonist (K_B) when $m = 1$. Curves were first fitted to the foregoing general model, allowing the parameter m to be estimated. Subsequently, if the estimated m parameter was not significantly different from unity, data were refitted with the model in which m was constrained to unity and, therefore, a K_B value could be estimated. The K_B value has been expressed as pK_B ($-\log K_B$), followed by 95% confidence limits. Calculations were performed with the data manipulation and analysis software RS1 (Bolt, Beranek, and Newman, Boston, MA).

3. Drugs and Solutions for Binding Experiments

[^{3}H]Glycine (NET 004, specific radioactivity 1620.6 GBq/mmol); [^{3}H]AMPA (NET 833, specific radioactivity 1961.0 GBq/mmol); [^{3}H]kainic acid (NET 875, specific radioactivity 2146.0

GBq/mmol); and [^{3}H]TCP (NET 886, specific radioactivity 1835.2 GBq/mmol) were from Du-Pont New England Nuclear (Boston, MA). GV 196771A was synthesized by the Medicinal Chemistry department of Glaxo Wellcome S.p.A, Verona. Glycine, glutamate, and various salts were from Sigma Chemical Co. (St. Louis, MO). All salts and reagents were of the highest analytical grade available.

B. Electrophysiological Recordings

We have employed the whole-cell patch-clamp–recording technique to measure macroscopic currents. The preparations used included primary cultures of rat embryonic neurons. Moreover, in parallel experiments, we have used extracellular recordings from the ventral root of isolated baby rat spinal cords to measure spinal cord windup.

1. Culture of Cortical, Hippocampal, and Spinal Cord Neurons

Cortical, hippocampal, and spinal cord neurons were prepared as previously described (35–37).

2. Isolation of Rat Neonatal Spinal Cords

Spinal cord samples were prepared from 4- to 10-day-old Sprague Dawley rats (Charles River), as described by Thompson et al. (38).

3. Electrical Recordings

Whole-cell patch-clamp recordings (39) were performed on cultured neurons after 1 week. The extracellular solution contained (mM): NaCl 140, KCl 5, $CaCl_2$ 1, HEPES 10, glucose 10, pH adjusted to 7.4. Tetrodotoxin (0.1 μM) was used to block spontaneous activity. The intracellular (pipette) solution contained (mM): CsCl 140, EGTA 11, $MgCl_2$ 4, Mg-ATP 2, HEPES 10, pH adjusted to 7.3. The recording chamber was placed on the stage of an inverted microscope and continuously superfused by gravity with the extracellular solution containing glycine and GV 196771A at the specified concentrations. Test NMDA solution was applied rapidly with the "U-tube" method, positioning the ejection hole within 100–200 μm of the cell. The cells were voltage-clamped at −60 mV. Only cells having a resting potential more negative than −40 mV were used. Currents were digitized (100 Hz), low-pass–filtered (40 Hz), and stored on-line using an IBM-compatible PC running pClamp (Axon Instruments, Foster City, CA).

Spinal windup was studied as follows: Closely fitting glass suction electrodes filled with Krebs solution were used for both stimulation and recording from dorsal and ventral roots, respectively (levels L4 or L5). For stimulation, an analogical stimulator (Grass Instruments, Quincy, MA) controlled by a personal computer (PC; see later) and coupled to a standard stimulus isolation unit (SIU; Grass Instruments) was used. For recording of the ventral root potential (VRP), an AXOPROBE-1A (Axon Instruments) was employed. The resulting signal was filtered at 0.2 kHz, digitized at 1 kHz using a TL-1 interface (Axon Instruments), and finally stored on PC hard disk. For stimulation, simultaneous data acquisition as well as off-line data analysis a personal computer employing custom-made software written in Axobasic (Axon Instruments) was used. Recruitment of the nociceptive afferent fibers (C-/group IV) in the dorsal root was achieved by applying rectangular electrical pulses with an amplitude of 50 V and a duration of 1 ms (38,40). Short trains (20 s; 1 Hz) of this type of stimuli produced cumulative synaptic responses from the corresponding ventral root, a phenomenon called *windup* (41). During the course of the experiment, the windup was evoked every 3 min. At least 1 h of recording in basal conditions (20 trains; aerated Krebs solution only) was allowed in each preparation, to test whether the windup remained stable. Subsequently, dimethyl sulfoxide (DMSO; 0.1%, the largest concentration employed in windup experiments; see following) was added to the Krebs solution used for the superfusion, and the windup recorded for another 30-min period. Only preparations with a stable level of windup during superfusion with both Krebs and DMSO in Krebs solutions were used. GV 196771A, D-AP5, or morphine were dissolved in ACSF from stock solution and superfused into the recording chamber at the same flow rate as control ACSF.

4. Data Analysis for Electrophysiology

Current amplitude was measured and analyzed with custom-made analysis software written in Axobasic (Axon Instruments). All current measurements, unless otherwise stated, refer to the steady-state value of the responses (Iss) and are the average of the last 3–4 s of agonist application. For the generation of the agonist CRC, values were expressed as a percentage and normalized to the maximal effect. Glycine CRCs were obtained in the presence of 100 μM NMDA, whereas NMDA CRCs were obtained in the presence of 3 or 10 μM glycine (as indicated). Data were fitted to Eq. (2), to estimate the response at the steady state:

$$I_{ss} = I_{min} + \frac{(I_{max} - I_{min})[A]^n}{[EC_{50}]^n + [A]^n} \tag{2}$$

where I_{min} is the response obtained in the absence of added agonist, I_{max} is the maximal response, $[A]$ is the agonist concentration, $[EC_{50}]$ is the agonist concentration that gives 50% of the maximal response and n is the Hill slope factor.

The effect of GV 196771A was measured using the maximal response to NMDA and glycine. Then, data were fitted to Eq. (3):

$$I_{ss} = I_{bmax} + \frac{(100 - I_{bmax})}{1 + ([B]/IC_{50})^n} \tag{3}$$

where I_{bmax} is the maximal inhibitory effect produced by the antagonist $[B]$, IC_{50} is the concentration of the antagonist that produces half-maximal inhibition, and n is the slope factor. Then, the equilibrium dissociation constant of the antagonist receptor complex (apparent K_B) was determined by using the Leff-Dougall (42) generalized form of the Cheng-Prusoff equation:

$$K_B = \frac{IC_{50}}{[2 + [A]/EC_{50})^{1/n} - 1} \tag{4}$$

where IC_{50} is as defined before, $[A]$ is the concentration of glycine used, $[EC_{50}]$ is its concentration that induces 50% of the maximal response and n is the Hill slope factor of the glycine CRC. All data are presented as mean ± SEM followed by the number of replications (n): pEC_{50} ($-\log EC_{50}$); pIC_{50} ($-\log IC_{50}$); and pK_B ($-\log$ apparent K_B) values are given followed by 95% confidence interval (95% CL).

5. Drug and Solution for Electrophysiological Studies

Morphine hydrochloride, NMDA, and glycine were purchased from Sigma, whereas L-AP5 from TOCRIS (Langford, UK). GV 196771A was stored at 10 mM either in a solution of 50% DMSO–50% distilled water (patch-clamp experiments), or 100% DMSO (windup experiments). The maximal concentration of DMSO present in the final solutions was 0.5% for patch-clamp experiments, and 0.1% for windup experiments. At these concentrations DMSO did not affect the measured responses.

C. Behavioral Studies

1. Effect of GV 196771A on Thermal Hyperalgesia in a Rat Model of Painful Mononeuropathy: Chronic Constriction Injury Model (CCI)

Male Sprague–Dawley rats (Charles River) weighing 200–300 g were used. Animals were housed in groups of two or three and fed with chow pellet diet with free access to water. They were fasted overnight before beginning the study and were allowed free access to water. Rats were anesthetized with pentobarbital sodium (50 mg/kg i.p.). The left common sciatic nerve was exposed, and proximal to the sciatic trifurcation, about 10 mm of nerve was freed of adhering tissue and four ligatures (3.0 chromic gut) were tied loosely around it, with about 1-mm spacing (43). Rats were tested for thermal hyperalgesia using a commercially available analgesimeter (Plantar test, Ugo Basile, Comerio, Italy) by applying a heat stimulus (50 W, 8 V) directed onto the plantar surface of each hindpaw and the paw withdrawal latency (s) was determined. Four latency measurements were taken for each hindpaw and averaged. The results were expressed as difference scores (DS) by subtracting the latency of the control side from the latency of the ligated side. Negative DSs indicated a lower threshold on the ligated side, supporting a hyperalgesic state. The animals developed thermal hyperalgesia within 14–21 days after surgery.

Two different protocols were followed:

1. *Prophylactic treatment*: GV 196771A (6 mg/kg) or vehicle was administered orally to animals on the day of surgery, at a dose volume of 10 ml/kg. Then, postoperatively 3 mg/kg GV 196771A or vehicle was administered twice a day for 10 days. Hyperalgesia was measured on days 0, 3, 9, 14, 21, and 30.
2. *Therapeutic treatment*: GV 196771A (1–10 mg/kg) or vehicle was administered orally to animals on days 14 or 21 after ligation, and the hyperalgesia was tested 1, 4, and 8 h after treatment.

2. Effect of GV 196771A on Pain Behavior in the Mouse Paw Formalin Test

Male albino CD mice (Charles River) weighing 25–30 g were used. Animals were housed in groups of five or six and fed with chow pellet diet with free access to water. They were fasted overnight before the study and were allowed free access to water.

The protocol used in this study is a modification of the method described by Dubuisson and Dennis (44). Before the formalin injection, mice were placed individually into clear Perspex cages, which serve as observation chambers. After 15 min of adaptation to the cage, 20 μL of 1% formalin was injected into the plantar surface of the left hindpaw. The amount of time, in seconds, that the animals spent licking the injected paw for the first 5 min (early phase; EP) and then from 20 to 60 min (late phase; LP) after formalin was used as measurement of the intensity of pain. GV 196771A (0.1–10 mg/kg, p.o.), or vehicle (0.5% Methocel) was administered in a dose volume of 10 mL/kg 1 h before formalin injection for GV 196771A. Five to ten animals for each group were used.

3. Effect of GV 196771A on Acute Inflammatory Pain Induced by Carrageenan

Carrageenan (100 mL; 2%) was injected intraplantar into the left hindpaw. Three hours later, the rats were tested for the development of thermal hyperalgesia, which was assessed as described by Hargreaves et al. (45) by using a commercially available analgesia meter (Plantar test, Ugo Basile). Thermal paw-flick latency (in seconds) was determined by focusing a heat beam (50 W, 8 V) on the plantar surface of the hindpaw of freely moving rats, in Perspex boxes. Four measurements were taken for each hindpaw and averaged. GV 196771A (0.3–10 mg/kg) or vehicle (0.5% Methocel) were administered orally in a dose volume of 10 mL/kg 30 min before carrageenan administration. Seven to twenty-two animals for each group were used.

4. Statistical Analysis for Behavioral Studies

For all experiments the data are expressed as mean ± SEM.

CCI Test: Prophylactic Treatment. Statistical analysis was performed within each group to compare DS calculated at each time point following ligation versus basal values before surgery. In addition, the time course of DS of the vehicle-treated group was compared with that of the GV 196771A-treated group. ANOVA one-way analysis followed by Dunnett's test, for which $p < 0.05$ was considered significant, were used.

CCI Test. Therapeutic Treatment. Statistical analysis was performed to compare DS of control response (vehicle) and GV 196771A-treated groups, taken at various times after administration, versus pretreatment values, using ANOVA one-way analysis followed by Dunnett's test, for which $p < 0.05$ was considered significant. Dose–response curve regression analysis was then performed to evaluate regression line parameters to calculate the ED_{50} (dose of GV 196771A in milligrams per kilogram, that reduced the thermal hyperalgesia by 50%).

Formalin Test. Statistical analysis was performed to compare control response (vehicle) with test response using ANOVA one-way analysis followed by Dunnett's test, for which $p < 0.05$ was considered significant. Dose–response curve regression analysis was then performed to evaluate regression line parameters to calculate the ED_{50} (dose of GV 196771A in milligrams per kilogram, that reduced the licking time by 50%).

Carrageenan Test. Statistical analysis was performed to compare control response (vehicle) with test response using ANOVA one-way analysis followed by Dunnett test, for which $p < 0.05$ was considered significant. Dose–response curve regression analysis was then performed to evaluate regression line parameters to calculate the ED_{50} (dose of GV 196771A, in milligrams per kilogram, that reduced the thermal hyperalgesia by 50%).

5. Drugs and Solutions for Behavioral Studies

GV 196771A was prepared as a stock solution of 1 mg/mL in 0.5% methylcellulose (Methocel); further dilutions were prepared in 0.5% Methocel.

III. RESULTS

A. Binding Experiments

1. [^{3}H]Glycine

To characterize GV 196771A as a glycine site antagonist, we studied its effects on the binding of glycine in rat cerebral cortex membranes; GV 196771A inhibited [^{3}H]glycine binding in a concentration-dependent fashion. Moreover, GV 196771A was able to completely suppress the specific binding of glycine (Fig. 2A). The resulting pK_i was 7.56 ± 0.09 (n = 5).

2. [^{3}H]TCP

Because TCP binds to only open NMDA receptors, labeled TCP can be used to measure the fraction of open channels independently from electrophysiological methods. In agreement with its expected behavior, very low specific [^{3}H]TCP binding to rat cerebral cortex membranes was observed in the absence of glycine and glutamate. After addition of glutamic acid (1 μM), increasing concentrations of glycine (0.1 nM–100 μM) progressively enhanced [^{3}H]TCP binding

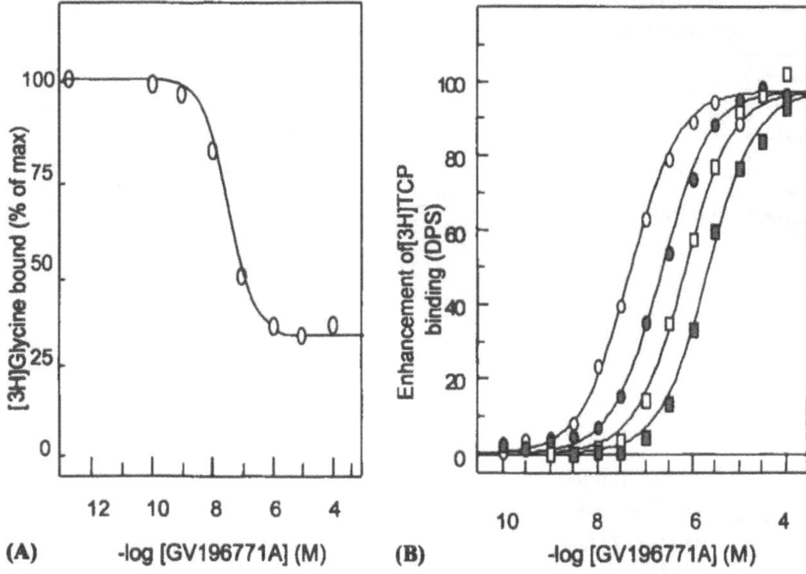

Figure 2 (A) Displacement binding curve of [^{3}H]glycine by GV 196771A in rat cortical membranes. (B) Antagonism of GV 196771A against glycine-induced enhancement of [^{3}H]TCP binding: control (○); GV 196771A, 0.3 μM (●); GV 196771A, 1 μM (□); and GV 196771A 3 μM (■). In [^{3}H]TCP-binding experiments a concentration of 1 μM glutamic acid was used.

until it reached a maximum. The glycine CRC had an estimated pEC_{50} of 7.32 (7.27–7.39; 95% CL). The action of GV 196771A was examined on TCP binding. In the presence of increasing concentrations of GV 196771A (0.3–3 μM), parallel rightward shifts of the glycine CRC could be observed (see Fig. 2B) with no significant depression of the maximal response. The Shild slope factor was not significantly different from unity (m = 1.09; 0.99–1.19; 95% CL), and a pK_B value of 7.13 (7.06–7.21; 95% CL) was estimated.

3. [^{3}H]AMPA and [^{3}H]Kainic Acid

GV 196771A did not displace [^{3}H]AMPA binding up to a concentration of 10 μM. Therefore, a pIC_{50} of less than 4 could be inferred for GV 196771A. In the same experiments, glutamic acid dose-dependently inhibited [^{3}H]AMPA binding with an estimated pIC_{50} of 6.64, in line with previous determinations (30).

Similarly, GV 196771A did not displace [^{3}H]kainic acid binding up to 1 μM. At 100 μM, 60% inhibition of specific [^{3}H]kainic acid binding was observed. A pK_I of 4.47 was calculated for GV 196771A, whereas, in the same experiment, a pK_I of 7.24 was obtained for glutamic acid.

B. Electrophysiological Recordings

1. GV 196771A Antagonizes NMDA- and Glycine-Induced Currents in Embryonic Rat Neurons

Because the NMDA receptor regulates the gating of an intrinsic ion channel, one can quantitatively study the effect of GV 196771A by measuring the currents flowing through this channel. In the primary cultures of cortical, hippocampal, and spinal neurons, NMDA (1–300 μM) and

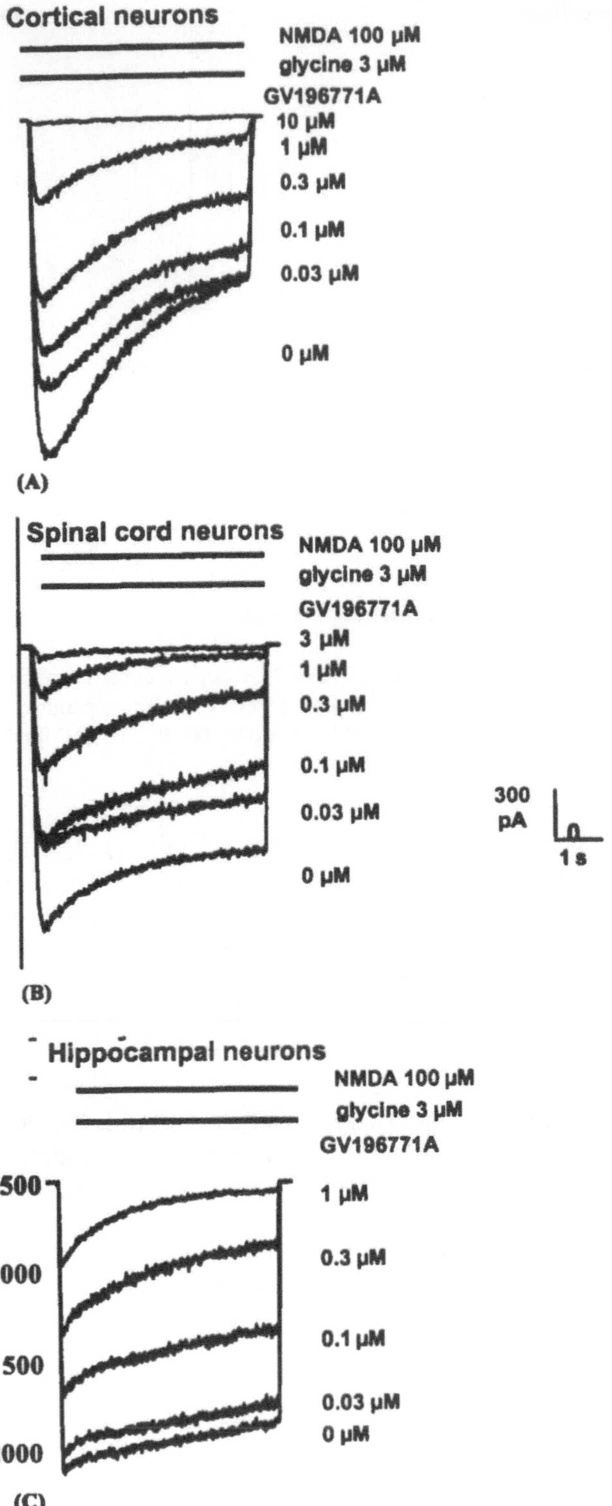

Figure 3 Trace recordings of NMDA (100 μM), glycine (3 μM)-induced currents from (A) rat cortical, (B) spinal cord, and (C) hippocampal neurons from embryonic rat. The concentrations of GV 196771A are described in the figure.

Table 1 pEC_{50}s (95% CL), Hill Slope Factors (*n*) for NMDA and Glycine, CRCs and pIC_{50} and pK_B Values (95% CL) for GV 196771A in Cortex, Spinal Cord, and Hippocampal Neurons from Embryonic Rat

	NMDA pEC_{50} (*n*)	Glycine pEC_{50} (*n*)	GV 196771A pIC_{50}	GV 196771A pK_B
Cortex	4.96 (4.89–5.04)	6.73 (6.57–6.98)	6.26	7.47
	1.4	1.1	(6.15–6.40)	(7.36–7.61)
Spinal cord	4.90 (4.86–4.95)	6.61 (6.50–6.77)	6.98	8.05
	1.7	1.4	(6.84–7.19)	(7.91–8.26)
Hippocampus	4.97 (4.85–5.15)	6.64 (6.57–6.72)	6.76	7.86
	1.7	1.3	(6.69–6.84)	(7.79–7.94)

glycine (10 nM–10 μM) induced currents in a concentration-dependent manner only in the presence of both agonists. Currents were characterized by the presence of two phases: a transient and a sustained phase (Fig. 3A–C). NMDA and glycine-activated currents were measured at steady state, and data were transformed into CRC. The agonist pEC_{50} and slope values are reported in Table 1.

The NMDA and glycine-activated currents were completely inhibited by GV 196771A (0.01–10 μM) in all three preparations (Fig. 4A). The estimated pIC_{50}, and the corresponded pK_Bs are reported in Table 1. The antagonism shown by GV 196771A appeared to be competitive because 1 μM of the compound shifted the glycine CRC to the right (in the presence of 100 μM NMDA) without modifying the agonist maximum response (see Fig. 4B). On the other hand, GV 196771A 1 μM (n = 5–6) showed an insurmountable antagonism of NMDA CRC obtained in the presence of glycine 10 μM (see Fig. 4C).

2. Suppression of Spinal Cord Windup by GV 196771A

The superfusion of isolated spinal cords with GV 196771A at 10 μM attenuated the amplitude of the "windup" (Fig. 5A; $n = 6$). On average, the windup was reduced by 25.5 ± 2% relative to controls. In parallel experiments, we confirmed that, in the same preparation, morphine (n = 2) or D-AP5 (n = 3) suppressed the windup (see Fig. 5B and C).

C. Antihyperalgesic Activity of GV 196771A

1. GV 196771A Reduces Thermal Hyperalgesia in CCI Model

Prophylactic Treatment. Before surgery, no significant difference between left and right thermally induced paw withdrawal latencies was detected in either vehicle-treated (mean ± SEM: 10.56 ± 0.51 s vs. 10.47 ± 0.52 s) or GV 196771A-treated (mean ± SEM: 10.60 ± 0.36 s vs. 10.48 ± 0.32 s) groups.

Following surgery, the vehicle-treated group showed a decrease in thermally induced paw withdrawal latency in the ligated paw. DSs were negative and significantly different ($p < 0.05$) from preoperative values from day 14 to day 30 after surgery (mean ± SEM: −1.33 ± 0.19; −1.44 ± 0.18 and −1.23 ± 0.49 on days 14, 21, and 30, respectively vs. 0.09 ± 0.18 on day 0), (Fig. 6A). The thermally induced paw withdrawal latency of the nonligated paw remained unchanged during the whole experiment (see Fig. 6B).

In GV 196771A-treated animals, a reduction in the latency of the operated on paw was observed during the whole experiment. However, DSs were not significantly different from

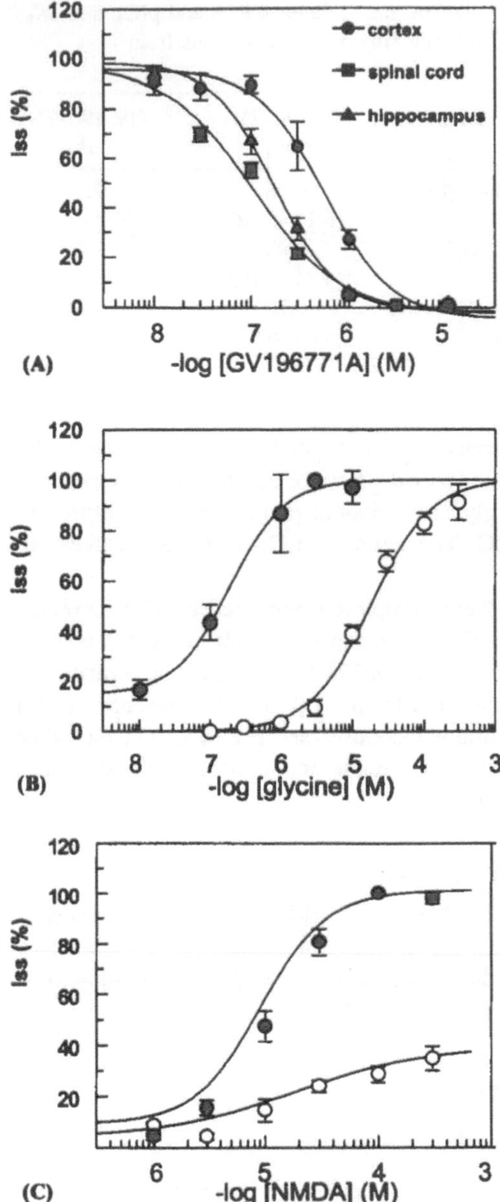

Figure 4 (A) Inhibitory effect of GV 196771A in rat cortical (●), spinal cord (■), and hippocampal (▲) neurons from embryonic rat. (B) CRC to a maximal concentration of NMDA (100 μM) in the presence of increasing concentrations of glycine. (C) CRC to a maximal concentration of glycine (10 μM) in the presence of increasing concentrations of NMDA. GV 196771A at 1 μM (○) antagonized in a competitive manner the glycine CRC (●; B) and in a noncompetitive way the NMDA CRC (●; C).

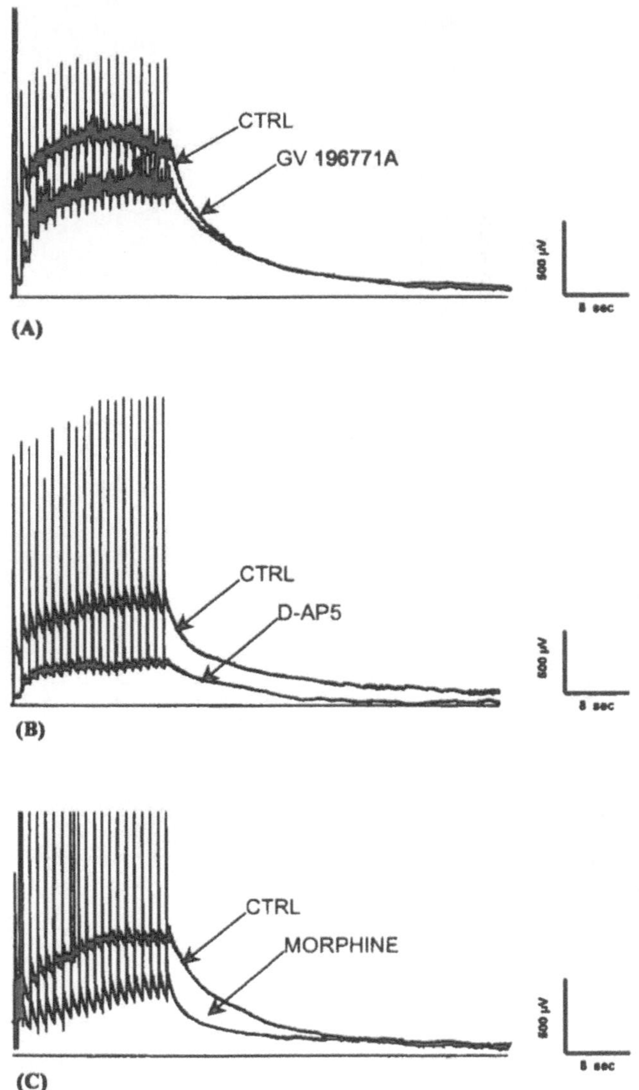

Figure 5 Suppressions of spinal cord windup by GV 196771A, morphine, and D-AP5: (A) effect of 1-h superfusion with GV 196771A (10 µM) dissolved in DMSO-containing (0.1%) Kerbs solution; (B) effect of a 20-min superfusion with D-AP5 (50 µM); (C) effect of a 30-min superfusion with morphine (3 M). Each panel shows two superimposed voltage records obtained from the same preparation before (*CTRL*) and during superfusion of the compounds indicated.

preoperative values (mean ± SEM: −0.64 ± 0.42; −0.98 ± 0.26; −0.64 ± 0.15; −0.58 ± 0.66; and −0.98 ± 0.24 on days 3, 9, 14, 21, and 30, respectively, vs. 0.12 ± 0.20 on day 0), (see Fig. 6A). Furthermore, DSs at days 14 and 21 in the GV 196771A-treated group were significantly lower ($p < 0.05$) compared with vehicle-treated animals at the same days, showing a complete protection from the development of the thermal hyperalgesia (see Fig. 6A).

In GV 196771A-treated animals, the thermally induced paw withdrawal latency of the nonligated paw remained unchanged during the whole experiment (see Fig. 6B).

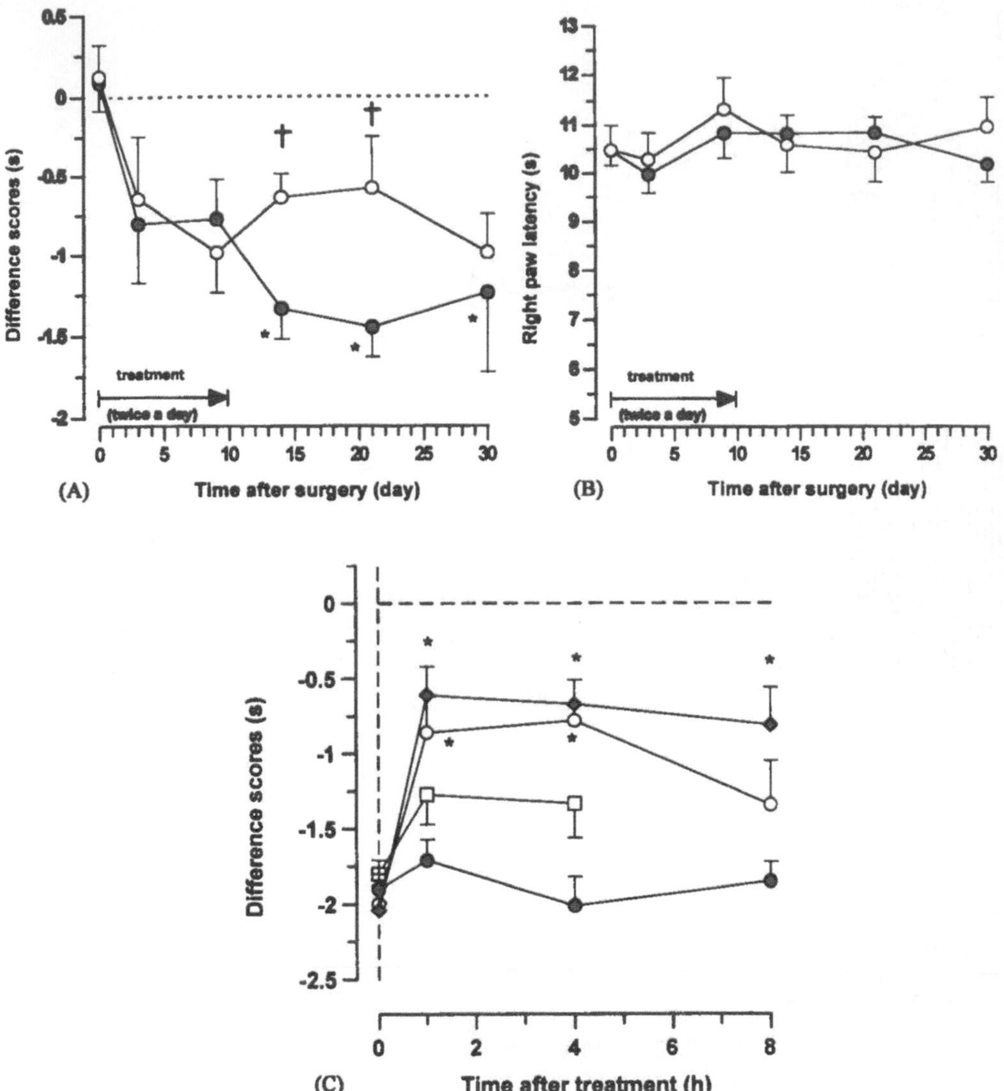

Figure 6 (A) Time course of thermal hyperalgesia after sciatic nerve ligation: In the vehicle-treated group (●; $n = 8$), DSs from day 14 to day 30 after surgery were negative and significantly different relative to the preoperative value (day 0; * denotes $p < 0.05$ vs. basal value). In the GV 196771A-treated group (3 mg/kg p.o.; ○ $n = 9$), no significant variation in DSs was observed during the whole experiment. Moreover, in GV 196771A-treated animals, DSs were significantly lower on days 14–21, compared with vehicle-treated animals († denotes $p < 0.05$ vs. vehicle-treated group. (B) Time course of the thermal hyperalgesia in the nonligated right paws. The graphs illustrate withdrawal latencies of the nonligated paws in prophylactically treated animals; no significant variations in either vehicle (●; $n = 8$) or GV 196771A groups (3 mg/kg p.o.; ○; $n = 9$) relative to the basal values (day 0) were observed during the whole experiment. (C) GV 196771A produces a decrease of thermal paw withdrawal latency in the therapeutic treatment. Control (●), GV 196771A at 1 (□), 3 (○), and 10 mg/kg, p.o. (◆); GV 196771A at 3 and 10 mg/kg reverses the thermal hyperalgesia at 1, 4, and 8 h after drug treatment (* denotes $p < 0.05$; $n = 6$–16 for each group).

Table 2 Percentage of Reduction of Thermal Hyperalgesia Measured 1, 4 and 8 h After Oral Treatment with GV 196771A in Neuropathic Rats (mean ± SEM)

Dose (mg/kg)	1 h (%)	4 h (%)	8 h (%)
1	31.1 ± 11	26.1 ± 12.7	ND
3	57 ± 12 (*)	61 ± 13.5 (*)	33 ± 14.5
10	71 ± 9.3 (*)	67.2 ± 7.8 (*)	60.3 ± 12.2 (*)

* $p < 0.05$; ND not determined.

Therapeutic Treatment. GV 196771A (1–10 mg/kg, p.o.) produced a dose-related reversal of thermal hyperalgesia by increasing the latency of the ligated paw. At 3 and 10 mg/kg, the reduction of thermal hyperalgesia was significant ($p < 0.05$), whereas it was not at 1 mg/kg p.o. (see Fig. 6C; Table 2). By measuring the analgesic effect at 1 h after treatment, an ED_{50} of 2.95 (1.50–8.44) mg/kg was calculated.

2. GV 196771A Reduces Pain Behavior in the Mouse Paw Formalin Test

In the vehicle-treated group, subcutaneous injection of formalin induced marked spontaneous nociceptive behaviors. The values of total licking time measured during the EP and the LP were 125.5 ± 7.2 s and 317.3 ± 42.8 s, respectively (Fig. 7).

GV 196771A (0.1–10 mg/kg p.o.) had no effect on the EP at all doses tested (see Fig. 7: left panel). On the other hand, a dose-related inhibition of the LP response was observed (amount of licking in seconds): 187.7 ± 38.9 at 0.1 mg/kg; 205.8 ± 42.2 at 0.3 mg/kg; 154.4 ± 24.4 at 1 mg/kg; 111.8 ± 25 at 3 mg/kg; 61.9 ± 10 at 10 mg/kg (see Fig. 7: right panel). The effects of GV 196771A were significant ($p < 0.05$) at 0.1, 1, 3, and 10 mg/kg. The calculated ED_{50} value was 0.6 (0.1–2.1) mg/kg p.o. No overt behavioral changes were observed at any dose tested.

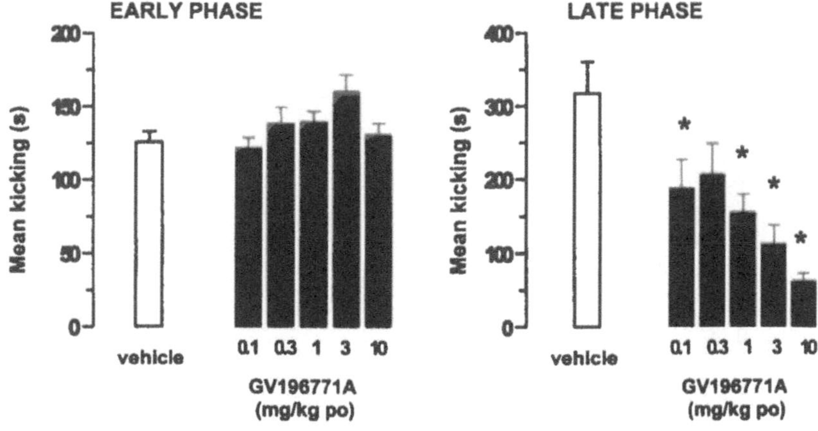

Figure 7 GV 196771A (0.1–10 mg/kg p.o.) produces inhibition of the LP of the formalin test in mice: $n = 7–19$ for each group; * denotes $p < 0.05$ vs. vehicle.

Table 3 Withdrawal Latencies (WL) of Carrageenan-Injected and Noninjected Paws in Rats Treated with Methocel 0.5% or GV 196771A (Mean ± SEM)

Treatment (mg/kg, p.o.)	WL Ipsilateral paw (s)	WL Contralateral paw (s)
Methocel 0.5%	6.13 ± 0.50	11.84 ± 0.27
GV 0.3	6.92 ± 0.74	11.39 ± 0.21
GV 1	7.97 ± 0.78 (*)	11.64 ± 0.28
GV 3	9.52 ± 0.70 (*)	11.82 ± 0.44
GV 10	8.32 ± 0.46 (*)	11.30 ± 0.27

* $p < 0.05$ vs. Methocel.

3. GV 196771A Reduces Acute Inflammatory Pain Induced by Carrageenan

In control animals, a decrease in thermal paw withdrawal latency was observed 3 h after application of intraplantar carrageenan into the inflamed (ipsilateral) paw, compared with the noninflamed (contralateral) paw (Table 3).

GV (0.3–10 mg/kg, p.o.) reduced thermal hyperalgesia in the inflamed paw without affecting the withdrawal latency of the contralateral, noninflamed paw (see Table 3). The effect was significant ($p < 0.05$) at 1, 3, and 10 mg/kg; the maximal response was reached at 3 mg/kg (59.7 ± 8.2% of suppression thermal hyperalgesia) (Fig. 8), and an ED_{50} of 2.3 (0.9–4.9) mg/kg was estimated.

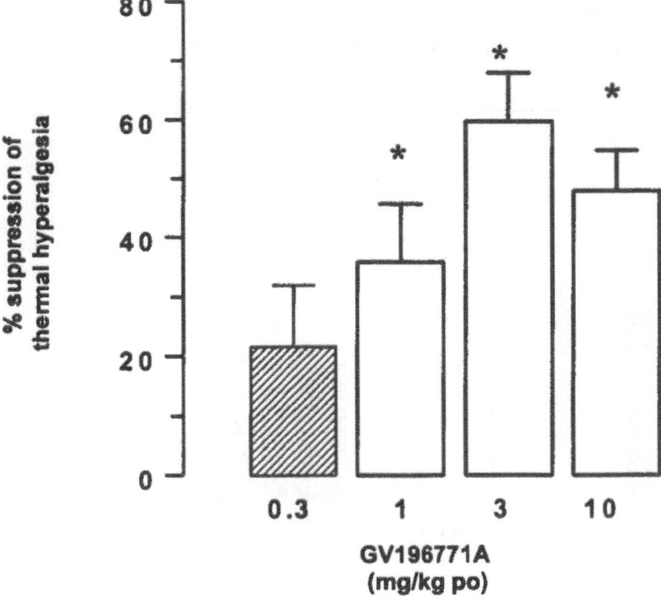

Figure 8 GV 196771A (0.3–10 mg/kg, p.o.) produces a dose-related suppression of thermal hyperalgesia following intraplantar injection of carrageenan: $n = 7–22$ for each group; * denotes $p < 0.05$.

IV. DISCUSSION

It is suggested that, in persistent pain, hyperalgesia and allodynia are the consequence of the prolonged stimulation of a specific sensory pathway, an event that is thought to recruit an NMDA-based detector of correlated activity (23,28,46–52). Several data have been reported indicating that NMDA receptor antagonists induce antinociception under conditions during which noxious inputs are tonically active, and when a modified excitability of the dorsal horn neurons occurs (21,24,53). Among the different classes of NMDA receptor antagonists, the ligands at the glycine site of the NMDA receptor have recently been reported to elicit antinociception against prolonged noxious stimulation in the absence of a marked influence on motor coordination (54). The results obtained with GV 1961771A further support the role of NMDA receptor in the development and maintenance of chronic pain and the analgesic effect of glycine site antagonists.

A. Inhibition of NMDA Receptors

GV 196771A possesses a high affinity (pK_i value of 7.56) for the glycine site located on the NMDA receptors present in the membranes of the cerebral cortex. In the same preparation, glycine in the presence of NMDA dose-dependently increased the binding of [^{3}H]TCP, which takes place only in open channels. As expected, [^{3}H]TCP could bind only when the NMDA receptor was activated by the simultaneous presence of the two agonists (see also Ref. 55). In these experiments GV 196771A showed a competitive behavior, because it displaced, in a parallel manner, the [^{3}H]TCP binding induced by glycine, with an apparent pK_B close to that obtained in displacement experiments (pK_B 7.13 vs. pK_i 7.56). These findings were confirmed and extended by functional studies using the patch–clamp technique on cortical, hippocampal, and spinal neurons in culture. Similar to the experiments with [^{3}H]TCP, activation of the inward currents required the simultaneous presence of the two agonists.

In marked contrast with another recently described glycine antagonist (56), GV 196771A was a very weak ligand for AMPA and kainate receptors. The measured affinity for these non-NMDA receptors was at least 1000 times lower than that estimated on the glycine-binding site of the NMDA receptors.

B. Electrophysiological Recordings: Patch–Clamp in Primary Cultures and Windup in Spinal Cord

In embryonic rat neurons, taken from the cortex, spinal cord, and hippocampus, the simultaneous presence of both NMDA and glycine induced currents flowing through the NMDA receptor channel. GV 196771A antagonized the NMDA–glycine-induced currents in all three preparations, with potencies close to the affinity values found in binding experiments, although in the spinal cord neurons the pK_B value of GV 196771A was higher (8.05) than in those found in cortical and hippocampal neurons (7.47 and 7.86, respectively). Also, in this study, GW 196771A was a competitive antagonist of the glycine-induced currents, whereas the antagonism of GV 196771A on NMDA-induced currents was not reversed by increasing the agonist concentration.

Repetitive low-frequency electrical stimulation of spinal cord dorsal roots using an intensity sufficient to recruit C-/group IV fibers, evokes a polysynaptic, compound electrical response in the corresponding ventral roots, known as windup (41). Because C-/group IV fibers carry the pain sensation centrally, the phenomenon of windup can be used as an index of central sensitization within the spinal cord (40). Our results show the activity of an NMDA glycine site antagonist in inhibiting the phenomenon of windup in isolated baby rat spinal cord, as previously described (38). The observed effect with D-AP5 agrees with the findings of Boxal et al. (57). GV 196771A depressed the windup, further demonstrating the involvement of NMDA receptors in the generation of this phenomenon (58). Moreover, the activity of GV 196771A was qualitatively similar to that observed with the standard opioid morphine.

C. Antihyperalgesic Activity

The effects of GV 196771A have been investigated in several animal pain models, including chronic neuropathic pain in rats (model of painful mononeuropathy; CCI) and in acute and sustained inflammatory pain (formalin test in mice and carrageenan test in rats).

The CCI in rats, which is effected by loose ligations of the sciatic nerve, reproduces in animals a neuropathic pain state (43).

By measuring the hyperalgesia to thermal stimulation, the results suggest that the compound was active when administered both pre- and postinjury. Indeed, GV 196771A, given before the nerve ligature, blocked the development of the hyperalgesia for a long period (at least 30 days). Moreover, it was able to reverse the hyperalgesia in animals that had already developed thermal hypersensitivity 14–21 days after the ligation of the sciatic nerve. The antinociceptive effect lasted for up to 4 and 8 h at 3 and 10 mg/kg, respectively, indicating a dose-related long-lasting activity.

NMDA receptors are located in the dorsal horns of the spinal cord where long-term changes in the processing of nociceptive information occur, and they contribute to the generation of central sensitization (59). This phenomenon is elicited by small-caliber, slowly conducting C-afferent fibers. A brief, low-frequency C-fiber-conditioning stimulus lasting 10 s can produce a central facilitation that lasts several hundred times longer. This facilitation is apparent as an expansion in the size of the cutaneous receptive fields of dorsal horn neurons, a drop in their threshold, and an increase in responsiveness, paralleling hypersensitivity. The increase in excitability induced by C afferents results in the previously subthreshold/subliminal inputs beginning to generate an output from the neuron (47). In addition, molecular changes, such as the synthesis of new receptors or higher expression of native receptors, can occur during central sensitization (60,61). The finding that GV 196771A is also active after the establishment of thermal hypersensitivity indicates that whatever the molecular mechanism that occurs in the spinal cord, it does not influence the activity of the compound. Moreover, the results support the hypothesis that NMDA receptors are involved in the development as well as in the maintenance of a hyperalgesic state, for GV 196771A prevents both the establishment of central sensitization and returns the spinal cord toward baseline levels of excitability, when given after central sensitization is already established. The antihypersensitivity effect of GV 196771A was specific, for the withdrawal latencies in the nonligated paw were unaffected by the treatment. This is consistent with the peculiarity of the NMDA receptor blockade, which affects only a pathological pain state without interfering with the physiological activity (59), in keeping with the hypothesis that the NMDA receptor enhances, rather than transmits, noxious information.

Formalin injected subcutaneously into the animal paw is a frequently used pain assay. Electrophysiological studies showed that formalin administration to a hindpaw excites primary C fibers in a biphasic manner, with a time course similar to that observed in behavioral studies (62). Indeed, there is an intense display of pain response for the first 5 min after formalin injection, followed by a lull in responding, and then a reemergence of pain response; namely, late phase, starting about 15 min after injection, which continues for about 45 min. Specifically, although the initial, early, phase of pain responding appears to be a direct result of chemical activation of primary nociceptive afferent fibers by formalin (63), there is evidence that the second phase is mediated largely by processes within the spinal cord. Consistent with the role of spinal NMDA receptors in tonic pain and hyperalgesia, the sensitization of spinal neurons thought to underlie the second phase of the formalin pain is mediated by NMDA receptors (64).

Oral administration of GV 196771A, 1 h before formalin injection, induce a dose-related inhibition of the late-phase formalin response, without acting on the early phase, supporting the concept that NMDA receptors are involved only in sustained nociceptive transmission. These results are in agreement with previous experiments using different NMDA antagonists, such as ketamine and dizocilpine (MK-801) (21), showing the selective reduction of dorsal horn activity during the late phase. Therefore, these findings suggest a dissociation between the ability of an NMDA antagonist to prevent central changes from occurring, without actually affecting the behavioral or spinal expression of the early phase.

The effect of GV 196771A in the carrageenan test further confirms the role of NMDA receptors in a sustained nociceptive transmission. Indeed, GV 196771A dose-dependently reduced thermal hyperalgesia associated with the inflamed paw. However, at the higher doses tested, GV 196771A did not completely reverse the hyperalgesic state. Moreover, also in this test, GV 196771A produced a specific effect on the hyperalgesic paw, as it did not modify the withdrawal latencies of the noninjected paw even at the highest dose used. This is consistent with the results previously obtained in the CCI model.

In conclusion, the results obtained with GV 196771A suggest that this compound is a potent NMDA glycine site antagonist that does not bind to the non-NMDA receptors. Moreover, the in vivo data indicate that GV 196771A may offer an innovative and safe way for the management of neuropathic pain and could offer a possible advantage for the clinical treatment of chronic pain.

REFERENCES

1. Hollmann M, Heinemann S. Cloned glutamate receptors. Annu Rev Neurosci 1994; 7:31–108.
2. Greenamyre JT, Porter HP. Anatomy and physiology of glutamate in the CNS. Neurology 1994; 44: S7–S13.
3. Pin JP, Duvoisin R. The metabotropic glutamate receptors: structure and functions. Neuropharmacology 1995; 34:1–26.
4. Choi DW. Glutamate receptors and the induction of excitotoxic neuronal death. Prog Brain Res 1994; 100:47–51.
5. Collingridge GL, Bliss TV. Memories of NMDA receptors and LTP. Trends Neurosci 1995; 18:54–56.
6. Mori H, Mishina M. Structure and function of the NMDA receptor channel. Neuropharmacology 1995; 34:1219–1237.
7. Nakanishi S. Molecular diversity of glutamate receptors and implications for brain function. Science 1992; 258:597–603.
8. Nakanishi S, Masu M. Molecular diversity and functions of glutamate receptors. Annu Rev Biophys Biomol Struct 1994; 23:319–348.
9. Kaczmarek L, Kossut M, Skangiel-Kramska J. Glutamate receptors in cortical plasticity: molecular and cellular biology. Physiol Rev 1997; 77:217–255.
10. Barnes JM, Henley JM. Molecular characteristics of excitatory amino acid receptors. Prog Neurobiol 1992; 39:113–133.

11. Moriyoshi K, Masu M, Ishi T, Shigemoto R, Mizuno N, Nakanishi S. Molecular cloning and characterization of the rat NMDA receptor. Nature 1991; 354:31–37.
12. Monyer HN, Sprengel R, Schoepfer A, Herb M, Higuchi H, Lomeli N, Burnashev B, Sakmann B, Seeburg PH. Heteromeric NMDA receptors: molecular and functional distinction of subtypes. Science 1992; 256:1217–1221.
13. Monyer HN, Burnashev B, Laurie DJ, Sakmann B, Seeburg PH. Development and regional expression in the rat brain and functional properties of four NMDA receptors. Neuron 1994; 12:529–540.
14. Nowak L, Bregestovski P, Ascher P, Herbet A, Prochiantz A. Magnesium gates glutamate-activated channels in mouse central neurones. Nature 1984; 307:462–465.
15. Mayer ML, Westbrook GL, Guthrie PB. Voltage-dependent block by Mg^{2+} of NMDA responses in spinal cord neurones. Nature 1984; 309:261–263.
16. Herron CE, Lester RA, Coan EJ, Collingridge GL. Frequency-dependent involvement of NMDA receptors in the hippocampus: a novel synaptic mechanism. Nature 1986; 322:265–268.
17. Ma QP, Woolf CJ. Noxious stimuli induce an *N*-methyl-D-aspartate receptor-dependent hypersensitivity of the flexion withdrawal reflex to touch: implications for the treatment of mechanical allodynia. Pain 1995; 61:383–390.
18. Dougherty PM, Willis WD. Modification of the responses of primate spinothalamic neurons to mechanical stimulation by excitatory amino acids and an *N*-methyl-D-aspartate antagonist. Brain Res 1991; 542:15–22.
19. Sluka KA, Westlund KN. An experimental arthritis in rats: dorsal horn aspartate and glutamate increases. Neurosci Lett 1992; 145:141–144.
20. Malmberg AB, Yaksh TL. Cyclooxygenase inhibition and the spinal release of prostaglandin E_2 and amino acids evoked by paw formalin injection: a microdialysis study in unanesthetized rats. J Neurosci 1995; 15:2768–2776.
21. Haley JE, Sullivan AF, Dickenson AH. Evidence for spinal *N*-methyl-D-aspartate receptor involvement in prolonged chemical nociception in the rat. Brain Res 1990; 518:218–226.
22. Davar G, Hama A, Deykin A, Vos B, Maciewicz R. MK-801 blocks the development of thermal hyperalgesia in a rat model of experimental painful neuropathy. Brain Res 1991; 553:327–330.
23. Mao J, Price DD, Mayer DJ, Lu J, Hayes RL. Intrathecal MK-801 and local nerve anesthesia synergistically reduce nociceptive behaviours in rats with experimental peripheral mononeuropathy. Brain Res 1992; 576:254–262.
24. Ren K, Hylden JLK, Williams G, Ruda MA, Dubner R. The intrathecal administration of excitatory amino acid receptor antagonists selectively attenuated carrageenan-induced behavioural hyperalgesia in rats. Eur J Pharmacol 1992; 219:235–243.
25. Jonhson JW, Asher P. Glycine potentiates the NMDA response in cultured mouse brain neurons. 1987; Nature 325:529–531.
26. Corsi M, Fina P, Trist DG. Co-agonism in drug–receptor activation: illustrated by the NMDA receptor. Trends Pharmacol Sci 1996; 17:220–222.
27. Dickenson AH, Aydar E. Antagonism at the glycine site on the NMDA receptor reduces spinal nociception in the rat. Neurosci Lett 1991; 121:263–266.
28. Leeson PD, Iversen LL. The glycine site on the NMDA receptor: structure–activity relationship and therapeutic potential. J Med Chem 1994; 37:4053–4067.
29. Mugnaini M, Antolini M, Corsi M, van Amsterdam FTM. [^{3}H]5,7-Dichlorokynurenic acid recognizes two binding sites in rat cerebral cortex membranes. J Recept Signal Transduct Res 1998; 18:91–112.
30. Giberti A, Ratti E, Gaviraghi G, Van Amsterdam FTM. Binding of DL-[^{3}H]-alpha-amino-3-hydroxy-5-methyl-isoxazole-4-propionic acid (AMPA) to rat cortex membranes reveals two sites or affinity states. J Recept Res 1991; 11:727–741.
31. Foster AC, Wong EMF. The novel anticonvulsant MK-801 binds to the activated state of the *N*-methyl-D-aspartate receptor in rat brain. Br J Pharmacol 1987; 91:403–409.
32. Munson PJ, Rodbard D. LIGAND: a versatile computerized approach for characterization of ligand-binding data. Anal Biochem 1980; 107:220–239.
33. De Lean A, Munson PJ, Rodbard D. Simultaneous analysis of families of sigmoidal curves: applica-

tion to bioassay, radioligand assay, and physiological dose–response curves. Am J Physiol 1978; 235:E97–E102.
34. Arunlakshana O, Schild HO. Some quantitative uses of drug antagonists. Br J Pharmacol 1959; 14: 48–58.
35. Tang L, Aizenman E. The modulation of *N*-methyl-D-aspartate receptors by redox and alkylating reagents in rat cortical neurones in vitro. J Physiol 1993; 465:303–323.
36. Goslin K, Banker G. Rat hippocampal neurons in low-density culture. In: Banker G, Goslin K, eds. Culturing Nerve Cells. Cambridge: MIT Press, 1991; 251–281.
37. Fitzgerald SC. Dissociated spinal cord and dorsal root ganglion cultures upon plastic tissue culture dishes, glass coverslips and wells. In: Shahar A, De Vellis J, Vernadakis A, Haber B, eds. A Dissection and Tissue Culture Manual of the Nervous System. New York: Alan Liss, 1989; 219–222.
38. Thompson SWN, Gerber G, Sivilotti LG, Woolf CJ. Long duration ventral root potentials in the neonatal rat spinal cord in vitro; the effects of ionotropic and metabotropic excitatory amino acids receptors antagonists. Brain Res 1992; 595:87–97.
39. Hamill OP, Marty A, Neher E, Sakmann B, Sigworth FJ. Improved patch–clamp techniques for high-resolution current recording from cells and cell-free membrane patches. Pflügers Arch 1981; 391:85–100.
40. Thompson SWN, Woolf CJ, Sivilotti LG. Small-caliber afferent inputs produce a heterosynaptic facilitation of the synaptic responses evoked by primary afferents A-fibers in the neonatal rat spinal cord in-vitro. J Neurophysiol 1993; 69:2116–2128.
41. Sivilotti LG, Thompson SWN, Woolf CJ. Rate of rise of the cumulative depolarization evoked by repetitive stimulation of small caliber afferents is a predictor action potential wind-up in rat spinal neurons in-vitro. J Neurophysiol 1993; 69:1621–1632.
42. Leff P, Dougall IG. Further concerns over Cheng–Prusoff analysis. Trends Pharmacol Sci 1993; 14: 110–112.
43. Bennett GJ, Xie YK. A peripheral mononeuropathy in the rat that produces disorders of pain sensation like those seen in man. Pain 1988; 33:87–107.
44. Dubuisson D, Dennis SG. The formalin test: a quantitative study of the analgesic effects of morphine, meperidine, and brain stem stimulation in rats and cats. Pain 1977; 4:161–174.
45. Hargreaves K, Dubner R, Brown F, Flores C, Joris J. A new method for measuring thermal nociception in cutaneous hyperalgesia. Pain 1988; 32:77–88.
46. Meldrum BS. Excitatory amino acid receptors and disease. Curr Opin Neurol Neurosurg 1992; 5: 508–513.
47. Woolf CJ, Doubell TP. The pathophysiology of chronic pain-increased sensitivity to low threshold A_β-fibre inputs. Curr Biol 1994; 4:525–534.
48. Dubner R, Ruda MA. Activity-dependent neuronal plasticity following tissue injury and inflammation. Trends Neurosci 1992; 15:96–103.
49. Urban L, Thompson SW, Dray A. Modulation of spinal excitability: co-operation between neurokinin and excitatory amino acid neurotransmitters. Trends Neurosci 1994; 17:432–438.
50. Mao J, Price DD, Mayer DJ. Mechanisms of hyperalgesia and morphine tolerance: a current view of their possible interactions. Pain 1995; 62:259–274.
51. Woolf CJ. An overview of the mechanisms of hyperalgesia. Pulm Pharmacol 1995; 8:161–167.
52. Dickenson AH, Chapman V, Green GM. The pharmacology of excitatory and inhibitory amino acid-mediated events in the transmission and modulation of pain in the spinal cord. Gen Pharmacol 1997; 28:633–638.
53. Yamamoto T, Yaksh TL. Spinal pharmacology of thermal hyperalgesia induced by constriction injury of sciatic nerve. Excitatory amino acid antagonists. Pain 1992; 49:121–128.
54. Millian MJ, Seguin L. Chemically-diverse ligands at the glycine B site coupled to *N*-methyl-D-aspartate (NMDA) receptors selectively block the late phase of formalin-induced pain in mice. Neurosci Lett 1994; 178:139–143.
55. Benavides J, Rivy J–P, Carter C, Scatton B. Differential modulation of [^{3}H]TCP binding to the NMDA receptor by L-glutamate and glycine. Eur J Pharmacol 1988; 149:67–72.
56. Woodward RM, Huettner JE, Guastella J, Keana JFW, Weber E. In vitro pharmacology of ACEA-

1021 and ACEA-1031: systematically active quinoxalinediones with high affinity and selectivity for *N*-methyl-D-aspartate receptor glycine site. Mol Pharmacol 1995; 47:568–581.

57. Boxall SJ, Thompson SWN, Dray A, Dickenson AM, Urban L. Metabotropic glutamate receptor activation contributes to nociceptive reflex activity in the rat spinal cord in-vitro. Neuroscience 1996; 74:13–20.
58. Dickenson AH. A cure for wind-up: NMDA receptor antagonists as potential analgesics. Trends Pharmacol 1990; 11:307–309.
59. Woolf CJ, Thompson SWN. The induction and maintenance of central sensitisation is dependent on NMDA receptor activation: implications for the treatment of post-injury pain hypersensitivity states. Pain 1991; 44:293–299.
60. Neumann S, Doubell TP, Leslie T, Woolf CJ. Inflammatory pain hypersensitivity mediated by phenotypic switch in myelinated primary sensory neurons. Nature 1996; 384:360–364.
61. Harris JA, Corsi M, Quartaroli M, Arban R, Bentivoglio M. Upregulation of spinal glutamate receptors in chronic pain. Neuroscience 1996; 74:7–12.
62. Dickenson AH, Sullivan A. Subcutaneous formalin-induced activity of dorsal horn neurones in the rat: differential response to an intrathecal opiate administered pre or post formalin. Pain 1987; 30: 349–360.
63. Heapy CG, Jamieson A, Russel NJW. Afferent C-fibre and A-delta activity in models of inflammation. Br J Pharmacol 1987; 90:164P.
64. Coderre TJ, Vaccarino AL, Melzack R. Central nervous system plasticity in the tonic pain response to subcutaneous formalin injection. Brain Res 1990; 535:155–158.

48

Voltage-Gated Sodium Channels and Pain

Recent Advances

Derek J. Trezise and Simon Tate
Glaxo Wellcome Research and Development, Stevenage, Hertfordshire, England

Chas Bountra
GlaxoSmithKline, Harlow, Essex, England

I. INTRODUCTION

Voltage-gated sodium (Na^+) channels (VGSCs) are complex, transmembrane proteins that have a role in governing electrical activity in excitable tissues. The Na^+ channel is activated in response to depolarization of the cell membrane that causes a voltage-dependent conformational change in the channel from a resting, closed conformation to an active conformation, the result of which increases the membrane permeability to Na^+ ions (1–3). VGSCs comprise a multisubunit complex consisting of a large (230- to 270-kDa), highly glycosylated α-subunit and one or two smaller accessory β-subunits (β_1 and β_2).

Most attention has been directed toward the α-subunit, and recent molecular studies have extended the α-subunit gene family to ten separate members that have been characterized in terms of their electrophysiological properties and tissue distribution profile (Figs. 1 and 2) (4–18). Based on the sensitivity to a toxin derived from puffer fish, tetrodotoxin (TTX), Na^+ currents can be subdivided as either being TTX-sensitive (TTXs) or TTX-resistant (TTXr) (19–24). The four brain-type Na^+ channels (brain I, II, III, and VI) which are predominantly found in the central nervous system (CNS) are inhibited by low nanomolar concentrations of TTX (5,7,11,13). PN-1, which is found in neuroendocrine tissues and in sensory nerves, is also TTX-sensitive (12,16), as is the skeletal muscle channel α-subunit (17). By contrast, there are three channels that are inhibited by only micromolar concentrations of TTX, the major cardiac channel h1/SKM2 (10) and two channels, SNS and SNS2 which are expressed only in sensory neurones (4,14,15,18).

II. MOLECULAR ADVANCES

The development of a range of α-subunit-specific probes, including riboprobes, antisense DNA oligonucleotides, and antipeptide antibodies, has advanced our understanding of the role of VGSCs in the pathogenesis of pain. Molecular distribution studies suggest that there is a dynamic expression of voltage-gated Na^+ channels in primary sensory (dorsal root ganglion; DRG) neurones that can change during development, response to injury, and on exposure to inflammatory mediators (25–37). When combined with electrophysiological data, the changes in Na^+ channel

Channel	Summary Tissue Distribution	Naïve DRG Cell Body Staining	Association with pain pathology
Brain Type I	SCN1a	6	Noda et al
Brain Type II	SCN2a/Type IIa	13	Noda et al, Auld et al
Brain Type III	SCN3a	4	Kayano et al
Brain Type VI	SCN8a/NaCH6/PN4	3	Burgess et al
Skeletal Muscle	SCN4a/SKM1	5	Trimmer et al
Cardiac	SCN5a/h1	2000	Gellens et al,
PN1	SCN9a/hNE/NaS	4	Klugbauer et al, Toledo-Aral et al
SNS	SCN10a/PN3	31000	Akopian et al, Sangameswaran et al
SNS2	SCN11a/NaN/PN5	1500	Tate et al, Dib-Hajj et al
Atypical Heart /Glial	SCN6a/nav2.3 SCN7a/NaG	?	Felipe et al, Akopian et al (1997)

(A)

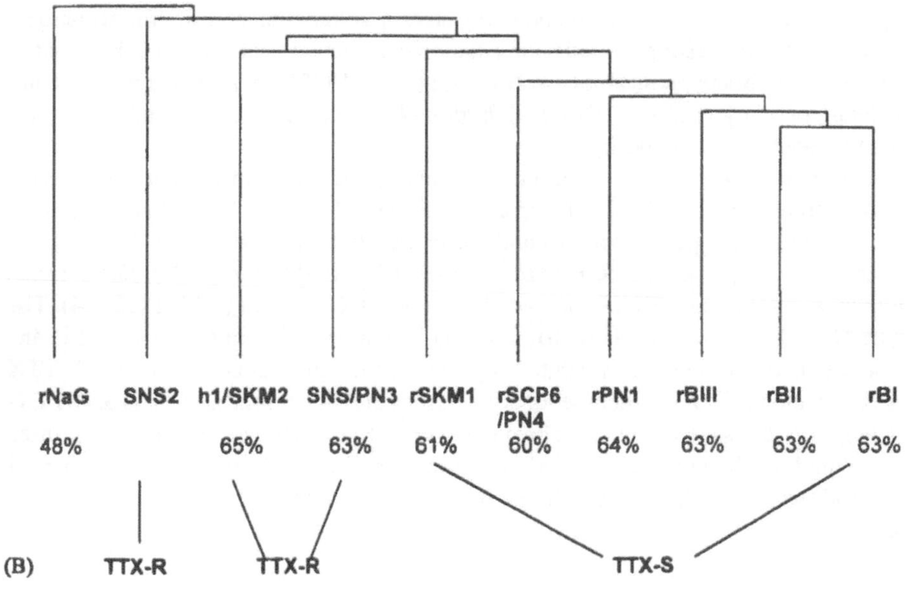

Figure 1 (A) Mammalian voltage-gated sodium channel gene family. (B) Relative homologies of the rat voltage-gated sodium channel gene family calculated by the Genetics Computer Group figure program and illustrated as a dendrogram. Percentages relate to sequence similarity with SNS2. Two major families can be seen: Those encoding the TTX-sensitive (TTXs) sodium channels (rSKM1, rSCP6/PN4, rBI, rBII, and rBIII) and those encoding the TTX-resistant (TTXr) channels (SNS/PN3 and h1/SKM2). SNS2 appears to form part of a new family related to both TTXr and TTXs sodium channels.

Channel	*Summary Tissue Distribution*	*Naïve DRG Cell Body Staining*	*Association with pain pathology*
Brain Type I	Brain, spinal cord, heart,	Weakly expressed Large>medium>small	Not known
Brain Type II	Brain, spinal cord, DRG	Low level expresison	Regulated by NGF
Brain Type III	Embryonic form in the rat, although expressed in human brain	Very low expression	Upregulated in rat DRG following axotomy
Brain Type VI	Brain, spinal cord, glial cells, DRG	Large>medium>small	Not known
Skeletal Muscle	Skeletal muscle	Not present	Not known
Cardiac	Heart	Not present	Not known
PN1	DRG, neuroendocrine cells, PC12 cells	Large=medium=small	Upregulated by NGF and inflammation Upregulated in SNS null mice
SNS	DRG only	Small>>medium>large	Re-distributed in neuropathic pain from cell body to site of injury. Upregulated in inflammatory pain models. Antisense reverses neuropathic and inflammatory hyperalgesia in rat models.
SNS2	DRG only	Small>>medium	Similar re-distribution of protein in neuropathic pain states as SNS.
Atypical Heart/Uterus (human)	Heart, Uterus, lung	Large=medium>small	Not known
Glial (rat)	DRG, glial cells	Large>medium>small	Not known

Figure 2 Summary tissue distribution for the voltage-gated sodium channel gene family, with extended detail for DRG tissue and possible links with pain pathology.

redistribution in peripheral neurons can be linked to the induction and maintenance of chronic pain pathologies.

For example, the type III Na^+ channel is barely expressed in the adult rat; however, following axotomy of the sciatic nerve, there is a large up-regulation of both type III mRNA and protein in the cell bodies of the DRG (26,27). It has been proposed that there may be a "molecular switch" in this particular rat model that causes a reversion back to a neonatal phenotype, in which the brain III channel is widely found. The mRNA for SNS channels is down-regulated in small DRG cell bodies after axotomy, a phenomenon that can be attenuated by treatment with nerve growth factor (38). These molecular changes coincide with a decrease in whole-cell TTXr current, an increase in total TTXs Na^+ current, and the appearance of a rapidly repriming Na^+ current not found in unlesioned neurons (30). The narrowing of the action potential, the decrease in firing threshold, and the spontaneous spikes that originate in the soma of some axotomized DRG neurons can all be explained by this change in Na^+ channel expression (39–41). Accumulation of Na^+ channel α-subunits at sites other than the soma, notably the injury site itself, may play a key role in the initiation and maintenance of ectopic discharges (31). Indeed, Matzner and Devor (42) demonstrated that there was a sufficient increase in Na^+ channel density at a neuroma to reduce the firing threshold to the point that damaged neurons would repetitively discharge.

Interestingly, following chronic constriction injury of the rat sciatic nerve, a more relevant animal model of clinical neuropathy than axotomy, the SNS protein translocates from the cell body to the peripheral axons (35,36). Antisense nucleotides directed against SNS reverse the behavioral symptoms of neuropathic pain in this model (36). Studies with SNS and SNS2 have been extended to DRG and peripheral nerve tissue removed from human patients with characterized painful neuropathies. After brachial plexus injury, both SNS and SNS2 α-subunits redistribute in DRG neurons (29). There is a sudden decrease of SNS and SNS2 protein in the sensory cell bodies of DRG, the central axons of which have been avulsed from the spinal cord and an increase in the staining intensity is observed in nerve fibers (Fig. 3). It is tempting to speculate that these molecular changes are sufficient to drive ectopic discharge from the damaged primary afferents which give rise to the parasthesias and hyperesthesias that these patients experience.

In certain inflammatory pain conditions, modulation of VGSCs may represent an important mechanism by which mediators released at a site of inflammation sensitize and activate primary afferent neurons. Proinflammatory agents, such as prostaglandin E_2(PGE_2) serotonin (5-HT), and adenosine lower the threshold for activation of TTXr in small DRG neurons and accelerate channel activation and inactivation (28,34,43). This translates to a reduced action potential firing threshold and a propensity to sustain burst discharges, rather than fire single spikes (43). For PGE_2, the second-messenger pathway-coupling receptor-binding to channel modulation involves cAMP-dependent protein kinase (43–44). Specific phosphorylation sites for this enzyme on the SNS channel have been identified (45). The SNS and SNS2 mRNA and protein are up-regulated in some DRG neurons following injection of complete Freund's adjuvant or carrageenan into the rat paw, adding further weight to the importance of these channels in inflammatory pain states (33,46).

The demonstration of two functional TTXr voltage-gated Na^2 channels in sensory neurons—SNS and SNS2—has provided a molecular basis for the heterogeneity of the TTXr sodium current recorded from DRG neurons (23,24). Most small DRG cells coexpress both SNS and SNS2 (37) and the relative abundance of SNS and SNS2 channels within any single neuron may determine the electrophysiological profile of the TTXr current recorded from a particular DRG cell body. The colocalization of the two channels in only small DRG cells, which are precisely those cells that are characterized by the presence of TTXr currents, suggests that they may have functional synergy. Whenever SNS has been expressed recombinantly, either in mam-

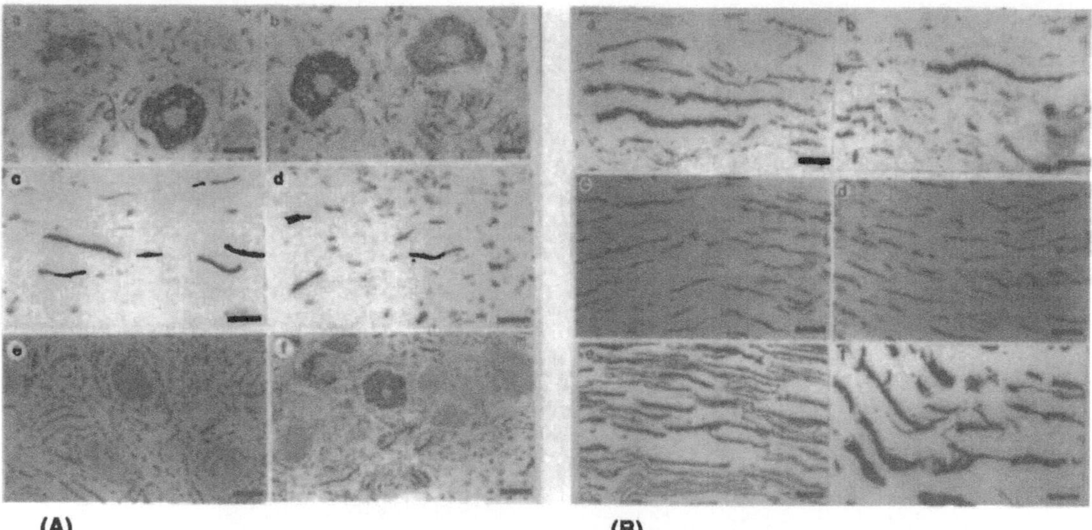

(A) (B)

Figure 3 (A) SNS (a, c, e) and SNS2 (b, d, f) immunoreactivity in postmortem DRG (a and b), avulsed DRG 4 days after injury (c and d), and avulsed DRG 3 months after injury (e and f). Scale bar = 25 μM in (a–d) and 50 μM in (e and f). (B) SNS (a and c) and SNS2 (b and d) immunoreactivity in injured nerve 4 days after injury (a and b) and in normal nerve (c and d). Immunostaining with antineurofilament antibody in normal nerve and injured nerve (4 days after injury) is given in (e and f), respectively.

malian cells or in *Xenopus* oocytes, the voltage dependence of activation is always more depolarized and the inactivation kinetics significantly slower than has ever been recorded for the native TTXr current in small DRG neurons. It is possible that the electrophysiological differences observed between recombinant SNS and native TTXr are either due to association with other accessory β-subunits or indeed by a functional association with SNS2. A significant percentage (13%) of small, SNS2-labeled cells did not coexpress SNS (47), and a functional correlate for these cells has recently been observed in DRG neurons (23). These cells have been named type D cells and similar to SNS2 currents have a much more hyperpolarized availability when compared with TTXr currents recorded from type B and C TTXr-containing cells. In these type B and C cells, the biophysical properties of TTXr are intermediate between SNS and SNS2, suggesting that the current results from a combination of the activity of both SNS2 and SNS channels.

III. ADVANCES IN PHARMACOLOGY

Many drugs that are used clinically to treat peripheral neuropathies, including some local anesthetics (e.g., lignocaine; lidocaine), antiarrythmics (e.g., mexiletine) and anticonvulsants (e.g., phenytoin and carbamazepine), are blockers of VGSCs (48–51). Numbers-needed-to-treat (NNT; i.e., the number of patients needed to treat with a certain drug to obtain one with a defined degree of pain relief) has been introduced as a useful method to examine analgesic efficacy (50–51). This method permits a clinically relevant comparison between different drugs.

Phenytoin and carbamazepine are widely used anticonvulsants. These drugs exert their membrane stabilizing properties in part by blocking sodium channels (52) and, thereby, reduce neuronal excitability in sensitized C-fiber nociceptors. In painful diabetic neuropathy, carbamazepine has an NNT of 3.3 (2–9.4) and phenytoin an NNT of 2.1 (1.5–3.6) (53). Although

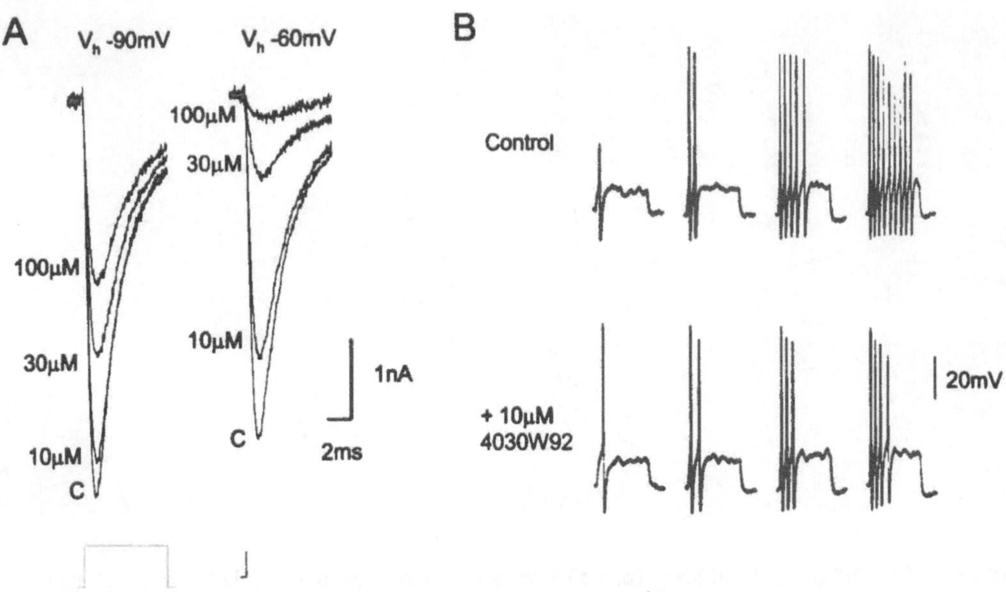

Figure 4 4030W92 blocks TTX-R channels in primary afferent neurones in a voltage-and use-dependent manner (panel A). In current clamp (panel B) this translates to preferential inhibition of the later spikes in a burst of action potentials evoked by current injection (modified from Trezise et al., 1998, with permission).

carbamazepine is frequently used in poststroke pain, it was not significantly better than placebo in a small study ($n = 14$) that showed a clear effect of the tricyclic antidepressant amitriptyline (54). However, the corresponding NNT of 3.4 (1.7–105) is quite acceptable, and the lack of statistical significance may simply be related to the small sample size. Carbamazepine is the treatment of choice for trigeminal neuralgia, and data from three controlled trials have been published (55–57). It is difficult to interpret the data from the latter study, which also failed to find an effect. For the two other studies, there is combined NNT of 2.6 (2.2–3.3) (51). It is reported that carbamazepine causes both a reduction in pain intensity—a reduction in pain paroxysms—and in triggers (57). There is only anecdotal data on oxcarbamazepine (58), a new carbamazepine-like anticonvulsant, acting by sodium channel blockade and characterized by a less bothersome side effect profile than carbamazepine.

Kastrup et al. (59) reported that infusions of lidocaine relieved painful diabetic neuropathy and the data from that study showed a favorable NNT of 3. Lidocaine is not convenient for prolonged treatment, because it cannot be dosed orally. Studies on its oral analogue mexiletine have, therefore, been carried out. Two studies with oral mexiletine established a beneficial effect (60,61), whereas two others reported no effect (62) or only an effect in subanalyses and not on primary effect variables (63). One trial studied the effect of mexiletine in chronic dysesthetic pain after spinal cord injury, but failed to find an effect (64).

Galer et al. (65) have recently reported on a study in which postherpetic neuralgia (PHN) patients obtained significantly more benefit from a topical adhesive patch impregnated with lidocaine than from application of a nonmediated topical adhesive patch. This study utilized a randomized, placebo-controlled, crossover design and recruited selected patients who had been using the lidocaine patch for at least 1 month, in an open-label compassionate use protocol (i.e., enriched enrollment). The median ''time to exit'' in the lidocaine patch phase was greater than

14 days, as compared with 3.8 days during the placebo phase ($p < 0.001$). Also 78% (25/32) of the subjects preferred the lidocaine patch treatment period, with 11 reporting "moderate relief," 11 "a lot of relief," and 7 "complete pain relief." Topical lidocaine treatment of PHN provides several distinct advantages over currently used oral agents, such as the tricyclic antidepressants, anticonvulsants, and opiates. The lidocaine patch produces clinically insignificant serum levels of lidocaine and is thought to relieve the constant pains and allodynia of PHN by reducing, via sodium channel blockade, ectopic discharges from damaged peripheral sensory nerves (66,67). Unlike the antidepressants, anticonvulsants, and opiates, the topical lidocaine patch does not cause any systemic side effects, does not result in any drug–drug interactions, and does not require dose titration. Also, once-daily application of topical patches is simple to use, without the need for dose titration or repeated dosing throughout the day.

Lamotrigine is a new anticonvulsant, which acts by stabilizing the slow-inactivated conformation of a subtype of sodium channel, and probably by this mechanism suppresses the neuronal release of glutamate. Anecdotal observations in patients with central pain (68) and an uncontrolled study in painful diabetic neuropathy (69) indicate that lamotrigine will relieve neuropathic pain. Lamotrigine has been tried as an add-on treatment to carbamazepine in trigeminal neuralgia (70), and in this setting it has a favourable NNT of 2.1 (1.3–6.1).

The precise mechanism of action of these agents remains unclear: there is compelling evidence from animal studies for both peripheral and spinal sites of action, and data to suggest that not all of these molecules behave in the same way. Recent studies have focused on further understanding the cellular actions of these established Na^+ channel blockers.

Unlike phenytoin and carbamazepine, lamotrigine (10–100 mg/kg^{-1} s.c.) is capable of reversing cold allodynia in the chronic constriction injury model (71) and of inhibiting PGE_2- and streptozocin-induced mechanical hyperalgesia (72). Interestingly, lamotrigine has no effect in the thermal tail-flick model or in other purely "nociceptive" paradigms, indicating that it somehow selects for hyperalgesia over normal sensory stimuli. A new more potent analogue of lamotrigine, 4030W92, is effective in a range of different animal models of pain, including complete Freund's adjuvant and CCI (73–75). Like lamotrigine, 4030W92 appears to be truly "antihyperalgesic," rather than simply antinociceptive. Plasma concentrations of 4030W92 ~2 μM) that do not affect normal nerve conduction in vivo are effective in suppressing the burst firing of spontaneously active fibers in rat sciatic neuromas (76).

This capacity to selectivity inhibit ectopic activity following neuronal injury is shared by other Na^+ channel blockers (77–82). The increase in Na^+ channel density at the injury site or DRG, which drives ectopic discharge, may be such that only a low concentration of blocker is required to normalize the available Na^+ channel population (83). A contributory factor is also likely to be the way in which these molecules inhibit Na^+ channels. Both lamotrigine and 4030W92 inhibit TTXr and TTXs Na^+ channels in small DRG neurons in a voltage- and use-dependent manner, by preferentially binding to a channel inactivation state (75,84). 4030W92 is 12-fold more potent than lamotrigine and has an estimated binding affinity for the inactivated state of TTXr of 3 μM, close to the effective plasma concentration. In dissociated neurones, state-dependent block translates to preferential inhibition of the later spikes in a train evoked by current injection and of spikes evoked at high compared with low frequency. Similar findings have recently been reported with phenytoin, carbamazepine, and the local anesthetics bupivacaine and lidocaine (85,86).

Inhibition of ecoptic discharge from damaged neurons presumably underlies the efficacy of Na^+ channel blockers in treating pains with paroxysmal, lancinating components. However, it seems unlikely that it is the sole site of action of these agents. A growing body of evidence suggests that Na^+ channel blockers also act spinally to produce analgesia. Mexiletine inhibits nociceptive responses to intrathecally administered algogenic agents (e.g., bradykinin) (87), whereas the second phase of the formalin response is attenuated by intrathecal lidocaine (88). These behavioral observations are reinforced by electrophysiological experiments. In decerebrate, spinalized rats, systemic lidocaine suppresses C-fiber–evoked polysynaptic reflexes without inhibiting peripheral nerve conduction (89). More directly, iontophoretic application of lidocaine or lamotrigine to the spinal cord inhibits dorsal horn neuron responses to noxious, and to lesser degree, innocuous stimuli (90–92). 4030W92 also has spinal actions, as evidenced by the inhibition of central sensitization produced by intrathecal administration of NMDA (Woolf CJ, unpublished observations). In spinal cord in vitro preparations, both lignocaine and 4030W92 suppress dorsal root-evoked ventral root potentials (93,94).

A common observation throughout these studies is that dorsal horn neuron responses to C-fiber inputs are generally more sensitive to inhibition than A–fiber-evoked potentials. An intriguing explanation for this, and perhaps the reason for preferential block of ectopic discharge by low concentrations of Na^+ channel blockers, is that some agents may exhibit selectivity for certain Na^+ channel isoforms over others (e.g., brain III, SNS, SNS2). At present, this area of research is in its infancy. Both phenytoin and carbamazepine produce a much more marked inhibition of native TTXs than of TTXr channels in DRG neurons (95,96). Similarly, 4030W92, lidocaine, and bupivicaine are three- to fivefold more potent at inhibiting TTXs than TTXr (22,75,86). The neuroprotective drug riluzole blocks TTXr and TTXs channels with comparable potency (97). WIN 17317-3 is a highly potent blocker of TTXr (IC_{50} value 250 nM) but also has profound K^+ channel-blocking effects (98). To our knowledge no compounds have been reported that select for TTXr over TTXs Na^+ channels.

The results of direct comparisons of current Na^+ channel blockers on recombinant human channels are eagerly awaited. The identification of new molecules with isoform-selective–blocking properties will permit determination of the important Na^+ channels in chronic pain state etiology and pathophysiology. Moreover, these may represent a new generation of analgesic drugs with improved efficacy and a wider therapeutic index.

REFERENCES

1. Catterall WA. Cellular and molecular biology of voltage-gated sodium channels. Physiol Rev 1992; 72:S15–S48.
2. Goldin AL. Ligand and Voltage-Gated Ion Channels. Vol. 2. Boca Raton, FL: CRC Press, 1994.
3. Hille B. Ionic Channels of Excitable Membranes. Sunderland, MA: Sinauer, 1984.
4. Akopian AN, Sivilotti L, Wood J. A tetrodotoxin-resistant voltage gated sodium channel expressed by sensory neurons. Nature 1996; 379:257–262.
5. Akopian AN, Souslova V, Sivilotti L, Wood JN. Structure and distribution of a broadly expressed atypical sodium channel. FEBS Lett 1997; 400:183–187.
6. Auld VJ, Goldin AL, Krafte DS, Marshall J, Dunn JM, Catterall WA, Lester HA, Davidson N, Dunn RJ. A rat brain Na^+ channel alpha subunit with novel gating properties. Neuron 1988; 1:449–461.
7. Burgess DL, Kohrman DC, Galt J, Plummer NW, Jones JM, Spear B, Meisler MH. Mutation of a new sodium channel gene, Scn8a, in the mouse mutant motor endplate disease. Nat Genet 1995; 10: 461–465.
8. Felipe A, Knittle TJ, Doyle KL, Tamkun MM. Primary structure and differential expression during development and pregnancy of a novel voltage-gated sodium channel in the mouse. J Biol Chem 1994; 269:30125–30131.
9. Fish LM, Sangameswaran L, Delgado SG, Koch BD, Jakeman LB, Kwan J, Herman RC. Cloning of a sodium channel α-subunit (PN-1) from rat dorsal root ganglia. Soc Neurosci Abstr 1995; 21: 1824.
10. Gellens ME, George AL Jr, Chen LQ, Chahine M, Horn R, Barchi RL, Kallen RG. Primary structure

and functional expression of the human cardiac tetrodotoxin-insensitive voltage-dependent sodium channel. Proc Natl Acad Sci USA 1992; 89:554–558.
11. Kayano T, Noda M, Flockerzi V, Takahashi H, Numa S. Primary structure of rat brain sodium channel III deduced from the cDNA sequence. FEBS Lett 1988; 228:187–94.
12. Klugbauer N, Lacinova L, Flockerzi V, Hofmann F. Structure and functional expression of a new member of the tetrodotoxin-sensitive voltage-gated sodium channel family from human neuroendocrine cells. EMBO J 1995; 14:1084–1090.
13. Noda M, Ikeda T, Suzuki H, Takahashi T, Kuno M, Numa S. Expression of functional sodium channels from cloned cDNA. Nature 1986; 322:826–888.
14. Sangameswaran L, Delgado SG, Fish LM, Koch BD, Jakeman LB, Stewart GR, Sze P, Hunter JC, Eglen RM, Herman RC. Structure and function of a novel voltage-gated, tetrodotoxin-resistant sodium channel specific to sensory neurons. J Biol Chem 1996; 271:5953–5956.
15. Tate S, Benn S, Hick C, Trezise D, John V, Mannion R, Costigan M, Plumpton C, Grose D, Gladwell Z, Kendall G, Dale K, Bountra C, Woolf C. Two sodium channels contribute to the TTX-R sodium current in primary sensory neurones. Nat Neurosci 1998; 1:653–655.
16. Toledo–Aral JJ, Moss BL, He Z, Koszowski AG, Whisenand T, Levinson SR, Wolf JJ, Silos–Santiago I, Halegoua S, Mandel G. Identification of PN-1, a predominant voltage-dependent sodium channel expressed principally in peripheral neurons. Proc Natl Acad Sci USA 1997; 94:1527–1532.
17. Trimmer JS, Cooperman SS, Tomiko SA, Zhou JY, Crean SM, Boyle MB, Kallen RG, Sheng ZH, Barchi RL, Sigworth FJ. Primary structure and functional expression of a mammalian skeletal muscle sodium channel. Neuron 1989; 3:33–49.
18. Dib–Hajj SD, Tyrrell L, Black JA, Waxman SG. NaN, a novel voltage-gated Na channel, is expressed preferentially in peripheral sensory neurons and down-regulated after axotomy. Proc Natl Acad Sci USA 1998; 95:8963–8968.
19. Caffrey JM, Eng DL, Black JA, Waxman SG, Kocsis JD. Three types of sodium channels in adult rat dorsal root ganglion neurons. Brain Res 1992; 592:283–297.
20. Elliott AA, Elliott JR. Characterization of TTX-sensitive and TTX-resistant sodium currents in small cells from adult rat dorsal root ganglia. J Physiol 1993; 463:39–56.
21. Rizzo MA, Kocsis JD, Waxman SG. Slow sodium conductances of dorsal root ganglion neurons: intraneuronal homogeneity and interneuronal heterogeneity. J Neurophysiol 1994; 72:2796–2815.
22. Roy ML, Narahashi T. Differential properties of tetrodotoxin-sensitive and tetrodotoxin-resistant sodium channels in rat dorsal root ganglion. J Neurosci 1992; 12:2104–2111.
23. Rush AM, Brau ME, Elliott AA, Elliott JR. Electrophysiological properties of sodium current subtypes in small cells from adult rat dorsal root ganglia. J Physiol (Lond) 1998; 511:771–789.
24. Scholz A, Appel N, Vogel W. Two types of TTX-resistant and one TTX-sensitive Na^+ channel in rat dorsal root ganglion neurons and their blockade by halothane. Eur J Neurosci 1998; 10:2547–2556.
25. Black JA, Dib–Hajj S, Mcnabola K, Jeste S, Rizzo MA, Kocsis, JD, Waxman SG. Spinal sensory neurons express multiple sodium channel α-subunit mRNAs. Mol Brain Res 1996; 43:117–131.
26. Black JA, Cummins TR, Plumpton C, Chen YH, Hormuzdiar W, Clare JJ, Waxman S. Upregulation of a silent sodium channel after peripheral, but not central, nerve injury in DRG neurons. Neurophysiol 1999; 82:2776–2785.
27. Black JA, Waxman SG. Sodium channel expression: a dynamic process in neurons and non-neuronal cells. Dev Neurosci 1996; 18:139–152.
28. Cardenas CG, Del Mar L, Cooper BY, Scroggs RS. 5-HT_4 receptors couple positively to tetrodotoxin-insensitive sodium channels in a subpopulation of capsaicin-insensitive rat sensory neurons. J Neurosci 1997; 17:7181–7189.
29. Coward K, Plumpton C, Facer P, Birch R, Carlstedt T, Tate S, Bountra C, Anand P. Immunolocalization of SNS/PN3 and NaN/SNS2 sodium channels in human pain states. Pain 2000; 85:41–50.
30. Cummins TR, Waxman SG. Downregulation of tetrodotoxin-resistant and upregulation of a rapidly repriming tetrodotoxin-sensitive sodium current in small spinal sensory neurons after nerve injury. J Neurosci 1997; 17:3503–3514.
31. Devor M, Govrin–Lippman R, Angelides K. Na^+ channel immunolocalization in peripheral mamma-

lian axons and changes following nerve injury and neuroma formation. J Neurosci 1993; 13:1976–1992.

32. Dib–Hajj S, Black JA, Felts P, Waxman SG. Down regulation of transcripts for Na^+ channel α-SNS in spinal sensory neurons following axotomy. Proc Natl Acad Sci USA 1996; 93:14950–14954.
33. Gold MS. Tetrodotoxin-resistant Na^+ currents and inflammatory hyperalgesia. Proc Natl Acad Sci USA 1999; 96:7645–7649.
34. Gold MS, Reichling DB, Shuster MJ, Levine JD. Hyperalgesic agents increase a tetrodotoxin-resistant Na^+ current in nociceptors. Proc Nat Acad Sci USA 1996; 93:1108–1112.
35. Novakovic SD, Tzoumaka E, McGivern JG, Haraguchi M, Sangameswaran L, Gogas KR, Eglen RM, Hunter JC. Distribution of the tetrodotoxin-resistant sodium channel PN3 in rat sensory neurons in normal and neuropathic conditions. J Neurosci 1998; 18:2174–2187.
36. Porreca F, Lai J, Bian D, Wegert S, Ossipov MH, Eglen RM, Kassotakis L, Novakovic S, Rabert DK, Sangameswaran L, Hunter JC. A comparison of the potential role of the tetrodotoxin-insensitive sodium channels PN3/SNS and NaN/SNS2, in rat models of chronic pain. Proc Natl Acad Sci USA 1999; 96:7640–7644.
37. Waxman SG, Kocsis JD, Black JA. Type III sodium channel mRNA is expressed in embryonic but not adult spinal sensory neurons, and is re-expressed following axotomy. J Neurophysiol 1994; 72: 466–470.
38. Fjell J, Cummins TR, Dib–Hajj S, Fried K, Black JA, Waxman SG. Differential role of GDNF and NGF in the maintenance of two TTX-resistant sodium channels in adult DRG neurons. Mol Brain Res 1999; 67:267–282.
39. Babbedge RC, Soper A, Gentry CT, Hood VG, Campbell EA, Urban L. In vitro characterization of a peripheral afferent pathway of the rat after chronic sciatic nerve section. J Neurophysiol 1996; 76: 3169–3177.
40. Study RE, Kral MG. Spontaneous action potential activity in isolated dorsal root ganglion neurons from rats with a painful neuropathy. Pain 1996; 65:235–242.
41. Stebbing MJ, Eschenfelder S, Habler H–J, Acosta MC, Janig W, McLachlan EM. Changes in the action potential in sensory neurones after peripheral axotomy in vivo. Neuroreport 1999; 10:201–206.
42. Matzner L, Devor M. Hyperexcitability at sites of nerve injury depends on voltage-sensitive Na^+ channels. J Neurophysiol 1994; 72:349–359.
43. England S, Bevan S, Docherty RJ. PGE_2 modulates the tetrodotoxin-resistant sodium current in neonatal rat dorsal root ganglion neurons via the cyclic AMP–protein kinase A cascade. J Physiol 1996; 495:429–440.
44. Gold MS, Levine JD, Correa AM. Modulation of TTX-R I_{Na} by PKC and PKA and their role in PGE_2-induced sensitization of rat sensory neurons in vitro. J Neurosci 1998; 18:10345–10355.
45. Fitzgerald EM, Okuse K, Wood JN, Dolphin AC, Moss SJ. cAMP-dependent phosphorylation of the tetrodotoxin-resistant voltage-dependent sodium channel SNS. J Physiol 1999; 516:433–466.
46. Tanaka M, Cummins TR, Ishikawaw K, Dib–Hajj SD, Black JA, Waxman SG. SNS Na^+ channel expression increases in dorsal root ganglion neurons in the carrageenan inflammatory pain model. Neuroreport 1998; 9:967–972.
47. Amaya F, Decosterd I, Samad T, Plumpton C, Tate S, Mannion RJ, Costigan M, Woolf C. Diversity of expression of the sensory neuron specific TTX-resistant voltage-gated sodium ion channels SNS and SNS2. Mol Cell Neurosci 2000; 4:331–342.
48. Tanelian DL, Brose WG. Neuropathic pain can be relieved by drugs that are use-dependent Na^+ channel blockers: lidocaine, carbamazepine and mexiletine. Anaesthesiology 1991; 74:949–951.
49. Upton N. Mechanisms of action of new antiepileptic drugs: rational design and serendipitous findings. Trends Pharmacol Sci 1994; 15:456–463.
50. Sindrup H, Jensen TS. Efficacy of pharmacological treatments of neuropathic pain: an update and effect related to mechanism of drug action. Pain 1999; 83:389–400.
51. McQuay HJ, Moore RA. An Evidence Based Resource for Pain Relief. Oxford: Oxford University Press, 1998.

52. Dray A. Agonists and antagonists of nociception. In: Jensen TS, Turner JA, Wiesenfeld–Hallin Z, eds. Proceedings of the 9th World Congress on Pain. Seattle: IASP Press, 1997:279–292.
53. McQuay H, Carroll D, Jadad AR, Wiffen P, Moore RA. Anticonvulsant drugs for the management of pain: a systematic review. Br Med 1995; 311:1047–1052.
54. Leijon G, Boivie J. Central post stroke pain—a controlled trial of amitriptyline and carbamazepine. Pain 1989; 36:27–36.
55. Campbell FG, Graham JG, Zilkha KJ. Clinical trial of carbamazepine (Tegretol) in trigeminal neuralgia. J Neurol Neurosurg Psychiatry 1996; 29:265–267.
56. Killian JM, Fromm JM. Carbamazepine in the treatment of neuralgia. Use of side effects. Arch Neurol 1986; 19:129–136.
57. Nicol CF. A four year double blind study of tegretol in facial pain. Headache 1969; 9:54–57.
58. Zakrzewska JM, Patsalos PN. Oxcarbazepine: a new drug in the management of intractable trigeminal neuralgia. J Neurol Neurosurg Psychiatry 1989; 52:472–476.
59. Kastrup J, Petersen P, Dejgard A, Angelo H, Hilsted J. Intravenous lidocaine infusion—a new treatment for chronic painful diabetic neuropathy? Pain 1987; 28:69–75.
60. Dejgard A, Petersen P, Kastrup J. Mexiletine for treatment of chronic painful diabetic neuropathy. Lancet 1988; 2:9–11.
61. Oskarsson P, Lins PE, Ljunggren JG. Efficacy and safety of mexiletine in the treatment of painful diabetic neuropathy. Diabetes Care 1997; 20:1594–1597.
62. Wright JM, Oki JC, Graves L. Mexiletine in the symptomatic treatment of diabetic peripheral neuropathy. Ann Pharmacother 1997; 31:29–34.
63. Stracke H, Meyer UF, Schumacher HF, Federlin K. Mexiletine in the treatment of diabetic neuropathy. Diabetes Care 1992; 15:1550–1555.
64. Chiou–Tan FY, Tuel SM, Johnson JC, Priebe MM, Hirsh DD, Strayer JR. Effect of mexiletine on spinal cord injury dysesthetic pain. Am J Physiol Med Rehabil 1996; 75:84–87.
65. Galer BS, Rowbotham MC, Perander J, Friedman E. Topical lidocaine patch relieves post herpetic neuralgia more effectively than a vehicle topical patch: results of an enriched enrollment study. Pain 1999; 80:533–538.
66. Rowbotham MC, Davies PS, Verkempinck CM, Galer BS. Lidocaine patch: double blind controlled study of a new treatment method for post herpetic neuralgia. Pain 1996; 65:39–44.
67. Rowbotham MC, Davies PS, Galer BS. Multicentre, double blind, vehicle controlled trial of long term use of lidocaine patches for postherpetic neuralgia. 8th World Congress of Pain—Abstracts. Seattle: IASP Press, 1996:274.
68. Canavero S, Bonicalzi V. Lamotrigine control of central pain. Pain 1996; 68:179–181.
69. Eisenberg E, Alon N, Ishay A, Daoud D, Yarnitsky D. Lamotrigine in the treatment of painful diabetic neuropathy. Eur J Neurol 1998; 5:167–173.
70. Zakrzewska JM, Chaudry Z, Nurmikko TJ, Patton DW, Mullens EL. Lamotrigine (Lamictal) in refractory trigeminal neuralgia: results from a double blind placebo controlled crossover trial. Pain 1997; 73:223–230.
71. Hunter JC, Gogas KR, Hedley LR, Jacobsen LO, Kassotakis L, Thompsen J, Fontana DJ. The effect of novel antiepileptic drugs in rat experimental models of acute and chronic pain. Eur J Pharmacol 1997; 324:153–160.
72. Nakamura–Craig M, Follenfant, RL. Effect of lamotrigine in the acute and chronic hyperalgesia induced by PGE_2 and in the chronic hyperalgesia in rats with streptozotocin-induced diabetes. Pain 1995; 63:33–37.
73. Clayton NM, Collins SD, Sargent R, Brown T, Nobbs M, Bountra C. The effects of the novel Na$^+$ channel blocker 4030W92 in models of acute and chronic inflammatory pain in the rat. Br J Pharmacol 1998; 123:79P.
74. Collins SD, Clayton NM, Nobbs M, Bountra C. The effects of 4030W92, a novel Na$^+$ channel blocker, on the treatment of neuropathic pain in the rat. Br J Pharmacol 1998.
75. Trezise DJ, John VH, Xie X. Voltage- and use-dependent inhibition of Na$^+$ channels in rat sensory neurones by 4030W92, a new antihyperalgesic agent. Br J Pharmacol 1998; 124:953–963.
76. Gardiner JC, Gupta P, Butler P, Pryke JG, Roffey SJ. The sodium channel modulators lamotrigine

and 4030W92 block ectopic discharge originating in rat sciatic neuromas. Br J Pharmacol 1998; 123: 21P.

77. Wall PD, Gutnick M. Properties of afferent nerve impulses originating from a neuroma. Nature 1974; 248:740–743.
78. Yaari Y, Devor M. Phenytoin suppresses spontaneous ectopic discharge in rat sciatic nerve neuromas. Neurosci Lett 1985; 58:117–122.
79. Chabal C, Russell L, Burchiel KJ. The effects of intravenous lidocaine, tocainide and mexiletine on spontaneously active fibers originating in rat sciatic neuromas. Pain 1989; 38:333–338.
80. Omana–Zapata I, Khabbaz MA, Hunter JC, Clarke DE, Bley KR. Tetrodotoxin inhibits neuropathic ectopic activity in neuromas, dorsal root ganglia and dorsal horn neurones. Pain 1997; 72:41–49.
81. Omano–Zapata I, Khabbaz MA, Hunter JC, Bley KR. QX-314 inhibits ectopic nerve activity associated with neuropathic pain. Brain Res 1997; 771:228–237.
82. Abdi S, Lee DH, Chung JM. The antiallodynic effects of amitryptiline, gabapentin and lidocaine in a rat model of neuropathic pain. Anesth Analg 1998; 87:1360–1366.
83. Matzner L, Devor M. Na^+ conductance and the threshold for repetitive neuronal firing. Brain Res 1992; 597:92–98.
84. Trezise DJ, John VH, Xie X. Electrophysiological studies on the effects of lamotrigine on rat dorsal root ganglion neurones in vitro. Br J Pharmacol 1997; 122:31P.
85. Backus KH, Pflimlin P, Trube G. Action of diazepam on the voltage-dependent Na^+ current. Comparison with the effects of phenytoin, carbamazepine, lidocaine and flumazenil. Brain Res 1991; 548: 41–49.
86. Scholz A, Kuboyama N, Hempelmann G, Vogel W. Complex blockade of TTX-resistant Na^+ currents by lidocaine and bupivacaine reduce firing frequency in DRG neurons. J Neurophysiol 1998; 79: 1746–1754.
87. Hitosugi H, Kashiwazaki T, Ohsawa M, Kamei J. Effects of mexiletine on algogenic mediator-induced nociceptive responses in mice. Methods Find Exp Clin Pharmacol 1999; 21:409–413.
88. Yashpal K, Mason P, McKenna JE, Sharma SK, Henry JL, Coderre TJ. Comparison of the effects of treatment with intrathecal lidocaine given before and after formalin on both nociception and Fos expression in the spinal cord dorsal horn. Anaesthesiology 1998; 88:157–164.
89. Woolf CJ, Wiesenfeld–Hallin Z. The systemic administration of local anaesthetics produces a selective depression of C-afferent fibre evoked activity in the spinal cord. Pain 1985; 23:361–374.
90. Fraser HM, Chapman V, Dickenson AH. Spinal local anaesthetic actions on afferent evoked responses and wind-up of nociceptive neurones in the rat spinal cord: combination with morphine produces marked potentiation of antinociception. Pain 1992; 49:33–41.
91. Luo L, Wiesenfeld–Hallin Z. Effects of intrathecal local anesthetics on spinal excitability and on the development of autotomy. Pain 1995; 63:212–214.
92. Blackburn–Munro G, Fleetwood–Walker SM. The effects of Na^+ channel blockers on somatosensory processing by rat dorsal horn neurones. Neuroreport 1997; 8:1549–1554.
93. Nagy I, Woolf CJ. Lignocaine selectively reduces C-fibre evoked neuronal activity in rat spinal cord in vitro by decreasing *N*-methyl-D-aspartate and neurokinin receptor-mediated post synaptic depolarizations; implications for the development of novel centrally acting analgesics. Pain 1995; 64:59–70.
94. Trew EA, Xie X, Trezise DJ. Modulation of synaptic transmission in the rat spinal cord in vitro by 4030W92, a novel antihyperalgesic agent. Br J Pharmacol 1998; 125:51P.
95. Song J–H, Huang C–S, Nagata K, Yeh JZ, Narahashi T. Differential action of riluzole on tetrodotoxin-sensitive and tetrodotoxin-resistant sodium channels. J Pharmacol Exp Ther 1997; 282:707–714.
96. Rush AM, Elliott JR. Phenytoin and carbamazepine: differential inhibition of Na^+ currents in small cells from adult rat dorsal root ganglia. Neurosci Letts 1997; 226:95–98.
97. Song J–H, Nagat K, Huang C–S, Yeh JZ, Narahashi T. Differential block of two types of sodium channels by anticonvulsants. Neuroreport 1996; 7:3031–3036.
98. Clark SA, Kaczorowski GJ, Wafford KA. Inhibition of the tetrodotoxin-resistant sodium current of acutely dissociated rat dorsal root ganglion neurones by WIN17317-3. J Physiol 1998; P168.

49
Calcium Channel Antagonists and the Control of Pain

Anthony H. Dickenson and Elizabeth A. Matthews
University College London, London, England

Alvaro M. Diaz
Universidad de Cantabria, Santander, Spain

I. INTRODUCTION

Calcium ions play an important role in neurotransmission, being essential for transmitter release from terminals. They also play a key role in neurons, linking receptors and enzymes, acting as intracellular signals, forming a channel-gating mechanism, and contributing to the degree of depolarization of the cell. Thus, calcium channels, the means by which calcium enters the neuron and terminal, are targets for a variety of neurotransmitters, neuromodulators, and drugs (1). This chapter will concentrate on the roles of calcium channels in the events that lead to pain. Most of our knowledge is based on the spinal cord.

II. DIFFERENT CALCIUM CHANNELS

Two families of voltage-dependent calcium channels (VDCCs) exist in vertebrate sensory and other neurons. This distinction has been made primarily on the basis of the well-defined electrophysiological properties of the two families of channels. The first type of channel is the low-threshold, rapidly inactivating, slowly deactivating channels (low-voltage activated; LVA; also referred to as T-type), whereas the others make up the group of high-threshold, slowly activating, fast-deactivating channels (high-voltage activated; HVA) (2). In the rat spinal cord, the existence of both families of VDCCs has been demonstrated by voltage clamp studies on sensory neurons (3).

The pharmacological tools for full investigation of the LVA are, as yet, not fully developed. By contrast, the availability of different ligands and toxins has allowed at least three main subtypes within the HVA channels to be distinguished. One, the L-type, has high affinity for dihydropyridines (DHP), phenylalkylamines (verapamil); and benzothiazepines (diltiazem); the N-type is selectively blocked by ω-conotoxin-GVIA, and the third, the P-type, is ω-agatoxin-IVA sensitive. Recently, other subtypes (sometimes termed O-, Q-, and R-type) have also been described (2,4,5) but as yet, little is known about their roles in pain-related transmission.

Within the spinal cord, L-type calcium channels are present in the dorsal horn, with a density comparable with a number of brain areas (6). N-type channels show the highest densities in the most superficial laminae I and II of the spinal cord, the areas at which the fine afferent fibers terminate (7,8). The spinal location of the P-type channel has not been studied. Selective antagonists of VDCCs have proved to be powerful pharmacological tools for identifying and characterizing calcium channels. A synthetic VDCC antagonist, SNX-230 (a derivative of ω-conopeptide; MVIIC), shows high-affinity binding to receptors in rat brain and blocks one or more high-threshold VDCCs that are neither L- nor N-type. The neuroanatomical distribution of these high-affinity non-L, non-N VDCC receptors for SNX-230 has been compared with the location of the N-type VDCCs. That distinct location of the two ligands was seen in cervical spinal cord suggests that there are calcium channels other than L- and N-types within it (8).

The influx of calcium into neurons would seem to be important in persistent pain models in which peripheral or central sensitization and plasticity are present (9). Thus, several studies have shown that behavioral responses to phasic nociceptive tests, such as the tail-flick and hot-plate during which brief stimuli are used, are not clearly affected by changes in the levels of calcium or its mobilization (10,11). However, when the stimulus is more prolonged, as in tonic nociceptive tests such as formalin and the writhing test, calcium channel blockers have effectiveness (10,12). The discovery of agents selective for the different channels has allowed the roles of particular types of channel to be assessed in different models of pain.

III. INFLAMMATORY PAIN

There are several models of persistent nociception produced by inflammation. The subcutaneous injection of dilute formalin has been used as a model to study peripheral and central spinal events after the induction of a peripheral inflammatory state. Formalin injected into the hindpaw produces an acute phase 1 and then a delayed persistent phase 2 that can be observed in both behavioral studies (13) and in electrophysiological studies of dorsal horn neurons (14–16). There is a remarkable concordance in the timing and magnitude of the responses using these different approaches. Several central neurotransmitter systems are involved in the formalin response. In particular, predominant actions of glutamate on the AMPA receptor underlie the first phase, whereas an important role of the *N*-methyl-D-aspartate (NMDA) receptor in phase 2, when peripheral inflammation is present, has led to the idea that this receptor facilitates nociception in the second phase (16–20). This response to formalin has therefore been used to study the effects of calcium channel antagonists on acute and more persistent behavior and neuronal activity at the spinal cord.

Blockade of VDCCs by the trivalent cations neodymium ($NdCl_3$) and lanthanum ($LaCl_3$) resulted in a dose-dependent suppression of both phases of the response to formalin (21,22). ω-Conopeptides, which selectively block N-type VDCC, also produced a dose-dependent inhibition of both the initial phase 1, when given by the intrathecal route; order of effectiveness: SNX-111 > SNX-185 > SNX-239 ≫ SNX-159; and phase 2: SNX-111 > SNX-185 > SNX-239 > SNX-159. In contrast, SNX-231, which is selective for a non-L/non-N–site present in the spinal cord, and also the L-type VDCC blockers nifedipine, nimodipine, verapamil, and diltiazem had minimal effects on either phase of the formalin test even at the high doses. By contrast, the P-type channel blocker ω-agatoxin IVA produced only a 40% inhibition of phase 1 at the highest dose, whereas phase 2 was suppressed in a dose-dependent fashion. High doses of the N-type VDCC produced characteristic shaking behavior, tail movements, and impaired coordination. A further study with SNX-111 showed dose-dependent suppression of both the acute phase 1 and tonic phase 2 of the formalin test when the N-type blocker was infused for 72 h immediately before testing. Phase 2 nociceptive responses were suppressed by bolus injections of SNX-111 injected spinally once the activity had been established. However, at antinociceptive doses there was no significant motor effect (22). Another study has reported that spinal L-type calcium channel blockers have at best, mild transient actions on the formalin test when given spinally (9).

A more recent electrophysiological study in vivo has examined the role of VDCCs in facilitated nociceptive processing at the level of the spinal cord (23). The effects of the intrathecal administration of different VDCC blockers were studied in the formalin model of inflammation, monitoring the responses of convergent dorsal horn neurons in rats under halothane anesthesia. Administration of the L-type calcium channel blocker verapamil before formalin injection had no significant effect on either the first or second phase of the formalin response. Pretreatment with the N-type calcium channel blocker ω-conotoxin-GVIA reduced both phases of the formalin response. The low dose of ω-conotoxin-GVIA significantly inhibited the first-phase response, whereas the high dose additionally significantly reduced the second phase. Pretreatment with the P-type calcium channel blocker ω-agatoxin-IVA had no effect on the first phase, whereas a marked dose-related reduction in the second phase of formalin response was found, with the high dose producing almost complete inhibition (23). An important point is the possible toxicity of these compounds, but in this study the doses used were 20-fold less those reported to produce toxicity in behavioral studies after spinal application (22). Remarkably, the results of this electrophysiological study agree almost entirely with the behavioral studies with this model (21,22).

These electrophysiological and behavioral results indicate that there is a distinct contribution of each type of spinal VDCC (L-, N-, and P-type calcium channels) to the two phases of the responses of dorsal horn neurons to the peripheral injection of formalin. The L-type channels appear to play minimal roles in the formalin response, whereas blockade of N- and P-type channels reduced the responses. The inhibitions of both phases produced by the N-type antagonist contrasted the marked and selective inhibition of the second phase seen after the P-type antagonist.

Another electrophysiological study addressed the involvement of VDCCs of the N- and L-type in the spinal processing of innocuous and noxious input from the knee joint, both under normal conditions and under inflammatory conditions induced in the knee joint by kaolin and carrageenan before the recordings (25). P-type channels were not studied here. The antagonist at N-type calcium channels, ω-conotoxin-GVIA, reduced the responses to both innocuous and noxious pressure applied to the knee joint in neurons with input from the normal joint and in neurons recorded with the inflamed joint (hyperexcitable neurons). Spinal nimodipine decreased the responses to innocuous and noxious pressure applied to the knee in neurons with input from the normal joint and in neurons with input from the inflamed knee joint (hyperexcitable neurons). The ionophoretic administration of the agonist at the L-type calcium channel, S(−)-Bay K 8644, enhanced the responses to mechanical stimulation of the knee joint in all neurons tested. These data show that VDCCs of both the N- and the L-type are important for the sensory functions of the spinal cord and are involved in the spinal processing of nonnociceptive as well as nociceptive mechanosensory input from the joint, under both normal and inflammatory conditions. These results differ from those with formalin in that L-type channels are reported to play a role, whereas the L-type calcium channel blocker verapamil did not affect either phase of the formalin response, even at high doses. The latter suggests that calcium influx through L-type VDCCs does not appear to be involved in the hyperexcitability of the dorsal horn neurons subsequent to formalin-evoked inflammation. In behavioral studies using the formalin test, antinociceptive effects of several L-type antagonists have been reported (26–28). In all studies, the L-type antagonists were administered systemically. In one of these studies (27), pretreatment with verapamil produced a potent and dose-dependent inhibition of both phases of the formalin-induced nociception. It is likely that these positive effects of systemic L-type calcium channel blockers could be explained by actions at peripheral or supraspinal sites. However, it also must be borne in mind that nonselective effects of these agents by the systemic route could interfere with the results.

Intradermal capsaicin injection causes primary hyperalgesia to heat and mechanical stimuli applied near the injection site, as well as secondary mechanical hyperalgesia (increased pain from noxious stimuli) and mechanical allodynia (pain from innocuous stimuli) in an area surrounding the site of primary hyperalgesia. A study in rats tested the hypothesis that the secondary hyperalgesia and allodynia observed following capsaicin was dependent on activation of VDCCs in the spinal cord (29). Animals were pretreated with L-type (nifedipine), N-type (ω-conotoxin-GVIA) or P-type (ω-agatoxin-IVA) calcium channel blockers to the spinal dorsal horn before the injection of capsaicin. None of the antagonists had any affect on normal sensory or motor responses, but all three blockers dose dependently prevented the development of secondary mechanical hyperalgesia and allodynia. These data suggest that all three calcium channels are important for the development of mechanical hyperalgesia and allodynia that occurs following capsaicin injection(29).

IV. NEUROPATHY

Another major pain state is that caused by damage to peripheral nerves. The results from the formalin studies show that the L-type channel plays a minor role at best, the N-type channel is needed for both phases, and the P-type channel makes an important and selective contribution to the second phase. This might allow the use of agents acting to block these channels in particular pain states and here a major issue is neuropathic pain. In a comparison of the effects of antagonists specific to the N-, L-, and P-type VDCCs, as well as an antagonist at a non-L-, non-N-type site, drugs were given by lumbar intrathecal, intravenous, or regional nerve block catheters implanted in rats with tactile allodynia induced by tight ligation of the fifth and sixth lumbar spinal nerves (30). Intrathecally delivered N-type VDCC blockers (ω-conopeptides SNX-239, SNX-159, and SNX-111) produced dose-dependent blockade of tactile allodynia (touch-evoked nocieptive behavior). Intrathecal L-type and non–N-, non–L-type ω-conopeptide SNX-230) and P-type (ω-agatoxin-IVA) VDCC antagonists had no effect on this behavior at the highest doses examined. No VDCC antagonist suppressed paw withdrawal when administered by other routes. These results emphasize the importance of N-type, but not L- or P-type, VDCCs in the spinal cord in systems mediating persistent tactile allodynia after nerve injury.

In a further study in rats with an experimentally induced painful peripheral neuropathy, intrathecal bolus injections of SNX-111 blocked mechanical allodynia in a dose-dependent manner. SNX-111 was given by continuous intrathecal infusion and produced a reversible blockade of mechanical allodynia without any sign of tolerance (24). These results show that selective N-type VDCC blockers are potent and efficacious antiallodynia agents when they are administered by the spinal route against neuropathic pain. The spontaneous pain-related behavior and the hyperalgesia that is also produced in these models needs to be studied.

Tactile allodynia induced by L-5/6 selective nerve ligation was dose-dependently blocked by intrathecal bolus administration of N-type selective synthetic conopeptide homologues SNX-111, SNX-239, and SNX-159, with no effect when administered intravenously or regionally to the nerve. ω-Agatoxin-IVA and SNX-230 (synthetic P/Q-type selective conopeptide homologue) were without effect (30). In the chronic constriction injury (CCI) model of nerve injury, SNX-111 and SNX-124 reduced heat hyperalgesia and mechanoallodynia when delivered directly to the site of injury, and these were without effect in the uninjured nerve (31). Mechanical hyperalgesia in rats with partial nerve ligation was reduced by subcutaneous injection of SNX-

111 into the receptive field, whereas SNX-230 had no effect. Neither compound had any effect in control animals (32).

Intrathecal administration of the selective N-type VDCC antagonist, ω-conotoxin-GVIA, produces inhibition of both electrically and naturally (innocuous and noxious) evoked neuronal responses, recorded from the rat dorsal horn. After the establishment of neuropathy the inhibitory effect of ω-conotoxin-GVIA, especially at low doses, was significantly enhanced. In contrast, intrathecal administration of the P-type VDCC antagonist, ω-agatoxin-IVA, did not significantly inhibit the electrically evoked dorsal horn neuronal responses, and its pharmacological profile was unaltered after nerve injury (33).

V. ROLES OF L-TYPE CALCIUM CHANNELS IN PAIN

Although DHP binding sites are found in the spinal cord (6), the involvement of L-type channels in the release of neurotransmitters from sensory neurons in the spinal cord is controversial (34,35), and not only is little or no transmitter release in the brain mediated by these channels, but also specific modulation of these channels by transmitters has only occasionally been reported (36). Even when L-type–dependent release of neurotransmitters has been demonstrated from dorsal root ganglion neurons, it is dependent on the type of stimulus. Thus, the L-type antagonist nifedipine attenuated potassium-stimulated release of substance P (SP) and calcitonin gene-related peptide (CGRP) from dorsal root ganglion, but not that evoked by more physiological stimuli, such as that produced by the inflammatory mediator bradykinin (37). As L-type VDCCs are primarily localized on cell bodies and dendrites of neurons of rat CNS (38), calcium influx through these channels may be more relevant to regulation of calcium-dependent intracellular events rather than transmitter release. For example, L-type calcium channels mediate synaptic activation of immediate early genes so that calcium influx through both L- and N-type calcium channels appear to be involved in the increase of spinal proenk mRNA levels induced by forskolin (39).

Thus, it could be suggested that even if changes in L-type calcium channels are contributing to neuronal plasticity or central sensitization after formalin, they appear to play minor roles in the neuronal and behavioral responses. Possibly, the situation could be different after more persistent nociception—several hours, rather than the 1–2 h of the formalin response, such as that produced by injection of carrageenan. In fact, results with this model, discussed earlier (25), support this idea, as do the studies using capsaicin as the stimulus (29).

VI. ROLES OF N-TYPE CALCIUM CHANNELS IN PAIN

The N-type antagonist ω-conotoxin-GVIA produces a clear inhibition of both phases of the formalin response (21–23), and this blocker that binds irreversibly to the N-type calcium channel is very similar in effect to ω-conopeptides, such as SNX-111, that bind reversibly with high affinity to N-type calcium channels. The latter possess fewer adverse behavioral effects at antinociceptive doses, especially when administered intraspinally (5).

ω-Conotoxin-GVIA selectively blocks N-type VDCCs in cell bodies and presynaptic terminals (40). N-type channels are located with high density in the superficial dorsal horn where small myelinated and unmyelinated nociceptive afferents terminate (7,8). This strategic location suggests that N-type channels play a key role in neurotransmitter release from small primary afferents. In vitro, the release of CGRP from rat spinal afferents is mediated by ω-conotoxin–sensitive calcium channels and N-type antagonists block the depolarization-coupled release of neuropeptides from capsaicin-sensitive spinal afferents as well as substance P release from primary sensory neurons in culture (35,41). All these data suggest that the reductions in phase 1 and phase 2 of the formalin response as seen with N-type antagonists could result from blockade of neuropeptide release from nociceptive afferents. However, glutamate release is another possibility. ω-Conopeptides are able to reduce depolarization-evoked glutamate release (42). Interestingly, presynaptic blockade of N-type channels by ω-conotoxin-GVIA inhibits glutamatergic synaptic transmission between dorsal root ganglion neurons and spinal cord neurons (43). Taken together, these results demonstrate that N-type calcium channels play a dominant role in glutamatergic sensory neurotransmission. They suggest, in addition, that modulation of N-channel activity may act to cause a presynaptic inhibition of synaptic transmission between DRG neurons and their targets in the intact spinal cord. Furthermore, ω-conotoxin–sensitive N-type channels play a major role in the spinal synaptic transmission that mediates monosynaptic and electrically evoked slow polysynaptic reflexes, and a lesser but still significant role in fast and capsaicin-evoked polysynaptic reflexes. L-type channels play a minor role (44).

The balance of the literature would therefore favor a control of both glutamate and peptide release by N-type channels. Both phases of the formalin response require glutamate release and activation of the AMPA and NMDA receptors, in the first and second phases, respectively, with an additional role of neuropeptides in the second phase, possibly to remove the magnesium block of the NMDA receptor (45). Consequently, ω-conotoxin-GVIA and the SNX compounds would appear to reduce release of both peptides and glutamate, which is likely to be the basis for their additional effectiveness against the tactile allodynia produced by nerve damage. Other evidence that implies an interneuronal site for the action of conopeptides on N-type VDCCs include the failure of peripherally applied N-type VDCC blockers applied to the site of injury to inhibit allodynia after spinal nerve ligation (SNL) suggesting spinal blockade of N-type channels affects interneuronal neurotransmitter release and not release from terminals of primary afferent fibers; N-type calcium channel blockers may well have broad effectiveness in both acute and more persistent inflammatory and neuropathic nociceptive transmission.

VII. P-TYPE CALCIUM CHANNELS

The P-type calcium channel blocker ω-agatoxin-IVA produces a potent dose-dependent reduction in the second phase of the formalin response, but no significant effect (only a weak inhibition) on the acute response (phase 1) (21–23). This, therefore, suggests that the P-type channel is involved in events only in the second phase. Indeed, the actions of ω-agatoxin-IVA resemble those of spinal NMDA antagonists in that they are selective for the prolonged or facilitated phase of the formalin response (14–18,20).

A number of studies reinforce the importance of ω-agatoxin-IVA–sensitive P-type channels in the regulation of glutamate release in the brain (41,42). Recently, evidence for the presence of P-type channels in the spinal cord has been provided by an in vitro study during which ω-agatoxin-IVA blocked a substantial fraction of current carried by HVA calcium channels in spinal cord interneurons (46).

Finally, it has been suggested that nitric oxide (NO) generated by neurons in the spinal cord in response to NMDA receptor activation could play a role during prolonged nociception (47). In fact, the second phase of the formalin response is reduced by nitric oxide synthase (NOS) inhibitors (48). The increased neuronal excitability produced by NMDA receptor activation requires the production of NO, which could act retrogradely onto presynaptic afferent fibers to further increase neurotransmitter release from C fibers (49). In fact, NMDA-induced NOS activity in rat frontal cortex is blocked by ω-agatoxin-IVA but not by L- and N-type antagonists (50).

Therefore, it could be hypothesized that the selective effects of ω-agatoxin-IVA on the second phase of the formalin response are a consequence of its block of P-type channels that are not only necessary for glutamate release, but also for NMDA receptor activation of NOS. Blockers of these channels may have high selectivity for persistent noxious hyperexcitable states, sparing acute transmission.

VIII. IMPLICATIONS

SNX-111 is one of the few new calcium channel blockers that has been given to patients, and it appears to be well tolerated in clinical studies when given as a neuroprotective agent (5). A key stage in the appraisal of the possible roles of these agents in pain therapy is a series of controlled trials in different pain states. Presumably, the initial studies will have to use the spinal route. The problem that many of the tools acting on calcium channels are based on toxins and so are limited to the spinal route may have been overcome by the finding that gabapentin, the antiepileptic drug effective in the treatment of neuropathy, may act through the modulation of these channels. A series of randomized, controlled trials of gabapentin have revealed its effectiveness. One, in patients with postherpetic neuralgia, concluded that gabapentin was effective in the treatment of this pain state (51). Furthermore, another controlled trial showed clear pain reductions in patients with diabetic neuropathy (52). These two studies are remarkable, as they are the first clinical trials to enroll large number of patients, more than 100 in each case. In addition, a preliminary study in a mixed group of patients reported that gabapentin was effective in pain caused by peripheral nerve injury and central lesions, with particular effectiveness on paroxysmal pain and allodynia, but with no effect on some other measures (53). In keeping with these studies in patients, both spinal and systemic gabapentin reduces heat hyperalgesia and mechano- and cold allodynia in the chronic constriction injury model of neuropathy (54), and a behavioral study reports that systemic gabapentin blocks mechanical allodynia in a rat model of diabetic neuropathy (55). In electrophysiological studies, gabapentin inhibits both innocuous- and noxious-evoked responses of spinal neurons of rats after spinal nerve ligation, although it also produced similar inhibitory effects on neuronal responses of sham-operated rats. The actions of gabapentin, therefore, are not specific for neuropathy and are apparent after general nerve or tissue damage (56–59). The weak actions or lack of effect of the drug in normal animals, but the novel actions after tissue or nerve damage, fit well with the profile of the characterized calcium channel blockers described previously in this chapter.

The mechanism of action of gabapentin is not established, but there are recent strong indications that the drug may interact with calcium channels. The so-called gabapentin-binding protein (GBP) is associated with the $\alpha 2\delta$-subunit of the calcium channel (60). This subunit of the channel, an accessory protein found in all calcium channels, may be the target for gabapentin—it has to be assumed that it acts as an antagonist at these channels. This mode of action would fit with the evidence that N-type calcium channel blockers are more effective in reducing behavioral and electrophysiological responses to sensory stimuli after both nerve injury and tissue damage (33). Very recent studies, at least after nerve damage, show that N-type calcium channels are up-regulated (61).

The early indications were solely on the potential of calcium channel blockers in therapy designed to alleviate the consequences of cerebral ischemia (62) and spinal cord injury (63). It is now clear that their therapeutic potential may also include pain. Thus, there is now a strong body of evidence supporting the role of calcium channels in a number of pain states and good evidence to support the concept of plasticity in their roles, in that blockers show enhanced actions after both tissue and nerve damage. The next challenge would be to produce systemically tolerated drugs that target these key channels. Whether side effects will compromise the therapeutic potential of these agents remains to be seen.

ACKNOWLEDGMENTS

This work is supported by the Wellcome Trust.

REFERENCES

1. Spedding M, Paoletti R. Classification of calcium channels and the sites of action of drugs modifying channel function. Pharmacol Rev 1992; 44:63–376.
2. Bertolino M, Llinás RR. The central role of voltage-activated and receptor-operated calcium channels in neuronal cells Annu Rev Pharmacol Toxicol 1992; 32:399–421.
3. Ryu PD, Randic M. Low- and high-voltage activated calcium currents in rat spinal dorsal horn neurons. J Neurophysiol 1990; 63:273–285.
4. Olivera BM, Miljanich GP, Ramachandran J, Adams ME. Calcium channel diversity and neurotransmitter release: the ω-conotoxins and ω-agatoxins. Annu Rev Biochem 1994; 63:823–867.
5. Miljanich GP, Ramachandran J. Antagonists of neuronal calcium channels: structure, function, and therapeutic implications. Annu Rev Pharmacol Toxicol 1995; 35:707–734.
6. Gandhi VC, Jones DJ. Identification and characterization of [^{3}H]nitrendipine binding sites in rat spinal cord. J Pharmacol Exp Ther 1998; 247:473–480.
7. Kerr LM, Filloux F, Olivera BM, Jackson H, Wamsley JK. Autoradiographic localization of calcium channels with [^{125}I]ω-Conotoxin in rat brain. Eur J Pharmacol 1998; 146:181–183.
8. Gohil K, Bell JR, Ramachandran J, Miljanich GP. Neuroanatomical distribution of receptors for a novel voltage-sensitive calcium channel antagonist, SNX-230 (ω-conopeptide MVIIC). Brain Res 1994; 653:258–266.
9. Coderre TJ, Melzack R. The role of NMDA receptor-operated calcium channels in persistent nociception after formalin-induced tissue injury. J Neurosci 1992; 12:3671–3675.
10. Chapman DB, Way EL. Modification of endorphin/enkephalin analgesia and stress induced analgesia by divalent cations, a cation chelator and an ionophore. Br J Pharmacol 1982; 75:89–96.
11. Contreras E, Tamayo L, Amigo M. Calcium channel antagonists increase morphine-induced analgesia an antagonize morphine tolerance. Eur J Pharmacol 1998; 148:463–466.
12. Del Pozo E, Caro G, Baeyens JM. Analgesic effects of several calcium channel blockers in mice. Eur J Pharmacol 1987; 137:155–160.
13. Porro CA, Cavazzuti M. Spatial and temporal aspects of spinal cord and brainstem activation in the formalin pain model. Prog Neurobiol 1993; 41:565–607.
14. Dickenson AH, Sullivan AF. Peripheral origins and central modulation of subcutaneous formalin-induced activity of dorsal horn neurones. Neurosci Lett 1987; 8:201–211.
15. Dickenson AH, Sullivan AF. Subcutaneous formalin-induced activity of dorsal horn neurones in the rat: differential response to an intrathecal opiate administered pre or post formalin. Pain 1987; 30: 349–360.
16. Haley JE, Sullivan AF, Dickenson AH. Evidence for spinal *N*-methyl-D-asparate receptor involvement in prolonged chemical nociception in the rat. Brain Res 1990; 518:218–226.
17. Yamamoto T, Yaksh TL. Comparison of the antinociceptive effects of pre- and posttreatment with intrathecal morphine and MK801, an NMDA antagonist, on the formalin test in the rat. Anesthesiology 1992; 77:757–763.
18. Vaccarino AL, Marek P, Kest B, Weber E, Keana JF, Liebeskind JC. NMDA receptor antagonists, MK-801 and ACEA-1011, prevent the development of tonic pain following subcutaneous formalin. Brain Res 1993; 615:331–334.

19. Hunter JC, Singh L. Role of excitatory amino acid receptors in the mediation of the nociceptive response to formalin in the rat. Neurosci Lett 1994; 174:217–221.
20. Millan MJ, Seguin L. Chemically-diverse ligands at the glycine B site coupled to *N*-methyl-D-aspartate (NMDA) receptors selectively block the late phase of formalin-induced pain in mice. Neurosci Lett 1994; 178:139–143.
21. Malmberg AB, Yaksh TL. Voltage-sensitive calcium channels in spinal nociceptive processing: blockade of N- and P-type channels inhibits formalin-induced nociception. J Neurosci 1994; 14: 4882–4890.
22. Malmberg AB, Yaksh TL. Effect of continuous intrathecal infusion of ω-conopeptides, N-type calcium channels blockers, on behaviour and antinociception in the formalin and hot-plate tests in rats. Pain 1995; 60:83–90.
23. Diaz A, Dickenson AH. Blockade of spinal N- and P-type, but not L-type, calcium channels inhibits the excitability of rat dorsal horn neurones produced by subcutaneous formalin inflammation. Pain 1997; 69:93–100.
24. Bowersox SS, Gadbois T, Singh T, Pettus M, Wang YX, Luther RR. Selective N-type neuronal voltage-sensitive calcium channel blocker, SNX-111, produces spinal antinociception in rat models of acute, persistent and neuropathic pain. J Pharmacol Exp Ther 1996; 279:1243–1249.
25. Neugebauer V, Vanegas H, Nebe J, Rumenapp P, Schaible HG. Effects of N- and L-type calcium channel antagonists on the responses of nociceptive spinal cord neurons to mechanical stimulation of the normal and the inflamed knee joint. J Neurophysiol 1996; 76:3740–3749.
26. Bustamante D, Miranda HF, Pelissier T, Paeile R. Analgesic action of clonixin, nifedipine and morphine using the formalin test. Gen Pharmacol 1989; 20:319–322.
27. Gürdal H, Sara Y, Tuluny FC. Effects of calcium channel blockers on formalin-induced nociception and inflammation in rats. Pharmacology 1992; 44:290–296.
28. Miranda HF, Bustamante D, Kramer V, Pelissier T, Saavedra H, Paeile C, Fernández E, Pinardi G. Antinociceptive effects of Ca^{2+} channels blockers. Eur J Pharmacol 1992; 217:137–141.
29. Sluka KA. Blockade of calcium channels can prevent the onset of secondary hyperalgesia and allodynia induced by intradermal injection of capsaicin in rats. Pain 1997; 71:157–164.
30. Chaplan SR, Pogrel JW, Yaksh TL. Role of voltage-dependent calcium channel subtypes in experimental tactile allodynia. J Pharmacol Exp Ther 1994; 269:1117–1123.
31. Xiao W-H, Bennett GJ. Synthetic ω-conopeptides applied to the site of nerve injury suppress neuropathic pains in rats. J Pharmacol Exp Ther 1995; 274:666–672.
32. White DM, Cousins MJ. Effect of subcutaneous administration of calcium channel blockers on nerve injury-induced hyperalgesia. Brain Res 1988; 801:50–58.
33. Matthews EA, Dickenson AH. Effects of spinally delivered N- and P-type voltage-dependent calcium channel antagonists on dorsal horn neuronal responses in a rat model of neuropathy. Pain 2001; 92: 235–246.
34. Perney TM, Hirning LD, Leeman SE, Miller RJ. Multiple calcium channels mediate neurotransmitter release from peripheral neurons. Proc Natl Acad Sci USA 1986; 83:6656–6659.
35. Holz GG, Dunlap K, Kream RM. Characterization of the electrically evoked release of substance P from dorsal root ganglion neurons: methods and dihydropyridine sensitivity. J Neurosci 1988; 8: 468–471.
36. Anwyl R. Modulation of vertebrate neuronal calcium channels by transmitters. Brain Res Rev 1991; 16:265–281.
37. Evans AR, Nicol GD, Vasko MR. Differential regulation of evoked peptide release by voltage-sensitive calcium channels in rat sensory neurons. Brain Res 1996; 712:265–273.
38. Ahlijanian MK, Westenbroek RE, Caterall WA. Subunit structure and localization of voltage sensitive calcium channels in mammalian brain, spinal cord, and retina. Neuron 1990; 4:819–832.
39. Ha TS, Kim YH, Song DK, Wie MB, Suh HW. Molecular mechanisms underlying the regulation of proenkephalin gene expression in cultured spinal cord cells. Neuropeptides 1996; 30:506–513.
40. McCleskey A, Fox AP, Cruz LJ, Olivera BM, Tsien RW, Yoshikami D. ω-Conotoxin: direct and persistent blockade of specific types of calcium channels in neurons but not in muscle. Proc Natl Acad Sci USA 1987; 84:4327–4331.
41. Maggi CA, Giuliani S, Santicioli P, Tramontana M, Meli A. Effect of omega conotoxin on reflex

responses mediated by activation of capsaicin-sensitive nerves of the rat urinary bladder and peptide release from the rat spinal cord. Neuroscience 1990; 34:243–250.
42. Dickie BGM, Davies JA. Calcium channel blocking agents and potassium-stimulated release of glutamate from cerebellar slices. Eur J Pharmacol 1992; 229:97–99.
43. Gruner W, Silva LR. ω-Conotoxin sensitivity and presynaptic inhibition of glutamatergic sensory neurotransmission in vitro. J Neurosci 1994; 14:2800–2808.
44. Bell JA. Selective blockade of spinal reflexes by omega-conotoxin in the isolated spinal cord of the neonatal rat. Neuroscience 1993; 52:711–716.
45. Dickenson AH. Mechanisms of central hypersensitivity. In: Dickenson AH, Besson JM, eds. The Pharmacology of Pain: Handbook of Experimental Pharmacology. Berlin: Springer, 1997:167–210.
46. Mintz IM, Adams ME, Bean BP. P-type calcium channels in rat central and peripheral neurons. Neuron 1992; 9:85–95.
47. Meller ST, Gebhart GF. Nitric oxide (NO) and nociceptive processing in the spinal cord. Pain 1993; 52:127–136.
48. Haley JE, Dickenson AH, Schachter M. Electrophysiological evidence for a role of nitric oxide in prolonged chemical nociception. Neuropharmacology 1992; 31:251–258.
49. Sorkin LS. NMDA evokes an L-NAME sensitive spinal release of glutamate and citrulline. Neuroreport 1993; 4:479–482.
50. Alagarsamy S, Johnson M. Voltage-dependent calcium channel involvement in NMDA-induced activation of NOS. Neuroreport 1995; 6:2250–2254.
51. Rowbotham MC, Harden N, Stacey B, Bernstein P, Magnus–Miller L. Gabapentin for the treatment of postherpetic neuralgia. JAMA 1998; 280:1837–1842.
52. Backonja M, Beydoun A, Edwards KR, et al. Gabapentin for the symptomatic treatment of painful neuropathy in patients with diabetes mellitus: a randomized controlled trial. JAMA 1998; 280:1831–1836.
53. Attal N, Brasseur L, Parker F, Chauvin M, Bouhassira D. Effects of gabapentin on the different components of peripheral and central neuropathic pain syndromes: a pilot study. Eur Neurol 1998; 40:191–200.
54. Hunter JC, Gogas KR, Hedley LR, Jacobson LO, Kassotakis L, Thompson J, Fontana DJ. The effect of novel anti-epileptic drugs in rat experimental models of acute and chronic pain. Eur J Pharmacol 1997; 324:153–160.
55. Field MJ, McCleary S, Hughes J, Singh L. Gabapentin and pregabalin, but not morphine and amitriptyline, block both static and dynamic components of mechanical allodynia induced by streptozozin in the rat. Pain 1999; 80:391–398.
56. Field MJ, Holloman EF, McCleary S, Hughes J, Singh L. Evaluation of gabapentin and *S*-(+)-isobutyl GABA in a rat model of postoperative pain. J Pharmacol Exp Ther 1997; 282:1242–1246.
57. Stanfa LC, Singh L, Williams RG, Dickenson AH. Gabapentin, ineffective in normal rats, markedly reduces C-fibre evoked responses after inflammation. Neuroreport 1997; 8:587–590.
58. Chapman V, Suzuki R, Chamarette HLC, Rygh LJ, Dickenson AH. An electrophysiological study of the inhibitory effects of systemic carbamazepine and gabapentin on spinal neuronal responses in spinal nerve ligated rats. Pain 1998; 75:261–273.
59. Jones DL, Sorkin LS. Systemic gabapentin and *S*-(+)-isobutylgamma-aminobutyric acid block secondary hyperalgesia. Brain Res 1998; 810:93–99.
60. Taylor CP, Gee NS, Su T, Kocsis JD, Welty DF, Brown JP, Dooley DJ, Boden P, Singh L. A summary of mechanistic hypotheses of gabapentin pharmacology. Epilepsy Res 1998; 29:233–249.
61. Cizkova D, Marsala M, Stauderman K, Yaksh TL. Calcium channel α 1B subunit in spinal cord/DRG of normal and nerve-injured rats. Proceedings 9th World Congress on Pain 1999:134.
62. Faden AI. Pharmacological treatment of central nervous system trauma. Pharmacol Toxicol 1996; 78:12–17.
63. Zeidman SM, Ling GS, Ducker TB, Ellenbogen RG. Clinical applications of pharmacologic therapies for spinal cord injury. J Spinal Disord 1996; 9:367–380.

50

Profile of Ziconotide (SNX-111)

A Neuronal N-Type Voltage-Sensitive Calcium Channel Blocker

S. Scott Bowersox, Martha Mayo, and Robert R. Luther
Elan Pharmaceuticals, Menlo Park, California, U.S.A.

I. INTRODUCTION

The aggressive and effective management of severe pain has been a relatively neglected part of overall medical practice. Because pain is not objectively measurable, it is a symptom vulnerable to being overlooked or underestimated in the assessment of health status. Even when the need for pain management is recognized by clinicians, treatment options are often limited by fears of prescription-narcotic analgesic abuse or addiction. Moreover, severe pain is often poorly responsive to existing treatment modalities. For example, of the approximately 9 million people worldwide who develop cancer each year, 60–90% suffer from moderate-to-severe pain (1). In severe pain, intraspinal opioid delivery may be required to obtain adequate relief; however, it has been reported that intraspinal opioids are ineffective in approximately 26% of such clinical situations (2), and even when effective, development of tolerance or adverse effects can lead to treatment failure. Moreover, noncancer patients with neuropathic pain arising from injury to peripheral nerves, spinal cord, or brain are often treatment-resistant or else require intolerably high or stupefying doses of opioids to achieve relief. Thus, a clear need exists for effective nonopioid analgesic agents with acceptable side effect profiles for long-term administration in both malignant and nonmalignant chronic pain settings.

Ziconotide (SNX-111), a member of a new class of nonopioid analgesic agents, developed by Elan Pharmaceuticals, is currently in clinical development for the treatment of severe pain resulting from both neuropathic and nonneuropathic (visceral and somatic) disease states. The nonclinical pharmacological profile of ziconotide, reviewed briefly in this chapter, provides a rational basis for understanding the potential clinical usefulness of this compound in the treatment of pain. Ziconotide is intended for clinical administration by spinal routes (e.g., intrathecal or epidural delivery).

II. MOLECULAR PHARMACOLOGY

A. Ziconotide Structure and Class

Ziconotide is the synthetic version of one of a group of small (24- to 29-amino acids) disulfide-rich peptides, termed ω-conotoxins, found in the venoms of predatory marine snails belonging

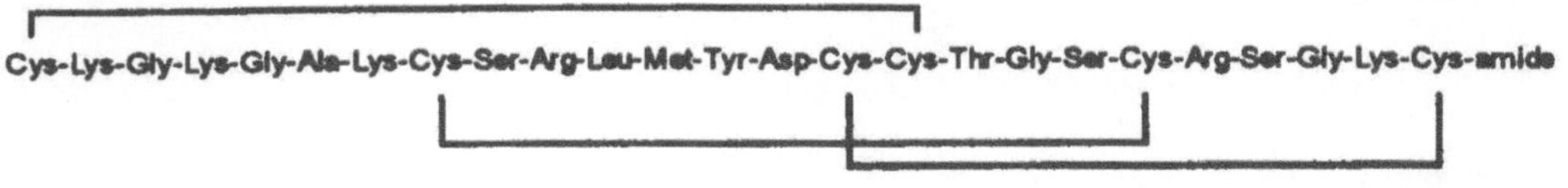

ω-conotoxin MVIIA (reduced), cyclic (1→16), (8→20), (15→25) tris (disulfide)

Chemical formula: $C_{102}H_{172}N_{36}O_{32}S_7$
Molecular weight: 2630.18 Daltons

Figure 1 Structure of ziconotide (SNX-111): Constituent amino acids are given in the standard three-letter code. The six cysteine residues are linked by disulfide bridges in the pattern 1–4, 2–5, 3–6.

to the genus *Conus* (Fig. 1) (3–5). Approximately 12 ω-conotoxins have been isolated from *Conus* snail venoms. All bind to voltage-sensitive calcium channels (VSCCs), although they differ greatly in their affinities for specific VSCC subtypes.

In the literature, ω-conotoxin often refers to one specific peptide, ω-conotoxin GVIA. This ω-conopeptide, the first to be described, was isolated from *C. geographicus* and has been extensively used as a standard ligand for characterizing voltage-sensitive calcium channels (6). Ziconotide is the synthetic form of another ω-conotoxin, MVIIA, originally isolated from the venom of *C. magus* (7). Although ziconotide has only 40% sequence homology to ω-conotoxin GVIA, both compounds have nearly the same binding affinity for neuronal N-type VSCCs; however, unlike ω-conotoxin GVIA, which binds virtually irreversibly to the N-type channel in in vitro-binding assays, ziconotide binding is reversible (8,9). This difference in apparent binding kinetics has also been observed in functional assays (10,11).

B. Molecular Target of Ziconotide—the N-Type Neuronal Calcium Channel

The therapeutic potential of ziconotide is related to its ability to block N-type VSCCs. The N-type channel is one of at least five classes of VSCC (designated L, N, T, P/Q, and R) that have been identified on the basis of electrophysiological and structural criteria (4). All share a common set of structural components: a central α_1-subunit containing the calcium-conducting pore, an α_2/δ-subunit, and a β-subunit. The α_1-subunit contains voltage-sensing elements and binding sites for calcium channel blockers. At least five different genes encode for α_1-subunits in neuronal VSCCs; the α_{1B}-subunit defines the N-type channel. Distinct variants of the N-type VSCC α_{1B}-subunit are differentially expressed in the mammalian brain and sympathetic neurons (12). Ziconotide binds with equal affinity to the dominant isoforms of the N-type VSCC in the peripheral and central nervous systems (Miller J, personal communication, 1998). The specificity of ziconotide for the N-type VSCC has been confirmed in both binding studies (8) and in electrophysiological studies carried out in clonal cell lines expressing α_{1B}-subunits (13). Ziconotide has no appreciable affinity for other ion channels, nor does it interact with cholinergic, monoaminergic, or peptidergic receptors (Bowersox S, unpublished findings, 1998). In competitive in vitro radioligand-binding studies, ziconotide binds weakly to the *N*-methyl-D-aspartate (NMDA) receptor and to potentiate ligand binding to the regulatory glycine-binding site on glutamate receptors (Bowersox S, unpublished findings, 1998). These interactions are unlikely to influence glutaminergic neurotransmission in vivo, because they are approximately six orders of magnitude weaker than the interaction of ziconotide with N-type VSCCs.

C. Anatomical Distribution of N-Type VSCCs

N-type VSCCs are found throughout the mammalian nervous system where they are expressed on neuronal somata, dendrites, dendritic shafts, and axon terminals (14,15). In the rat brain, N-type VSCCs are particularly dense in regions that are rich in synaptic connections (16). In the rat spinal cord, autoradiographic binding studies with [^{125}I]ziconotide have indicated that N-type VSCCs are confined to Rexed's laminae I and II of the dorsal horn (16), sites that receive most of their input from primary peripheral nociceptive afferent fibers (17). More precise localization of N-type VSCCs by immunostaining with antibodies against the α_{1B}-subunit has confirmed that N-type channels are the predominant VSCCs associated with primary nociceptive afferents in the rat spinal cord, although recent studies indicate that N-type channels are distributed more evenly throughout the dorsal horn than initially thought (18).

D. Ziconotide Interactions with N-Type VSCCs

Ziconotide blocks depolarization-induced calcium influx, and by this action, affects a variety of intracellular calcium-dependent processes, including the modulation of neuronal excitability, release of neurotransmitters, activation of second-messenger systems, and gene transcription. The dominant pharmacological effect of ziconotide at the cellular level is the blockade of neurotransmitter release from presynaptic nerve terminals (4). In general, neurotransmission at specific synapses depends on the concerted actions of more than one type of VSCC (19–22), and the relative importance of particular VSCC subtypes varies from one synapse to the next. Although several VSCC subtypes pass calcium currents necessary for triggering neurotransmitter release from central and peripheral neuron terminals (4), evidence suggests that N-type VSCCs specifically regulate this process in neuronal populations responsible for the spinal processing of noxious somatosensory stimuli and endogenous neuropathic pain signals (18,23–26).

III. ANALGESIC PROPERTIES OF ZICONOTIDE

A. Nonclinical Findings

1. Acute and Persistent Pain

Ziconotide is antinociceptive in animal models of acute pain when it is administered by spinal routes. Athermal (heat) stimulus is used in two rat models of acute nociceptive pain, the hot-plate test and the tail-immersion test. Ziconotide administered by either intrathecal (i.t.) bolus injection or continuous i.t. infusion produces analgesic effects in rats using the hot-plate test (27–30). The analgesic effect is both greater and more sustained with i.t. infusion as compared with i.t. bolus dosing. In contrast, in the tail-immersion model, i.t. infusion is not effective at the dose that produces analgesia in the hot-plate test (Wang J, personal communication, 1998). A third model, the rat paw pressure test, employs a mechanical stimulus to produce nociception. In this model, i.t. bolus injection of ziconotide is antinociceptive at doses that also elicit mild stereotypic-shaking behavior (30).

The antinociceptive effects of ziconotide in the hot-plate test are unaltered when the compound is administered subacutely by i.t. infusion, suggesting an absence of tolerance or tachyphylaxis (28). Tolerance and tachyphylaxis also are not observed in rodent models of persistent and neuropathic pain (28–30). These findings contrast sharply with those obtained with opioid analgesics, such as morphine, for which analgesic potency declines substantially with subacute and chronic use (28).

Persistent pain is relevant to the potential therapeutic application of ziconotide in the treatment of severe, intractable chronic pain. Persistent (tonic) as well as acute pain states are modeled in the formalin test (31). In this model, a small amount of dilute formalin is injected subcutaneously into the dorsal hindpaw of a rat or mouse and the number of hindpaw flinches is counted periodically at regular intervals during a 60- to 90-min observation period. Formalin injection induces a characteristic biphasic nociceptive response. The acute phase (phase 1) occurs during the first 10 min after formalin injection; the tonic phase (phase 2) occurs from 10 to 90 min after formalin injection.

The formalin test has been employed in rats and mice to investigate the acute and tonic antinociceptive activity of ziconotide when administered by i.t. bolus injection and continuous infusion, as well as by intracerebroventricular (i.c.v.) and intravenous (i.v.) bolus injections. Effects of i.t. ziconotide on acute phase 1 responses are variable, whereas tonic phase 2 responses are blocked consistently (27,29). Species differences are demonstrated when ziconotide is administered intracerebroventricularly. In mice, i.c.v. ziconotide has greater analgesic potency than i.t. ziconotide (32); however in rats, i.c.v. ziconotide does not suppress nociceptive responses (Bowersox S, unpublished observation, 1998). Nociceptive responses are decreased in phases 1 and 2 when high doses (1 mg/rat) of ziconotide are given intravenously; however, at lower i.v. doses, a lack of overall antinociceptive effect may be attributed to pharmacokinetic variables affecting distribution into the CNS (Tenorio E., personal communication, 1998). The positive response to i.c.v. ziconotide in mice suggests that ziconotide may inhibit supraspinal nonciceptive-signaling pathways under some conditions, in addition to blocking pain-signaling pathways at the level of the spinal cord.

2. Neuropathic Pain

Severe neuropathic pain is extremely difficult to manage in the clinical setting, as conventional drug therapies drug therapies typically fail to provide adequate relief. Ziconotide has been investigated in three rat models of neuropathic pain that involve ligation of either L5/L6 spinal nerves or all or part of the sciatic nerve. In the Kim and Chung model (33) (ligation of L5/L6 spinal nerves), i.t.-bolus injections and i.t., epidural, and i.v. infusions of ziconotide all diminish mechanical allodynic effects (29,34,35), whereas epidural and local bolus injections of ziconotide are not antiallodynic (34). In the Bennett and Xie model (36) of neuropathic pain (loose ligation of the sciatic nerve), perineurally administered ziconotide attenuates mechanical allodynia and heat hyperalgesia, but not mechanical hyperalgesia (37). In contrast, in the Seltzer model (38) (partial ligation of the sciatic nerve), mechanical hyperalgesia is reduced in a dose-dependent fashion by subcutaneous injection of ziconotide into tissue innervated by the injured nerve (39).

Other observations from these studies in animal models of neuropathic pain include the following:

1. Maximal analgesic effects of ziconotide are observed at comparable i.t.- and epidural-infusion doses.
2. Intrathecally administered ziconotide suppresses mechanical and cold allodynia, but does not appear to affect the course of its development.

3. The antiallodynic effects of intravenously administered ziconotide develop more slowly and take longer to subside after treatment, compared with the effects of i.t. infusion.

B. Clinical Findings

1. Safety and Efficacy Studies in Patients with Chronic Pain

Intrathecally administered ziconotide is effective clinically in both nonneuropathic (visceral and somatic) and neuropathic pain in patients with cancer and acquired immune deficiency syndrome (AIDS) and in patients with nonmalignant neuropathic pain. A phase I/II open-label feasibility trial and two, phase II/III pivotal trials have been conducted in patients with pain caused by cancer and AIDS, as well as in patients with neuropathic pain caused by nonmalignant conditions. Results of the phase I/II feasibility trial suggested that ziconotide provided clinically relevant pain relief (40). A total of 259 patients were enrolled at 47 investigative centers in the pivotal nonmalignant pain trial, and a total of 112 patients were enrolled at 38 investigative centers in the pivotal malignant pain trial. Analyses of both trials showed clinically and statistically significant differences in pain relief between the placebo and ziconotide treatment groups (Luther R, personal communication; 41).

2. Pilot Studies in Perioperative Patients

Two pilot studies have been conducted to evaluate the feasibility of use of ziconotide for the management of perioperative pain when administered by the i.t. or epidural route. A total of 30 patients were enrolled at four investigative centers in a study of the safety and efficacy of i.t. ziconotide in the management of perioperative pain (42). Twenty-six of the patients were eligible for the efficacy analysis. Between 24 and 48 h after initiation of study treatment, significantly less patient-controlled analgesia (PCA) morphine was used by the combined ziconotide treatment groups (0.7 and 7.0 μg/h ziconotide) than by the placebo treatment group. A second study was undertaken to assess the safety and effectiveness of ziconotide when administered epidurally to patients with acute postoperative pain (43). A total of 25 patients were enrolled at five investigative centers; 24 of the patients were eligible for the efficacy analysis. During the first 24 h after initiation of study treatment, patients in the 7.0-μg/h ziconotide treatment group used significantly less PCA morphine than did patients in the placebo treatment group. Mean use of PCA morphine by patients in the 0.7-μg/h ziconotide treatment group was also lower than with placebo treatment.

IV. CONCLUSIONS

Nonclinical studies have shown that the selective N-type VSCC blocker, ziconotide, is a potent analgesic agent in rodent models of acute, persistent, and neuropathic pain when administered intrathecally. Based on its favorable preclinical pharmacodynamic and safety profile, the results of which have been encouraging, ziconotide has been advanced to clinical testing. Ziconotide may well constitute the first of a new class of medicinal agent that targets neuronal N-type VSCCs for the treatment of severe chronic pain of malignant and nonmalignant origin as well as acute perioperative pain.

REFERENCES

1. Von Roenn JH, Cleeland CS, Gonin R, Hatfield AK, Pandya KJ. Physician attitudes and practice in cancer pain management. A survey from the Eastern Cooperative Oncology Group. Ann Intern Med 1993; 119:121–126.
2. Ventafridda V, Spoldi E, Caraceni A, De Conno F. Intraspinal morphine for cancer pain. Acta Anaesthesiol Scand Suppl 1987; 85:47–53.
3. Olivera BM, Rivier J, Clark C, Ramilo CA, Corpuz GP, Abogadie FC, Mena EE, Woodward SR, Hillyard DR, Cruz LJ. Diversity of *Conus* neuropeptides. Science 1990; 249:257–263.
4. Olivera BM, Miljanich GP, Ramachandran J, Adams ME. Calcium channel diversity and neurotransmitter release: the ω-conotoxins and ω-agatoxins. Annu Rev Biochem 1994; 63:823–867.
5. Miljanich GP, Ramachandran J. Antagonists of neuronal calcium channels: structure, function, and therapeutic implications. Annu Rev Pharmacol Toxicol 1995; 35:707–734.
6. Olivera BM, McIntosh JM, Cruz LJ, Luque FA, Gray WR. Purification and sequence of a presynaptic peptide toxin from *Conus geographus* venom. Biochemistry 1984; 23:5087–5090.
7. Olivera BM, Gray WR, Zeikus R, McIntosh JM, Varga J, Rivier J, de Santos V, Cruz LJ. Peptide neurotoxins from fish-hunting cone snails. Science 1985; 230:1338–1343.
8. Olivera BM, Cruz LJ, de Santos V, et al. Neuronal calcium channel antagonists. Discrimination between calcium channel subtypes using omega-conotoxin from *Conus magus* venom. Biochemistry 1987; 26:2086–2090.
9. Kristipati R, Nadasdi L, Tarczy–Hornoch K, Lau K, Miljanich GP, Ramachandran J, Bell JR. Characterization of the binding of omega-conopeptides to different classes of non–L-type neuronal calcium channels. Mol Cell Neurosci 1994; 5:219–228.
10. Vega T, De Pascual R, Bulbena O, Garcia AG. Effects of omega-toxins on noradrenergic neurotransmission in beating guinea pig atria. Eur J Pharmacol 1995; 276:231–238.
11. Hirata H, Albillos A, Fernandez F, Medrano J, Jurkiewicz A, Garcia AG. omega-Conotoxins block neurotransmission in the rat vas deferens by binding to different presynaptic sites on the N-type Ca^{2+} channel. Eur J Pharmacol 1997; 321:217–223.
12. Lin Z, Haus S, Edgerton J, Lipscombe D. Identification of functionally distinct isoforms of the N-type Ca^{2+} channel in rat sympathetic ganglia and brain. Neuron 1997; 18:153–166.
13. Rock DM, Horne WA, Stoehr J, Hashimoto C, Zhou M, Cong R, Palma A, Hidayetoglu D, Offord J. Does α_{1E} code for T-type calcium channels? A comparison with GH3 pituitary T-type and recombinant α_{1B} calcium channels. In: Tsien RW, Clozel J–P, Nargeot J, eds. Low–Voltage-Activated-Type Calcium Channels. Proceedings from the International Electrophysiology Meeting, Montpellier, 21–22 Oct 1996. Chester, England: Adis International, 1998:279–289.
14. Westenbroek RE, Hell JW, Warner C, Dubel SJ, Snutch TP, Catterall WA. Biochemical properties and subcellular distribution of an N-type calcium channel alpha 1 subunit. Neuron 1992; 9:1099–1115.
15. Mills LR, Niesen CE, So AP, Carlen PL, Spigelman I, Jones OT. N-type Ca^{2+} channels are located on somata, dendrites, and a subpopulation of dendritic spines on live hippocampal pyramidal neurons. J Neurosci 1994; 14(11 pt2):6815–6824.
16. Gohil K, Bell JR, Ramachandran J, Miljanich GP. Neuroanatomical distribution of receptors for a novel voltage-sensitive calcium-channel antagonist, SNX-230 (omega-conopeptide MVIIC). Brain Res 1994; 653:258–266.
17. Cervero F, Iggo A. The substantia gelatinosa of the spinal cord: a critical review. Brain 1980; 103: 717–772.
18. Westenbroek RE, Hoskins L, Catterall WA. Localization of Ca^{2+} channel subtypes on rat spinal motor neurons, interneurons, and nerve terminals. J Neurosci 1998; 18:6319–6330.
19. Luebke JI, Dunlap K, Turner TJ. Multiple calcium channel types control glutamatergic synaptic transmission in the hippocampus. Neuron 1993; 11:895–902.
20. Regehr WG, Mintz IM. Participation of multiple calcium channel types in transmission at single climbing fiber to Purkinje cell synapses. Neuron 1994; 12:605–613.

21. Wheeler DB, Randall A, Tsien RW. Changes in action potential duration alter reliance of excitatory synaptic transmission on multiple types of Ca^{2+} channels in rat hippocampus. J Neurosci 1996; 16: 2226–2237.
22. Gaur S, Newcomb R, Rivnay B, Bell JR, Yamashiro D, Ramachandran J, Miljanich GP. Calcium channel antagonist peptides define several components of transmitter release in the hippocampus. Neuropharmacology 1994; 33:1211–1219.
23. Diaz A, Dickenson AH. Blockade of spinal N- and P-type, but not L-type, calcium channels inhibits the excitability of rat dorsal horn neurones produced by subcutaneous formalin inflammation. Pain 1997; 69:93–100.
24. Neugebauer V, Vanegas H, Nebe J, Rumenapp P, Schaible HG. Effects of N- and L-type calcium channel antagonists on the responses of nociceptive spinal cord neurons to mechanical stimulation of the normal and the inflamed knee joint. J Neurophysiol 1996; 76:3740–3749.
25. Maggi CA, Tramontana M, Cecconi R, Santicioli P. Neurochemical evidence for the involvement of N-type calcium channels in transmitter secretion from peripheral endings of sensory nerves in guinea pigs. Neurosci Lett 1990; 114:203–206.
26. Santicioli P, Del Bianco E, Tramontana M, Geppetti P, Maggi CA. Release of calcitonin gene-related peptide-like immunoreactivity induced by electrical field stimulation from rat spinal afferents is mediated by conotoxin-sensitive calcium channels. Neurosci Lett 1992; 136:161–164.
27. Malmberg AB, Yaksh TL. Voltage-sensitive calcium channels in spinal nociceptive processing: blockade of N- and P-type channels inhibits formalin-induced nociception. J Neurosci 1994; 14: 4882–4890.
28. Malmberg AB, Yaksh TL. Effect of continuous intrathecal infusion of ω-conopeptides, N-type calcium channel blockers, on behavior and antinociception in the formalin and hot-plate tests in rats. Pain 1995; 60:83–90.
29. Bowersox SS, Gadbois T, Singh T, Pettus M, Wang Y–X, Luther RR. Selective N-type neuronal voltage-sensitive calcium channel blocker, SNX-111, produces spinal antinociception in rat models of acute, persistent, and neuropathic pain. J Pharmacol Exp Ther 1996; 279:1243–1249.
30. Bowersox SS, Tich N, Mayo M, Luther R. SNX-111: antinociceptive agent N-type voltage senstive calcium channel blocker. Drugs Future 1998; 23:152–160.
31. Dubuisson D, Dennis SG. The formalin test: a quantitative study of the analgesic effects of morphine, meperidine, and brain stem stimulation in rats and cats. Pain 1977; 4:161–174.
32. Hynansky A, Elliott KJ, Inturrisi CE. The omega conopeptide SNX-111 is antinociceptive in the mouse formalin test. 12th Annual Scientific Meeting. American Pain Society, Orlando, FL, Nov 4–7, 1993.
33. Kim SH, Chung JM. An experimental model for peripheral neuropathy produced by segmental spinal nerve ligation in the rat. Pain 1992; 50:355–363.
34. Chaplan SR, Pogrel JW, Yaksh TL. Role of voltage-dependent calcium channel subtypes in experimental tactile allodynia. J Pharmacol Exp Ther 1994; 269:1117–1123.
35. Wang Y–X, Pettus M, Singh T, Bowersox SS, Luther RR. Effects of subacute intravenous SNX-111 infusion on mechanical allodynia in a rat model of painful peripheral neuropathy [abstr]. Soc Neurosci Abstr 1996; 22:511.
36. Bennett GJ, Xie Y–K. A peripheral mononeuropathy in rat that produces disorders of pain sensation like those seen in man. Pain 1988; 33:87–107.
37. Xiao WH, Bennett GJ. Synthetic ω-conopeptides applied to the site of nerve injury suppress neuropathic pains in rats. J Pharmacol Exp Ther 1995; 274:666–672.
38. Seltzer Z, Dubner R, Shir Y. A novel behavioral model of neuropathic pain disorders produced in rats by partial sciatic nerve injury. Pain 1990; 3:205–218.
39. White DM, Cousins MJ. Effect of subcutaneous administration of calcium channel blockers on nerve injury-induced hyperalgesia. Brain Res 1998; 801:50–58.
40. Brose W, Pfeifer B, Hassenbusch S, Burchiel K, Byas–Smith M, Krames E, McGuire D, Tich N, Luther RR. Analgesia produced by SNX-111 in patients with morphine-resistant pain. 15th Annual Scientific Meeting. American Pain Society. Washington, DC, Nov 14–17, 1996.

41. Presley R, Charapata S, Ferrar–Brechner T, et al. Chronic opioid-resistant, neuropathic pain: marked analgesic efficacy of intrathecal ziconotide. 17th Annual Scientific Meeting. American Pain Society. San Diego, CA, Nov 5–8, 1998.
42. Atanassoff PG, Hartmannsgruber MWB, Sturaitis M, Otellin A. A new N-type calcium channel blocker SNX-111 administered intrathecally for acute postoperative pain [abstr]. European Society of Anaesthesiologists—Annual Congress: Royal College of Anaesthetists, UK; 1998; 80 (suppl 1): A628.
43. Atanassoff PG, Wallace MS, Wendel D, Edell TA, Ross M, Mayo M, Singh T, Luther R, McGuire D. Analgesic efficacy of epidural ziconotide in acute postoperative pain. 17th Annual Scientific Meeting. American Pain Society. San Diego, CA, Nov 5–8, 1998.

51

Nitric Oxide Synthase Inhibitors and the Role of Nitric Oxide in Nociception

Kate J. Bradley and P. Max Headley
University of Bristol, Bristol, England

I. INTRODUCTION

Since the discovery of nitric oxide (NO) as a physiological mediator of vasodilation (1) there has been an explosion in the literature on this ubiquitous mediator. It is an endogenous molecule that is involved in many physiological functions, including those of the cardiovascular, immune, and nervous systems. In the peripheral nervous system, NO is one of the many mediators released by "nonadrenergic, noncholinergic" (NANC) nerve fibers that may mediate certain gastrointestinal, genitourinary, and respiratory functions. The discovery of its synthetic enzyme in the central nervous system (CNS) and evidence that NO can mediate the synthesis of cyclic guanosine monophosphate (cGMP) (2) triggered a search for functional roles of NO in the CNS, where it has since been implicated as a neuromediator of many functions, including learning, memory, and coordination of neuronal activity with local blood flow. Among these nervous system functions, it appears to have a role in nociception, both centrally and peripherally, as investigated largely by Gebhart's and Ferreira's laboratories respectively. The very large literature that has subsequently emerged cannot be fully surveyed in this short chapter, but we attempt here to indicate the rather bewildering range of effects on nociceptive processing that NO appears to either mediate or modulate.

II. DETERMINING THE ROLES OF NO IN THE CNS: SYNTHESIS, SYNTHESIS INHIBITORS, AND DONORS OF NO

Nitric oxide is synthesized from L-arginine by the enzyme nitric oxide synthase (NOS), of which three isoforms are known to exist: endothelial NOS (eNOS), neuronal NOS (nNOS), and inducible NOS (iNOS). Of these isoforms, eNOS and nNOS are constitutively expressed, whereas the expression of iNOS is induced in a wide range of cell types by immune or inflammatory stimuli. In the CNS, nNOS is the predominant form, although eNOS is also located in certain neuronal populations of the brain as well as in blood vessels. However, neuronal NOS is not confined to the CNS, having also been detected in skeletal muscle and the epithelium of the trachea and bronchi. More recently, it has been demonstrated, by antisense mapping, that two isoforms of nNOS, formed by alternative splicing of mRNA, appear to differ functionally in their effect on morphine analgesia and tolerance (3) (see Sec. IV), and their existence may lead to difficulties in interpreting previous experimental data.

The reaction catalyzed by NOS involves the conversion of L-arginine to citrulline and NO; many cofactors are required for this reaction, including NADPH, FAD, FMN, and, with the constitutive forms, calmodulin. Both nNOS and eNOS, therefore, are calcium-dependent, being activated, by calmodulin, by an influx of calcium into the cell. In the CNS, this can occur following the activation of *N*-methyl-L-aspartate (NMDA) receptors. NO itself is a very short-lived molecule (half-life of milliseconds to seconds); however, models of its diffusional spread suggest that a point source synthesizing NO for 1–10 s would lead to a 200-μm sphere of influence: in the brain this volume could encompass 2 million synapses (4). Actions of NO are mediated by the activation of soluble guanylate cyclase and consequent increase in levels of cGMP in target cells (2).

Experimentally, the main techniques used to investigate the endogenous role of NO have been the use of NOS inhibitors and NO donors. The first inhibitor of NOS, N^{ω}-monomethyl-L-arginine (L-NMMA), was identified approximately 10 years ago (5); since then over 100 NOS inhibitors have been reported in the literature. These are predominantly either derivatives of L-arginine, or heterocyclic compounds, such as the nitroindazole group of fused heterocycles and imidazole plus its substituted derivatives (see Ref. 6 for review). The main pitfall in the use of most of these compounds has been the lack of selectivity, as all three isoforms of the enzyme are inhibited. Because NO causes vasodilation, inhibition of eNOS can lead to extreme hypertension, which may influence experimental results. This is most relevant in tests of thermal nociception, in which reduced blood flow to the periphery alters thermal gradients and so changes the activation of thermal nociceptors. A few of the compounds are claimed to have a selective action on the neuronal and inducible forms of the enzyme. For example 7-nitroindazole (7-NI), although it shows no selectivity in vitro, appears selective in vivo, having minimal cardiovascular effects (7), and 1-(2-trifluoromethylphenyl) imidazole (TRIM), which demonstrates selectivity both in vitro and in vivo (8,9). The explanation for the discrepancy of the in vitro and in vivo activity of 7-NI is unclear. L-*N*6-(1-iminoethyl)lysine (L-NIL) has been reported to be selective for the inducible form of NOS (10), and has been used to demonstrate that this form of the enzyme is mainly responsible for generating NO in the late phase of the inflammatory response (11).

Nitric oxide donors include the organic nitrates and nitrites and inorganic nitroso compounds (e.g. sodium nitroprusside; SNP). These have been less widely used to investigate the role of NO in the nervous system; however, they have been extensively used clinically as vasodilators and may find other clinical applications in thrombotic, gastrointestinal, genitourinary, and respiratory disorders, for their potential in mimicking nitrergic nerve-mediated responses. Other techniques that have been used to investigate the role of NO are the use of "scavengers" of NO, such as hemoglobin (Hb), and inhibitors of soluble guanylate cyclase, such as methylene blue (MB). L-Arginine, the substrate for NO synthesis, has also been widely used to show "reversal" of effects induced by NOS inhibitors; however, this approach is not unequivocal as L-arginine is also the substrate for both kyotorphin, a releaser of the endogenous opioid metenkephalin, which in turn is antinociceptive (12), and for agmatine, which binds to both α_2-adrenoceptors and imidazoline receptors (13).

"Knockouts" of nNOS have also been made to investigate the endogenous role of NO in the nervous system, but have not provided a definitive answer because some residual NOS activity remained.

III. POSSIBLE ROLES OF NO IN NOCICEPTION

There is much controversy and conflicting evidence surrounding the possible role of NO in the transmission of nociceptive information. Some reports suggest that NO has a pronociceptive action, whereas other evidence suggests an antinociceptive role.

Nitric oxide may influence nociceptive processing at many levels in the system, and may potentially have different effects, depending on the site and the concentration (14) of NO. NO has also been extensively investigated to determine whether it affects or mediates the action of commonly used analgesic drugs, such as opioid agonists, α_2-adrenoceptor agonists and nonsteroidal anti-inflammatory drugs (NSAID). Experimental evidence on the role of NO in nociception is presented in the following sections.

A. NO: A Pronociceptive Molecule?

The discovery that activation of NMDA receptors resulted in an increase in cGMP through the production of a labile substance later identified as NO (15), coupled with existing knowledge of the role of NMDA receptors in long-term changes in neuronal excitability (16), has led to much research into the role of NO in nociception, particularly its potential role in hyperalgesic states. However, evidence using knockout mice, which exhibited normal behavioral responses in the formalin test of nociception, that were unaffected by the NOS inhibitor N^{ω}-nitro-L-arginine methyl ester (L-NAME), suggested that NO is not essential for the development of hyperalgesia (17), although evidence from other studies suggests that it may still have a role to play.

1. Intracerebroventricular (i.c.v.) Administration of NOS Inhibitors

NOS inhibitors administered i.c.v. have been used to elucidate the role of supraspinal NO in nociceptive processing; most of the experimental evidence points to a pronociceptive role for NO. Behavioral models of pain that have been used include the tail-flick test, where L-NAME was antinociceptive (an effect reversed by cGMP) (12), the paw-pressure test, in which L-NAME increased withdrawal latencies, and the formalin test during which L-NAME i.c.v. attenuated paw licking (18). These studies support a pronociceptive role for NO, as inhibition of its synthesis leads to analgesia.

In a model of neuropathic pain produced by ligation of the sural nerve, both L-NAME and MB, administered either supraspinally or spinally, decreased the resultant thermal hyperalgesia (19), suggesting that NO is also involved in nociceptive processing of neuropathic pain at both spinal and higher levels.

2. Intrathecal (i.t.) Administration of NOS Inhibitors

More experimental effort has gone into addressing the role of NO in the spinal cord. At a neurochemical level, the NO donor SNP led to release of calcitonin gene-related peptide (CGRP) and substance P from the dorsal horn in vitro (20). The expression of c-*fos* in response to noxious mechanical stimulation (21) and intraplantar formalin (22) was reduced by i.t. pretreatment with L-NAME.

Functionally, both behavioral and electrophysiological studies have addressed the role of spinal NO in nociception, where a function for NO in the normal, noninflamed state is questionable (23–25). The main role for NO appears to be in mediating hyperalgesia, rather than baseline reflexes; for example L-NAME (26) and MB (27) preadministration blocked thermal hyperalgesia induced by i.t. NMDA, whereas alone they did not affect baseline tail-flick latency. This is supported by the evidence that the NO donor SNP, directly caused hyperalgesia, which was reduced by coadministration of Hb (26). In an inflammatory model of hyperalgesia, L-NAME i.t. blocked the thermal hyperalgesia for 3 h, although there was no effect on edema; however, L-NAME did not change thermal or mechanical latencies in a normal paw (24). In another study, however, inflammation did not alter the ability of 7-NI (i.t.) to inhibit NMDA receptor-mediated windup and postdischarge of DH neurones in response to electrical stimulation (28). This suggests that as long as a stimulus is adequate to activate NMDA receptors, the presence of peripheral inflammation is not necessary for the involvement of NO.

Nitric oxide also appears to have a role spinally in mediating neuropathic pain; following ligation of the sciatic nerve, L-NAME and MB blocked thermal hyperalgesia, whereas in sham-operated animals neither L-NAME or MB had any effect (29).

The route of administration of NOS inhibitors may influence their actions, suggesting that NO may have different roles according to its location. For example, in an electrophysiological study of the responses of DH neurons to electrical stimulation and formalin, L-NAME applied topically to the spinal cord reduced the responses of the cells to Aβ- and C- fiber inputs, but had no effect when it was Aβ- and C- fiber injected intravenously (i.v.) or directly into the receptive field (30). In the formalin test, L-NAME applied onto the spinal cord reduced both the first and second phases; by i.v. or intraplantar (i.pl.) administration, it reduced only the second-phase responses.

3. Systemic Administration of NOS Inhibitors

Systemic administration of NOS inhibitors tends to have an antinociceptive effect, which is likely to be a balance of peripheral, spinal, and supraspinal actions. L-NAME given systemically blocked hyperalgesia from i.t. NMDA (26) and elicited antinociception in the formalin, hot-plate, and acetic acid abdominal constriction tests (18). 7-NI (7,31) and TRIM (8,9), which are both devoid of cardiovascular effects, elicited a dose-dependent antinociceptive behavior in mice, inhibiting both licking behavior in the late phase of the formalin test and acetic acid-induced abdominal constrictions following i.p. administration.

4. Peripheral Actions of NOS Inhibitors

Following peripheral administration, NOS inhibitors blocked the edema associated with intraplantar carrageenan (32), phospholipase A_2 (33), and substance P (34), suggesting an endogenous role for NO at the site of acute inflammation in modulating the inflammatory response and edema. In the acute phase of skin inflammation there is also induction of iNOS (35), which is to the isoform responsible for generating NO during the late phase of the inflammatory response (11).

5. Mechanical Versus Thermal Hyperalgesia?

Some studies have suggested that NO is involved in mediating thermal (24,27,29), but not mechanical (24), hyperalgesia, whereas other studies have demonstrated a role for NO in modulation of mechanical nociception (21,25,36). However, it must be remembered that the extreme hypertension that accompanies the administration of most NOS inhibitors (with the exception of 7-NI and TRIM) could lead to artifactual changes, particularly in tests of thermal nociception. In one study in which methoxamine was used to mimic the blood pressure changes, the apparent antinociception caused by L-NAME was equalled by methoxamine, suggesting that it was a consequence of the cardiovascular changes, as methoxamine has no known antinociceptive effect (25).

B. Nitric Oxide: an Antinociceptive Role?

There is some evidence suggesting that NO can play an antinociceptive role. For example, central administration of the NO donor SIN-1 caused dose-dependent analgesia in the paw-pressure test, under conditions of prostaglandin (PG)E_2-induced hyperalgesia (37). However, the literature suggesting an antinociceptive function for NO is far smaller than that supporting a pronociceptive function, suggesting that the latter is the dominant role for central NO under most conditions. The situation is apparently different when it comes to the antinociceptive activity of other agents. For example, in the periphery the antinociceptive actions of opioids are mediated by NO (see Sec. IV.A) and the analgesic actions of endogenous opioids, acetylcholine, and of α_2-adrenoceptor agonists may all involve NO in an antinociceptive role.

IV. NITRIC OXIDE INTERACTIONS WITH OPIOID MECHANISMS (ENDOGENOUS OR EXOGENOUS)

A. Short-Term Opioid Administration

The evidence for the involvement of NO in the mediation or modulation of brief opioid analgesia is contradictory. L-NAME i.t. potentiated the antinociceptive action of morphine i.t. in the tail-flick and paw-pressure tests in rats, an effect that could be reversed by the NO donor SIN-1 (38). This suggests that NO plays a pronociceptive role in the spinal cord, interfering with the antinociceptive action of exogenous opioid agonists. This study was later extended by the demonstration that inhibition of spinal NOS potentiated μ- and δ-, and, to a lesser extent, κ-opioid–mediated spinal antinociception in several pain models (39). In a similar study, N^{ω}-nitro-L-arginine (L-NA), Hb, and MB given i.t. potentiated the action of morphine given i.c.v., again suggesting a pronociceptive role for NO at the spinal level (40). In an electrophysiological study, L-NAME (i.v.) increased the potency of systemic fentanyl in anesthetized rats, which also suggests a pronociceptive role for NO (41). In contrast, in another study in which morphine was administered systemically, i.t. administration of a NOS inhibitor caused a dose-dependent decrease in antinociception; in this case suggesting that NO may mediate opioid antinociception at the spinal level (42).

The evidence concerning interactions of supraspinal NO with opioid mechanisms is also confusing. One early study found that i.c.v. morphine antinociception was unaffected by N^{δ}-iminoethyl-L-ornithine (L-NIO) i.c.v., but was prevented by MB, suggesting that the analgesia was dependent on cGMP generation by NO-independent mechanisms (37). This is contradicted by another study (39) that showed that coadministration of L-NAME with morphine i.c.v. potentiated the analgesia. However, in another study when MB or the NOS inhibitor L-NA were administered i.t., both potentiated the antinociceptive action of i.c.v. morphine (40).

The central site of NOS inhibition appears important in determining the outcome of opioid analgesia; L-NA given i.t. lowers systemic and i.t. morphine analgesia, suggesting an antinociceptive role for NO at the spinal level; whereas, given i.c.v., it increases both systemic and i.c.v. morphine analgesia (3). In the same study an antisense probe (i.t. or i.c.v.) targeting nNOS-2 reduced morphine analgesia, shifting the morphine dose–response curve twofold to the right. This would fit with the existence of two isoforms of NOS, one form that inhibits opioid analgesia predominating supraspinally and another system that facilitates opioid actions predominating at the spinal level.

Chronic treatment with L-arginine (i.p.) reduces both morphine antinociception and levels of morphine found in certain brain sites and the spinal cord following subcutaneous administration (43); activity of NOS in the midbrain was also increased (44). Administration of L-NA before each injection of L-arginine prevented the effects on both central morphine levels and on the degree of antinociception (43). These data suggest that L-arginine reduced the antinociceptive effect of morphine by either increasing brain NOS activity, which suggests a pronociceptive role for NO, or decreasing the entry of morphine into central sites by NO-dependent mechanisms.

In the periphery, most of the evidence points to an antinociceptive role for NO in modulating opioid analgesia; this contrasts with the evidence suggesting that NO has a proinflammatory role in the periphery. Antinociception resulting from peripheral administration of morphine was antagonized both by the NOS inhibitors L-NIO and L-NMMA, and by MB (45); i.pl. administration of the NO donor SIN-1 alone caused a dose-dependent analgesia.

B. Prolonged Opioid Administration

Although there is no change in the level of NOS following prolonged opioid administration, administration of a NOS inhibitor prevented the development of tolerance to morphine, whereas L-arginine accelerated the development of tolerance (46). Numerous reports indicate that NMDA receptor antagonists block the development of tolerance, an effect that could be explained if decreased NO synthesis results. nNOS-1, which predominates at the supraspinal level, is likely to be responsible for the development of tolerance, because antisense probes against it prevented the onset of tolerance to morphine in mice (3).

C. Endogenous Opioids

The degree of involvement of NO in modulating the antinociception caused by endogenous opioids is also nuclear. The antinociceptive effects of β-endorphin given i.c.v. were attenuated by L-NA given i.t.; this attenuation was reversed by L-arginine, which was ineffective alone (40); this suggests that the actions of endogenous opioids may be mediated by NO playing an antinociceptive role in the spinal cord. This contrasts with morphine i.c.v. which, in the same study, was potentiated by spinal NOS inhibition. Consistent with this, β-endorphin antinociception was potentiated both by L-arginine (47) and by NO donors (SNP, SIN-1) (48) i.c.v., but was unaffected by L-arginine i.t. (47); the antinociception elicited by μ-, δ-, and κ-opioid agonists was unaffected (47). A more recent study tied things together by suggesting that the antinociceptive actions of β-endorphin i.c.v. were mediated by spinal metenkephalin release that was NO-dependent, as spinal L-NA attenuated the antinociception, whereas i.c.v. it was without effect (49).

V. NITRIC OXIDE: CHOLINERGIC–ADRENERGIC INTERACTIONS

Muscarinic agonists applied to the rostroventral medulla of rats are antinociceptive in the hot-plate and paw-pressure tests; this antinociception can be reversed by the NOS inhibitor L-NA and by MB, which alone had no effect on response latencies (50). This suggests that the antinociception caused by muscarinic stimulation of the RVM is mediated by the L-arginine–NO–cGMP cascade, with NO having an antinociceptive role. This is supported by another study in which the antinociceptive effect of i.c.v. carbachol was reversed by both MB and L-NIO (37). Release of acetylcholine (ACh) by superfusion of the forebrain in rats was reduced by L-NA, but increased by a NO donor, suggesting that NO can enhance release of ACh centrally (51).

At the level of the spinal cord, intrathecal administration of L-NA similarly had no effect alone, but inhibited the antinociception caused by a muscarinic agonist in the hot-plate and tail-flick tests (52). The muscarinic antagonist, atropine (i.t.) caused a sensitization of mechanical responses that was enhanced and prolonged by NOS inhibitors (53), again suggesting that the antinociceptive role of ACh involves NO.

In the periphery the analgesic effects of ACh in a rat paw made hyperalgesic with PGE_2 were mimicked by the NO donor SNP, were enhanced by an inhibitor of cGMP phosphodiesterase, and were blocked by L-NMMA and MB (54), suggesting that NO–cGMP is also responsible for mediating the analgesic actions of ACh in the periphery.

Interactions between NO, cholinergic, and adrenergic mechanisms have also been reported; i.t. clonidine, an α_2-adrenoceptor agonist, caused a dose-dependent antinociception to mechanical pressure in sheep. This was enhanced by neostigmine, but antagonized by a NOS inhibitor (36,55), suggesting that antinociception following activation of spinal α_2-adrenoceptors involves cholinergic mechanisms that are mediated by NO.

VI. NO INTERACTIONS WITH PROSTANOIDS

Many recent studies have examined possible links between the NO and prostanoid pathways, and there is good evidence for interactions between the two, with NO assuming a proinflammatory role. Interleukin-1_β can induce both NOS and cyclooxygenase (COX) expression (56) and NO can increase the synthesis and release of prostanoids (57). Some NSAIDs, for example indomethacin, which inhibit COX, are also able to decrease the generation of NO (58). NOS inhibitors in vivo wereable to inhibit, whereas NO donors increased prostaglandin formation (59); this was not by direct inhibition of the COX enzyme, but may reflect a NO-driven production of prostaglandins. In contrast, another study showed that NO inhibited both COX-2 induction and activity in macrophages, whereas metabolites of COX had no effect on iNOS activity (60); however, in the same study, when production of endogenous NO was inhibited, small amounts of exogenous NO did increase the activity of COX-2.

Some evidence suggests that there may be an ongoing requirement for NO generation in the allodynia caused by prostanoids. Administration of PGE_2 (i.t.) to conscious mice caused an allodynia that was prevented by simultaneous treatment with L-NAME, dizodilpine (MK = 801; an NMDA receptor antagonist), and a PGE receptor antagonist; however, 5 min after PGE_2 administration only L-NAME was able to block the allodynia (61).

VII. POTENTIAL CLINICAL USE OF MODULATORS OF ENDOGENOUS NO

There are problems with the currently available NOS inhibitors. Most lack adequate specificity for NOS isoforms, and by inhibiting eNOS cause major vasoconstriction that can obscure any underlying effects on the nervous system. Those agents showing some selectivity for nNOS lack satisfactory solubility. NO donors affect all systems and are inherently very unstable molecules; NO scavengers are similarly too nonspecific in their actions. Consequently, the role of NO in nociception has yet to be defined accurately. In addition, NO is a ubiquitous molecule that appears to have many functions. It is highly likely that it is able to act in opposing roles, depending on the location of its release and the local conditions that prevail. Therefore, there cannot be any clinical applications, in the field of pain, for the current generation of agents that modulate NO levels. Any such use would be dependent on the development of more specific inhibitors of NOS and further characterization of the complex roles and sites of action of NO in the processing of nociceptive messages in both peripheral and central nervous systems.

ACKNOWLEDGMENTS

This review was written while the authors were supported by the Wellcome Trust (KJB, ref. 033838/D/91/Z) and NIH (PMH, ref. GM35523).

Abbreviations

ACh	acetylcholine
cGMP	cyclic guanosine monophosphate
CNS	central nervous system
COX	cyclooxygenase
DH	dorsal horn
FAD	flavin adenine dinucleotide
FMN	flavin mononucleotide
HB	hemoglobin
i.c.v.	intracerebroventricular
i.pl.	intraplantar
i.t.	intrathecal
i.v.	intravenous
L-NA	N^{ω}-nitro-L-arginine
L-NAME	N^{ω}-nitro-L-arginine methyl ester
L-NIL	*L-N*6-(1-iminoethyl)lysine
L-NIO	N^{δ}-iminoethyl-L-ornithine
L-NMMA	N^{ω}-monomethyl-L-arginine
MB	methylene blue
NADPH	reduced nicotine adenine dinucleotide phosphate
NANC	nonadrenergic, noncholinergic
7-NI	7-nitroindazole
NMDA	*N*-methyl-D-aspartate
NO	nitric oxide
NOS	nitric oxide synthase
NSAID	nonsteroidal anti-inflammatory drug
PG	prostaglandin
RVM	rostroventral medulla
SIN-1	3-morpholino-sydnonimine
SNP	sodium nitroprusside
TRIM	1-(2-trifluoromethylphenyl) imidazole

REFERENCES

1. Palmer RM, Ferrige AG, Moncada S. Nitric oxide release accounts for the biological activity of endothelium-derived relaxing factor. Nature 1987; 327:524–526.
2. Garthwaite J, Charles SL, Chess-Williams R. Endothelium-derived relaxing factor release on activation of NMDA receptors suggests role as intercellular messenger in the brain. Nature 1988; 336: 385–388.
3. Kolesnikov YA, Pan Y, Babey A, Jain S, Wilson R, Pasternak GW. Functionally differentiating two neuronal nitric oxide synthase isoforms through antisense mapping: evidence for opposing NO actions on morphine analgesia and tolerance. Proc Natl Acad Sci USA 1997; 94:8220–8225.
4. Wood J, Garthwaite J. Models of the diffusional spread of nitric oxide: implications for neural nitric oxide signalling and its pharmacological properties. Neuropharmacology 1994; 33:1235–1244.
5. Hibbs JB Jr, Traintor RR, Zavrin Z. Macrophage cytotoxicity: role for L-arginine deiminase and imino nitrogen oxidation to nitrite. Science 1987; 235:473–476.
6. Moore PK, Handy RLC. Selective inhibitors of neuronal nitric oxide synthase—is no NOS really good NOS for the nervous system? Trends Pharmacol Sci 1997; 18:204–211.

7. Moore PK, Babbedge RC, Wallace P, Gaffen ZA, Hart SL. 7-Nitro indazole, an inhibitor of nitric oxide synthase, exhibits anti-nociceptive activity in the mouse without increasing bloodpressure. Br J Pharmacol 1993; 108:296–297.
8. Handy RLC, Wallace P, Gaffen ZA, Whitehead KJ, Moore PK. The antinociceptive effect of 1-(2-trifluoromethylphenyl)imidazole (TRIM), a potent inhibitor of neuronal nitric oxide synthase in vitro, in the mouse. Br J Pharmacol 1995; 116:2349–2350.
9. Handy RLC, Harb HL, Wallace P, Gaffen Z, Whitehead KJ, Moore PK. Inhibition of nitric oxide synthase by 1-(2-trifluoromethylphenyl) imidazole (TRIM) in vitro: antinociceptive and cardiovascular effects. Br J Pharmacol 1996; 119:423–431.
10. Moore MW, Webber RK, Jerome GM, Tjoeng FS, Misko TP, Currie MG. L-*N*6-(1-iminoethyl)lysine: a selective inhibitor of inducible nitric oxide synthase. J Med Chem 1994; 37:3886–3888.
11. Handy RLC, Moore PK. A comparison of the effects of L- NAME, 7-NI and L-NIL on carrageenan-induced hindpaw oedema and NOS activity. Br J Pharmacol 1998; 123:1119–1126.
12. Kawabata A, Umeda N, Takagi H. L-Arginine exerts a dual role in nociceptive processing in the brain: involvement of the kyotorphin–met-enkephalin pathway and NO–cyclic GMP pathway. Br J Pharmacol 1993; 109:73–79.
13. Li G, Regunathan S, Barrow CJ, Eshraghi J, Cooper R, Reis DJ. Agmatine: an endogenous clonidine-displacing substance in the brain. Science 1994; 263:966–969.
14. Kawabata A, Manabe S, Manabe Y, Takagi H. Effect of topical administration of L-arginine on formalin-induced nociception in the mouse: a dual role of peripherally formed NO in pain modulation. Br J Pharmacol 1994; 112:547–550.
15. Garthwaite J, Garthwaite G, Palmer RMJ, Moncada S. NMDA receptor activation induces nitric oxide synthesis from arginine in rat brain slices. Eur J Pharmacol 1989; 172:413–416.
16. Coderre TJ, Fisher K, Fundytus ME. The role of ionotropic and metabotropic glutamate receptors in persistent nociception. In: Jensen TS, Turner JA, Wiesenfeld–Hallin Z, eds. Proceedings of the 8th World Congress on Pain. 1997:259–275.
17. Crosby G, Marota JJA, Huang PL. Intact nociception-induced neuroplasticity in transgenic mice deficient in neuronal nitric oxide synthase. Neuroscience 1995; 69:1013–1017.
18. Moore PK, Oluyomi AO, Babbedge RC, Wallace P, Hart SL. L-*N*(G)-Nitro arginine methyl ester exhibits antinociceptive activity in the mouse. Br J Pharmacol 1991; 102:198–202.
19. Salter M, Strijbos PJLM, Neale S, Duffy C, Follenfant RL, Garthwaite J. The nitric oxide–cyclic GMP pathway is required for nociceptive signalling at specific loci within the somatosensory pathway. Neuroscience 1996; 73:649–655.
20. Garry MG, Richardson JD, Hargreaves KM. Sodium nitroprusside evokes the release of immunoreactive calcitonin gene-related peptide and substance P from dorsal horn slices via nitric oxide-dependent and nitric oxide-independent mechanisms. J Neurosci 1994; 14:4329–4337.
21. Lee JH, Wilcox GL, Beitz AJ. Nitric oxide mediates Fos expression in the spinal cord induced by mechanical noxious stimulation. Neuroreport 1992; 3:841–844.
22. Roche AK, Cook M, Wilcox GL, Kajander KC. A nitric oxide synthesis inhibitor (L-NAME) reduces licking behavior and Fos-labeling in the spinal cord of rats during formalin-induced inflammation. Pain 1996; 66:331–341.
23. Malmberg AB, Yaksh TL. Spinal nitric oxide synthesis inhibition blocks NMDA-induced thermal hyperalgesia and produces antinociception in the formalin test in rats. Pain 1993; 54:291–300.
24. Meller ST, Cummings CP, Traub RJ, Gebhart GF. The role of nitric oxide in the development and maintenance of the hyperalgesia produced by intraplantar injection of carrageenan in the rat. Neuroscience 1994; 60:367–374.
25. Semos ML, Headley PM. The role of nitric oxide in spinal nociceptive reflexes in rats with neurogenic and nonneurogenic peripheral inflammation. Neuropharmacology 1994; 33:1487–1497.
26. Kitto KF, Haley JE, Wilcox GL. Involvement of nitric oxide in spinally mediated hyperalgesia in the mouse. Neurosci Lett 1992; 148:1–5.
27. Meller ST, Dykstra C, Gebhart GF. Production of endogenous nitric oxide and activation of soluble guanylate cyclase are required for *N*-methyl-D-aspartate-produced facilitation of the nociceptive tail-flick reflex. Eur J Pharmacol 1992; 214:93–96.

28. Stanfa LC, Misra C, Dickenson AH. Amplification of spinal nociceptive transmission depends on the generation of nitric oxide in normal and carrageenan rats. Brain Res 1996; 737:92–98.
29. Meller ST, Pechman PS, Gebhart GF, Maves TJ. Nitric oxide mediates the thermal hyperalgesia produced in a model of neuropathic pain in the rat. Neuroscience 1992; 50:7–10.
30. Haley JE, Dickenson AH, Schachter M. Electrophysiological evidence for a role of nitric oxide in prolonged chemical nociception in the rat. Neuropharmacology 1992; 31:251–258.
31. Moore PK, Wallace P, Gaffen Z, Hart SL, Babbedge RC. Characterization of the novel nitric oxide synthase inhibitor 7-nitro indazole and related indazoles: antinociceptive and cardiovascular effects. Br J Pharmacol 1993; 110:219–224.
32. Ialenti A, Ianaro A, Moncada S, Di Rosa M. Modulation of acute inflammation by endogenous nitric oxide. Eur J Pharmacol 1992; 211:177–182.
33. Cirino G, Cicala C, Sorrentino L, Regoli D. Effects of bradykinin antagonists, N^G-monomethyl-L-arginine and L-N^G-nitroarginine on phospholipase A_2 induced oedema in rat paw. Gen Pharmacol 1991; 22:801–804.
34. Hughes SR, Williams TJ, Brain SD. Evidence that endogenous nitric oxide modulates oedema formation induced by substance P. Eur J Pharmacol 1990; 191:481–484.
35. Vane JR, Mitchell JA, Appleton I, Tomlinson A, Bishop–Bailey D, Croxtall J, Willoughby DA. Inducible isoforms of cyclooxygenase and nitric-oxide synthase in inflammation. Proc Natl Acad Sci USA 1994; 91:2046–2050.
36. Lothe A, Li P, Tong C, Yoon Y, Bouaziz H, Detweiler DJ, Eisenach JC. Spinal cholinergic alpha-2 adrenergic interactions in analgesia and hemodynamic control: role of muscarinic receptor subtypes and nitric oxide. J Pharmacol Exp Ther 1994; 270:1301–1306.
37. Duarte IDG, Ferreira SH. The molecular mechanism of central analgesia induced by morphine or carbachol and the L-arginine–nitric oxide–cGMP pathway. Eur J Pharmacol 1992; 221:171–174.
38. Przewlocki R, Machelska H, Przewlocka B. Inhibition of nitric oxide synthase enhances morphine antinociception in the rat spinal cord. Life Sci 1993; 53:PL1–PL5.
39. Machelska H, Labuz D, Przewlocki R, Przewlocka B. Inhibition of nitric oxide synthase enhances antinociception mediated by mu, delta and kappa opioid receptors in acute and prolonged pain in the rat spinal cord. J Pharmacol Exp Ther 1997; 282:977–984.
40. Xu JY, Tseng LF. Nitric oxide/cyclic guanosine monophosphate system in the spinal cord differentially modulates intracerebroventricularly administered morphine- and beta-endorphin-induced antinociception in the mouse. J Pharmacol Exp Ther 1995; 274:8–16.
41. Bradley KJ, Headley PM. Effects of NOS inhibition on the spinal potency of a μ-opioid agonist in the anaesthetised rat. J Physiol 1997; 504:105P.
42. Eisenach JC, Song HK, Pan J. IV morphine produces antinociception by a spinal action involving nitric oxide. Soc Neurosci Abstr 1997; 23:1021.
43. Bhargava HN, Bian JT. *N*(G)-nitro-L-arginine reverses L-arginine induced changes in morphine antinociception and distribution of morphine in brain regions and spinal cord of the mouse. Brain Res 1997; 749:351–353.
44. Bhargava HN, Bian JT, Kumar S. Mechanism of attenuation of morphine antinociception by chronic treatment with L-arginine. J Pharmacol Exp Ther 1997; 281:707–712.
45. Ferreira SH, Duarte IDG, Lorenzetti BB. The molecular mechanism of action of peripheral morphine analgesia: stimulation of the cGMP system via nitric oxide release. Eur J Pharmacol 1991; 201:121–122.
46. Babey AM, Kolesnikov Y, Cheng J, Inturrisi CE, Trifilletti RR, Pasternak GW. Nitric oxide and opioid tolerance. Neuropharmacology 1994; 33:1463–1470.
47. Xu JY, Tseng LF. Increase of nitric oxide by L-arginine potentiates beta-endorphin- but not mu-, delta- or kappa-opioid agonist-induced antinociception in the mouse. Eur J Pharmacol 1993; 236: 137–142.
48. Xu JY, Pieper GM, Tseng LF. Activation of a NO-cyclic GMP system by NO donors potentiates beta-endorphin-induced antinociception in the mouse. Pain 1995; 63:377–383.
49. Tseng LF, Wang HQ, Xu JY. Inhibition of spinal nitric oxide synthase by *N*(omega)-nitro-L-arginine

blocks the release of met-enkephalin and antinociception induced by supraspinally administered beta-endorphin in the rat. Neuroscience 1997; 78:461–467.
50. Iwamoto ET, Marion L. Pharmacological evidence that nitric oxide mediates the antinociception produced by muscarinic agonists in the rostral ventral medulla of rats. J Pharmacol Exp Ther 1994; 269:699–708.
51. Prast H, Philippu A. Nitric oxide releases acetylcholine in the basal forebrain. Eur J Pharmacol 1992; 216:139–140.
52. Iwamoto ET, Marion L. Pharmacologic evidence that spinal muscarinic analgesia is mediated by an L-arginine/nitric oxide/cyclic GMP cascade in rats. J Pharmacol Exp Ther 1994; 271:601–608.
53. Zhuo M, Meller ST, Gebhart GF. Endogenous nitric oxide is required for tonic cholinergic inhibition of spinal mechanical transmission. Pain 1993; 54:71–78.
54. Duarte IDG, Lorenzetti BB, Ferreira SH. Peripheral analgesia and activation of the nitric oxide–cyclic GMP pathway. Eur J Pharmacol 1990; 186:289–293.
55. Xu Z, Li P, Tong C, Figueroa J, Tobin JR, Eisenach JC. Location and characteristics of nitric oxide synthase in sheep. spinal cord and its interaction with alpha$_2$-adrenergic and cholinergic antinociception. Anesthesiology 1996; 84:890–899.
56. Tetsuka T, Daphna–Iken D, Srivastava SK, Baier LD, DuMaine J, Morrison AR. Cross-talk between cyclooxygenase and nitric oxide pathways: prostaglandin E_2 negatively modulates induction of nitric oxide synthase by interleukin 1. Proc Natl Acad Sci USA 1994; 91:
57. Sautebin L, Ialenti A, Ianaro A, Di Rosa M. Modulation by nitric oxide of prostaglandin biosynthesis in the rat. Br J Pharmacol 1995; 114:323–328; 12168–12172.
58. Pang L, Hoult JRS. Induction of cyclooxygenase and nitric oxide synthase in endotoxin-activated J774 macrophages is differentially regulated by indomethacin: enhanced cyclooxygenase-2 protein expression but reduction of inducible nitric oxide synthase. Eur J Pharmacol 1996; 317:151–155.
59. Salvemini D, Settle SL, Masferrer JL, Seibert K, Currie MG, Needleman P. Regulation of prostaglandin production by nitric oxide; an in vivo analysis Br J Pharmacol 1995; 114:1171–1178.
60. Swierkosz TA, Mitchell JA, Warner TD, Botting RM, Vane JR. Co-induction of nitric oxide synthase and cyclooxygenase: interactions between nitric oxide and prostanoids. Br J Pharmacol 1995; 114: 1335–1342.
61. Minami T, Onaka M, OkudaAshitaka E, Mori H, Ito S, Hayaishi O. L-NAME, an inhibitor of nitric oxide synthase, blocks the established allodynia induced by intrathecal administration of prostaglandin E_2. Neurosci Lett 1995; 201:239–242.

52
Adenosine and Pain

Michael J. Sheehan
Glaxo Wellcome Research and Development, Stevenage, Hertfordshire, England

Chas Bountra
GlaxoSmithKline, Harlow, Essex, England

I. INTRODUCTION

The endogenous nucleoside adenosine performs multiple functions within the body. It can be progressively phosphorylated to generate the high-energy molecules adenosine mono-, di-, and triphosphate (AMP, ADP, and ATP), and from ATP may be further modified to generate the intracellular second-messenger cyclic-AMP (cAMP). More recently, it has become apparent that adenosine also acts as a chemical-signaling agent or local hormone in its own right. The diversity of responses that are mediated by adenosine in this signaling context is also wide, but as a rule, its effects are generally inhibitory: for example, it reduces heart rate, inhibits fatty acid release from adipocytes, down-regulates the immune response, and acts as a central nervous system (CNS) depressant. The latter response is particularly relevant in understanding the role of adenosine in the physiology of pain.

A. Origin and Removal of Endogenous Adenosine

As a cell becomes ischemic, either through increased activity or restriction of blood supply, there is depletion in levels of ATP and ADP and a rise in AMP, which is then dephosphorylated to adenosine by the enzyme 5′-nucleotidase. Equilibrative transporters facilitate adenosine release across the cell membrane into the extracellular space, to the extent that under severe hypoxic conditions the concentration of adenosine may rise 100-fold (Müller and Scior, 1993). However, even increased neuronal activity can give rise to measurable increases in extracellular levels (Ballarin et al., 1987). Once released into the intracellular space, adenosine is removed by reuptake via equilibrative and sodium-dependent transporters, and is metabolized by the enzymes adenosine deaminase, *ecto*-5′-nucleotidase, and adenosine kinase.

B. Adenosine Receptors

Adenosine exerts most of its hormonal effects by acting at cell-surface receptors of the G protein-coupled type. To date, four receptor subtypes have been identified, the pharmacological characteristics and distribution of which are summarized in Table 1. Although the A_1 and A_{2a} receptors are relatively well-characterized, the A_3 receptor was cloned only in 1992, and selective pharmacological tools are just being developed. Similarly, the A_{2b} receptor still awaits the development of selective agonists and antagonists, and tends to be identified pharmacologically only by elimi-

Table 1 Characteristics of Adenosine Receptors

	Receptor subtype			
	A_1	A_{2a}	A_{2b}	A_3
Distribution	Brain; sympathetic nerve terminals; heart (sinoatrial node and myocytes); adipocytes	Brain (especially dopamine-rich areas); inflammatory cells, including neutrophils and eosinophils; vasculature	Brain; gut; vasculature; skin fibroblasts; immune cells	Mast cells; brain; testis; spleen; heart
Consequences of activating receptor	Inhibition of neuronal activity and neurotransmitter release; antinociception; bradycardia; reduction in metabolism; inhibition of lipolysis	Anti-inflammatory action; hypotension	Hypotension	Stimulation of mast cell mediator release?
Second-messenger[a]	↓ cAMP; ↑ gK^+; ↑ PI; ↑ MAPK	↑ cAMP	↑ cAMP	↓ cAMP; ↑ PI
Nonselective[b] agonist	NECA	NECA	NECA	NECA
Selective agonists[b]	CPA, CCPA, R-PIA GR79236	CGS 21680; CV-1808	None	IB-MECA
Relatively nonselective antagonists[b]	8PT; CGS15943	8PT; CGS15943	8PT; CGS15943	CGS15943
Selective antagonists[b]	DPCPX; PACPX	ZM241385; DMPX	None	I-ABOPX

[a] Abbreviations for second-messengers: cAMP, cyclic 3′,5′ adenosine monophosphate; gK^+, potassium ionic conductance; PI, phosphatidyl inositol turnover; MAPK, mitogen-activated protein kinase.

[b] Abbreviations for compounds: NECA (5′-*N*-ethylcarboxamidoadenosine); 8-PT, 8-phenyltheophylline; CGS15943, 9-chloro-2-(2-furyl)[1,2,4]-triazolo [1,5-c]quinazolin-5-amine; CPA, N^6-cyclopentyladenosine; CCPA, 2-chloro-N^6-cyclopentyladenosine; R-PIA, *R*-N^6-(phenyl-2-isopropyl)adenosine; GR79236, *N*[1*S*, *trans*)-2-hydroxycyclopentyl]adenosine; DPCPX, 8-cyclopentyl-1,3-dipropylxanthine; PACPX, 1,3-dipropyl-8-(2-amino-4-chlorophenyl)-xanthine; CGS21680, [[2-[4-(2-carboxyethyl)phenyl]ethyl]amino]-*N*: ethylcarboxamidoadenosine; CV-1808, 2-phenylaminoadenosine; ZM241385, 4-(2-[7-amino-2-(2-furyl)[1,2,4]triazolo[2,3-a][1,3,5]triazin-5-ylamino]ethyl)phenol; DMPX, 3,7-dimethyl-1-propargylxanthine; IB-MECA, *N*-^{6}-(3-iodobenzyl)-5′-methylcarboxamidoadenosine; I-ABOPX, 1-propyl-3-(3-iodo-4-aminobenzyl)-8-(4-oxyacetate)phenylxanthine.

nating the effects of the other three receptors and assuming that what remains is A_{2b}-mediated. Until recently, the literature on the pharmacology of adenosine and pain has been confounded by the use of poorly selective compounds and a lack of awareness of species differences in adenosine receptor pharmacology.

II. ANTINOCICEPTIVE EFFECTS OF ADENOSINE AGONISTS

Adenosine receptor agonists can be highly effective antinociceptive agents in a wide variety of standard tests when administered systemically, intrathecally, or centrally to rodents (see Sawynok and Sweeney, 1989, for a review of the early experimental data). The breadth of antinociceptive activity is similar to, but not identical with, that of opioids: both classes of compound are effective against thermal nociceptive stimuli; opioids tend to be more efficacious against mechanical nociception, whereas adenosine agonists are more efficacious against inflammatory and neuropathic pain (see Secs. III and IV for more details).

Early studies suggested that adenosine agonists were effective in antinociceptive tests mainly by acting as general CNS or cardiovascular depressant agents. However, it is possible to observe maximal antinociception at doses lower than those causing sedation and motor impairment, demonstrating that the antinociceptive effect is not merely secondary to CNS depression. Nevertheless, the therapeutic window is usually less than tenfold (Post, 1984; Sosnowski et al., 1989).

The adenosine A_1 receptor is the predominant subtype through which antinociceptive effects are mediated. The evidence for this assignation is partly the rank order of potency of agonists (Sawynok et al., 1986), but also the ability of selective A_1 antagonists such as PACPX and DPCPX to block the response to agonists (Aley and Levine, 1997; our own unpublished data). However, sometimes, there may be an additional component mediated by activation of A_{2a} receptors (see Sec. VII).

As with opioid analgesics, it is possible to demonstrate tolerance to adenosine-mediated antinociception (Aley et al., 1995; Aley and Levine, 1997). Our own experience, however, is that tolerance to adenosine A_1 agonists is difficult to induce unless very high doses of agonist are continuously administered, and so may not be a problem when considering their clinical use. Biochemical studies show that the A_1 receptor itself is extremely resistant to mechanisms of desensitization (Palmer et al., 1996).

III. ADENOSINE AGONISTS IN NEUROPATHIC PAIN

One of the differences in the spectrum of antinociceptive activity between opioid analgesics and adenosine agonists is that opioids are relatively ineffective in clinical conditions involving central neuropathic pain, as well as in animal models of such neuropathies, but adenosine agonists show better efficacy, at least in the animal models. For example, the A_1 agonist R-PIA inhibited allodynia induced by sciatic nerve ligation or intrathecal strychnine administration in rat, models in which opioids are only poorly effective (Sosnowski and Yaksh, 1989; Sjolund et al., 1996). Adenosine itself has been infused intravenously in human subjects with peripheral neuropathic pain and found to be effective (Belfrage et al., 1995). Indeed, intrathecally administered adenosine was reported to exert an analgesic effect of surprisingly long duration in patients with neuropathic pain (>24 h in some patients) (Sawynok, 1998). Given the very short metabolic half-life of adenosine, this finding implies that it may be able to trigger an adaptive response in neurons that persists long after the compound itself has disappeared.

IV. MECHANISMS OF ADENOSINE ANTINOCICEPTION

Adenosine agonists (especially A_1 receptor agonists) are antinociceptive when administered either locally at a peripheral site, intrathecally, or directly into the cerebral ventricles, and it is possible to show by using antagonists that do not enter the CNS, or by judicious choice of dose, that these are independent mechanisms. It is thus probably naïve to expect there to be a single neurochemical mechanism that underlies all of these actions. Nevertheless, in common with many other pharmacological agents with antinociceptive properties, A_1 agonists share the ability to act at presynaptic receptors to inhibit neuronal transmission. There is a great deal of redundancy in these neurochemical mechanisms: for example, there is synergism between adenosine and α_2-adrenoceptor agonists or $GABA_B$ agonists, whereas adenosine antagonists attenuate the antinociceptive effects of senotonin (5-HT; 5-hydroxytryptamine) (Aran and Proudfit, 1990; Sabetkasai and Zarrindast, 1993; Sawynok and Reid, 1991).

Even more intriguing is the relation between adenosine and opioid analgesia. Especially in the spinal cord, adenosine may be a major mediator of the analgesic action of morphine. μ-Opioid agonists can induce release of adenosine from spinal cord synaptosomes (Cahill et al., 1995), whereas intrathecal administration of the adenosine antagonist 8-phenyltheophylline blocked the effects of morphine injected into the periaqueductal gray in the hot-plate test (but not in the tail-flick test). However, Aley and Levine (1997) found that antagonists of μ-opioid receptors, α_2-adrenoceptors, and adenosine A_1 receptors, all blocked antinociception induced by all three classes of agonist. These findings demonstrate that a putative pathway, such as *morphine → adenosine release → antinociception*, is too simplistic, and that the reality is likely to involve a network of mutually interacting pathways.

The mechanistic link between adenosine- and opioid-induced analgesia raises the question of whether both mechanisms are subject to tolerance and withdrawal. Aley et al. (1995) were able to demonstrate cross-tolerance to the A_1 agonist CPA and the μ-opioid agonist DAMGO, and also elicited cross-withdrawal with appropriate antagonists. However, our own experience suggests that analgesia induced by adenosine A_1 agonists is much less susceptible to tolerance than morphine-induced analgesia.

The current working hypothesis, therefore, is that adenosine, acting at A_1 receptors, can presynaptically inhibit activity in nociceptive afferent neurons projecting to the spinal cord, and probably also at later stages in the pain pathway. One strong candidate for the neurochemical mechanism by which A_1 agonists cause presynaptic inhibition is hyperpolarization by opening ATP-sensitive potassium channels (Ocana and Baeyens, 1994). However, in view of the multiplicity of second messengers, which A_1 receptors can activate (see Table 1), it would not be surprising to find alternative mechanisms in different parts of the pathway.

V. STUDIES IN HUMAN SUBJECTS

In this section we summarize the published clinical data specifically concerning the use of adenosine as an algesic or analgesic agent, but excluding cardiac pain (discussed in Sec. VI). Adenosine itself is used clinically by the intravenous route for terminating paroxysmal supraventricular tachycardia, and it is the only direct-acting agonist that is generally available for use in humans. Its ultrashort plasma half-life (a few seconds) and cardiovascular depressant effect make it far from ideal as a pharmacological tool for investigating mechanisms of analgesia, but until selective and stable agonists enter clinical testing we are limited to drawing tentative conclusions from the available data.

Paradoxically, adenosine can act either as an algesic or an analgesic agent, depending on the study design. Intra-arterial injection induces muscle pain similar to that caused by ischemia (Sylven et al., 1988; Gaspardone et al., 1995); pain is also induced by cutaneous administration, either to the blister base (Bleehen and Keele, 1977) or on intradermal injection (Pappagallo et al., 1993). As with cardiac pain, there is evidence that adenosine released in ischemic muscle tissue induces pain, which could be construed as a protective response, reducing muscle activity and preventing further damage. These studies thus suggest that adenosine may be an endogenous mediator of certain pain responses in peripheral tissues, perhaps similar to prostanoids, 5-HT or bradykinin. Indeed, Bleehen and Keele (1977) found significant synergy between pain induced by adenosine and 5-HT in the blister base, although not with bradykinin. The argument appears to be confirmed by the ability of the adenosine antagonists theophylline (nonselective for any adenosine receptor type) and bamiphylline (supposedly A_1-selective, but see later discussion) to block ischemia-induced pain in the forearm and adenosine-induced intradermal pain, respectively (Jonzon et al., 1989; Pappagallo et al., 1993). It may also partly explain why the weak adenosine antagonist caffeine is sometimes included in proprietary analgesic compounds.

Despite the foregoing observations, the role of adenosine as an algesic mediator is by no means certain. As discussed later for cardiac pain, there is a poor correlation between the degree of ischemia (which is likely to be directly responsible for adenosine release) and reported pain. Furthermore, there is a growing literature demonstrating that adenosine can act as an analgesic agent in human studies. For example, Segerdahl and colleagues have shown that i.v. adenosine infusion attenuates the perception of heat pain or allodynia induced by mustard oil in healthy volunteers, and reduces spontaneous neuropathic pain and tactile allodynia in patients with neuropathic pain (Bellfrage et al., 1995; Ekblom et al., 1995; Segerdahl et al., 1995; Sollevi et al., 1995). Furthermore, despite the reports just quoted suggesting that adenosine may be a mediator of ischemic pain, a recent study in eight volunteers demonstrated that intra-arterial infusion of adenosine delayed the onset of ischemic muscle pain in a theophylline-reversible manner (Eriksson et al., 1997).

These apparently contradictory results may potentially be reconciled by resolving the data into three types of study. First, there is clear evidence for an antinociceptive effect of adenosine in neuropathic pain states or models thereof, and the weight of evidence indicates that this effect is mediated by A_1 receptor activation. The second group comprises models in which pain is induced by local injection of adenosine (or nucleotide precursors that break down to adenosine in situ). In these studies, the high local concentrations of adenosine will activate all adenosine receptors in the vicinity, potentially leading to release of mast cell or other inflammatory cell mediators by A_{2b} or A_3 receptor activation (Feoktistov and Biaggioni, 1997). Although some xanthine antagonists have been used to block local nociceptive responses to adenosine, there is very limited pharmacological data available concerning their selectivity at human adenosine receptor subtypes (and there is considerable species variability in this). In our opinion, therefore, the role of A_1 receptor activation in causing pain in these situations has not been proved. Finally, the remaining group of studies implicated adenosine in mediating ischemic pain in muscle. This issue will be discussed in the following section on cardiac pain, to which it is closely related.

VI. ADENOSINE AND CARDIAC (ANGINAL) PAIN: THE ENDOGENOUS MEDIATOR?

Cardiac pain or angina pectoris originates when the metabolic demand for oxygen outstrips the ability of the coronary vasculature to supply it, a situation that is most commonly caused by atherosclerosis in the coronary arteries. Ischemia may also be deliberately induced during cardiac surgery, as during balloon angioplasty to restore flow in stenosed coronary arteries, and the periods of ischemia during balloon inflation are associated with intense pain for the patients who are conscious during the procedure. However, there may be a poor correlation between the degree of pain and the degree of ischemia, as demonstrated by angina patients undergoing continuous electrocardiographic monitoring where periods of so-called silent ischemia may be revealed that did not give rise to symptoms.

Because adenosine is released from cardiac cells during ischemic episodes, it is a potential mediator of the associated pain. The evidence has been reviewed extensively by Tomai et al. (1993) and Sylven (1993), and may be summarized as follows. Bolus injection of adenosine, either intravenously or directly into the coronary circulation, causes chest pain that is perceived by the subject as being angina-like (Sylven et al., 1986, 1989; Lagerqvist et al., 1992). This pain can be attenuated by an adenosine antagonist, aminophylline, which can also reduce pain induced by balloon angioplasty (Hashino et al., 1996). Importantly, adenosine infusion induces pain without causing ischemia in its own right (Crea et al., 1990), supporting its role as a primary nociceptive mediator. The mechanism may be through direct stimulation by adenosine of cardiac afferent nerves (Crea et al., 1992).

Although adenosine may induce pain during severe cardiac ischemia, it can have other effects on heart muscle without causing pain. For example, a recent preliminary study on the cardioprotective effects of adenosine reported reductions in infarct size, but no painful side effects were reported (Mahaffey et al., 1997). Thus, the algesic response to adenosine may perhaps be dose-dependent: low doses seem to be adequate to elicit its cardioprotective effects, but high local concentrations are necessary to induce pain. This suggestion is supported by the observation that the adenosine-uptake blocker, dipyridamole, potentiated adenosine-induced cardiac pain (Sylven et al., 1986). The same phenomenon of dose-dependence of response may also hold true for ischemic pain in muscle. If so, there is currently insufficient evidence to determine whether a single adenosine receptor subtype mediates different responses at different levels of occupancy, or whether separate subtypes with varying affinity for adenosine are involved.

VII. A_{2A}, A_{2B}, AND A_3 ADENOSINE RECEPTORS AND ANTINOCICEPTION

The evidence discussed in the foregoing clearly demonstrates that A_1 adenosine agonists are effective antinociceptive agents. What is the role, if any, of the other adenosine receptor subtypes? The answer, in brief, seems to be: very little.

Selective A_{2a} agonists have little or no antinociceptive effect; occasional reports that they are slightly hyperalgesic may be because A_{2a} receptor activation leads to vasodilation, which can potentiate inflammatory stimuli (Poon and Sawynok, 1998; Karlsten et al., 1992). Apparently contradictory data comes from the recent report describing a strain of transgenic mice lacking the adenosine A_{2a} receptor (Ledent et al., 1997), in which one phenotypic change observed was a tendency to hypoalgesia, manifested as a slowness in reaction to algesic stimuli. On the whole, however, it seems unlikely that the A_{2a} receptor plays as prominent a role as the A_1 receptor in nociceptive transmission (although see Sec. IX on adenosine and migraine).

To our knowledge there is no evidence for or against an involvement of A_{2b} receptors in nociceptive transmission, nor, in the absence of selective ligands (see Table 1), is such evidence likely to emerge. For the A_3 adenosine receptor, it is possible to show in the rat that A_3 agonists induce mast cell degranulation, which leads to a local inflammatory response (Sawynok et al., 1997; Reeves et al., 1997). However, although the human mast cell can degranulate in response to high local concentrations of adenosine, the A_3 receptor does not appear to mediate the response.

VIII. INHIBITION OF ADENOSINE KINASE OR ADENOSINE DEAMINASE

The role of endogenous adenosine in pain pathways may be investigated by using inhibitors of the enzymes adenosine kinase or adenosine deaminase. In brief, the results from rodent studies show that an adenosine kinase inhibitor, such as 5′-amino-5′-deoxyadenosine can be antinociceptive in its own right when injected intrathecally, whereas adenosine deaminase inhibitors, such as deoxycoformycin and erythro-9-(2-hydroxy-3-nonyl)adenine (EHNA), are weak or ineffective (Keil and DeLander, 1994; Poon and Sawynok, 1995, 1998). However, it would be unwise to translate such data into expectations of activity in humans. The redundancy of mechanisms for the removal of adenosine may well lead to species differences in the predominant mechanism, and there may even be variation across different parts of the CNS in a single species. Furthermore, there is no certainty that there would be adequate tonic adenosine release in the appropriate regions to allow these enzyme inhibitors to enhance its action. The results of trials with novel adenosine kinase inhibitors such as GP-3269 (reported to be undergoing phase I clinical trials as an analgesic agent) may provide the evidence to justify or reject these caveats.

IX. ADENOSINE AND MIGRAINE

The evidence for a link between adenosine and migraine is largely circumstantial, but nonetheless intriguing. Adenosine mediates vasodilation by acting through A_{2a} or A_{2b} receptors (depending on the location of the vascular bed and the species being studied) and therefore, might contribute to cranial vessel dilation during a migraine attack. In support of this hypothesis, adenosine infusion in humans, has been reported to cause intense headache (Sollevi, 1986) or induce migraine attacks in a susceptible subject (Brown and Waterer, 1995). Substantially elevated plasma levels of adenosine were measured in migraineurs during a migraine attack (Guieu et al., 1998). These observations would suggest that an appropriate adenosine antagonist might be an effective antimigraine treatment, but no clinical data are yet available. We incline to be rather pessimistic about this hypothesis on the basis of the poor effectiveness of the weak adenosine antagonist caffeine in treating migraine.

More speculatively, the ability of adenosine A_1 agonists to reduce neurogenic inflammation, at least in the extremities (e.g., Honore et al., 1998), suggests that they might also be capable of inhibiting the release of vasoactive peptides in the cranial vasculature, and thereby inhibit a primary cause of migraine attacks. To our knowledge this is a hypothesis that has yet to be tested.

X. THERAPEUTIC IMPLICATIONS

One main conclusion from this review is that adenosine A_1 agonists may offer a new approach to treating pain, particularly of the neuropathic type. The problem with such treatments is that there would be a strong likelihood of mechanism-related side effects. Although A_1 agonists are antinociceptive at low doses, higher doses cause cardiovascular and CNS side effects, and the therapeutic window is narrow (certainly less than tenfold). Unless a dosing mechanism could be devised to deliver accurately controlled plasma levels, this problem would militate against their widespread use.

One alternative possibility would be to use A_1 agonists as an adjunct to opioid therapy as a possible way of minimizing the necessary dose of both compounds. This attractive idea is unfortunately not supported by our own animal studies, where no synergy was observed, nor by an anecdotal report of a clinical trial with adenosine which failed to demonstrate opiate-sparing activity (Sawynok, 1998).

The potential for using adenosine analogues in treating migraine is also yet to be explored. We suggest that A_1 agonists may be effective in reducing neurogenic vasodilation originating from the release of vasoactive peptides, such as CGRP, from trigeminal neurons.

Section VI summarized the evidence for adenosine being the mediator of ischemic pain. Another superficially attractive idea might, therefore, be to block this pain with an adenosine antagonist. However, cardiac (anginal) pain has a survival benefit in that it prevents the sufferer from continuing to put excessive metabolic demand on the myocardium, and the adenosine that is released locally also confers a protective effect against further ischemic damage. Clearly, it would be undesirable to remove these factors without simultaneously modifying the underlying disease process. In contrast, for critical limb ischemia, there is a case to be made for allowing the patient to tolerate a greater degree of painful muscle ischemia, because there is some evidence to suggest that adenosine may act as a stimulus to neovascularization (e.g., Fischer et al., 1997).

In summary, adenosine and adenosine receptors appear to play a fundamental role in nociceptive pathways, offering opportunities for totally new analgesic therapies. However, this must be considered as a high-risk strategy where the benefit may have to be balanced against the likelihood of side effects.

REFERENCES

Aley KO, Levine JD. (1997) Multiple receptors involved in peripheral alpha 2, mu, and A1 antinociception, tolerance, and withdrawal. J Neurosci 17:735–744.

Aley KO, Green PG, Levine JD. (1995) Opioid and adenosine peripheral antinociception are subject to tolerance and withdrawal. J Neurosci 15:8031–8038.

Aran S, Proudfit HK. (1990) Antinociceptive interactions between intrathecally administered alpha noradrenergic agonists and 5′-*N*-ethylcarboxamide adenosine. Brain Res 519:287–293.

Ballarin M, Herrera–Marschitz M, Casas M, Ungerstedt U. (1987) Striatal adenosine levels measured "in vivo" by microdialysis in rats with unilateral dopamine denervation. Neurosci Lett 83:338–344.

Belfrage M, Sollevi A, Segerdahl M, Sjolund KF, Hansson P. (1995) Systemic adenosine infusion alleviates spontaneous and stimulus evoked pain in patients with peripheral neuropathic pain. Anesth Analg 81:713–717.

Bleehen T, Keele CA. (1977) Observations on the algogenic actions of adenosine compounds on the human blister base preparation. Pain 3:367–377.

Brown SGA, Waterer GW. (1995) Migraine precipitated by adenosine. Med J Aust 162:389.

Cahill CM, White TD, Sawynok J. (1995) Spinal opioid receptors and adenosine release: neurochemical and behavioral characterization of opioid subtypes. J Pharmacol Exp Ther 275:84–93.

Crea F, Pupita G, Galassi AR, el-Tamimi H, Kaski JC, Davies G, Maseri A. (1990) Role of adenosine in pathogenesis of anginal pain. Circulation 81:164–172.

Crea F, Gaspardone A, Kaski JC, Davies G, Maseri A. (1992) Relation between stimulation site of cardiac afferent nerves by adenosine and distribution of cardiac pain: results of a study in patients with stable angina. J Am Coll Cardiol 20:1498–1502.

Ekblom A, Segerdahl M, Sollevi A. (1995) Adenosine increases the cutaneous heat pain threshold in healthy volunteers. Acta Anaesthesiol Scand 39:717–722.

Eriksson B, Svedenhag J, Sylvan C. (1997) Analgesic effects of intraarterially administered adenosine in the ischemic forearm test. Circulation 96(suppl I):I–632.

Feoktistov I, Biaggioni I. (1997) Adenosine A_{2B} receptors. Pharmacol Rev 49:381–402.

Fischer S, Knoll R, Renz D, Karliczek GF, and Schaper W. (1997). Role of adenosine in the hypoxic induction of vascular endothelial growth factor in porcine brain derived microvascular endothelial cells. Endothelium 5:155–165.

Gaspardone A, Crea F, Tomai F, Versaci F, Iamele M, Gioffre G, Chiariello L, Gioffre PA. (1995) Muscular and cardiac adenosine-induced pain is mediated by A_1 receptors. J Am Coll Cardiol 25:251–257.

Guieu R, Devaux C, Henry H, Bechis G, Pouget J, Mallet D, Sampien F, Juin M, Gola R, Rochat H. (1998) Adenosine and migraine. Can J Neurol Sci 25:55–58.

Hashino T, Ikeda H, Ueno T, and Imaizumi T. (1996) Aminophylline reduces cardiac ischemic pain during percutaneous transluminal coronary angioplasty. J Am Coll Cardiol 28:1725–1731.

Honore P, Buritova J, Chapman V, Besson JM. (1998). UP 202-56, an adenosine analogue, selectively acts via A_1 receptors to significantly decrease noxiously-evoked spinal *c-fos* protein expression. Pain 75:281–293.

Jonzon B, Sylven C, Kaijser L. (1989) Theophylline decreases pain in the ischemic forearm test. Cardiovasc Res 23:807–809.

Karlsten R, Gordh T, Post C. (1992) Local antinociceptive and hyperalgesic effects in the formalin test after peripheral administration of adenosine analogues in mice. Pharmacol Toxicol 70:434–438.

Keil GJ 2nd, DeLander GE. (1994) Adenosine kinase and adenosine deaminase inhibition modulate spinal adenosine- and opioid agonist-induced antinociception in mice. Eur J Pharmacol 271:37–46.

Lagerqvist B, Sylven C, Hedenstrom H, Waldenstrom A. (1990) Intravenous adenosine but not its first metabolite inosine provokes chest pain in healthy volunteers. J Cardiovasc Pharmacol 16:173–176.

Ledent C, Vaugeois JM, Schiffmann SN, Pedrazzini T, El Yacoubi M, Vanderhaeghen JJ, Costentin J, Heath JK, Vassart G, Parmentier M. (1997) Aggressiveness, hypoalgesia and high blood pressure in mice lacking the adenosine A_{2a} receptor. Nature 388:674–678.

Mahaffey KW, Puma JA, Barbagelata A, et al. (1997) Does adenosine in combination with thrombolysis reduce infarct size? Results from the controlled, randomized AMISTAD trial. Circulation 96 (suppl 1):I–206.

Müller CE, Scior T. (1993) Adenosine receptors and their modulators. Pharm Acta Helv 68:77–111.

Ocana M, Baeyens JM. (1994) Role of ATP-sensitive K^+ channels in antinociception induced by R-PIA, an adenosine A_1 receptor agonist. Naunyn-Schmiedeberg Arch Pharmacol 350:57–62.

Palmer TM, Benovic JL, Stiles GL. (1996) Molecular basis for subtype-specific desensitization of inhibitory adenosine receptors. Analysis of a chimeric A_1–A_3 adenosine receptor. J Biol Chem 271: 15272–15278.

Pappagallo M, Gaspardone A, Tomai F, Iamele M, Crea F, Gioffre PA. (1993) Analgesic effect of bamiphylline on pain induced by intradermal injections of adenosine. Pain 53:199–204.

Poon A, Sawynok J. (1995) Antinociception by adenosine analogs and an adenosine kinase inhibitor: dependence on formalin concentration. Eur J Pharmacol 286:177–184.

Poon A, Sawynok J. (1998) Antinociception by adenosine analogs and inhibitors of adenosine metabolism in an inflammatory thermal hyperalgesia model in the rat. Pain 74:235–245.

Post C. (1984) Antinociceptive effects in mice after intrathecal injection of 5′-*N*-ethylcarboxamide adenosine. Neurosci Lett 51:325–330.

Reeves JJ, Jones CA, Sheehan MJ, Vardey CJ, Whelan CJ. (1997) Adenosine A_3 receptors promote degranulation of rat mast cells both in vitro and in vivo. Inflamm Res 46:180–184.

Sabetkasai M, Zarrindast MR. (1993) Antinociception: interaction between adenosine and GABA systems. Arch Int Pharmacodyn Ther 322:14–22.

Sawynok J. (1998) Adenosine and pain [abstr]. Presented at 6th International Symposium on Adenosine and Adenine Nucleotides, Ferrara, Italy, May 19–24, 1998. Drug Dev Res 43:36.

Sawynok J, Reid A. (1991) Noradrenergic and purinergic involvement in spinal antinociception by 5-hydroxytryptamine and 2-methyl-5-hydroxytryptamine. Eur J Pharmacol 204:301–309.

Sawynok J, Sweeney MI. (1989) The role of purines in nociception. Neuroscience 32:557–569.

Sawynok J, Sweeney MI, White TD. (1986) Classification of adenosine receptors mediating antinociception in the rat spinal cord. Br J Pharmacol 88:923–930.

Sawynok J, Zarrindast MR, Reid AR, Doak GJ. (1997) Adenosine A_3 receptor activation produces nociceptive behaviour and edema by release of histamine and 5-hydroxytryptamine. Eur J Pharmacol 333: 1–7.

Segerdahl M, Ekblom A, Sjolund KF, Belfrage M, Forsberg C, Sollevi A. (1995) Systemic adenosine attenuates touch evoked allodynia induced by mustard oil in humans. Neuroreport 6:753–756.

Sjolund KF, Sollevi A, Segerdahl M, Hansson P, Lundeberg T. (1996) Intrathecal and systemic *R*-phenylisopropyl-adenosine reduces scratching behaviour in a rat mononeuropathy model. Neuroreport 7: 1856–1860.

Sollevi A. (1986). Cardiovascular effects of adenosine in man: possible clinical implications. Prog Neurobiol 27:319–349.

Sollevi A, Belfrage M, Lundeberg T, Segerdahl M, Hansson P. (1995) Systemic adenosine infusion: a new treatment modality to alleviate neuropathic pain. Pain 61:155–158.

Sosnowski M, Stevens CW, Yaksh TL. (1989) Assessment of the role of A_1/A_2 adenosine receptors mediating the purine antinociception, motor and autonomic function in the rat spinal cord. J Pharmacol Exp Ther 250:915–922.

Sosnowski M, Yaksh TL. (1989) Role of spinal adenosine receptors in modulating the hyperesthesia produced by spinal glycine receptor antagonism. Anesth Analg 69:587–592.

Sylven C. (1993) Mechanisms of pain in angina pectoris—a critical review of the adenosine hypothesis. Cardiovasc Drugs Ther 7:745–759.

Sylven C, Beermann B, Jonzon B, Brandt R. (1986) Angina pectoris-like pain provoked by intravenous adenosine in healthy volunteers. Br Med J 293:227–230.

Sylven C, Jonzon B, Fredholm B, Kaijser L. (1988) Adenosine injection into the brachial artery produces ischemia-like pain or discomfort in the forearm. Cardiovasc Res 22:674–678.

Sylven C, Jonzon B, Edlund A. (1989) Angina pectoris-like pain provoked by i.v. bolus of adenosine: relationship to coronary sinus blood flow, heart rate and blood pressure in healthy volunteers. Eur Heart J 10:48–54.

Tomai F, Crea F, Gaspardone A, Versaci F, Esposito C, Chiariello L, Gioffre PA. (1993) Mechanisms of cardiac pain during coronary angioplasty. J Am Coll Cardiol 22:1892–1896.

53

Adenosine Kinase Inhibition as a Therapeutic Approach to Analgesia

Elizabeth A. Kowaluk
Abbott Laboratories, Abbott Park, Illinois, U.S.A.

I. INTRODUCTION

The endogenous purine nucleoside adenosine (ADO) activates discrete extracellular receptors (termed P_1 receptors) to serve as an inhibitory modulator of cellular and tissue function (1,2). ADO has been characterized as a "homeostatic" or "retaliatory" modulator of cellular activity (3). Tissue levels of extracellular ADO increase locally during periods of pathophysiological stress (e.g., tissue trauma and inflammation, ischemia, or seizures). Extracellular ADO accumulation may reflect the direct release of ADO itself or the release of ATP, which is degraded by extracellular nucleotidases to ADO (4) (Fig. 1). ADO in the extracellular space activates P_1 receptors to elicit a variety of responses that tend to counteract the initial adverse stimulus, thereby restoring cellular function toward normal (5,6). ADO is rapidly inactivated in extracellular fluids (a half-life on the order of seconds) (7), and its endogenous actions are highly localized. Four subtypes of the P_1 family of G–protein-coupled receptors have been identified and cloned: A_1, A_{2A}, A_{2B}, and A_3.

There is now abundant evidence to suggest that ADO is an endogenous modulator of antinociceptive and anti-inflammatory processes, and that opportunities exist for therapeutic intervention based on mimicking or potentiating its actions as a modulator of cellular activity. Recently, potentiation of the concentration and actions of extracellular endogenously released ADO using inhibitors of the ADO-metabolizing enzyme, ADO kinase (AK) (see Fig. 1), has emerged as an approach to the development of ADO-based pharmaceutical agents. This chapter provides a brief summary of the role of ADO in antinociception and inflammation, followed by a discussion of the rationale for AK inhibition as an approach to developing novel analgesic and anti-inflammatory agents, a review of the properties of the enzyme, and a discussion of the antinociceptive and anti-inflammatory properties of AK inhibitors reported to date.

II. ROLE OF ADENOSINE IN PAIN AND INFLAMMATION

There is considerable evidence for a role of ADO in modulating pain transmission at the level of the spinal cord. ADO-containing neurons have been localized to the substantia gelatinosa of the dorsal horn of the spinal cord (8). In addition, ADO A_1 and A_{2A} receptors have been localized to the spinal cord (9–12), as well as to the cell bodies of dorsal root ganglion cells (13). The

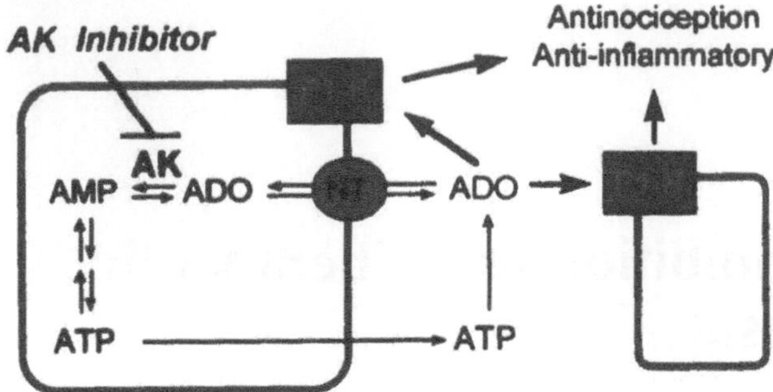

Figure 1 Mechanism of action of adenosine and modulation by AK inhibitors: AK inhibitors potentiate the concentrations and actions of endogenously released extracellular ADO, which traverses the cell membrane by a bidirectional, facilitated diffusion transporter (NT). Extracellular ADO elicits antinociceptive and anti-inflammatory effects by activating specific extracellular P_1 receptors (P_1-R).

ADO-metabolizing enzymes, ADO deaminase (ADA) (14) and AK (Kowaluk EA, et al., unpublished results), and ADO transport sites (15) have also been localized to the spinal cord. ADO is well known to serve as an inhibitory neuromodulator in the central nervous system (CNS) (4). Activation of ADO A_1 receptors results in inhibition of cyclic-AMP production, increased K^+ currents, and decreased Ca^{2+} currents. Presynaptically, ADO inhibits neurotransmitter and neuropeptide release, including glutamate, substance P, and calcitonin-gene related peptide (CGRP) (16,17). Postsynaptically, ADO suppresses sensory transmission as a result of the activation of K^+ conductances and membrane hyperpolarization (18,19). ADO receptor agonists inhibit pain behaviors elicited by spinal injection of substance P and the glutamate agonist *N*-methyl-D-aspartate (NMDA) (20), potentially reflecting the direct postsynaptic actions of ADO. ADO A_1 agonists also reduced cerebrospinal fluid (CSF) substance P levels, in parallel with pain relief in rats (21). As later described, intrathecal ADO, ADO receptor agonists, and AK inhibitors elicit antinociceptive effects in animal models, and these effects are blocked by systemic or intrathecal ADO receptor antagonists such as theophylline (22), further supporting a spinal site for ADO-mediated antinociception.

There is also evidence for the contribution of supraspinal and peripheral mechanisms to antinociception by ADO and ADO analogues, although these have been less extensively evaluated than spinal pathways. The intracisternal or intracerebroventricular administration of ADO and ADO analogues elicits antinociception in animal models (23,24), suggesting a potential role of supraspinal ADO in antinociception. ADO A_1 and A_{2A} receptors, ADA, AK, and ADO transport sites, all are localized in the brain (25–27). Although the role of ADO in modulation of nociception in the periphery appears to be complex (28), studies with AK inhibitors (29) indicate a peripheral site of action in inflammatory and persistent pain states. The actions of endogenously released ADO to inhibit peripheral neurotransmitter release (30) and to attenuate inflammatory processes may contribute to the modulation of antinociception by ADO in the periphery. ADO is released at sites of inflammation (31) and exerts anti-inflammatory effects through multiple mechanisms (32). It modulates neutrophil function (A_{2A} receptor) (33), endothelial cell permeability (A_1 and A_{2A} receptors) (34), tumor necrosis factor-α (TNF-α) production in vitro (A_3 receptor) and in vivo (35,36), and collagenase (MMP-1) production and gene expression on synoviocytes in vitro (A_{2B} receptor) (37). Accordingly, ADO receptor agonists and AK inhibitors have efficacy in various animal models of inflammation (32,35,38–41). Local, peripheral mechanisms at the site of injury appear to mediate the anti-inflammatory effects of systemically administered AK inhibitors, as these effects were blocked by the peripheral ADO receptor antagonist,

8-(*p*-sulfophenyl)theophylline, and by local application of exogenous ADA (to degrade endogenously released ADO) at sites of inflammation (31). The CNS may also play a role in the anti-inflammatory actions of ADO (42). Thus, intrathecal A_1 ADO receptor stimulation suppressed neutrophil accumulation at peripheral sites of inflammation, potentially by deactivating the NMDA–receptor-signaling pathway which, in turn, modulated tissue ADO levels at the peripheral inflamed site. These observations suggest that overlapping molecular mechanisms may contribute to the modulation of pain and inflammation by ADO analogues.

The role of ADO in antinociception is supported by behavioral evidence from a spectrum of animal pain models. Direct-acting ADO receptor agonists and AK inhibitors are active in classic models of acute nociceptive pain such as the mouse hot-plate test (43) and the mouse tail-flick assay (44). In addition, ADO receptor agonists and AK inhibitors provide antinociceptive activity in models of chemically induced persistent pain, including the rat formalin test (45) and the mouse abdominal constriction assay (46). Spinally administered ADO agonists are also effective in rat models of neuropathic pain, including the thermal hyperalgesia induced by constriction injury of the sciatic nerve (Bennett model) (47), the tactile allodynia evoked by spinal glycine receptor antagonism (48), and the tactile allodynia induced by L5–L6 spinal nerve ligation (Chung model) (49). More recently, the efficacy of a systemically administered AK inhibitor has been demonstrated in a rat model of diabetic neuropathic pain (50). In addition, UP-202-56, an ADO analogue acting selectively through A_1 receptors, provided antinociception in several animal models of inflammatory and neuropathic pain and significantly decreased carrageenan-evoked spinal c-Fos protein expression (51). In clinical studies, intravenous ADO infusion improved pain symptoms in several experimental clinical pain models at doses that exhibited no overt cardiovascular effects (52–54). ADO infusion was also superior to placebo in reducing pain symptoms in patients with neuropathic pain (55). The beneficial effects of ADO were reported to persist for many hours after termination of the ADO infusion. Interestingly, intrathecal administration of a single dose of ADO has also demonstrated long-lasting (>24 h) attenuation of tactile allodynia in an animal model of neuropathic pain (56). In addition, perioperative low-dose ADO infusion reduced the requirement for inhalation anesthetic during surgery and reduced the need for postoperative opioid analgesia (57). Spinal administration of the ADO A_1 agonist, (*R*)-phenylisopropyladenosine (*R*-PIA), relieved allodynia in a patient with intractable neuropathic pain (58).

III. ADENOSINE KINASE INHIBITION AS A THERAPEUTIC APPROACH TO ANALGESIA AND INFLAMMATION

A. Potentiation of Adenosine by AK Inhibition

Inhibition of the key ADO-regulating enzyme, ADO kinase (AK), has emerged as a method for taking advantage of the effects of endogenous ADO for therapeutic benefit. AK is a key intracellular enzyme regulating intra- and extracellular ADO concentrations (59) (see Fig. 1). AK rapidly phosphorylates ADO, maintaining intracellular ADO concentrations at low levels. ADO passes to and from the extracellular environment by a nonconcentrative, bidirectional, facilitated diffusion transporter. Because ADO uptake is driven by its concentration gradient, inhibition of AK indirectly decreases cellular reuptake of ADO (60), potentiating the local concentration and the effects of ADO in the extracellular compartment. As the actions of endogenous ADO are highly localized and AK inhibition may be more effective in cells undergoing accelerated ADO release (61). It has been proposed that the effects of AK inhibitors may be more pronounced in tissue sites at which pathophysiological events result in enhanced ADO production from ATP (see Fig. 1), thereby potentially limiting systemic side effects.

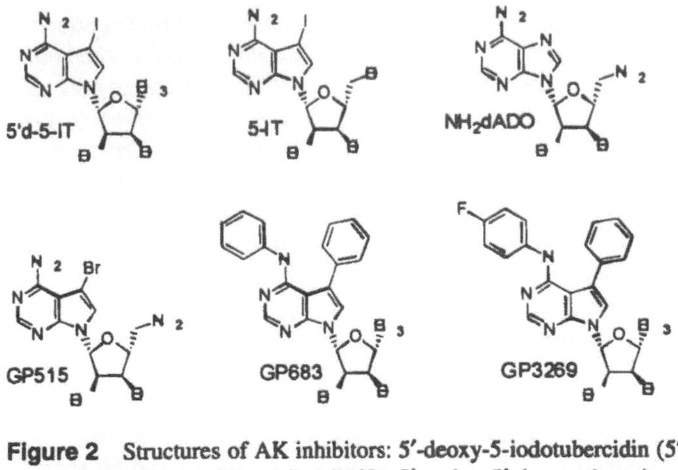

Figure 2 Structures of AK inhibitors: 5′-deoxy-5-iodotubercidin (5′d-5IT; AK IC_{50} = 0.8 nM); 5-iodotubercidin (5-IT; AK IC_{50} = 5 nM)(68); 5′-amino-5′-deoxyadenosine (NH_2dADO; AK IC_{50} = 8 nM)(68); GP515 (AK IC_{50} = 4.6 nM)(74); GP683 (AK IC_{50} = 0.5 nM)(74); GP3269 (AK IC_{50} = 11 nM)(76).

The augmentation of ADO availability by AK inhibitors has been demonstrated in several systems in vitro, including hippocampal and spinal cord slices (62,63), as well as during excitotoxic insults to rat striatum in vivo (64). In the latter study, the excitotoxin, kainic acid (KA), was unilaterally perfused into one striatum of rats that were implanted bilaterally with striatal microdialysis probes. KA perfusion produced a local increase in extracellular ADO levels in the ipsilateral injured striatum, but not in the contralateral control, artificial CSF-perfused striatum. Systemic administration of the potent and selective AK inhibitor 5′-deoxy-5-iodotubercidin (5′d-5IT; Fig. 2) enhanced the KA-evoked ADO release, without altering basal extracellular ADO levels in the contralateral control striatum, lending support to the hypothesis that AK inhibition may selectively enhance the actions of ADO at tissue sites where pathophysiological events result in increased ADO production.

The behavioral effects of potent and selective AK inhibitors in a variety of animal pain and inflammation models are blocked or reversed by ADO receptor antagonists, consistent with the potentiation of endogenous ADO which, in turn, activates its receptors, as an underlying mechanism mediating the effects of AK inhibitors in vivo (see Sec. IV). ADO metabolism also proceeds by deamination by ADA. However, an intrathecally administered ADA inhibitor failed to produce antinociception in vivo in the mouse tail-flick assay (44), in the rat formalin test (45), and in rat carrageenan-induced thermal hyperalgesia (65), under conditions that an AK inhibitor was efficacious. Similar results have also been reported relative to the anticonvulsant actions of AK versus ADA inhibitors (66). Thus, AK appears to play a more prominent role in regulating ADO levels in the CNS than does ADA.

B. Enzymology and Molecular Biology of Adenosine Kinase

Adenosine kinase (ATP:adenosine-5′-phosphotransferase; EC 2.7.1.20) is a cytosolic enzyme that catalyzes the phosphorylation of ADO to AMP, with ATP serving as the phosphate source. Magnesium is also required for AK activity, and the true AK cosubstrate is probably the $MgATP^{2-}$ complex (67). The enzyme appears to be monomeric, with a molecular weight in the range of 38–56 kDa. The AK gene has been cloned and expressed from rat (68) and human (68,69) tissues. The enzyme lacks a "classic" ATP-binding motif, and it appears to be distinct from other well-characterized nucleoside kinases. However, the AK cDNA contains two regions with sequence similarity to several plant and microbial sugar kinases (68,69). Two isoforms of

AK mRNA have been identified in human tissues (68). The two mRNAs encode proteins that are identical in sequence except at the amino terminus, where the first 4 residues of one are replaced by 21 residues in the other. The two isoforms appear to arise as a result of differential splicing of a single transcriptional product, but their physiological significance has not yet been defined. Both isoforms were expressed in *Escherichia coli* to provide soluble, active protein that exhibited the enzymatic characteristics of AK. No differences were observed in the gross enzymatic properties of the two AK isoforms. Both isoforms were inhibited by the classic AK inhibitors, 5-iodotubercidin (5-IT) and 5′-amino-5′-deoxyadenosine (NH_2dADO) (see Fig. 2), with potency similar to that observed between isozymes (68). The structure of AK, determined by X-ray crystallography, has been reported recently (70). The enzyme structure consists of two α-helix–β sheet domains, with the active site lying between the two domains. The overall structure is similar to that of *E. coli* ribokinase, consistent with earlier predictions based on the gene sequence (68,69).

IV. ADENOSINE KINASE INHIBITORS AND ANALGESIA

Adenosine kinase inhibitors exhibit efficacy in a variety of animal pain models, mirroring the broad spectrum of effectiveness that has been described for ADO and ADO receptor agonists (see Sec. II).

A. Brief Nociception

Intrathecal administration of the potent AK inhibitor NH_2dADO (see Fig. 2) induced antinociception in the mouse tail-flick assay (44). NH_2dADO was a more effective antinociceptive agent in this model than the ADA inhibitor, deoxycoformycin, as has also been reported in animal seizure models (66). The effects of intrathecal NH_2dADO were blocked by intrathecal coadministration of the nonselective ADO receptor antagonist, theophylline, consistent with a mechanism of action for NH_2dADO of potentiating ADO to activate its receptors in the spinal cord. The efficacy of systemically administered AK inhibitors, including NH_2dADO, 5′d-5IT, and 5-IT (see Fig. 2), have been demonstrated in the mouse hot-plate test (71). The antinociceptive effects of 5′d-5IT were blocked by the centrally and peripherally acting ADO receptor antagonist, theophylline, but not by the peripheral ADO receptor antagonist, 8-(*p*-sulfophenyl)-theophylline. In addition, antinociception by 5′d-5IT was blocked completely by the selective A_1 adenosine receptor antagonist DPCPX, modestly by the A_{2A} selective antagonist ZM 241385, and not blocked at all by the opioid antagonist naloxone. Together these data suggest a nonopioid, predominantly central, A_1 receptor-mediated effect underlying the actions of 5′d-5IT to relieve acute thermal nociception. The antinociceptive effects of 5′d-5IT were additive with morphine, and they were maintained following subchronic administration.

B. Chemically Induced Persistent Pain

The AK inhibitors also provide efficacy in animal models of persistent pain. Intrathecally administered NH_2dADO was effective in the persistent phase (phase 2) of the rat formalin test (45). The effects of NH_2dADO were inhibited by intrathecal administration of the nonselective ADO receptor antagonist caffeine, consistent with a mechanism of enhanced ADO levels acting by activation of ADO receptors in the spinal cord. NH_2dADO also produced antinociception following intraplantar administration with formalin in the rat formalin test (29). These peripheral effects of NH_2dADO to evoke antinociception also appeared to be due to the accumulation of ADO and activation of ADO receptors because they were blocked by intraplantar coadministration of the ADO receptor antagonist caffeine. The antinociceptive effects of NH_2dADO were observed at doses that exhibited no signs of motor impairment or reduced locomotor activity (29). Although both spinal and peripheral (intraplantar) actions of AK inhibitors have been demonstrated with local administration, the efficacy of a systemically administered AK inhibitor has not been reported. The relative contributions of the spinal and peripheral sites' action on the effects of a systemically administered AK inhibitor also remain to be defined. The ADA inhibitor, deoxycoformycin was ineffective after either intrathecal or intraplantar administration under similar conditions (29,45), again suggesting a more prominent role of AK than ADA in regulating endogenous ADO in the spinal cord and at peripheral sites of tissue injury. In addition, systemically administered 5′d-5IT also provided antinociception in the phenyl-*p*-quinone-induced abdominal constriction assay of persistent chemical pain (71).

C. Inflammatory Pain

Intrathecal NH_2dADO and 5-IT provided dose-dependent antinociception in the rat carrageenan-induced inflammatory pain model (65). Both agents elicited antinociception more potently in the inflamed paw in than in the noninflamed paw. As also reported in the formalin model, the effects of the AK inhibitors were superior to that of the ADA inhibitor, deoxycoformycin, which was ineffective, although deoxycoformycin enhanced the antinociceptive effects of threshold doses of NH_2dADO. The effects of intrathecal NH_2dADO were inhibited by intrathecal administration of the nonselective ADO receptor antagonist caffeine, and by the A_1 adenosine receptor selective antagonist CPT, but not the A_{2A} receptor antagonist DMPX, consistent with a role of amplification of endogenous ADO and activation of spinal A_1 receptors in antinociception by the AK inhibitor. The efficacy of a systemically administered AK inhibitor has also been demonstrated in this model. The potent and selective AK inhibitor 5′d-5IT relieved carrageenan-induced thermal hyperalgesia after intraperitoneal administration (72). 5′d-5IT was an order of magnitude more potent in relieving thermal hyperalgesia of the inflamed paw than in relieving acute thermal nociception in the contralateral noninflamed paw. 5′d-5IT was also fully effective in blocking carrageenan-induced thermal hyperalgesia at doses that had no effect on rotorod performance, a measure of motor impairment. The antihyperalgesic effects of 5′d-5IT were apparently not secondary to its anti-inflammatory actions, because 5′d-5IT was more potent in attenuating carrageenan-induced hyperalgesia than in reducing the accompanying paw edema. A similar conclusion was drawn from studies of the effects of intrathecal NH_2dADO on carrageenan-induced hyperalgesia and edema (65). The antihyperalgesic actions of intraperitoneal 5′d-5IT (72) were blocked by systemic administration of the adenosine A_1 selective receptor antagonist CPT, and of the adenosine A_{2A} receptor selective antagonist DMPX, suggesting that the activation of both receptor subtypes by endogenous ADO contributes to the antihyperalgesic actions of the systemically administered AK inhibitor.

D. Neuropathic Pain

Systemically administered 5′d-5IT also attenuated tactile allodynia in streptozocin-injected rats, a model of diabetic neuropathic pain (73). Pretreatment with the nonselective ADO receptor antagonist theophylline significantly reduced the antiallodynic effects of 5′d-5IT, consistent with the potentiation of endogenous ADO and activation of its receptors as a mechanism of action for 5′d-5IT in this model.

The AK inhibitors may also have a use as analgesic and anesthetic-sparing agents during the perioperative period, as previously demonstrated with ADO itself (57). The AK inhibitor GP683 (Metabasis Therapeutics; see Fig. 2) decreased the desflurane anesthetic requirement in dogs, without producing adverse effects on the cardiovascular system (74,75). GP3269 (Metabasis Therapeutics; see Fig. 2), an analogue of GP683, is entering phase II clinical development for pain and epilepsy. This compound is a potent AK inhibitor that is reported to have good oral bioavailability, although its efficacy has been reported only in preclinical seizure models (76). Its efficacy in preclinical pain models has not been reported.

V. ADENOSINE KINASE INHIBITORS AND INFLAMMATION

The AK inhibitors are also effective in various animal models of inflammation. The potent and selective AK inhibitor GP515 (Metabasis Therapeutics; see Fig. 2) significantly improved survival in two models of septic shock: murine endotoxic shock and a rat model of bacterial peritonitis (38). Improved survival by the AK inhibitor in the latter model suggests that the anti-inflammatory actions of ADO do not suppress the normal immune response to infection, because in this particular model sepsis results from an infectious process (32,38). GP515 and other AK inhibitors also decreased carrageenan-induced pleurisy and paw edema, as well as neutrophil accumulation into air pouches and into the skin of rodents after local injection of inflammatory mediators such as carrageenan and other proinflammatory agents (31,32,34,39). The in vivo anti-inflammatory effects of GP515 were reversed by administration of ADO receptor antagonists, consistent with a role of endogenous ADO and activation of ADO receptors in the action of GP515. An AK inhibitor of undisclosed structure (AKI-2; Gensia) demonstrated efficacy in the rat adjuvant arthritis model, which exhibits histopathological and clinical features similar to those seen in rheumatoid arthritis (32). The AK inhibitor reduced paw edema and decreased bone and cartilage damage as indicated by a radiographic analysis (32), supporting a potential disease-modifying action. The effects of the compounds were reversed by coadministration of an ADO receptor antagonist. Anti-inflammatory efficacy was observed even when treatment with the AK inhibitor was initiated several days after the onset of arthritis. The effects of the AK inhibitor on bone protection observed in the rat adjuvant arthritis model may reflect actions of ADO on MMP regulation (37) and on modulation of TNF-α production (35,36) (see Sec. II).

VI. SUMMARY

The antinociceptive effects of ADO and ADO analogues have been known for many years. However, recent advances in the understanding of the neurobiology of pain, and a growing body of evidence implicating ADO as an endogenous modulator of pain and inflammation, have led to a further appreciation of the potential of ADO as a target for the development of analgesic and anti-inflammatory agents. In particular, AK inhibition has emerged as a novel therapeutic approach to harnessing the effects of endogenous ADO for therapeutic benefit. As detailed in the foregoing, preclinical evidence indicates that AK inhibitors may potentially have usefulness as analgesic agents in a broad spectrum of pain types. Progression of these agents into clinical studies over the next several years will provide an understanding of their potential as part of a therapeutically useful new class of analgesic and anti-inflammatory agents.

REFERENCES

1. Burnstock G. A basis for distinguishing two types of purinergic receptor. In: Bolis L, Straub RE, eds. Cell Membrane Receptors for Drugs and Hormones. New York: Raven, 1978; 107–118.

2. Williams M. Adenosine: the prototypical modulator. Neurochem Int 1989; 14:249–264.
3. Newby AC. Adenosine and the concept of "retaliatory metabolites." Trends Biochem Sci 1984; 2: 42–44.
4. Brundege JM, Dunwiddie TV. Role of adenosine as a modulator of synaptic activity in the central nervous system. Adv Pharmacol 1997; 39:353–391.
5. Bruns RF. Role of adenosine in energy supply/demand balance. Nucleosides Nucleotides 1991; 10: 931–943.
6. Miller LP, Hsu C. Therapeutic potential for adenosine receptor activation in ischemic brain injury. J Neurotrauma 1992; 9:S563–S577.
7. Moser GH, Schrader J, Deussen A. Turnover of adenosine in plasma of human and dog blood. Am J Physiol 1989; 25:C799–C806.
8. Braas KM, Newby AC, Wilson VS, Snyder SH. Adenosine-containing neurons in the brain localized by immunocytochemistry. J Neurosci 1986; 6:1952–1961.
9. Goodman RR, Snyder SH. Autoradiographic localization of adenosine receptors in rat brain using [^{3}H]cyclohexyladenosine. J Neurosci 1980; 2:1230–241.
10. Choca JI, Proudfit HK, Green RD. Identification of A_1 and A_2 adenosine receptors in the rat spinal cord. J Pharmacol Exp Ther 1987; 242:905–910.
11. Geiger JD, Labella FS, Nagy LL. Characterization and localization of adenosine receptors in rat spinal cord. J Neurosci 1984; 4:2303–2310.
12. Choca JI, Green RD, Proudfit HK. Adenosine A_1 and A_2 receptors of the substantia gelatinosa are located predominantly on intrinsic neurons: an autoradiography study. J Pharmacol Exp Ther 1988; 247:757–764.
13. MacDonald RL, Skerritt JH, Werz MA. Adenosine agonists reduce voltage-dependent calcium conductance of mouse sensory neurons in cell culture. J Physiol 1986; 370:75–90.
14. Geiger JD, Nagy JI. Distribution of adenosine deaminase activity in rat brain and spinal cord. J Neurosci 1986; 6:2707–2714.
15. Geiger JD, Nagy JI. Localization of [^{3}H]-nitrobenzylthioinosine binding sites in rat spinal cord and primary afferent neurons. Brain Res 1985; 34:321–327.
16. Vasko MR, Ono H. Adenosine analogs do not inhibit the potassium-stimulated release of substance P from rat spinal cord slices. Naunyn Schmiedebergs Arch Pharmacol 1990; 342:441–446.
17. Santicioli P, Del Bianco E, Tramontana M, Maggi CA. Adenosine inhibits action potential-dependent release of calcitonin gene-related peptide- and substance P-like immunoreactivities from primary afferents in rat spinal cord. Neurosci Lett 1992; 144:211–214.
18. Salter MW, De Koninck Y, Henry JL. Physiological roles of adenosine and ATP in synaptic transmission in the spinal dorsal horn. Prog Neurobiol 1993; 41:125–56.
19. Li E, Perl E. Adenosine inhibition of synaptic transmission in the substantia gelatinosa. J Neurophysiol 1994; 4:1611–1621.
20. Delander GE, Wahl JJ. Behaviour induced by putative nociceptive neurotransmitters is inhibited by adenosine or adenosine analogs coadministered intrathecally. J Pharmacol Exp Ther 1988; 246:565–570.
21. Sjolund KF, Sollevi A, Segerdahl M, Lundberg T. Intrathecal adenosine analog administration reduces substance P in cerebrospinal fluid along with behavioural effects that suggest antinociception in rats. Anesth Analg 1997; 85:627–632.
22. Sawynok J, Sweeney MI, White TD. Classification of adenosine receptors mediating antinociception in the rat spinal cord. Br J Pharmacol 1986; 88:923–930.
23. Herrick–Davis K, Chippari S, Luttinger D, Ward SJ. Evaluation of adenosine agonists as potential analgesics. Eur J Pharmacol 1989; 162:365–369.
24. Yarbrough GG, McGuffin–Clineschmidt JC. In vivo behavioral assessment of central nervous system purinergic receptors. Eur J Pharmacol 1981; 76:137–144.
25. Jarvis M, Williams M. Adenosine in central nervous system function. In: Williams M, ed. Adenosine and Adenosine Receptors. Clifton, NJ: Humana Press, 1990;423–474.
26. Geiger JD, Nagy JI. Adenosine and [^{3}H]nitrobenzylthioinosine as markers of adenosine metabolism

and transport in central purinergic systems. In: Williams M, ed. Adenosine and Adenosine Receptors. Clifton, NJ: Humana Press, 1990:225–288.
27. Geiger JD, Parkinson FE, Kowaluk EA. Regulators of endogenous adenosine levels as therapeutic agents. In: Jacobson KA, Jarvis MF, eds. Purinergic Approaches in Experimental Therapeutics. New York: Wiley–Liss, 1997;55–84.
28. Doak GJ, Sawynok J. Complex role of peripheral adenosine in the genesis of the response to subcutaneous formalin in the rat. Eur J Pharmacol 1995; 281:311–318.
29. Sawynok J, Reid A, Poon A. Peripheral antinociceptive effect of an adenosine kinase inhibitor with augmentation by an adenosine deaminase inhibitor, in the rat formalin test. Pain 1998; 74:75–81.
30. Fredholm BB, Dunwiddie TV. How does adenosine inhibit transmitter release? Trends Pharmacol Sci 1988; 9:130–134.
31. Cronstein BN, Naime ED, Firestein G. The antiinflammatory effects of an adenosine kinase inhibitor are mediated by adenosine. Arthritis Rheum 1995; 38:1040–1045.
32. Firestein GS. Anti-inflammatory effects of adenosine kinase inhibitors in acute and chronic inflammation. Drug Dev Res 1996; 39:371–376.
33. Firestein GS, Bullough DA, Erion MD, Jimenez R, Ramirez–Weinhouse M, Barankiewicz J, Smith CW, Gruber HE, Mullane KM. Inhibition of neutrophil adhesion by adenosine and an adenosine kinase inhibitor. The role of selectins. J Immunol 1995; 154:326–334.
34. Rosengren S, Bong GW, Firestein GS. Anti-inflammatory effects of an adenosine kinase inhibitor: decreased neutrophil accumulation and vascular leakage. J Immunol 1995; 154:5444–5451.
35. Parmely MJ, Zhou WW, Edwards CK, Borcherding DR, Silverstein R, Morrison DC. Adenosine and a related carbocyclic nucleoside analogue selectively inhibit tumor necrosis factor-alpha production and protect mice against endotoxin challenge. J Immunol 1993; 151:389–396.
36. Sajjadi FG, Takabayashi K, Foster AC, Domingo RC, Firestein GS. Inhibition of TNF-alpha expression by adenosine: role of A_3 adenosine receptors. J Immunol 1996; 156:3435–3442.
37. Boyle DL, Sajjadi FG, Firestein GS. Adenosine receptor stimulation inhibits synoviocyte collagenase gene expression. Arthritis Rheum 1996; 39:923–930.
38. Firestein GS, Boyle D, Bullough DA, Gruber HE, Sajjadi FG, Montag A, Sambol B, Mullane KM. Protective effects of an adenosine kinase inhibitor in septic shock. J Immunol 1994; 152:5853–5859.
39. Cottam HB, Wasson DB, Shih C, Raychaudri A, Di Pasquale G, Carson D. New adenosine kinase inhibitors with oral anti-inflammatory activity: synthesis and biological evaluation. J Med Chem 1993; 36:3424–3430.
40. Lesch ME, Ferin MA, Wright CD, Schrier DJ. The effects of (*R*)-*N*-(1-methyl-2-phenylethyl)-adenosine (L-PIA), standard A_1-selective adenosine agonist, on rat acute models of inflammation and neutrophil function. Agents Actions 1991; 34:25–27.
41. Schrier DJ, Lesch ME, Wright CD, Gilbertson RB. The antiinflammatory effects of adenosine receptor agonists on the carrageenan-induced pleural inflammatory response in rats. J Immunol 1990; 145: 1874–1879.
42. Bong GW, Rosengren S, Firestein GS. Spinal cord adenosine receptor stimulation in rats inhibits dermal neutrophil accumulation: the role of *N*-methyl-D-aspartate receptors. J Clin Invest 1996; 98:1–7.
43. Holmgren M, Hedner J, Mellstrand T, Nordberg G, Hedner TH. Characterization of the antinociceptive effects of some adenosine analogues in the rat. Naunyn-Schmiedeberg/Arch Pharmacol 1986; 334:290–293.
44. Keil GJ, Delander GE. Spinally mediated antinociception is induced in mice by an adenosine kinase, but not an adenosine deaminase inhibitor. Life Sci 1992; 51:171–176.
45. Poon A, Sawynok J. Antinociception by adenosine analogs and an adenosine kinase inhibitor: dependence on formalin concentration. Eur J Pharmacol 1995; 286:177–184.
46. Ahlijanian MK, Takemori AE. Effects of (−)-N^6-(*R*-phenylisopropyl)adenosine and caffeine on nociception and morphine-induced analgesia, tolerance and dependence. Eur J Pharmacol 1985; 112: 171–179.
47. Yamamoto T, Yaksh TL. Spinal pharmacology of thermal hyperesthesia induced by constriction injury of sciatic nerve. Excitatory amino acid antagonists. Pain 1992; 49:121–128.

48. Sosnowski M, Yaksh TL. Role of spinal adenosine receptors in modulating the hyperesthesia produced by spinal glycine receptor antagonism. Anesth Analg 1989; 69:587–592.
49. Lee YL, Yaksh TL. Pharmacology of the spinal adenosine receptor which mediates the antiallodynic action of intrathecal adenosine agonists. J Pharmacol Exp Ther 1996; 277:1642–1648.
50. Lynch JJ, Jarvis MF, Kowaluk EA. An adenosine kinase inhibitor attenuates tactile allodynia in a rat model of diabetic neuropathic pain. Eur J Pharmacol 1999; 364:141–146.
51. Honore P, Buritova J, Chapman V, Besson J–M. UP 202-56, an adenosine analogue, selectively acts via A_1 receptors to significantly decrease noxiously-evoked spinal c-Fos protein expression. Pain 1998; 75:281–293.
52. Segerdahl M, Ekblom A, Sollevi A. The influence of adenosine, ketamine, and morphine on experimentally induced ischemic pain in healthy volunteers. Anesth Analg 1994; 79:787–791.
53. Segerdahl M, Ekblom A, Sjolund KF. Systemic adenosine attenuates touch evoked allodynia induced by mustard oil in humans. Neuroreport 1995; 6:753–756.
54. Ekblom A, Segerdahl M, Sollevi A. Adenosine increases the cutaneous heat pain threshold in healthy volunteers. Acta Anesth Scand 1995; 39:717–722.
55. Bellfrage M, Sollevi A, Segerdahl M. Systemic adenosine infusion alleviates spontaneous and stimulus evoked pain in patients with peripheral neuropathic pain. Anesth Analg 1995; 81:713–717.
56. Lavand'homme PM, Eisenach JC. Exogenous and endogenous adenosine enhance the spinal antiallodynic effects of morphine in a rat model of neuropathic pain. Pain 1999; 80:31–36.
57. Segerdahl M, Irestedt L, Sollevi A. Antinociceptive effect of perioperative adenosine infusion in abdominal hysterectomy. Acta Anesth Scand 1997; 41:180–185.
58. Karlsten R, Gordh T. An A_1-selective adenosine agonist abolishes allodynia elicited by vibration and touch after intrathecal injection. Anesth Analg 1995; 80:844–847.
59. Arch JRS, Newsholme EA. The control of the metabolism and the hormonal role of adenosine. Essays Biochem 1978; 14:82–123.
60. Davies LP, Jamieson DD, Baird–Lambert JA, Kazlauskas R. Halogenated pyrrolopyrimidine analogues of adenosine from marine organisms: pharmacological activities and potent inhibition of adenosine kinase. Biochem Pharmacol 1984; 33:347–355.
61. Newby AC, Holmquist AC, Illingworth J, Pearson D. The control of adenosine concentration in polymorphonuclear leukocytes, cultured cells and isolated perfused heart from the rat. Biochem J 1983; 214:317–323.
62. Pak MA, Haas HL, Decking UKM, Schrader J. Inhibition of adenosine kinase increases endogenous adenosine and depresses neuronal activity in hippocampal slices. Neuropharmacology 1994; 33: 1049–1053.
63. Golembiowska K, White TD, Sawynok J. Adenosine kinase inhibitors augment release of adenosine from spinal cord slices. Eur J Pharmacol 1996; 307:157–162.
64. Britton DR, Mikusa J, Lee C–H, Jarvis MF, Williams M, Kowaluk EA. Site and event specific increase in striatal adenosine release by adenosine kinase inhibition in rats. Neurosci Lett 1999; 266: 93–96.
65. Poon A, Sawynok J. Antinociception by adenosine analogs and inhibitors of adenosine metabolism in an inflammatory thermal hyperalgesia model in the rat. Pain 1998; 74:235–245.
66. Zhang G, Franklin PH, Murray TF. Manipulation of endogenous adenosine in the rat prepiriform cortex modulates seizure susceptibility. J Pharmacol Exp Ther 1993; 264:1415–1424.
67. Palella TD, Andres CM, Fox IH. Human placental adenosine kinase, kinetic mechanism and inhibition. J Biol Chem 1980; 255:5264–5269.
68. McNally T, Helfrich RJ, Cowart M, Dorwin SA, Meuth JL, Idler KB, Klute KA, Simmer RL, Kowaluk EA, Halbert DN. Cloning and expression of the adenosine kinase gene from rat and human tissues. Biochem Biophys Res Commun 1997; 231:645–650.
69. Spychala J, Datta NS, Takabayashi K, Datta M, Fox IH, Gribbin T, Mitchell BS. Cloning of human adenosine kinase cDNA: sequence similarity to microbial ribokinases and fructokinases. Proc Natl Acad Sci USA 1996; 93:1232–1237.
70. Matthews II, Erion MD, Ealick SE. Structure of human adenosine kinase at 1.5 A resolution. Biochemistry 1998; 37:15607–15620.

71. Kowaluk EA, Kohlhaas K, Bannon A, Gunther K, Lynch JJ, Jarvis MF. Characterization of the effects of adenosine kinase inhibitors on acute thermal nociception in mice. Pharmacol Biochem Behav 1999; 63:83–91.
72. Kowaluk EA, Mikusa J, Wismer C, Jarvis MF. An adenosine kinase inhibitor attenuates carrageenan-induced hyperalgesia and inflammation in the rat. Drug Dev Res 1998; 43:39.
73. Lynch JJ, Jarvis MF, Kowaluk EA. An adenosine kinase inhibitor attenuates tactile allodynia in a rat model of diabetic neuropathic pain. Eur J Pharmacol 1999; 364:141–146.
74. Wiesner JB, Ugarkar BG, Castellino AJ, Barankiewicz J, Dumas DP, Gruber HE, Foster AC, Erion MD. Adenosine kinase inhibitors as a novel approach to anticonvulsant therapy. J Pharmacol Exp Ther 1999; 289:1669–1677.
75. Wang B, Rang J, White PF, Foster AC, Grettenberger HM, Kopcho J, Wender RH. The effect of GP683, an adenosine kinase inhibitor, on the desflurane anesthetic requirement in dogs. Anesth Analg 1997; 85:675–680.
76. Erion MD, Wiesner JB, Dare J, Kopcho J, Ugarkar. GP3269: an adenosine regulating agent with anticonvulsant activity. Nucleosides Nucleotides Ther Biol Appl 1996; 1(Suppl28).

54

P2X Purinergic Receptors for ATP in Nociception

Philip A. Bland-Ward
GlaxoSmithKline, Stevenage, Hertfordshire, and Glaxo Institute of Applied Pharmacology, University of Cambridge, Cambridge, England

Iain P. Chessell and Patrick P. A. Humphrey
Glaxo Institute of Applied Pharmacology, University of Cambridge, Cambridge, England

I. INTRODUCTION

It has been established for some years that nucleotides and nucleosides can have algogenic effects when applied to blister-base preparations in humans (1) and that ATP can be released by antidromic stimulation of sensory nerves (2). Only recently, however, has evidence been obtained that purines can activate sensory nerve endings directly and can modulate the transmission of nociceptive information. In this chapter we review the evidence suggesting that P_2 receptors for ATP play a role in the initiation and processing of pain and discuss the possibility that antagonists at certain P_2 receptor types may represent an important new class of analgesic agents.

Purinoceptors for ATP fall into two broad groups: ionotropic receptors, which are termed P2X, and metabotropic receptors, termed P2Y (3). Currently, there is little evidence that P2Y receptors play a role in pain, although their possible importance should not be dismissed. There is also a wealth of evidence that the ultimate breakdown product of ATP, adenosine, plays a role in nociceptive processing (4), and it may be that P2X and adenosine (P_1) receptors act together as physiological regulators of nociceptive traffic. Seven P2X receptor subunits have been cloned (P2X1–P2X7), with each subunit, when expressed homomerically, able to form functional channels. Importantly, two of these subunits (P2X2 and P2X3) are able to form a functional heteropolymeric combination (5) with P2X3, and thus also the heteromeric combination, expressed selectively at high levels in sensory C-fiber neurons. The expression of these receptors in sensory neurons corresponds to numerous reports of ATP-evoked depolarization and calcium influx in isolated dorsal root ganglia cells (6–8). The localization of P2X receptors on nociceptive dorsal root ganglia cells is supplemented by data showing that these receptors can have effects upstream from the spinal inputs. Thus, ATP excites a subpopulation of dorsal horn neurons in the cord (9), and also can modulate synaptic transmission in the substantia gelatinosa of the spinal cord (10). The functional relevance of these receptors is supported by findings that some P_2 antagonists have antinociceptive effects when intrathecally administered in rats (11).

A critical question is whether ATP itself initiates pain at the level of the sensory nerve ending. Clearly, the presence of the receptors themselves on nerve endings, and a mechanism for the release of ATP with which to activate them is essential for this hypothesis to be valid. For the former, there is evidence that supports the presence of P2X receptors at the level of the nerve ending, which includes observation of P2X3 immunoreactivity on nociceptive sensory nerve endings (12) and functional studies, described in the following. The sources of ATP to activate these sensory nerve terminals are diverse. First, ATP can be coreleased with norepinephrine (noradrenaline) following sympathetic stimulation (13), which may underlie the maintenance of "sympathetic pain," as well as by antidromic stimulation of sensory nerves (2). Sympathetic activity is often associated with painful stimulation, and it has been proposed that this contributes to the pain of arthritis (14)—an interesting observation given that P2X receptors appear to be localized to nociceptive nerve endings in the joint capsule (see subsequent discussion). Another obvious source of ATP is from damaged cells, which could underlie the pain associated with tissue trauma. Release of ATP from platelet dense-granules may also occur in trauma (15). Vascular endothelial cells also appear to release ATP readily, without any concomitant cellular lysis (16). It is clear, therefore, that numerous sources of extracellular ATP can become involved when traumatic events occur. Here we focus in more detail on the evidence supporting a role for P2X receptors on primary afferent neurons and the possibility that P2X receptors are critically present on the peripheral terminals of sensory nerves.

II. EVIDENCE THAT P2X RECEPTORS ARE FUNCTIONALLY EXPRESSED ON SENSORY AFFERENTS

With use of the neonatal rat isolated tail–spinal cord preparation in vitro, Trezise and Humphrey (17) compared the ability of ATP and α, βmeATP to elicit discharge of cutaneous sensory neurons innervating the tail, measured indirectly by the magnitude of evoked ventral root depolarizations. Application of either ATP or α, βmeATP to the denuded tail surface resulted in rapidly developing (< 5 s) and concentration-related responses (ATP EC_{50} = 4.0 mM vs. α, βmeATP EC_{50} = 0.4 mM), whereas UTP (an agonist at non-P2X receptors) and L-β, γ-meATP (a P2X1 receptor agonist) were inactive. These data suggest that neonatal rat tail cutaneous sensory neurons are stimulated by the action of α, βmeATP on homomeric P2X3 receptors or on a heteromeric P2X receptor containing P2X3 subunits (e.g., P2X2/3). Furthermore, α, βmeATP appeared to be specific in its action on P_2 receptors in these experiments, as evinced by the demonstration that α, βmeATP-evoked responses were abolished by preincubation with the P_2 antagonist pyridoxal-5-phosphate (P-5-P) (Fig. 1).

Further evidence for the existence of P2X receptors on sensory nerve terminals has been provided by a recent study by Dowd et al. (18), during which the effects of nucleotide analogues on afferents innervating the knee joint of the rat were examined. Afferents were characterized by their conduction velocity and capsaicin sensitivity, and approximately half of all polymodal C fibers studied increased their firing rate when α, βmeATP or ATP was applied by either intra-articular or close-arterial injection. The increase in firing rate was transient with ATP, indicating rapid breakdown by *ecto*-nucleotidase (Fig. 2). Importantly, the increases in afferent discharge evoked by both ATP and α, βmeATP were significantly inhibited by the antagonist PPADS; a dose of 16 μg/kg PPADS increased the mean ED_{50} value for α, βmeATP from 31 ± 12 to 258 ± 84 nmol, confirming the involvement of P_2 receptors. Given that responses of these native sensory neurons resemble those observed at the P2X2/3 heteromer (5), and the responses observed in this study did not desenitize within milliseconds, it is likely that nociceptor activation in the rat knee joint by P2X agonists occurs by activation of the P2X2/3 heteromeric receptor.

Finally, the results of a recent behavioral study indicate that activation of P2X receptors on hindpaw sensory neurons is perceived as a noxious stimulus by conscious animals. Thus, subplantar administration of either ATP or α, βmeATP elicited a pattern of behavior in conscious

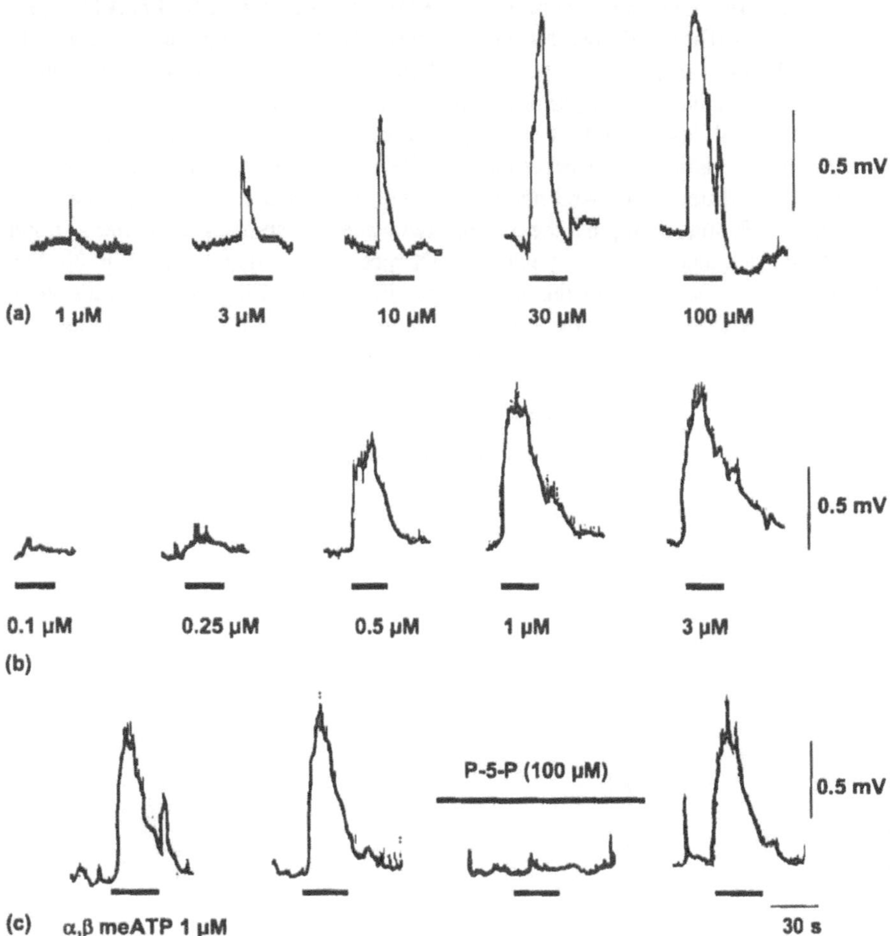

Figure 1 Representative traces showing ventral root depolarization responses evoked in the neonatal rat tail–spinal cord preparation by 30-s application of (a) ATP and (b) α, βmeATP. The lower trace (c) shows inhibition of responses evoked by 30-s application of α, βmeATP with the P_2 receptor antagonist, pyridoxal-5-phosphate (P-5-P; 100 μM). (From Ref. 17.)

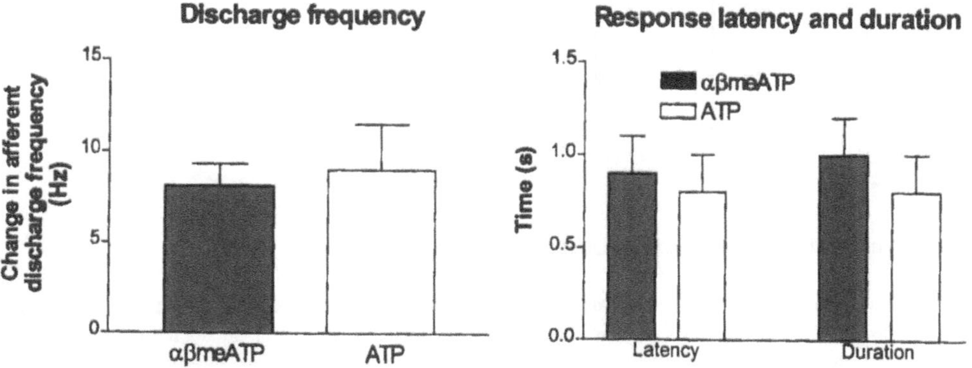

Figure 2 Increases in nociceptor discharge (left panel), latency to onset of excitation and duration of response (right panel) following i.a. injection of α, βmeATP (60 nmol; n = 14) or ATP (2000 nmol; n = 7). (From Ref. 18.)

rats that is strongly indicative of acute nociception (19). Following subplantar α, βmeATP injection (100–1000 nmol), rats displayed dose-related hindpaw-lifting and licking activity, which, following a dose of 200 nmol α, βmeATP, was immediate in onset, monophasic, and of short (< 20 min) duration. Such behavior was partially inhibited by systemic morphine pretreatment and was abolished after local desensitization of hindpaw nociceptors with subplantar capsaicin, confirming the nociceptive nature of the behavioral profile evoked by subplantar α, βmeATP injection. Interestingly, α, βmeATP-evoked nociception was also abolished by subplantar pretreatment with α, βmeATP, suggesting that the progressive wane of responses seen after a single injection may be the consequence of sensory neuron P2X receptor desensitization (Fig. 3). The rapid onset of behavioral nociception (in the absence of hindpaw swelling) supports the view that α, βmeATP exerts its algesic effect by virtue of a direct action on P2X receptors present on hindpaw sensory neurons. These receptors presumably comprise P2X1 or P2X3 subunits, the only P2X subunits activated by α, βmeATP. Because neither adenosine nor adenosine diphosphate (ADP) exhibited algesic activity after subplantar injection, sensory nerve activation does not appear to occur because of nonspecific actions of α, βmeATP at purinoceptors other than the P2X type.

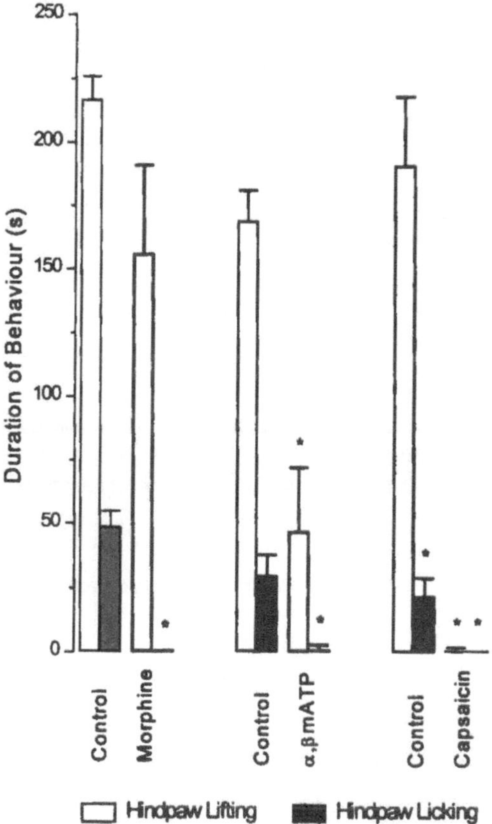

Figure 3 Results of three separate experiments showing the effect of pretreatment with morphine (3 mg/kg, i.v.), α, βmeATP (600 nmol, subplantar) or capsaicin (100 μg, subplantar) on nociceptive behaviors evoked by subsequent subplantar injection of α, βmeATP (600 nmol). Columns indicate mean ± S.E. mean hindpaw-lifting (open columns) or licking (filled columns) behavior during the 5 min after subplantar injection, (n = 5–8 animals per group). *$P < 0.01$ compared with appropriate control group. (From Ref. 19.)

III. SUMMARY

The combined electrophysiological and behavioral evidence considered in this chapter provides compelling support for the existence of functional P2X receptors on peripheral sensory nerve endings, including capsaicin-sensitive nociceptors. Moreover, it is evident that activation of such P2X receptors evokes a discharge of peripheral nociceptors that is subsequently interpreted as a noxious stimulus by supraspinal centers. In this context, the P2X receptor must be considered an important candidate as a target for pharmacological intervention in the treatment of nociceptive pain.

REFERENCES

1. Bleehan T, Keele CA. Observations on the algogenic actions of adenosine compounds on the human blister base preparation. Pain 1977; 3:367–377.
2. Holton P. The liberation of adenosine triphosphate on antidromic stimulation of sensory nerves. J Physiol 1959; 145:494–504.
3. Fredholm BB, Abbracchio MP, Burnstock G, Daly JW, Harden K, Jacobson KA, Leff P, Williams M. VI. Nomenclature and classification of purinoceptors. Pharmacol Rev 1994; 46:143–156.
4. Sawynok J, Sweeney MI. The role of purines in nociception. Neuroscience 1989; 32:557–569.
5. Lewis C, Neidhart S, Holy C, North RA, Buell G, Surprenant A. Coexpression of $P2X_2$ and $P2X_3$ receptor subunits can account for ATP-gated currents in sensory neurons. Nature 1995; 377:432–435.
6. Bean BP. ATP-activated channels in rat and bullfrog sensory neurons. concentration dependence and kinetics. J Neurosci 1990; 10:1–10.
7. Bouvier MM, Evans ML, Benham CD. Calcium influx induced by stimulation of ATP receptors on neurons cultured from rat dorsal root ganglia. Eur J Neurosci 1990; 3:285–291.
8. Robertson SJ, Rae MG, Rowan EG, Kennedy C. Characterization of a P2X-purinoceptor in cultured neurones of the rat dorsal root ganglia. Br J Pharmacol 1996; 118:951–956.
9. Jahr CE, Jessell TM. ATP excites a subpopulation of dorsal horn neurones. Nature 1983; 304:730–733.
10. Li J, Perl ER. ATP modulation of synaptic transmission in the spinal substantia gelatinosa. J Neurosci 1995; 15:3357–3365.
11. Driessen B, Reimann W, Selve N, Friderichs E, Bultmann R. Antinociceptive effect of intrathecally administered P_2-purinoceptor antagonists in rats. Brain Res 1994; 666:182–188.
12. Cook SP, Vulchanova L, Hargreaves KM, Elde R, McCleskey EW. Distinct ATP receptors on pain-sensing and stretch-sensing neurons. Nature 1997; 387:505–508.
13. Burnstock G. Noradrenaline and ATP as contransmitters in sympathetic nerves. Neurochem Int 1990; 17:357–368.
14. Levine JD, Goetzl EJ, Basbaum AL. Contribution of the nervous system to the pathophysiology of rheumatoid arthritis and other polyarthritides. Pathol Chronic Inflamm Arthritis 1987; 13:3698–383.
15. Gordon JL. Extracellular ATP: effects, sources and fate. Biochem J 1986; 233:309–319.
16. Pearson JD, Gordon JL. Vascular endothelial and smooth muscle cells in culture selectively release adenine nucleotides. Nature 1979; 281:384–386.
17. Trezise DJ, Humphrey PPA. Activation of cutaneous afferent neurons by adenosine triphosphate in the neonatal rat tail–spinal cord preparation in vitro. In: Olesen J, Edvinsson L, eds. Headache Pathogenesis: Monoamines, Neuropeptides, Purines and Nitric Oxide. New York: Lippincott–Raven, 1997:111–116.
18. Dowd E, McQueen DS, Chessell IP, Humphrey PPA. Activation by P2X purinoceptor agonists of sensory nerves innervating the rat knee joint (abstr). Br J Pharmacol 1997; 122:286P.
19. Bland–Ward PA, Humphrey PPA. Acute nociception mediated by hindpaw P2X receptor activation in the rat. Br J Pharmacol 1997; 122:365–371.

55

Somatostatin Receptors in Analgesia

Gareth A. Hicks
GlaxoSmithKline, Harlow, Essex, England

Marcus Schindler
Boehringer Ingelheim Pharma KG, Biberach, Germany

Wasyl Feniuk and Patrick P. A. Humphrey
Glaxo Institute of Applied Pharmacology, Cambridge, England

I. INTRODUCTION

The hypothalamic peptide somatostatin (SRIF), originally discovered because of its ability to inhibit the release of growth hormone from the pituitary (1), is widely distributed in peripheral organs as well as the brain and spinal cord. The immunohistochemical localization of SRIF in sensory afferent axons terminating in the substantial gelatinosa of the dorsal horn of the spinal cord (2,3), spinal interneurons (4), as well as important pain-regulating centers in the brain, such as periaqueductal gray (5), cingulate cortex (6), and spinal trigeminal nucleus (7), have implicated this neuropeptide as an endogenous regulator of pain transmission. Because SRIF may also be released from the peripheral terminals of capsaicin-sensitive primary afferent neurons (8), sensory neuromodulation may occur at peripheral as well as central loci. The analgesic effect of exogenously administered SRIF was first demonstrated in rats following i.c.v. administration (9), and subsequent studies in humans have demonstrated effective pain relief following intravenous infusions in patients with cluster headache (10), as well as following intrathecal or epidural injections of SRIF to patients with postoperative (11) and cancer pain (12). However, as a consequence of its short half-life, the clinical usefulness of SRIF is limited and metabolically more stable analogues have been developed. The cyclic octapeptide analogues of SRIF, octreotide and vapreotide (RC-160), have been used in clinical as well as animal studies and analgesic activity has been demonstrated following either central or peripheral administration (13–15). For vapreotide, the antinociceptive activity in rats involved an indirect central opioidergic mechanism (15). The widespread distribution of SRIF in the gastrointestinal tract and its presence in the peripheral terminals of sensory afferent neurons has also prompted investigations into the effect of octreotide in patients with irritable bowel syndrome (IBS) who have lowered visceral sensory thresholds. In IBS patients, octreotide caused a significant increase in the threshold for visceral pain perception during colonic distension, to values similar to those obtained in healthy subjects, without modifying colonic compliance (16,17). This suggests that octreotide increases visceral sensory thresholds by inhibiting peripheral nociceptors located in the gut wall,

Table 1 Ligand-Binding Profile of SRIF Analogues on CHO-K1 Cell Membranes Expressing Human Recombinant SRIF Receptors[a]

	sst_1	sst_2	sst_3	sst_4	sst_5
SRIF	9.17	9.97	9.10	8.90	9.88
SRIF-28	9.13	8.87	9.20	8.62	9.28
Octreotide	6.20	9.37	8.10	5.61	7.68
Vapreotide	6.37	9.77	7.59	6.65	7.97
BIM-23027	<5	9.77	7.70	5.47	7.45
L-362855	6.35	9.00	8.20	7.27	9.55
BIM-23056	6.67	6.98	7.30	7.10	7.83

[a] Values are pIC_{50} determined from inhibition of specific $[^{125}I]$BIM-23027 (sst_2) or $[^{125}I]Tyr^{11}$-SRIF binding.

the afferent pathways to the central nervous system (CNS), or possibly within the CNS itself. However, in these studies a peripheral site of action seems more likely.

Somatostatin produces its biological effects by activating specific receptors belonging to the seven-transmembrane superfamily of G protein-coupled receptors (18). The genes coding for five distinct somatostatin receptor types (sst_1–sst_5) have now been cloned and these show a widespread and overlapping distribution both in the brain and periphery (18). Several mechanisms in the periphery, brain, and spinothalamic tract may be involved in producing the analgesic effect of SRIF or its analogues (19), but the nature of the receptors that mediate these effects are still largely unknown.

II. RECEPTOR SELECTIVITY OF SRIF ANALOGUES

We have determined the receptor affinity of SRIF and other peptide analogues on membranes from CHO-K1 cells expressing human recombinant sst_1–sst_5 receptors to define their receptor selectivity (Table 1). As many of the analgesic effects of SRIF have been mimicked in subsequent clinical and animal studies with octreotide, it is clearly tempting to speculate that the analgesic effects of SRIF are mediated, at least partly, by activation of sst_2 receptors because octreotide has high affinity and is clearly selective for this SRIF receptor type. However, the possibility that other SRIF receptors may also be involved in mediating the analgesic effect of SRIF cannot be excluded.

In view of the selectivity of octreotide for the sst_2 receptor type, and the possible involvement of this receptor in mediating the analgesic actions of SRIF, further studies have been carried out to determine the immunohistochemical localization of sst_2 receptors at sites involved in pain regulation using a selective anti-sst_2 receptor antibody (20).

III. IMMUNOHISTOCHEMISTRY

Although some workers have explored the distribution of the mRNA for each SRIF receptor type in the brain and spinal cord (18), such studies may not reflect the distribution of the receptor protein. Autoradiographic studies do map the protein distribution (21), but have been hampered by a lack of high-affinity selective ligands for all the SRIF receptor types. Using specific anti-sst_2 receptor antisera, sst_2 receptors have been localized in several regions of the rat brain involved in the processing of noxious information (20). Such areas include the superficial laminae of the dorsal horn of the spinal cord (substantial gelatinosa), the periaqueductal gray, and the anterior cingulate cortex (Fig. 1). In the dorsal horn, strong immunoreactivity could still be detected

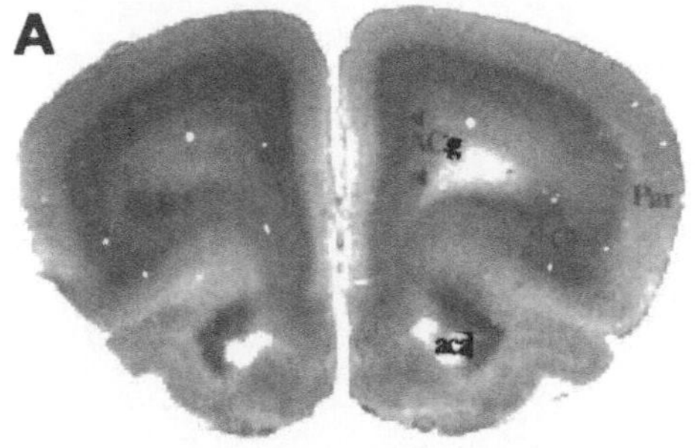

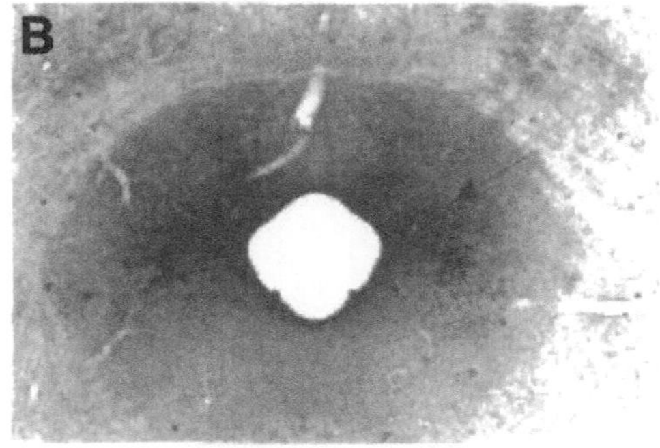

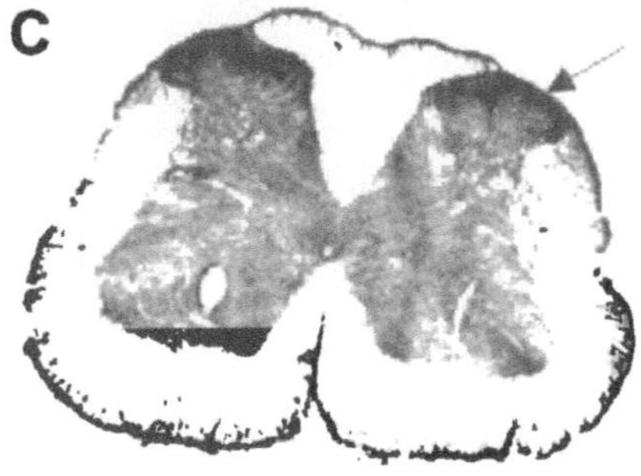

Figure 1 Immunohistochemical localization of $sst_{(2A)}$ receptors in sites involved in pain processing: (A) Labeling was observed in the deep layers of the anterior cingulate cortex (ACg) in which receptors were found on pyramidally shaped neuronal cell bodies and ascending dendrites. (B,C) Dense labeling (indicated by arrows) was also found in the dorsolateral part of the (B) periaqueductal gray and (C) the substantia gelatinosa of the spinal cord.

following dorsal root rhizotomy (at level L4 and L5) suggesting that the receptors are not localized on primary afferent neurons and are localized postsynaptically (20). This conclusion is consistent with the observed hyperpolarizing action of SRIF and reduction in spontaneous firing of dorsal horn neurons in rat isolated spinal cord slice preparations (22). The immunoreactive neurons labeled by the anti-sst_2 receptor antibody in the dorsolateral periaqueductal gray were mostly projection neurons with axons ascending to the thalamus (20). We have found (26) that these neurons hyperpolarize in response to both SRIF and the selective sst_2 receptor ligand BIM-23027 (see Table 1), suggesting that the receptors identified immunohistochemically by the anti-

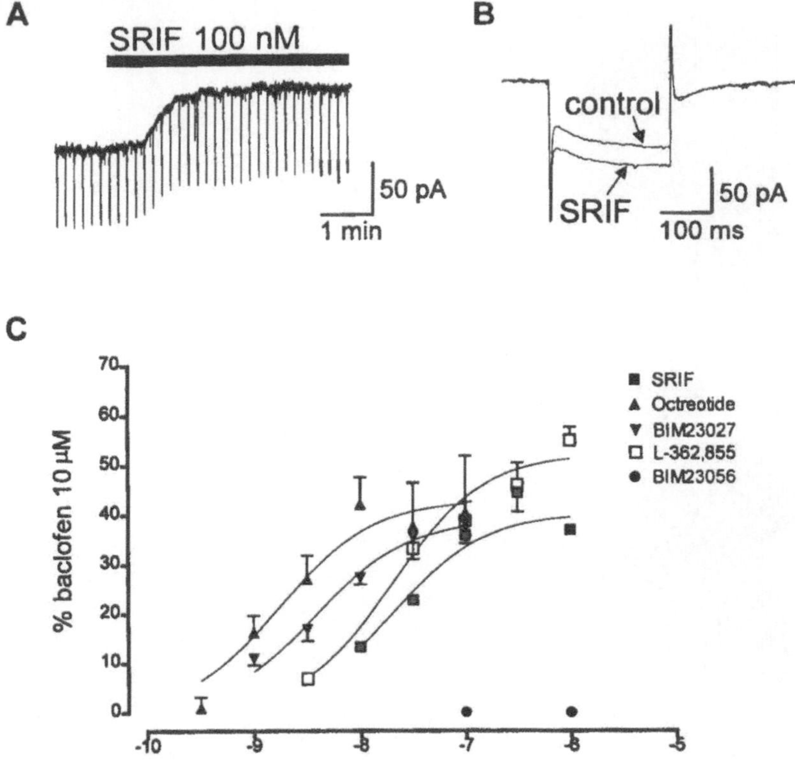

Figure 2 Outward current produced by sst_2 receptor activation in the deep layer pyramidal neurons of the anterior cingulate cortex: (A) Outward current in response to SRIF (100 nM; solid bar) is accompanied by (B) an increase in whole-cell conductance. Downward deflections show the membrane current response to 500-ms-long 10-mV–hyperpolarizing steps. The traces in (B) show the average of ten such steps before drug application ("control"), and during the peak of the response ("SRIF"). (C) Concentration–effect curves for SRIF and related analogues (see legend) for activation of outward currents in rat anterior cingulate cortex neurons. Peak current amplitudes are expressed as the percentage of the response to baclofen (10 μM) in the same neuron. Each data point is the mean ± SE mean from three to five experiments. (From Ref. 26.)

sst_2 receptor antisera are functionally active. In the anterior cingulate cortex, deep layer pyramidal neuron cell bodies, and ascending dendrites were labeled by the anti-sst_2 receptor antibody. Activation of the anterior cingulate cortex has, for many years, been thought to mediate the affective response to pain (23), and recent functional-imaging studies support the view that this area of the brain is a major pain-processing area (24,25). However, little is known about the functional effects of SRIF in this important brain region. We have recently carried out a detailed investigation into the effects of SRIF and some receptor-selective ligands (see Table 1) on rat anterior cingulate pyramidal cells in vitro.

IV. SRIF AND RAT ANTERIOR CINGULATE PYRAMIDAL CELLS IN VITRO

The effects of SRIF have been studied using whole-cell patch-clamp recordings from deep-layer, pyramidal cells of the rat anterior cingulate cortex, visualized in isolated brain slices

(25). SRIF produced a concentration-dependent, Ba^{2+}-sensitive, outward current, which was associated with an increase in membrane conductance (Fig. 2A,B). In the presence of the γ-aminobutyric acid B ($GABA_B$) agonist, baclofen, SRIF produced no further current. These observations suggested that the outward current activated by SRIF was carried by K^+ions. The effect of SRIF was mimicked by several sst_2 receptor analogues, including octreotide and BIM-23027 (see Table 1 and Fig. 2C), suggesting that the response was a consequence of activation of sst_2 receptors. This was confirmed by the antagonistic activity of the sst_2 receptor-blocking drug, Cyn-154806 (27). It is tempting to speculate that inhibition of anterior cingulate neuronal activity that would be produced by the sst_2–receptor-mediated outward current would produce analgesia in vivo.

V. CONCLUDING REMARKS

The identification of sst_2 receptors at both central and peripheral sites involved in the transmission of nociceptive information, together with the reported analgesic actions of SRIF and octreotide, suggests that a selective, nonpeptidic and centrally acting sst_2 agonist would be analgesic. It is also possible that a peripherally acting agonist might also ameliorate the pain associated with such conditions as irritable bowel syndrome and cluster headache (see foregoing). Although in the past, advances in SRIF receptor research have been hampered by the lack of good drug tools, the recent identification of the first potent sst_2–receptor-blocking drug (27) and the identification of the first potent nonpeptidic somatostatin receptor agonist (28) suggests that novel and selective drugs acting at somatostatin receptors may soon be identified and offer novel therapeutic advances in the future.

REFERENCES

1. Brazeau P, Vale W, Burgus R, Ling N, Butcher M, Rivier J, Guillemin R. Hypothalamic polypeptide that inhibits the secretion of immunoreactive pituitary growth hoormone. Science 1973; 179:77–79.
2. Hokfelt T, Elde R, Johansson O, Luft R, Nilsson G, Arimura A. Immunohistochemical evidence for separate populations of somatostatin-containing and substance P-containing primary afferent neurons in the rat. Neuroscience 1976; 1:131–136.
3. Dalsgaard CJ, Hokfelt T, Johansson O, Elde R. Somatostatin immunoreactive cell bodies in the dorsal horn and the parasympathetic intermediolateral nucleus of the rat spinal cord. Neurosci Lett 1981; 27:335–339.
4. Elde R, Johansson O, Hokfelt T. Immunocytochemical studies of somatostatin neurons in brain. Adv Exp Med Biol 1985; 188:167–181.
5. Finley JC, Maderdrut JL, Roger LJ, Petrusz P. The immunocytochemical localization of somatostatin-containing neurons in the rat central nervous system. Neuroscience 1981; 6:2173–2192.
6. Finley JC, Grossman GH, Dimeo P, Petrusz P. Somatostatin-containing neurons in the rat brain: widespread distribution revealed by immunocytochemistry after pretreatment with pronase. Am J Anat 1978; 153:483–488.
7. Lazarov N, Chouchkov C. Localization of somatostatin-like immunoreactive fibres in the trigeminal principal sensory nucleus of the cat. Acta Histochem 1990; 89:91–97.
8. Szolcsanyi J, Helyes Z, Oroszi G, Nemeth J, Pinter E. Release of somatostatin and its role in the mediation of the anti-inflammatory effect induced by antidromic stimulation of sensory fibres of rat sciatic nerve. Br J Pharmacol 1998; 123:936–942.
9. Rezek M, Havlicek V, Leybin L, La Bella FS, Friesen H. Opiate-like naloxone-reversible actions of somatostatin given intracerebrally. Can J Physiol Pharmacol 1978; 56:227–231.
10. Sicuteri F, Geppetti P, Marabini S, Lembeck F. Pain relief by somatostatin in attacks of cluster headache. Pain 1984; 18:359–365.

11. Taura P, Planella V, Balust J, Beltran J, Anglada T, Carrero E, Burgues S. Epidural somatostatin as an analgesic in upper abdominal surgery: a double-blind study. Pain 1994; 59:135–140.
12. Mollenholt P, Rawal N, Gordh T Jr, Olsson Y. Intrathecal and epidural somatostatin for patients with cancer. Analgesic effects and postmortem neuropathologic investigations of spinal cord and nerve roots. Anesthesiology 1994; 81:534–542.
13. Penn RD, Paice JA, Kroin JS. Octreotide: a potent new non-opiate analgesic for intrathecal infusion. Pain 1992; 49:13–19.
14. Williams G, Ball JA, Lawson RA, Joplin GF, Bloom SR, Maskill MR. Analgesic effect of somatostatin analogue (octreotide) in headache associated with pituitary tumours. Br Med J 1987; 295:247–248.
15. Betoin F, Ardid D, Herbet A, Aumaitre O, Kemeny JL, Duchene-Marullaz P, Lavarenne J, Eschalier A. Evidence for a central long-lasting antinociceptive effect of vapreotide, an analog of somatostatin, involving an opioidergic mechanism. J Pharmacol Exp Ther 1994; 269:7–14.
16. Bradette M, Delvaux M, Staumont G, Fioramonti J, Bueno L, Frexinos J. Octreotide increases thresholds of colonic visceral perception in IBS patients without modifying muscle tone. Dig Dis Sci 1994; 39:1171–1178.
17. Mertz H, Walsh JH, Sytnik B, Mayer EA. The effect of octreotide on human gastric compliance and sensory perception. Neurogasroenterol Mot 1995; 7:175–185.
18. Schindler M, Humphrey PPA, Emson PC. Somatostatin receptors in the central nervous system. Prog Neurobiol 1996; 50:9–47.
19. Humphrey PPA. Somatostatin receptor activation and analgesia. In: Sandler M, Ferrari M, Harnett S. eds. Migraine: Pharmacology and Genetics. Chapman & Hall, 1996:221–232.
20. Schindler M, Holloway S, Hathway G, Woolf CJ, Humphrey PPA, Emson PC. Identification of somatostatin sst2(a) receptor expressing neurones in central regions involved in nociception. Brain Res 1998; 798:25–35.
21. Holloway S, Feniuk W, Kidd EJ, Humphrey PPA. A quantitative autoradiographical study on the distribution of somatostatin sst_2 receptors in the rat central nervous system using $[^{125}I]$BIM-23027. Neuropharmacology 1996; 35:1109–1120.
22. Murase K, Nedeljkov V, Randic M. The actions of neuropeptides on dorsal horn neurons in the rat spinal cord slice preparation: an intracellular study. Brain Res 1982; 234:170–176.
23. Vogt BA, Sikes RW, Vogt LJ. Anterior cingulate cortex and the medial pain system. In: Vogt BA, Gabriel M, eds. Neurobiology of Cingulate Cortex and Limbic Thalamus: A Comprehensive Handbook. Boston, Birkhauser. 1993:313–344.
24. Vogt BA, Derbyshire S, Jones AK. Pain processing in four regions of human cingulate cortex localized with co-registered PET and MR imaging. Eur J Neurosci 1996; 8:1461–1473.
25. Rainville P, Duncan GH, Price D, Carrier B, Bushnell C. Pain affect encoded in human anterior cingulate but not somatosensory cortex. Science 1997; 277:968–971.
26. Hicks GA, Feniuk W, Humphrey PPA. Outward current produced by somatostatin (SRIF) in rat anterior cingulate pyramidal cells in vitro. Br J Pharmacol 1998; 124:252–258.
27. Bass RT, Buckwalter BL, Patel BP, Pausch MH, Price LA, Strnad J, Hadcock JR. Identification and characterization of novel somatostatin antagonists. Mol Pharmacol 1996; 50:709–715.
28. Ankersen M, Crider M, Liu S, Ho B, Andersen H, Stidsen C. Discovery of a novel non-peptide somatostatin agonist with SST4 selectivity. J Am Chem Soc 1998; 120:1368–1373.

56
Cannabinoids

Roger G. Pertwee
University of Aberdeen, Aberdeen, Scotland

I. INTRODUCTION

Many of the effects of cannabinoids are mediated by specific cannabinoid receptors, two types of which have so far been identified: CB_1, cloned in 1990, and CB_2, cloned in 1993 (1,2). Both these receptor types are negatively coupled to adenylate cyclase through $G_{i/o}$ proteins and positively coupled to mitogen-activated protein kinase. In addition, CB_1 receptors are positively coupled to inwardly rectifying and A-type potassium channels and negatively coupled to N-type and P/Q-type calcium channels, again through $G_{i/o}$ proteins. Other effector systems for the CB_1 receptor have also been proposed (1,2). CB_1 receptors are present in the central nervous system (CNS) as well as in certain neuronal and nonneuronal peripheral tissues. Their distribution in brain and spinal cord is heterogeneous and unlike that for any other receptor type, with central areas expressing CB_1 receptors, including some that are implicated in the processing of nociceptive stimuli (1,3). At the neuronal level, some central and peripheral CB_1 receptors are located at nerve terminals where they probably modulate neurotransmitter release when activated (1–3). In contrast, CB_2 receptors are found mainly in cells of the immune system. Another important recent discovery has been that mammalian tissues produce cannabinoid receptor agonists, the most important of which are arachidonoyl ethanolamide (anandamide) and 2-arachidonoyl glycerol (1,2). Endogenous cannabinoids and their receptors constitute the endogenous cannabinoid system.

This chapter reviews the evidence that cannabinoid receptor agonists are analgesic. Both animal and human data are considered. Much of this research has been conducted with (−)-Δ^9-tetrahydrocannabinol (Δ^9-THC), the main psychotropic constituent of cannabis, and with structural analogues of this cannabinoid, for example bicyclic or tricyclic compounds such as CP-55,940 and L-nantradol that lack the pyran ring of Δ^9-THC (1). Other cannabinoid receptor agonists used for this research include the aminoalkylindole, (+)-WIN 55212, and anandamide (1). Δ^9-THC and CP-55,940 exhibit little difference in their affinities for CB_1 and CB_2 receptors, whereas anandamide exhibits modest selectivity for CB_1 receptors, and (+)-WIN 55212 modest selectivity for CB_2 receptors (2). Unlike CP-55,940 and (+)-WIN 55212, both Δ^9-THC and anandamide seem to have significantly less efficacy at CB_2 than at CB_1 receptors (2). WIN55212, Δ^9-THC and its analogues contain chiral centers and exhibit marked stereoselectivity in both binding assays and functional tests (1,2). For WIN 55212, it is the (+)-enantiomer that is the more active, whereas it is the (−)-enantiomers of Δ^9-THC and its analogues that have the greater activity. The anandamide molecule does not contain any chiral centers. Two other important cannabinoid receptor ligands to be mentioned in this chapter are SR 141716A, a potent and selective CB_1 receptor antagonist (1) and SR 144528, a potent and selective CB_2 receptor antagonist (4). Although there is some evidence that cannabinoids have anti-inflammatory properties (1,2,5), this aspect of cannabinoid pharmacology has not been dealt with here. Also excluded is any discussion of the analgesic or anti-inflammatory effects of Δ^9-tetrahydrocannabinol-11-oic acid and its more potent dimethylheptyl analogue, CT_3 (6–8), as these compounds have been the subject of a recent review (9).

II. ANIMAL EXPERIMENTS

A. Cannabinoid-Induced Antinociception

As shown in Table 1 for Δ^9-THC, cannabinoid receptor agonists have long been known to exhibit antinociceptive activity in a range of animal tests. This activity is shared by many other cannabinoid receptor agonists including CP-55940 and analogues of Δ^9-THC and CP-55940 (65–71; also see Sec. II.B), (+)-WIN 55212 and related compounds (65,69,71–75 see Sec. II.B), the endogenous cannabinoids, anandamide and 2-arachidonoyl glycerol (60,76–82), and analogues of anandamide (69,77,79,81,83–85). At antinociceptive doses, cannabinoids usually also depress motor activity and deep body temperature. However, it is unlikely that there is any cause-and-effect relation between these additional effects and cannabinoid-induced antinociception. Thus, there are reports that when administered intrathecally, some pharmacological agents (yohimbine, norbinaltorphimine, and antisera to dynorphin A) can attenuate cannabinoid-induced antinociception in the rat or mouse tail-flick test without affecting cannabinoid-induced hypomotility, catalepsy, or hypothermia (40,76,86,87). Additionally, there is one report that intraperitoneal administration of the *N*-methyl-D-aspartate (NMDA) antagonist dizocilpine (MK-801)-attenuates Δ^9-THC-induced antinociception in the mouse tail-flick test without affecting Δ^9-THC-induced hypothermia (34), and another that direct administration of CP-55940 into the rat caudate nucleus produces catalepsy, but no antinociception in the tail-flick test (88). There are also reports that cannabinoid-induced antinociception in the mouse tail-flick test is still detectable when hypothermia is prevented by elevating ambient temperature to about 38°C (23), and that it has proved possible in some experiments to render mice tolerant to Δ^9-THC-induced antinociception (by pretreatment with an opioid or with antisense oligodeoxynucleotide to the κ_1-receptor) without also making them tolerant to Δ^9-THC-induced hypomotility, catalepsy, or hypothermia (16,86,89). It is unlikely that cannabinoid-induced depression of the mouse tail-flick response arises from changes in tail skin temperature (23).

B. Antinociception and Cannabinoid CB_1 Receptors

There is good evidence that cannabinoids can induce antinociception through the activation of CB_1 receptors and this may be summarized as follows:

1. The antinociceptive potencies of several different cannabinoid receptor agonists are no less than the potencies of other types of analgesic agent already known to act through receptors. For example, Martin (25) reported intravenous ED_{50} values in the mouse abdominal stretch test, tail-flick test, and hot-plate test to be 0.2, 1.0, and 5.1 mg/kg, respectively, for Δ^9-THC and 0.3, 3.5, and 1.2 mg/kg, respectively, for morphine sulfate. Equipotency between Δ^9-THC and morphine for antinociception has also been observed in rats or mice after oral or intraperitoneal administration (17,47). Some cannabinoid receptor agonists are even more potent than Δ^9-THC as antinociceptive agents [e.g., CP-55940 ($ED_{50} = 0.09$ mg/kg i.v. in the mouse tail-flick test; 18) and (−)-11-OH Δ^8-THC-dimethylheptyl ($ED_{50} = 0.009$ mg/kg i.v. in the mouse tail-

Table 1 Animals Tests in Which Δ^9-THC Shows Antinociceptive Activity When Administered Orally or by Systemic Injection

Noxious stimulus	Response	Species	Effective routes[a]	Refs.
Clamp or clip on tail	Biting at clip, etc.	Mouse	p.o.	10
		Rat	s.c.	11, 12
Clamp on tail	Minimum alveolar concentration (MAC) of cyclopropane required to prevent motor response	Rat	i.p.	13
Clamp on tail	Minimum alveolar concentration (MAC) of halothane required to prevent motor response	Dog	i.v.	14
Thermal to tail	Tail-flick	Mouse	i.v., i.p., s.c.	11, 15–36
		Rat	i.v., i.p.	17, 32, 37–43
Thermal to feet (hot plate)	Paw-lick, jumping, or escape	Mouse	i.v., i.p., s.c., p.o.	6, 10, 17, 20, 21, 25, 29, 30, 32, 33, 44–49
		Rat	i.p., s.c., i.v.	17, 37, 38, 43, 45, 50
Thermal to an area of back	Skin-twitch reflex	Dog (chronic spinal)	i.v.	51
Noxious agent into peritoneum	Abdominal-stretching	Mouse	i.v., s.c., p.o.	10, 20–22, 25, 45, 47, 52–57
		Rat	s.c.	45
		Cat	s.c.	45
Formalin into hindpaw (subplantar) after Δ^9-THC treatment	Limping, paw-lifting, etc. using a rating scale	Rat	p.o.	58
Pressure to hindpaw	Vocalization or motor responses	Rat	i.p., p.o.	10, 47, 59, 60
Pressure to toe	Flexor reflex	Dog (chronic spinal)	i.v.	51
Electrical to feet	Motor response	Rat	s.c.	11, 12
Electrical to feet or brain sites	Vocalization or motor responses	Rat	i.p.	61
Electrical to feet	Lever-pressing	Monkey	i.p.	62
Electrical to sciatic nerve	Vocalization or motor responses	Rabbit	Not specified	63
Electrical to tooth (dentine)	Vocalization or motor responses	Dog	i.v.	64

[a] Cannabinoids are also antinociceptive when administered intrathecally, intracerebrally, or intracerebroventricularly (see text).

flick test; 90). It is noteworthy that subcutaneously, Δ^9-THC is significantly less potent than morphine in both rats and mice (11,16,25,49).

2. A graded relation exists between cannabinoid dose and the degree of antinociception produced, as is well-illustrated by the data obtained from Δ^9-THC experiments with mice and rats (i.v., i.p., or s.c.) using the tail-flick and hot-plate tests (17,18,23,26,29,32,35).

3. The antinociceptive potencies of cannabinoid receptor agonists are structure-dependent and correlate well with their binding affinities for CB_1 receptors. This has been most fully demonstrated in the mouse tail-flick test using the intravenous route (91,92). Subcutaneous po-

tency values for analogues of CP-55940 in the mouse abdominal-stretch test have also been reported to correlate well with CB_1-binding affinity (93).

4. Enantiomeric pairs of chiral cannabinoid receptor agonists exhibit a marked degree of stereoselectivity as antinociceptive agents, the more active member of each pair usually being the one with the higher affinity for the CB_1 receptor. Examples include the notably greater systemic potencies shown by (+)-than (−)-WIN 55212 in mouse or rat tail-flick or formalin paw tests (72,94), and by the (−)-than the (+)-enantiomers of Δ^8-THC in the mouse hot-plate test (49), of nantradol, CP-55940, CP-55244, 11-OH-Δ^8-THC-dimethylheptyl and 11-OH-hexahydrocannabinol-dimethylheptyl in the mouse tail-flick test (22,24,90,95) and of nantradol in the mouse abdominal-stretch test (22). Cannabinoids also show stereoselectivity as antinociceptive agents when injected directly into the CNS. Here, however, the more potent isomer of an enantiomeric pair is not always the one with the higher affinity for CB_1 receptors (see following statement 6).

5. The CB_1 receptor antagonist, SR 141716A, prevents the antinociceptive effects of a number of different cannabinoid receptor agonists and does this selectively at an appropriately high potency. For example, Compton et al. (96) have reported ED_{50} values for SR 141716A of 0.16 mg/kg i.v. and 0.38 mg/kg i.p. against i.v. THC in the mouse tail-flick test and of 2.7 mg/kg i.p. against i.v. Δ^9-THC in the mouse abdominal-stretch test. The lower potency shown by SR 141716A in the abdominal-stretch test than the tail-flick test may point to the existence of multiple mechanisms for cannabinoid-induced antinociception (96). Similarly, there are reports (30) that i.p. SR 141716A (0.04–2 mg/kg) antagonizes antinociception induced by i.v. Δ^9-THC in the mouse tail-flick or hot-plate tests; also that i.p. SR 141716A (ED_{50} = 1.62 mg/kg) antagonizes antinociception induced by i.v. (+)-WIN 55212 in the mouse tail-flick test (97) and that in the rat tail-flick test, i.p. SR 141716A (10 and 30, but not 3, mg/kg) antagonizes i.v. THC and i.c.v. (intracerebroventricular) SR 141716A (100 or 300 μg) antagonizes i.c.v. THC (42). Additionally, SR 141716A attenuates antinociception induced by (−)-11-OH-Δ^8-THC-dimethylheptyl in the rat tail-flick test when these agents are coadministered into the rostral ventromedial medulla, a brain area that receives input from the periaqueductal gray and projects to the dorsal horn of the spinal cord (98). SR 141716A antagonizes cannabinoids in the rat or mouse tail-flick test at doses that do not to attenuate morphine-induced antinociception (42,96).

6. Cannabinoids induce antinociception when injected directly into areas of the CNS that are known to contain CB_1 receptors. Although there are a few reports that cannabinoid receptor agonists are active in the hot-plate test when administered to rats or mice intrathecally or intracerebroventricularly (38,82,99,100), most studies have been carried out using the tail-flick test. These have shown cannabinoid receptor agonists to be active in rats when injected stereotaxically into the posterior ventrolateral periaqueductal gray area (88) or rostral ventromedial medulla (98), and in mice and rats when injected intrathecally (31,41,99–101) or intracerebroventricularly (88,101,102). It seems likely that the predominant site of action of cannabinoids was within the brain when they were injected intracerebroventricularly (102) and within the spinal cord when the intrathecal route was used (31,41). There is good evidence that the antinociception observed in these experiments is mediated by CB_1 receptors. In particular, when injected into the brain, cerebral ventricles, or spinal cord, cannabinoids are readily antagonized by centrally administered SR 141716A (42,98) or by drugs expected to impair CB_1 receptor signaling (see following paragraph 7). Cannabinoids administered by these routes also exhibit stereoselectivity (88,98,100,101,103) and show potencies that are appropriately high and that usually correlate positively with their binding affinities for CB_1 receptors (88,98,100,101,103) and negatively with their lipid solubilities (103). Additionally, intracerebroventricular pretreatment with an antisense oligodeoxynucleotide directed against the CB_1 receptor has been reported to attenuate antinociception induced by i.c.v. CP55940 in a "warm water" mouse tail-flick test (104). It is

noteworthy that there are some injection sites in rat brain at which cannabinoids do not suppress the tail-flick response. These include the caudate nucleus, in which CP-55940 produces catalepsy but not antinociception (88), the posterior dorsolateral and anterior ventrolateral periaqueductal gray area (88), and areas dorsal to the rostral ventromedial medulla (98). Interestingly, although the antinociceptive potency of cannabinoids usually correlates positively with binding affinity for CB_1 receptors, this is not always so. Thus, after i.c.v. injection, CP-56667 has been reported by Welch et al. (101) to show 16-fold greater potency in the mouse tail-flick test than its (−)-enantiomer, CP-55940, even though it has less affinity for the CB_1 receptor than CP-55940. Why this should be remains to be established.

7. The antinociceptive activities of cannabinoid receptor agonists can be attenuated by some agents expected to impair CB_1 receptor signaling. Thus, Welch et al. (101) have reported that antinociception induced in the mouse tail-flick test by i.c.v. administration of Δ^9-THC, Δ^8-THC, or CP-55940 can be reduced or abolished by intrathecal pretreatment with pertussis toxin, calcium, or thapsigargin (increases intracellular calcium), although not by forskolin, 8-(4-chlorophenylthio)-cAMP, dibutyryl-cAMP, or apamin (blocks low-conductance, calcium-gated potassium channels). When all injections were made intrathecally, cannabinoid-induced antinociception was attenuated by pertussis toxin, forskolin, 8-(4-chlorophenylthio)-cAMP and apamin, but not by dibutyryl-cAMP, calcium, or thapsigargin (79,101). Pretreatment with pertussis toxin but not dibutyryl-cAMP also attenuated antinociception in the tail-flick test induced by CP-55940 when the injection site was the rat posterior ventrolateral periaqueductal gray area (88).

C. Pathways and Neurotransmitter Systems Mediating Antinociception Induced by Cannabinoid Receptor Agonists

There is evidence from two investigations that activation of cannabinoid receptors leads to a selective inhibition of processing of nociceptive stimuli both in the spinal cord and the ventroposterolateral nucleus of the thalamus. In one of these studies, Tsou et al. (94) found intraperitoneal (+)-WIN 55212 to decrease c-*fos* expression that had been evoked in the spinal ventral horn and in the superficial and neck regions of the spinal dorsal horn by injection of formalin into the plantar surface of the rat hindpaw. No such changes in c-*fos* expression were detected after (−)-WIN 55212 administration, and neither enantiomer affected c-*fos* expression in the nucleus proprius. In the other study, Martin et al. (105) found that when injected intravenously, (+)-, but not (−)-WIN 55212 suppressed neuronal activity in the ventroposterolateral nucleus of the thalamus that had been induced in urethane-anesthetized rats by application of a noxious stimulus (pressure) to the contralateral hindpaw. In contrast, (+)-WIN 55212 did not suppress the activation of nonnociceptive mechanosensitive neurons of the ventroposterolateral nucleus.

The ability of intravenously administered Δ^9-THC to elevate tail-flick latency can be attenuated by injection of yohimbine into the lumbar region of the rat spinal cord (40), suggesting that antinociception induced by cannabinoid receptor activation depends at least partly on the release from descending neurons of norepinephrine, acting on spinal α_2-adrenoceptors. The spinal component of cannabinoid-induced antinociception may also depend to some extent on the release of opioid peptides onto spinal κ-receptors. Support for this hypothesis comes from several types of experiments. First, there are reports that the ability of certain cannabinoid receptor agonists to produce antinociception in the mouse tail-flick or hot-plate test following their systemic or intrathecal administration can be attenuated by intrathecal injection of the selective κ-receptor antagonist, norbinaltorphimine (30,36,76,101); of antiserum for the endogenous selective κ-receptor agonists dynorphin A_{1-8} and dynorphin A_{1-17}; or of α-neoendorphin antiserum (30,87,106). In contrast, no such attenuation has been detected after intrathecal injections of the selective δ-receptor antagonist ICI-174864, or of the opioid antagonist naloxone, which has some selectivity for μ-opioid receptors (100,101). Second, Pugh et al. (107) have found that intrathecal injection of an antisense oligodeoxynucleotide directed against the κ_1-receptor reduces antinociception induced in the mouse tail-flick test by intrathecal Δ^9-THC. The same oligodeoxynucleotide also blocked the antinociceptive effect of a κ-receptor agonist (U-50488), but not that of selective μ-(DAMGO) or δ-(DPDPE) receptor agonists. Third, Corchero et al. (108) have detected increases in prodynorphin and proenkephalin gene expression in the spinal cords of rats that had received daily injections of Δ^9-THC (5 mg/kg i.p.) for 5 days. Repeated cannabinoid administration to rats also elevates proenkephalin gene expression in certain regions of the brain, including the periaqueductal gray area (109). Finally, there is a report that repeated subcutaneous treatment with a selective κ-opioid receptor agonist (U-50488 or C 1977) renders mice tolerant to the antinociceptive effects in the tail-flick test of intrathecal challenges not only with U-50488 or C 1977 but also with Δ^9-THC (86). Also repeated subcutaneous treatment of mice with Δ^9-THC can induce tolerance to the antinociceptive effects in the tail-flick test both of intrathecal Δ^9-THC and of intrathecal U-50488, C 1977, or dynorphin A_{1-17} (86,106). The same pretreatment with Δ^9-THC did not induce tolerance to the antinociceptive effects of intrathecally injected agonists for μ-(DAMGO) or δ-opioid receptors (DPDPE) (86).

Pretreatment with an opioid (morphine) can also render mice and rats tolerant to the antinociceptive effect of Δ^9-THC when it is administered systemically instead of intrathecally (16,35,39). Similarly, Δ^9-THC can induce tolerance to the antinociceptive effect in mice and rats of systemically administered morphine as well as to its own antinociceptive effect (35,39,45,110). Supraspinal opioid pathways may also be involved in cannabinoid-induced antinociception, as Δ^9-THC can be antagonized in the rat hot-plate test by i.c.v. injected β-chlornaltrexamine (50).

D. Synergism Between Cannabinoids and Opioids

Experiments with mice or rats using the tail-flick or hot-plate test have shown that cannabinoids can interact synergistically with opioid receptor agonists in the production of antinociception. This synergism seems to be receptor-mediated, for it can be blocked by both cannabinoid and opioid receptor antagonists (29,100,111). Although such synergism can occur when a cannabinoid and an opioid are coadministered systemically (29,45,111,112), it can also occur when the cannabinoid and opioid are both given intrathecally (36,87,100) or when both drugs or just the opioid are given i.c.v. (29,101). This would suggest that cannabinoid–opioid synergism has both spinal and supraspinal components. As far as the putative spinal component is concerned, one possibility is that it stems from the combined abilities of opioids to activate spinal μ- or δ-opioid receptors directly and of cannabinoids to activate spinal κ-receptors indirectly through the release of κ-opioids (see foregoing Sec. II.C) (87,106). In line with this hypothesis, it is opioid receptor agonists with μ/δ-selectivity (morphine or DPDPE) as opposed to κ-selectivity (U-50488) that interact synergistically with cannabinoids when injected intrathecally (36). Moreover, in mice, synergism between Δ^9-THC and morphine can be blocked by intrathecal injections of naloxone, of the κ-selective antagonist, norbinaltorphimine, of the δ-receptor antagonist, naltrindol, or of antisera for the κ-selective endogenous opioid peptides, dynorphin A_{1-8}, dynorphin A_{1-13}, and dynorphin A_{1-17} (29,87,100). One apparent anomaly is that unlike several other cannabinoid receptor agonists, CP 55940 does not enhance morphine-induced antinociception in the mouse tail-flick test when it is injected intrathecally (100,101,106). This raises the intriguing possibility that mouse spinal cord contains a novel type or subtype of cannabinoid receptor (106). Note, however, that synergism between CP-55940 and morphine has been detected in the mouse tail-flick test when both drugs are injected i.c.v. (101).

E. Suppression of Thermal and Mechanical Hyperalgesia and Allodynia

There have been several reports that cannabinoids can suppress responses to thermal or mechanical stimuli when these are applied to the hindpaws of rats that have been made hyperalgesic, for example by intradermal injection of a noxious agent. In two investigations, no differences were detected between the ability of cannabinoids to suppress responses to paw pressure in such animals than in normal animals. More specifically, Kosersky (59) reported that oral administration of Δ^9-THC, albeit at the rather high dose of 100 mg/kg, suppressed vocalization of rats in response to pressure applied to a paw that had been injected with yeast or carrageenan. This dose was equally effective against vocalization elicited by pressure application to an uninjected paw. Δ^9-THC and anandamide, injected intraperitoneally, are both antihyperalgesic in a rat model of arthritic pain in which the hindpaw is rendered hypersensitive to a pressure stimulus by intradermal injection of Freund's complete adjuvant (60). Neither cannabinoid seemed to be more or less potent in preventing motor responses to pressure when applied to paws that had been injected with Freund's adjuvant than when applied to uninjected paws.

In other investigations, cannabinoids have suppressed responses to pressure or thermal stimuli more readily when these stimuli are applied to a paw that has been made hyperalgesic than when they are applied to a normal paw. In experiments with rats, orally administeıed Δ^9-THC suppressed paw pressure-induced vocalization and motor responses at lower doses when the pressure was applied to a yeast-injected paw (e.g., ED_{50} = 4 mg/kg) than to a normal paw (e.g., ED_{50} = 32 mg/kg) (10,47). Thermal hyperalgesia induced in rats by intraplantar injection of carrageenan into the hindpaw could be suppressed by anandamide administered either directly into a carrageenan-treated paw (10 pg) or intrathecally (0.024 and 0.24 pg) (113,114). The same intrathecal doses of anandamide were not antinociceptive in rats with carrageenan-free hindpaws. Because of the rather low doses used in these experiments, it is likely that anandamide was acting close to the injection site and, consequently, that it can suppress thermal hyperalgesia by acting at sites outside as well as within the CNS. The antihyperalgesic effect of intraplantar anandamide (10 ng) was significantly attenuated by SR 141716A, coadministered at a reasonably low dose (100 ng), suggesting that this effect is CB_1 receptor-mediated (113). Herzberg et al. (115) investigated the antihyperalgesic activity of the cannabinoid receptor agonist, (+)-WIN 55212, in a rat model of neuropathic pain in which the right hindpaw is rendered hyperalgesic by the application of four loose ligatures around the trunk of the sciatic nerve. At doses of 0.43–4.3 mg/kg i.p., this cannabinoid delayed withdrawal responses of the hindpaw ipsilateral to the sciatic ligation to heat and cold stimuli (suppression of thermal hyperalgesia), to a pinprick (suppression of mechanical hyperalgesia) and, to pressure from a von Frey hair (suppression of mechanical allodynia), without affecting withdrawal responses to the same stimuli of the other hindpaw or of either hindpaw of sham-operated rats. The ability of (+)-WIN 55212 to suppress mechanical allodynia and thermal hyperalgesia was significantly attenuated when SR 141716A was coadministered (0.5 or 5 mg/kg i.p.). However, when given by itself, SR 141716A (0.5 mg/kg i.p.) exacerbated both the allodynia and the hyperalgesia (see also Sec. II. G).

Anandamide can inhibit potassium- and capsaicin-evoked release of immunoreactive calcitonin gene-related peptide (CGRP) from tissue obtained from the dorsal half of the lumbar enlargement of rat spinal cord, and this effect can be readily abolished by SR 141716A (114). The same research group also found anandamide to inhibit capsaicin-evoked release of CGRP from an in vitro preparation of rat hind paw skin (113). These findings together with evidence that there are cannabinoid-binding sites not only in the spinal cord (1,79,114,116,117), but also on the terminals of primary afferent fibers in rat trigeminal ganglia (114), opens up two possible mechanisms for anandamide-induced inhibition of evoked CGRP release from primary afferent fibers. Thus, anandamide could produce this effect (and antinociception–antihyperalgesia) by acting through CB_1 receptors located on the peripheral terminals of capsaicin-sensitive primary afferent nociceptive fibers and by acting through CB_1 receptors located spinally or supraspinally (114).

F. Palmitoylethanolamide

Calignano et al. (82) have compared the antinociceptive properties of anandamide with those of another endogenous fatty acid amide, palmitoylethanolamide. They found that palmitoylethanolamide shares the ability of anandamide to suppress behavioral responses induced by injecting formalin into the hindpaws of mice (licking and flexing of the injected limb). Both acylethanolamides were active at low doses (50 μg) when injected into the hindpaws together with formalin, as were methanandamide (50 μg) and (+)-WIN 55212 (500 μg). Additional experiments with the CB_1 antagonist SR 141716A, and the CB_2 antagonist SR 144528, showed that the antinociceptive effect of anandamide was blocked only by SR 141716A, whereas that of palmitoylethanolamide was blocked only by SR 144528. Combined injections of equal doses of anandamide and palmitoylethanolamide into the hindpaws (0.1 μg) induced antinociception with a potency approximately 100 times greater than that of either compound administered alone. This synergism could be blocked by pretreatment with either SR 141716A or SR 144528. The results of Calignano et al. (82) lend further support to the hypothesis that anandamide can suppress nociception by acting through peripheral CB_1 receptors in the skin (see Sec. II.E) and suggest that palmitoylethanolamide can also produce this effect by interacting directly with cutaneous tissue, in this case through "CB_2-like" receptors. Additionally, formalin-induced hyperalgesia can be suppressed in mice by intravenous palmitoylethanolamide or anandamide (82) and in rats by intraperitoneal palmitoylethanolamide (119), and palmitoylethanolamide (and anandamide) can attenuate signs of persistent pain induced by inflammation of the rat urinary bladder (119). The status of palmitoylethanolamide as a cannabinoid receptor ligand is currently unclear. Thus, Facci et al. (118) have found that at low concentrations, palmitoylethanolamide inhibits 5-HT release from a cell line known to express CB_2 receptors (RBL-2H3 cells), and that it readily displaces [^{3}H](+)-WIN 55212 from specific-binding sites on membranes obtained from these cells. On the other hand, Showalter et al. (69) have reported that palmitoylethanolamide has little affinity for cloned human CB_2 receptors, and there are also several reports that it does not bind to CB_1 receptors (1).

G. The Role of the Endogenous Cannabinoid System in Pain Perception

The evidence that cannabinoid CB_1 receptors can mediate antinociception raises the possibility that the endogenous cannabinoid system has a physiological or pathophysiological role in pain perception. One strategy for investigating this possibility is to explore the effect of a cannabinoid receptor antagonist on nociception and, indeed, some experiments have already been performed with SR 141716A and SR 144528. As these agents seem to be inverse agonists, rather than pure antagonists (4,120,121), there are at least two ways in which they might affect any component of nociception that is being actively regulated by the endogenous cannabinoid system through cannabinoid receptors. One of these would be to antagonize an endogenously released cannabinoid receptor agonist (pharmacological antagonism) and the other, to reduce the number of any constitutively active CB_1 receptors (inverse agonism).

In line with the notion that the endogenous cannabinoid system does tonically regulate thermal nociceptive thresholds, Richardson et al. (116,122) have shown that hot plate latencies can be decreased in drug-free mice both by a single intrathecal injection of SR 141716A and by repeated intrathecal administration of an antisense oligodeoxynucleotide directed against CB_1

cannabinoid receptor mRNA. The hypernociceptive effect of SR 141716A was dose-dependently blocked by two NMDA receptor antagonists, D-AP-5 and MK-801, suggesting that the effect may be NMDA-dependent (116). [MK-801 has also been reported to attenuate antinociception induced by Δ^9-THC in the mouse tail-flick test (34)]. Calignano et al. (82) found that behavioral signs of nociception provoked by injecting formalin into the hind paws of mice were enhanced by intraplantar or intravenous injection of SR 141716A or SR 144528. Their finding that rat paw skin contains five to ten times more anandamide and palmitoylethanolamide than rat brain or plasma is consistent with their hypothesis that SR 141716A and SR 144528 were not acting as inverse agonists, but rather, by blocking the actions of endogenously produced anandamide and palmitoylethanolamide. Herzberg et al. (115) have obtained evidence that SR 141716A enhances thermal hyperalgesia and mechanical allodynia in rats by showing it to increase the sensitivity to thermal and mechanical stimuli of hindpaws that have been rendered hyperalgesic by sciatic nerve ligation. As the dose of SR 141716A used (0.5 mg/kg i.p.) did not alter the sensitivity of unlesioned paws to these stimuli, the data from this investigation provide support for a role for the endogenous cannabinoid system in the regulation of nociceptive thresholds for hyperalgesic, but not nonhyperalgesic tissue. In a number of other investigations, however, SR 141716A, by itself, has lacked any detectable effect on nociception in either normal or "hyperalgesic" animals. Smith et al. (60) found that SR 141716A (10 mg/kg i.p.) did not alter motor responses of rats to pressure applied to their hindpaws, irrespective of whether the paws had been made hypersensitive by injection with Freund's complete adjuvant. Richardson et al. (113) reported that the motor response to a thermal stimulus applied to rat hindpaws that had been rendered hypersensitive by an intraplantar injection of carrageenan was unaffected by SR 141716A, injected directly into the paw at a dose known to block the antihyperalgesic effect of anandamide. There are also reports that systemic administration of SR 141716A does not produce any detectable decrease in mouse tail-flick latency (97). Such negative results with SR 141716A do not necessarily rule out a physiological role for the endogenous cannabinoid system in pain perception. Thus there are reports that although the endogenous cannabinoid, anandamide, is an established CB_1 cannabinoid receptor agonist, its antinociceptive effect in some animal models is not susceptible to antagonism by SR 141716A (60,77). Additional differences between the antinociceptive properties of anandamide and other cannabinoid receptor agonists, such as Δ^9-THC also exist and these are detailed elsewhere (76,79,88).

III. HUMAN STUDIES

As shown in Table 2, the effect of cannabinoids on the perception of experimentally induced pain by human subjects is far from clear. Thus, although there are some data suggesting that cannabis or Δ^9-THC may reduce perception of this type of pain (125,128), there are other data that indicate that cannabis or Δ^9-THC have no detectable effect (123,124,127,128), or that cannabis can increase sensitivity to and reduce tolerance of experimental pain (123–125). As to other types of acute pain, Jain et al. (130) obtained good evidence that intramuscular injection of the potent cannabinoid receptor agonist, L-nantradol, can reduce postoperative pain (see Table 2). However, it is unclear from the data of Regelson et al. (129) whether this kind of pain was reduced by oral Δ^9-THC in their clinical study (see Table 2).

Several anecdotal accounts of the ability of cannabis to relieve chronic pain are to be found in the book by Grinspoon and Bakalar (131). To these may be added the responses to a questionnaire distributed to multiple sclerosis patients who self-medicate with cannabis (132). Of the 112 subjects in this survey who were experiencing the following symptoms, the percentage reporting improvement after taking cannabis was 96.5% for spasticity at sleep onset, 95.1%

Table 2 Effects of Cannabinoids on Experimental or Acute Postoperative Pain in Humans

Subjects	Treatment	Stimulus and study design	Measured analgesic response	Result	Refs.
Male cannabis users (n = 26)	Smoked cannabis (n = 20)	Ascending and descending electrical current to fingers	Pain tolerance and detection of ascending pain and descending touch sensation	Hyperalgesia	123, 124
	Placebo (n = 6)	[P]		No effect	
Male cannabis users (n = 16)	Smoked cannabis (1) moderate dose (2) high dose	Twenty thermal stimuli of nine intensities (heat) in random order [ol]	Subjective rating	(1) Hyperalgesia (2) Analgesia?	125
Male and female cannabis users and nonusers (n = 32)	Smoked cannabis	Thermal to forearm (heat) [db, r, co, P]	Time between stimulus onset and reported pain sensation	No effect	126
	Placebo			No effect	
Male (n = 5)	Δ^9-THC 25 mg p.o.	Thermal to hand (icy water) [db, r, co, P]	Time between stimulus onset and (1) Pain onset (2) Pain intolerable	No effect No effect	127
Healthy males after removal of four impacted third molars from each subject on four separate occasions (n = 10)	Δ^9-THC before surgery (1) 0.22 or (2) 0.44 mg/kg i.v.	Pressure to forehead and electrical to shoulder after operation [db, r, co, P]	(1) Pain detection (2) Pain tolerance	Analgesia No effect	128
		Postoperative pain [db, r, co, P]	Patient ranking of pain severity: THC vs. P and diazepam	(1) Analgesia (n = 3) (1) No effect (n = 6) (2) Hyperalgesia (n = 10)	
Patients with advanced cancer (n = 27)	Δ^9-THC 2.5 or 5 mg p.o. capsules 0.1 mg/kg t.i.d.[b]	Postoperative pain [db, r, co, P]	Medical records and verbal reports	No effect (n = 13) Analgesia (n = 14)	129
	Placebo			No effect (n = 18) Analgesia (n = 9)[a]	
Male and female patients with acute postoperative pain (n = 56)	L-Nantradol 1.5–3 mg i.m.	Postoperative pain [db, r, st, P]	Subjective-rating scale	Analgesia	130

[a] Seven of these patients had just completed a treatment period with Δ^9-THC, raising the possibility that this apparent placebo effect may have been produced by residual Δ^9-THC.
[b] Dose subsequently halved or doubled, depending on side effects.
sb, single blind; db, double-blind; c, crossover; P, placebo-controlled; r, randomized; st, stratified; ol, open-label.

for pain in muscles, 93.2% for spasticity when waking at night, 92.3% for pain in the legs at night, 90.7% for tremor of arms or head, and 90.6% for depression. The numbers of subjects reporting these symptoms were, respectively, 86, 61, 59, 52, 43, and 74. In an earlier survey of ten spinal cord-injured patients, there are also claims that cannabis can reduce spasticity and pain (133). In addition, results from a case study with one amputee indicate that orally administered Δ^9-THC (dronabinol) is markedly more effective than conventional drug treatments in reducing the incidence of phantom limb pain episodes (134). The ability of cannabinoids to relieve chronic pain has also been investigated in placebo-controlled clinical trials using either Δ^9-THC or nabilone (Table 3). Relatively few such studies have been carried out. Even so, the clinical data that have been obtained suggest that cannabinoids are capable of bringing about relief from continuous moderate pain arising from cancer or from pain associated with multiple sclerosis or spinal cord injury. Holdcroft et al. (135) have found oral administration of a cannabis extract reduced the requirement for morphine by a patient suffering from severe chronic abdominal pain (see Table 3). Whether this relates to the apparent ability of cannabinoids to enhance opioid-induced antinociception in animals (see Sec. II.D) remains to be established. In a study that compared the efficacy of oral Δ^9-THC and codeine for relief of advanced cancer pain, Noyes et al. (137) found 10 mg of Δ^9-THC to be slightly less effective than 60 mg of codeine, and 20 mg of Δ^9-THC was slightly more effective than 120 mg of codeine. However, the higher of these doses of Δ^9-THC induced unwanted symptoms that were judged to be of sufficient severity to rule out the use of this dose in the clinic. The most commonly reported of these symptoms were dizziness, sedation, and dry mouth (more than 75% of subjects); blurred vision (65% of subjects); mental clouding (53% of subjects); and ataxia, numbness, disorientation, disconnected thought, slurred speech, muscle twitching, and impaired memory (27–44% of subjects). The side effects of the lower, less analgesic dose of Δ^9-THC (10 mg p.o.) were relatively mild and of brief duration and, therefore, acceptable. In an investigation (130) into the effect of intramuscular L-nantradol on acute postoperative pain (see Table 3), the most frequently reported side effect was drowsiness–sedation (18 out of 40 patients after 1.5–3 mg). There were three reports of mild hallucinations and two of a moderate dysphoric reaction to L-nantradol.

Some individuals may be more at risk from the adverse effects of cannabinoids than others. For example, cannabis may aggravate existing psychoses (141) and can elevate heart rate (142). Consequently, it would be unwise to give psychotropic cannabinoids to patients with schizophrenia (overt or latent), coronary arteriosclerosis, or congestive heart failure. The clinical significance of the ability of cannabinoids to retard fetal development, to induce fetal resorption in animals, or to suppress immune function remains to be established (142,143). Withdrawal of cannabis or of psychotropic cannabinoid administration can precipitate abstinence signs in humans. However, these are both transient and mild, and their significance when cannabinoids are used clinically remains to be established (110,142,144).

Tolerance to many of the pharmacological effects of cannabinoids can be induced readily and rapidly in animals (see foregoing) and humans and this tolerance appears to be largely pharmacodynamic (1,110). Most tolerance studies with human subjects have been conducted without double-blind or placebo treatments. This is an important limitation because there is evidence that certain responses to cannabis can be markedly influenced by the "expectation" of subjects. An additional interpretational difficulty associated with many of those studies in which the development of tolerance has been followed in the laboratory arises from the practice of allowing dose levels and frequency of administration to be decided by the subjects themselves. It is noteworthy, therefore, that the production of tolerance by oral Δ^9-THC has been clearly demonstrated in one set of experiments with 12 human subjects in which drug administrations were made double-blind and in which placebo treatments and predetermined drug regimens were used (145). Rather large oral doses of Δ^9-THC were used in this study (initially 70 mg/

Table 3 Effects of Cannabinoids in Humans on Abdominal Pain, Cancer Pain, or Pain Associated with Muscle Spasms

Subjects	Treatment	Type of pain and study design	Measured analgesic response	Result	Ref.
Male with familial Mediterranean fever ($n = 1$)	Cannabis extract (p.o.) 16–38 mg Δ^9-THC/day	Continuous severe abdominal pain [db, r, co, P]	Need for morphine	Analgesia	135
Male and female patients with advanced cancer ($n = 10$)	Δ^9-THC (p.o.) 5-, 10-, 15-, or 20-mg capsules once daily in the morning	Cancer pain [db, r, co, P]	Subjective-rating scales	5 mg: no analgesia 10 mg: analgesia? >10 mg: analgesia	136
Male and female patients with advanced cancer ($n = 36$)	Δ^9-THC (p.o.) 10- or 20-mg capsules once daily in the morning	Cancer pain [db, r, co, P]	Subjective-rating scales	10 mg: analgesia? 20 mg: analgesia	137
Male with spinal cord injury ($n = 1$)	Δ^9-THC (p.o.) 5 mg[a] once daily in the evening	Painful spasticity [db, r, co, P]	Subjective visual analog scale	Analgesia	138
Male with multiple dysmorphy and cervical myelopathy with progressive spastic tetraparesis ($n = 1$)	Δ^9-THC (p.o.) 10 mg or Δ^9-THC hemisuccinate per rectum 5 mg once daily	Painful spasticity [ol]	Self-rated and need for other analgesics	Analgesia (slight)	139
Male with multiple sclerosis ($n = 1$)	Nabilone (p.o.) 1 mg on alternate days	Painful spasticity [db, co, P]	Subjective visual analog scale	Analgesia	140

[a] Δ^9-THC and placebo were taken with baclofen (40 mg) and clonazepam (1 mg).
sb, single-blind; db, double-blind; c, crossover; P, placebo-controlled; r, randomized; st, stratified; ol, open-label.

24 h in divided doses of 10 mg every 4 h plus 20 mg at bedtime; and later 210 mg/24 h). Consequently, the important question of whether cannabinoid tolerance to sought-after effects develops significantly in humans when "clinically relevant" dose regimens are used still needs to be addressed.

When taken orally, Δ^9-THC seems to undergo somewhat variable absorption from the gastrointestinal tract and to have a rather narrow "therapeutic window" (146). This makes it difficult to predict an oral dose of a cannabinoid that will be both effective and tolerable to a patient and points to a need for better cannabinoid formulations and modes of administration. Such absorption difficulties may account for anecdotal claims that cannabis is superior to Δ^9-THC as a medicine because the comparison is usually between smoked cannabis (fast, reliable absorption) and oral Δ^9-THC (slower, less reliable absorption). However, it is also possible that, in addition to Δ^9-THC, there are other constituents of cannabis that contribute to its putative beneficial effects either directly or by modulating the effects of Δ^9-THC. In line with this possibility, there are reports that the antinociceptive effect of Δ^9-THC in mice can be modulated by cannabidiol, a nonpsychotropic constituent of cannabis. The nature of this interaction seems to vary both with the antinociceptive test used and with the route of administration. Thus, cannabidiol potentiates the effect of intraperitoneal Δ^9-THC in the mouse hot-plate test (147), but attenuates (57) or has no effect (55) on antinociception induced by oral Δ^9-THC in abdominal-stretch tests. The existence of interactions between Δ^9-THC and two other constituents of cannabis, cannabichromene and cannabinol, has also been sought. Intraperitoneal cannabichromene has been reported to potentiate antinociception in the mouse tail-flick test, 120 min but not 30 or 60 min after intraperitoneal Δ^9-THC (19), whereas the antinociceptive effects of Δ^9-THC and cannabinol appear to be additive (48,57).

Following administration by some routes (e.g., oral), but not others (e.g., inhalation), cannabinoids will undergo first-pass hepatic metabolism. This too could explain why the nature and intensity of the effects of cannabis and Δ^9-THC might vary with the route of administration used, as there is evidence that, when injected subcutaneously, intravenously, or intrathecally, the primary metabolite of Δ^9-THC, 11-hydroxy-Δ^9-THC, is 2.5–12.9 times more potent as an antinociceptive agent than its parent compound in mouse hot-plate, tail-flick, or abdominal-stretch tests (26,49,56,100). Whether, because of the 11-hydroxy-metabolite's greater polarity, there are also pharmacologically significant differences between the distribution patterns of these two cannabinoids in the body that remain to be established. Even though 11-hydroxy-Δ^9-THC has greater antinociceptive potency than Δ^9-THC, there are reports that the ability of Δ^9-THC to induce antinociception in mice and rats is enhanced by pharmacological or surgical treatments expected to inhibit enzymic formation of the 11-hydroxy-metabolite (32,45).

IV. CONCLUSIONS

There is little doubt from results obtained in animal experiments that cannabinoids are antinociceptive. Some of the data also suggest that cannabinoids suppress responses to noxious stimuli more readily in animals that have been made hypersensitive to such stimuli than in normal animals. Why this should be has yet to be established. The antinociceptive effect of cannabinoids can be achieved, at least partly, through the activation of CB_1 receptors located in brain and spinal cord. Cannabinoids may also induce this effect by acting outside the CNS to inhibit secretion from nociceptive neurons. It will be important to follow up evidence that there are additional types of cannabinoid receptors through which cannabinoids can produce antinociception. In particular, there is a need for further experiments that explore the role of CB_2/CB_2-like receptors in nociception more fully.

In some animal models, SR 141716A does not block anandamide-induced antinociception even though it is effective against the antinociceptive effects of other cannabinoid receptor agonists in the same models. One possible explanation for this apparent anomaly is that the anandamide molecule is not chiral and so is not subject to the same stereochemical constraints as other cannabinoids that do possess chiral centers. Thus, it may be that anandamide shares pharmacological properties both with cannabinoid receptor agonists and with the noncannabimimetic enantiomers of these agonists. Already there is a report that, in rats, one noncannabimimetic enantiomer (HU211) of a potent cannabinoid receptor agonist (HU210) can suppress autotomy, a behavioral model of neuropathic pain, and that it may do this by blocking NMDA receptors (148). It could be, therefore, that anandamide-induced antinociception stems from a combination of HU210-like (cannabimimetic) and HU211-like (noncannabimimetic) actions and that it is resistant to antagonism by SR 141716A in some animal models because of a prominent HU211-like component in these models.

Evidence is beginning to emerge that the endogenous cannabinoid system has a physiological role in pain perception: the tonic regulation of thermal nociceptive thresholds. This intriguing possibility requires confirmation. If true, it will be important to establish whether "analgesic tone" in the endogenous cannabinoid system arises from the presence of constitutively active cannabinoid receptors or from the ongoing release of anandamide or 2-arachidonoyl glycerol, as this could help identify new strategies for pain management; for example, the production of analgesia with drugs that inhibit the tissue uptake or metabolism of endogenous cannabinoids (149). The question of whether the antinociceptive effect of the endogenous fatty acid amide, palmitoylethanolamide, is mediated by any type of cannabinoid receptor, known or undiscovered, also needs to be further explored.

In line with the animal data, there are limited clinical data to suggest that cannabinoids are effective against at least some types of pain in humans. These are postoperative, cancer, and phantom limb pain, as well as pain associated with multiple sclerosis and spinal cord injury. There is sufficient evidence from these studies to warrant further clinical investigations with cannabinoids. These should be directed at providing objective and conclusive answers to the following questions. First, do cannabinoids have efficacy against pain that is of clinical significance and, if so, against what type(s) of pain are they most effective? Second, what is the clinical significance both of the known adverse effects of cannabinoids and of the ability of these drugs to induce tolerance? Third, will it prove possible to develop strategies that can separate the analgesic effect of cannabinoids from their psychotropic effect? Given the evidence that cannabinoids can relieve pain by acting outside the CNS, one such strategy could be to design cannabinoid receptor agonists that cannot cross the blood–brain barrier, yet can still gain access to cannabinoid receptors in peripheral tissues. Another strategy may be to exploit the synergism between opioids and cannabinoids that has been observed in animal models of antinociception. Whether such synergism would confer any therapeutic advantage will depend on the relative extents to which the sought-after and unwanted effects of these drugs are augmented in patients by combined cannabinoid–opioid administration. It is also possible that the synergism between palmitoylethanolamide and anandamide that has been reported to exist for antinociception in mice has therapeutic potential.

V. IMPORTANT RECENT ADVANCES

Since the completion of this chapter in 1998, several reviews have been published on cannabinoids and pain (150–152). There have also been a number of important new findings. Walker et al. (153) have reported that subcutaneous injection of formalin into the rat hindpaw causes the release of increased amounts of anandamide in the periaqueductal gray area. This finding suggests that the signs of enhanced tonic activity of the endocannabinoid system that have been observed previously in animals models of hyperalgesia (see Sec. II. G), may depend, at least partly, on increased endogenous cannabinoid release. Martin et al.(154) have identified additional sites in rat brain at which cannabinoids can induce antinociception. By using the tail-flick test and applying (+)-WIN 55212 through implanted cannulae, they showed that the submedius and lateral posterior nuclei of the thalamus, the superior colliculus, the central and basolateral nuclei of the amygdala, and the A5 noradrenergic group in the brain stem were cannabinoid-sensitive sites. Several brain areas were also identified in which (+)-WIN 55212 did not elicit an antinociceptive response. Meng et al. (155) have investigated the effect of intravenous (+)-WIN 55212 on the activity of subpopulations of neurons in the rat rostral ventromedial medulla (RVM). These are neurons that exhibit either a pause in activity ("off" cells) or a burst of activity ("on" cells) just before the tail is withdrawn in response to a noxious radiant heat stimulus. Both the activity pause of off neurons and the activity burst of on neurons were eliminated by (+)-WIN 55212 in anesthetized rats, and this effect could be reversed by intravenous injection of the CB_1-selective antagonist SR 141716A. Spinal nociceptive neurotransmission is facilitated by the on cells and inhibited by the off cells that project to the dorsal horn. Consequently, these results suggest that (+)-WIN 55212 may induce antinociception by acting through CB_1 receptors to modulate descending control exerted on spinal nociceptive neurons by the RVM. A similar mechanism has been proposed for opioids. However, results from experiments with naloxone suggest that the effects of (+)-WIN 55212 on the activity of neurons of the RVM are not mediated by endogenous opioids (155). By itself, intravenous SR 141716A produced a hyperalgesic response in the tail-flick test and prolonged the activity pause of off neurons, further evidence that the endogenous cannabinoid system can exhibit tonic activity in pain pathways. Other evidence that cannabinoids modulate the activity of neurons projecting from the brain stem to spinal cord comes from an investigation by Hohmann et al. (156). They showed that i.c.v. injections of (+)-WIN 55212 suppressed activity evoked in spinal wide-dynamic–range neurons of the lumbar dorsal horn of anesthetized rats by the application of noxious heat to the hindpaw. They also found that the ability of intravenous (+)-WIN 55212 to suppress noxious heat-evoked activity of these neurons could be abolished by spinal transection.

Hohmann et al. (157) have obtained further evidence that CB_1 receptors that can mediate an antinociceptive effect are present on neurons in the dorsal horn of the spinal cord. Direct administration of (+)-WIN 55212 to the dorsal surface of the lumbar spinal cord of anesthetized rats suppressed responses evoked in wide-dynamic–range neurons in the lumbar dorsal horn by the application of noxious heat to the ipsilateral hindpaw. This effect appeared to be CB_1-mediated as it could be attenuated by SR 141716A (1 mg/kg i.v.), and it was not produced by the inactive enantiomer of (+)-WIN 55212. Even more recently, Hohmann and Herkenham (158,159) used in situ hybridization histochemistry to demonstrate the presence of CB_1, but not CB_2 receptor mRNA in primary afferent neurons. Their results suggest that CB_1 receptor mRNA is present in 10–15% of all neurons in adult rat dorsal root ganglia. Of these, 24% coexpressed substance P mRNA. The same incidence of coexpression (24%) was observed for CB_1 and CGRP mRNA, raising the possibility that CB_1 receptors are present in neurons that synthesize both neuropeptides. In contrast, the incidence of colocalization of CB_1 and somatostatin mRNA was minimal. Thus, most of the CB_1 mRNA was in dorsal root ganglion neurons that did not contain substance P, CGRP, or somatostatin. These could include large-diameter neurons that are known to express glutamate (158).

It has been suggested that most primary afferent neurons that express CB_1 receptors are not C fibers but, rather, larger-diameter neurons such as Aβ- or Aδ-fiber neurons. This hypothesis is based on a comparison of the extent to which Aβ-, Aδ-, and C-fiber primary afferent neurons express substance P, CGRP, somatostatin, and CB_1 receptors (158) and on the observation that selective depletion of sensory C fibers with neonatal capsaicin produces only a 16% decrease in cannabinoid receptor density in the rat superficial lumbar dorsal horn (160). The presence of CB_1 receptors on medium- and large-diameter primary afferent neurons would support a role for CB_1 receptors in neuropathic pain (158). Results obtained in this and another investigation also revealed signs of significant differences between the neuronal distribution patterns and densities of cannabinoid and opioid receptors in the spinal cord (158,161). An observation that unilateral dorsal rhizotomy across successive spinal segments from C3 to T1 or T2 induces marked ipsilateral loss of cannabinoid-binding sites in the superficial dorsal horn provides further evidence for the presence of cannabinoid receptors at the central terminals of primary afferent neurons (161). A considerable number of cannabinoid-binding sites remained in the dorsal horn after this rhizotomy-induced deafferentation, suggesting that there is a large population of cannabinoid receptors on the terminals of neurons that project from the brain to the spinal cord or on intrinsic spinal neurons (161).

Some evidence that CB_1 receptors are present not only on central, but also on peripheral, terminals of primary afferent neurons has already been described (see Secs. II.E and II.F). This is now supported by more recent data from sciatic nerve ligation experiments that showed that, in rats, cannabinoid receptors are transported from dorsal root ganglia toward the peripheral terminals (159). Further support comes from the results of experiments with rhesus monkeys subjected to a tail-immersion test (162). These experiments showed that thermal hyperalgesia induced by injection of capsaicin into the end of the tail could be suppressed by injection of low doses of Δ^9-THC into the same site and that this effect of Δ^9-THC could be prevented by SR 141716A when this was injected into the tail as well. It was also found that the highest dose of Δ^9-THC used in these experiments was not antinociceptive in nonhyperalgesic monkeys. This finding is in line with previous reports that cannabinoids are more effective as antinociceptive agents in animals sensitized to noxious stimuli than in unsensitized animals (see Sec. II.E) as are results obtained recently by Li et al. (163) in rat experiments with (+)-WIN 55212.

Recent data obtained by Strangman and Walker (164) suggest one possible cause for the higher antinociceptive potency of cannabinoids in animals sensitized to noxious stimuli. They investigated the effect of (+)-WIN 55212 on windup, a centrally mediated increase in both the frequency and duration of spinal nociceptive responses that is induced by repetitive low-frequency noxious electrical stimulation of C fibers and that may possibly contribute to the development of hyperalgesia and allodynia associated with chronic pain. They found that intravenous (+)-WIN 55212 inhibited the windup of wide-dynamic range and nociceptive-specific neurons of the lumbar dorsal horn of anesthetized, laminectomized rats that had been induced by repeated noxious transcutaneous electrical stimulation. This could be done at a dose that was subeffective for inhibiting responses of nociceptive-specific neurons to single stimuli. Use of a similar animal model has also yielded further evidence for the tonic control of spinal nociceptive processing through spinal CB_1 cannabinoid receptors (see Sec. II.G). Thus, Chapman (165) has reported that spinal administration of SR 141716A to anesthetized rats potentiates C-fiber-mediated responses of dorsal horn neurons to transcutaneous electrical stimulation.

There is now convincing evidence that the eicosanoid cannabinoids, anandamide and methanandamide, are agonists for vanilloid VR1 receptors in sensory neurons, a property not shared by noneicosanoid cannabinoids (166; see 152 and 167 for further discussion).

Finally, there have been two independent reports concerning results obtained with two different strains of CB_1 receptor-knockout mice. One of these strains exhibited normal nociception in tail-immersion, tail-pressure, hot-plate, and abdominal-stretching tests (168). The other strain showed normal nociception in the tail-flick test, but reduced sensitivity to noxious stimuli in the formalin paw test and the hot-plate test (169). Further experiments are required to establish the bases both for the different results obtained with the two CB_1 knockout strains and for the unexpected observation that CB_1 receptor-knockout mice exhibit signs of hypoalgesia, rather than hyperalgesia in some tests.

REFERENCES

1. Pertwee RG. Pharmacology of cannabinoid CB_1 and CB_2 receptors. Pharmacol Ther 1997; 74:129–180.
2. Pertwee RG. Advances in cannabinoid receptor pharmacology. In: Brown D, ed. Cannabis. The Genus *Cannabis*. Harwood Academic, 1998:125–174.
3. Tsou K, Brown S, Sañudo–Peña MC, Mackie K, Walker JM. Immunohistochemical distribution of cannabinoid CB_1 receptors in the rat central nervous system. Neuroscience 1998; 83:393–411.
4. Rinaldi–Carmona M, Barth F, Millan J, Derocq J–M, Casellas P, Congy C, Oustric D, Sarran M, Bouaboula M, Calandra B, Portier M, Shire D, Brelière J–C, Le Fur G. SR 144528, the first potent and selective antagonist of the CB_2 cannabinoid receptor. J Pharmacol Exp Ther 1998; 284:644–650.
5. Dewey WL. Cannabinoid pharmacology. Pharmacol Rev 1986; 38:151–178.
6. Doyle SA, Burstein SH, Dewey WL, Welch SP. Further studies on the antinociceptive effects of Δ^6-THC-7-oic acid. Agents Actions 1990; 31:157–163.
7. Burstein SH, Audette CA, Breuer A, Devane WA, Colodner S, Doyle SA, Mechoulam R. Synthetic nonpsychotropic cannabinoids with potent antiinflammatory, analgesic, and leukocyte antiadhesion activities. J Med Chem 1992; 35:3135–3141.
8. Burstein SH, Friderichs E, Kogel B, Schneider J, Selve N. Analgesic effects of 1′,1′dimethylheptyl-Δ^8-THC-11-oic acid (CT_3) in mice. Life Sci 1998; 63:161–168.
9. Burstein SH. The cannabinoid acids: nonpsychoactive derivatives with therapeutic potential. Pharmacol Ther 1999; 82:87–96.
10. Sofia RD, Nalepa SD, Harakal JJ, Vassar HB. Anti-edema and analgesic properties of Δ^9-tetrahydrocannabinol (THC). J Pharmacol Exp Ther 1973; 186:646–655.
11. Melvin LS, Johnson MR, Harbert CA, Milne GM, Weissman A. A cannabinoid derived prototypical analgesic. J Med Chem 1984; 27:67–71.
12. Weissman A, Milne GM, Melvin LS. Cannabimimetic activity from CP-47, 497, a derivative of 3-phenylcyclohexanol. J Pharmacol Exp Ther 1982; 223:516–522.
13. Vitez TS, Way WL, Miller RD, Eger EI. Effects of delta-9-tetrahydrocannabinol on cyclopropane MAC in the rat. Anesthesiology 1973; 38:525–527.
14. Stoelting RK, Martz RC, Gartner J, Creasser C, Brown DJ, Forney RB. Effects of delta-9-tetrahydrocannabinol on halothane MAC in dogs. Anesthesiology 1973; 38:521–524.
15. Bhargava HN, Matwyshyn GA. Influence of thyrotropin releasing hormone and histidyl-proline diketopiperazine on spontaneous locomotor activity and analgesia induced by Δ^9-tetrahydrocannabinol in the mouse. Eur J Pharmacol 1980; 68:147–154.
16. Bloom AS, Dewey WL. A comparison of some pharmacological actions of morphine and Δ^9-tetrahydrocannabinol in the mouse. Psychopharmacology 1978; 57:243–248.
17. Buxbaum DM. Analgesic activity of Δ^9-tetradrocannabinol in the rat and mouse. Psychopharmacologia 1972; 25:275–280.
18. Compton DR, Johnson MR, Melvin LS, Martin BR. Pharmacological profile of a series of bicyclic cannabinoid analogs: classification as cannabimimetic agents. J Pharmacol Exp Ther 1992; 260: 201–209.
19. Davis WM, Hatoum NS. Neurobehavioral actions of cannabichromene and interactions with Δ^9-tetrahydrocannabinol. Gen Pharmacol 1983; 14:247–252.
20. Dewey WL, Harris LS, Howes JF, Kennedy JS, Granchelli FE, Pars HG, Razdan RK. Pharmacology of some marijuana constituents and two heterocyclic analogues. Nature 1970; 226:1265–1267.
21. Dewey WL, Harris LS, Kennedy JS. Some pharmacological and toxicological effects of *l-trans-*

Δ^8- and *l-trans*-Δ^9-tetrahydrocannabinol in laboratory rodents. Arch Int Pharmacodyn 1972; 196: 133–145.

22. Koe BK, Milne GM, Weissman A, Johnson MR, Melvin LS. Enhancement of brain [^{3}H]flunitrazepam binding and analgesic activity of synthetic cannabimimetics. Eur J Pharmacol 1985; 109: 201–212.
23. Lichtman AH, Smith FL, Martin BR. Evidence that the antinociceptive tail-flick response is produced independently from changes in either tail-skin temperature or core temperature. Pain 1993; 55:283–295.
24. Little PJ, Compton DR, Johnson MR, Melvin LS, Martin BR. Pharmacology and stereoselectivity of structurally novel cannabinoids in mice. J Pharmacol Exp Ther 1988; 247:1046–1051.
25. Martin BR. Charaterization of the antinociceptive activity of intravenously administered delta-9-tetrahydrocannabinol in mice. In: Harvey DJ, ed. Marihuana '84. Oxford: IRL Press, 1985:685–692.
26. Martin BR. Structural requirements for cannabinoid-induced antinoceptive activity in mice. Life Sci 1985; 36:1523–1530.
27. Martin BR, Compton DR, Semus SF, Lin S, Marciniak G, Grzybowska J, Charalambous A, Makriyannis A. Pharmacological evaluation of iodo and nitro analogs of Δ^8-THC and Δ^9-THC. Pharmacol Biochem Behav 1993; 46:295–301.
28. Pertwee RG, Browne SE, Ross TM, Stretton CD. An investigation of the involvement of GABA in certain pharmacological effects of delta-9-tetrahydrocannabinol. Pharmacol Biochem Behav 1991; 40:581–585.
29. Reche I, Fuentes JA, Ruiz–Gayo M. Potentiation of Δ^9-tetrahydrocannabinol-induced analgesia by morphine in mice: involvement of μ- and κ-opioid receptors. Eur J Pharmacol 1996; 318:11–16.
30. Reche I, Fuentes JA, Ruiz–Gayo M. A role for central cannabinoid and opioid systems in peripheral Δ^9-tetrahydrocannabinol-induced analgesia in mice. Eur J Pharmacol 1996; 301:75–81.
31. Smith PB, Martin BR. Spinal mechanisms of Δ^9-tetrahydrocannabinol-induced analgesia. Brain Res 1992; 578:8–12.
32. Sofia RD, Barry H. The effects of SKF 525-A on the analgesic and barbiturate-potentiating activity of Δ^9-tetrahydrocannabinol in mice and rats. Pharmacology 1983; 27:223–236.
33. Spaulding TC, Ford RD, Dewey WL, McMillan DE, Harris LS. Some pharmacological effects of phenitrone and its interaction with Δ^9-THC. Eur J Pharmacol 1972; 19:310–317.
34. Thorat SN, Bhargava HN. Effects of NMDA receptor blockade and nitric oxide synthase inhibition on the acute and chronic actions of Δ^9-tetrahydrocannabinol in mice. Brain Res 1994; 667:77–82.
35. Thorat SN, Bhargava HN. Evidence for a bidirectional cross-tolerance between morphine and Δ^9-tetrahydrocannabinol in mice. Eur J Pharmacol 1994; 260:5–13.
36. Welch SP. Blockade of cannabinoid-induced antinociception by norbinaltorphimine, but not *N, N*-diallyl-tyrosine-Aib-phenylalanine-leucine, ICI 174,864, or naloxone in mice. J Pharmacol Exp Ther 1993; 265:633–640.
37. Bhattacharya SK, Sen AP, Mohan, Rao PJR, Dasgupta G. Role of prostaglandins in some neuropharmacological actions of gD^9-tetrahydrocannabinol (THC) in the rat. Asia Pac J Pharmacol 1989; 4: 179–188.
38. Gallager DW, Sanders–Bush E, Sulser F. Dissociation between behavioural effects and changes in metabolism of cerebral serotonin following Δ^9-tetrahydrocannabinol. Psychopharmacologia 1972; 26:337–345.
39. Hine B. Morphine and Δ^9-tetrahydrocannabinol: two-way cross tolerance for antinociceptive and heart-rate responses in the rat. Psychopharmacology 1985; 87:34–38.
40. Lichtman AH, Martin BR. Cannabinoid-induced antinociception is mediated by a spinal α_2-noradrenergic mechanism. Brian Res 1991; 559:309–314.
41. Lichtman AH, Martin BR. Spinal and supraspinal components of cannabinoid-induced antinociception. J Pharmacol Exp Ther 1991; 258:517–523.
42. Lichtman AH, Martin BR. The selective cannabinoid antagonist SR 141716A blocks cannabinoid-induced antinociception in rats. Pharmacol Biochem Behav 1997; 57:7–12.
43. Novelli GP, Peduto VA, Bertol E, Mari F, Pieraccioli E. Analgesic interaction between nitrous oxide and delta-9-tetrahydrocannabinol. Br J Anaesth 1983; 55:997–1000.

44. Burstein SH, Hull K, Hunter SA, Latham V. Cannabinoids and pain response: a possible role for prostaglandins. FASEB J 1988; 2:3022–3026.
45. Kaymakcalan S, Deneau GA. Some pharmacologic properties of synthetic delta-9-tetrahydrocannabinol. Acta Med Turc Suppl 1972; 1:5–27.
46. Segelman AB, Sofia RD, Segelman FP, Harakal JJ, Knobloch LC. *Cannabis sativa* L. (marijuana) V: pharmacological evaluation of marijuana aqueous extract and volatile oil. J Pharm Sci 1974; 63:962–964.
47. Sofia RD, Vassar HB, Knobloch LC. Comparative analgesic activity of various naturally occurring cannabinoids in mice and rats. Psychopharmacologia 1975; 40:285–295.
48. Takahashi RN, Karniol IG. Pharmacological interaction between cannabinol and Δ^9-tetrahydrocannabinol. Psychopharmacologia 1975; 41:277–284.
49. Wilson RS, May EL. Analgesic properties of the tetrahydrocannabinols, their metabolites and analogs. J Med Chem 1975; 18:700–703.
50. Tulunay FC, Ayhan IH, Portoghese PS, Takemori AE. Antagonism by chlornaltrexamine of some effects of Δ^9-tetrahydrocannabinol in rats. Eur J Pharmacol 1981; 70:219–224.
51. Gilbert PE. A comparison of THC, nantradol, nabilone, and morphine in the chronic spinal dog. J Clin Pharmacol 1981; 21:311S–319S.
52. Formukong EA, Evans AT, Evans FJ. Analgesic and antiinflammatory activity of constituents of *Cannabis sativa* L. Inflammation 1988; 12:361–371.
53. Jackson DM, Malor R, Chesher GB, Starmer GA, Welburn PJ, Bailey R. The interaction between prostaglandin E, and Δ^9-tetrahydrocannabinol on intestinal motility and on the abdominal constriction response in the mouse. Psychopharmacology 1976; 47:187–193.
54. Osgood PF, Howes JF, Razdan RK, Pars HG. Drugs derived from cannabinoids. 7. Tachycardia and analgesia structure–activity relationships in Δ^9-tetrahydrocannabinol and some synthetic analogues. J Med Chem 1978; 21:809–811.
55. Sanders J, Jackson DM, Starmer GA. Interactions among the cannabinoids in the antagonism of the abdominal constriction response in the mouse. Psychopharmacology 1979; 61:281–285.
56. Watanabe K, Kijima T, Narimatsu S, Nishikami J, Yamamoto I, Yoshimura H. Comparison of pharmacological effects of tetrahydrocannabinols and their 11-hydroxy-metabolites in mice. Chem Pharm Bull 1990; 38:2317–2319.
57. Welburn PJ, Starmer GA, Chesher GB, Jackson DM. Effect of cannabinoids on the abdominal constriction response in mice: within cannabinoid interactions. Psychopharmacologia 1976; 46:83–85.
58. Moss DE, Johnson RL. Tonic analgesic effects of Δ^9-tetrahydrocannabinol as measured with the formalin test. Eur J Pharmacol 1980; 61:313–315.
59. Kosersky DS, Dewey WL, Harris LS. Antipyretic, analgesic and anti-inflammatory effects of Δ^9-tetrahydrocannabinol in the rat. Eur J Pharmacol 1973; 24:1–7.
60. Smith FL, Fujimori K, Lowe J, Welch SP. Characterization of Δ^9-tetrahydrocannabinol and anandamide antinociception in non-arthritic and arthritic rats. Pharmacol Biochem Behav 1998; 60:183–191.
61. Parker JM, Dubas TC. Automatic determination of the pain threshold to electroshock and the effects of Δ^9-THC. Int J Clin Pharmacol Ther Toxicol 1973; 7:75–81.
62. Scheckel CL, Boff E, Dahlen P, Smart T. Behavioral effects in monkeys of racemates of two biologically active marijuana constituents. Science 1968; 160:1467–1469.
63. Bicher HI, Mechoulam R. Pharmacological effects of two active constituents of marihuana. Arch Int Pharmacodyn 1968; 172:24–31.
64. Kaymakcalan S, Türker RK, Türker MN. Analgesic effect of Δ^9-tetrahydrocannabinol in the dog. Psychopharmacologia 1974; 35:123–128.
65. Martin BR, Thomas BF, Razdan RK. Structural requirements for cannabinoid receptor probes. In: Pertwee RG, ed. Cannabinoid Receptors. London: Academic, 1995:35–85.
66. Martin BR, Compton DR, Prescott WR, Barrett RL, Razdan RK. Pharmacological evaluation of dimethylheptyl analogs of Δ^9-THC: reassessment of the putative three-point cannabinoid-receptor interaction. Drug Alcohol Depend 1995; 37:231–240.
67. Singer M, Dutta AK, Compton DR, Martin BR, Razdan RK. Synthesis and pharmacology of (*R*)- and (*S*)-4′-hydroxy-Δ^9-tetrahydrocannabinols. Eur J Med Chem 1997; 32:165–170.

68. Wiley JL, Compton DR, Gordon PM, Siegel C, Singer M, Dutta A, Lichtman AH, Balster RL, Razdan RK, Martin BR. Evaluation of agonist–antagonist properties of nitrogen mustard and cyano derivatives of Δ^8-tetrahydrocannabinol. Neuropharmacology 1996; 35:1793–1804.
69. Showalter VM, Compton DR, Martin BR, Abood ME. Evaluation of binding in a transfected cell line expressing a peripheral cannabinoid receptor (CB_2): identification of cannabinoid receptor subtype selective ligands. J Pharmacol Exp Ther 1996; 278:989–999.
70. Huffman JW, Yu S, Showalter V, Abood ME, Wiley JL, Compton DR, Martin BR, Bramblett RD, Reggio PH. Synthesis and pharmacology of a very potent cannabinoid lacking a phenolic hydroxyl with high affinity for the CB_2 receptor. J Med Chem 1996; 39:3875–3877.
71. Huffman JW, Lainton JAH. Recent developments in the medicinal chemistry of cannabinoids. Curr Med Chem. 1996; 3:101–116.
72. Compton DR, Gold LH, Ward SJ, Balster RL, Martin BR. Aminoalkylindole analogs: cannabimimetic activity of a class of compounds structurally distinct from Δ^9-tetrahydrocannabinol. J Pharmacol Exp Ther 1992; 263:1118–1126.
73. Kumar V, Alexander MD, Bell MR, Eissenstat MA, Casiano FM, Chippari SM, Haycock DA, Luttinger DA, Kuster JE, Miller MS, Stevenson JI, Ward SJ. Morpholinoalkylindenes as antinociceptive agents: novel cannabinoid receptor agonists. Bioorg Med Chem Lett 1995; 5:381–386.
74. Wiley JL, Compton DR, Dai D, Lainton JAH, Phillips M, Huffman JW, Martin BR. Structure–activity relationships of indole- and pyrrole-derived cannabinoids. J Pharmacol Exp Ther 1998; 285: 995–1004.
75. Dutta AK, Ryan W, Thomas BF, Singer M, Compton DR, Martin BR, Razdan RK. Synthesis, pharmacology, and molecular modeling of novel 4-alkyloxy indole derivatives related to cannabimimetic aminoalkyl indoles (AAIs). Bioorg Med Chem 1997; 5:1591–1600.
76. Smith PB, Compton DR, Welch SP, Razdan RK, Mechoulam R, Martin BR. The pharmacological activity of anandamide, a putative endogenous cannabinoid, in mice. J Pharmacol Exp Ther 1994; 270:219–227.
77. Adams IB, Compton DR, Martin BR. Assessment of anandamide interaction with the cannabinoid brain receptor: SR 141716A antagonism studies in mice and autoradiographic analysis of receptor binding in rat brain. J Pharmacol Exp Ther 1998; 284:1209–1217.
78. Mechoulam R, Ben-Shabat S, Hanus L, Ligumsky M, Kaminski NE, Schatz AR, Gopher A, Almog S, Martin BR, Compton DR, Pertwee RG, Griffin G, Bayewitch M, Barg J, Vogel Z. Identification of an endogenous 2-monoglyceride, present in canine gut, that binds to cannabinoid receptors. Biochem Pharmacol 1995; 50:83–90.
79. Welch SP, Dunlow LD, Patrick GS, Razdan RK. Characterization of anandamide- and fluoroanandamide-induced antinociception and cross-tolerance to Δ^9-THC after intrathecal administration to mice: blockade of Δ^9-THC-induced antinociception. J Pharmacol Exp Ther 1995; 273:1235–1244.
80. Fride E, Mechoulam R. Pharmacological activity of the cannabinoid receptor agonist, anandamide, a brain constituent. Eur J Pharmacol 1993; 231:313–314.
81. Adams IB, Ryan W, Singer M, Thomas BF, Compton DR, Razdan RK, Martin BR. Evaluation of cannabinoid receptor binding and in vivo activities for anandamide analogs. J Pharmacol Exp Ther 1995; 273:1172–1181.
82. Calignano A, La Rana G, Giuffrida A, Piomelli D. Control of pain initiation by endogenous cannabinoids. Nature 1998; 394:277–281.
83. Abadji V, Lin S, Taha G, Griffin G, Stevenson LA, Pertwee RG, Makriyannis A. (*R*)-Methanandamide: a chiral novel anandamide possessing higher potency and metabolic stability. J Med Chem 1994; 37:1889–1893.
84. Barg J, Fride E, Hanus L, Levy R, Matus–Leibovitch N, Heldman E, Bayewitch M, Mechoulam R, Vogel Z. Cannabinomimetic behavioral effects of and adenylate cyclase inhibition by two new endogenous anandamides. Eur J Pharmacol 1995; 287:145–152.
85. Ryan WJ, Banner WK, Wiley JL, Martin BR, Razdan RK. Potent anandamide analogs: the effect of changing the length and branching of the end pentyl chain. J Med Chem 1997; 40:3617–3625.
86. Smith PB, Welch SP, Martin BR. Interactions between Δ^9-tetrahydrocannabinol and kappa opioids in mice. J Pharmacol Exp Ther 1994; 268:1381–1387.

87. Pugh G, Smith PB, Dombrowski DS, Welch SP. The role of endogenous opioids in enhancing the antinociception produced by the combination of Δ^9-tetrahydrocannabinol and morphine in the spinal cord. J Pharmacol Exp Ther 1996;279:608–616.
88. Lichtman AH, Cook SA, Martin BR. Investigation of brain sites mediating cannabinoid-induced antinociception in rats: evidence supporting periaqueductal gray involvement. J Pharmacol Exp Ther 1996; 276:585–593.
89. Rowen DW, Embrey JP, Moore CH, Welch SP. Antisense oligodeoxynucleotides to the $kappa_1$ receptor enhance Δ^9-THC-induced antinociceptive tolerance. Pharmacol Biochem Behav 1998; 59: 399–404.
90. Little PJ, Compton DR, Mechoulam R, Martin BR. Stereochemical effects of 11-OH-Δ^8-THC-dimethylheptyl in mice and dogs. Pharmacol Biochem Behav 1989; 32:661–666.
91. Martin BR, Compton DR, Thomas BF, Prescott WR, Little PJ, Razdan RK, Johnson MR, Melvin LS, Mechoulam R, Ward SJ. Behavioral, biochemical, and molecular modeling evaluations of cannabinoid analogs. Pharmacol Biochem Behav 1991; 40:471–478.
92. Compton DR, Rice KC, de Costa BR, Razdan RK, Melvin LS, Johnson MR, Martin BR. Cannabinoid structure–activity relationships: correlation of receptor binding and in vivo activities. J Pharmacol Exp Ther 1993; 265:218–226.
93. Melvin LS, Milne GM, Johnson MR, Subramaniam B, Wilken GH, Howlett AC. Structure–activity relationships for cannabinoid receptor-binding and analgesic activity: studies of bicyclic cannabinoid analogs. Mol Pharmacol 1993; 44:1008–1015.
94. Tsou K, Lowitz KA, Hohmann AG, Martin WJ, Hathaway CB, Bereiter DA, Walker JM. Suppression of noxious stimulus-evoked expression of fos protein-like immunoreactivity in rat spinal cord by a selective cannabinoid agonist. Neuroscience 1996; 70:791–798.
95. Yan G, Yin D, Khanolkar AD, Compton DR, Martin BR, Makriyannis A. Synthesis and pharmacological properties of 11-hydroxy-3-(1′,1′-dimethylheptyl)hexahydrocannabinol: a high-affinity cannabinoid agonist. J Med Chem 1994; 37:2619–2622.
96. Compton DR, Aceto MD, Lowe J, Martin BR. In vivo characterization of a specific cannabinoid receptor antagonist (SR 141716A): inhibition of Δ^9-tetrahydrocannabinol-induced responses and apparent agonist activity. J Pharmacol Exp Ther 1996; 277:586–594.
97. Rinaldi–Carmona M, Barth F, Héaulme M, Shire D, Calandra B, Congy C, Martinez S, Maruani J, Néliat G, Caput D, Ferrara P, Soubrié P, Brelière JC, Le Fur G. SR 141716A, a potent and selective antagonist of the brain cannabinoid receptor. FEBS Lett 1994; 350:240–244.
98. Martin WJ, Tsou K, Walker JM. Cannabinoid receptor-mediated inhibition of the rat tail-flick reflex after microinjection into the rostral ventromedial medulla. Neurosci Lett 1998; 242:33–36.
99. Yaksh TL. The antinociceptive effects of intrathecally administered levonantradol and desacetyllevonantradol in the rat. J Clin Pharmacol 1981; 21:334S–340S.
100. Welch SP, Stevens DL. Antinociceptive activity of intrathecally administered cannabinoids alone, and in combination with morphine, in mice. J Pharmacol Exp Ther 1992; 262:10–18.
101. Welch SP, Thomas C, Patrick GS. Modulation of cannabinoid-induced antinociception after intracerebroventricular versus intrathecal administration to mice: possible mechanisms for interaction with morphine. J Pharmacol Exp Ther 1995; 272:310–321.
102. Martin WJ, Lai NK, Patrick SL, Tsou K, Walker JM. Antinociceptive actions of cannabinoids following intraventricular administration in rats. Brain Res 1993; 629:300–304.
103. Lichtman AH, Smith PB, Martin BR. The antinociceptive effects of intrathecally administered cannabinoids are influenced by lipophilicity. Pain 1992; 51:19–26.
104. Edsall SA, Knapp RJ, Vanderah TW, Roeske WR, Consroe P, Yamamura HI. Antisense oligodeoxynucleotide treatment to the brain cannabinoid receptor inhibits antinociception. Neuroreport 1996; 7:593–596.
105. Martin WJ, Hohmann AG, Walker JM. Suppression of noxious stimulus-evoked activity in the ventral posterolateral nucleus of the thalamus by a cannabinoid agonist: correlation between electrophysiological and antinociceptive effects. J Neurosci 1996; 16:6601–6611.
106. Pugh G, Mason DJ, Combs V, Welch SP. Involvement of dynorphin B in the antinociceptive effects of the cannabinoid CP55,940 in the spinal cord. J Pharmacol Exp Ther 1997; 281:730–737.

107. Pugh G, Abood ME, Welch SP. Antisense oligodeoxynucleotides to the κ-1 receptor block the antinociceptive effects of Δ^9-THC in the spinal cord. Brain Res 1995; 689:157–158.
108. Corchero J, Avila MA, Fuentes JA, Manzanares J. Δ^9-Tetrahydrocannabinol increases prodynorphin and proenkephalin gene expression in the spinal cord of the rat. Life Sci 1997; 61:PL39–PL43.
109. Manzanares J, Corchero J, Romero J, Fernandez-Ruiz JJ, Ramos JA, Fuentes JA. Chronic administration of cannabinoids regulates proenkephalin mRNA levels in selected regions of the rat brain. Mol Brain Res 1998; 55:126–132.
110. Pertwee RG. Tolerance to and dependence on psychotropic cannabinoids. In: Pratt JA, ed. The Biological Bases of Drug Tolerance and Dependence. London: Academic, 1991:231–263.
111. Smith FL, Cichewicz D, Martin ZL, Welch SP. The enhancement of morphine antinociception in mice by Δ^9-tetrahydrocannabinol. Pharmacol Biochem Behav 1998; 60:559–566.
112. Ghosh P, Bhattacharya SK. Cannabis-induced potentiation of morphine analgesia in rat—role of brain monoamines. Ind J Med Res 1979; 70:275–280.
113. Richardson JD, Kilo S, Hargreaves KM. Cannabinoids reduce hyperalgesia and inflammation via interaction with peripheral CB_1 receptors. Pain 1998; 75:111–119.
114. Richardson JD, Aanonsen L, Hargreaves KM. Antithyperalgesic effects of spinal cannabinoids. Eur J Pharmacol 1998; 345:145–153.
115. Herzberg U, Eliav E, Bennett GJ, Kopin IJ. The analgesic effects of *R*(+)-WIN 55,212-2 mesylate, a high affinity cannabinoid agonist, in a rat model of neuropathic pain. Neurosci Lett 1997; 221: 157–160.
116. Richardson JD, Aanonsen L, Hargreaves KM. Hypoactivity of the spinal cannabinoid system results in NMDA-dependent hyperalgesia. J Neurosci 1998; 18:451–457.
117. Welch SP. Blockade of cannabinoid-induced antinociception by naloxone benzoylhydrazone (NalBZH). Pharmacol Biochem Behav 1994; 49:929–934.
118. Facci L, Dal Toso R, Romanello S, Buriani A, Skaper SD, Leon A. Mast cells express a peripheral cannabinoid receptor with differential sensitivity to anandamide and palmitoylethanolamide. Proc Natl Acad Sci USA 1995; 92:3376–3380.
119. Jaggar SI, Hasnie FS, Sellaturay S, Rice ASC. The anti-hyperalgesic actions of the cannabinoid anandamide and the putative CB_2 receptor agonist palmitoylethanolamide in visceral and somatic inflammatory pain. Pain 1998; 76:189–199.
120. Bouaboula M, Perrachon S, Milligan L, Canat X, Rinaldi-Carmona M, Portier M, Barth F, Calandra B, Pecceu F, Lupker J, Maffrand J-P, Le Fur G, Casellas P. A selective inverse agonist for central cannabinoid receptor inhibits mitogen-activated protein kinase activation stimulated by insulin or insulin-like growth factor 1. Evidence for a new model of receptor/ligand interactions. J Biol Chem 1997; 272:22330–22339.
121. MacLennan SJ, Reynen PH, Kwan J, Bonhaus DW. Evidence for inverse agonism of SR 141716A at human recombinant cannabmoid CB_1 and CB_2 receptors. Br J Pharmacol 1998; 124:619–622.
122. Richardson JD, Aanonsen L, Hargreaves KM. SR 141716A, a cannabinoid receptor antagonist, produces hyperalgesia in untreated mice. Eur J Pharmacol 1997; 319:R3–R4.
123. Hill SY, Schwin R, Goodwin DW, Powell BJ. Marihuana and pain. J Pharmacol Exp Ther 1974; 188:415–418.
124. Hill SY, Goodwin DW, Schwin R, Powell B. Marijuana: CNS depressant or excitant? Am J Psychiatry 1974; 131:313–315.
125. Clark WC, Janal MN, Zeidenberg P, Nahas GG. Effects of moderate and high doses of marihuana on thermal pain: a sensory decision theory analysis. J Clin Pharmacol 1981; 21:299S–310S.
126. Milstein SL, MacCannell KL, Karr GW, Clark S. Marijuana produced changes in cutaneous sensitivity and affect: users and non-users. Pharmacol Biochem Behav 1974; 2:367–374.
127. Karniol IG, Shirakawa I, Takahashi RN, Knobel E, Musty RE. Effects of Δ^9-tetrahydrocannabinol and cannabinol in man. Pharmacology 1975; 13:502–512.
128. Raft D, Gregg J, Ghia J, Harris L. Effects of intravenous tetrahydrocannabinol on experimental and surgical pain. Psychological correlates of analgesic response. Clin Pharmacol Ther 1977; 21:26–33.
129. Regelson W, Butler JR, Schultz J, Kirk T, Peek L, Green ML, Zalis MO. Δ^9-Tetrahydrocannabinol

as an effective antidepressant and appetite-stimulating agent in advanced cancer patients. In: Braude MC, Szara S, eds. Pharmacology of Marihuana. New York: Raven, 1976:763–776.

130. Jain AK, Ryan JR, McMahon FG, Smith G. Evaluation of intramuscular levonantradol and placebo in acute postoperative pain. J Clin Pharmacol 1981; 21:320S–326S.
131. Grinspoon L, Bakalar JB. Marihuana, the Forbidden Medicine. New Haven: Yale University Press, 1993.
132. Consroe P, Musty R, Rein J, Tillery W, Pertwee R. The perceived effects of smoked cannabis on patients with multiple sclerosis. Eur Neurol 1997; 38:44–48.
133. Dunn M, Davis R. The perceived effects of marijuana on spinal cord injured males. Paraplegia 1979; 12:175.
134. Finnegan–Ling D, Musty RE. Marinol and phantom limb pain: a case study. Proc Int Cannabinoid Res Soc 1994; 53.
135. Holdcroft A, Smith M, Jacklin A, Hodgson H, Smith B, Newton M, Evans F. Pain relief with oral cannabinoids in familial Mediterranean fever. Anaesthesia 1997; 52:483–488.
136. Noyes R, Brunk F, Baram DA, Canter A. Analgesic effect of Δ^9-tetrahydrocannabinol. J Clin Pharmacol 1975; 15:139–143.
137. Noyes R, Brunk SF, Avery DH, Canter A. The analgesic properties of delta-9-tetrahydrocannabinol and codeine. Clin Pharmacol Ther 1975; 18:84–89.
138. Maurer M, Henn V, Dittrich A, Hofmann A. delta-9-Tetrahydrocannabinol shows antispastic and analgesic effects in a single case double-blind trial. Eur Archs Psychiatry Clin Neurosci 1990; 240: 1–4.
139. Brenneisen R, Egli A, ElSohly MA, Henn V, Spiess Y. The effect of orally and rectally administered Δ^9-tetrahydrocannabinol on spasticity: a pilot study with 2 patients. Int J Clin Pharmacol Ther 1996; 34:446–452.
140. Martyn CN, Illis LS, Thom J. Nabilone in the treatment of multiple sclerosis. Lancet 1995; 345: 579.
141. McGuire PK, Jones P, Harvey I, Williams M, McGuffin P, Murray RM. Morbid risk of schizophrenia for relatives of patients with cannabis-associated psychosis. Schizophrenia Res 1995; 15:277–281.
142. Hollister LE. Health aspects of cannabis. Pharmacol Rev 1986; 38:1–20.
143. Munson AE, Fehr KO. Immunological effects of cannabis. In: Fehr KO, Kalant H, eds. Adverse Health and Behavioral Consequences of Cannabis Use. Toronto: Addiction Research Foundation, 1983:257–353.
144. Jones RT. Cannabis tolerance and dependence. In: Fehr KO, Kalant H, eds. Toronto: Addiction Research Foundation, 1983; 617–689.
145. Jones RT, Benowitz N. The 30-day trip—clinical studies of cannabis tolerance and dependence. In: Braude MC, Szara S, eds. The Pharmacology of Marihuana. New York: Raven, 1976:627–642.
146. Pertwee RG. Cannabis and cannabinoids: pharmacology and rationale for clinical use. Pharm Sci 1997; 3:539–545.
147. Karniol IG, Carlini EA. Pharmacological interaction between cannabidiol and Δ^9-tetrahydrocannabinol. Psychopharmacologia 1973; 33:53–70.
148. Zeltser R, Seltzer Z, Eisen A, Feigenbaum JJ, Mechoulam R. Suppression of neuropathic pain behavior in rats by a non-psychotropic synthetic cannabinoid with NMDA receptor-blocking properties. Pain 1991; 47:95–103.
149. Pertwee RG. Pharmacological, physiological and clinical implications of the discovery of cannabinoid receptors. Biochem Soc Tran 1998; 26:267–272.
150. Martin BR, Lichtman AH. Cannabinoid transmission and pain perception. Neurobiol Dis 1998; 5: 447–461.
151. Walker JM, Hohmann AG, Martin WJ, Strangman NM, Huang SM, Tsou K. The neurobiology of cannabinoid analgesia. Life Sci 1999; 65:665–673.
152. Pertwee RG. Cannabinoid receptors and pain. Prog Neurobiol 2001; 63:569–611.
153. Walker JM, Huang SM, Strangman NM, Tsou K, Sañudo-Peña MC. Pain modulation by release of the endogenous cannabinoid anandamide. Proc Natl Acad Sci USA 1999; 96:12198–12203.

154. Martin WJ, Coffin PO, Attias E, Balinsky M, Tsou K, Walker JM. Anatomical basis for cannabinoid-induced antinociception as revealed by intracerebral microinjections. Brain Res 1999; 822:237–242.
155. Meng ID, Manning BH, Martin WJ, Fields HL. An analgesia circuit activated by cannabinoids. Nature 1998; 395:381–383.
156. Hohmann AG, Tsou K, Walker JM. Cannabinoid suppression of noxious heat-evoked activity in wide dynamic range neurons in the lumbar dorsal horn of the rat. J Neurophysiol 1999; 81:575–583.
157. Hohmann AG, Tsou K, Walker JM. Cannabinoid modulation of wide dynamic range neurons in the lumbar dorsal horn of the rat by spinally administered WIN 55,212-2. Neurosci Letts 1998; 257:119–122.
158. Hohmann AG, Herkenham M. Localization of central cannabinoid CB_1 receptor messenger RNA in neuronal subpopulations of rat dorsal root ganglia: a double-label in situ hybridization study. Neuroscience 1999; 90:923–931.
159. Hohmann AG, Herkenham M. Cannabinoid receptors undergo axonal flow in sensory nerves. Neuroscience 1999; 92:1171–1175.
160. Hohmann AG, Herkenham M. Regulation of cannabinoid and mu opioid receptors in rat lumbar spinal cord following neonatal capsaicin treatment. Neurosci Lett 1998; 252:13–16.
161. Hohmann AG, Briley EM, Herkenham M. Pre- and postsynaptic distribution of cannabinoid and mu opioid receptors in rat spinal cord. Brain Res 1999; 822:17–25.
162. Ko M–C, Woods JH. Local administration of Δ^9-tetrahydrocannabinol attenuates capsaicin-induced thermal nociception in rhesus monkeys: a peripheral cannabinoid action. Psychopharmacology 1999; 143:322–326.
163. Li J, Daughters RS, Bullis C, Bengiamin R, Stucky MW, Brennan J, Simone DA. The cannabinoid receptor agonist WIN 55,212–2 mesylate blocks the development of hyperalgesia produced by capsaicin in rats. Pain 1999; 81:25–33.
164. Strangman NM, Walker JM. Cannabinoid WIN 55,212–2 inhibits the activity-dependent facilitation of spinal nociceptive responses. J Neurophysiol 1999; 82:472–477.
165. Chapman V. The cannabinoid CB_1 receptor antagonist, SR 141716A, selectively facilitates nociceptive responses of dorsal horn neurones in the rat. Br J Pharmacol 1999; 127:1765–1767.
166. Zygmunt PM, Petersson J, Andersson DA, Chuang H, Sfrgård M, Di Marzo V, Julius D, Högestätt ED. Vanilloid receptors on sensory nerves mediate the vasodilator action of anandamide. Nature 1999; 400:452–457.
167. Pertwee RG, Ross RA. Cannabinoid receptors and their ligands. Prostaglandins, Leukotrienes and Essential Fatty Acids. 2002; 66:101–121.
168. Ledent C, Valverde O, Cossu C, Petitet F, Aubert L–F, Beslot F, Böhme GA, Imperato A, Pedrazzini T, Roques BP, Vassart G, Fratta W, Parmentier M. Unresponsiveness to cannabinoids and reduced addictive effects of opiates in CB_1 receptor knockout mice. Science 1999; 283:401–404.
169. Zimmer A, Zimmer AM, Hohmann AG, Herkenham M, Bonner TI. Increased mortality, hypoactivity, and hypoalgesia in cannabinoid CB_1 receptor knockout mice. Proc Natl Sci USA 1999; 96: 5780–5785.

57

Antinociceptive Effects of Centrally Administered Neurotrophic Factors

Judith A. Siuciak
Pfizer Inc., Groton, Connecticut, U.S.A.

I. INTRODUCTION

In recent years, extensive research has shown that small proteins, collectively called the neurotrophins, have profound influences on the development, survival, regulation of function, and plasticity of diverse neuronal populations in both the central and peripheral nervous system (1,2). The neurotrophins comprise a family of homologous proteins which includes nerve growth factor (NGF), brain-derived neurotrophic factor (BDNF), neurotrophin-3 (NT-3), and neurotrophin-4/5 (NT-4/5). Despite the 50–55% similarity in the amino acid composition of these (3,4), the neurotrophins differ in terms of their spatial and temporal distribution, target specificity, and they operate through different high-affinity membrane receptors.

A family of tyrosine kinases, the Trks, function as specific and high-affinity receptors for these factors (5,6) Three *trk* family genes, designated *trk* A, *trk* B, and *trk* C have now been identified. Transcripts produced by each of the *trk* genes encode full-length (140- to 145-kDa) tyrosine kinase receptors (TrkA, TrkB, and TrkC, respectively). Each of these receptors includes an extracellular ligand-binding domain, a transmembrane domain, and an intracellular tyrosine kinase domain. NGF, BDNF, or NT-4/5, and NT3 bind with high affinity to and induce phosphorylation of, TrkA, TrkB, and TrkC, respectively. NT-3 can also bind to and phosphorylate TrkB, but with at least a tenfold lower affinity than to TrkC. Thus, the neurotrophins exhibit distinct, but occasionally, overlapping specificities for the Trk receptors.

Classic studies of these proteins have long focused on their trophic influences on the survival of various neuronal populations during development. A large amount of recent research has also addressed the potential therapeutic role of the neurotrophins in neurodegenerative diseases such as Alzheimer's, Parkinson's, and amyotrophic lateral sclerosis (ALS). However, notwithstanding their potential effects in development or degeneration, there is growing evidence suggesting that the neurotrophins may have a broader range of actions in the intact, adult central nervous system (CNS). The aim of the present chapter is to review recent studies addressing the neurochemical and behavioral effects of neurotrophic factors following central administration, with particular emphasis on actions related to the analgesic effects of these compounds.

II. DISTRIBUTION OF [^{125}I]-BDNF– AND [^{125}I]-NT-3–BINDING SITES

The studies summarized in the current chapter arose from experiments addressing the distribution of iodinated NT-3- and BDNF-binding sites in the intact, adult rat brain. In contrast with the relatively limited distribution of [^{125}I]-NGF binding, [^{125}I]-NT-3- and [^{125}I]-BDNF-binding sites were more numerous and much more widely distributed (7–9). Figure 1 shows the binding of [^{125}I]-NT-3 in a coronal section of the rat brain that includes the periaqueductal gray (PAG) area. Of particular interest to the present studies was the finding that binding sites for both NT-3 and BDNF were located in the periaqueductal gray, the raphe nuclei, and the dorsal spinal cord, areas that are known to play a role in the processing of nociceptive information. Studies addressing the distribution of *trk* mRNA in rat brian by in situ hybridization have also reported transcripts for trkB and trkC, the signal-transducing receptors for BDNF and NT-3, respectively, in the dorsal and median raphe nuclei (10) and in the midbrain periaqueductal gray (11). The presence of binding sites for the neurotrophic factors throughout areas comprising a well characterized nociceptive pathway, led us to question the potential role these factors might play in modulating nociceptive transmission. Furthermore, binding sites were also found throughout the various raphe nuclei, areas containing the largest population of serotonergic cell bodies within the central nervous system. A large body of evidence implicates serotonin in nociception and the analgesic action of morphine (12,13), thus the possible neuromodulatory actions of BDNF and NT-3 on serotonergic function was also of interest.

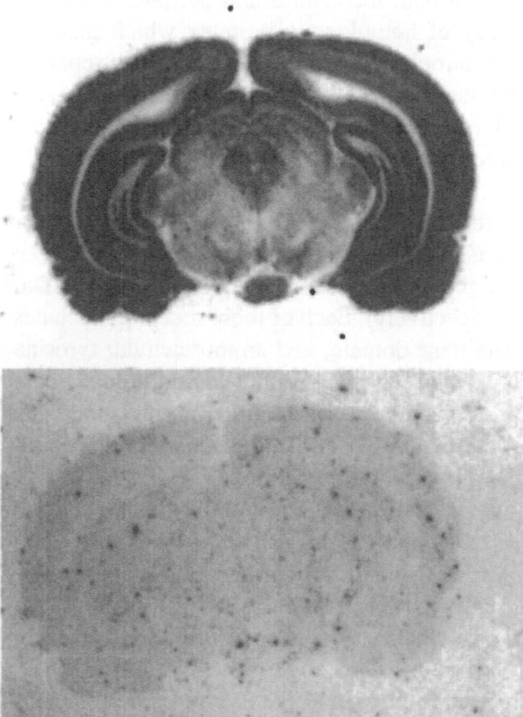

Figure 1 Autoradiographs showing the distribution of [^{125}I]-NT-3-binding sites in a coronal section of an adult rat brain: (top) total binding using 300 pM [^{125}I]-NT-3; (bottom) nonspecific binding obtained in the presence of 10 nM NT-3.

III. BEHAVIORAL EFFECTS OF CENTRALLY ADMINISTERED NEUROTROPHIC FACTORS

The neurotrophic proteins exist functionally as homodimers, with molecular weights of approximately 26 kDa; thus, their size prevents diffusion across the blood–brain barrier. All of the studies summarized in this chapter that address the neurochemical and behavioral effects of neurotrophic factors involve the direct intraparenchymal delivery of these proteins. Unless otherwise noted, these proteins were infused into the midbrain, adjacent to the PAG and dorsal/median raphe nuclei, using a permanent indwelling catheter attached to an osmotic minipump (14,15). These pumps infused either a phosphate-buffered saline (PBS) vehicle or neurotrophic factor for up to 14 days, during which time the animal was freely moving, and its behavior could be monitored. At the end of the infusion period, animals were sacrificed and the brains removed and processed for neurochemistry using high-performance liquid chromatography (HPLC) coupled to electrochemical detection or radioimmunoassay.

Our initial experiments demonstrated that central administration of BDNF into the midbrain was effective in producing analgesia in the tail-flick and hot-plate tests, two models employing a phasic, high-intensity nociceptive stimulus (14). The effect of BDNF administration in the Randall–Selitto paw pressure test is shown in Fig. 2. Midbrain BDNF infusion significantly increased the paw pressure threshold (117% increase, $p < 0.001$). Thus, BDNF is also effective in producing analgesia in an animal model utilizing a mechanical nociceptive stimulus.

BDNF administration also produced analgesia in the formalin test (15), an animal model of moderate, continuous pain which has been suggested to be a more clinically relevant pain model (16–18). The formalin test has been suggested as a model for the screening of mild analgesics [i.e., weak analgesics such as the nonsteroidal anti-inflammatory drugs (NSAIDs)]

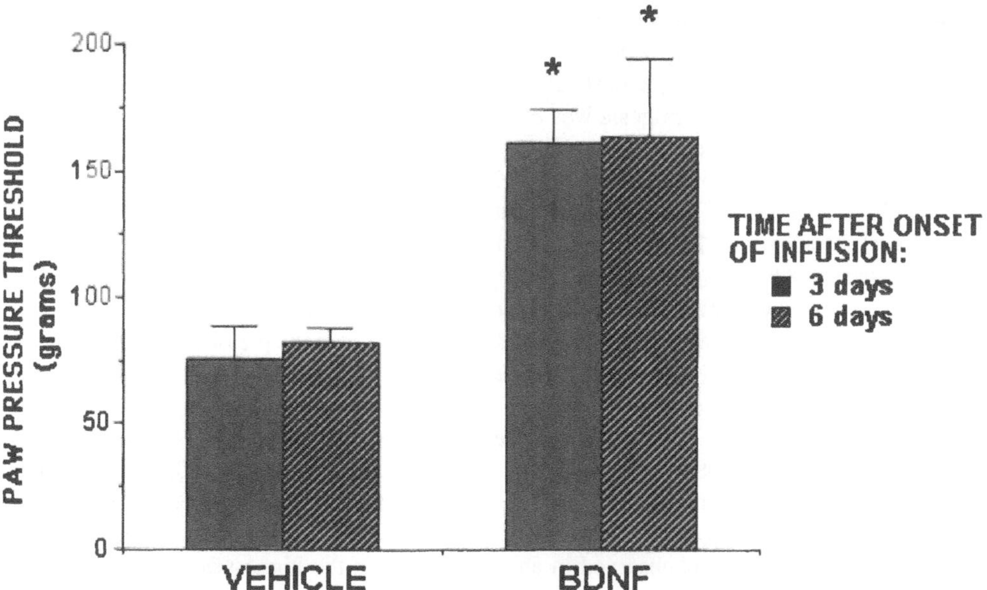

Figure 2 Analgesic effect of BDNF in the Randall–Selitto paw pressure test: Rats received midbrain infusions of PBS vehicle (12 μL/day) or BDNF (12 μg/day) and paw pressure thresholds (g) were assessed on day 8. Values shown are mean ± SEM for eight rats per group.

that have little or no effect in animal models using acute-phasic stimuli such as the tail-flick or hot-plate test (19–22). Midbrain infusion of BDNF decreased the behavioral paw flinch response to subcutaneous formalin injection in both the early and late phases of the test. Although the effect of midbrain-infused BDNF (12 μg/day) on the tail-flick was modest (i.e., an increase of several seconds), the use of formalin as a nociceptive stimulus revealed a more pronounced antinociceptive effect.

We have also assessed the effects of centrally administered BDNF in an animal model of peripheral mononeuropathic pain. This model displays many chronic pain symptoms similar to those found in humans, including *allodynia* (an innocuous stimulus perceived as painful), *hyperalgesia* (an exaggerated response to noxious stimulus), and signs of spontaneous pain (23,24). In the following experiments, the effect of BDNF administration was determined following loose ligation of the sciatic nerve that resulted in mechanical allodynia and hyperalgesia to thermal and mechanical stimuli. Ligation of the sciatic nerve was performed on day 1. Animals were tested using a thermal paw stimulator, von Frey hairs, or Randall–Selitto paw pressure apparatus. Withdrawal latencies to a noxious thermal and mechanical stimuli decreased significantly on the ligated side within 1 week after nerve ligation, indicating hindpaw hyperalgesia on the nerve-injured side compared with control hindpaw latencies. Hyperalgesia continued to persist for up to 4 weeks following nerve ligation surgery. Mechanical allodynia was also observed within the first 3 days after ligation of the sciatic nerve and persisted for a similar time frame.

On day 14, 2 weeks after the nerve ligation surgery, animals were infused with either PBS or BDNF into the midbrain. This time frame for surgery and BDNF infusion was chosen for two reasons: first, to allow for the behavioral assessment and removal of animals that did not show hyperalgesia and allodynia from the study. The remaining animals were randomly assigned to VEH or BDNF infusion groups. Second, we wished to utilize a time period when the behavioral response (hyperalgesia and allodynia) was stable. Mechanical and thermal hyperalgesia and mechanical allodynia were assessed on days 17 and 24 after surgery (3 and 10 days after the onset of infusion of vehicle or BDNF, respectively).

Figure 3 demonstrates that 2 weeks postsurgery, sciatic nerve ligation (lx) resulted in thermal hyperalgesia ($F_{1,36} = 5.8$; $p < 0.02$; sham/VEH = 11.03 ± 0.71 s; lx/VEH = 8.49 ± 0.58 s). However, thermal hyperalgesia was completely eliminated in animals receiving BDNF infusions, and withdrawal latencies returned to control levels as early as 3 days following the onset of infusion (day 17 after nerve ligation; 49% increase lx/BDNF vs. lx/VEH-infused rats). These beneficial effects were maintained without decrement or apparent tolerance for an additional week of infusion (day 24 after nerve ligation; lx/BDNF rats showed a 49% increase vs. lx/VEH-infused rats). Similar results were found when testing for mechanical hyperalgesia using the Randall–Selitto paw pressure test (Fig. 4), or mechanical allodynia using von Frey hairs (Fig. 5). Ligation of the sciatic nerve produced a decrease in paw pressure and withdrawal thresholds when compared with the sham-operated control rats, and infusion of BDNF reversed these decrements.

Additional studies have further characterized BDNF-induced analgesia using the tail-flick test. Animals infused with either PBS or BDNF at concentrations of 6, 12, 60, or 116 μg/day and tested on the tail-flick on days 1, 5, and 11 showed a dose-dependent increase in the tail-flick latency (Fig. 6). As the concentration of BDNF was increased, however, hyperreactivity and significant weight loss was observed in animals receiving the highest dose of BDNF (116 μg/day).

The onset and duration of action of BDNF is also shown in Fig. 6. Maximum analgesia was reached within 24 h and remained stable for the duration of the infusion, indicating no

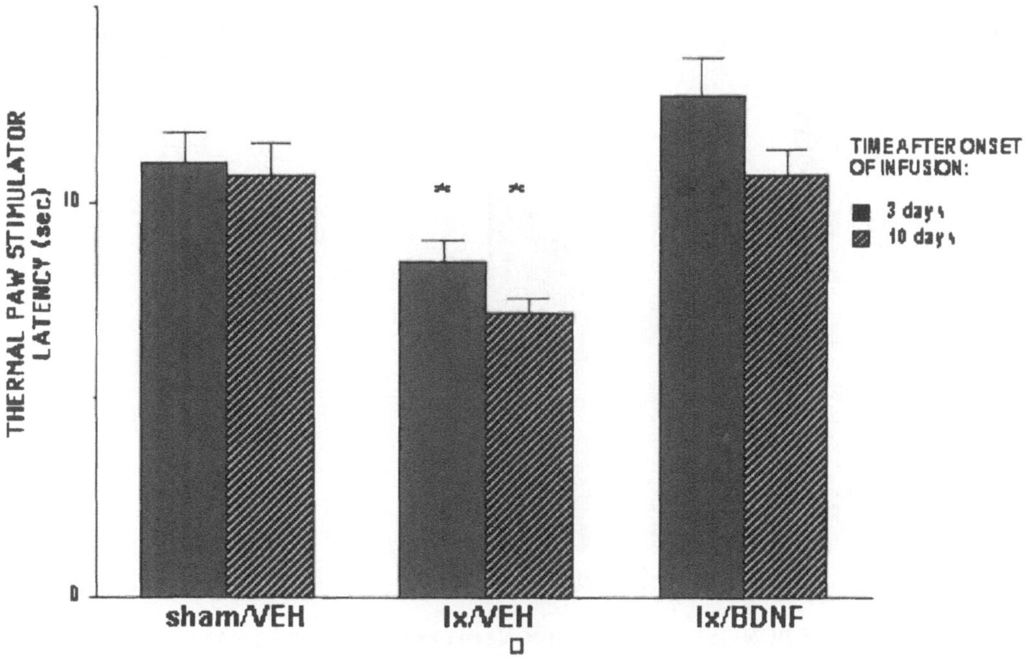

Figure 3 Effect of BDNF on thermal hyperalgesia associated with ligation of the sciatic nerve: Sciatic nerve ligation (lx) or sham surgery was performed 2 weeks before drug administration. Rats received midbrain infusions of PBS vehicle (12 μL/day) or BDNF (12 μg/day), and paw withdrawal latencies (s) were assessed at 3 and 10 days after the onset of infusion. Values shown are mean ± SEM for 7–13 rats per group.

development of tolerance. This time course was similar for all doses examined. In our previous studies, we have observed analgesia on the tail-flick test as early as 4 h after the onset of the BDNF infusion (15).

Previous studies have also shown that the BDNF-induced increase in tail-flick latency was reversible following cessation of the infusion (14). In these experiments, rats were infused with either BDNF or PBS vehicle for 11 days, at which time the infusion was terminated by removal of the osmotic pump. Within 24 h after pump removal, tail-flick latencies returned to normal baseline levels and remained stable when tested again 48 h after pump removal. Figure 7 shows the distribution of BDNF after midbrain infusion in animals that were receiving BDNF infusion at the time of sacrifice (see Fig. 7a) and animals in which the pump had been removed 24 h earlier (see Fig. 7b). In animals with active pumps, the spread of immunoreactivity following infusion of BDNF included the PAG, the dorsal and median raphe, and a large portion of the adjacent tegmentum. In contrast, when the pump was removed before sacrifice, the amount of immunoreactivity was greatly diminished. This decrease in BDNF following termination of the infusion paralleled the decrease in the analgesic response observed in the tail-flick test.

Other members of the neurotrophin family were also examined for their potential analgesic effects. Figure 8 compares the tail-flick latencies of rats receiving infusions of NGF, NT-3, BDNF, or NT-4. All neurotrophins were delivered at a concentration of 12 μg/day and the animals were tested on day 11 after the onset of infusion. No differences were seen between

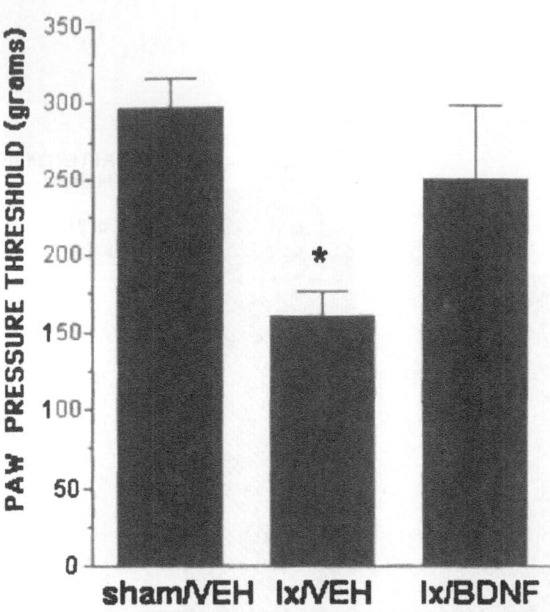

Figure 4 Effect of BDNF on mechanical hyperalgesia associated with ligation of the sciatic nerve: Sciatic nerve ligation (lx) or sham surgery was performed 2 weeks before drug administration. Rats received midbrain infusions of PBS vehicle (12 μL/day) or BDNF (12 μg/day) and paw pressure thresholds (g) were assessed at 10 days after the onset of infusion. Values shown are mean ± SEM for 7–13 rats per group.

vehicle and NGF-infused rats, although these data were limited to a single concentration of the neurotrophic factors. NT-4 and BDNF, which are both high-affinity ligands for the trkB site, showed equivalent effects on the tail-flick test and produced a greater analgesic effect than NT-3. This smaller effect of NT-3 paralleled the lower affinity of NT-3 at the trkB site, suggesting the analgesic effect of the neurotrophins may be mediated by the trkB receptor. Although not shown here, the analgesic effect of NT-3 and NT-4 in the tail-flick test showed an onset and duration of action similar to that observed with BDNF.

Several alternative sites of infusion for BDNF have been examined. Intracerebroventricular (i.c.v.) delivery increased tail-flick latencies similar to that seen with infusion near the PAG/dorsal raphe; however, the weight loss observed at this site was more severe, most probably due to other periventricular sites such as the hypothalamus (25). Infusions into the spinal cord, locus coeruleus, hippocampus, or cortex produced no analgesia on the tail-flick test (unpublished observations). The midbrain infusion site, near the PAG and dorsal and median raphe nuclei, permits BDNF access to the largest number of serotonergic cell bodies within the central nervous system. However, as seen in Fig. 7a and b, following midbrain infusion, BDNF diffusion is restricted to the areas immediately adjacent to the cannula. In contrast to the localized midbrain delivery, infusion of BDNF into the lateral ventricle permits BDNF access to a wide range of periventricular areas, including, but not restricted to, the PAG. The lack of an analgesic effect at sites distant from the PAG and raphe nuclei is most likely related to the poor distribution of BDNF within the parenchyma and failure of the protein to reach analgesia-sensitive sites.

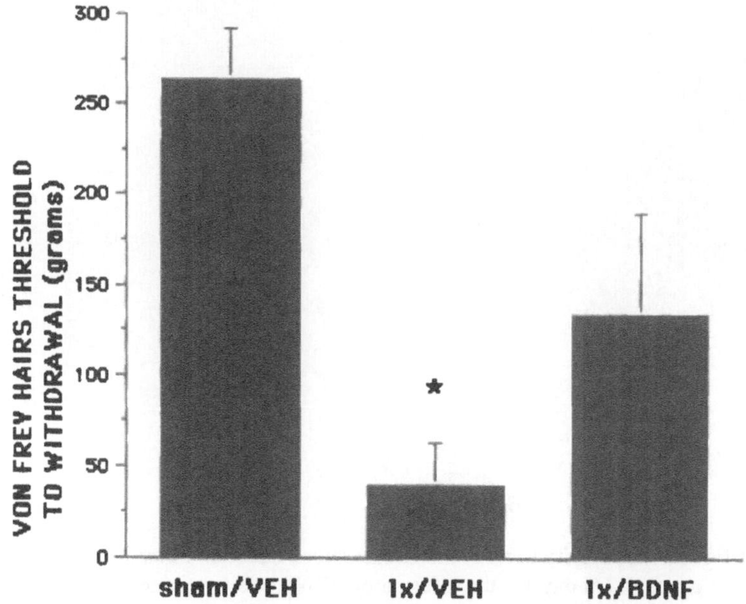

Figure 5 Effect of BDNF on mechanical allodynia associated with ligation of the sciatic nerve: Sciatic nerve ligation (lx) or sham surgery was performed 2 weeks before drug administration. Rats received midbrain infusions of PBS vehicle (12 μL/day) or BDNF (12 μg/day) and withdrawal responses to von Frey hairs (g) were assessed 10 days after the onset of infusion. Values shown are mean ± SEM for 7–13 rats per group.

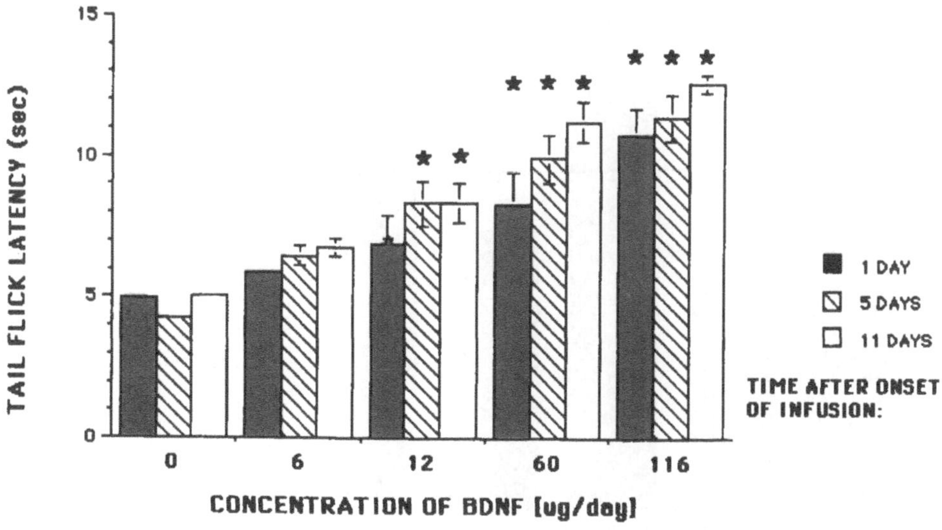

Figure 6 Dose–response to BDNF in the tail-flick test: Rats received midbrain infusions of PBS vehicle (12 μL/day) or BDNF (6–116 μg/day) and tail-flick latencies (s) were assessed on days 1, 5, and 11. Values shown are mean ± SEM for 10–12 rats per group.

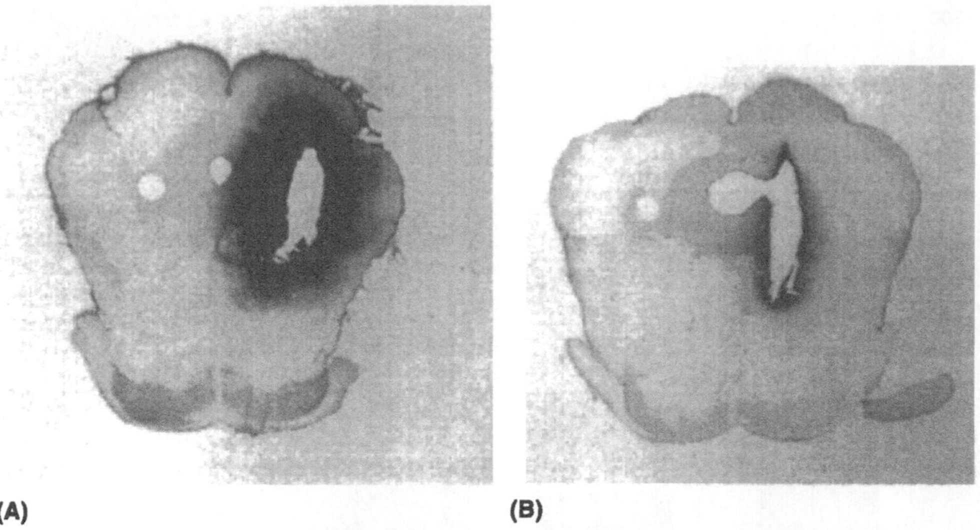

Figure 7 Distribution of BDNF immunoreactivity in rat brain: Rats received midbrain infusions of PBS vehicle (12 μL/day) or BDNF (12 μg/day). On day 11, the infusion of BDNF was terminated in half of the animals by removal of osmotic minipumps (B), whereas the osmotic pumps in the remaining animals were allowed to remain functional (A). Animals were sacrificed 24 h later and distribution of exogenously delivered BDNF was determined by BDNF immunocytochemistry.

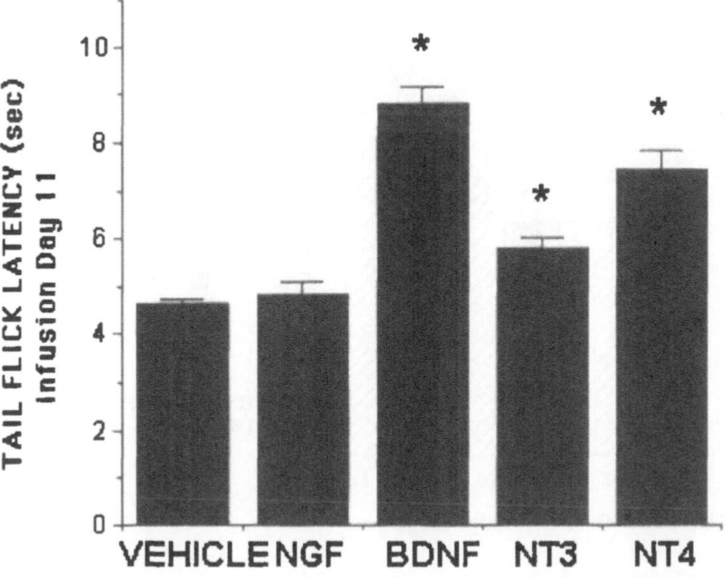

Figure 8 Comparison of the analgesic effects of neurotrophic factors in the tail-flick test: Rats received midbrain infusions of PBS vehicle (12 μL/day) or neurotrophic factor (12 μg/day) and tail-flick latencies (s) were assessed on day 11. Values shown are mean ± SEM for 8–12 rats per group.

IV. NEUROCHEMICAL EFFECTS OF CENTRALLY ADMINISTERED BDNF

A. Effects on Monoaminergic Systems

Given our initial observation of [^{125}I]-NT-3- and BDNF-binding sites within serotonergic areas of the brain, such as the raphe nuclei, additional studies were performed to determine the potential neurochemical effects of central BDNF. Figure 9 shows the levels of serotonin (5-HT) and 5-hydroxyindoleacetic acid (5-HIAA) in the PAG following infusion of PBS vehicle, BDNF, or NT-3. BDNF administration resulted in a significant increase in 5-HT (40%) and 5-HIAA (80%) levels, as well as an increase in serotonin turnover as measured by the 5-HIAA/5-HT ratio (20%) (14). Similar effects were seen in the dorsal and median raphe.

The serotonergic neurons in the dorsal and median raphe have widespread projections throughout the brain and spinal cord. Table 1 summarizes the neurochemical effects following midbrain infusion of BDNF. Alterations in 5-HT activity were observed in every brain area examined (25). Changes in 5-HT were limited to the site of the infusion, the PAG and dorsal and median raphe, as well as in the cortex. However, changes in 5-HIAA and the 5-HT/5-HIAA ratio were found in virtually every area examined, including the NRM and lumbar spinal cord, which together with the PAG, comprise a well-characterized descending pathway involved in the processing of nociceptive information. Forebrain areas, such as the cortex and hippocampus, also showed significant increases in serotonergic activity. Changes in dopaminergic activity were also seen, although these were not as robust as the 5-HT increases and were limited to increases in the metabolites dihydroxyphenylacetic acid (DOPAC) and homovanillic acid (HVA). No changes in norepinephrine or amino acids were observed in any of the brain areas examined (25).

Although it was clear that BDNF has a dramatic effect on serotonergic activity within the CNS, the mechanism of action on serotonin neurons was unclear. Our initial experiments were designed to determine whether BDNF had an effect on serotonin reuptake. However, infusion of BDNF into the midbrain had no significant effect on [^{3}H]5-HT uptake in either the PAG, DR, cortex, or spinal cord (Siuciak JA, unpublished observations). In the course of other experi-

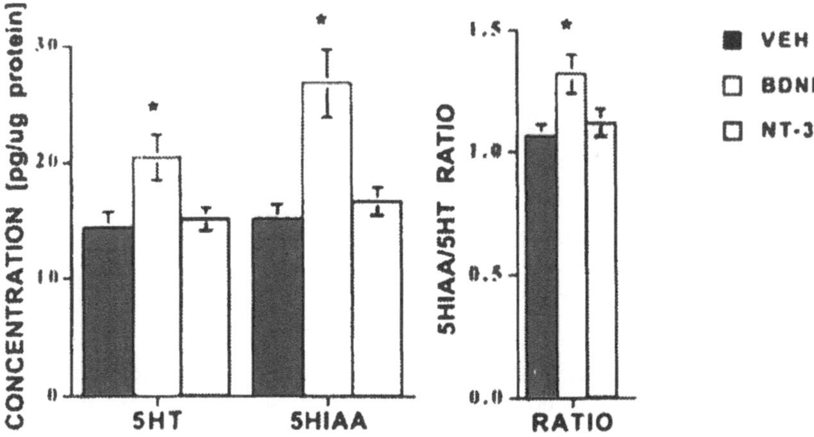

Figure 9 Effect of BDNF and NT-3 on serotonergic activity in the PAG: 5-HT and 5-HIAA concentrations (pg/μg protein) and 5HIAA/5HT ratio in the PAG of rats that received 14 days of continuous infusion of PBS vehicle (12 μL/day), or BNDF or NT-3 (12 μg/day). Values shown are mean ± SEM for 6–8 rats per group.

Table 1 Neurochemical Effects of BDNF[a]

Increased 5-HT levels
PAG
Dorsal/median raphe
Cortex
Increased 5-HIAA levels and increased 5-HIAA/5-HT ratio
PAG
Dorsal/median raphe
Nucleus raphe magnus
Dorsal spinal cord
Hippocampus
Cortex
Striatum
N. accumbens
Hypothalamus
Increased DOPAC and HVA levels
Cortex
Striatum

[a] Brain areas were obtained from rats that were continuously infused with either PBS vehicle (12 μL/day) or BNDF (12 μg/day) into the midbrain, near the PAG and dorsal/median raphe.
Source: Ref. 25.

ments in which alternative areas of the brain have been infused with BDNF, we have also failed to see an effect of BDNF on 5-HT uptake (26).

An alternative mechanism we have recently explored is the effect of BDNF on tryptophan hydroxylase (TPH), the rate-limiting enzyme in the synthesis of 5-HT. TPH converts tryptophan to 5-HT and is found only in cells that synthesize 5-HT. An increase in TPH levels or activity would be expected to result in an increase in 5-HT biosynthesis and availability, assuming sufficient availability of the precursor tryptophan and the tetrahydrobiopterin cofactor.

In these studies (27), TPH mRNA levels in the PAG/dorsal raphe taken from rats continuously infused with BDNF in vivo were measured using quantitative competitive reverse transcription polymerase chain reaction (RT-PCR). Midbrain BDNF infusion increased TPH expression by 13-fold as early as 24 h after the onset of infusion, and this increased expression remained elevated throughout the duration of the infusion (11 days), consistent with the prolonged elevation of tail-flick latencies. This increase in TPH mRNA levels was also seen following BDNF administration in the RN46A serotonergic cell line derived from raphe neurons, indicating a direct effect of BDNF on raphe neurons (27). Thus, BDNF may augment 5-HT synthesis in vivo by directly affecting steady-state TPH mRNA levels.

B. Effects on Peptidergic Systems

In addition to the serotonergic projections of the midbrain, substantial nonserotonergic projections from the PAG to the NRM or spinal cord, or both also exist. Several peptides localized in these projections are thought to play a role in nociception and analgesia. Thus, the modulation of neuropeptide systems by BDNF, whether a direct or indirect effect, may contribute to the antinociceptive effects of this protein. Additional studies have examined peptide levels within the brain and spinal cord following midbrain infusion of BDNF. Because our previous experiments had demonstrated naloxone reversibility of BDNF-induced analgesia (14), the endogenous opioid peptides, β-endorphin and metenkephalin were obvious candidates. Levels of β-endorphin were significantly increased in both the PAG (63%) and in the dorsal spinal cord (97%) (15). No changes in β-endorphin were found in the ventral spinal cord, striatum, or in the hypothalamus, where the cell bodies of these β-endorphin neurons are located. Metenkephalin levels in the PAG or striatum were unaffected by BDNF; however, there was a trend toward increased content of metenkephalin in the dorsal spinal cord (15). Whether the effect of BDNF on β-endorphin levels is direct or indirect, these studies have demonstrated a selective effect on intrinsic pools of β-endorphin within nociceptive areas (i.e., the PAG and dorsal spinal cord) without concomitant changes in other brain areas. Selectivity was also seen, in that within the PAG, increases in β-endorphin activity were not accompanied by alterations in levels of the other opioid peptide, metenkephalin. Thus, activation of β-endorphin pathways may underlie, at least in part, the analgesia elicited from midbrain infusion of BDNF in the rat.

Opioid receptors in the rat brain are also modulated following midbrain BDNF administration (28). In these studies, rat brain sections were hybridized with [^{33}P]-labeled riboprobes for μ-, δ-, or κ-opioid receptors. Image analysis was performed on autoradiograms containing areas of either the ventromedial/ventrolateral PAG at the site of the infusion (within a 0.3-mm radius) or adjacent (0.3–0.5 mm from infusion site) to the infusion site, as well as in the striatum. Comparison of the levels of mRNA for opioid receptor mRNA in PBS- and BDNF-treated rats indicated that BDNF administration significantly increased μ-receptors in the ventral/ventrolateral PAG areas at the site of infusion (ratio infused/uninfused side: VEH = 91.1 ± 2.6; BDNF = 117.8 ± 7.5, 29% increase; $p < 0.022$). However, adjacent ventral/ventrolateral PAG areas (ratio infused/uninfused side: VEH = 99.0 ± 4.2; BDNF = 112.3 ± 4.9; $p < 0.106$), showed no significant changes in μ-receptor mRNA. δ-Receptor mRNA in the PAG was upregulated by 29 and 14% at the site of infusion and adjacent areas (site of infusion, VEH = 101.0 ± 1.9; BDNF = 130.8 ± 5.4, $p < 0.001$; adjacent, VEH = 97.9 ± 1.5; BDNF = 112.0 ± 4.0; $p < 0.017$).

Prolonged midbrain infusion of BDNF also altered levels of substance P, a neurotransmitter associated with the transmission of nociceptive information from peripheral receptive fields into the CNS. Analgesic agents, such as morphine, act partly by inhibiting the release of substance P from primary nociceptive afferents (29–31). BDNF treatment resulted in a 113% increase in substance P levels in the dorsal spinal cord. No changes were found in the PAG, ventral spinal cord, or striatum (15).

Neuropeptide Y (NPY) is another widely distributed neuropeptide present in fibers and cell bodies in the dorsal horn of the spinal cord, and it has been reported to play a role in the modulation of nociceptive transmission (32,33). Following BDNF administration, NPY levels were increased in the dorsal spinal cord (64%) and striatum (93%), but unchanged in the PAG and ventral spinal cord (15). Previous studies have also reported BDNF-induced changes in NPY levels after hippocampal administration (34).

Thus, BDNF has a modulatory effect on relevant neuropeptides within areas of the brain and spinal cord involved in the processing of nociceptive information. Alterations in these neuropeptides by BDNF, either directly or indirectly, may play a role in the analgesia resulting from central BDNF administration.

V. CONCLUSION

The studies summarized in this chapter demonstrate that midbrain BDNF administration produces analgesia in several animal models of acute and chronic pain. We have also presented data indicating BDNF may be effective in alleviating symptoms of painful peripheral neuropathy. Furthermore, although long-term or repeated exposure to exogenously administered opioids may result in diminished therapeutic efficacy or tolerance, the beneficial effects of BDNF did not appear to diminish with continued infusion.

The underlying mechanism by which BDNF produces analgesia appears to involve, at least partly, changes in serotonergic activity, which reflect activation of supraspinal as well as descending serotonergic pathways, and parallels the antinociceptive actions of these neurotrophins. However, modulation of neuropeptides such as β-endorphin, may also be involved.

Relative to CNS applications of these molecules, the difficulty of delivering large proteins across the blood–brain barrier remains a problem. Implanted pumps and cannulae have been used to deliver several agents to the human central nervous system; however, the long-term delivery of proteins using these devices is without precedent. Furthermore, these factors have a limited diffusion following central administration, a problem that would be increased as brain size increased. These limitations appear to necessitate the development of second-generation approaches, such as carrier delivery systems (35), small molecule mimetics, effectors that regulate neurotrophic factor levels, or modulate their signal transduction mechanisms, or implantation of cells that have been genetically modified to secrete neurotrophic factors.

Additional problems may be found in terms of their selectivity. TrkB receptors, which mediate the actions of BDNF and other neurotrophins, are expressed by the vast majority of brain neurons, thus making it difficult to target these factors to selective brain populations. Even more problematic may be the effects of these neurotrophic factors on nonneuronal populations. Long-term administration could also lead to immunological responses, although for central administration, this would seem to be a minor problem.

REFERENCES

1. Lewin GR, Bard YA. Physiology of the neurotrophins. Annu Rev Neurosci 1996; 19:289–317.
2. Lindsay RM, Wiegand SJ, Altar CA, DiStefano PS. Neurotrophic factors: from molecule to man. Trends Neurosci 1994; 17:182–190.
3. Hohn A, Leibrock J, Bailey K, Barde Y–A. Identification and characterization of a novel member of the nerve growth factor/brain-derived neurotrophic factor family. Nature 1990; 344:339–341.
4. Maisonpierre PC, Belluscio L, Squinto S, Ip NY, Furth ME, Lindsay RM, Yancopoulos GD. NT-3; a neurotrophic factor related to NGF and BDNF. Science 1990; 247:1446–1451.
5. Barbacid M. The trk family of neurotrophin receptors. J Neurobiol 1994; 7:1484–1494.
6. Bothwell M. Functional interactions of neurotrophins and neurotrophin receptors. Annu Rev Neurosci 1995; 18:223–253.
7. Altar CA, Burton LE, Bennet G, Dugich–Djordjevic M. Recombinant human NGF is biologically active and labels novel high affinity binding sites in rat brain. Proc Natl Acad Sci USA 1991; 88: 281–285.
8. Altar CA, Siuciak JA, Wright P, Ip NY, Lindsay RM, Wiegand SJ. In situ hybridization of trkB and trkC receptor mRNA in rat forebrain and association with high-affinity binding of [^{125}I]-BNDF, NT-4/5 and NT-3. Eur J Neurosci 1994; 6:1389–1405.
9. Raivich G, Kruetzberg GW. The localization and distribution of high affinity nerve growth factor binding sites of the adult rat. A light microscopic autoradiographic study using [^{125}I]-NGF. Neuroscience 1987; 20:23–36.
10. Richardson RM, Verge VMK, Riopelle RJ. Distribution of neuronal receptors for nerve growth factor in the rat. J Neurosci 1986; 6:2312–2321.
11. Merlio JP, Ernfors P, Jaber C, Persson H. Molecular cloning of rat trkC and distribution of cells expressing mRNA for members of the trk family in the rat central nervous system. Neuroscience 1992; 51:513–532.
12. Richardson BR. Serotonin and nociception. Ann NY Acad Sci 1990; 600:511–525.
13. Sawynok J. The 1988 Merck Frost Award. The role of ascending and descending noradrenergic and

serotonergic pathways in opioid and non-opioid antinociception as revealed by lesion studies. Can J Physiol Pharmacol 1989; 67:975–988.

14. Siuciak JA, Altar CA, Wiegand SJ, Lindsay RM. Antinociceptive effect of brain-derived neurotrophic factor and neurotrophin-3. Brain Res 1994; 633:326–330.
15. Siuciak JA, Wong V, Pearsall D, Wiegand SJ, Lindsay RM. BDNF produces analgesia in the formalin test and modifies neuropeptide levels in rat brain and spinal cord areas associated with nociception. Eur J Neurosci 1995; 7:663–670.
16. Dubuisson D, Dennis SG. The formalin test: a quantitative study of the analgesic effects of morphine, meperidine and brain stem stimulation in rats and cats. Pain 1977; 4:161–174.
17. Abbott FV, Franklin KB, Ludwick RJ, Melzack R. Apparent lack of tolerance in the formalin test suggests different mechanisms for morphine analgesia in different types of pain. Pharmacol Biochem Behav 1981; 15:737–640.
18. Abbott FV, Melzack R, Samuel C. Morphine analgesia in the tail-flick and formalin pain tests is mediated by different neural systems. Exp Neurol 1982; 75:644–651.
19. Hunskaar S, Fasmer OB, Hole K. Antinociceptive effects of orphenadrine citrate in mice. Eur J Pharmacol 1985; 111:221–226.
20. Hunskaar S, Hole K. The formalin test in mice: dissociation between inflammatory and non-inflammatory pain. Pain 1987; 30:103–114.
21. Rosland JH, Tjolsen A, Maehle B, Hole K. The formalin test in mice: effect of formalin concentration. Pain 1990; 42:235–242.
22. Tjolsen A, Lund A, Hole K. Antinociceptive effect of paracetamol in rat is partly dependent on spinal serotonergic systems. Eur J Pharmacol 1991; 193:193–201.
23. Bennett GJ, Kajander KC, Sahara Y, Iadarola MJ, Sugimoto T. Neurochemical and anatomical changes in the dorsal horn of rats with an experimental painful peripheral neuropathy. In: Cervero F, Bennet GJ, Headly PM, eds. Processing of Sensory Information in the Superficial Dorsal Horn of the Spinal Cord. New York: Plenum, 1989; 463–471.
24. Bennett GJ, Xie YK. A peripheral mononeuropathy in rat that produces disorders of pain sensation like those seen in man. Pain 1988; 33:87–107.
25. Siuciak JA, Boylan C, Fritsche M, Lindsay RM. BDNF increases monoaminergic activity in rat brain following intracerebroventricular or intraparenchymal administration. Brain Res 1996; 633:326–330.
26. Mamounas LA, Blue ME, Siuciak JA, Altar CA. BDNF promotes the survival and sprouting of serotonergic axons in rat brain. J Neurosci 1995; 15:7929–7939.
27. Siuciak JA, Clark MS, Rind HB, Whittemore SR, Russo AF. BDNF induction of tryptophan hydroxylase mRNA levels in the rat brain. J Neurosci Res 1998; 52:149–158.
28. Siuciak JA, Lewis DR, Lindsay RM, Williams FG. BDNF increases opioid receptor mRNA expression in the PAG. Soc Neurosci Abstr 1996; 22:993.
29. Jessell TM, Iversen LL. Opiate analgesics inhibit substance P release from rat trigeminal nucleus. Nature 1977; 268:549–551.
30. Yaksh TL, Jessel TM, Gamse R, Mudge AW, Leeman SE. Intrathecal morphine inhibits substance P release from mammalian spinal cord in vivo. 1980; 286:155–157.
31. Brodin E, Gazelius B, Panopoulus P, Olgart L. Morphine inhibits substance P release from peripheral sensory nerve endings. Acta Physiol Scand 1983; 117:567–576.
32. Duggan AW, Hope PJ, Lang CW. Microinjection of NPY into the superficial dorsal horn reduces stimulus evoked release of immunoreactive substance P in the anesthetized cat. Neuroscience 1991; 44:733–740.
33. Hua XY, Boublik JH, Spicer MA, Rivier JE, Brown MR, Yaksh TL. The antinociceptive effects of spinally administered NPY in the rat: systematic studies on structure activity relationships. J Pharmacol Exp Ther 1991; 258:243–248.
34. Croll SD, Eidgand SJ, Anderson KD, Lindsay RM, Nawa H. Neuropeptide regulation by BDNF and NGF in adult rat forebrain. Eur J Neurosci 1994; 6:1343–1353.
35. Croll SD, Chesnutt CR, Rudge JS, Ryan TE, Siuciak JA, DiStephano PS, Wiegand SJ, Lindsay RM. Co-infusions with a trkB-Fc receptor body carrier enhances BDNF distribution in the adult rat brain. Exp Neurol 1998; 152:20–33.

58
Peripheral Neurotrophic Factors and Pain

Lorne M. Mendell
State University of New York at Stony Brook, Stony Brook, New York, U.S.A.

I. INTRODUCTION

One of the hallmarks of nociceptive afferents is their sensitization following stimuli that cause inflammation. Sensitization is characterized by a lowering of the threshold of individual nociceptive afferents, as well as their increased firing frequency at a given stimulus level. The result is inflammatory hyperalgesia, the persistence of which can represent a serious clinical problem requiring therapeutic attention. The mechanisms underlying this sensitization are complex (see later discussion), but it now seems clear that substances released into the injured region play an important role in this action. The ability of these substances to contribute to sensitization depends not only on their appearance or up-regulation as a result of injury, but also on the availability of appropriate receptors on cells, including the nociceptive afferents themselves. One of the striking findings is the number of substances that contribute to peripheral sensitization (e.g., prostaglandin E_2 [PGE_2], serotonin, and bradykinin (1)). It has now become apparent that peripherally released nerve growth factor (NGF) also contributes to hyperalgesia during inflammation (2).

This has come as somewhat of a surprise because NGF was originally thought to be a prenatal survival factor for small-diameter nociceptive sensory neurons expressing peptides such as substance P or calcitonin gene-related peptide (CGRP) (3) and terminating in the superficial dorsal horn (4). However, with the discovery of the high-affinity receptor for NGF, trkA, and the availability of antibodies to permit its localization (5), several interesting facts have emerged. Most importantly for the present discussion, the high-affinity receptors for NGF are present on many small-diameter neurons in the adult rat (6). This suggests that the role of NGF is more extensive than its developmental role that was previously well established. In this chapter we concentrate on the role of peripherally administered neurotrophins on inflammatory pain mechanisms, and then briefly discuss their role in neuropathic pain.

II. NGF AND INFLAMMATORY PAIN

Two lines of evidence came together to suggest a role for NGF in inflammatory pain. The first of these was that NGF is up-regulated in the skin after inflammatory injury (7). This up-regulation begins virtually immediately after injury and lasts for several hours. A second finding was that administration of exogenous NGF to animals, either systemically (8) or locally (9,10), leads to hyperalgesia. Similar experiments in humans as part of clinical trials confirmed that NGF administered exogenously either systemically (11) or locally (12) is sufficient to cause pain. In animals it was determined that the onset of inflammatory thermal hyperalgesia has a rapid onset, within about 30 min (8,13). After systemic injection thermal hyperalgesia lasts several days (8); after local injection (Fig. 1) the duration is of the order of hours to 1 day (10). Thus, although NGF has local peripheral effects, it undoubtedly affects other systems that can act to prolong the thermal hyperalgesia. Systemic administration of NGF also elicits mechanical hyperalgesia, but this effect differs from thermal hyperalgesia in having an onset latency of several hours, rather than several minutes (8). There is also evidence that NGF can elicit allodynia that is associated with a novel ability of large-diameter fibers both to express substance P (14) and to evoke "windup" of motoneuron responses that can be prevented by application of antagonists to the neurokinin-1 receptor (15).

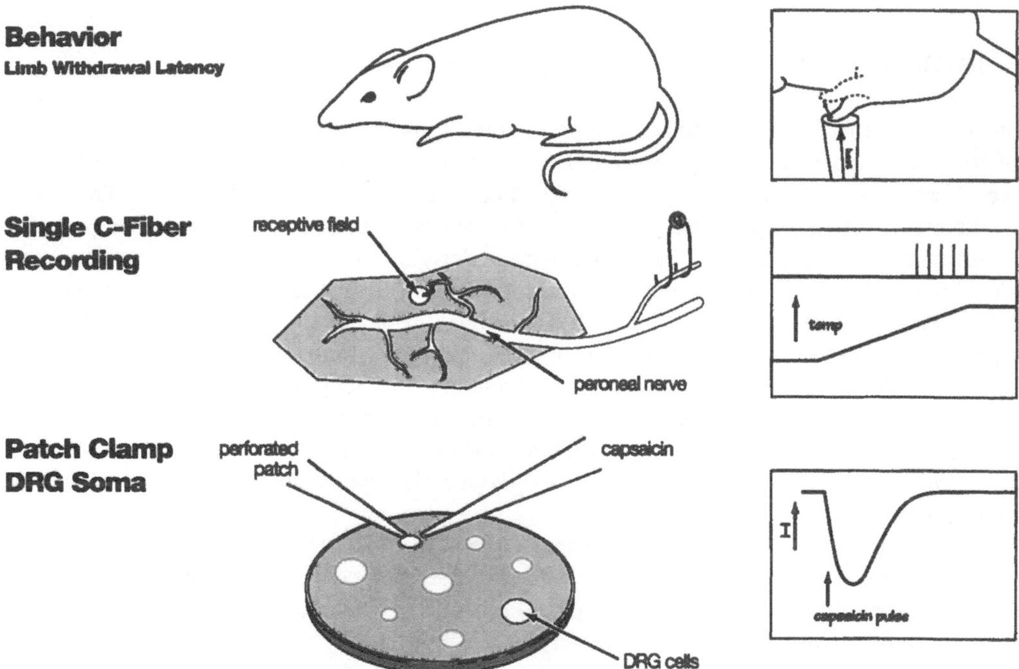

Figure 1 Different experimental approaches to the study of sensitization of nociceptive afferents by neurotrophins, (e.g., NGF): Behavioral experiments are depicted (top) in which a local application of a noxious heat stimulus leads to withdrawal of the limb. The latency to withdrawal is an indication of sensitivity to noxious heat (Hargreaves method). Comparison of mean withdrawal latency of a hindlimb treated by microinjection with a substance such as NGF and the contralateral limb treated with a placebo provides an index of the sensitizing effect of the substance. (Middle row) the in vitro isolated skin–nerve preparation. Heating the skin on its epidermal surface (below) leads to discharge of afferent fibers isolated on the recording nerve strand. Application of NGF or other sensitizing agent to the receptive field of the unit on the surface of the corium can result in increased sensitivity of the unit to heat, measured as a decrease in threshold temperature. (Bottom row) perforated patch recording from a DRG cell isolated in dissociated cell culture. A second electrode filled with capsaicin is placed close to the patched cell and the response to a brief puff of capsaicin is measured as an inward current (I) in voltage clamp. NGF can rapidly condition this response to capsaicin. For further details see text and references noted therein.

III. NGF AND PERIPHERAL SENSITIZATION

Behavioral studies opened the possibility that NGF is able to sensitize individual sensory afferents to noxious heat stimulation. This was confirmed by recording from individual small-diameter cutaneous afferents in the in vitro skin preparation (16). When NGF was placed into the solution bathing the corium surface of the isolated skin, the response of most individual small-diameter afferents to noxious heat was sensitized as determined by a reduction in their threshold (see Fig. 1). In these experiments the search stimulus was mechanical, and so some small-diameter units were found that were not sensitive to the noxious heat stimulus. In some of these cases the "silent" fibers became sensitive to the noxious thermal stimulus after treatment with NGF. These data indicate that NGF sensitizes small-diameter afferents to noxious heat. No sensitization to mechanical stimuli was observed. This agrees with the lack of a rapid sensitization to mechanical stimulation measured behaviorally (8). In effect these differences argue for two mechanisms of sensitization, one peripheral, as demonstrated directly by recording from individual afferent fibers (16), and the other nonperipheral and, thus presumably, central (Fig. 2).

A. Role of Mast Cells

Behavioral experiments revealed more details concerning the peripheral and central mechanisms of NGF-induced hyperalgesia. A role for mast cells was established for peripheral sensitization because prior degranulation of mast cells by application of 48/80 delayed the appearance of NGF-induced sensitization to noxious heat (9,13). A similar finding was made in electrophysiological studies of individual afferents (16). The membrane of mast cells expresses the trkA receptor (17) and NGF can elicit degranulation of mast cells (18). It was suggested that the degranulation products, specifically serotonin, sensitized nociceptive afferents (13). Prior mast cell degranulation did not prevent the development of the later component of hyperalgesia. This

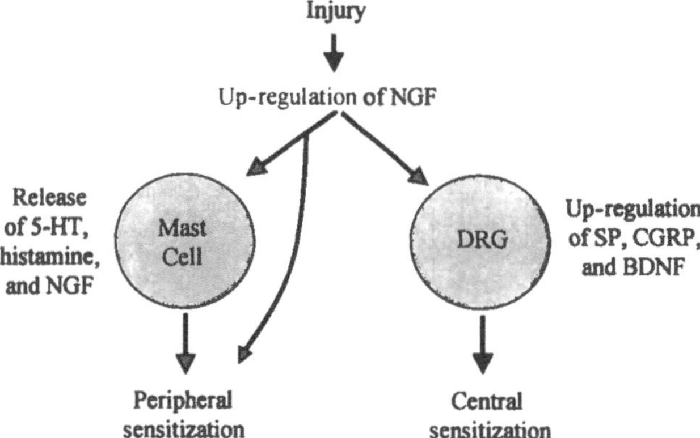

Figure 2 Scheme to illustrate peripheral and central effects of NGF in producing inflammatory hyperalgesia: Injury by traumatic events, such as burns, results in up-regulation of NGF by the action of cytokines, such as TNF-α and IL 1-β (Left): NGF can act either directly on terminals of trkA-expressing neurons (i.e., nociceptive afferents) or on mast cells that release sensitizing agents, such as serotonin, histamine, or NGF itself, to produce peripheral sensitization. The action of NGF on these sensory afferents also results in up-regulation of peptides and BDNF in DRG cell bodies which increases the activation of NMDA receptors on cells in the spinal cord, producing central sensitization.

was eliminated by prior systemic treatment with dizicilpine (MK-801) (13), suggesting that it involved the *N*-methyl-D-aspartate (NMDA) receptor in the spinal cord.

B. Direct Effects of NGF on Nociceptive Afferents

Recent experiments have added considerable detail to these mechanisms. In the periphery, events leading to the upregulation of NGF depend on prior up-regulation of the cytokines TNF-α and interleukin (IL)-1β (19). However, although degranulation of mast cells could reduce or even eliminate the early component of NGF-induced sensitization, sensitization could occur under some conditions despite prior degranulation of mast cells (20). This has been taken to suggest that NGF might have a direct sensitizing effect on primary nociceptive afferents known to express trkA receptors. Consistent with this is that mast cells themselves contain NGF (21) that might play a role in mast cell-induced sensitization of nociceptive afferents to noxious thermal stimulation.

Recent experiments have provided evidence that NGF can directly sensitize responses of small-diameter sensory afferents. Sensory neuron cell bodies were studied in dissociated cell culture to avoid the ambiguity that would result from investigation of afferent terminals in the skin where many other cell types that potentially contribute to the response are present (see Fig. 1). A receptor for noxious heat is the VR-1 receptor that also responds to capsaicin (22). Administration of capsaicin elicits thermal pain in human subjects (23). Thus, the response of sensory neurons to capsaicin was studied as a substitute for noxious heat (24). NGF acutely sensitized the response of the cell body to capsaicin and reversed the tachyphylaxis (25) exhibited by the second of two responses to brief puffs of capsaicin delivered 10 min after the first. This action of NGF was very rapid, within minutes, similar to the rapid sensitization to noxious heat by NGF observed behaviorally. It exhibited a dependency on the concentration of NGF in the medium that ranged between 2 and 100 ng/mL (24). Although these actions were on DRG cell bodies, the short latency of the response indicates that it does not involve transcription and thus is independent of the nucleus. Thus, what was observed in the cultured cell body could also be expected to occur in the sensory terminals, indicating the potential for a direct effect of NGF in sensitizing the response of nociceptive neurons to noxious heat.

IV. NGF AND CENTRAL SENSITIZATION

The NMDA-mediated central component of behavioral sensitization was originally believed (13) to be the result of NGF-induced up-regulation of peptide levels in nociceptive neurons previously shown to take place (Fig. 2) (9,26). This was assumed to increase release of these neuropeptides from the central terminals of nociceptive afferents. This would lead indirectly to greater activation of the NMDA receptors in superficial laminae of the spinal cord owing to their greater level of peptide-induced depolarization and subsequent relief from magnesium blockade (27). More recently, activation of trkA in the peripheral terminals of nociceptive afferents by NGF has been found to enhance levels of another neurotrophin, brain-derived neurotrophic factor (BDNF), in their cell bodies (28–30). Exogenous administration of the immunoadhesin molecule trkB-IgG reduces the effects of nociceptive stimulation consistent with the notion that BDNF is released into the spinal cord to activate nociceptive interneurons (30,31). Recent evidence suggests that BDNF can directly enhance the response of NMDA receptors in motoneurons in neonatal rats (Arvanian and Mendell, 2001), and thus presumably in the superficial dorsal horn where trkB receptors are expressed in adults (30).

V. ROLE OF trkB AGONISTS IN PERIPHERAL SENSITIZATION

BDNF and the other trkB agonist NT-4/5 also have a hyperalgesic effect in the periphery (10). Electrophysiological studies on single afferents confirm the sensitization by these agents (10,16), and the effects of NT-4/5 can be prevented by prior mast cell degranulation. This suggests either that mast cells also express trkB receptors (32) or that NT-4/5 can activate trkA receptors (33). NT-4/5 also can condition the response to capsaicin currents measured in dissociated cell culture (24). In both the behavioral and electrophysiological investigations NT-3, the agonist for the trkC receptor, failed to elicit any signs of hyperalgesia (10,24).

VI. NGF AS A NECESSARY COMPONENT OF INFLAMMATORY HYPERALGESIA

The studies just discussed illustrate that administration of NGF is sufficient to induce hyperalgesia. Because NGF is up-regulated after inflammation, a significant question is whether it is necessary for inflammatory hyperalgesia. This question has been approached by asking whether preventing the up-regulation of NGF can reduce the hyperalgesia accompanying experimentally induced inflammation. This has been accomplished in two ways: first, by administering an antibody to NGF in association with the experimental inflammatory agent (9,13), and second, by administering the immunoadhesin trkA-IgG to neutralize any free NGF (34). Both treatments virtually abolished hyperalgesia measured by means of the Hargreaves test.

In certain respects this is a surprising finding, for numerous hyperalgesic agents such as bradykinin and PGE_2 are up-regulated after inflammation, and it might have been expected that these would have continued to induce hyperalgesia, although at a reduced level (35). The implication of these findings is that these agents interact at some level (i.e., their effects are not independent). Such interactions are known to take place (e.g., NGF interacts with the bradykinin system) (36; see review in 35). Furthermore, each of these agents work through the second-messenger systems at the level of the primary afferent or perhaps other cells as well; hence, it is not unreasonable to expect that abolishing one of the components would prevent the others from exerting their normal effect.

VII. JOINT AND VISCERAL AFFERENTS

This chapter has concentrated on the effects of neurotrophins on inflammatory hyperalgesia transmitted from the skin by impulses in cutaneous afferent fibers. It is important to acknowledge that these agents might also play important roles in the inflammatory hyperalgesia from other structures, such as viscera, joints, and muscle. Neurotrophins are up-regulated in the inflamed bladder (37) and NGF sensitizes the response of bladder afferents to mechanical stimulation (38). In agreement with this administration of trkA-IgG abolishes the hyperreflexia associated with bladder inflammation (39). Experimental models of arthritis lead to increased discharges of joint nociceptors and previously ''silent'' nociceptors begin to exhibit activity (40). Both acute (16) and systemic (41) treatments with NGF result in increased sensitivity of noxious thermoreceptors innervating the skin, and thresholds are increased if NGF levels are artificially lowered (42). The finding that NGF levels are elevated in the synovial fluid of arthritic joints (43), coupled with the changes observed in the bladder, suggest that NGF's role in inflammatory hyperalgesia is probably quite general.

VIII. NGF AND NEUROPATHIC PAIN

Finally, it is important to point out a possible role for NGF in reversing the changes that may account for neuropathic pain after peripheral nerve injury. Several mechanisms have been implicated in the pain that accompanies these injuries. Of specific interest here is the allodynia that occurs whereby stimuli that are normally not painful become painful, often excruciatingly so. One mechanism thought to be important in this change is the accumulation of sodium channels in the membrane of the central cut end of the damaged fibers (i.e., in the neuroma) (44). This may enhance the sensitivity of these fibers to mechanical activation of their cut end. The central terminals of large fibers in the damaged nerve sprout from the deeper laminae in the dorsal horn into the more superficial ones to potentially activate cells important in transmission of nociceptive stimuli (45,46). This sprouting probably results from the lack of some message coming from the damaged nonmyelinated fibers normally innervating these superficial laminae which themselves do not degenerate because they are cut in the periphery (47). Provision of NGF to the cut end prevents this sprouting response (48) and thus might be expected to reduce neuropathic pain (49).

An additional consequence of peripheral nerve damage is the invasion of sympathetic axons into ganglion cells (50) that would enhance the potential for hyperalgesia and allodynia. NGF delivered directly to the dorsal root ganglion enhances this sprouting, and provision of anti-NGF inhibits it (51). Thus, the effect of NGF on persistent pain following nerve damage is likely to be complex because it initiates changes that can increase or decrease the painful consequences.

IX. CONCLUSION

We have summarized the effects of peripherally administered NGF on inflammatory and neuropathic pain. In inflammation the situation appears to be relatively simple because NGF elicits sensitization, either peripheral or central, which always enhances the painful quality of a stimulus. Thus, reduction of NGF levels locally at the site of inflammation would be expected to have therapeutic value, all other factors being equal. In neuropathic pain the situation is more complex because changes induced by NGF can have opposite effects. However, even here it might be possible to selectively activate the beneficial effects of NGF; for example, by applying it to the cut end of the nerve, rather than intrathecally. These studies also indicate that NGF administered for other purposes might have some pain-producing side effects that would contraindicate its use, or at least require countermeasures.

At a more basic level these findings indicate the close linkage between developmental neurobiology and pain physiology in that a molecule whose role in development is as a survival factor is also "used" in adults as an inflammatory mediator and as a stimulant of axonal sprouting. These multiple roles for the same molecule point to complex intracellular-signaling mechanisms whose elucidation will almost certainly provide new insights into pain mechanisms and the role of neurotrophins in modulating them.

Note added in Proof: It has now been demonstrated that MAPkinase and PKC do not contribute to the interaction between trkA and VR1; however, the effect of NGF can be reduced by inhibitors of PKA (52). Phospholipase C has recently been shown to be a major mediator of the interaction between trkA and VR1 (53; Shu and Mendell, unpublished observations). The effect of NGF on the membrane currents induced in sensory neurons by noxious heat is similar to its effect on the inward currents produced by capsaicin (54).

ACKNOWLEDGMENTS

The author's work described in this chapter was supported primarily by NS-32264 and by NS-14899 from NINDS–NIH. Additional support was provided by NS 16996 (Javits Neuroscience Award) and a grant from the Christopher Reeve Paralysis Foundation.

REFERENCES

1. Kress M, Reeh P. Chemical excitation and sensitization in nociceptors. In: Belmonte C, Cervero F, eds. The Neurobiology of Nociceptors. Oxford: Oxford University Press, 1996:258–297.
2. Lewin GR, Mendell LM. Nerve growth factor and nociception. Trends Neurosci 1993; 16:353–359.
3. Goedert M, Otten U, Hunt SP, Bond A, Chapman D, Schlumpf M, Lichtensteiger W. Biochemical and anatomical effects of antibodies against nerve growth factor on developing rat sensory ganglia. Proc Natl Acad Sci USA 1984; 81:1580–1584.
4. Ruit KG, Elliott JL, Osborne PA, Yan Q, Snider WD. Selective dependence of mammalian dorsal root ganglion neurons on nerve growth factor during embryonic development. Neuron 1992; 8:573–587.
5. Mendell LM. Neurotrophic factors and the specification of neural function. Neuroscientist 1995; 1: 26–34.
6. McMahon SB, Armanini MP, Ling LH, Phillips HS. Expression and coexpression of trk receptors in subpopulations of adult primary sensory neurons projecting to identified peripheral targets. Neuron 1994; 12:1161–1171.
7. Donnerer J, Schuligoi R, Stein C. Increased content and transport of substance P and calcitonin gene-related peptide in sensory nerves innervating inflamed tissue: evidence for a regulatory function of nerve growth factor in vivo. Neuroscience 1992; 49:693–698.
8. Lewin GR, Ritter AM, Mendell LM. Nerve growth factor-induced hyperalgesia in the neonatal and adult rat. J Neurosci 1993; 13:2136–2148.
9. Woolf CJ, Safieh–Garabedian B, Ma Q–P, Crilly P, Winter J. Nerve growth factor contributes to the generation of inflammatory sensory hypersensibility. Neuroscience 1994; 62:327–331.
10. Shu X, Llinas A, Mendell LM. Effects of trkB and trkC neurotrophin receptor agonists on thermal nociception: a behavioral and electrophysiological study. Pain 1999; 80:463–470.
11. Petty BG, Cornblath DR, Aldornato BT, Chaudhry V, Flexner C, Wachsman M, Sinicropi D, Burton LE, Peroutka SJ. The effect of systemically administered recombinant human nerve growth factor in healthy human subjects. Ann Neurol 1994; 36:244–246.
12. Dyck PJ, Peroutka S, Rask C, Burton E, Baker MK, Lehman KA, Gillen DA, Hokanson JL, O'Brien PC. Intradermal recombinant human nerve growth factor induces pressure allodynia and lowered heat-pain threshold in humans. Neurology 1997; 48:501–505.
13. Lewin GR, Rueff A, Mendell LM. Peripheral and central mechanisms of NGF-induced hyperalgesia. Eur J Neurosci 1994; 6:1903–1912.
14. Neumann S, Doubell TP, Leslie T, Woolf CJ. Inflammatory pain hypersensitivity mediated by phenotypic switch in myelinated primary sensory neurons. Nature 1996; 384:360–364.
15. Thompson SWN, Dray A, McCarson KE, Krause JE, Urban L. Nerve growth factor induces mechanical allodynia associated with novel A fiber-evoked spinal reflex activity and enhanced neurokinin-1 receptor activation in the rat. Pain 1995; 62:219–231.
16. Rueff A, Mendell LM. Nerve growth factor and NT-5 induce increased thermal sensitivity of cutaneous nociceptors in vitro. J Neurophysiol 1996; 76:3593–3596.
17. Horigome K, Pryor JC, Bullock ED, Johnson, EM Jr. Mediator release from mast cells by nerve growth factor. J Biol Chem 1993; 268:14881–14887.
18. Mazurek N, Weskamp G, Erne P, Otten U. Nerve growth factor induces mast cell degranulation without changing intracellular calcium levels. FEBS Lett 1986; 198:315–320.
19. Woolf CJ, Ma QP, Allchorne A, Poole S. Peripheral cell types contributing to the hyperalgesic action of nerve growth factor in inflammation. J Neurosci 1996; 16:2716–2723.

20. Amann R, Schuligoi R, Herzeg G, Donnerer J. Intraplantar injection of nerve growth factor into the rat hind paw: local edema and effects on thermal nociceptive threshold. Pain 1995; 64:323–329.
21. Leon A, Buriani A, Dal Toso R, Fabris M, Romanello S, Aloe L, Levi-Montalcini R. Mast cells synthesize, store, and release nerve growth factor. Proc Natl Acad Sci USA 1994; 91:3739–3743.
22. Caterina MJ, Schumacher MA, Tominaga M, Rosen TA, Levine JD, Julius D. The capsaicin receptor: a heat activated ion channel in the pain pathway. Nature 1997; 389:816–824.
23. LaMotte R, Lundberg LE, Torebjork HE. Pain, hyperalgesia and activity in nociceptive C units in humans after intradermal injection of capsaicin. J Physiol (Lond) 1992; 448:749–764.
24. Shu X, Mendell LM. Nerve growth factor acutely sensitizes the response of adult rat sensory neurons to capsaicin. Neurosci Lett 1999; 274:159–162.
25. Koplas PA, Rosenberg RL, Oxford GS. The role of calcium in the desensitization of capsaicin responses in rat dorsal root ganglion neurons. J Neurosci 1997; 17:3525–3537.
26. Lindsay RM, Harmar AJ. Nerve growth factor regulates expression of neuropeptide genes in adult sensory neurons. Nature 1989; 337:362–364.
27. McMahon SB, Lewin GR, Wall PD. Central hyperexcitability triggered by noxious inputs. Curr Opin Neurobiol 1993; 3:602–610.
28. Apfel SC, Wright DE, Wiideman AM, Dormia C, Snider WD, Kessler JA. Nerve growth factor regulates the expression of brain-derived neurotrophic factor mRNA in the in the peripheral nervous system. Mol Cell Neurosci 1996; 7:134–142.
29. Michael GJ, Averill S, Nitkunan A, Rattray M, Bennett DLH, Yan Q, Priestley JV. Nerve growth factor treatment increases brain derived neurotrophic factor selectively in trkA-expressing dorsal root ganglion cells and in their central terminations within the spinal cord. J Neurosci 1997; 17:8476–8490.
30. Mannion RJ, Costigan M, Decosterd I, Amaya F, Ma QP, Holstege JC, Ji RR, Acheson A, Lindsay RM, Wilkinson GA, Woolf CJ. Neurotrophins: peripherally and centrally acting modulators of tactile stimulus-induced inflammatory pain hypersensitivity. Proc Natl Acad Sci USA 1999; 96:9385–9390.
31. Kerr BJ, Bradbury EJ, Bennett DL, Trivedi PM, Dassan P, French J, Shelton DB, McMahon SB, Thompson SW. Brain-derived neurotrophic factor modulates nociceptive sensory inputs and NMDA-evoked responses in the rat spinal cord. J Neurosci 1999; 19:5138–5148.
32. Tam SY, Tsai M, Yamaguchi M, Yano K, Butterfield JH, Galli SJ. Expression of functional TrkA receptor tyrosine kinase in the HMC-1 human mast cell line and in human mast cells. Blood 1997; 90:1807–1820.
33. Berkemeier LR, Winslow JW, Kaplan DR, Nikolics K, Goeddel DV, Rosenthal A. Neurotrophin-5: a novel neurotrophic factor that activates trkA and trkB. Neuron 1991; 7:857–866.
34. McMahon SB, Bennett DL, Priestley JV, Shelton DL. The biological effects of endogenous nerve growth factor on adult sensory neurons revealed by a trkA–IgG fusion molecule. Nat Med 1995; 1:774–780.
35. Levine JD, Taiwo Y. Inflammatory Pain. In: Wall PD, Melzack R, eds. Textbook of Pain. Edinburgh: Churchill Livingstone, 1994:45–56.
36. Rueff A, Dawson AJ, Mendell LM. Characteristics of nerve growth factor induced hyperalgesia in adult rats: dependence on enhanced bradykinin-1 receptor activity but not neurokinin-1 receptor activation. Pain 1996; 66:359–372.
37. Oddiah D, Anand P, McMahon SB, Rattray M. Rapid increase of NGF, BDNF and NT-3 mRNAs in inflamed bladder. Neuroreport 1998; 9:1455–1458.
38. Dmitrieva N, McMahon SB. Sensitisation of visceral afferents by nerve growth factor in the adult rat. Pain 1996; 66:87–97.
39. Dmitrieva N, Shelton D, Rice ASC, McMahon SB. The role of nerve growth factor in a model of visceral inflammation. Neuroscience 1997; 78:449–459.
40. Schaible HG, Schmidt RF. Effects of an experimental arthritis on the sensory properties of fine articular afferent units. J Neurophysiol 1985; 54:1109–1122.
41. Lewin GR, Mendell LM. Regulation of cutaneous C-fibre nociceptors by nerve growth factor in the developing rat. J Neurophysiol 1994; 71:941–949.

42. Bennett DL, Koltzenburg M, Priestley JV, Shelton DL, McMahon SB. Endogenous nerve growth factor regulates the sensitivity of nociceptors in the adult rat. Eur J Neurosci 1998; 10:1282–1291.
43. Aloe L, Tuveri MA, Carcassi U, Levi–Montalcini R. Nerve growth factor in the synovial fluid of patients with chronic arthritis. Arthritis Rheum 1992; 35:351–355.
44. Devor M. The pathophysiology of damaged peripheral nerves. In: Wall PD, Melzack R, eds. Textbook of Pain. Edinburgh: Churchill Livingstone, 1994:79–100.
45. Mannion RJ, Doubell TP, Coggeshall RE, Woolf CJ. Collateral sprouting of uninjured primary afferent A-fibers into the superficial dorsal horn of the adult rat spinal cord after topical capsaicin treatment to the sciatic nerve. J Neurosci 1996; 16:5189–5195.
46. Koerber HR, Mirnics K, Brown PB, Mendell LM. Central sprouting and functional plasticity of regenerated primary afferents. J Neurosci 1994; 14:3655–3671.
47. Mannion RJ, Doubell TP, Gill H, Woolf CJ. Deafferentation is insufficient to induce sprouting of A-fibre central terminals in the rat dorsal horn. J Comp Neurol 1998; 393:135–144.
48. Bennett DL, French J, Priestley JV, McMahon SB. NGF but not NT-3 or BDNF prevents the A fiber sprouting into lamina II of the spinal cord that occurs following axotomy. Mol Cell Neurosci 1996; 8:211–220.
49. Ren K, Thomas DA, Dubner R. Nerve growth factor alleviates a painful peripheral neuropathy in rats. Brain Res 1995; 699:286–292.
50. Lee BH, Yoon YW, Chung K, Chung JM. Comparison of sympathetic sprouting in sensory ganglia in three animal models of neuropathic pain. Exp Brain Res 1998; 120:432–438.
51. Ramer MS, Bisby MA. Adrenergic innervation of rat sensory ganglia following proximal or distal painful sciatic neuropathy: distinct mechanisms revealed by anti-NGF treatment. Eur J Neurosci 1999; 11:837–846.
52. Shu X, Mendell LM. Acute sensitization by NGF of the response of small-diameter sensory neurons to capsaicin. J Neurophysiol 2001; 86:2931–2938.
53. Chuang Hh, Prescott ED, Kong H, Shields S, Jordt SE, Basbaum AI, Chao MV, Julius D. Bradykinin and nerve growth factor release the capsaicin receptor from PtdIns(4,5)P2-mediated inhibition. Nature 2001; 411:957–962.
54. Galoyan SM, Mendell LM. NGF potentiates heat activated currents in small DRG cells isolated from adult rat. Neurosci Abstr 2001; 27: Program No. 926.11.
55. Arvanian VL, Mendell LM. Acute modulation of synaptic transmission to neurons by BDNF in the neonatal rat spinal cord. Eur J Neurosci 2001; 141:1800–1808.

59
Profile of Tramadol and Tramadol Analogues

Robert B. Raffa
Temple University School of Pharmacy, Philadelphia, Pennsylvania, U.S.A.

Elmar Friderichs
Grünenthal GmbH, Aachen, Germany

I. OVERVIEW

Tramadol hydrochloride, (1*RS*, 2*RS*)-2-[(dimethylamino)methyl]-1-(3-methoxyphenyl)-cyclohexanol HCl (tramadol) (Fig. 1), is a centrally acting synthetic analgesic widely used throughout the world. Tramadol appears to produce its analgesic effect through two mechanisms (1–6). One mechanism relates to weak affinity for μ-opioid receptors (about 6000-fold less than morphine, 100-fold less than *d*-propoxyphene, and about the same as dextromethorphan). An active metabolite (*O*-desmethyltramadol) binds to opioid receptors with greater affinity than the parent compound and might contribute to this component (7). In most animal tests and in human clinical trials (8–10), the analgesic effect of tramadol is only partially blocked (<50%) by the opioid antagonist naloxone, suggesting a significant nonopioid mechanism. The nonopioid mechanism appears related to tramadol's ability to enhance synaptic levels of the neurotransmitters 5-hydroxytryptamine (5-HT; serotonin) and norepinephrine (NE). Several lines of evidence suggest that the two mechanisms combine in a complementary fashion and sometimes greater-than-additive (synergistic) manner to produce antinociception, but only in an additive, or less than additive, manner in several side effect measures (10). This proposed duality in mechanism of action is consistent with, and forms the basis for understanding, tramadol's clinical attributes. Analogues of tramadol have been designed that emphasize one or the other of tramadol's mechanisms of action.

II. THE HISTORY OF TRAMADOL AND ANALOGUES

A. Discovery and Development

Over the years tramadol has gained a growing worldwide reputation as an effective, safe, and well-tolerated drug for inhibition of moderate to severe pain. In contrast to its now rapidly increasing use, the compound was widely overlooked by the medical community for more than two decades. The compound dates back to 1962 when it was discovered by chemists of the German pharmaceutical company Grünenthal (11), who were looking for new structures with

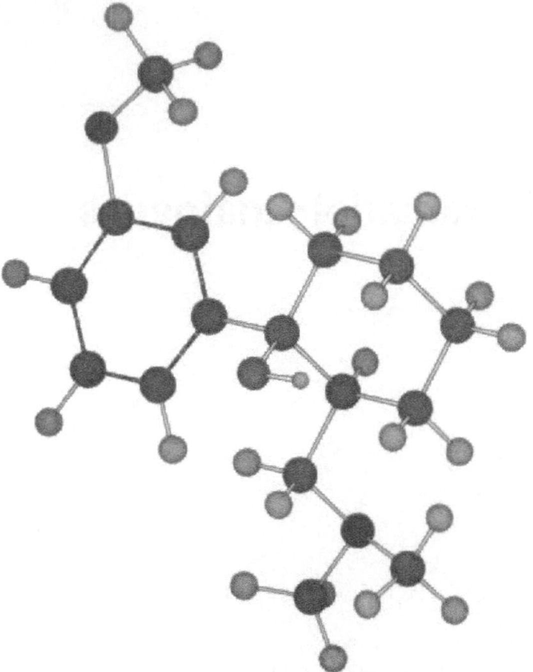

Figure 1 Chemical structure of tramadol (CS Chem 3D Pro software; CambridgeSoft Corp.).

spasmolytic and antiallergic–antihistaminic properties. The pharmacological-screening program at the company revealed an appreciable antinociceptive activity and central nervous system (CNS) effects, such as Straub tail and hyperlocomotion, reminiscent of opioid-like compounds. The original compound comprised *S*- and *R*-enantiomers (*cis–trans* mixture) that could easily be separated by solubility differences. The pharmacological testing of the individual enantiomers (12) showed the *R*-enantiomer was a much stronger analgesic, therefore, all efforts were concentrated on this compound, which in the first stereochemical elucidation was erroneously attributed to the *trans*-configuration (Fig. 2) and the compound was therefore named *tra*madol.

Clinical investigations performed in Germany between 1965 and 1970 (13–15) confirmed a substantial analgesic potential combined with a very low level of opioid-type side effects (such as respiratory depression, constipation, or induction of euphoria) (16). At that time the company was not very interested in marketing analgesics; therefore, the compound became available for licensing. Negotiations with one major U. S. drug company were unsuccessful, but a Japanese company conducted a major preclinical research program (17–19) that validated and extended the findings of Grünenthal, especially by evaluating the preclinical opioid-type tolerance or dependence potential of the compound (20,21). Despite excellent results and a quick introduction of an injectable form into the Japanese market, the drug had only limited success (the reasons for which are still unknown). In Germany, the injectable form was likewise registered for marketing, but was not actively pursued.

Ongoing clinical investigations confirmed the high oral availability of the compound. The increasing popularity of orally active weak opioids with a low, or at least limited, dependence potential prompted Grünenthal to develop a capsule formulation of tramadol, registered under the brand name Tramal. Tramal competed favorably with the weak opioids and became increasingly successful. Repeated application in chronic pain treatment confirmed the low tolerance or

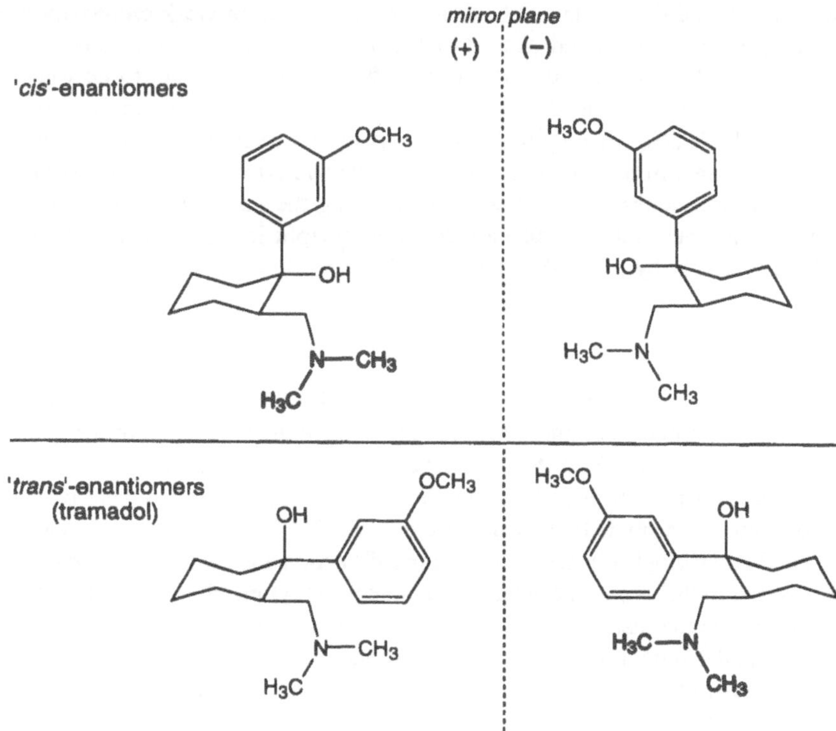

Figure 2 Enantiomers of tramadol.

dependence potential, and despite experimentation use by opioid abusers, the compound did not replace opioids and never significantly penetrated into the drug-abuse scene. This was in contrast with other weak opioids, and in 1985, when pentazocine, tilidine, and buprenorphine were subjected to narcotic scheduling, tramadol retained its normal prescription status. At that time, tramadol became the only centrally acting monoanalgesic in Germany available without narcotic prescription. This position reinforced the use of the compound in various acute and chronic pain situations (22–24), and tramadol filled the gap on the WHO "analgesics ladder" between the weak analgesics of the nonsteroidal anti-inflammatory drugs (NSAID) and acetaminophen (paracetamol) type and the strong opioids of the morphine type.

B. The Question of Mechanism

The understanding of opioid-induced pain inhibition was strongly advanced by the discovery of opioid receptors and their subtypes. Radioligand-binding experiments became available and tramadol was investigated in such experiments, but the compound showed only a modest affinity. Only one metabolite of tramadol, the *O*-desmethyl derivative (M1), had an appreciable binding affinity and selectivity for the μ-opioid subtype. The low-binding affinity made it very unlikely that tramadol itself was responsible for the opioid component of its mechanism of action. It was speculated that similar to the methoxy compound codeine, which is metabolically converted to morphine, tramadol might be demethylated by the microsomal P450 enzymes to the active metabolite *O*-desmethyl tramadol responsible for analgesia and opioid-type side effects. At first glance this explanation appeared reasonable, but it could not explain the discrepancy between the strong analgesic potency and the low level of respiratory depression or weak propensity to induce tolerance and dependence. A mixed agonist–antagonist action profile was ruled out; therefore, it became more and more clear that the key to the action profile had to be found outside the opioid properties of the compound. First hints were found during the pharmacological reevaluation at the end of the 1980s, when tramadol was prepared for approval in several European countries beyond Germany. In pain models, the antinociceptive effect was partly resistant to inhibition by the opioid antagonist naloxone, and in exploring the potential mechanism of this nonopioid component, it turned out that tramadol increased synaptic levels of the neurotransmitters NE and 5-HT, apparently by re-uptake inhibition (25,26).

C. Licensing

In 1989 the compound was licensed in the United States by the Johnson & Johnson company McNeil Pharmaceutical. A fruitful collaboration resulted in a refined understanding of the pharmacological action profile of the compound (5,10). Tramadol is marketed as a racemic mixture of two optical isomers, and part of the investigations dealt with the question: To what extent do the individual enantiomers contribute to the analgesic effect (27)? The experiments revealed both enantiomers to be pharmacologically active. The "opioid" action and 5-HT–reuptake inhibition is predominantly due to the (+)-enantiomer and its *O*-desmethyl metabolite, whereas the NE–reuptake inhibition is predominantly due to the (−)-enantiomer. Isobolographic analysis of the enantiomers confirmed that both contributed additively and in some models even synergistically to the overall analgesic effect. Thus, tramadol is one of the rare examples for which the use of a racemic drug is superior to the use of one enantiomer alone. Tramadol is now marketed worldwide under a variety of trade names either alone or in combination with another analgesic.

III. CLINICAL PROFILE

A. Pharmacokinetics

1. Routes of Administration

Tramadol is available for virtually all routes of administration in a variety of formulations (28). Availability within individual countries might be limited, such as in the United States where Ultram is presently available only by the oral route.

2. Absorption and Distribution

Racemic tramadol is rapidly and almost completely absorbed after oral administration, with an absolute bioavailability (100-mg dose) of about 75%, not significantly affected by food. Its plasma-protein binding is about 20%, and its volume of distribution about 2.7 L/kg. Analgesic activity in humans begins within 1 h after oral administration and peaks in approximately 2–3 h after administration.

3. Metabolism

Tramadol is extensively metabolized after oral administration, more so in humans (≥60%) than in some animal species. The major metabolic pathways involve *N*- and *O*-demethylation and glucuronidation or sulfation in the liver. The M1 metabolite (*O*-desmethyl tramadol) pathway is catalyzed by the CYP2D6 isozyme of cytochrome P-450, which is subject to metabolic inhibition or induction by other drugs. There is no evidence of self-induction in humans. Metabolism is reduced in patients with advanced hepatic disease (dose adjustment is recommended in cirrhotic patients).

4. Elimination

Tramadol and its metabolites are excreted primarily in the urine. The mean terminal plasma elimination half-life of tramadol is about 6.3 h. Linear pharmacokinetics have been observed following multiple doses of 50 and 100 mg to steady-state. The plasma elimination half-life of racemic tramadol increases slightly (about 1 h) after multiple dosing. Impaired renal function results in decreased elimination (dose adjustment is recommended when creatinine clearance is <30 mL/min). Consideration of dose adjustment is recommended for patients older than 75 years.

B. Indications

Tramadol is used to treat moderate to severe pain of a variety of acute and chronic conditions. Its relative merit in each of these situations depends on the benefit/risk ratio for each individual patient.

C. Adverse Effect Profile

The following is a synopsis. Consult the appropriate labeling for prescribing information.

1. Adverse Reactions

In the double-blind or open-label extension periods in U.S. studies of 550 patients with chronic nonmalignant pain, the overall incidence rates of adverse experiences were similar to the active control groups: acetaminophen (300 mg) with codeine phosphate (30 mg); or aspirin (325 mg) with codeine phosphate (30 mg). Tramadol does not inhibit cyclooxygenase activity. Hence, NSAID-induced effects are not seen. The most common effects occurred under the combined category of dizziness/vertigo/nausea/vomiting.

2. Contraindications, Warnings, and Precautions

Tramadol is contraindicated in patients with known allergic reactions or hypersensitivity toward tramadol (or its excipients) and in cases of acute intoxication with CNS depressants or with other psychotropic drugs, and in patients who are receiving monoamine oxidase (MAO) inhibitors. Precaution is advisable in situations of respiratory depression, increased intracranial pressure or head trauma, acute abdominal conditions, renal or hepatic disease, patients physically dependent on opioids, and other situations, such as concomitant medications: carbamazepine (enzymatic induction of tramadol metabolism); quinidine (selective inhibitor of CYP2D6), and others noted in the foregoing. Seizures have been reported at doses higher than the recommended dose range, but some have been reported at doses within the recommended range. Seizure risk might be enhanced in patients receiving CNS drugs that reduce seizure threshold, such as tricyclics, selective serotonin-reuptake inhibitors (SSRIs), monoamine oxidase inhibitors (MAOIs), or neuroleptics.

3. Drug Abuse–Dependence

Tramadol has some potential for abuse, and dependence may occur. Symptoms of withdrawal may include agitation, anxiety, nervousness, insomnia, hyperkinesia, tremor, and gastrointestinal effects. In patients with a tendency to drug abuse, a history of drug dependence, or who are chronically using opioids, tramadol is not recommended or may be used only with particular caution. The results of a postmarketing survey of the United States experience have been reported (29).

IV. PRECLINICAL PROFILE

A. In Vitro Tests

1. Opioid Receptor Binding

The affinity of tramadol for μ-opioid receptors (K_i value) is in the micromolar (μM) range, and it has even weaker affinity for δ- and κ-opioid receptors (5,30) (Table 1). Tramadol does not bind (at concentrations up to 10 or 100 μM) to other receptor sites, and it is not an inhibitor of arachidonate metabolism. Tramadol's relatively low-binding affinity at the μ-opioid receptor (about 100-fold less than that of *d*-propoxyphene) does not appear sufficient to explain its preclinical antinociceptive potency, which is typically between that of codeine and morphine. The M1 metabolite binds with about 200-fold higher affinity for the μ-opioid receptor than does the parent compound.

2. Monoamine-Reuptake Inhibition

Tramadol, unlike codeine or morphine, also inhibits the neuronal reuptake of NE and 5-HT (see Table 1). It does not inhibit the uptake of other neurotransmitters. The ability of tramadol to inhibit the neuronal reuptake of NE and 5-HT is in the same concentration range that it binds to μ-opioid receptors. As in μ-opioid binding, the relatively low affinity of tramadol for 5-HT- and NE-reuptake sites (about two orders of magnitude less than imipramine) seems insufficient by itself to explain its antinociceptive potency.

B. In Vivo Tests

1. Naloxone

In several tests in mice and rats, tramadol-induced antinociception is only partially blocked by the opioid antagonist naloxone, whereas morphine and codeine are completely blocked (Fig. 3).

Table 1 In Vitro Activity of Tramadol, M1 Metabolite, Enantiomers and Reference Compounds (Values are K_i in μM)

Compound	μ	δ	κ	NE	5-HT
Morphine	0.00034	0.092	0.57	IA	IA
d-Propoxyphene	0.034	0.38	1.22	IA	IA
Codeine	0.2	5.1	6.0	IA	IA
Dextromethorphan	1.28	11.5	7.0	0.24	0.023
Tramadol	2.1	57.6	42.7	0.78	0.99
Imipramine	3.7	12.7	1.8	0.0066	0.021
Tramadol enantiomers					
(+) Enantiomer	1.3	62.4	54.0	2.51	0.53
(−) Enantiomer	24.8	213	53.5	0.43	2.35
Tramadol metabolite					
(±) M1	0.0121	0.911	0.242	1.52	5.18

NE, norepinephrine; M1, mono-*O*-desmethyltramadol; IA, inactive at 10 μM.
Source: Ref. 4.

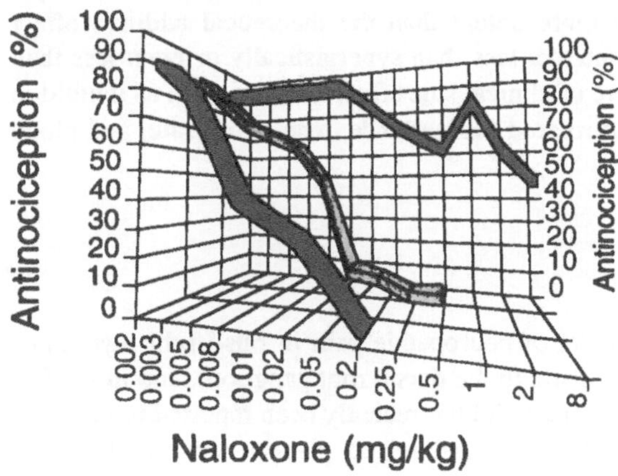

Figure 3 Representation of the incomplete inhibition of i.p. tramadol-induced antinociception (rear curve) by s.c. naloxone, compared with the complete inhibition of antinociception induced by codeine (middle curve) and morphine (near curve) in the mouse abdominal constriction test. (From Ref. 5.)

Naloxone totally blocks tramadol-induced antinociception only in the tail-flick test. In humans also, there appears to be a clinically relevant nonopioid component to tramadol-induced analgesia. In a randomized, crossover study in humans (8), tramadol-induced analgesia against transcutaneous electrical stimulation of the sural nerve was attenuated 26% (as measured by R-III spinal reflex) or 31% (as measured by visual analog scale) by naloxone (0.8 mg, i.v.). The contribution of a monoaminergic component to tramadol analgesia in humans, and minimal contribution of M1, has been reported (31).

2. Cross-Tolerance

In mice, pretreatment with morphine resulted in only about a 3-fold rightward shift of the i.p. tramadol dose–response curve compared with about 16-fold for morphine (32). Extended twice-daily pretreatment with tramadol resulted in only about a 4-fold rightward shift of the morphine dose–response curve. In the arthritic rat model, no cross-tolerance to i.v. tramadol was observed in morphine-tolerant animals (9). In rats, opioid-like subjective effects of tramadol are less than those predicted by its analgesic potency relative to morphine (33).

3. Yohimbine and Ritanserin

The i.p. administration of 1.0 mg/kg of the adrenoceptor antagonist yohimbine or the 5-HT receptor antagonist ritanserin have no effect on the antinociceptive action of morphine administered spinally (intrathecally), but they significantly reduce the antinociceptive action of tramadol (5). This suggests that the ability of tramadol to inhibit the reuptake of 5-HT and NE in vitro is translated into a physiologically significant ability to contribute to the antinociceptive effect of tramadol in vivo.

C. Analgesic Synergy

The (+) enantiomer of tramadol binds to μ-opioid receptors and inhibits 5-HT reuptake more potently than does the (−) enantiomer, whereas the (−) enantiomer is the more potent inhibitor of NE reuptake. The (+) and (−) enantiomers individually produce centrally mediated (spinal) antinociception in mice. In several tests, the combination of enantiomers is more potent than either enantiomer alone and is significantly more potent than the theoretical additive effect (thus, is synergistic) (10). The enantiomers interact less than synergistically or even less than additively in several preclinical tests predictive of clinical side effect liability, such as inhibition of colonic propulsive motility, impairment of rotarod performance, respiratory rate, and blood pressure.

V. NEUROPATHIC PAIN

Tramadol has an antiallodynic effect in a model of neuropathic pain in rats (tight ligation of the L5 and L6 nerve roots of the sciatic nerve distal to the dorsal root ganglion), and this effect is only partially antagonized by naloxone (34). Tramadol has recently been reported to be effective for the pain of diabetic neuropathy in a multicenter randomized, placebo-controlled double-blind study (35).

VI. ANALOGUES

The success of tramadol stimulated extensive investigations of the structure–activity relation; more than 2000 derivatives were synthesized and submitted to biochemical and pharmacological investigations. Molecular modeling revealed which part of the chemical structure was responsible for the opioid component and which one for the inhibition of NE and 5-HT reuptake. The systematic variation of the basic structure resulted in molecules that were pure uptake inhibitors and others being pure strong μ-opioid agonists, with a potency in the range of fentanyl. A further goal of these investigations was to select compounds that, in contrast to tramadol, had uptake inhibition and μ-opioid activity combined in one enantiomer. These efforts were successful; the first compounds of this new type are under clinical investigation.

A. Grünenthal

During early investigations of tramadol it became clear that the chemical structure of the molecule was sufficiently flexible to fit into the general models of opioid-like compounds, as elaborated by Beckett and Casy (36,37) and Janssen and Van der Eycken (38). According to their conception, the essential parameters for "opioid" properties are an aromatic ring system substituted by an O-containing group in *meta*-position, which is linked to a central carbon and a two-carbon chain, followed by a basic N with at least one CH_3 group. In the tramadol molecule, the central C and one C of the ethyl chain is incorporated into a cyclohexane ring system. Unlike the rigid morphine molecule, the cyclohexane ring allows a certain degree of flexibility. On the one hand, this reduces opioid-receptor affinity by impairing the fit to the complementary shape of the opioid receptor but, on the other hand, allows a certain degree of nonopioid effect. Tramadol has two asymmetric C atoms, each containing two optical isomers, a (+) form and a (−) form. The best fit to the opioid receptor is the (+) form of the *R*-enantiomer, whereas the mirror-image (−) form shows a better fit to the NE transporter.

Opioid receptor affinity of the (+)-enantiomer is increased by two orders of magnitude by replacing the–OCH_3 by the free–OH, which occurs during metabolic conversion. Analogues (C) in which the methoxy-substituent was replaced by homologous groups (e.g., ethoxy, propoxy, phenoxy, or benzyloxyl) had tramadol-like low affinity for opioid receptors. Such compounds were metabolically desalkylated to the same *O*-hydroxy derivative as tramadol, which was the prerequisite for opioid-like analgesic activity. Compared with tramadol, the higher homologues showed an increased toxicity. Shift of the O-group of the phenyl ring from the *meta*- to *ortho*- or *para*-position, or adding additional ring substituents, reduced analgesic activity and abolished opioid-receptor binding. The same occurred with substitution of CH_3 of the basic *N* by higher homologues or incorporating the N into a five- or six-membered ring system. In contrast to modifications at the aromatic ring, substitution of –OH of the cyclohexyl by halogen or even H had only a weak influence on opioid receptor affinity, as did splitting-off the –OH and introducing a 1,2- or 1,6-double bond.

Derivatives in which a methylene group was placed between the central C and the aromatic ring completely lost their opioid-receptor affinity, but inhibition of NE and 5-HT reuptake was essentially increased, and the compounds retained antitussive properties (39,40). A hydrogen in the 2-, 3-, or 4-position of the cyclohexane ring could be replaced by $-CH_3$ or –OH without, as a rule, essential loss of opioid properties. A free –OH in the 4-position moderately decreased activity, but substitution with an alkyl-, benzyl-, or phenylethylether group strongly increased opioid receptor binding and analgesic potency. Efforts to further simplify the basic structure of the tramadol molecule by breaking up the cyclohexane ring into a noncyclic phenylpropylamine chain were very successful.

B. Johnson & Johnson

In separate efforts, fusion of one *N*-methyl with the cyclohexane ring resulted in nonopioid antinociceptive agents (41). These 4-aryloctahydroisoindoles comprise four diastereomeric families and each diastereomer consists of a pair of enantiomers (Fig. 4). In general, hydroxyl substituents at the 4-position of the isoindole system retained or enhanced activity, substituents (methyl- or pheny-) at the 5 and 7a positions retained activity, a phenyl substituent at the 7 position diminished activity and unsaturation at either the 5,6- or the 6,7-position was tolerated. Lipophilic substituents on the aryl ring tended to increase, whereas large substituents on *N* decreased potency in some tests. Compounds from related ring systems were also active. The antinociceptive activity of these compounds in the mouse abdominal-constriction test might be by a different mechanism than that in the 48°C hot-plate test.

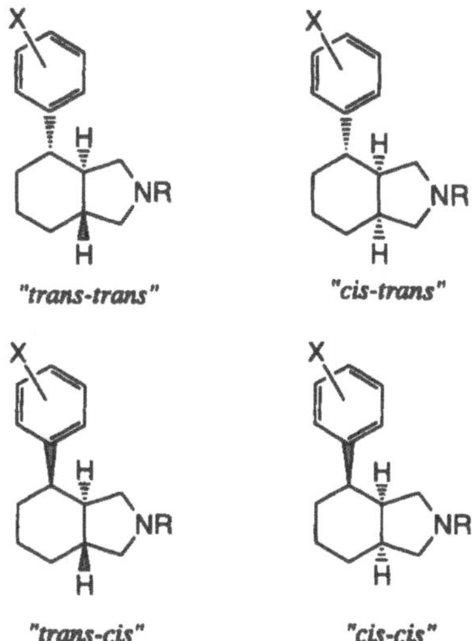

Figure 4 Structures of arylisoindoles. (From Ref. 41.)

VII. SUMMARY

Tramadol appears to produce analgesia by both opioid (predominantly at the μ-receptor) and nonopioid (related to its ability to affect the neuronal release or reuptake of NE and 5-HT) mechanisms. The overall analgesic action probably derives from the different pharmacologies of its two enantiomers, and to some extent on its M1 metabolite. The enantiomers appear to interact in a complementary and synergistic manner in the analgesic endpoint, but only in a simple additive or counteractive manner on nonanalgesic (side effect) endpoints. The clinical profile of tramadol apparently results from the fortuitous combinations and interactions of its component parts.

ACKNOWLEDGMENTS

The authors have summarized the collaborative effort of investigators at Grünenthal GmbH, McNeil Pharmaceutical, the R. W. Johnson Pharmaceutical Research Institute, and external investigators. The authors gratefully acknowledge all of their many contributions.

REFERENCES

1. Lee CR, McTavish D, Sorkin EM. Tramadol: a preliminary review of its pharmacodynamic and pharmacokinetic properties, and therapeutic potential in acute and chronic pain states. Drugs 1993; 46:313–340.
2. Raffa RB, Nayak RK, Liao S, Minn FL. The mechanism(s) of action and pharmacokinetics of tramadol hydrochloride. Rev Contemp Pharmacother 1995; 6:485–497.
3. Raffa, RB, Friderichs E. The basic science aspect of tramadol hydrochloride. Pain Rev 1996; 3:249–271.
4. Raffa RB. A novel approach to the pharmacology of analgesics. Am J Med 1996; 101(suppl 1A): 40S–46S.
5. Raffa RB, Friderichs E, Reimann W, Shank RP, Codd EE, Vaught JL. Opioid and nonopioid components independently contribute to the mechanism of action of tramadol, an "atypical" opioid analgesic. J Pharmacol Exp Ther 1992; 260:275–285.
6. Friderichs E, Felgenhauer F, Jongschaapp P, Osterloh G. Pharmacological studies on analgesia, dependence on and tolerance of tramadol, a potent analgetic drug. Arzneimittelforschung 1978; 28: 122–134.
7. Hennies H-H, Friderichs E, Schneider J. Receptor binding, analgesic and antitussive potency of tramadol and other selected opioids. Arzneimittelforschung 1988; 38:877–880.
8. Collart L, Luthy C, Dayer P. Partial inhibition of tramadol antinociceptive effect by naloxone in man. Br J Clin Pharmacol 1993; 35:73P.
9. Kayser V, Besson J-M, Guilbaud G. Evidence for a noradrenergic component in the antinociceptive effect of the analgesic agent tramadol in an animal model of clinical pain, the arthritic rat. Eur J Pharmacol 1992; 224:83–88.
10. Raffa RB, Friderichs E, Reimann W, Shank RP, Codd EE, Vaught JL, Jacoby HI, Selve N. Complementary and synergistic antinociceptive interaction between the enantiomers of tramadol. J Pharmacol Exp Ther 1993; 267:331–340.
11. Flick K, Frankus E, Friderichs E. Untersuchungen zur chemischen Struktur und analgetischen Wirkung von phenylsubstituierten Aminomethylcyclohexanolen. Arzneimittelforschung 1978; 28:107–113.
12. Frankus E, Friderichs E, Kim SM, Osterloh G. Über die Isomerentrennung, Strukturaufklärung und pharmakologische Charakterisierung von 1-(*m*-methoxyphenyl)-2-(dimethylaminomethyl)-cyclohexan-l-ol. Arzneimittelforschung 1978; 28:114–121.

13. Flohé L, Arend I, Cogal A, Richter W, Simon W. Clinical study on the development of dependency after long-term treatment with tramadol. Arzneimittelforschung 1978; 28:213–217.
14. Schenck EG, Arend I. Klinische Prüfung von Tramadol nach dem Paarlingskarten-system. Arzneimittelforschung 1978; 28:196–199.
15. Rost A, Schenck EG. Beeinflussung der Schmerzschwelle an der Zahnpulpa durch Tramadol und andere Analgetika. Arzneimittelforschung 1978; 28:181–183.
16. Richter W, Barth H, Flohé L, Giertz H. Clinical investigation on the development of dependence during oral therapy with tramadol. Arzneimittelforschung 1985; 35:1742–1744.
17. Mitsushima T, Kawazura H, Ishii T, Kitano T, Hemmi, Z. Pharmacological studies on a new analgesic drug, 1-(*m*-methoxyphenyl)-2-dimethylaminomethylcyclohexanol (1) hydrochloride (K-315). (3rd report) Relationship between monoamine in brain levels and analgesic action of K-315 in mice. Folia Pharmacol Jpn 1973; 69:437–445.
18. Henmi Z, Horii D, Mitsushima T, Kawazura, H, Hayashi H, Mori M, Sano N, Shimizu S, Horikomi K, Shino K. Pharmacological studies on the new analgesic: 1-(*m*-methoxyphenyl)-2-dimethylaminomethylcyclohexanol (1) hydrochloride (K-315). Report 1: Analgesic and general pharmacologica properties of K-315. Folia Pharmacol Jpn 1972; 68:102–113.
19. Kitano T, Hayashi H, Ishii T, Henmi Z. Pharmacological studies on the new analgesic drug 1-(*m*-methoxyphenyl)-2-dimethylaminomethylcyclohexanol (1) hydrochloride (2nd report). Effect of K-315 on EEG and afferent pathways. Folia Pharmacol Jpn 1972; 68:114–128.
20. Murano T, Yamamoto H, Endo N, et al. Studies of dependence on tramadol in rats Arzneimittelforschung 1978; 28:152–158.
21. Yanagita T. Drug dependence potential of 1-(*m*-methoxyphenyl)-2-(dimethylaminomethyl)cyclohexan-1-ol hydrochloride (tramadol) tested in monkeys. Arzneimittelforschung 1978; 28:158–163.
22. Cossmann M, Wilsmann KM. Anwendung der Tramadol- Injektionslösung (Tramal) beim akuten Schmerz. Offene Prüfung zur Beurteilung der Akutwirkung und der Verträglichkeit bei einmaliger perenteraler Anwendung. Münch Med Wochenschr 1988; 130:633–636.
23. Cossmann M, Wilsmann KM. Behandlung länger andauernder Schmerzsyndrome. Beurteilung der Wirkung und Verträglichkeit von Tramadol (Tramal) bei mehrmaliger Gabe. Münch Med Wochenschr 1987; 129:851–854.
24. Cossmann M, Wilsmann KM. Wirkung und Begleitwirkungen von Tramadol. Offene Phase-IV-Prüfung mit 7198 Patienten. Therapiewoche 1987; 37:3475–3485.
25. Driessen B, Reimann W, Giertz H. Effects of the central analgesic tramadol on the uptake and release of noradrenaline and dopamine in vitro. Br J Pharmacol 1993; 108:806–811.
26. Driessen B, Reimann W. Interaction of the central analgesic, tramadol, with the uptake and release of 5-hydroxytryptamine in the rat brain in vitro. Br J Pharmacol 1992; 105:147–151.
27. Friderichs E, Reimann W, Selve N. Contribution of both enantiomers to antinociception of the centrally acting analgesic tramadol. Naunyn-Schmiedeberg Arch Pharmacol 1992; 346(suppl 1):R36.
28. Physicians' Desk Reference. 52nd ed. Montvale, NJ: Medical Economics, 1990:2064–2066.
29. Goodman A. Postmarketing surveillance program finds little abuse potential with tramadol. Anesthesiol News 1997; Dec:15–16.
30. Lai J, Ma S–W, Porreca F, Raffa RB. Tramadol, M1 metabolite and enantiomer affinities for cloned human opioid receptors expressed in transfected HN9.10 neuroblastoma cells. Eur J Pharmacol 1996; 316:369–372.
31. Desmeules J, Piguet V, Collart L, Dayer P. Contribution of monoaminergic modulation to the analgesic effect of tramadol. Br J Clin Pharmacol 1996; 41:7–12.
32. Mattia A, Vanderah T, Raffa RB, Vaught JL, Tallarida RJ, Porreca F. Characterization of the unusual antinociceptive profile of tramadol in mice. Drug Dev Res 1993; 28:176–182.
33. Preston KL, Jasinski DR, Testa M. Abuse potential and pharmacological comparison of tramadol and morphine. Drug Alcohol Depend 1991; 27:7–17.
34. Bian D, Nichols ML, Ossipov MH, Porreca F. Antiallodynic effects of tramadol in a model of neuropathic pain in rats. Analgesia 1996; 2:57–62.
35. Harati Y, Gooch C, Swenson M, Edelman S, Greene D, Raskin P, Donofrio P, Cornblath D, Sachdeo

R, Siu CO, Kamin M. Double-blind randomized trial of tramadol for the treatment of the pain of diabetic neuropathy. Neurology 1998; 50:1842–1846.

36. Beckett AH, Casy AF. Synthetic analgesics: stereochemical considerations. J Pharm Pharmacol 1954; 6:986–999 [discussion 999–1001].
37. Beckett AH. Stereochemical factors in biological activity. In: Jucker E, ed. Progress in Drug Research. Vol 1. Basel: Birkhäuser-Verlag, 1959:455–530.
38. Janssen PAJ, Van der Eycken CAM. The chemical anatomy of potent morphine-like analgesics. In: Burger A, ed. Drugs Affecting the Central Nervous System. Vol. 2. New York: Marcel Dekker, 1968:25–60.
39. Englberger W, Friderichs E, Reimann W, Schneider J. Analgesic and antitussive properties of EM 405. Agents Actions 1991; 32:62–64.
40. Selve N. EM 405: a new substance with an uncommon profile of anti-inflammatory activity. Agents Actions 1991; 32:59–61.
41. Carson JR. Non-opioid antinociceptive agents structurally related to tramadol. IBC Symposium: Novel Targets in the Treatment of Pain. Washington DC, Oct 6–7, 1997.

60

Sumatriptan and Related 5-HT$_{1B/1D}$ Receptor Agonists

Novel Treatments for Migraine

Helen E. Connor
Glaxo Wellcome R&D, Stevenage, Hertfordshire, England

Reijo Salonen
Glaxo Wellcome, Inc., Research Triangle Park, North Carolina, U.S.A.

Patrick P. A. Humphrey
Glaxo Institute of Applied Pharmacology, University of Cambridge, Cambridge, England

I. INTRODUCTION

Sumatriptan, a serotonin (5-HT)$_{1B/1D}$ receptor agonist, is the first of a novel class of drugs for the short-term treatment of migraine. The efficacy of sumatriptan in alleviating both the headache and the associated symptoms of a migraine attack is now well established by data from many rigorously designed, placebo-controlled clinical trials (1,2). Sumatriptan was first made widely available in Europe for the short-term treatment of migraine and cluster headache in 1991. Sumatriptan has now been used worldwide by more than 9 million patients in the treatment of more than 180 million attacks of migraine. In addition to oral tablets, subcutaneous, intranasal, and suppository formulations of sumatriptan are available for those patients who have severe nausea and vomiting, or who require a very rapid onset of headache relief. In the last 2 years, several other 5-HT$_{1B/1D}$ receptor agonists (colloquially known as *triptans*) have also become available (e.g., zolmitriptan, naratriptan, or rizatriptan) (3). These have a pharmacological profile broadly similar to sumatriptan, but differ slightly in terms of their physicochemical or pharmacokinetic properties.

II. SUMATRIPTAN: SUMMARY OF PHARMACOLOGICAL PROFILE

Sumatriptan is a selective agonist for 5-HT$_{1B}$, 5-HT$_{1D}$, and 5-HT$_{1F}$ receptors, with lower affinity for other 5-HT$_1$ receptor subtypes (5-HT$_{1A}$ and 5-HT$_{1E}$), and little or no significant activity at other 5-HT (including 5-HT$_{2A}$, 5-HT$_3$, and 5-HT$_7$) and non–5-HT receptors (see Refs. 4 and 5 for details). Sumatriptan causes a selective contraction of cranial blood vessels (e.g., canine and human isolated basilar artery; human isolated dural vasculature) with little or no contractile effect in a variety of peripheral vessels (4). In anesthetized dogs, sumatriptan selectively constricts the carotid vasculature, with little or no effect on blood pressure (4). This craniovascular selectivity is due to the 5-HT_1 receptor selectivity of sumatriptan and the differential distribution of 5-HT receptors mediating vasoconstriction. Hence, 5-HT_{1B} receptors predominantly mediate constriction in the cranial vasculature (6), whereas 5-HT_{2A} receptors predominantly mediate constriction in peripheral vascular beds. The presence of a small population of contractile 5-HT_{1B} receptors in human large coronary arteries (7) has, however, led to the labeling restrictions for sumatriptan and other 5-$HT_{1B/1D}$ receptor agonists whereby this class of drug is contraindicated in patients with coronary artery disease.

In addition to a vasoconstrictor effect, sumatriptan has an inhibitory effect on some nerves through activation of prejunctional inhibitory 5-HT_1 receptors (4). This action is thought to account for the inhibitory effect of sumatriptan on development of neurogenic plasma protein extravasation in the dura mater of rodents following stimulation (electrical and chemical) of the trigeminal nerve. This inhibitory effect appears to be specific for the cranial circulation (8).

III. MECHANISM OF ACTION IN MIGRAINE

Three possible mechanisms are proposed to explain the clinical efficacy of sumatriptan in migraine. Each of these involve the interaction of sumatriptan with the trigeminovascular system to result in inhibition of afferent trigeminal nerve firing (Fig. 1). Despite much preclinical and clinical research to pinpoint the important mechanism, however, it is still not clear how much each one of the following actions actually contributes to the clinical efficacy of sumatriptan. Indeed, it may be that a combination of actions accounts for the effective alleviation of migraine symptoms.

1. Vasoconstriction of distended, pain-sensitive intracranial arteries to normalize vessel diameter and thereby reduce afferent firing of the trigeminal nerve. This probably involves an action of sumatriptan at the level of the large cerebral or meningeal arteries, or both, and is mediated by activation of 5-HT_{1B} receptors on the vascular smooth muscle. The ability of sumatriptan to constrict large cerebral and meningeal arteries in humans has been demonstrated in several clinical studies (for example, 9,10).
2. Inhibition of neuropeptide release from peripheral terminals of perivascular trigeminal

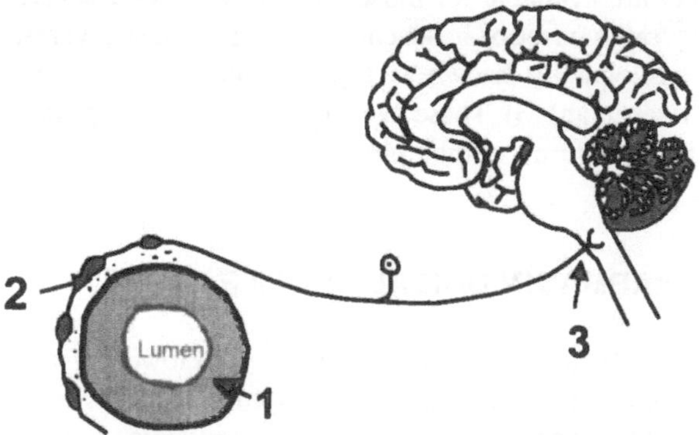

Figure 1 Schematic diagram to illustrate the three possible mechanisms of action of sumatriptan in migraine: (1) selective constriction of large intracranial arteries; (2) inhibition of neuropeptide release from peripheral trigeminal nerve terminals; and (3) central inhibition of trigeminal nerve firing. See text for more details.

nerve terminals in the dural vasculature, leading to a reduction in edema formation–neurogenic inflammation, and an associated reduction in afferent trigeminal firing. A clinically effective dose of sumatriptan reduces cranial venous levels of calcitonin gene-related peptide (CGRP) in migraineurs (11).

3. An action, either pre- or postsynaptically, within the trigeminal nucleus caudalis, the first central site of termination for trigeminal fibers arising from the cranial vasculature, to inhibit synaptic transmission and, thereby, inhibit activation of second-order fibers. This latter action requires penetration of the blood–brain barrier (12,13).

Recent preclinical data have suggested that both 5-HT_{1D} and 5-HT_{1F} receptors mediate peripheral and central inhibition of the trigeminal nerve (6,14,15). Furthermore, a possible role for 5-HT_{1B} receptors in this effect has not been excluded. Hence, it is not yet clear which receptor mechanism is most important for the trigeminal inhibitory effects of sumatriptan and related compounds.

IV. EFFECT OF SUMATRIPTAN IN OTHER PAIN STATES

Sumatriptan has been evaluated in several other types of headache. The compound shows very good efficacy in the treatment of cluster headache (16). Efficacy of sumatriptan in the treatment of chronic–tension-type headache was, however, described as modest (17). However, tension-type headaches in diagnosed migraineurs seem to respond to sumatriptan as well as migraine headaches (18). Whether sumatriptan has any clinical usefulness in nonheadache pain states in humans has not been fully evaluated, although a pilot study in atypical facial pain showed sumatriptan to be no better than placebo (19). Preclinical data suggests that sumatriptan has a specific effect against trigeminovascular pathways, and has no activity in animal models of nociceptive pain (20).

V. MAJOR CURRENT ISSUES FOR $5\text{-HT}_{1B/1D}$ RECEPTOR AGONISTS: NOVEL SHORT-TERM TREATMENTS

A. 5-HT_{1D} and 5-HT_{1F} Receptor Agonists as Nonvasoconstrictor Treatments for Migraine

Research effort has recently been focused at identifying selective agonists for 5-HT_{1D} or 5-HT_{1F} receptors to achieve inhibition of the trigeminal nerve without accompanying vasoconstrictor effects. This could have safety and tolerability benefits over current $5\text{-HT}_{1B/1D}$ agonists. Such compounds, (for example, LY334370 and PNU-142633, 5-HT_{1F} and 5-HT_{1D} receptor-selective agonists, respectively (15,21)), are effective at blocking dural neurogenic inflammation in the rodent model. Clinical efficacy data with these compounds have recently been reported. PNU-142633, a highly selective and potent 5-HT_{1D} receptor agonist, was ineffective in the brief treatment of migraine (21). It was reported that this compound did not penetrate very effectively into the CNS. Hence, these clinical data indicate that peripheral 5-HT_{1D} receptors, at least, are not a good target for effective treatment of migraine, and further question the predictive validity of the rat cranial neurogenic inflammation model (see subsequent discussion).

Interestingly, this selective 5-HT_{1D} agonist caused "triptan-like" side effects in some patients (21). This suggests that the characteristic triptan side effects reported with all compounds of this class (1–3) may, at least partly, be mediated by 5-HT_{1D} receptors, and hence, they are not solely attributable to peripheral 5-HT_{1B} receptor vasoconstrictor mechanisms. LY334370, a

5-HT_{1F} receptor agonist, had efficacy in the brief treatment of migraine. However, this was accompanied by a high incidence of CNS side effects, such as asthenia, dizziness, and somnolence (22). Whether these CNS side effects were mediated by activation of central 5-HT_{1F} receptors, or by some other mechanism, is still unclear. However, any advantage of targeting 5-HT_{1F} receptors to quickly treat migraine is dependent on separating efficacy from CNS side effects.

B. The Importance of Cranial Neurogenic Inflammation to the Pathophysiology of Migraine

Neurogenic inflammation has not yet been shown to occur in humans during a migraine attack (for example, 23). Several compounds that were effective in the rodent cranial neurogenic inflammation model have subsequently been ineffective clinically in the treatment of established migraine headache [for example, NK_1 receptor antagonists (24) and an endothelin antagonist (25)]. Hence, the rodent cranial neurogenic inflammation model is probably not a good predictor of clinical efficacy. This may relate to species differences or, more likely, indicate that the antidromic method of gross electrical stimulation of the trigeminal nerve and the measurement of dural extravasation do not adequately reflect what happens during a migraine headache.

C. The Importance of a Central Site of Action for $5\text{-HT}_{1B/1D}$ Receptor Agonists

In preclinical experiments, sumatriptan has inhibitory effects on neuronal cell firing in the feline trigeminal nucleus caudalis only after disruption of the blood–brain barrier (26). However, some of the more recent $5\text{-HT}_{1B/1D}$ receptor agonists (for example, zolmitriptan, naratriptan) are more lipophilic, and more readily gain access to this central site (12). Whether this confers any clinical advantage is a subject of debate. There is a fine balance between lipophilicity and CNS side effects, such that highly lipophilic drugs of this class would be expected to be undesirable as migraine treatments. It has also been suggested that the blood–brain barrier is disrupted during a migraine attack, allowing less lipophilic drugs, such as sumatriptan, to gain access to the trigeminal nucleus caudalis pathologically.

D. Recurrence of Migraine Headache

Clinical data suggest that sumatriptan does not modify the underlying disease process in a migraine attack, despite effectively inhibiting the symptoms. Sumatriptan has a pharmacokinetic half-life of approximately 24h (27). It is perhaps not surprising that in some patients with long attacks, migraine headache recurs (2). However, plasma half-life may not be the most important factor, and more understanding is needed about what factors are key to reducing headache recurrence (28). Whether any of the more recent $5\text{-HT}_{1B/1D}$ agonists (for example, naratriptan) (29) have lower recurrence rates will become clear with clinical use and experience.

REFERENCES

1. Tfelt–Hansen P. Efficacy and adverse events of subcutaneous, oral, and intranasal sumatriptan used for migraine treatment: a systematic review based on number needed to treat. Cephalalgia 1998; 18: 532–538.
2. Perry CM, Markham A. Sumatriptan. An updated review of its use in migraine. Drugs 1998; 55: 889–922.

3. Goadsby PJ. 5-$HT_{1B/1D}$ agonists in migraine: comparative pharmacology and its therapeutic implications. CNS Drugs 1998; 10:271–286.
4. Beattie DT, Connor HE, Feniuk W, Humphrey PPA. The pharmacology of sumatriptan. Rev Contemp Pharmacother 1994; 5:285–294.
5. Connor HE, Beattie DT. 5-Hydroxytryptamine receptor subtypes: relation to migraine. In: Edvinsson L, ed. Migraine Pathophysiology. London, Martin Dunitz, 2000, in press.
6. Longmore J, Shaw D, Smith D, Hopkins R, McAllister G, Pickard JD, Sirinathsinghji DJ, Butler AJ, Hill RG. Differential distribution of $5HT_{1D}$- and $5HT_{1B}$-immunoreactivity within the human trigemino-cerebrovascular system: implications for the discovery of new antimigraine drugs. Cephalalgia 1997; 17:833–842.
7. Maassen VanDenBrink A, Reekers M, Bax WA, Ferrari MD, Saxena PR. Coronary side-effect potential of current and prospective antimigraine drugs. Circulation 1998; 98:25–30.
8. Buzzi MG, Moskowitz MA. The antimigraine drug, sumatriptan (GR43175), selectively blocks neurogenic plasma extravasation from blood vessels in dura mater. Br J Pharmacol 1990; 99:202–206.
9. Caekebeke JF, Ferrari MD, Zwetsloot CP, Jansen J, Saxena PR. Antimigraine drug sumatriptan increases blood flow velocity in large cerebral arteries during migraine attacks. Neurology 1992; 42: 1522–1526.
10. Henkes H, May A, Kuhne D, Berg–Dammer E, Diener HC. Sumatriptan: vasoactive effect on human dural vessels, demonstrated by subselective angiography. Cephalalgia 1996; 16:224–230.
11. Edvinsson L, Goadsby PJ. Neuropeptides in migraine and cluster headache. Cephalalgia 1994; 14: 320–327.
12. Hoskin KL, Goadsby PJ. Comparison of more and less lipophilic serotonin ($5HT_{1B/1D}$) agonists in a model of trigeminovascular nociception in cats. Exp Neurol 1998; 150:45–51.
13. Storer RJ, Goadsby PJ. Microiontophoretic application of serotonin $(5HT)_{1B/1D}$ agonists inhibits trigeminal cell firing in the cat. Brain. 1997; 120:2171–2177.
14. MacLeod AM, Street LJ, Reeve AJ, Jelley RA, Sternfeld F, Beer MS, Stanton JA, Watt AP, Rathbone D, Matassa VG. Selective, orally active 5-HT_{1D} receptor agonists as potential antimigraine agents. J Med Chem 1997; 40:3501–3503.
15. Johnson KW, Schaus JM, Durkin MM, Audia JE, Kaldor SW, Flaugh ME, Adham N, Zgombick JM, Cohen ML, Branchek TA, Phebus LA. 5-HT_{1F} receptor agonists inhibit neurogenic dural inflammation in guinea pigs. Neuroreport 1997; 8:2237–2240.
16. Gobel H, Lindner V, Heinze A, Ribbat M, Deuschl G. Acute therapy for cluster headache with sumatriptan: findings of a one-year long-term study. Neurology 1998 51:908–911.
17. Brennum J, Kjeldsen M, Olesen J. The 5-HT_1-like agonist sumatriptan has a significant effect in chronic tension-type headache. Cephalalgia. 1992; 12:375–379.
18. Cady RK, Gutterman D, Saiers JA, Beach ME. Responsiveness of non-IHS migraine tension-type headache to sumatriptan. Cephalalgia 1997; 17:588–590.
19. Harrison SD, Balawi SA, Feinmann C, Harris M. Atypical facial pain: a double-blind placebo-controlled crossover pilot study of subcutaneous sumatriptan. Eur Neuropsychopharmacol 1997; 7:83–88.
20. Skingle M, Birch PJ, Leighton GE, Humphrey PP. Lack of antinociceptive activity of sumatriptan in rodents. Cephalalgia 1990; 10:207–212.
21. McCall R. Preclinical and clinical studies in migraine using the selective 5-HT_{1D} receptor agonist PNU-142633. Presented at IBS 3rd Annual Conference on Migraine. Philadelphia, May 1999.
22. Goldstein DJ, Roon KI, Offen WW, Phebus LA, Johnson KW, Schaus JM, VanLaar T, Ferrari MD. Migraine treatment with selective 5-HT_{1F} receptor agonist (SSOFRA) LY334370. Cephalalgia 1999; 19:318.
23. May A, Shepheard SL, Knorr M, Effert R, Wessing A, Hargreaves RJ, Goadsby PJ, Diener HC. Retinal plasma extravasation in animals but not in humans: implications for the pathophysiology of migraine. Brain 1998; 121:1231–1237.
24. Goldstein DJ, Wang O, Saper JR, Stoltz R, Silberstein SD, Mathew NT. Ineffectiveness of neurokinin-1 antagonist in acute migraine: a crossover study. Cephalalgia 1997; 17:785–790.

25. May A, Gijsman HJ, Wallnofer A, Jones R, Diener HC, Ferrari MD. Endothelin antagonist bosentan blocks neurogenic inflammation, but is not effective in aborting migraine attacks. Pain 1996; 67: 375–378.
26. Kaube H, Hoskin KL, Goadsby PJ. Inhibition by sumatriptan of central trigeminal neurones only after blood–brain barrier disruption. Br J Pharmacol 1993; 109:788–792.
27. Lacey LF, Hussey EK, Fowler PA. Single dose pharmacokinetics of sumatriptan in healthy volunteers. Eur J Clin Pharmacol 1995; 47:543–548.
28. Dahlof C. Would any acute treatment for migraine demonstrate recurrence? Cephalalgia 1997: 17(suppl 17):17–19 [discussion 19–20].
29. Mathew NT, Asgharnejad M, Peykamian M, Laurenza A. Naratriptan is effective and well tolerated in the acute treatment of migraine. Results of a double-blind, placebo-controlled, crossover study. The Naratriptan S2WA3003 Study Group. Neurology 1997; 49:1485–1490.

61
Cholinergic Approaches to Pain Therapy

Stephen P. Arneric
DuPont Pharmaceutical Company, Wilmington, Delaware, U.S.A.

I. INTRODUCTION

It has been estimated that nearly one-half billion cases of pain are reported each year, and over 50% of individuals seeking treatment are unsatisfied with current treatment modalities (1–3). A major challenge in biomedical research is the identification of new compounds that more effectively treat both acute and chronic pain states and that lack the side effects associated with the use of morphine and its congeners (e.g., tolerance, abuse, respiratory depression, or constipation). Similarly, compounds that have the anti-inflammatory, analgesic, and antipyretic actions of the nonsteroidal, anti-inflammatory drugs (NSAIDs) without their gastrointestinal side effects remained elusive entities until the identification of the inducible NSAID target enzyme, cyclooxygenase-2 (COX-2), and the commercialization of compounds such as celecoxib or roecoxib (Vioxx) (4). Thus, efforts to identify and develop safer, more efficacious analgesic therapeutics, especially for neuropathic pain, for which no fully effective therapy exists, is a primary research objective for the field of pain management (5).

Modulation of the cholinergic system has been receiving increasing attention as a neurochemical approach used to achieve improved pain therapies. This has been achieved by targeting three primary mechanisms on drug classes: enhancement of acetylcholine (ACh) transmission by inhibition of ACh esterase (AChEase), direct activation of muscarinic ACh receptors (mAChRs), and modulation of nicotinic ACh receptors (nAChRs).

The focus of this chapter will be to give a brief overview of the biology and pharmacology associated with each cholinergic mechanism, describe the lastest advances toward achieving a viable therapy, and highlight the issues associated with further successful development. Each of these molecular approaches have entered at least phase II trials and, with favorable outcomes, may be anticipated to lead to the introduction of novel analgesics by the early portion of the next decade. Because of the more recent advances in understanding nAChR-mediated pharmacology, emphasis will be giving to this mechanism.

II. BACKGROUND: CHOLINERGIC SYSTEMS AND RECEPTORS RELATED TO THE PAIN PATHWAYS

Cholinergic systems are found throughout the neural axis of the pain pathway. ACh and related congeners, as previously described for the opioids, can be algogenic or antinociceptive (6–9), depending on the site of administration and subtype of receptor activated. Before describing the anatomical localization of the cholinergic receptor systems, a synopsis of the the nomenclature for subtypes of nAChRs and mAChRs will follow.

Briefly, nAChRs are ligand-gated ion channels (LGICs), and mAChR families are seven-transmembrane domain (7TM)-coupled metabotropic receptors. mAChRs exist as five specific gene products (M_1, M_2, M_3, M_4, and M_5) that are negatively coupled to adenylate cyclase (M_2, M_4), or positively coupled to phosphatidylinositol phosphate (M_1, M_3, M_5) (10). Neuronal nAChR subunit genes, similar to those found at the neuroskeletal junction, form a pentameric channel composed of various subunits (11) that can gate ions including Na^+, K^+, and Ca^{2+}, depending on the subunit combination. Of the neuronal genes cloned across species, eight (α_2–α_9) code for α subunits (see 12, 13) based on the presence of adjacent cysteine residues in the predicted protein sequences, in a region homologous to the putative agonist-binding site of the muscle α-subunit (α_1). A conserved lysine in the N-terminal extracellular domain of these subunits is believed to be important in the binding of ChCMs (i.e., compounds that active or inhibit nAChR function). Three neuronal non–α-subunits have been identified (β_2–β_4). As a group, however, β-subunits are as different from each other as they are from α-subunits. Rat, human, and chick nAChR genes of the same name are highly homologous (>70% amino acid identity) (12). Of all the subunits cloned across species, only α_6 and α_8 have not been identified in human tissue. Continued cloning efforts are anticipated to result in the identification of novel nAChR subtypes. Thus, the potential for receptor diversity is much greater for nAChRs than for mAChRs.

At the level of somatic nociceptors in the skin, ACh is synthesized, stored, and released from keratinocytes, where it may have a role in either modulating nociceptor sensitivity or promoting wound healing (14). Local injection of ACh or nicotine into the skin of animals and humans, similar to capsaicin, is well known for its painful algesic response (15–17). In skin, little is known about the pharmacology of cholinergic receptor activation. However, it is known that α_3-, α_4-, α_9-, β_2-, and β_4-subunits are present. In addition, activation of nAChRs by nicotine can enhance the release of nociceptive transmitters, such as calcitonin gene-related peptide (CGRP), and result in eliciting an axon reflex at the peripheral end of C fibers (6). This raises the possibility that topical application of compounds that desensitize nAChRs present in skin may have use, as has capsaicin for vanilloid receptors, to produce pain relief. mAChRs within skin may also have a role in skin physiology (14).

In dorsal root ganglian (DRG) and trigeminal ganglion a variety of nAChR subunits exist including α_2-, α_3-, α_4-, α_5-, α_7-, β_2-, and β_4-subunits (18–20). In trigeminal ganglion the two major subtypes that exist, based on immunoprecipitation experiments, are the $\alpha_4\alpha_5\beta_2$ and $\alpha_3\alpha_5\beta_4$-subtypes of nAChRs (18). These combinations of nAChRs are similarly found in sympathetic ganglion (20). The presence of mAChR immunoreactivity is restricted to the small to medium-sized neurons of the DRG as well as the central and peripheral branches of their unmyelinated fibers, suggesting that these receptors are involved in modulating the transduction of noxious stimuli from the periphery (21).

Spinal intrinsic cholinergic inhibitory pathways represent a key modulating system in pain processing: mAChRs are concentrated in the superficial laminae of the dorsal horn of the spinal cord (22), the primary relay area of noxious sensory processing, whereas nAChRs are present with the superficial laminae as well as in medial aspects of the neck of the dorsal horn (23). The source of the innervation of these receptors arises from cholinergic neurons with cell bodies deep within the neck of the dorsal horn (22). Although some reports suggest a nociceptive effect of spinally applied nAChR agonists that may be mediated by activation of primary afferents (24) and enhanced release of glutamate (24), most reports indicate that enhancing cholinergic transmission in spinal cord is antinociceptive and that this antinociception is dependent on mAChRs activation (6,26,27). Intrathecally administered AChEase inhibitors and nonselective cholinergic agonists are entirely attenuated by mAChR, but not nAChR, antagonists (26–28).

The efficacy of several major pain relievers is mediated by cholinergic mechanisms. For example, the antinociception of opioids and the antimigraine agent, sumatriptan, are dependent on the release of ACh to interact with mAChRs. The antinociceptive effect of sumatriptan in mice was prevented by depletion of ACh stores with hemicholinium, or by the mAChR antagonist atropine (29). Intravenous administration of morphine increases the release of norepinephrine (NE) and ACh in dorsal horn dialysates, an effect inhibited by intravenous naloxone or cervical spinal cord transection (30). The spinal release of ACh by morphine, a consequence of indirect α_2-adrenergic activation from descending spinal noradrenergic pathways, results in the synthesis of nitric oxide (NO) that serves as a further positive feedback to locally released NE (30). Thus, recent data support the concept that the analgesic effects of opioids depend, in part, on the spinal release of ACh and nitric oxide. Similarly, pharmacological evidence indicates that spinal muscarinic antinociception is also dependent on an L-arginine–nitric oxide–cyclic GMP cascade in rats (31).

More than one type of mAChR may mediate these antinociceptive actions of AChEase inhibitors and mAChR agonists. Some reports suggest that spinal M_1 and M_3 mAChRs mediate antinociception in the rat (32), whereas subsequent data suggest that M_1 mAChR subtype is not a requirement for antinociceptive activity (33). Further adding to this complexity is the recent report that the antinociceptive effects of muscarinic activation are diminished in M_2 mAChR knockouts (34). Although not yet considered a governing event in the antinociceptive action of ChCMs, nAChR activation at the central end of C fibers can result in decreased release of the nociceptive transmitters' substance P (SP) and CGRP from slices of rat dorsal horn (6,18,35). This is an intriguing finding because in other systems these peptides regulate the phosphorylation state (hence, the rate of rate of receptor activation and desensitization) of nAChRs, suggesting a potential for reciprocal regulation (36). The subunits of nAChRs present at this level of the spinal cord are complementary to those of the DRG, suggesting that the pharmacology of this region could be complex. This diversity may, in many aspects, parallel the complexity seen with μ-, δ-, and κ- opioid receptors that differentially modulate pain processing (37,38).

Relatively little is known about the subtypes of nAChRs that might be involved in antinociception. The ability of the nAChR antagonist DHβE to block nAChR-mediated antinociceptive effects suggests that β_2-containing (perhaps $\alpha_4\beta_2$) nAChR subtypes may play a role, whereas the lack of effect with lower doses of MLA makes it likely that α_7-containing nAChRs do not (9,39). Consistent with this pharmacology, recent antisense knockdown experiments suggest that a significant component of the antinociception mediated by A-85380, a potent nAChR activator (40), is due to activation of α_4-containing neurons in the region of the nucleus raphe magnus (41,42). In addition, homologous recombinant experiments, which have knockedout the α_4-subunit of the nAChR in mice, suggest that this prevents some, but not all, of the antinociceptive actions of (−)-nicotine (42a). Because the remaining antinociceptive actions were in another model of nociception, and these effects were also ablated by the nonselective antagonist mecamylamine, these findings suggest that multiple nAChR subtypes are involved in modulating nociceptive input. Adding to the complexity is that nAChR agonists, such as epibatidine, can produce behavioral signs of both irritation and antinociception when they are injected intrathecally, and the pharmacology of these two actions is distinct (9). This raises the possibility that nonselective nAChR activation induces release of both nociceptive neurotransmitters (e.g., glutamate, SP, and CGRP) (6) and antinociceptive neurotransmitters (e.g., ACh, 5-HT, and NE) (42,43). As these effects are likely mediated by actions at different nAChR subtypes, it may be possible to improve on the efficacy of epibatidine by developing compounds that selectively increase release of inhibitors of pain signaling, or decrease the release of nociceptive transmitters (e.g., SP or CGRP).

Although activation of cholinergic mechanisms in the brain stem and higher centers can be either algogenic (9) or antinociceptive (44,45), the predominant systemic effect of AChEase inhibitors, mAChR agonists, and ChCMs are antinociceptive (6,28,33). Moreover, activation of sites rostral to the brain stem have so far uncovered only mAChR-mediated, not nAChR-mediated, descending inhibitory mechanisms (46,47). Nonetheless, other processes contribute to a response that is ultimately antinociceptive.

For example, take the antinociceptive actions of (−)-nicotine, for which a variety of other neurotransmitter systems with inhibitory influences on pain signaling play an important role in the antinociceptive effects of nAChR agonists. Intrathecal administration of mAChR, 5-HT, α_2-adrenergic, but not opioid, antagonists can attenuate the antinociceptive effects of nAChR activation (43,48). Similarly, lesions that deplete NE or 5-HT attenuate nAChR-mediated antinociception (39,49). From these experiments, it appears that activation of nAChRs can produce antinociception through the release of multiple neurotransmitters. Given that interference with any single one of these other neurotransmitters is insufficient to produce complete blockade of the effect (41,43,48,49), it appears that several contribute in parallel, rather than in series. The ability of intrathecal administration of antagonists of these neurotransmitters to reduce the antinociceptive effects of systemically injected (−)-nicotine suggests that the spinal cord is an important site for neurotransmitter release (48). However, intrathecal mecamylamine only modestly attenuates the antinociceptive effects of systemic (−)-nicotine, and direct injection of any of several nAChR agonists into the brain stem can produce antinociception (8,42,48,49). These data suggest that activation of descending inhibition originating in brain stem sites, such as the nucleus raphe magnus, plays an important role in nAChR-mediated antinociception (41). Indeed, recent colocalization studies indicate that α_4-containing nAChRs are present on serotonergic neurons in the raphe magnus (41), an important component of the pain modulating system (50).

III. ACETYLCHOLINESTERASE INHIBITORS

Administration of AChEase inhibitors such as neostigmine (Fig. 1) will produce antinociception when given centrally (28). Until recently, whether peripheral sites of antinociceptive action exist for AChEase inhibitors has been unexplored. Buerkle and co-workers (51) demonstrated in a rat inflamed knee joint model that intra-articular administration of neostigmine results in dose-dependent thermal and mechanical antinociception, as can be seen with intrathecal neostigmine. In an analogous study, the clinical analgesic action of intra-articular neostigmine was determined after patients had undergone knee arthroscopy. Intra-articular administration of 500 μg of neostigmine produced moderate analgesia that was substantially longer in duration when compared with 2 mg of intra-articular morphine (52). An intriguing aspect of AChEase inhibitors is that their efficacy is enhanced during chronic pain states in which pain itself leads to increased descending NE neurotransmission and spinal ACh release (28). Thus, AChEase inhibitors may be especially effective in chronic pain states, particularly when combined with opioids, α_2-agonists, or antidepressants (53,54). These studies provide preclinical and clinical support of the concept that activation of peripheral and central mAChRs can provide therapeutically meaningful benefit when given alone or as adjunctive therapy.

The primary issue with systemic AChEase inhibitors is related to their ability to nonselectivity increase cholinergic transmission. At low doses they can lead to generalized gastrointestinal distress, including nausea and emesis and, at higher doses, the classic "SLUD syndrome"

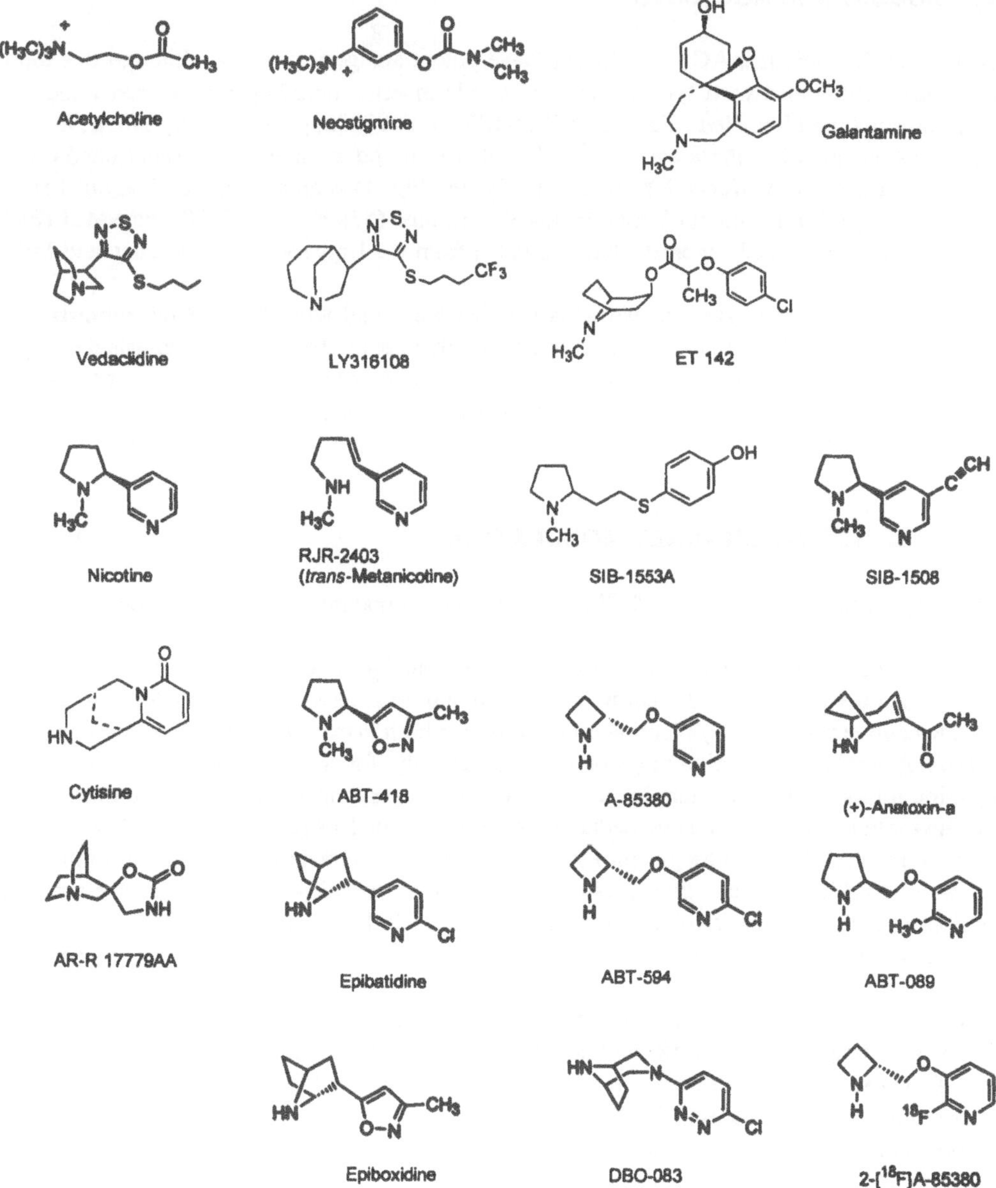

Figure 1 Structures of currently developed AChEase inhibitors that may be of use in pain management.

(*s*alivation, *l*acrimation, *u*rination, *d*efecation) as well as central sympathetic stimulation can be observed to increase blood pressure (55). Although, many of these effects can be limited by intrathecal or local administration, this delivery requirement clearly reduces their broad therapeutic usefulness.

Will the better-tolerated AChEase inhibitors currently developed for the treatment of Alzheimer's disease (e.g., donepezil [Aricept] or galantamine; see Fig. 1) (56) find secondary markets for pain management? It remains to be explored whether the doses used for Alzheimer's disease treatment are sufficient as a pain therapy.

IV. MUSCARINIC AGONISTS

Agonists at the various mAChRs (M_1–M_4) have potent analgesic activity, although this too is frequently confounded with typical muscarinic side effects, including pronounced effects on gastrointestinal motility. Vedaclidine (NNC 11-1053, LY297802; phase II; Lilly/Nova Nordisk) is the most advanced of these agents (33,57), but is rumored to have been discontinued owing to gastrointestinal side effects. LY 316108 (Lilly; see Fig. 1) is another mAChR agonist at the preclinical stage for treatment of irritable bowel syndrome (57). ET 142, SS20, and SM21 (FID-72021; Fidia) are mAChR agonists that originated from the Universities of Florence and Milan (58).

Many of the same gastrointestinal issues that are found with the mAChR agonists used for the treatment of Alzheimer's disease (56) are likely to apply for mAChR agonists developed as pain therapies. However, should one of these agents become available, in contrast to nAChR agonists, they are not anticipated to have any Controlled Substances Act-scheduling liabilities associated with them.

V. CHOLINERGIC CHANNEL MODULATORS

Cholinergic channel modulators (ChCMs) are compounds that modulate the function of nAChRs (13).

Reports indicating that (−)-nicotine may have analgesic activity date back to the early 1930s when it was shown that nicotine was effective in treating visceral pain (59). This modest antinociceptive action of (−)-nicotine is demonstrable both in experimental animals and humans (60,61). A single site of action of (−)-nicotine is unlikely, for antinociception is observed after injection into several brain stem locations (8,42). However, consistent effects are obtained by injecting into the lateral tegmental peducular pontine and nucleus raphe magnus where it stimulates the release of ACh, norepinephrine, and serotonin to activate descending pain inhibitory pathways (31,43,62). Alternatively, nAChR activation in the spinal cord can produce antinociception by a process that involves an increase in intracellular calcium (63–65).

However, it was not until the discovery of the frog alkaloid, epibatidine, by Daly and coworkers (66–69), that the tools were available to more precisely characterize the nAChR approach to pain modulation. Epibatidine is 100–200 times more potent than morphine as an analgesic, acting through nAChRs and not antagonized by the opioid receptor antagonist, naloxone. This alkaloid is nonselective in its actions at several nAChRs, including the ganglionic ($\alpha_3\beta_x$) and neuromuscular ($\alpha_1\ \beta_{1\delta\gamma\epsilon}$) subtypes (68). As a consequence, there is a very narrow window between the beneficial analgesic actions of the compound and its toxic and ultimately lethal effects on the cardiorespiratory system (70).

Nonetheless, epibatidine has provided some key insights into the therapeutic potential of the nAChR approach. For example, the involvement of spinal nAChRs in the modulation of inflammatory responses was established in a model of acute arthritis in rats. Following administration of epibatidine to the dorsal horn with a microdialysis fiber, the inflammation caused by a mixture of kaolin and carrageenan injected into the knee joint was reduced (71). Outcome measures of heat hyperalgesia, knee joint circumference, and temperature, all were reduced, supporting a role of ChCMs to treat persistent inflammatory pain and neurogenic inflammation.

Critically, it was shown that, in contrast to (−)-nicotine, the antinociceptive actions of epibatidine are not necessarily tolerated with repeated dosing. Although both enantiomers of epibatidine have equivalent affinities for nAChRs and similar antinociceptive potencies and efficacy, only one enantiomer achieves this lack of tolerance (72). This key feature has been incorporated into some of the follow-on compounds in clinical development (73–76).

ABT-594 (Abbott) is an azetidine bioisostere of (−)-nicotine (see Fig. 1) that retains the analgesic actions associated with this class of compound while showing a reduced propensity toward the toxic side effects seen with epibatidine (35,49,77–80). ABT-594 is approximately 100 times more potent than morphine in a spectrum of pain models and, unlike morphine, shows no evidence of developing tolerance or opioid-like dependence liability, nor does it have effects on respiration or gastrointestinal motility (49,79). Interestingly, ABT-594 exerts neuroprotective effects in spinal cord cultures against substance P- or glutamate-induced toxicities (80) and is effective in models of neuropathic pain (78). The observation that ABT-594 does not tolerate with repeated dosing is encouraging to its potential success for treating chronic pain syndromes, without leading to some of the known effects that are induced by tolerance with ChCMs (73,81).

DBO-83 ((82,83); University of Milan), RJR-2403 (84,85; RJR/Targacept), and CMI 980 (Cytomed) represent other novel ChCMs. ABT-594 is the only ChCM reported to be in clinical development for the treatment of pain.

Although compounds similar to ABT-594 have a superior preclinical side-effect profile relative to epibatidine (49,79), there are still no reports on the general tolerability of this compound in patients. Gastrointestinal side effects have been the plague of all previous cholinergic approaches and may remain an issue for the clinical success of ChCMs.

Another less-recognized issue is genotype-dependent differences in analgesic responsiveness to therapies. Recently it is becoming apparent that opioids can demonstrate robust strain-selective potencies in preclinical models of antinociception (86). Although there are clear patient-to-patient variations in the responsiveness to opioids, these variations have not negatively affected their usefulness. Genotype-dependent differences can also be shown for sensitivity to ChCMs. For example, the acute analgesic potency of cytisine measured by the tail-flick assay differed by more than 3200-fold between CD-1 and CF-1 outbred strains of mice (87). This was not a generalized pharmacological difference in sensitivity to ChCMs, as inhibition of locomotor activity and induction of seizures and lethality to cytisine did not differ between strains. It remains to be determined whether similar sensitivities to ChCMs will be reflected in clinical studies.

VI. FUTURE DIRECTIONS, PERSPECTIVES, AND ISSUES

Although the concept of cholinergic-mediated analgesia is more than half a century old, it is uncertain whether any of the three major mechanisms—AChEase inhibition, mAChR agonism, or ChCM modulation—will lead to clinically viable treatments of pain. Efforts are underway by several pharmaceutical companies to verify the usefulness of these approaches (refer to Table 1 for a synopsis). Issues that must be resolved include:

1. What is the clinical efficacy of these agents against various forms of acute and neuropathic pain? Are they broad, or limited?
2. What are the clinical side effect profiles of these agents? What are the drug–drug interactions?
3. Will ChCMs require DEA scheduling?

AChEase inhibitors may find utility as powerful adjuncts to other existing therapies when given intrathecally (53), but they may be limited to this route of administration. The approval of oral AChEase inhibitors for the treatment of other indications, such as Alzheimer's disease,

Table 1 Potential Cholinergic Therapies to Treat Pain

Compounds	Company	Phase	Indication: comments	Refs.
AChEase inhibitors				
Neostigmine		II	Acute joint pain; postoperative pain	28,51,52
Galantamine	J&J	III—pain preclinical	Alzheimer's disease—a well-tolerated cholinesterase inhibitor with weak nAChR activity—line extension to pain?	56
mAChR agonists				
Vedaclidine	Lilly/Novo Nordisk	II	Acute and inflammatory pain	33,57
LY 316108	Lilly	Preclinical	Acute pain; irritable bowel syndrome	57
ET-142	Univ. Milan	Preclinical	Acute pain	Investigational Drug Database
ChCMs				
ABT-594	Abbott	II	Acute and neuropathic pain	35,49,77,78,79,80
RJR-2403	Targacept	I	Acute pain	84,85
Iodinated; epibatidine	NIDA	Preclinical	Potential PET ligands	90,91
A-85380 and fluorinated derivatives	Abbott/NIDA	Preclinical	A-85380 and fluorinated derivatives are being explored as PET ligand tools	40,93
RJR-2557	Targacept	Preclinical	Acute pain	Investigational Drug Database
CMI-980	CytoMed	Preclinical	Acute pain: epibatidine analogues	Investigational Drug Database
DBO-083	Univ. Milan/Abbott	Preclinical	Acute pain: novel structure	82,83
Epiboxidine	Novo Nordisk	Preclinical	Epibatidine analogue	94
ABT-418	Abbott	Phase II—pain preclinical?	Attention deficit hyperactivity disorder: modest efficacy in acute preclinical pain model	45,95
ABT-089	Abbott	Phase I—pain preclinical?	Attention deficit hyperactivity disorder: modest efficacy in acute preclinical pain model	96,97,98
SIB 1508Y	Sibia	Phase II—pain preclinical?	Parkinson's disease: efficacy in pain models not reported	99
SIB 1553A	Sibia	Phase II—pain preclinical?	Alzheimer's disease: efficacy in pain models not reported	99
AR-R 17779AA	Astra	Preclinical	Best available, novel α_7 selective full agonist: does it modify nociceptive processing?	100

could pave the way to expanding the acceptability of this approach. Less encouraging is the mAChR agonist approach since it has been so difficult to avoid the side effect liabilities of these agents as demonstrated by the side effect profiles of nAChR agonists for treating Alzheimer's disease. Each of these targets, especially the ChCM approach seem to have utility to treat a broad spectrum of pain states, including neuropathic as well as acute inflammatory pain. In addition, ChCMs have opioid-sparing potential that represent a beneficial drug–drug interaction. Yet interactions with other clinically used agents, such as anesthetics, could be detrimental and must still be defined (88,89). The use of positron emmision tomography (PET) ligands to label nAChRs and possibly serve as a means of establishing central receptor occupancy may facilitate clinical research in this area (90–92). However, the potential for side effects and the looming possibility for scheduling of these agents, regardless of physical dependence liabilities (93), could limit commercial success. Despite these caveats, there is sufficient promise that in the new millennium there will be one or more of these powerful new approaches to meet the unmet medical needs in fighting against various pain states.

REFERENCES

1. Erickson D. Progress against pain. Start-up. Windhover's Rev Emerg Med Ventures 1997; 2:8–3.
2. Engberg G, Orzepowski L. Beyond pain. New approaches to pain relief. New York Times Chicago Life, Supplement, Sunday, November, 23, 1997. pp. 25/66–69.
3. Brownlee S, Schrof JM. The quality of mercy. U.S. News World Report, March 17, 1997, 54–67.
4. Lipsky PE. Specific COX-2 inhibitors in arthritis, oncology and beyond: where is the science headed? J Rheumatol 1999; 56:25–30.
5. Millan MJ. The induction of pain: an integrative review. Prog Neurobiol 1999; 57:1–164.
6. Flores CM, Hargreaves KM. Neuronal nicotinic receptors: new targets in the treatment of pain. In: Arneric SP, Brioni JD, eds. Neuronal Nicotinic Receptors: Pharmacology and Therapeutic Opportunities. New York: Wiley–Liss, 1999; 359–377.
7. Iwamoto ET, Marion L. Characterization of the antinociception produced by intrathecally administered muscarinic agonists in rats. J Pharmacol Exp Ther 1993; 266:329–338.
8. Iwamoto ET. Characterization of the antinociception induced by nicotine administration into the pedunculopontine tegmental nucleus and raphe magnus. J Pharmacol Exp Ther 1991; 257:120–133.
9. Khan IM, Buerkle H, Taylor P, Yaksh TL. Nociceptive and antinociceptive responses to intrathecal administered nicotinic agents. Neuropharmacology 1998; 37:1515–1525.
10. Brown JH, Taylor P. Muscarinic receptor agonists and antagonists. In: Gilman AG, Rall TW, Nies AS, Taylor P, eds. Goodman and Gilman's Pharmacological Basis of Therapeutics. 9th ed. New York: McGraw-Hill, 1996; 141–160.
11. Lindstrom J. Nicotinic acetylcholine receptors in health and disease. Mol Neurobiol 1997; 15:193–222.
12. McGehee DS, Role LW. Physiological diversity of nicotinic acetylcholine receptors expressed by vertebrate neurons. Annu Rev Physiol 1995; 57:521–546.
13. Arneric SP, Holladay MW. Agonists and antagonists of nicotinic acetylcholine receptors. In: Clementi F, Gotti C, Fornasari D, eds. Neuronal Nicotinic Receptors. Handbook of Experimental Pharmacology. Heidelberg: Springer-Verlag, 1999; Chap. 14.
14. Grando SA. Biological functions of keratinocyte cholinergic receptors. J Investi Dermatol Symp Proc 1997; 2:41–48.
15. Armstrong D, Dry RML, Keele CA, Makham JW. Observations on chemical exitants of cutaneous pain in man. J Physiol 1953; 120:326–351.
16. Keele CA, Armstrong D. Substances Producing Pain and Itch. London: Edward Arnold, 1964; 107–123.
17. Steen KH, Reeh PW. Actions of cholinergic agonists and antagonists on sensory nerve endings in rat skin, in vitro. J Neurophysiol 1993; 70:397–405.

18. Puttfarcken PS, Manelli AM, Arneric SP, Donnelly–Roberts DL. Evidence for nicotinic receptors potentially modulating nociceptive transmission at the level of the primary sensory neuron: studies with F11 cells. J Neurochem 1997; 69:930–938.
19. Flores CM, DeCamp RM, Kilo S, Rogers SW, Hargreaves KM. Neuronal nicotinic receptor expression in sensory neurons of the rat trigeminal ganglion: demonstration of alpha$_3$beta$_4$, a novel subtype in the mammalian nervous system. J Neurosci 1996; 16:7892–7901.
20. Ramirez–Latorre J, Crabtree G, Turner J, Role L. Molecular composition and biophysical characteristics of nicotinic receptors. In: Arneric SP, Brioni JD, eds. Neuronal Nicotinic Receptors: Pharmacology and Therapeutic Opportunities. New York: Wiley–Liss, 1999; 43–64.
21. Bernardini N, de Stefano ME, Tata AM, Biagioni S, Augusti–Tocco G. Neuronal and non-neuronal cell populations of the avian dorsal root ganglia express muscarinic acetylcholine receptors. Int J Dev Neurosci 1998; 16:365–77.
22. Barber RP, Phelps PE, Houser CR, Crawford GD, Salvatetra PM. The morphology and distribution of neurons containing choline acetyltransferase in the adult rat spinal cord: an immunocytochemical study. Comp Neurol 1984; 229:329–346.
23. Khan IM, Yaksh TL, Taylor P. Epibatidine binding sites and activity in the spinal cord. Brain Res 1997; 753:269–282.
24. Roberts RGD, Stevenson JE, Westerman RA, Pennefather J. Nicotinic acetylcholine receptors on capsaicin-sensitive nerves. Neuroreport 1995; 6:1578–1582.
25. Khan IM, Marsala M, Printz MP, Taylor P, Yaksh TL. Intrathecal nicotinic agonist-elicited release of excitatory amino acids as measured by in vivo spinal microdialysis in rats. J Pharmacol Exp Ther 1996; 278:97–106.
26. Green PG, Kitchen I. Antinociception opioids and the cholinergic system. Prog Neurobiol 1986; 26:119–146.
27. Pert A. Cholinergic and catecholaminergic modulation of nociceptive reactions. Pain Headache 1987; 9:1–63.
28. Eisenbach JC. Muscarinic-mediated analgesia. Life Sci 1999; 64:549–554.
29. Ghelardini C, Galeotti N, Nicolodi M, Donaldson S, Sicuteri F, Bartolini A. Involvement of central cholinergic system in antinociception induced by sumatriptan in mouse. Int J Clin Pharmacol Res 1997; 17:105–109.
30. Xu Z, Tong C, Pan HL, Cerda SE, Eisenbach JC. Intravenous morphine increases release of nitric oxide from spinal cord by an alpha-adrenergic and cholinergic mechanism. J Neurophysiol 1997; 78:2072–2078.
31. Iwamoto ET, Marion L. Pharmacologic evidence that spinal muscarinic analgesia is mediated by an L-arginine/nitric oxide/cyclic GMP cascade in rats. J Pharmacol Exp Ther 1994; 271:601–608.
32. Naguib M, Yaksh TL. Characterization of muscarinic receptor subtypes that mediate antinociception in rat spinal cord. Anesth Analg 1997; 85:847–853.
33. Sheardown MJ, Shannon HE, Swedberg MD, Suzdak PD, Bymaster FP, Olesen PH, Mitch CH, Ward JS, Sauerberg P. M_1 receptor agonist activity is not a requirement for muscarinic antinociception. J Pharmacol Exp Ther 1997; 281:868–875.
34. Gomez J, Shannon H, Kostenis E, Felder C, Zhang L, Brodkin J, Grinberg A, Sheng H, Wess J. Pronounced pharmacologic deficits in M_2 muscarinic acetylcholine receptor knockouts. Proc Natl Acad Sci USA 1999; 96:1692–1697.
35. Donnelly–Roberts D, Puttfarken PS, Kunztweiler TA, Briggs CA, Anderson DJ, Campbell JE, Piatonni–Kaplan M, McKenna DG, Wasicak JT, Holladay MW, Williams M, Arneric SP. 5-[(2*R*)-azetidinylmethoxy]-2-chloropyridine (ABT-594): a novel, orally effective antinociceptive agent acting via neuronal nicotinic acetylcholine receptors. I. In vitro characterization. J Pharmacol Exp Ther 1998; 285:777–786.
36. Mulle C, Benoit P, Pinset C, Roa M, Changeux JP. Calcintonin gene-related peptide enhances the rate of densensitization of the nicotinic acetylcholine receptor in cultured mouse muscle cells. Proc Natl Acad Sci USA 1988; 85:5728–5732.
37. Cherney NI. Opioid analgesics. Comparative features and prescribing guidelines. Drugs 1996; 51: 713–717.

38. Reisine T, Pasternak. Opioid analgesics and antagonists. In: Hardman JG, Limbird, LE, Molinoff PB, Ruddon RW, Gilman AG, eds. Goodman and Gilman's the Pharmacological Basis of Therapeutics. 9th ed. New York: McGraw Hill, 1996; 521–555.
39. Rao TS, Correa LD, Reid RT, Lloyd GK. Evaluation of anti-nociceptive effects of neuronal nicotinic acetylcholine receptor (nAChR) ligands in the rat tail-flick assay. Neuropharmacology 1996; 35: 393–405.
40. Sullivan, JP, Donnelly–Roberts D, Briggs CA, Anderson DJ, Gopalakrishnan M, Piattoni–Kaplan M, Campbell JE, McKenna DG, Molinari E, Hettinger AM, Garvey DS, Wasicak J, Holladay MW, Williams M, Arneric SP. A-85380 [3-(2(*S*)-azetidinylmethoxy)pyridine]: in vitro pharmacological properties of a novel, high affinity $\alpha_4\beta_2$ nicotinic acetylcholine receptor ligand. Neuropharmacology 1996; 35:725–734.
41. Bitner RS, Nikkel AL, Curzon P, Arneric SP, Bannon AW, Decker MW. Role of the nucleus raphe magnus in antinociception produced by ABT-594: immediate early gene responses possibly linked to neuronal nicotinic acetylcholine receptors on serotonergic neurons. J Neurosci 1998; 18:5426–5432.
42. Iwamoto ET. Antinociception of nicotine administration into the mesopontine tegmentum of rats: evidence for muscarinic actions. J Pharmacol Exp Ther 1989; 251:412–421.
42a. Marubio LM, Del Mar Arroyo–Jimenez M, Cordero–Erausquin M, Lena C, LeNovere N, De Kerchove D'Exaerde A, Huchet M, Damaj MI, Changeux J–P. Reduced antinociception in mice lacking neuronal nicotinic receptor subunits. Nature 1999; 398:805–810.
43. Iwamoto ET, Marion L. Adrenergic, serotonergic and cholinergic components of nicotine antinociception in rats. J Pharmacol Exp Ther 1993; 265:777–789.
44. Damaj MI, Glassco W, Dukat M, May EL, Glennon RA, Martin BR. Pharmacology of novel nicotinic analogs. Drug Dev Res 1996; 38:177–187.
45. Damaj MI, Fei–Yin M, Dukat M, Glassco W, Glennon RA, Martin BR. Antinociceptive responses to nicotinic acetylcholine receptor ligands after systemic and intrathecal administration in mice. J Pharmacol Exp Ther 1998; 284:1058–1065.
46. Franco AC, Prado WA. Antinociceptive effects of stimulation of discrete sites in the rat hypothalamus: evidence for the participation of the lateral hypothalamus area in descending pain suppression mechanisms. Braz. J Med Biol Res 1996; 29:1531–1541.
47. Oliveira MA, Prado WA. Antinociception induced by stimulating amygdaloid nuclei in rats: changes produced by systemically administered antagonists. Braz J Med Biol Res 1998; 31:681–690.
48. Roger DT, Iwamoto ET. Multiple spinal mediators in parenteral nicotine-induced antinociception. J Pharmacol Exp Ther 1993; 267:341–349.
49. Decker MW, Curzon P, Holladay MW, Nikkel AL, Bitner SR, Bannon AW, Donnelly–Roberts DL, Puttfarken PS, Kuntzweiler TA, Briggs CA, Williams M, Arneric SP. The role of neuronal nicotinic acetylcholine receptors in antinociception: effects of ABT-594. J Physiology (Paris) 1998; 92:221–224.
50. Wang Q–P, Nakai Y. The dorsal raphe: an important nucleus in pain modulation. Brain Res Bull 1994; 34:575–585.
51. Buerkle H, Boschin M, Marcus MA, Brodner G, Wusten R, Van Aken H. Central and peripheral analgesia mediated by the acetylcholinesterase-inhibitor neostigmine in the rat inflamed knee joint model. Anesth Analg 1998; 86:1027–1032.
52. Yang LC, Chen LM, Wang CJ, Buerkle H. Postoperative analgesia by intra-articular neostigmine in patients undergoing knee arthroscopy. Anesthesiology 1998; 88:334–339.
53. Abram SE, Winne RP. Intrathecal acetyl cholinesterase inhibitors produce analgesia that is synergistic with morphine and clonidine in rats. Anesth Analg 1995; 81:501–507.
54. Eisenbach JC, Gebhart GF. Intrathecal amitriptyline. Antinociceptive interactions with intravenous morphine and intrathecal clonidine, neostigmine, and carbamylcholine in rats. Anesthesiology 1995; 83:1036–1045.
55. Taylor P. Anticholinesterase agents. In: Gilman AG, Rall TW, Nies AS, Taylor P, eds. Goodman and Gilman's Pharmacological Basis of Therapeutics. 9th ed. New York: McGraw-Hill, 1996:161–176.

56. Grundman M, Corey–Bloom J, Thal LJ. Perspectives in clinical Alzheimer's disease research and the development of antidementia drugs. J Neural Transm Suppl 1998; 53:255–75.
57. Mitch C. Discovery and investigation of muscarinic agonists with potent antinociceptive activity, In: New Methods in Pain Control, Gordon Conference, Aug 3, 1998.
58. Gualtieri F, Bottalico C, Calandrella A, et al. Presynaptic cholinergic modulators as potent cognition enhancers and analgesic drugs. 2. 2-Phenoxy, 2-(phenylthio)-, and 2-(phenylamino)alkanoic acid esters. J Med Chem 1994; 37:1712–1719.
59. Davis L, Pollock LJ, Stone TT. Visceral pain. Surg Gynecol Obstet 1932; 55:418–426.
60. Tripathi HL, Martin BR, Aceto MD. Nicotine-induced antinociception in mice and rats: correlation with nicotine brain levels. J Pharmacol Exp Ther 1982; 221:91–96.
61. Pomerleau OF. Nicotine as a psychoactive drug: anxiety and pain reduction. Psychopharm Bull 1986; 22:865–869.
62. Hunt TE, Wu WH, Zbuzek VK. The effects of serotonin biosynthesis inhibition on nicotine and nifedipine-induced analgesia in rats. Anesth Analg 1998; 87:1109–1112.
63. Damaj MI, Welch SP, Martin BR. Involvement of calcium and L-type channels in nicotine-induced antinociception. J Pharmacol Exp Ther 1993; 266:1330–1338.
64. Rathouz BDKMM. Synaptic-type acetylcholine receptors raise intracellular calcium levels in neurons by two mechanisms. J Neurosci 1994; 14:6935–6945.
65. Bannon AW, Gunther KL, Decker MW, Arneric SP. The influence of Bay K 8644 treatment on (+/−)-epibatidine-induced analgesia. Brain Res 1995; 678:244–250.
66. Spande TF, Garraffo HG, Edwards MW, Yeh HJC, Pannell L, Daly JW. Epibatidine: a novel (chloropyridyl)azabicycloheptane with potent analgesic activity from an Ecuadoran poison frog. J Am Chem Soc 1992; 114:3475–3478.
67. Badio B, Daly JW. Epibatidine, a potent analgetic and nicotinic agonist. Mol Pharmacol 1994; 45: 563–569.
68. Gerzanich V, Peng X, Wang F, Wells G, Anand R, Fletcher S, Lindstrom J. Comparative pharmacology of epibatidine: a potent agonist for neuronal nicotinic acetylcholine receptors. Mol Pharmacol 1995; 48:774–782.
69. Perry DC, Kellar KJ. [^{3}H]Epibatidine labels nicotinic receptors in rat brain: an autoradiographic study. J Pharmacol Exp Ther 1995; 275:1030–1034.
70. Sullivan JP, Decker MW, Brioni JD, Donnelly–Roberts D, Anderson DJ, Bannon AW, Kang C–H, Adams P, Piattoni–Kaplan M, Buckley MJ, Gopalakrishnan M, Williams M, Arneric SP. (±)-Epibatidine elicits a diversity of in vitro and in vivo effects mediated by nicotinic acetylcholine receptors. J Pharmacol Exp Ther 1994; 271:1–8.
71. Lawand NB, Lu Y, Westlund KN. Nicotinic cholinergic receptors: potential targets for inflammatory pain relief. Pain 1999; 80:291–299.
72. Damaj MI, Creasy KR, Grove AD, Rosecrans JA, Martin BR. Pharmacologic effects of epibatidine optical enantiomers. Brain Res 1994; 664:34–40.
73. Decker MW, Brioni JD, Bannon AW, Arneric SP. Diversity of neuronal nicotinic acetylcholine receptors: lessons from behavior and implications for CNS therapeutics. Life Sci 1995; 56:545–570.
74. Glennon RA, Dukat M. Nicotinic cholinergic receptor pharmacophores In: Arneric SP, Brioni JD, eds. Neuronal Nicotinic Receptors: Pharmacology and Therapeutic Opportunities. New York: Wiley–Liss, 1999;271–284.
75. Holladay MW, Dart MJ, Lynch JK. Neuronal nicotinic acetylcholine receptors as targets for drug discovery. J Med Chem 1997; 40:4169–4194.
76. Holladay MW, Wasicak JT, Lin N–H, He Y, Ryther KB, Bannon AW, Buckley MJ, Kim DJB, Decker MW, Anderson DJ, Campbell JE, Kuntzweiler TA, Donnelly–Roberts DL, Piattoni–Laplan M, Briggs CA, Williams M, Arneric SP. Identification and structure–activity relationships of (*R*-5-(2-azetidinylmethoxy)-2-chloropyridine (ABT-594), a potent, orally active analgesic agent acting via neuronal nicotinic acetylcholine receptors. J Med Chem 1998; 41:407–412.
77. Decker MW, Bannon AW, Buckley MJ, Kim DJB, Holladay MW, Ryther KB, Lin NH, Wasicak JT, Williams M, Arneric SP. Antinociceptive effects of the novel neuronal nicotinic acetylcholine receptor agonist, ABT-594, in mice. Eur J Pharmacol 1998; 346:23–33.

78. Bannon AW, Decker MW, Kim DJB, Campbell JE, Arneric SP. ABT-594, a novel cholinergic channel modulator, is efficacious in nerve ligation and diabetic neuropathy models of neuropathic pain. Brain Res 1998; 801:158–163.
79. Bannon AW, Decker MW, Holladay MW, Curzon P, Donnelly–Roberts D, Puttfarcken PS, Bitner RS, Pauly JL, Diaz A, Porsolt R, Dickenson AH, Williams M, Arneric SP. Broad-spectrum, nonopioid analgesic activity by selective modulation of neuronal nicotinic acetylcholine receptors. Science 1998; 279:77–81.
80. Donnelly–Roberts D, Puttfarcken P, Jacobs IX, Kuntzweiler T, Arneric SP. ABT-594: neuroprotective effects in spinal cord (sc) cultures by a broad spectrum analgesic acting via nicotinic acetylcholine receptors (nAChRs). Soc Neurosci, New Orleans, LA Oct 1997.
81. Marks MJ. Desensitization and the regulation of neuronal nicotinic receptors In: Arneric SP, Brioni JD, eds. Neuronal Nicotinic Receptors: Pharmacology and Therapeutic Opportunities. New York: Wiley–Liss, 1999;65–80.
82. Barlocco D, Cignarella G, Tondi D, Vianello P, Villa S, Bartolini A, Ghelardini G, Galeotti N, Anderson DJ, Kuntzweiler TA, Colombo D, Toma L. Mono- and disubstituted-3,8-diazabicyclo[3.2.1]octane derivatives as analgesics structurally related to epibatidine: synthesis, activity, and modeling. J Med Chem 1998; 41:674–681.
83. Ghelardini C, Galeotti N, Barlocco D, Bartolini A. Antinociceptive profile of the new nicotinic agonist DBO-83. Drug Dev Res 1997; 40:251–258.
84. Bencherif M, Lovette ME, Fowler KW, Arrington S, Reeves L, Caldwell WS, Lippiello PM. RJR-2403: a nicotinic agonist with CNS selectivity I. In vitro characterization. J Pharmacol Exp Ther 1996; 279:1413–1421.
85. Lippiello PM, Bencherif M, Gray JA, Peters S, Grigoryan G, Hodges H, Collins AC. RJR-2403: a nicotinic agonist with CNS selectivity II. In vivo characterization. J Pharmacol Exp Ther 1996; 279:1422–1429.
86. Mogul et al. 1999.
87. Seale TW, Nael R, Singh S, Basmadjian G. Inherited, selective hypoanalgesic response to cytisine in the tail-flick test in CF-1 mice. Neuroreport 1998; 9:201–205.
88. Flood P, Ramirex–Latorre J, Role L. $\alpha_4\beta_2$ neuronal nicotinic acetylcholine receptors in the central nervous system are inhibited by isoflurane and propofol, but α_7-type nicotinic receptors are unaffected. Anesthesiology 1997; 86:859–865.
89. Yost SC, Dodson BA. Inhibition of nicotinic acetycholine receptor by barbiturates and by procaine: do they act at different sites? Cell Mol Neurobiol 1993; 13:159–172.
90. Liang F, Navarro HA, Abraham P, Kotian P, Ding Y–S, Fowler J, Volkow N, Kuhar MJ, Carroll FI. Synthesis and nicotinic acetylcholine receptor binding properties of exo-2-(2′-fluoro-5′-pyridinyl)-7-azabicyclo[2.2.1]heptane: a new positron emission tomography ligand for nicotinic receptors. J Med Chem 1997; 40:2293–2295.
91. Musachio JL, Horti A, London ED, Dannals RF. Synthesis of radioiodinated analog of epibatidine: (+)-exo-2-(2-iodo-5-pyridyl)-7-azabicyclo[2.2.1]heptane for in vitro and in vivo studies of nicotinic acetylcholine receptors. J Label Comp Radiopharm 1997; 39:39.
92. Villemagne ML, Musachio JL, Scheffel U. Nicotine and related compounds as PET and SPECT ligands. In: Arneric SP, Brioni JD, eds. Neuronal Nicotinic Receptors: Pharmacology and Therapeutic Opportunities. New York: Wiley–Liss, 1999;235–250.
93. Williams M, Arneric SP. Beyond the tobacco debate: dissecting out the therapeutic potential of nicotine. Exp Opin Invest Drugs 1996; 5:1035–1045.
94. Badio B, Garraffo M, Plummer CV, Padgett WL, Daly JW. Synthesis and nicotinic activity of epiboxidine: an isoxazole analogue of epibatidine. Eur J Pharmacol 1997; 321:189–194.
95. Arneric SP, Anderson DJ, Bannon AW, Briggs CA, Buccafusco JJ, Brioni JD, Cannon JG, Decker MW, Gopalakrishnan M, Holladay MW, Kyncl J, Marsh KC, Pauly J, Radek R, Rodrigues AD, Sullivan JP. Preclinical pharmacology of ABT-418: a prototypical cholinergic channel activator for the potential treatment of Alzheimer's disease. CNS Drug Rev 1995; 1:1–26.
96. Decker MW, Bannon AW, Curzon P, Gunther KL, Brioni JD, Holladay MW, Lin N–H, Li Y, Daanen JF, Buccafusco JF, Prendergast MA, Jackson W, Arneric SP. ABT-089 [2-methyl-3-(2-

(*S*)-pyrrolidinylmethoxy)pyridine dihydrochloride]: II. A novel cholinergic channel modulator with effects on cognitive performance in rats and monkeys. J Pharmacol Exp Ther 1997; 283:247–258.

97. Sullivan JP, Donnelly–Roberts D, Briggs CA, Gopalakrishnan M, Hu I, Campbell JE, Anderson DJ, Piattoni–Kaplan M, Molinari E, McKenna DG, Gunn DE, Lin N–H, Ryther KB, He Y, Holladay MW, Williams M, Arneric SP. ABT-089 [2-methyl-3-(2-(*S*)-pyrrolidinylmethoxy)pyridine dihydrochloride]: a potent and selective cholinergic channel modulator with cytoprotective properties. J Pharmacol Exp Ther 1997; 283:235–246.

98. Arneric SP, Campbell JE, Carroll S, Daanen JF, Holladay MW, Johnson P, Lin N–H, Marsh KC, Peterson B, Qui Y, Roberts EM, Rodrigues AD, Sullivan JP, Trivedi J, Williams M. ABT-089 [3-(2(*S*)-pyrrolidinylmethoxy)-2-methylpyridine]: an orally effective cholinergic channel modulator with potential once-a-day dosing and cardiovascular safety. Drug Dev Res 1997; 41:31–43.

99. Menzaghi F, McClure DE, Lloyd KG. Subtype-selective nAChR agonists for the treatment of neurological disorders: SIB-1508Y and SIB-1553A. In: Arneric SP, Brioni JD, eds. Neuronal Nicotinic Receptors: Pharmacology and Therapeutic Opportunities. New York: Wiley–Liss, 1999;379–394.

100. Kaiser F, Hudzik T, Borrelli A, Awere S, Cramer C, Widzowski D. AR-R17779: a selective α_7-nicotinic agonist, has anxiolytic and sensory gating-enhancing properties and reduced nicotine-like side effects. Soc Neurosci Abstr 1998; 331:11.

62

Analgesic Effects of Vedaclidine, a Mixed Agonist–Antagonist at Muscarinic Receptor Subtypes

Harlan E. Shannon, Daniel E. Womer, Frank P. Bymaster, David O. Calligaro, Neil W. DeLapp, Charles H. Mitch, and John S. Ward
Eli Lilly and Company, Indianapolis, Indiana, U.S.A.

Michael D. B. Swedberg, Malcolm J. Sheardown, Anders Fink-Jensen, Preben H. Olesen, and Per Sauerberg
Health Care Discovery, Novo Nordisk A/S, Måløv, Denmark

I. INTRODUCTION

Currently available drugs for the treatment of pain, including the treatment of acute or nociceptive pain as well as for persistent or neuropathic pain, are clearly efficacious, but their clinical usefulness is limited by a variety of side effects. Often, the first line of therapy, particularly for mild to moderate pain, is aspirin and related nonsteroidal anti-inflammatory drugs (NSAIDs) or acetaminophen (paracetamol). For moderate to severe pain, NSAIDs still are the drugs of choice in most regions of the world, whereas opioid agonists and mixed agonist–antagonists are also used in the United States. Each of these classes of drugs has the potential to produce highly undesirable side effects. The currently available NSAIDs, which inhibit both cyclooxygenase 1 and 2 (COX 1 and 2) can produce gastrointestinal lesions and potentially fatal bleeding if used long enough at sufficiently high doses. Newer NSAIDs that selectively inhibit COX-2 may avoid the gastrointestinal lesions of the older compounds. However, there appears to be a ceiling to the maximal pain relief that can be achieved with NSAIDs, including, and perhaps particularly, COX-2 inhibitors. Opioids are effective in relieving even severe pain, but the use of opioids is markedly constrained throughout the world because of their abuse liability and potential to produce physical dependence after repeated administration. Even with brief administration, opioids produce side effects such as constipation, respiratory depression, and changes in sensorium, which can be quite problematic and place limitations on their clinical use. Additional pharmacological approaches for the treatment of pain are clearly needed.

Several lines of evidence indicate that the muscarinic–cholinergic system plays a prominent role in the processing of pain-related information. First, a substantial body of literature, spanning at least 50 years, has demonstrated that muscarinic cholinergic agonists as well as cholinesterase inhibitors produce antinociception in a variety of species and in a variety of tests for antinociception (1–6). Interestingly, muscarinic agonists are as efficacious as full opioid agonists in more stringent antinociceptive tests such as the mouse tail-flick procedure (3,7), a test in which mixed agonist–antagonist opioids are inactive. Moreover, the cholinesterase inhibitors physostigmine and tacrine have been reported to produce analgesia in humans as well as to potentiate the analgesic effects of morphine in humans (8,9). Moreover, it has recently been demonstrated that the cholinesterase inhibitor neostigmine produces analgesia in humans after intrathecal administration (10,11). Direct-acting muscarinic agonists have not, to our knowledge, been evaluated in humans for their analgesic properties, presumably because of the prominent parasympathomimetic effects of currently available muscarinic agonists. Taken together, however, the data suggest that the development of a muscarinic agonist that does not produce parasympathomimetic effects might provide clinically useful analgesia.

A_δ and C fibers, which carry nociceptive information from nociceptors, enter the spinal cord in the dorsal horn and synapse in Rexed's laminae I, II, III, IV, and V, particularly in the substantia gelatinosa (lamina II). The secondary neurons in these pathways project through the spinothalamic tract, among other pathways, to the ventrobasal nucleus of the thalamus. From the thalamus, neurons convey nociceptive information to the somatosensory cortex. Descending and centrifugal pathways are also important in modulating nociceptive information. Muscarinic receptors are abundant throughout these pathways. In the spinal cord, muscarinic receptors are present in laminae II and III and have been identified as being of the pharmacological M_1 and M_2 subtypes (12). However, with in vitro autoradiography, Höglund and Baghdoyan (13) found that M_2- and M_3-binding sites were localized in the superficial laminae of the dorsal horn in rats where nociceptive A_δ and C fibers terminate. There was also evidence for the presence of M_4 receptors in the cord, but no evidence for M_1 receptors was obtained (13). In the thalamus, the predominant muscarinic receptor is the M_2 subtype for which both mRNA (14) and protein (15) have been found. However, in addition to M_2 receptors, protein for M_1 and M_4 (15) as well as mRNA for M_1, M_3, M_4, and M_5 (14) receptors have been found in the thalamus. In the cortex, M_1 and M_4 protein as well as mRNA are particularly abundant (14–16). Thus, muscarinic receptors are located throughout pain pathways, suggesting the possibility that muscarinic agonists could act at all levels of the central nervous system (CNS) to modulate nociceptive information.

Parasympathomimetic effects, such as bradycardia, hypotension, diarrhea, urination, salivation, and lacrimation, are most likely primarily mediated by peripheral M_2 and M_3 receptors. M_2 receptors constitute approximately 90% of the muscarinic receptors in the heart, and they are also abundant in the ileum and lung (17,18). M_3 receptors occur predominantly in secretory glands and on smooth muscle, such as ileum and bladder, (16,17,19); whereas, M_1 receptors also occur in the periphery in sympathetic ganglia, gastrointestinal tissue, and salivary glands (17, 20, 21) and, thus, may also contribute to some of the peripheral side effects of muscarinic–cholinergic drugs. Peripheral M_4 same receptors have been identified in lung, uterus, and ileum (16, 17); however, it is currently unknown what role, if any, these peripheral M_4 receptors play in mediating undesirable parasympathomimetic effects. To date, M_5 receptors have not been described in peripheral tissues. Thus, a muscarinic agonist devoid of activity at M_2, M_3, and possibly M_1 receptors might be expected to be relatively free of peripheral parasympathomimetic effects.

From extensive structure–activity relation studies (22), vedaclidine (butylthio[2.2.2], LY297802/NNC11-1053; Fig. 1) was chosen for development as a muscarinic agonist that produces analgesia and is relatively devoid of parasympathomimetic side effects. The present report summarizes the pharmacology of vedaclidine.

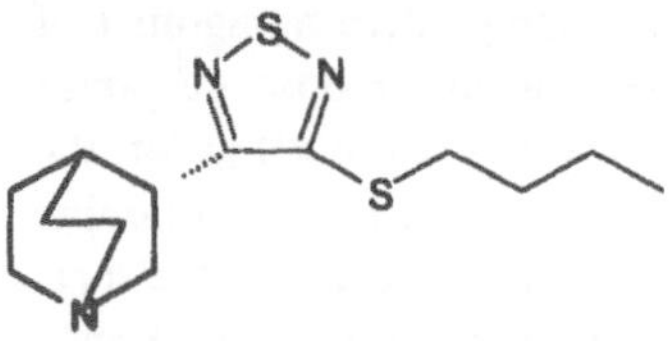

Figure 1 Chemical structure of vedaclidine: (+)-3(*S*)-3-[4-butylthio-1,2,5-thiadiazol-3-yl]-1-azabicyclo[2.2.2]octane (butylthio[2.2.2]; LY297802/NNC11-1053).

II. IN VITRO PHARMACOLOGY OF VEDACLIDINE

In vitro, vedaclidine has high affinity for muscarinic receptors in brain homogenates. The K_i values for inhibiting [^{3}H]oxotremorine-M (agonist-binding sites), [^{3}H]pirenzepine (M_1 receptors), and [^{3}H]QNB (M_2 receptors) were 0.32, 1.4, and 11 nM, respectively (23). Vedaclidine inhibited [^{3}H]cytisine binding to nicotinic receptors, with an IC_{50} of 3120 nM; however, it had little or no affinity for other neurotransmitter receptors and uptake sites. In isolated tissues, vedaclidine was an agonist with high affinity for M_1 receptors in the rabbit vas deferens, but it was an antagonist at M_2 receptors in guinea pig atria and at M_3 receptors in guinea pig urinary bladder. These data indicate that in vitro vedaclidine is highly selective for muscarinic receptors and is an agonist at pharmacological M_1 receptors, but an antagonist at pharmacological M_2 and M_3 receptors (23).

III. ANALGESIC EFFECTS OF VEDACLIDINE

The immediate antinociceptive profile of vedaclidine was assessed in the mouse using the grid-shock, tail-flick, hot-plate, and writhing tests (24). Its ED_{50} values ranged from approximately 0.2 to 1.5 mg/kg s.c. (Table 1) and 1.5 to 12.2 mg/kg p.o., yielding p.o./s.c. ratios ranging from 7 to 27. In contrast the ED_{50} values for producing salivation and tremor were higher than 30 and 12 mg/kg s.c., and >60 and >60 mg/kg p.o., yielding therapeutic ratios of more than 130 × and 54 × s.c., and 40 × and 40 × p.o. Motor impairment or lethality were seen only at doses approximately 100 and 250 times higher than the antinociceptive doses after p.o. and s.c. administration, respectively. In all antinociceptive tests, vedaclidine was equieffective to, and approximately 3- to 25-fold more potent than, morphine. Its duration of action was similar

Table 1 Potencies of Vedaclidine and Morphine in Producing Antinociceptive Effects After s.c. Administration in the Mouse

Test	Vedaclidine ED_{50}(mg/kg)	Morphine ED_{50}(mg/kg)
Writhing	0.19	0.69
Grid shock	0.23	2.2
Tail-flick	0.39	9.2
Hot plate	1.5	3.8

to that of morphine. The muscarinic antagonist scopolamine was a competitive antagonist of vedaclidine in that scopolamine produced dose-related shifts to the right in the dose–response curve for vedaclidine. In contrast, the opioid antagonist naltrexone was without effect on the antinociceptive effects of vedaclidine. The quaternary muscarinic antagonist metscopolamine did not antagonize it at doses equimolar to scopolamine, indicating that its analgesic effects were mediated centrally. After 6.5 days of repeated dosing in mice, there was marked tolerance to the antinociceptive effects of morphine, but minimal if any tolerance to vedaclidine. Taken together, these data indicate that vedaclidine is a potent and efficacious antinociceptive agent, with a very favorable therapeutic window (24).

The concomitant administration of an opioid, such as morphine, and an NSAID, such as ibuprofen, produce synergistic analgesic effects. However, it is unknown whether muscarinic agonists are additive or synergistic with NSAIDs in producing analgesia. To investigate possible interactions between vedaclidine and an NSAID, vedaclidine and ibuprofen were administered alone and concomitantly in a fixed-dose ratio of 1:10 in the mouse acetic acid-induced writhing test. When administered alone, both vedaclidine and ibuprofen produced dose-related decreases in writhing (Fig. 2; closed symbols). When administered concomitantly in a fixed-dose ratio of 1 part to 10 parts ibuprofen, the combination also inhibited writhing. Plotting the dose–response curve for the combination twice (i.e., as a function of the dose of each drug in the combination

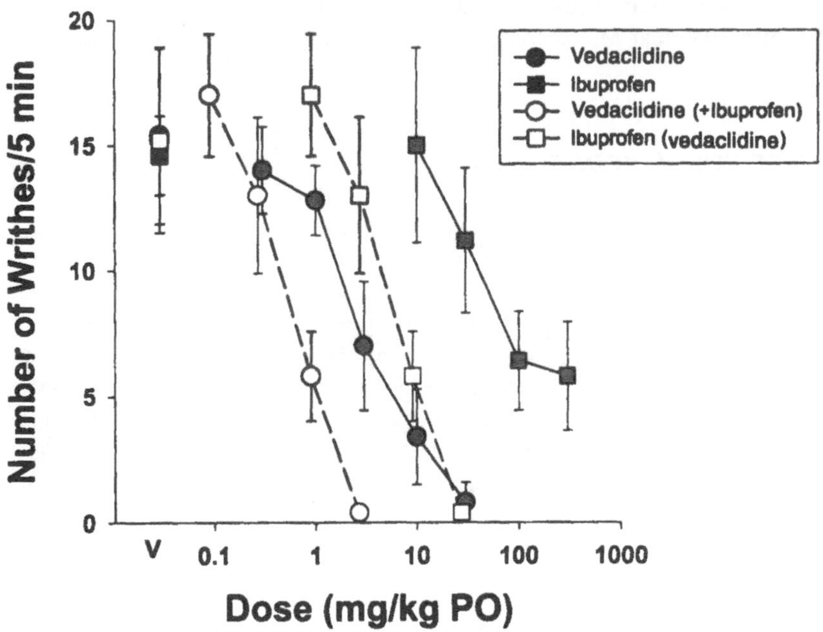

Figure 2 Dose–response curves for vedaclidine alone, ibuprofen alone, and vedoclidine in combination with ibuprofen (1:10) in the mouse acetic acid–induced writing assay. Vehicle or drug was administered p.o. 25 min before acetic acid. Beginning 5 min later, the number of writhes was counted for 5 min. Abscissa: dose of vedaclidine or ibuprofen, or total dose of vedaclidine plus ibuprofen (mg/kg) in a ratio of 1:10 administered p.o. Ordinate: number of writhes during 5 min. Vertical lines represent ±SEM and are absent when smaller than the size of the point. The dose–response curve for the 1:10 combination (open symbols) was plotted twice; that is, as a function of the relative doses of vedaclidine and ibuprofen. Points above V represent the effects of vehicle or vehicle + vehicle.

separately; (see Fig. 2; open symbols) demonstrated that the dose–response curve for each drug when administered in the combination was shifted three- to tenfold to the left of the dose–response curve for either drug administered alone. When plotted as an isobologram (data not shown), the effects of the concomitant administration of vedaclidine and ibuprofen were highly synergistic.

The central sensitization of spinal neurons can lead to altered pain states. One method of producing central sensitization is to administer an inflammatory agent, such as carrageenan. After the development of inflammation produced by the administration of carrageenan, responses to noxious stimuli become exaggerated, a condition known as hyperalgesia, and normally nonnoxious stimuli can produce nocifensive responses, a condition known as allodynia. To determine if vedaclidine could reverse preexisting central sensitization, its dose–response curve was determined 2 h after the administration of carrageenan and 30 min after vedaclidine's s.c. administration. The response latency to a thermal stimulus was determined for both the injured and the uninjured paw, and the data were expressed as the difference between the two paws. As may be seen in Fig. 3, vedaclidine produced a dose-related antithermal hyperalgesia effect in the carrageenan model of central sensitization. Thus, the muscarinic–cholinergic system is involved not only in modulating the processing of acute nociceptive stimuli, but it can also modulate altered processing of sensory stimuli under conditions of central sensitization. Further experiments are needed to determine whether muscarinic agonists such as vedaclidine can prevent the development of central sensitization by administering it before the administration of carrageenan. Moreover, it would be of interest to determine whether muscarinic agonists can reverse or prevent allodynia, particularly mechanical allodynia, as measured by changes in

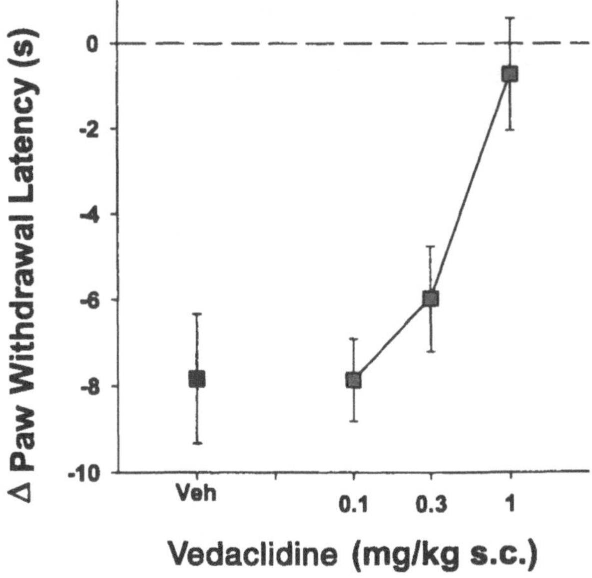

Figure 3 Dose-related reversal of thermal hyperalgesia produced by vedaclidine in the carrageenan model in rats. Vehicle or a dose of vedaclidine was administered 90 min after carrageenan and response latencies to a thermal stimulus was determined 30 min later. Abscissa: dose (mg/kg) of vedaclidine administered s.c. Ordinate: difference (Δ) in paw withdrawal latency in seconds between the inflamed and noninflamed paw. Vertical lines represent ±SEM and are absent when less than the size of the point. Points above Veh represents the effects of vehicle.

the threshold produced by carrageenan or capsaicin to mechanical stimuli such as von Frey hairs.

IV. RECEPTOR SUBTYPES INVOLVED IN PRODUCING ANALGESIA AND THEIR LOCUS

The muscarinic receptor subtype(s) involved in producing acute antinociception are controversial. Although it has been suggested previously that M_1 receptors mediate the antinociceptive effects of muscarinic agonists (25–27), Höglund and Baghdoyan (13) were unable to find autoradiographic evidence for the presence of M_1 receptors in the spinal cord. Therefore, the antinociceptive effects of vedaclidine were compared with two arecoline analogues, propoxy-TZTP (Table 2) and 3-Cl-propylthio-TZTP (28), which are relatively devoid of M_1 receptor agonist activity in vitro (see Table 2); (see also Ref. 28). Propoxy-TZTP and 3-Cl-propylthio-TZTP inhibited [^{3}H]oxotremorine–M binding in rat brain homogenates with IC_{50} values of 1.6 and 1.4 nM, respectively. All three compounds produced antinociception, but none of the compounds stimulated PI hydrolysis in cells expressing human M_1 receptors. Thus, M_1 agonist activity is not required for producing antinociception.

Muscarinic M_2 and M_4 receptors are coupled through pertussis toxin-sensitive G proteins ($G_{i/o}$) to the inhibition of adenylate cyclase. Therefore, we administered pertussis toxin intrathecally (i.t.) to mice to determine if the inactivation of inhibitory G proteins would block the antinociceptive effects of muscarinic agonists. In mice treated with vehicle, vedaclidine produced dose-related antinociceptive effects in the tail-flick test. In mice treated with 0.3 μg of pertussis toxin, the antinociceptive effects of oxotremorine and vedaclidine were completely blocked (data not shown). The blockade of muscarinic antinociception by pertussis toxin demonstrates that M_2 or M_4, or both receptors mediate antinociception. Vedaclidine is an M_2 receptor weak partial agonist and an M_4 agonist, suggesting that either M_2 or M_4 receptors or both mediate antinociception in vivo.

Both spinal and supraspinal sites are involved in mediating analgesia. To investigate the involvement of spinal and supraspinal sites in the analgesic effects produced by vedaclidine, dose–response curves were determined for oxotremorine and vedaclidine in the mouse tail-flick test after both intrathecal (i.t.) and intracerebroventricular (i.c.v.) administration. After i.t. administration, both oxotremorine and vedaclidine produced dose-related antinociception in the tail-flick test (Fig. 4; left panel). However, after i.c.v. administration, oxotremorine but not vedaclidine produced dose-related antinociception in the tail-flick test (see Fig. 4; right panel). Thus, whereas the nonselective muscarinic agonist oxotremorine produced antinociception at both spinal and supraspinal sites in the tail-flick test, vedaclidine produced antinociception in

Table 2 Comparison of the M_1 Efficacy and Antinociceptive Activity of Vedaclidine and Propoxy-TZTP

Compound	Writhing ED_{50}(mg/kg)	Grid shock ED_{50}(mg/kg)	M_1PI[a] Max (%)	M_1PI[a] EC_{50}(μM)
Vedaclidine	0.19	0.23	18	>100
Propoxy-TZTP[b]	0.41	0.75	25	>100

[a] Inositol phosphate hydrolysis in BHK cells transfected with human M_1 receptors.
[b] TZTP: thiadiazole tetrahydropyridine.

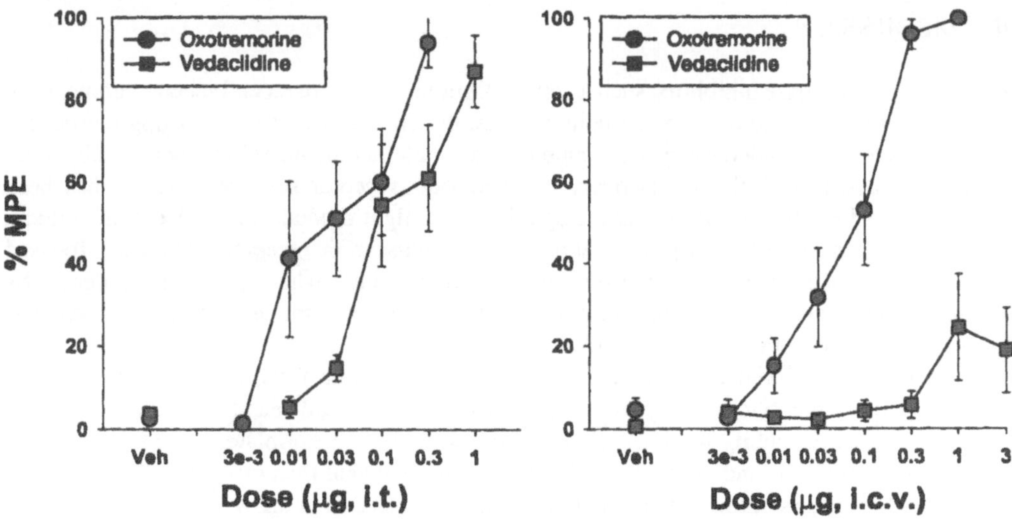

Figure 4 Dose–response curves for oxotremorine and vedaclidine in the mouse tail-flick test after either intrathecal (i.t.) administration (left panel) or after intracerebroventricular (i.c.v.) administration. Abscissa: dose of drug in micrograms per mouse. Ordinate: %MPE, %+ maximum possible effect. Points above Veh represent the effects of vehicle.

this test only at spinal sites. In contrast, in the hot-plate test, which is mediated primarily by supraspinal sites, both oxotremorine and vedaclidine produced antinociception after i.c.v. administration (data not shown).

V. FURTHER IN VIVO PHARMACOLOGY OF VEDACLIDINE

The pharmacology of vedaclidine was further characterized in vivo (23). To assess activity at M_2 receptors, the drug's effects on heart rate and brain levels of acetylcholine were examined. Vedaclidine produced only marginal increases in heart rate, but antagonized the negative chronotropic effects carbachol. Similarly, it was without effect on acetylcholine levels in rat brain. Taken together, these data indicate that vedaclidine is a weak partial agonist at pharmacological M_2 receptors in vivo over the therapeutic-dose range. To assess the relative contribution of M_3 receptors, the effects of vedaclidine administered alone and in combination with oxotremorine in producing salivation were examined. Administered alone, the magnitude of the salivation produced by vedaclidine was less than that of oxotremorine. Moreover, vedaclidine decreased the salivation produced by oxotremorine more than that of vedaclidine alone. Thus, vedaclidine appears to be a weak partial agonist at pharmacological M_3, as well as at M_2, receptors in vivo.

Undesirable side effects produced by opioids include constipation and respiratory depression (29). Vedaclidine had no effect on charcoal meal transit in mice at doses that produced antinociception, whereas morphine produced the expected decrease in charcoal meal transit (23). Furthermore, in guinea pigs, morphine produced dose-related decreases in ventilatory tidal volume, as expected. Vedaclidine decreased tidal volume at lower doses, but at higher doses stimulated respiration. Taken together, these data suggest that vedaclidine is less likely to produce constipation and respiratory depression than morphine and thus may have an improved therapeutic profile over opioids.

VI. DISCUSSION

Although cholinesterase inhibitors, such as physostigmine and, more recently, neostigmine, have been demonstrated to produce analgesia in humans, the clinical use of direct-acting muscarinic agonists has been precluded by their prominent parasympathomimetic effects such as salivation, tremor, and diarrhea. With the discovery of muscarinic receptor subtypes, interest has been kindled in the development of muscarinic agonists that might produce antinociception, without parasympathomimetic effects, by acting at one or a few muscarinic receptor subtypes. A focused drug discovery effort has led to the discovery of vedaclidine, which produces analgesia by actions at muscarinic receptors, but does not produce parasympathomimetic effects at efficacious doses and has a wide therapeutic window.

Vedaclidine showed efficacy in a wide range of analgesia tests, ranging from tests for acute antinociception to tests of hyperresponsivity owing to central sensitization. In acute antinociception tests, including writhing, grid shock, tail-flick, and hot-plate, vedaclidine was as efficacious as morphine and as much as 10–25 times more potent than morphine. The NSAIDs, which are clinically useful in mild to moderate pain, are effective in the writhing test, but not in the more stringent grid-shock, tail-flick, and hot-plate tests. Similarly, mixed agonist–antagonist opioids, such as pentazocine and nalbuphine, which are clinically useful in the treatment of mild to moderate pain, are generally inactive in the hot-plate and tail-flick tests. Only opioid agonists, such as morphine, that are clinically useful in treating severe pain are efficacious in all four of these acute nociception tests. Therefore, vedaclidine might be expected to have more efficacy than NSAIDs or opioid mixed agonist–antagonists, and possibly as much efficacy as opioid agonists, such as morphine, in the treatment of nociceptive pain.

In addition to efficacy in acute nociceptive tests, vedaclidine also reversed thermal hyperalgesia produced by carrageenan. These latter results are of potential importance for several reasons. First, our results demonstrate that vedaclidine can produce analgesia, not only in acute pain models, but also in a model of inflammatory pain. Second, because carrageenan produces a state of central sensitization as measured by thermal hyperalgesia, these results indicate that vedaclidine may directly influence central sensitization. It would be of interest to determine whether this agent also reverses electrophysiological measures of central sensitization.

Vedaclidine was highly synergistic with the NSAID ibuprofen in the mouse-writhing test. To our knowledge, this is the first demonstration that muscarinic analgesics can potentiate the analgesic effects of NSAIDs. The clinical value of NSAIDs is limited in a number of ways. For example, NSAIDs that inhibit both COX-1 and COX-2 produce significant gastrointestinal ulcers and bleeding with continued use, most likely as a direct consequence of COX-1 inhibition. Second, the magnitude of the efficacy of NSAIDs is limited in that they are ineffective in moderate to severe pain, particularly when that pain is relatively unrelated to inflammation. In early toxicology studies, vedaclidine did not produce gastrointestinal lesions, nor did it potentiate COX-1 or COX-2 in vitro (unpublished observations); therefore, this agent is unlikely to produce or potentiate gastrointestinal lesions produced by NSAIDs in humans. In the present studies, it was demonstrated that although a 300-mg/kg dose of ibuprofen administered alone was unable to completely inhibit writhing, a dose of 30 mg/kg of ibuprofen in the presence of a dose of vedaclidine completely inhibited writhing. Thus, when given in combination with vedaclidine, the dose of an NSAID could be lowered below a dose that might be expected to produce gastrointestinal ulceration or other side effects, yet the combination would produce effective analgesia. Because vedaclidine and NSAIDs have different mechanisms of action, the combination also might provide greater analgesia in a broader variety of pain states.

Muscarinic receptors are abundant in pain pathways, including the substantia gelatinosa of the dorsal horn of the spinal cord, the ventrobasal nucleus of the thalamus, and the cortex. Thus, muscarinic agonists could modulate nociceptive information at any or all of these levels.

The muscarinic receptor subtype involved in vivo has been previously suggested to be of the pharmacological M_1 subtype based on blockade by muscarinic antagonists (25–27). However, we identified two arecoline analogues, propoxy-TZTP and 3-Cl-propylthio-TZTP, which are relatively devoid of M_1 agonist activity, but were quite efficacious in tests of antinociception. The selectivity of M_1 antagonists, such as pirenzepine, for cloned muscarinic receptors in CHO cells is only approximately 10- to 30-fold (30), suggesting that effects mediated by pharmacological M_1 receptors could be composed of actions at both genetically defined M_1 and M_4 receptors. Muscarinic M_4, as well as M_2, receptors are coupled to the pertussis toxin-sensitive G proteins G_I and G_0. The intrathecal administration of pertussis toxin completely blocked the antinociceptive effects of systemically administered oxotremorine and vedaclidine in the tail-flick test. Vedaclidine is a weak partial M_2 agonist, the blockade by pertussis toxin suggests that the antinociceptive effects of muscarinic agonists such as vedaclidine may be mediated at least partly by M_4 receptors in the spinal cord.

Both the nonselective muscarinic agonist oxotremorine and the mixed agonist–antagonist vedaclidine produced analgesia in the tail-flick test after intrathecal administration, but only oxotremorine produced analgesia after i.c.v. administration. On the other hand, both oxotremorine and vedaclidine produced analgesia in the hot-plate test after both i.c.v. and i.t. administration. These findings demonstrate that both oxotremorine and vedaclidine act at both the spinal and supraspinal levels to produce anitinociception. In addition, our findings demonstrate that oxotremorine, but not vedaclidine can apparently stimulate a descending cholinergic inhibitory pathway (31–33). However, further experiments are required to specifically address this possibility. Further research is needed defining spinal, supraspinal, and descending muscarinic–cholinergic pathways that may be involved in mediating analgesia.

Vedaclidine appears to have a wide therapeutic window relative to nonselective muscarinic agonists, NSAIDs, and opioids. Its therapeutic index for producing antinociception relative to salivation or tremor was 50- to 100-fold, respectively. In contrast to NSAIDs, vedaclidine did not produce gastrointestinal lesions in early toxicology studies. Similarly, it produced minimal changes in heart rate over the antinociceptive dose range. Short-term use of opioids is primarily limited by their propensity to produce tolerance, respiratory depression, and constipation. In the present studies, the repeated administration of vedaclidine produced little if any tolerance, whereas the repeated administration of morphine produced the expected tolerance. Furthermore, vedaclidine did not produce respiratory depression at higher doses and had no effect on charcoal meal transit, in contrast to morphine that depressed respiration and decreased charcoal meal transit at doses that produced antinociception. Thus, vedaclidine, at analgesic doses, might be expected to be relatively devoid of the most problematic side effects of NSAIDs and opioids.

In summary, vedaclidine is a novel muscarinic receptor ligand that produces analgesia similar in magnitude to that produced by NSAIDs and opioids. Moreover, it produces analgesia at doses that do not produce parasympathomimetic effects. It is efficacious in a variety of diverse pain models, ranging from acute to persistent pain. Moreover, vedaclidine does not appear to produce the most serious side effects of either NSAIDs (GI ulceration) or opioids (constipation and tolerance), as well as being synergistic with NSAIDs. Thus, this agent may have therapeutic use in the treatment of pain as an alternative to NSAIDs and opioids and, in addition, it may have clinical use in a broader range of pain states than either NSAIDs or opioids.

REFERENCES

1. Chen G. The anti-tremorine effect of some drugs as determined by Hoffner's method of testing analgesia in mice. J Pharmacol Exp Ther 1958; 124:73–76.

2. Herz A. Actions of arecoline on the central nervous system. Naunyn Schmiedebergs Arch Exp Pathol Pharmacol 1962; 242:414–429.
3. Harris LS, Dewey WL, Howes JF, Kennedy JS, Pars H. Narcotic-antagonist analgesics: interactions with cholinergic systems. J Pharmacol Exp Ther 1969; 169:17–22.
4. Metys J, Wagner N, Metysova J, Herz A. Studies in central antinociceptive action of cholinomimetic agents. Int J Neuropharmacol 1969; 8:413–425.
5. Ireson JD. A comparison of the antinociceptive actions of cholinomimetic and morphine-like drugs. Br J Pharmacol 1970; 40:92–101.
6. Swedberg MDB. The mouse grid-shock analgesia test: pharmacological characterization of latency to vocalization threshold as an index of antinociception. J Pharmacol Exp Ther 1994; 269:1021–1028.
7. Howes JF, Harris LS, Dewey WL, Voyda CA. Brain acetylcholine levels and inhibition of the tail-flick reflex in mice. J Pharmacol Exp Ther 1969; 169:23–28.
8. Flodmark S, Wramner T. The analgetic action of morphine, eserine and prostigmine studied by a modified Hardy–Wolff–Goodell method. Acta Physiol Scand 1945; 9:88–96.
9. Peterson J, Gordh TE, Hartvig P, Wiklund L. A double-blind trial of the analgesic properties of physostigmine in postoperative patients. Acta Aneasthesiol Scand 1986; 30:283–288.
10. Hood DD, Eisenach JC, Tuttle R. Phase I safety of intrathecal neostigmine methylsulfate in humans. Anesthesiology 1995; 82:331–343.
11. Chung CJ, Kim JS, Park HS, Chin YJ. The efficacy of intrathecal neostigmine, intrathecal morphine, and their combination for post-cesarean section analgesia. Anesth Analg 1998; 87:341–346.
12. Gillberg PG, Askmark H. Changes in cholinergic and opioid receptors in the rat spinal cord, dorsal root and sciatic nerve after ventral and dorsal root lesion. J Neural Transm 1991; 85:31–39.
13. Höglund AU, Baghdoyan HA. M_2, M_3 and M_4 but not M_1 muscarinic receptor subtypes are present in rat spinal cord. J Pharmacol Exp Ther 1997; 281:470–477.
14. Buckley NJ, Bonner TI, Brann MR. Localization of a family of muscarinic receptor mRNAs in rat brain. J Neurosci 1988; 8:4646–4652.
15. Levey AI, Kitt CA, Simonds WF, Price DL, Brann MR. Identification and localization of muscarinic acetylcholine receptor proteins in brain with subtype specific antibodies. J Neurosci 1991; 11:3218–3226.
16. Levey AI. Immunological localization of M_1–M_5 muscarinic acetylcholine receptors in peripheral tissues and brain. Life Sci 1993; 52:441–448.
17. Dörje F, Levey AI, Brann M. Immunological detection of muscarinic receptor subtype proteins (M_1–M_5) in rabbit peripheral tissues. Mol Pharmacol 1991; 90:459–462.
18. Barnes PJ. Muscarinic receptor subtypes: implications for lung. Thorax 1989; 44:161–167.
19. Noronha-Blob L, Lowe V, Patton A, Canning B, Costello D, Kinnier WJ. Muscarinic receptors: relationships among phosphoinositide breakdown, adenylate cyclase inhibition, in vitro detrusor muscle contractions and in vivo cystometrogram studies in guinea pig bladder. J Pharmacol Exp Ther 1989; 249:843–851.
20. Brown DA, Fatherazi S, Garthwaite J, White RD. Muscarinic receptors in rat sympathetic ganglia. Br J Pharmacol 1980; 70:577–592.
21. North RA, Black BE, Suprenant AM. Muscarinic M_1 and M_2 receptors mediate depolarization and presynaptic inhibition in guinea pig enteric nervous system. J Physiol 1985; 368:435–452.
22. Olesen PH, Sauerberg P, Treppendahl S, Larsson O, Sheardown MJ, Suzdak PD, Mitch CH, Ward JS, Bymaster FP, Shannon HE, Swedberg MDB. 3-(3-Alkylthio-1,2,5-thiadiazolyl-4-yl)-1-azabicycles. Structure–activity relationships for antinociception mediated by central muscarinic receptors. Eur J Med Chem 1996; 31:221–230.
23. Shannon HE, Sheardown MJ, Bymaster FP, Calligaro DO, DeLapp NW, Gidda J, Mitch CH, Sawyer BD, Stengel PW, Ward JS, Olesen PH, Suzdak PD, Sauerberg P, Swedberg MDB. Pharmacology of butylthio[2.2.2] (LY297802/NNC11-1053): a novel analgesic with mixed muscarinic receptor agonist and antagonist activity. J Pharmacol Exp Ther 1997; 281:884–894.
24. Swedberg MDB, Sheardown MJ, Sauerberg P, Olesen PH, Suzdak PD, Hansen KT, Bymaster FP, Ward JS, Mitch CH, Calligaro DO, DeLapp NW, Shannon HE. Butylthio[2.2.2] ((+)-3(*R*)-[4-(butyl-

thio)-1,2,5-thiadiazol-3-yl]-1-azabicyclo[2.2.2]octane): an antinociceptive orally active muscarinic agonist in mouse and rat. J Pharmacol Exp Ther 1997; 281:876–883.

25. Ghelardini L, Fanetti L, Malcangio M, Malmberg A, Aiello OP, Giotti A, Bartonini A. Central muscarinic analgesia is mediated by M_1 receptors. Eur J Pharmacol 1990; 183:1941–1942.
26. Iwamoto ET, Marion L. Characterization of the antinociception produced by intrathecally administered muscarinic agonists in rats. J Pharmacol Exp Ther 1993; 266:329–339.
27. Naguib M, Yaksh TL. Characterization of muscarinic receptor subtypes that mediate antinociception in the rat spinal cord. Anesth Analg 1997; 85:847–853.
28. Sheardown MJ, Shannon HE, Swedberg MDB, Suzdak PD, Bymaster FP, Olesen PH, Mitch CH, Ward JS, Sauerberg P. M_1 receptor agonist activity is not a requirement for muscarinic antinociception. J Pharmacol Exp Ther 1997; 281:868–875.
29. Jaffe JH, Martin WR. Opioid analgesics and antagonists. In: Gilman AG, Rall TW, Niles AS, Taylor P, eds. Goodman and Gilman's The Pharmacological Basis of Therapeutics. New York: Pergamon Press, 1990:485–521.
30. Buckley NJ, Bonner TI, Buckley CM, Brann MR. Antagonist binding properties of five cloned muscarinic receptors expressed in CHO-K1 cells. Mol Pharmacol 1989; 35:469–479.
31. Iwamoto ET. Antinociception after nicotine administration into the mesopontine tegmentum of rats: evidence for muscarinic actions. J Pharmacol Exp Ther 1989; 251:412–421.
32. Iwamoto ET. Characterization of the antinociception induced by nicotine in the pedunculopontine nucleus and the nucleus raphe magnus. J Pharmacol Exp Ther 1991; 257:120–133.
33. Chiang C-Y, Zhuo M. Evidence for the involvement of a descending cholinergic pathway in systemic morphine analgesia. Br Res 1989; 478:293–300.

63
Gabapentin and Related Compounds

Mark J. Field and Lakhbir Singh
Parke-Davis Neuroscience Research Centre, Cambridge University Forvie Site, Cambridge, England

M. Isabel Gonzalez
GlaxoSmithKline, Harlow, Essex, England

I. INTRODUCTION

Gabapentin [1-(aminomethyl)cyclohexaneacetic acid; Neurontin] is a cyclic γ-aminobutyric acid (GABA) analogue with ability to penetrate into the CNS. However, it does not interact with GABA receptors (1). It was originally synthesized to treat spasticity, but is currently in clinical use as an add-on therapy in patients with partial and generalized tonic–clonic seizures refractory to conventional therapies (2). Recent studies have shown that gabapentin has much broader therapeutic usefulness than previously realized: Gabapentin and related compounds are effective in animal models of chronic pain and anxiety disorders. In this chapter, we review the pharmacology of gabapentin in preclinical models of pain.

II. PHARMACOLOGY OF GABAPENTIN

The mechanism of action of gabapentin is still not completely understood and may involve different sites of action to account for all of its pharmacological actions. However, a single highly specific [^{3}H]gabapentin-binding site has been described in the brain (3). Further work carried out in our laboratories identified this to be the $\alpha_2\delta$-subunit of voltage-dependent calcium channels (4). To date, gabapentin and pregabalin [formally (*S*)-3-isobutylgaba; CI-1008] are the most active compounds that interact with this site. (*R,S*)-3-Isobutylgaba stereoselectively inhibits [^{3}H]gabapentin binding to brain membranes, with the (*S*)-enantiomer showing an affinity similar to gabapentin, whereas the corresponding (*R*)-enantiomer is ten times weaker (5). Consistent with these binding studies, in animal models of pain (Table 1) and epilepsy, gabapentin and pregabalin show similar potency. In contrast, (*R*)-isobutylgaba either is inactive or is weakly active at ten times higher doses (see Table 1). The mechanism of action of gabapentin, therefore, may be associated with the modulation of certain types of Ca^{2+} currents. Furthermore, it has been reported that gabapentin can block calcium currents in rat cortical neurons (6). However, the involvement of other mechanisms cannot yet be ruled out (for review, see 1).

Table 1 Comparison of Antihyperalgesic Actions of Pregabalin, Gabapentin, and *R*-3-Isobutylgaba in Models of Inflammatory Pain with Their $\alpha_2\delta$ Binding and Sedative/Ataxic Action

		Minimum effective dose			
Compound	$\alpha_2\delta$ Binding IC_{50} (μM)	Formalin test	Carrageenan mechanical hyperalgesia	Carrageenan thermal hyperalgesia	Rota-rod
Pregabalin	0.04	10	3	3	100
Gabapentin	0.08	30	10	30	300
R-3-Isobutylgaba	0.62	100	>100	>100	>100

Source: Refs. 3, 5, 7.

III. EFFECT OF GABAPENTIN IN ANIMAL MODELS OF PAIN

A. Acute Pain Tests

Recent studies indicate that neither gabapentin nor pregabalin affect transient acute pain responses induced by chemical, thermal, or mechanical stimulation (7–9).

B. Inflammatory Models of Pain

Gabapentin and pregabalin also have no effect on the nocifensive behaviors observed during the acute phase of the formalin test (7,9,10). However, both blocked the development of the late phase (7,9,10), indicating a selective antihyperalgesic action. Both compounds also blocked maintenance of carrageenan-induced thermal and mechanical hyperalgesia (7). Furthermore, the antihyperalgesic action of gabapentin is centrally mediated, and it can block the maintenance of carrageenan-induced sensitization of dorsal horn neurons (11). It is also an effective antihyperalgesic agent in a model of acute arthritis induced by administration of kaolin and carrageenan into a knee joint (12).

C. Models of Neuropathic Pain

Gabapentin and pregabalin are also effective in animal models of neuropathic pain. Both compounds show activity in the chronic constriction injury (CCI), Chung, and streptozocin models of neuropathic pain. Both of them blocked the maintenance of mechanical and thermal hyperalgesia, and also allodynia (8,13,14) as well as the abnormal neuronal responses (15). Mechanical allodynia is one of the most debilitating symptoms of neuropathic pain. Clinical studies have reported the presence of at least two distinct types of mechanical allodynia in neuropathic patients: first, static allodynia that is evoked by application of increasing pressure to the skin, and second, a dynamic type that is induced by lightly stroking the surface of the skin (16,17). Our recent studies show that both types of allodynia can also be detected in a rat model of diabetic neuropathy induced by a single dose of the pancreatic β-cell toxin streptozocin (18). In these studies, gabapentin and pregabalin blocked the maintenance of both types of allodynia (19). In contrast, morphine and amitriptyline, which is the first-line treatment for painful diabetic neuropathy (20), were effective only against static allodynia (19). These data indicate that gabapentin and pregabalin possess a superior antiallodynic profile compared with current therapies.

D. Surgical Pain

Evaluation of gabapentin and pregabalin in a recently developed animal model of surgical pain revealed that these compounds possess preemptive analgesic activity. This model involves an incision of the plantar surface of the hindpaw. This incision leads to static allodynia and thermal hyperalgesia lasting several days, which appears to follow a time course similar to that seen in the clinic following surgery (21,22). A single preemptive administration of gabapentin or pregabalin dose-dependently blocked the development of both static allodynia and thermal hyperalgesia for over 48 h (22). The administration of a similar dose of pregabalin at one h after the incision produced a similar degree of antiallodynic and antihyperalgesic actions. However, consistent with its pharmacokinetic half-life, the duration of action was much shorter (4–5 h) (22). These data suggest that, in this model, the main afferent input responsible for prolonged hypersensitivity is over within 1 h of the initial incision. The blockade of this activity prevents development of hypersensitivity. These data indicate that prevention of the induction of hyperalgesia and allodynia is of paramount importance for the effective treatment of postoperative pain.

IV. SITE OF ACTION

Most of the research to date suggests a central mechanism of action for gabapentin. Thus, it has been demonstrated that direct intraplantar administration of gabapentin has no effect on carrageenan-induced thermal hyperalgesia or diabetes-induced static allodynia (7,19). However, gabapentin has been active following intrathecal administration in inflammatory and neuropathic pain models. This is also true in thermal injury and substance P-induced hyperalgesia models (9,13,23,24). Gabapentin also has no effect on the afferent discharges of injured afferents in the Chung model (14). Although these data suggest a central site of action for gabapentin, one study reports that a local intraplantar administration of gabapentin is effective in the formalin test (25). Therefore, a peripheral site of action cannot yet be completely ruled out.

V. CONCLUSION

Gabapentin represents a new class of antihyperalgesic and antiallodynic drugs with a central and opioid-independent mechanism of action. It is clear that gabapentin and related compounds do not block physiological pain. They appear to be effective only against hypersensitivity induced by tissue damage or neuropathy and, as such, should be referred to as antihypersensitive agents. This profile of action is very different from morphine, which is analgesic and blocks both physiological and pathophysiological pain. The efficacy of gabapentin from animal models of pain has translated into the clinic. It has been found that gabapentin can block pain produced by various chronic disorders (e.g., RSD, diabetic neuropathy, and PHN) (26–28). Taken together with its favorable side effect profile, such as lack of constipation, tolerance, and dependence, gabapentin offers an improved treatment for chronic pain syndromes.

REFERENCES

1. Taylor CP, Gee NS, Su T-Z, Kocsis JD, Welty DF, Brown JP, Dooley DJ, Boden P, Singh L. A summary of mechanistic hypotheses of gabapentin pharmacology. Epilepsy Res 1998; 29:233–249.

2. Goa KL, Sorkin EM. Gabapentin: a review of its pharmacological properties and clinical potential in epilepsy. Drugs 1993; 46:409–427.
3. Suman–Chauhan N, Webdale L, Hill DR, Woodruff N. Characterisation of [^{3}H]gabapentin binding to a novel site in rat brain: homogenate binding studies. Eur J Pharmacol 1993; 244:293–301.
4. Gee NS, Brown JP, Dissanayake VUK, Offord J, Thurlow R, Woodruff GN. The novel anticonvulsant drug, gabapentin (Neurontin), binds to the $\alpha_2\delta$ subunit of a calcium channel. J Biochem 1996; 271: 5768–5776.
5. Taylor CP, Vartanian MG, Yuen P, Bigge C, Suman–Chauhan N, Hill DR. Potent and stereospecific anticonvulsant activity of 3-isobutyl GABA relates to in vitro binding at a novel site labelled by tritiated gabapentin. Epilepsy Res 1993; 14:11–15.
6. Stefani A, Spadoni F, Berardi G. Gabapentin inhibits calcium currents in isolated rat brain neurons. Neuropharmacology 1998; 37:83–91.
7. Field MJ, Oles RJ, Lewis AS, McCleary S, Hughes J, Singh L. Gabapentin (Neurontin) and *S*-(+)-3-isobutylgaba represent a novel class of selective antihyperalgesic agents. Br J Pharmacol 1997; 121:1513–1522.
8. Hunter JC, Gorgas KR, Hedley LR, Jacobson LO, Kassotakis L, Thompson J, Fontana DJ. The effect of novel anti-epileptic drugs in rat experimental models of acute and chronic pain. Eur J Pharmacol 1997; 324:153–160.
9. Shimoyama N, Shimoyama M, Davis AM, Inturrisi CE, Elliott KJ. Spinal gabapentin is antinociceptive in the rat formalin test. Neurosci Lett 1997; 222:65–67.
10. Singh L, Field MJ, Ferris P, Hunter JC, Oles RJ, Williams RG, Woodruff GN. The antiepileptic agent gabapentin (Neurontin) possesses anxiolytic-like and antinociceptive actions that are reversed by D-serine. Psychopharmacology 1996; 127:1–9.
11. Stanfa LC, Singh L, Williams RG, Dickenson AH. Gabapentin (Neurontin), ineffective in normal animals, markedly reduces C-fibre evoked responses after inflammation. Neuroreport 1997; 8:587–590.
12. Houghton AK, Lu Y, Westlund KN. *S*-(+)-3-Isobutylgaba and its stereoisomer reduces the amount of inflammation and hyperalgesia in an acute arthritis model in the rat. J Pharmacol Exp Ther 1998; 285:533–538.
13. Hwang JH, Yaksh TL. Effect of subarachnoid gabapentin on tactile-evoked allodynia in a surgically induced neuropathic model in the rat. Reg Anaesth 1997; 22:249–256.
14. Abdi S, Lee DH, Chung JM. The antiallodynic effects of amitriptyline, gabapentin and lidocaine in a rat model of neuropathic pain. Anesth Analg 1998; 87:1360–1366.
15. Chapman V, Suzuki R, Chamarette HLC, Rygh LJ, Dickenson AH. Effects of systemic carbamazepine and gabapentin on spinal neuronal responses in spinal nerve ligated rats. Pain 1998; 75:261–272.
16. Koltzenburg M, Lundberg LER, Torebjörk HE. Dynamic and static components of mechanical hyperalgesia in human hairy skin. Pain 1992; 51:207–219.
17. Ochoa J, Yarnitsky D. Mechanical hyperalgesias in neuropathic pain patients; dynamic and static subtypes. Ann Neurol 1993; 33:465–472.
18. Courteix C, Eschalier A, Lavarenne J. Streptozocin-induced diabetic rats: behavioural evidence for a model of chronic pain. Pain 1993; 53:81–88.
19. Field MJ, McCleary S, Hughes J, Sing L. Gabapentin and pregabalin can block both static and dynamic components of mechanical allodynia induced by diabetes in the rat. Pain 1999; 80:391–398.
20. James JS, Page JC. Painful diabetic peripheral neuropathy. A stepwise approach to treatment. J Am Pediatr Med Assoc 1994; 8:439–447.
21. Brennan TJ, Vandermeulen EP, Gebhart GF. Characterisation of a rat model of incisional pain. Pain 1996; 64:493–501.
22. Field MJ, Holloman EF, McCleary S, Hughes J, Singh L. Evaluation of gabapentin and *S*-(+)-isobutylgaba in a rat model of postoperative pain. J Pharmacol Exp Ther 1997; 282:1242–1246.
23. Partridge BJ, Chaplan SR, Sakamoto E, Yaksh TL. Characterization of the effects of gabapentin and 3-isobutyl-γ-aminobutyric acid on substance P-induced thermal hyperalgesia. Anesthesiology 1998; 88:196–205.

24. Jun JH, Yaksh TL. The effect of intrathecal gabapentin and 3-isobutyl-γ-aminobutyric acid on the hyperalgesia observed after thermal injury in the rat. Anesth Analg 1998; 86:348–354.
25. Carlton SM, Zhou S. Attenuation of formalin-induced nociceptive behaviors following local peripheral injection of gabapentin. Pain 1998; 76:201–207.
26. Mellick GA, Mellick LB. Reflex sympathetic dystrophy treated with gabapentin. Arch Phys Med Rehabil 1997; 78:98–105.
27. Backonja M, Beydoun A, Edwards KR, Schwartz SL, Fonseca V, Hes M, LaMoreaux L, Garofalo E. Gabapentin for the treatment of painful neuropathy in patients with diabetes mellitus. JAMA 1998; 280:1831–1836.
28. Rowbotham M, Harden N, Stacey B, Bernstein P, Magnus-Miller L. Gabapentin for the treatment of postherpetic neuralgia. JAMA 1998; 280:1837–1842.

64

The Role of Gabapentin in the Management of Neuropathic Pain

Howard Rosner
Cedars Sinai Medical Center, Los Angeles, California, U.S.A.

Sudhir Diwan
New York Presbyterian Hospital, Cornell University, New York, New York, U.S.A.

I. INTRODUCTION

The successful management of neuropathic pain has long been elusive. Over the years many treatments have been suggested, including medical management, neuroaugmentation techniques, such as spinal cord stimulation, and neural ablative techniques, such as rhizotomy or chordotomy. No one technique or combination of treatments has been shown to be ideal and, in fact, each patient responds in a different fashion to similar treatments applied in apparently the same clinical setting.

II. PAIN CHARACTERISTICS

Many diverse neuropathic pain syndromes present with similar complaints. This presents one of the major challenges in the treatment of pain of neurogenic origin. Examples of neuropathic pain include various neuralgias and neuropathies which include mono- and polyneuropathies, postherpetic neuralgia, diabetic neuropathy, drug-induced neuropathy, deafferentation neuropathy, nerve transection or compression injury, "failed back syndrome" with radicular pain, plexopathies, complex regional pain syndromes types I and II (causalgia and reflex sympathetic dystrophy), HIV-related neuropathies, and cancer-induced neuropathic pain.

The characteristics of neuropathic pain are usually described as burning, tingling, or shooting, and are clinically described as hyperesthesia, hyperalgesia, hyperpathia, or allodynia, to describe patient's complaints. Although the precipitating event can be different in each presentation of neuropathic pain, the underlying etiology for each presentation is damage to either the peripheral or central nervous system. Conventional management techniques tend to fail because the pain is usually opiate-resistant at clinical doses, without producing significant side effects. Centrally there appears to be a participatory role of the *N*-methyl-D-aspartate (NMDA) receptor complex that differentiates this syndrome from more classic nociceptive pain.

By contrast, the classic pain transmission and perception system, involving nociceptive pain, is mediated by thermo-, mechano-, or chemoreceptors, all of which are subtypes of nociceptors. Nociceptors have a widespread systemic distribution and are found throughout cutaneous and connective tissue, bone, muscle, and viscera. Activation of nociceptors produces normal

Table 1 Analgesic Adjuvants for Chronic Pain and Neuropathies

Adjuvant	Indication
Tricyclic antidepressants	Neuropathic pain
Antiepileptic drugs	Neuropathic pain
Phenothiazines	Neuropathic pain, anxiety, delirium, nausea

expected responses to stimuli, which are described as "sharp, dull, aching, or throbbing." In contrast to neuropathic pain, nociceptive pain is usually opiate-sensitive at clinical doses without causing undo side effects. Some examples of nociceptive pain include pain elicited by (nonneural) tissue injury, such as traumatic pain, postoperative pain, cancer pain, and pressure or bone pain.

III. MANAGEMENT OF NEUROPATHIC PAIN

The approach to management of neuropathic pain, therefore, has involved many different techniques, often used in combination. The more elusive the problem, the larger the number of medications that may be tried and ultimately used. In addition, intractable neuropathic pain may involve the implantation of a spinal cord stimulator or intrathecal morphine. At the outset, a mild opiate analgesic may be adequate to treat the pain of neurogenic origin. However, when treating neuropathic pain, an adjuvant medication must be used from the outset. The reason that additional or adjuvant medications must be used is that neuropathic pain may be resistant to narcotic medications alone. The WHO ladder, recommended for patients with cancer pain stresses the early use of narcotic analgesics and the late use of analgesic adjuvants. Therefore, for primary neuropathic problems, the analgesic ladder needs to be modified from the outset: (1) tricyclic antidepressants, (2) antiseizure agents, and (3) antipsychotic agents. Table 1 lists the adjuvant medications most commonly used for management of neuropathic pain, and Table 2 lists some of the specific antidepressant medications used to help manage neuropathic pain.

Table 2 Tricyclic Antidepressants (TCIs) for Chronic Pain and Neuropathies

Generic and (trade) name	Starting dose and route of administration (mg p.o.q.d.)	Dose range for analgesia (mg/day)	Duration of action (h)	Comments
Amitriptyline (Elavil, Endep)	10–25 mg q.d.	75–150	24	[a]
Desipramine (Norpramin)	10–25 mg q.d.	75–150	24	[a]
Doxepin (Sinequan)	10–25 mg q.d.	75–150	24	[a]
Imipramine (Tofranil)	10–25 mg q.d.	75–150	24	Also available as an IM preparation
Nortriptyline (Pamelor)	10–25 mg q.d.	75–150	24	[a]

[a] Common side effects are sedation and dry mouth (anticholinergic). May cause orthostatic hypotension. Paroxitine (Paxil) is the only SSRI (selective serotonin reuptake blocker) with any degree of analgesia, usually started at 20 mg/day and advanced as high as 60 mg/day. Trazadone (Desyrel) has minimal analgesic activity; however, it can be used as a sleep aid and antidepressant adjuvant to TCs and SSRs in a single bedtime dose of 25–150 mg.

Table 3 Conventional Antiseizure Medications

Carbamazepine	Phenytoin
Clonazepam	Primidone
Ethosuxamide	Valproate
Phenobarbital	

Neuropathic pain syndromes are managed first with a tricyclic antidepressant (TCA) given once daily, usually at bedtime (1). It is important for pain patients to lead as normal a day–night cycle as possible, and these drugs not only help manage neuropathic pain, but most are also sedating enough to be used as a sleep aid. Although the majority of literature promotes the use of amitriptyline as the first-line TCA, the side effects and excess sedation of this and the other first-generation TCAs (doxepin and imipramine) limit their usefulness, particularly in elderly patients. Most patients find the metabolites of amitriptyline and imipramine—nortriptiline or desipramine—to be as effective in neuropathic pain control as the first-generation TCAs, with fewer deleterious side effects. Some newer antidepressants, including the selective serotonin reuptake blocker paroxetine, and venlefaxine, which behaves similarly to a "clean" tricyclic, have been advocated as substitutes for TCAs. Often, the TCA alone is inadequate to manage neuropathic pain, and additional agents must be employed. Antiepileptic drugs, such as carbamazepine and phenytoin, can be helpful, but both have significant side effects and toxicities that may make them inadvisable.

Antiseizure medications have also been widely used for management of neuropathic pain (2–5). Medications such as carbamazepine have been the gold standard for management of trigeminal neuralgia for many years: clonazepam has been used for neuropathies and spasm, phenytoin for various neuropathies, and valproate/divalproex for migraine headache and spasticity. Their toxicities and side effects have limited the therapeutic use of these drugs (6).

Table 3 lists the conventional antiseizure medications currently available. However, not all antiseizure medications have been effective in management of pain. Table 4 lists the conventional antiseizure medications that have been used to manage neuropathic pain and the specific syndromes for which they have been indicated. Much interest has been devoted to newer antiepileptic medications over the past several years in an effort to deliver equal or improved potency with reduced side effects. Tables 5 and 6 lists the antiepileptic drugs that have been developed

Table 4 Conventional Antiseizure Medications for Chronic Pain and Neuropathies

Carbamazepine (trigeminal neuralgia)
Clonazepam (neuropathies and spasm)
Phenytoin (neuropathies)
Valproate/divalproex (migraine headache, spasticity)

Table 5 Newer Antiseizure Medications

Felbamate	Tiagabine
Gabapentin	Topiramate
Lamotrigine	Vigabatrin
Oxycarbazepine	Pregabalin (in development)

Table 6 Newer Antiseizure Medications and Pain Management

Felbamate (experimental pain)
Gabapentin (clinical reports; blinded studies underway)
Lamotrigine (anecdotal)

and released in recent years, and Table 7 the specific antiseizure medications and recommended doses currently in use for the management of neuropathic pain.

Of the myriad medications that have been used to manage neuropathic pain, perhaps the one that has shown the most promise has been gabapentin. Gabapentin adds to the armamentarium available for the management of neuropathic pain; however, there remains substantial literature to support the use of the older, conventional antiepileptic medications; therefore, they should not yet be abandoned. Much interest has been focused on the use of gabapentin for management of neuropathic pain because of its degree of effectiveness coupled with its high patient tolerance and low side effect profile.

IV. PROFILE OF GABAPENTIN

Gabapentin is a 1-(aminomethyl)cyclohexaneacetic acid, with a molecular weight of 171.24 and the chemical formula $C_9H_{17}NO_2$. It is structurally related to γ-aminobutyric acid (GABA). It is not ionized, and as it does not bind to plasma proteins, it remains lipid-soluble and readily crosses the blood–brain barrier. It neither interacts with GABA receptors nor does it inhibit GABA uptake or degradation. The potential metabolic conversion of gabapentin to GABA or other agonists is unknown (7–9).

A. Gabapentin Pharmacokinetics

Gabapentin is rapidly absorbed orally, with maximum plasma concentrations reached within 3 h of administration. Food has no effect on absorption, so the drug can be given at any time.

Table 7 Antiseizure Medications for Chronic Pain and Neuropathies

Generic and (trade) name	Starting dose and route of administration (mg p.o.)	Dosage range for analgesia (mg/day)	Duration of action (h)	Comments[a]
Carbamazepine (Tegretol)	100 t.i.d.	300–1200	8	May cause aplastic anemia and agranulocytosis
Clonazepam (Klonopin)	0.25 t.i.d.–q.i.d.	0.75–6	6–8	May cause amnesia; anxiolytic
Gabapentin (Neurontin)	100 t.i.d.	300–3600	8	Very few side effects
Phenytoin (Dilantin)	100 q.d.	100–300	24	IV preparation available
Valproate (Depakene, Depakote)	125 t.i.d.	375–1000	8	Depakote preparation has better GI uptake. May cause hepatic dysfunction.

[a] Common side effects are sedation, imbalance, and dysphoria; may cause orthostatic hypotension.

Gabapentin passes the blood–brain barrier, does not bind plasma proteins, and is not metabolized. It has dose-dependent linear kinetics at doses up to 1200 mg, and has a direct correlation between dose and blood level. The drug is primarily eliminated unchanged by the kidneys at a constant rate regardless of the dose. Gabapentin neither induces nor inhibits its own metabolism through any feedback mechanisms. Uricosuric agents, such as probenecid or aspirin, do not affect renal excretion. Its clearance correlates linearly with the serum creatinine level. Serum steady state is achieved in 48–72 h after starting a given dose. Gabapentin has no known drug interactions with other antiepileptic medications; therefore, it can be used alone or in conjunction with other antiepileptics, such as phenytoin, valproate, or carbamazepine, to achieve maximal effect. In elderly patients, gabapentin causes mild sedation and minimally blunts motor and cognitive functioning during the initial period of treatment. Because of very low side effects profile, no plasma concentration monitoring is required (10,11).

B. Gabapentin Side Effects

Gabapentin has become very popular in both neurology and pain management because of its efficacy coupled with its very low side effect profile. The most common side effects are somnolence, dizziness, fatigue, sedation, fluid retention (ankle swelling and congestive heart failure in patients with compromised cardiac functions), nystagmus, and motor dyscoordination. Less common side effects are tremors, rhinitis, diplopia, amblyopia, and gingivitis. No morbidity, serious side effects, hypersensitivity, or systemic reactions have yet been reported with the exception of a single case report by Gould (12) documenting a new painful polyneuropathy in a patient being treated with gabapentin.

C. Gabapentin Mechanism of Action

The anticonvulsant effect of gabapentin has been studied in different animal models (13,14), but the exact mechanism of action remains unknown. In spite of its structural similarities to GABA, it has no affinity to either $GABA_a$ or $GABA_b$ receptors. The only indirect evidence that might indicate that gabapentin possesses some gabaergic effect is derived from experimental studies in which gabapentin exerted inhibitory actions on the release of catecholamines similar to the $GABA_a$ and $GABA_b$ receptor agonist baclofen. Gabapentin significantly increases aminooxyacetic acid (AOAA)-induced GABA accumulation in different regions of brain (15).

Gabapentin does not interact with any known antiepileptic drug receptor sites. It does not exhibit affinity for common CNS receptors, including adrenergic (α_1, α_2, or β), cholinergic (muscarinic or nicotinic), dopaminergic (D_1 or D_2), histamine, serotonin (S_1 or S_2), nor opiate (μ, δ, or κ) receptors (11).

D. Gabapentin as an Antiepileptic Drug

Epilepsy is a progressive condition that may affect cognitive skills and, eventually, can become a medically resistant condition, with development of intractable seizures. Suppression of seizures, drug tolerability, and quality of life of patients determine medical management of epilepsy. Gabapentin used as an add-on antiepileptic medication significantly reduces the frequency of partial seizures and secondarily generalized tonic–clonic seizures (16). The efficacy of gabapentin in the treatment of other seizures is not yet well defined. Recently, gabapentin has been advocated as a first-line, single-agent therapy for some types of seizures.

As a relatively new antiepileptic drug, gabapentin has been effective in decreasing the frequency of seizures with partial or generalized epilepsy (17). It is also effective in medically resistant cases. A single high-affinity–binding site for gabapentin in the rat brain has been described (18). Most antiepileptic medications exert their effect by modulating the activity of basic mediators of neuronal excitability. For gabapentin, $\alpha_2\delta$ Ca_2^{2+} channel subunit may be the critical target for antiepileptic actions (19). Nicholus et al. have purified and characterized a high-affinity [3H]+ gabapentin-binding protein from pig brain membrane that interacts with the $\alpha_2\delta$-subunit to exert antiepileptic effects. Kocsis et al. (20) postulated an electrophysiological effect that gabapentin mediated by increasing $GABA_a$ receptor activation, and suggested that the anticonvulsant effects of gabapentin may be related to enhanced GABA release in different regions of the brain. Honmou and colleagues (21) reported that gabapentin may increase free GABA levels in hippocampal cells.

E. Gabapentin in Neuropathic Pain

The etiology of neuropathic pain syndrome remains unclear; however, the underlying pathological characteristics seem to include abnormal activation of neurons within the nociceptive system. The pathological neurons spread excessive excitation to neighboring normal neurons and alter them to produce excessive discharges. Although the exact mechanism of action is unknown, gabapentin may be responsible for preventing the pathological spread of abnormal activation of neighboring neurons. Hunter et al. (22) evaluated the effect of the antiepileptic drugs on rat experimental models of acute and chronic pain and have suggested that newer antiepileptic drugs have the potential to be effective alternatives to either carbamazepine or phenytoin in the treatment of neuropathic pain. In his study, only gabapentin was able to ameliorate both cold and touch hyperesthesias.

Hwang and Yaksh (23) have studied the effect of subarachnoid gabapentin on tactile-evoked allodynia in a surgically induced neuropathic pain model in the rat. Spinal GABA receptors to modulate nerve injury-induced allodynia. Subarachnoid injection of gabapentin resulted in dose-dependent antagonism of allodynia. Failure to reverse the effect by $GABA_a$ or $GABA_b$ antagonists suggests that gabapentin is involved in the modulation of spinal receptors that do not represent either $GABA_a$ or $GABA_b$ sites. Gabapentin does not have a clear dose range for maximum efficacy, which is why the dose is increased as tolerated until pain relief is achieved. Gabapentin works synergistically with other antiepileptic drugs such as clonazepam or carbamazepine.

F. Gabapentin in Specific Pain Syndromes

1. Trigeminal Neuralgia

Trigeminal neuralgia is a syndrome of paroxysms of electric shock-like pain that lasts from several seconds to a few minutes afflicting the area of face supplied by one or more divisions of the trigeminal nerve. Carbamazepine is the first-line treatment for trigeminal neuralgia. Phenytoin and baclofen are also effective medications. Recently, there have been anecdotal reports from many practitioners who have noted satisfactory pain relief with the use of gabapentin. Because of serious side effects of carbamazepine (agranulocytosis and liver toxicity), gabapentin has the potential for becoming an important adjuvant and, perhaps, first-line treatment.

Sist et al. (24) reported two cases of idiopathic trigeminal neuralgia managed with gabapentin. The first was an 88-year-old woman with sharp and shooting paroxysms of pain lasting 30 s or less in V2. The patient self-report rated the pain at 10/10 on a 0–10 verbal scale, and allodynia was noted at one discrete spot above the right upper lip. A local anesthetic injection was performed at the trigger site and the patient was started on a regimen of baclofen, 10 mg q.i.d. She reported pain relief to 1/10 but subsequently returned to the clinic with a new paroxysm having discontinued baclofen because of dizziness. She was then given gabapentin, 300 mg t.i.d., and 1 week later her pain relief was again 1/10. At 6-month follow-up, the patient remained pain-free.

The second patient was an 84-year-old woman with an approximate 20-year history of idiopathic second-division trigeminal neuralgia with allodynia restricted to a small area overlying the right zygoma. She had rejected neurosurgical interventions and agreed to try gabapentin, 300 mg t.i.d. After 1 week, her paroxysmal pain was abated, but for no more than 3–4 h/dose. Her dosage was adjusted to 300 mg every 3 h over the next several days, after which she no longer experienced paroxysms. At 4-month follow-up, the patient was still pain-free, with no appreciable side effects at a dosage of 2400 mg/day.

2. Diabetic and Peripheral Neuropathic Pain

This type of pain can respond to anticonvulsant therapy. Phenytoin trials have been effective; prospective studies have also demonstrated the effectiveness of gabapentin. Backonja et al. (25,26) reported results of an 8-week double-blind, placebo-controlled, parallel group multicenter study of gabapentin in patients with peripheral diabetic neuropathy ($N = 165$). Patients had pain attributed to diabetic neuropathy for 1–5 years. The majority of patients in each group had type-2 diabetes with lower extremity neuropathies. The trial consisted of gabapentin versus placebo for an 8-week period. Of 165 patients studied, 84 received gabapentin and 81 placebo. The gabapentin group started with a 4-week–titration period (week 1: 900 mg/day; week 2: 1800 mg/day; week 3: 2400 mg/day; week 4: 3600 mg/day). Daily dosing was on a t.i.d. regimen. The final 4 weeks of treatment was at a fixed dosage equal to the maximum daily tolerable dosage achieved. All patients were titrated up to 3600 mg/day if tolerated, regardless of pain relief at lower dosages. If intolerable side effects occurred, the dose was titrated down by steps to a tolerable level.

Significant differences between the control and gabapentin groups were noted after the 8-week–study period. Measurements of mean daily pain score, mean sleep interference score, total pain score, visual analog scale, and present pain score, all demonstrated improvement in pain with gabapentin.

Rowbotham et al. (27) reported results of an 8-week, double-blind, placebo-controlled, parallel design, multicenter ($N = 229$) study of gabapentin in patients with postherpetic neuralgia (PHN). Patients had pain for 3 months or more, after healing of a herpes zoster skin rash, a visual analog scale value of 40/100 mm or more, a daily diary pain score of 4 or more on an 11-point Likert scale (0 = no pain, 10 = worst possible pain), and completion of 4 days or more of patient diaries in 7 days before baseline. Muscle relaxants, anticonvulsants, mexiletine, topical analgesics, and antiviral agents were discontinued more than weeks before screening. Previously prescribed tricyclic antidepressants (TCAs), or narcotics, or both could be continued if therapy was stabilized before study entry and remained constant throughout the study.

An 8-week gabapentin versus placebo trial period consisted of an initial 4-week–titration period (week 1: 900 mg/day; week 2: 1800 mg/day; week 3: 2400 mg/day; week 4: 3600 mg/day) dosed t.i.d. In the final 4 weeks of the study patients took gabapentin at a dose equal to the maximum tolerable dosage attained. All patients were titrated to tolerability up to 3600 mg/day regardless of efficacy achieved at the lower dosages. If intolerable side effects occurred, patients were titrated down by steps to a tolerable dose. Of the 229 patients randomized, 113 received gabapentin and 116 received placebo. Eighty-nine (78.8%) gabapentin patients and 95 (81.9%) placebo patients completed the study. Eighty patients (65%) of the gabapentin patients achieved the maximal 3600 mg/day dose. Differences in gabapentin and placebo were significant at 8 weeks for mean daily pain score. This mean pain score reduction with gabapentin started at week 2 with further reductions at week 4. At week 8, the pain reduction was maintained at the week 4 level. Gabapentin showed significant improvement over placebo for average daily sleep-rating scores, total pain, and psychological parameters. Sixteen percent of the gabapentin patients had a rating of no pain at the final week versus 8.8% of placebo patients.

Given the results of their studies as well as available data from other studies, Backonja and Rowbotham suggest that gabapentin should be considered in the treatment of neuropathic pain as a first-line agent. There are several case studies in the literature that support this view. Segal and Rordor (28) reported the use of gabapentin in a 77-year-old hospitalized woman with postherpetic neuralgia refractory to medical management, including the opiate analgesics oxcodone/APAP, morphine, and fentanyl, and analgesic adjuvants including oral desipramine and mexiletine, topical capsaicin cream, and injected bupivacaine. All of these drugs were either ineffective or produced intolerable side effects. On the 10th day of her hospitalization, the patient was started on gabapentin, 300 mg t.i.d. for pain. On day 3 of gabapentin therapy, the patient noted a significant decrease in the level of pain, from 8/10 to 4/10. On day 5, the pain had decreased to a mild level of 1/10. One month later, the pain was still 1/10; the patient was subsequently lost to follow-up. Rosner et al. (29) presented four case reports of patients with intractable neuropathic pain described as deafferentation neuropathy of the face, mixed sympathetically maintained and sympathetically independent pain, postherpetic neuralgia, and bilateral lower extremity HIV-related neuropathy. Patients ranged from 38 to 82 years. All were receiving other pain medications without satisfactory relief. Gabapentin as adjuvant therapy was added in doses ranging from 300 to 2000 mg/day. The patients were able to discontinue or decrease doses of one of the concurrent medications.

3. Complex Regional Pain Syndromes Types I (Reflex Sympathetic Dystrophy; RSD) and II (Causalgia)

These two syndromes are characterized by burning pain, allodynia, hyperpathia, edema, vasomotor and sudomotor changes, skin, bone, and soft-tissue changes. Sustained pain control and early evidence of disease reversal is noted in many patients (30). The mechanism of pain relief is unknown, but initial clinical experience with gabapentin in the management of RSD is promising, mandating randomized, blinded prospective clinical trials.

Mellick et al. have published four reports including nine RSD patients who have been treated with gabapentin (31–34). There were two men and seven women whose ages ranged from 42 to 68 years. Pain was localized to the upper and lower extremities. Gabapentin dosing was 900–2400 mg/day. Eight patients were maintained on t.i.d. dosing, and one patient was started on t.i.d. dosing and then advanced to q.i.d. dosing. Duration of treatment ranged from 2 to 6 months. Pain was assessed through patient self-report based on a 10-point scale. Eight patients reported that their pain relief was excellent (0–3) and one patient reported that it was good (3–5.5) with gabapentin administration. The authors also noted reversal of dystrophic signs, including corrections in skin temperature and color, relief from allodynia, and gradual reduction of changes in soft tissue. Four of the nine patients reported pain relief starting from 2 h to 12 days after institution of gabapentin therapy.

4. Neuropathic Pain Syndromes

Cheville et al. (35) described successful treatment of pain associated with chronic progressive radiation myelopathy in a 55-year-old woman with breast cancer and spinal metastases. Her pain developed after a course of radiation therapy deemed well within the safe range. After a 3-month course of doxorubicin (Adriamycin) for progressive bony metastases, the patient developed paresthesias, dysesthesias, and spastic paraparesis. Medical therapy with multiple adjuvant analgesics and opiates failed to relieve the pain or caused unacceptable side effects. The patient was then given gabapentin with good response.

De Jong (36), in an editorial, provided insight into the indications for gabapentin for neuropathic pain. He termed the efficacy of gabapentin as "remarkably consistent" in complex regional pain syndrome (CRPS), type I (reflex sympathetic dystrophy); phantom limb pain; postherpetic neuralgia; CRPS, type II (causalgia); diabetic neuropathy; postlaminectomy ("failed back") syndrome; syringomyelia; and "encouraging" in migraine headaches, fibromyalgia, multiple sclerosis, meralgia paresthetica, postradiation plexalgia, poststroke ("central") pain, and brachial plexus traction injury.

Mackin (37) reviewed the medical and pharmacological management of upper extremity neuropathic pain syndromes and reported that about half obtained worthwhile partial analgesia; several patients discontinued therapy because of side effects. His opinion was that if patients reported no benefit at a dose of 1000 mg/day they will probably not achieve benefit at higher doses. Those patients who obtain benefit in the 900- to 1200-mg/day range may benefit from further increases to 2000 mg and rarely to 3000 mg/day. Rosenberg et al. (38) performed a retrospective review of 122 patients who took gabapentin for pain relief for at least 30 days. There was a significant decrease in the visual analog pain score in the neuropathic pain group and possibly in the myofascial pain group. He noted no significant improvement for the low-back pain group. Patients with postherpetic neuralgia had a 53% decrease and the diabetic neuropathy group had a 19% decrease in pain scores. All patients with the greatest percentage improvement in pain scores were from the neuropathic pain group. In addition to diabetic neuropathy and postherpetic neuralgia pain, the neuropathic pain group included sympathetically maintained pain, phantom limb pain, and other neuropathic pain, all of which showed a decrease in pain score with gabapentin. Of the patients with more than a 75% decrease in pain score, nine had direct nerve injury and one had postherpetic neuralgia. There was no significant difference in opiate use with gabapentin in any group. In patients with neuropathic pain taking gabapentin without opiates, 45% had a 50% or more reduction in pain score compared with 25% of the patients taking opiates and gabapentin. The authors speculated that this may be due to opioids attenuating GABA release by decreasing calcium channel activity or from direct postsynaptic GABA antagonism by opioids. Concomitant antidepressant use did not have any significant effect on pain score changes. There were no significant differences in pain score changes with TCAs versus SSRIs.

Hansen (39) studied 62 patients with low-back pain who were treated with gabapentin for a minimum of 4 weeks. The average pain perception improved 46%, and the activity of daily living index improved 38% of function. Most patients were able to eliminate at least one prescribed medication.

Cheville et al. (40) reported five patients with refractory central and peripheral neuropathic pain treated with gabapentin. All patients failed prior analgesic therapy; several underwent invasive procedures designed to provide pain relief with deleterious results. The specific types of pain syndromes reported included chronic progressive radiation myelopathy, C6 tetraplegia, facial neuralgia, cervical radiculopathy, and hereditary sensory–motor neuropathy. All the patients experienced a 50–95% reduction of pain and reported an improvement in ambulation and activities of daily living. Two patients were able to return to work.

Huyhn et al. (41) reported one adult male patient with dysesthetic pain with T12 paraplegia from a prior gunshot wound. The patient had since developed burning dysesthetic pain below the level of injury which was worse at night. The pain was unresponsive to conventional treatments, including physical therapy, antidepressant and anticonvulsant medications (carbamazepine, phenytoin), opiate analgesics, and transcutaneous electrical nerve stimulation (TENS). The patient was treated with gabapentin and reported improvement in all measured pain-related indices.

Schachter and Carrazana (42) reported nine patients age 31–83, who were treated with gabapentin for refractory facial pain. Anatomical pathology was identified in four patients (pituitary tumor, meningioma, right-sided Bell's palsy, and acoustic neuroma). The remaining five were diagnosed with trigeminal neuralgia, multiple sclerosis, probable vascular etiology, and unidentified etiology. Each patient had significant relief of pain in the dosage range of 900–1800 mg/day for up to 12 months. The authors speculated that gabapentin enhances GABA and suppresses glutamate in the trigeminal nucleus and, thereby, decreases pain messages ascending from the trigeminal nucleus and thalamus to the cortex. They further postulated that gabapentin exerts complimentary analgesic actions by simultaneous effects at GABA and glutamate at two sites.

Newshan (43) reported three persons with AIDS whose distal sensory polyneuropathy pain was treated with gabapentin. The first, a 53-year-old man, complained of burning in his feet subsequent to stavudine treatment. The pain did not decrease despite dose reductions and finally discontinuation of stavudine. Amitriptyline and acetaminophen with codeine were unsuccessful. Gabapentin was then initiated, and by the fourth day, the patient reported a 50% reduction in pain. Ultimately, the pain was completely eliminated with gabapentin titration. The second patient was a 35-year-old man with Kaposi's sarcoma. He complained of sharp pain (8/10) in his feet and lower legs, where he had extensive Kaposi's lesions, and persistent burning and numbness in his feet, which made walking difficult. The patient tried oxycodone with acetaminophen, fentanyl patch, amitriptyline, and then desipramine unsuccessfully. Amitriptyline and desipramine also caused undue sedation. Gabapentin, 300 mg, was initiated at bedtime and was increased to t.i.d. The patient reported 100% relief of symptoms after the first dose, experiencing his first full night of sleep in weeks, and was able to walk freely with no pain. He continued to experience little to no pain at 1-month follow-up. The third patient was a 41-year-old man who complained of sharp tingling and burning in his feet that interfered with walking. Carbamazepine was unsuccessful in managing his pain, so gabapentin, 300 mg t.i.d., was initiated, which resulted in partial relief. The dose was doubled and the patient reported nearly complete relief from his symptoms and remained comfortable 2 months later.

Sist et al. (44) studied the effect of gabapentin in ten patients with neuropathic pain in the head and neck. Pain intensity was measured on a 10-point scale, and pain quality was measured on the McGill Pain Questionnaire (MPQ). Postsurgical pain ($n = 7$), trigeminal neuralgia ($n = 2$), and postherpetic neuralgia (C2 distribution, $n = 1$) were studied. The duration of pain ranged from 1.5 to 36 months. Five patients had exclusive neuropathic pain, three also had myofacial pain, one had recurrent tumor pain, and one had chronic osteoarthritic pain. Six patients had burning pain, seven had allodynia, and all ten had lancinating pain. Each patient was instructed to take 300 mg of gabapentin on day 1, then 300 mg b.i.d. on day 2, and 300 mg t.i.d. on day 3 and thereafter, unless further titration was required. The ultimate gabapentin dose range was 900–2400 mg/day. Three patients received gabapentin monotherapy; the other seven patients received concurrent medications that included amitriptyline, tramadol, oxycodone, hydrocodone, fentanyl, or acetaminophen. Three of these seven received neurolytic nerve blocks and one received a nondestructive local anesthetic diagnostic block. The follow-up period was 5–10 months. The median pain level in eight patients had decreased to 0/10 and MPQ values decreased from a mean of 4/5 to 0/5; two patients failed to attain complete neuropathic pain relief. Gabapentin was able to relieve steady and lancinating pain, as well as allodynia. None of the patients reported changes in their somatic pain complaints.

5. Postpoliomyelitis Pain

Zapp (45) described a 47-year-old woman with long-standing poliomyelitis who presented with severe left hip and lower back pain and moderate pain in the shoulders and neck. She also suffered from severe kyphoscoliosis and was confined to a wheelchair. Her major complaint was of continuous shooting and burning pain which kept her awake at night. An intravenous lidocaine challenge improved her pain so she was started on oral mexiletine which produced good analgesia. Therapy was discontinued secondary to gastrointestinal side effects. She was then started on a regimen of 300 mg of gabapentin twice daily, which gave her good analgesia. After 3 months, the patient's pain remained well controlled with only a mild ache and no adverse effects.

6. Central Pain

Schacter and Sauter (46) reported three patients with central pain treated with gabapentin. First was a 63-year-old woman who had diffuse right-sided pain which was partially (25% decrease) controlled with carbamazepine. Gabapentin was added at 300 mg b.i.d., and in less than 1 week, 70% of the pain was eliminated. Gabapentin was increased to 900 mg/day and the patient continued to have good pain relief 5 months after carbamazepine was discontinued. The second case was a 67-year-old man with persistent burning dysesthesias on his entire right side. No relief was experienced with carbamazepine, imipramine, thiorizadine, or clonazepam, but moderate relief was experienced with 900 mg/day of gabapentin. The third was an 82-year-old woman who had left periorbital and maxillary pain after a stroke. The patient did not respond to perphenazine/amitriptyline, notriptyline, carbamazepine, oxycodone, or baclofen. Gabapentin, 1800 mg/day, was then given and resulted in complete resolution of the pain.

7. Migraine Headaches

Mathew and Lucker (47) evaluated the efficacy and safety of gabapentin in the prophylactic treatment of migraine headaches in a 3-month open-label study. Doses ranging from 900 to 1800 mg/day reduced the severity and frequency of headaches. Nicoldi and Sicuteri (48) also evaluated the efficacy of gabapentin in the prophylactic treatment of chronic migraine. After a 1-month–washout period (except for analgesics) from previous antimigraine maintenance therapy, 17 patients (7 men and 10 women) who were partially or totally refractory to conventional antimigraine treatments were treated with gabapentin from 400 to 1200 mg/day for 1 month. Patients reported significant relief of headache severity and frequency when compared with both the baseline and washout period.

8. Erythromelalgia

McGraw and Kosek (49) reported two patients with erythromelalgia (pain in an erythematous area) treated with gabapentin. The first was a 42-year-old woman, with multiple sclerosis admitted to the hospital with severe bilateral leg pain, allodynia, and hyperpathia, improved only with cold compresses. Previous therapies of aspirin, oxycodone/APAP, intravenous morphine and prednisone, had failed. Gabapentin, 100 mg t.i.d., and imipramine, 10 mg h.s., were started. Pain relief was sustained after the dosage was increased to 400 mg t.i.d. At the time the report was written, the patient had remained pain-free for 4 months.

The second patient was a 9-year-old girl with incapacitating, burning, and stinging foot pain persisting around the clock and causing interruption of sleep. The pain was most intense in the feet, but also present in the hands. It was unrelieved by aspirin, opiates, or benzodiazepines. Relief could be achieved only by immersing the feet in buckets of ice water. Epidural local anesthetic was effective, but psychologically intolerable. Eventually she was started on gabapentin, 100 mg t.i.d., along with amitryptyline. The gabapentin dosage was increased to 300 mg t.i.d. The patient's symptoms improved, and after 1 month, she eventually became pain-free. The patient was maintained on this regimen for 4 months and subsequently tapered from both medications. At the time the report was written, the patient had remained pain-free for 6 months.

Wakim et al. (50) reported a case of a 9-year-old girl with erythromelalgia manifested by debilitating bilateral foot pain, burning, and itching that was relieved only by standing in cold water. The patient also had poor growth, bizarre posturing, tachycardia, hypertension, and elevated plasma and urinary catecholamines (pheochromocytoma-negative). She failed to respond to aspirin, propranolo, verapamil, and chelation therapy for suspected mercury toxicity. When the patient was given an epidural anesthetic along with gabapentin, she became pain-free, her heart rate nomalized, blood pressure decreased, and plasma and urine catecholamines became normal. She was discharged on a regimen of gabapentin, 100 mg b.i.d., and naproxen. Seven months after discharge that patient was doing well and off of all medications.

9. Multiple Sclerosis

Samkoff et al. (51) reported a 36-year-old woman who at the age of 27 developed right leg weakness that was eventually diagnosed as multiple sclerosis (MS). An MRI subsequently revealed multiple brain white matter lesions consistent with MS. After several years, the patient developed dysesthesias in both legs; described as intermittent, "tight," and "burning," and after several months, the pain became constant. She was initially treated with baclofen, amitriptyline, and carbamazepine with minimal success and adverse effects. Eventually, gabapentin was initiated at 300 mg daily and then increased to 300 mg t.i.d. Her pain control improved and at the time the report was written, the patient was experiencing pain relief for 6 months at 900 mg/day.

F. Gabapentin in Pregnancy

No serious malformations have been reported at gabapentin doses up to 3600 mg/day in humans; however, no study of gabapentin in pregnant humans has ever been performed. In animal reproductive studies, gabapentin produced delayed ossification of multiple bones and renal abnormalities; including hydroureter and hydronephrosis. According to the U.S. Food and Drug Administration (FDA) drug classification, gabapentin is a category C drug (i.e., safety or risk of the drug is not identified in pregnancy). Only nine cases of gabapentin use in pregnancy have been reported in the drug manufacturer's information booklet. Four of nine patients opted for termination of pregnancy, four delivered healthy babies at full term, and one baby was born with respiratory distress, pyloric stenosis, and an inguinal hernia. Gabapentin was not mutagenic in vivo or in vitro in standard assays. In September 1990, clinical development of gabapentin was temporarily suspended by the FDA after a statistically increased incidence of pancreatic acinar cell adenocarcinoma was found in male rats receiving high doses of gabapentin; however, the study was resumed after the FDA found that the tumors were species- and gender-specific.

V. FUTURE DRUG DEVELOPMENT

The next generation of anticonvulsants currently under development includes BW 534U87, ganaxolone, levetiracetam, MDL-27192, pregabalin, ralitoline, remacemide, retigabine, rufinamide, SB 204269, and TV 1901. Most interesting for pain management is pregabalin, a drug closely related to gabapentin. Pregabalin has now been studied in over 8000 patients worldwide as an analgesic, antiepileptic, and anxiolytic. Its chemical name is (*S*)-3-isobutylgaba and it is also known as CI-1008 and PD 144723. Personal communication from pain centers using the medication in clinical trials report that the analgesia obtained is similar to that of gabapentin. Clinical trials have indicated efficacy in diabetic neuropathy and other studies are ongoing for other types of pain.

VI. SUMMARY

The antiepileptic drug gabapentin has been demonstrated effective in a wide range of neuropathic pain syndromes in blinded clinical studies and multiple clinical case reports. Its effectiveness and low side effect profile make this an exciting addition to the armamentarium of medications for neuropathic pain. The safe use of gabapentin in pregnancy has not yet been established and is not recommended.

REFERENCES

1. Digregorio GJ, Kozin SH. Adjuvant drug therapy for pain. AFP Clin Pharmacol 1986; 33:227–232.
2. Swerdlow M. Anticonvulsant drugs and chronic pain. Clin Neuropharmacol 1984; 7:51–82.
3. Bruni J, Wilder BJ. Valproic acid: review of a new antiepileptic drug. Arch Neurol 1979; 36:393–398.
4. Burchiel KJ. Carbamazepine inhibits spontaneous activity in experimental neuromas. Exp Neurol 1988; 102:249–253.
5. Bouckoms AJ, Litman RE. Clonazepam: the treatment of neurologic pain syndrome. Psychosomatics 1985; 26:933–936.
6. Reynolds EH, Trimble MR. Adverse neuropsychiatric effects of anticonvulsant drugs. Drugs 1985; 29:570–581.
7. Chadwick D. Gabapentin [Comment]. Lancet 1993; 343:89–91.
8. Gabapentin Study Group. Lancet 1990; 335:1114–1117.
9. Schmidt B. Gabapentin. In: Levy R, ed. Antiepileptic Drugs. vol 3. New York: Raven Press, 1989; 925–935.
10. Morris GL III. Efficacy and tolerability of gabapentin in clinical practice. Clin Ther 1995; 17:891–900.
11. Beydoun A, Uthman BM, Sackellares C. Gabapentin: pharmacokinetics, efficacy and safety. Clin Neuropharmacol 1995; 18:469–481.
12. Gould HJ. Gabapentin induced polyneuropathy. Pain 1998; 74:341–343.
13. Brown DA, Marsh S. Axonal GABA receptors in mammalian peripheral nerve trunks. Brain Res 1 1978; 56:187–191.
14. Wamil AW, Taylor CP, McLean MJ. Effects of gabapentin on repetitive firing of action potentials and GABA responses of mouse central neurones in cell culture (abstr). Epilepsia 1991; 32(suppl 3):20.
15. Loscher W, Honack D, Taylor CP. Gabapentin increases aminooxyacetic acid-induced GABA accumulation in several regions of rat brain. Neurosci Lett 1991; 121:150–154.
16. McLean MJ, Ramsay RE, Leppik IE, et al. Gabapentin as add-on therapy in refractory partial epilepsy. Neurology 1993; 43:2292–2298.
17. Goa KL, Sorkin EM. Gabapentin: a review of its pharmacological properties and clinical potential in epilepsy. Drugs 1993; 46:409–427.
18. Suman-Chauhan N, Webdale L, Hill DR, Woodruff GN. Eur J Pharmacol 1993; 244:293–301.
19. Gee NS, Brown JP, Dissanayake V UK, et al. The novel anticonvulsant drug gabapentin (Neurontin) binds to the alpha-2-delta subunit of a calcium channel. J Biol Chem 1996; 271:5768–5776.
20. Kocsis JD, Honmou O. Gabapentin increases GABA-induced depolarization in rat neonatal optic nerve. Neurosci Lett 1994; 169:181–184.
21. Honmou O, Oyelese AA, Kocsis JD. The anticonvulsant gabapentin enhances promoted release of GABA in hippocampus: a field potential analysis. Brain Res 1995; 692:273–277.
22. Hunter JC, Gogas KR, Hedley LR, et al. The effect of novel anti-epileptic drugs in rat experimental models of acute and chronic pain. Eur J Pharmacol 1997; 324:153–160.
23. Hwang JH, Yaksh TL. Effect of subarachnoid gabapentin on tactile-evoked allodynia in a surgically induced neuropathic pain model in the rat. Reg Anesth 1997; 22:249–256.
24. Sist T, Filadora V, Miner M, et al. Gabapentin for idiopathic trigeminal neuralgia: report of two cases. Neurology 1997; 48:1467.

25. Backonja M, Hes MS, LaMoreaux LK, et al. Gabapentin (GBP; Neurontin) reduced pain in diabetics with painful peripheral neuropathy: results of a double-blind, placebo-controlled clinical trial (945-210). American Pain Society: 16th Annual Scientific Meeting, New Orleans, LA, Oct 23–26, 1997; abstr 654.
26. Backonja M, Beydoun A, Edwards S, et al. Gabapentin for the symptomatic treatment of painful neuropathy in patients with diabetes mellitus: a randomized controlled trial. JAMA 1998; 280:1831–1836.
27. Rowbotham M, Harden N, Stacey B, et al. Gabapentin for the treatment of post-herpetic neuralgia: results of a randomized controlled trial. JAMA 1998; 280:1837–1842.
28. Segal AZ, Rordorf G. Gabapentin as a novel treatment for postherpetic neuralgia. Neurology 1996; 46:1175–1176.
29. Rosner H, et al. Gabapentin: adjunctive therapy in neuropathic pain states. Clin J Pain 1996; 12:56–58.
30. Wahren LK, Torebjork E, Nystrom B. Quantitative sensory testing before and after regional guanethidine block in patients with neuralgia in the hand. Pain 1991; 46:23–30.
31. Mellick LB, Mellick GA. Successful treatment of reflex sympathetic dystrophy with gabapentin. Am J Emerg Med 1995; 13:96.
32. Mellick GA, Seng ML. The use of gabapentin in the treatment of reflex sympathetic dystrophy and a phobic disorder. Am J Pain Manage 1995; 5:7–9.
33. Mellick GA, Mellick LB. Gabapentin in the management of reflex sympathetic dystrophy. J Pain Sympt Manage 1995; 10:265–266.
34. Mellick GA, Mellick LB. Reflex sympathetic dystrophy treated with gabapentin. Arch Phys Med Rehabil 1997; 78:98–105.
35. Cheville A, et al. Neuropathic pain in radiation myelopathy: a case report Program Book, American Pain Society, 14th Annual Scientific Meeting, 1995; abstract 95823; p A-115.
36. De Jong, RH. Neurontin: pie in the sky or pie on the plate? Pain Dig 1996; 6:143–144.
37. Mackin GA. Medical and pharmacological management of upper extremity neuropathic pain syndromes. J Hand Ther 1997; 10:96–109.
38. Rosenberg JM, Harrel C, Ristic H, et al. The effect of gabapentin of neuropathic pain. Clin J Pain 1997; 13:251–255.
39. Hansen HC. Use of gabapentin in the management of low back pain. South Med J 1997; 90:S11.
40. Cheville AL, Pomeranz BA, Narcessian EJ. Gabapentin: a promising new therapy. Am Acad Phys Med Rehabil. 58th Annual Meeting, Chicago, IL. Oct 10–13, 1996; 78 (abstr P).
41. Huynh CH, Preibe MM. Gabapentin for the treatment of neuropathic pain in spinal cord injury. Am Acad Phys Med Rehabil 58th Annual Meeting, Chicago, IL. Oct 10–13, 1996;106 (abstract P104).
42. Schacter SC, Carrazanna EJ. Treatment of facial pain with gabapentin: case reports. J Epilepsy 1997; 10:148–150.
43. Newshan G. HIV neuropathy treated with gabapentin. AIDS 1998; 12:219–221.
44. Sist TC, Filadora VA, Miner M, et al. Experience with gabapentin for neuropathic pain in the head and neck: report of ten cases. Reg Anesth 1997; 22:473–478.
45. Zapp JJ. Postpoliomyelitis pain treated with gabapentin. Am Fam Phys 1996; 53:2442–2445.
46. Schacter S, Sauter M. Treatment of central pain with gabapentin: case reports. J Epilepsy 1996; 9: 223–226.
47. Mathew NT, Lucker C. Gabapentin in migraine prophylaxis: a preliminary open label study. Neurology 1996; 46:A169 [abstr S09.004].
48. Nicoldi M, Sicuteri F. A NMDA modulator, gabapentin, clearly facilitates resolution of chronic migraine. Pharmacol Res 1997; 35 (suppl):64.
49. McGraw T, Kosek P. Erythromelalgia pain managed with gabapentin. Anesthesiology 1997; 86:988–990.
50. Wakim ME, Zeltzer L, Roberts RL, et al. Management of erythromelalgia with epidural bupivacaine and fentanyl and oral gabapentin. J Invest Med 1997; 45:138a [abstr].
51. Samkoff LM, Daras M, Tuchman A, et al. Amelioration of refractory dysesthetic limb pain in multiple sclerosis by gabapentin. Neurology 1997; 49:304–305.

65
New Local Anesthetic Analgesics

Anisa Sabrine and Gordon Lyons
St. James's University Hospital, Leeds, England

I. INTRODUCTION

Local anesthetics have been used to provide pain relief in labor and for a variety of operations. Local anesthetics may be administered by a number of different routes to provide anesthesia: by local infiltration, intravenous regional anesthesia, field block, nerve plexus block, or central regional block. As well as facilitating intra- and postoperative analgesia, some postoperative complications, in particular thromboembolism, have been reduced in hip, urological, knee, and vascular surgery (1). High-risk surgical patients have a reduced incidence of cardiovascular failure, major infections, show a reduced stress response, and incur lower hospital costs (2). In obstetrics, maternal anesthetic mortality has been reduced by the increased use of regional anesthesia for cesarean section in preference to general anesthesia (3).

II. LOCAL ANESTHETICS

Local anesthetics may be used either as the sole method of anesthesia or to provide intraoperative analgesia in conjunction with general anesthesia. Continuous techniques are also an effective means of providing postoperative analgesia, usually in conjunction with opioid administration.

A. Licensed Local Anesthetics

The choice of drug is influenced by several factors: onset and duration of action, degree of sensory and motor blockade, central nervous system (CNS) toxicity and cardiotoxicity (Table 1).

III. RESEARCH AND DEVELOPMENT IN NEW LOCAL ANESTHETICS

A. Problems with Bupivacaine

The most serious adverse effects of local anesthetics involve the cardiovascular and central nervous systems and are usually the result of accidental intravascular or intrathecal injections. Accidental intravascular injection of toxic doses may result in central nervous system (CNS) symptoms which, for most local anesthetic drugs, occur at a lower concentration than that required for cardiac arrest.

Table 1 Onset, Duration, and Toxicity of Commonly Used Local Anesthetic Drugs

	Onset	Duration	Dose required to produce signs of CNS toxicity (mg/kg) in humans	Cardiac output in dogs (50%↓) (mg/kg)
Chloroprocaine	Very fast	Short	22.8	30
Lidocaine	Fast	Moderate	6.4	30
Mepivacaine	Fast	Moderate	9.8	40
Etidocaine	Fast	Long	3.4	20
Bupivacaine	Moderate	Long	1.6	10
Ropivacaine	Moderate	Long	—	—

Source: Refs. 4–6.

Bupivacaine has been widely used since the 1960s. Accidental intravenous injection may result in seizures and ventricular tachycardia and fibrillation without antecedent hypoxia. Deaths associated with the use of 0.75% bupivacaine in pregnant women in the United States (7), and with the use of bupivacaine for intravenous regional anesthesia in children in the United Kingdom (8), have prompted a search for local anesthetic agents that are less cardiotoxic.

B. Stereoisomerism

Most modern local anesthetics are chiral drugs, each possessing an asymmetric carbon atom and existing as two enantiomers (Figs. 1 and 2); that is, they are optically active stereoisomers (9).

There are two systems of terminology (Table 2).

The properties of enantiomers of local anesthetics, although similar, show important differences in many respects. These include differences in systemic toxicity, vasoactivity, and differential blockade, together with a potential difference in potency.

Bupivacaine is a racemic mixture containing equal amounts of the *R*(+)- and *S*(−)-isomers. The severe CNS and cardiac toxicity associated with this drug has prompted both the development of its pure *S*(−)-enantiomer, which is known to be less toxic, and the development of a new local anesthetic, ropivacaine, also a pure *S*(−)-enantiomer. Both are members of the group of local anesthetic compounds known as *N*-substituted pipecholylxylidines. Ropivacaine, the *S*(−)-enantiomer of the monohydrate of the hydrochloride salt of 1-propyl-2′,6′-pipecoloxy-

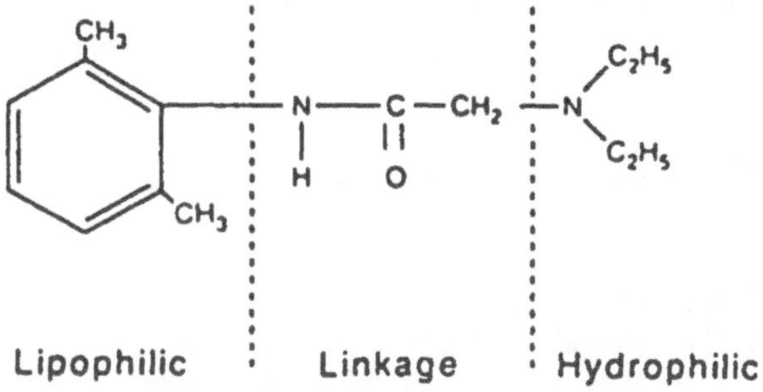

Lipophilic Linkage Hydrophilic

Figure 1 General structure of local anesthetics showing a lipophilic portion (aromatic ring), a hydrophilic portion (tertiary amine), and a linking chain (either amide or ester) containing the asymmetrical carbon atom: The amide local anesthetic agent lidocaine is shown as an example. (From Ref. 9.)

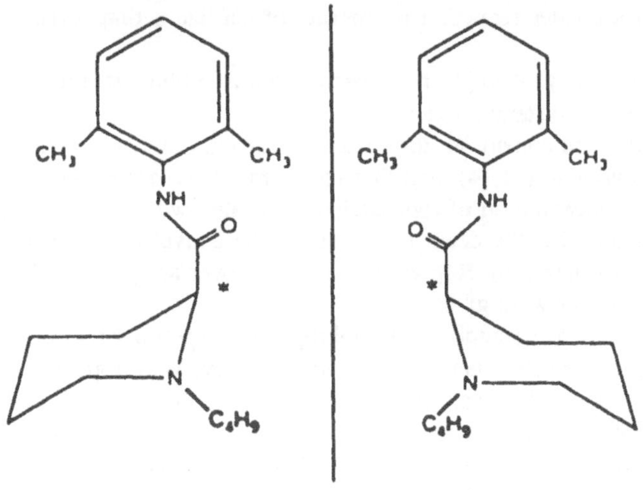

S-(-)-Bupivacaine R-(+)-Bupivacaine

Figure 2 The enantiomers of bupivacaine: The position of the asymmetrical carbon atom is indicated. (From Ref. 9.)

lidide, is currently used to provide anesthesia and analgesia for several types of surgery. *S*(−)-Bupivacaine is not yet licensed for clinical use and clinical trials are still being undertaken.

C. *S*(−)-Bupivacaine and Ropivacaine

1. Systemic Toxicity

Isolated Muscle Preparations. Local anesthetics inhibit depolarization of the nerve cell and thus propagation of a nerve impulse by preventing the influx of sodium ions through ion-specific channels in the cell membrane (10). Sodium channels exhibit a degree of stereoselectivity and *R*-enantiomers are better at blocking sodium flux than *S*-enantiomers. This should confer on *R*-enantiomers, in general, greater potency than their *S*-counterparts (11). In support of this, when molar concentrations are considered, *S*(−)-bupivacaine is 13% less potent than racemic bupivacaine when given epidurally to women in labor (12).

For sodium ions to enter the nerve cell, the channels must be opened by the action potential. Repeated stimulation provides multiple action potentials with increasing opportunity for the local anesthetic to enter the sodium channel. This kind of block is called frequency-dependent block. It is also seen in cardiac muscle fibers that exhibit stereoselectivity of ion channels. Consequently, the *R*(+)-enantiomer of bupivacaine produces not only a denser frequency-depen-

Table 2 Terminology of Stereoisomers

Definition	Enantiomer
Rotation of polarized light	+ or − *dextro* (*d*) or *levo* (*l*)
3-D structure	Rectus (*R*) or sinister (*S*)

dent block than the $S(-)$, but also a greater reduction in the rate of cardiac action potential depolarization and duration (13).

Animal Studies. From the foregoing, it might be expected that $S(-)$-bupivacaine and ropivacaine would display differences in systemic toxicity.

Animal studies have shown that the convulsant dose was significantly and substantially higher for $S(-)$-than for $R(+)$-bupivacaine (11,14), and that the former was less cardiotoxic than the latter (15). In addition, the concentration of ropivacaine associated with seizures was actually lower than that of bupivacaine, but the death rate at twice the convulsant dose was higher for bupivacaine than for ropivacaine (16). Ropivacaine caused fewer arrhythmias than racemic bupivacaine when the same doses were given (17).

Human Studies. In human studies, $S(-)$-bupivacaine and ropivacaine produce fewer cardiovascular changes than racemic bupivacaine when infused intravenously. With ropivacaine and racemic bupivacaine, when cardiovascular changes are seen, they are the same for both drugs (18,19). The alleged benefits of reduced toxicity of new local anesthetics compared with bupivacaine do not take into account differences in potencies. Although a local anesthetic might demonstrate a reduced toxicity in the laboratory, if it is less potent in the clinical setting, this advantage may disappear. This is because the dose given in clinical practice will have to be increased to offset deficiencies in potency.

2. Selectivity

For pain relief in labor, it is considered desirable to avoid motor blockade, while maintaining adequate analgesia. In animal studies, there has been no consistent difference between duration of sensory and motor block for either isomer of bupivacaine (11), despite the generally observed clinical effect that epidural racemic bupivacaine is relatively selective for sensory fibers. Zaric investigated the dose–response of sensory and motor block during continuous epidural infusion of 0.1, 0.2, and 0.3% ropivacaine in human volunteers. He found that ropivacaine 0.1% produced limited analgesia and minimal motor block, whereas with 0.2 and 0.3% ropivacaine, analgesia was more extensive, and motor block was considered moderate (20).

Claims for reduced motor block are also vulnerable to dose adjustments required to compensate for loss of potency.

3. Vasoactivity

All synthetic local anesthetics cause vasodilation at high concentration, but there is a tendency for the $S(-)$-enantiomers, in particular, to produce vasoconstriction at lower concentration. Aps and Reynolds found an increase in the intradermal potency of $S(-)$-bupivacaine in humans compared with racemic bupivacaine at higher drug concentrations (0.48–3.84 mmol/L). This could be explained by the increased vasoconstrictor effect described (21).

Studies of the effect on cutaneous capillary bloodflow in pigs suggest that ropivacaine appears to be a vasoconstrictor even at high concentration, potentially enhancing local anesthetic blockade in vivo (22). This may be important for field and plexus blocks, but might be less so for epidural blockade (23).

IV. USE OF NEW LOCAL ANESTHETICS

Clinical studies with ropivacaine and $S(-)$-bupivacaine have been conducted in the following surgical subspecialties: orthopedics, abdominal surgery, plastic surgery, urology, gynecology, ophthalmology, and obstetrics, using peripheral and central neural blockade. Some of the studies use experimental techniques (local anesthetic, epidural infusion, and patient-controlled administration of opioid) that are not seen in day-to-day clinical practice. The aims of these are to establish, first, that new local anesthetics can achieve anesthesia and analgesia in the required clinical setting and, second, to note differences in duration and differential between sensory and motor block.

Almost invariably, the concentrations chosen are sufficient to block Aα motor fibers, with the result that the differential nature of blockade and potency differences are both concealed. High concentrations are required to provide anesthesia for surgery, and anything less than this would be inhumane. Essentially, the message from studies of this nature is that local anesthesia is effective, and this is true for both ropivacaine and *S*(−)-bupivacaine, but there are insufficient data to support other claims.

Lower concentrations are appropriate when analgesia, rather than anaesthesia, is required. Comparisons of local anesthetics on the steep, rather than the flat upper part of the concentration–response curve are more explicit and are likely to reveal differences between agents. What is critical here is that comparisons are made with equipotent concentrations, corresponding to the same point on the curve. Clearly if compared concentrations do not produce equivalent analgesia, comparative statements about efficacy and differential blockade are invalid. The only areas in clinical practice that could permit studies of this kind are postoperative analgesia and obstetrics.

When given to women in labor, ropivacaine appears to have 60% and *S*(−)-bupivacaine 98% of the potency of racemic bupivacaine (12,24). Consequently, it may be necessary to administer a larger dose of ropivacaine to the patient to be effective, reducing the margin of safety.

V. WORK IN PROGRESS

Both ropivacaine and *S*(−)-bupivacaine are currently undergoing further clinical trials to investigate their efficacy both as a local anesthetic when used alone, and when used with other additives. Initial studies have shown improved efficacy when *S*(−)-bupivacaine with the addition of fentanyl was compared with *S*(−)-bupivacaine alone to provide intra- and postoperative epidural analgesia for lower extremity orthopedic procedures.

S(−)-Bupivacaine combined with clonidine has been more effective than either agent alone when given as a postoperative epidural infusion following total hip replacement surgery (25).

VI. SPECULATION ON FUTURE DEVELOPMENTS

In summary, it seems that, as a local anesthetic agent, ropivacaine is as effective as bupivacaine when used in high concentrations, the only difference being an increase in the duration of the sensory blockade (26). It remains to be seen whether the claims for reduced toxicity will survive the upward dose adjustment required in clinical practice because of its reduced potency. Few studies have been conducted comparing low concentrations of these drugs. The commercial preparation of *S*(−)-bupivacaine has been similar to the racemate in terms of its potency and, when licensed, has the potential to provide the anesthetist with a local anesthetic that is at least as potent as bupivacaine while maintaining a higher margin of safety.

The relatively new minimum local analgesic concentration (MLAC) method may permit the calculation of the therapeutic ratios for epidural local anesthetics allowing a more complete assessment of their suggested improved safety.

Currently, there are no new developments for more local anesthetics, and it is likely that only one of the new local anesthetics, ropivacaine or $S(-)$-bupivacaine will survive commercially. A license for intrathecal use might be hard to justify as their suggested benefits, principally reduced cardiotoxicity, do not play a part in this route of administration, because the risk of direct intravascular injection is almost negligible.

REFERENCES

1. Kehlet H. The rationale for regional anaesthesia—effects on stress, blood loss, thromboembolism and mental function. In: Kehlet H, ed. Practice in Postoperative Pain: Effect of Regional Anaesthesia and Pain Management on Surgical Outcome. Kent: Wells Medical, 1992:5–8.
2. Yeager MP, Glass DD, Neff RK, Brinck-Johnsen T. Epidural anesthesia and analgesia in high risk surgical patients. Anesthesiology 1987; 66:729–736.
3. Department of Health. Report on confidential enquiries into maternal deaths in the United Kingdom 1985–87. London: Her Majesty's Stationery Office (HMSO), 1991.
4. Difazio DA. Adjuvant techniques to improve the success of regional anesthesia: mixtures. In: Raj PP, ed. Clinical Practice of Regional Anesthesia. New York: Churchill Livingstone, 1991:154–160.
5. Cousins MJ, Bromage PR. Epidural neural blockade. In: Cousins MJ, Bridenbaugh PO, eds. Neural Blockade in Clinical Anesthesia and Management of Pain. 2d ed. Philadelphia: Lippincott, 1988: 253–360.
6. Covino BG. General considerations toxicity and complications of local anaesthesia. In: Nimmo WS, Smith G, eds. Anaesthesia. 1st ed, Vol 2. Oxford: Blackwell Scientific, 1989:1011–1033.
7. Albright GA. Cardiac arrest following regional anesthesia with etidocaine or bupivacaine. Anesthesiology 1979; 51:285–287.
8. Heath M. Deaths after intravenous regional anaesthesia. Br Med J 1982; 285:913–914.
9. Sidebotham DA, Schug SA. Stereochemistry in anaesthesia. Clin Exp Pharmacol Physiol 1997; 24: 126–130.
10. De Jong RH. Local Anesthetics. St Louis: Mosby, 1994:48.
11. Aberg G. Toxicological and local anaesthetic effects of optically active isomers of two local anaesthetic compounds. Acta Pharmacol Toxicol 1972; 31:273–286.
12. Lyons G, Columb MO, Wilson RC, Johnson RV. Epidural pain relief in labour. Br J Anaesth 1998; 81:280P–281P.
13. Vanhoutte F, Vereecke J, Verbeke N, Carmeliet E. Stereoselective effects of the enantiomers of bupivacaine on the electrophysiological properties of the guinea pig papillary muscle. Br J Pharmacol 1991; 103:1275–1281.
14. Luduena FP, Bogado EF, Tullar BF. Optical isomers of mepivacaine and bupivacaine. Arch Int Pharmacodyn 1972; 200:359–369.
15. Mazoit JX, Boico O, Samii K. Myocardial uptake of bupivacaine: II. Pharmacokinetics and pharmacodynamics of bupivacaine enantiomers in the isolated perfused rabbit heart. Anesth Analg 1993; 77:311–316.
16. Feldman HS, Arthur GR, Covino BG. Comparative systemic toxicity of convulsant and supraconvulsant doses of intravenous ropivacaine, bupivacaine and lidocaine in the conscious dog. Anesth Analg 1989; 69:794–801.
17. Ericson A-C, Avesson M. Effects of ropivacaine, bupivacaine and $S(-)$-bupivacaine on the ECG after rapid i.v. injection in conscious rats [abstr]. Nice: The International Monitor. XV Annual ESRA Congress, 1996;51.
18. Gristwood R, Bardsley H, Baker H, Dickens J. Reduced cardiotoxicity of levobupivacaine compared with racemic bupivacaine (Marcaine): new clinical evidence. Exp Opin Invest Drugs 1994; 3:1209–1212.
19. Scott DB, Lee A, Fagan D, Bowler GMR, Bloomfield P, Lundh R. Acute toxicity of ropivacaine compared with that of bupivacaine. Anesth Analg 1989; 69:563–569.

20. Zaric D, Nydahl PA, Phillipson L, Samuelsson L, Heierson A, Axelsson K. The effect of continuous epidural infusion of ropivacaine (0.1%, 0.2%, and 0.3%) and 0.25% bupivacaine on sensory and motor block in volunteers: a double blind study. Reg Anesth 1996; 21:14–25.
21. Aps C, Reynolds F. An intradermal study of the local anaesthetic effects of the isomers of bupivacaine. Br J Clin Pharmacol 1978; 6:63–68.
22. Kopacz DJ, Carpenter RL, Mackey DC. Effect of ropivacaine on cutaneous capillary blood flow in pigs. Anesthesiology 1989; 71:69–74.
23. Santos AC, Pederson H, Finster M. Local anesthetics. In: Chestnut DH, ed. Obstetric Anesthesia: Principles and Practice. St Louis: Mosby, 1994:202–226.
24. Capogna G, Celleno D, Lyons G, Columb M. Determination of the minimum local analgesic concentration of epidural ropivacaine in labour. Br J Anaesth 1998; 80(suppl):148.
25. Levobupivacaine. Summary of Pre-clinical and Clinical Experience. Cambridge: Chiroscience, 1998.
26. Wolff AP, Hasselström L, Kerkkamp HE, Gielen MJ. Extradural ropivacaine and bupivacaine in hip surgery. Br J Anaesth 1995; 74:458–460.

66

Spinal α_2-Adrenergic Agonists for Intractable Cancer Pain

Patricia Lavand'homme
Université Catholique de Louvain, Brussels, Belgium

James C. Eisenach
Wake Forest University School of Medicine, Winston-Salem, North Carolina, U.S.A.

I. INTRODUCTION

Pain as a complication of cancer is a common and challenging clinical problem. The World Health Organization (WHO) estimates that 30% of cancer patients experience chronic pain from their cancer or related to its treatment. Gratefully, acceptable control of pain can be achieved in more than 90% of these patients by using a combination of oral medications (WHO stepladder approach). However, in some patients, this option is not possible because long-term therapy, either owing to a high rate of side effects, eventual loss of efficacy of systemic medications, or inability to use the oral route of administration (intractable nausea and vomiting, bowel irradiation, or surgery). An alternative in these cases to oral treatment involves intraspinal (epidural or intrathecal) catheter insertion for long-term central delivery of medications.

Morphine remains the gold standard for spinal analgesia, although its prolonged administration often results in side effects, especially nausea, vomiting, constipation, and mood alteration. Among the common fears expressed by patients and some physicians with long-term morphine use are central respiratory depression, which is infrequent with extended administration, and development of pharmacological tolerance, which is less likely the cause of dose escalation than is pain increase from disease progression. Finally, a major concern and limiting factor for the use of large doses of spinal or systemic opioids is sedation and psychomotor and cognitive dysfunction, which clearly diminish patient's quality of life.

Although morphine is without question effective in relieving nociceptive and visceral pain, the responsiveness of neuropathic and deafferentation pain to opioids is less certain (1). Unfortunately, the cancer patient population carries a high prevalence of such painful conditions subsequent to surgery, radiotherapy, or chemotherapy, as well as from the cancer itself. Common therapeutic alternatives when systemic use of spinal opioids fail include addition of antidepressants or antiepileptics, available orally; spinal local anesthetics, which cause unwanted motor blockade and hypotension; or spinal α_2-adrenergic agonists. The latter, highly effective against neuropathic pain, represent a hopeful approach for intractable pain because they may permit patients to avoid destructive neurolytic procedures, which entail permanent side effects and in some cases, worsening pain.

α_2-Adrenergic mechanisms of regional analgesia have been clinically exploited for more than 10 years, and complete toxicological assessment has suggested that clonidine is safe for intraspinal use (2). Most publications on clonidine refer to its use in acute postoperative or obstetric pain, focusing on efficacy when administered alone or in combination with other analgesics. Commonly cited benefits provided by α_2-adrenergic agonists for spinal analgesia, especially for intractable cancer pain, include analgesia devoid of opioids' harmful side effects, sympatholysis (which may be particularly beneficial in neuropathic pain), synergy with other central analgesics, and lack of tolerance and especially no cross-tolerance with morphine and other opioids.

II. SPINAL MECHANISMS OF ANALGESIA MEDIATED BY α_2-ADRENERGIC AGONISTS

Spinally administered α_2-adrenergic agonists produce analgesia by mimicking activation of descending noradrenergic pathways: noradrenergic nuclei in the brain stem can be activated by opioids or by noxious stimuli, resulting in release of norepinephrine in the dorsal horn of the spinal cord (Fig. 1). Local application of norepinephrine in the spinal cord produces analgesia, independent of opioid receptor activation by stimulating α_2-adrenergic receptors (3). Thus, more selective α_2-adrenergic agonists, such as clonidine or dexmedetomidine, induce spinal analgesia directly, either by a postsynaptic inhibition and hyperpolarization, thereby decreasing excitability in the dorsal horn neurons, or by a presynaptic inhibition of primary afferents, thereby reducing the release of pain-related neurotransmitters such as substance P and glutamate. α_2-Adrenoceptors are coupled to G proteins and affect cAMP and Ca^{2+} availability (4).

Studies of mRNA have revealed the message for α_{2A}- and α_{2B}-adrenoreceptor subtypes diffusely distributed in human dorsal horn spinal cord, whereas there is little or no message for α_{2B}-adrenoceptors in the rat (5). α_{2A}-Adrenoceptors are likely responsible for analgesia in the

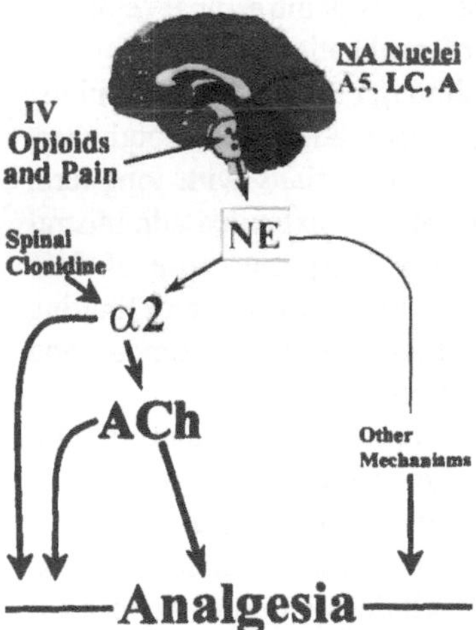

Figure 1 Spinal noradrenergic mechanisms of analgesia: Noradrenergic (NA) nuclei in the brain stem are activated by intravenous opioids and pain, leading to release of norepinephrine (NE) in the spinal cord. This NE causes pain relief by stimulating α_2-adrenergic receptors, which, in turn, act through many mechanisms. At least one of these is stimulation of cholinergic interneurons in the spinal cord to cause release of acetylcholine (ACh) for analgesia.

rat, but at present, no α_2-adrenergic agonist is completely selective for any subtype, and the subtype responsible for analgesia in humans is unknown. Animal and human studies have demonstrated that a part of the analgesia from spinal α_2-adrenergic agonist administration is mediated by activation of cholinergic inhibitory interneurons in the dorsal horn (see Fig. 1). Thus, epidural and intrathecal, but not intravenous clonidine increases acetylcholine (ACh) concentrations in human cerebrospinal fluid (CSF) (6). In addition, intrathecal injection of the cholinesterase inhibitor neostigmine, enhances analgesia from epidural and intrathecal clonidine (7). Spinally released ACh acts primarily on muscarinic receptors which, in turn, stimulate nitric oxide synthesis to contribute to analgesia (8).

Analgesia from α_2-adrenergic agonists is related to their CSF concentration, implying that their site of action resides in the spinal cord. Pharmacokinetic and pharmacodynamic studies demonstrate a relatively poor correlation between clonidine concentrations in blood and analgesia. In contrast, there is a strong relation between CSF clonidine concentration and analgesia from epidural clonidine, with an EC_{95} of approximately 130 ng/mL (9). Samso et al. compared epidural clonidine (300 μg) with the same dose administered intramuscularly, and showed no difference between the two routes for anesthesia-sparing effect or hormonal changes from operative stress, yet only the epidural route produced postoperative analgesia (10). Similarly, Bernard et al. demonstrated that clonidine is nearly twice as potent epidurally as intravenously (11). Intrathecal injection increases the duration of analgesia in comparison with intramuscular or epidural clonidine administration (12) (Fig. 2). Taken together, these findings confirm that clonidine is more effective after neuraxial than systemic administration and it exerts a predominant effect at the spinal cord level; therefore, it should be administered by intraspinal routes for analgesia. Epidural clonidine alone requires a large dose (ED_{50} = 300 μg) to obtain good analgesia in postoperative patients, although its effect is brief and necessitates a continuous infusion for sustained analgesia; the optimal rate of infusion in postoperative patients is approximately 40 μg/h (13).

There is a close relation between the injected epidural dose and plasma concentration of clonidine, and systemic absorption accounts for most of this drug's side effects. Clonidine and dexmedetomidine are lipophilic substances and their systemic absorption after spinal administra-

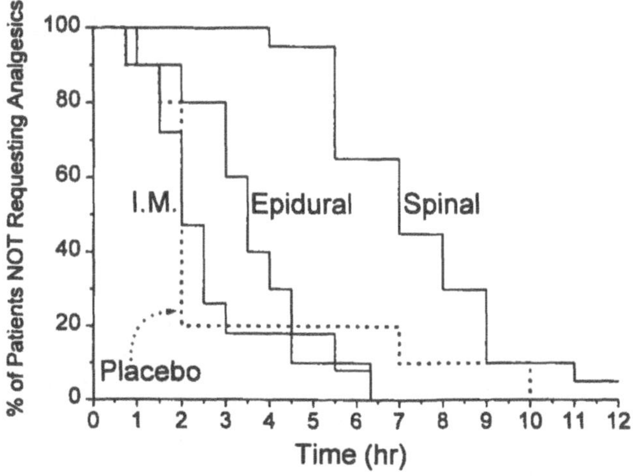

Figure 2 Clonidine produces analgesia by a spinal action: Duration of analgesia, defined as percentage of patients following surgery who do not request other analgesics, when 150 μg clonidine is injected intramuscularly (IM), epidurally, or spinally. IM administration does not differ from placebo.

tion is rapid, leading to their two major effects, hemodynamic depression and sedation. The main cardiovascular effect is reduced sympathetic nervous system activity which results from actions at multiple sites. In the brain stem, a postsynaptic effect on α_2-adrenoceptors reduces sympathetic drive. In addition, imidazoline structures, such as clonidine, can activate nonadrenergic, imidazoline-binding sites in the brain stem, producing hypotension and bradycardia and an antiarrythmogenic effect. In the periphery, activation of presynaptic α_2-adrenoceptors on sympathetic terminals decreases norepinephrine release and causes vasodilation. Finally, spinal administration directly inhibits sympathetic preganglionic neurons in the spinal cord, and this effect is more pronounced after injection along the neuroaxis with the highest density of such neurons (thoracic sites) (14). Cardiac effects are also complex, mainly bradycardia, but also a decrease in myocardial oxygen demand, at least when heart failure is not present. Thus, α_2-adrenergic agonists mainly reduce heart rate and blood pressure, the latter being of greater magnitude in hypertensive than in normotensive subjects. Central and peripheral sympatholysis may represent a part of the analgesic efficacy of α_2-adrenergic agonists in patients with neuropathic pain states that are sympathetically maintained.

Sedation commonly follows the use of α_2-adrenergic agonists and is related to an action in a brain stem nucleus, the locus caeruleus. This action is most likely due to systemic absorption, rather than cephalad migration in CSF, for delayed onset of sedation has not been observed from epidural or spinal clonidine. Sedation from epidural clonidine occurs rapidly, is dose-dependent over the range 50–900 μg, and can be antagonized by α_2-adrenergic antagonists. However, this sedative and, to a lesser degree, anxiolytic effect of α_2-adrenergic agonists is not accompanied by respiratory depression. In addition, α_2-adrenergic agonists do not potentiate respiratory depression from opioids (15). Clonidine does not alter minute ventilation, although there are occasional reports of intermittent upper airway obstruction during deep sedation following large doses of clonidine. Lack of respiratory depression makes α_2-adrenergic agonists desirable as analgesics, alone or combined with opioids or local anesthetics, but does not exclude careful patient monitoring, at least at the initiation of therapy. α_2-Adrenergic agonists can also alter hormone secretion: they reduce, but do not absolutely suppress, the neurohormonal response associated with stress (increased norepinephrine, epinephrine, corticotropin [ACTH], and cortisol) (16). α_2-Adrenergic agonists stimulate growth hormone release and in some circumstances, can inhibit insulin release. However, these effects are short-lasting and do not seem to have clinical importance in humans, unlike the hormonal effects produced by prolonged exposure to opioids. Other common side effects include dry mouth and dizziness, but unlike opioids, α_2-adrenergic agonists do not cause urinary retention or constipation (17).

III. ANALGESIC SYNERGY WITH CURRENTLY AVAILABLE SPINAL ANALGESICS

Spinally administered α_2-adrenergic agonists are effective alone only in large doses, at least in perioperative situations, and these doses are associated with sedation and hypotension. Consequently, these drugs are typically combined with other agents. Spinal injection of α_2-adrenergic agonists intensifies and prolongs sensory and motor blockade from local anesthetics: 150 μg clonidine increases by 100% the duration of a 50-mg–epidural or a 5-mg–intrathecal dose of bupivacaine (18), and smaller doses of clonidine (0.75–1 μg/kg) are also effective for this purpose. Because the motor blockade associated with local anesthetic limits their usefulness in chronic pain, more interesting is the combination with opioids. In animals, μ-opioid agonists interact synergistically with α_2-adrenergic agonists for analgesia (19). In humans, many studies have focused on this combination, and the effects are generally additive, rather than synergistic (20). An epidural clonidine bolus of 75–150 μg or an infusion rate of 20 μg/h enhances fentanyl and sufentanil analgesia duration or reduces opioid drug use (21,22). The effect is less clear with spinal morphine, which has a much longer duration of action than clonidine. In summary, small doses of α_2-adrenergic agonists added to μ-opioid agonists decrease analgesia onset and allow a 50% reduction in the opioid dose, thereby limiting side effects.

The cascade of α_2-adrenergic agonists stimulating ACh release leading to nitric oxide (NO) synthesis can also be manipulated to intensify analgesia (see Fig. 1). Thus, intrathecal injection of the cholinesterase inhibitor, neostigmine (50–200 μg), enhances analgesia from epidural clonidine in humans (7). In addition, the sympathetic stimulation from cholinergic receptor activation may decrease hypotension secondary to α_2-adrenergic agonist injection.

IV. SPECIFIC α_2-ADRENERGIC AGONISTS: CLONIDINE VERSUS DEXMEDETOMIDINE

There are two α_2-adrenergic agonists currently in human use: clonidine, which has received approval for systemic and epidural use; and dexmedetomidine, which is under clinical development for systemic administration. Medetomidine is a specific α_2-adrenergic agonist with a higher selectivity than clonidine (1620:1 for α_2:α_1 adrenergic receptor binding, compared with 220:1 for clonidine), and is widely used in veterinarian practice (4). Dexmedetomidine is the pharmacologically active *d*-isomer in the racemic mixture, and shares the same anesthetic and analgesic properties as clonidine. In humans, systemic dexmedetomidine has been examined as premedication before minor gynecological procedures (0.33–0.67 μg/kg) and as an adjuvant in abdominal surgery. Dexmedetomidine alleviates visceral pain and reduces intraoperative anesthetic and postoperative opioid requirements, but carries a high rate of side effects, mainly sedation, hypotension, and bradycardia (23,24). In contrast, respiratory rate and blood oxygen saturation are unaffected by dexmedetomidine. In human volunteers, the analgesic effect of a 1-μg/kg–i.v. bolus of dexmedetomidine is not significantly different from placebo or 2-μg/kg i.v. of fentanyl on dental pain, but does reduce tourniquet-induced ischemic pain (25). Dexmedetomidine's duration of action is short: the mean elimination half-life is 2.3 h for dexmedetomidine compared with 7.7 h for clonidine. After i.v. infusion in postoperative patients, the dexmedetomidine concentration in CSF corresponding to the unbound fraction is only 8% of blood concentration (versus 50% for clonidine). Heart rate, blood pressure, and plasma catecholamine concentrations decrease during dexmedetomidine infusion, reflecting a sympatholytic effect (26). Spinal dexmedetomidine has been studied in rats and in sheep, the latter with a spinal cord more similar in size to humans. It is argued that dexmedetomidine's selectivity for α_2-adrenergic receptors, being three to four times greater than clonidine's, should result in better spinal analgesia, despite its lipophilicity being 3.5 times greater than clonidine's. In sheep, single cervical intrathecal, or epidural boluses of 100 μg dexmedetomidine, a dose comparable with 300 μg of clonidine, result in plasma concentrations that are very low, with bioavailability in CSF after epidural injection of 22% (27). Blood pressure, but not heart rate, reductions followed epidural or intrathecal injection, with analgesia lasting approximately 1.5 h. As an α_2-adrenergic agonist, dexmedetomidine also acts in part by ACh release in the spinal cord dorsal horn: greater concentrations of ACh are obtained in spinal cord microdialysates after intrathecal dexmedetomidine administration than with clonidine in sheep and, similar to clonidine, intrathecal dexmedetomidine is also potentiated by neostigmine (6,28). In conclusion, dexmedetomidine might represent an interesting alternative to clonidine for analgesia, especially with epidural use. Only a few reports mention epidural injection in humans, but 2 μg/kg produced 4- to 6-h analgesia and reduced by 70% postoperative analgesic drug requirements during the first 24 h in one study (29). Blood pressure and heart rate were decreased by 20 and 25%, respectively, by dexmedetomidine.

V. α_2-ADRENERGIC AGONISTS AS ALTERNATIVES TO SPINAL OPIOIDS: TOLERANCE AND CROSS-TOLERANCE

One major limiting factor to long-term spinal opioid treatment is the development of some degree of tolerance, although causes for dose escalation in cancer patients often reflect other processes, such as disease progression and the development of an opioid-resistant neuropathic pain type. Because α_2-adrenergic agonists and opioids exert analgesic effects by different receptors and pathways in the spinal cord, there is a strong rationale for using α_2-adrenergic agonists to provide a "drug holiday" or in combination with opioids to reduce development of tolerance from the latter. This assumes that there is no cross-tolerance between opioids and α_2-adrenergic agonists. Many animal studies have explored tolerance and cross-tolerance of these agents, and suggest that any cross-tolerance between these classes of agents, if present, is minor (30).

In comparison with clonidine, dexmedetomidine possesses a higher intrinsic activity, implying a larger receptor reserve, longer infusion time before tolerance induction, and smaller degree of tolerance (31). In addition, increased intrinsic activity suggests that dexmedetomidine might be effective in the face of tolerance to clonidine. In contrast to spinal use, systemic injection of α_2-adrenergic agonists produces tolerance to the hypnotic effects, but minimally to the analgesic and sympatholytic effects; systemic dexmedetomidine retains its analgesic effect in rats tolerant to morphine (32). These findings are close to those reported in the human literature, in which tolerance and cross-tolerance do not appear to represent clinical problems. Epidural and intrathecal clonidine have been successfully administered in chronic pain and cancer patients during long periods of continuous infusion (5–12 months) and retain efficacy against pain that was previously resistant to opioids without evidence of tolerance development or neurotoxicity (33,34).

VI. AN ALTERNATIVE TO OPIOID-RESISTANT NEUROPATHIC PAIN

Numerous laboratory studies have been conducted in established animal models of peripheral and central neuropathic pain to examine therapeutic alternatives to opioids. In all of these models, α_2-adrenergic agonists have demonstrated efficacy in relieving mechanical allodynia or thermal hyperalgesia. In the spinal nerve-ligation rat model, which is insensitive to spinal opioids, clonidine and dexmedetomidine reduce mechanical allodynia with a better effect when injected spinally, near the affected dermatomes (35). Spinal dexmedetomidine totally relieves hyperalgesia in the sciatic nerve ligation model (36), and intrathecal clonidine suppresses autotomy after sciatic nerve section (37). In the latter model, intrathecal clonidine is ineffective in preventing development of presumed neuropathic pain, in contrast with spinal morphine, but clonidine is completely effective in treating established pain, again, in contrast to spinal morphine (38). Spinal clonidine delays thermal hyperalgesia in the sciatic nerve-ligation model by preventing spinal facilitation and also by reducing sympathetic outflow (39). Finally, intrathecal clonidine is much more effective than systemic clonidine in relieving mechanical allodynia after spinal cord ischemia in rats (40). These results reinforce the concept of a spinal site of action for α_2-adrenergic agonists in decreasing central sensitization. In addition, a peripheral and central sympatholytic effect may contribute to their efficacy.

In human volunteers, intradermal capsaicin injection produces temporary pain, with characteristics similar to neuropathic pain, including zones of primary heat hyperalgesia and secondary mechanical hyperalgesia, owing to a central sensitization process. Spinal, but not systemic clonidine significantly reduces capsaicin-induced pain and areas of hyperalgesia (41) (Fig. 3).

In patients with chronic pain in whom perceived risks of addiction and tolerance to prolonged opioid exposure are major concerns, α_2-adrenergic agonists have been tested as an alternative, especially in patients with neurogenic pain. Glynn et al., in a randomized, double-blind study, reported that a 150-μg epidural bolus of clonidine was equivalent to 5 mg of epidural morphine, for chronic pain treatment, and that clonidine was more effective than morphine when the pain was neurogenic (42). However, the same group, in a subsequent double-blind investigation, failed to find any difference between i.v. and epidural injection of a small dose of clonidine and questioned clonidine's usefulness (43). In a case of deafferentation pain that was unresponsive to sympathetic blocks, 150-μg–epidural clonidine produced total and long-lasting pain relief (44). Small doses (bolus of 25- to 75-μg)–epidural clonidine completely but transiently relieve postherpetic neuralgia. An epidural infusion of 150 μg of clonidine combined with opioids and local anesthetics before limb amputation has been reported to prevent the development of phantom limb pain (45). Rauck et al., in a double-blind clinical trial, demonstrated the efficacy of epidural clonidine alone to alleviate severe sympathetic dystrophy pain (46). In that study, a bolus of 300- or 700-μg–epidural clonidine was clearly superior to placebo, providing 6 h of pain relief, and a continuous infusion (average 30 μg/h) remained effective for 8 months. These high doses did not produce greater analgesia, nor did they produce greater

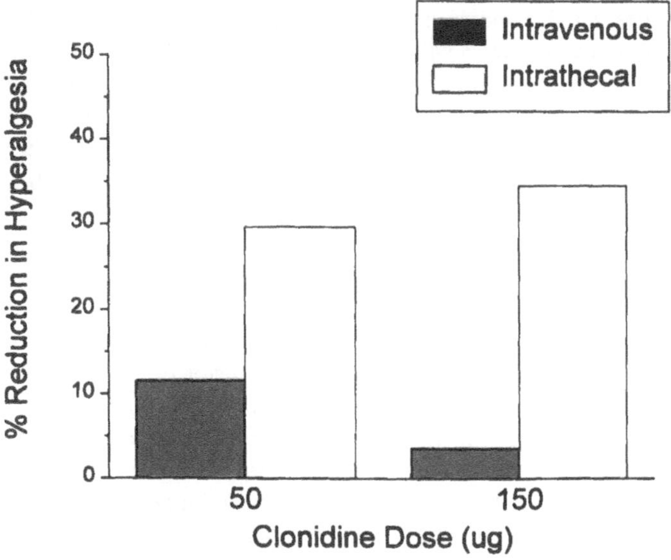

Figure 3 Clonidine reduces hyperalgesia by a spinal action: percentage reduction in area of hyperalgesia following intradermal injection of capsaicin in volunteers receiving intravenous or intrathecal clonidine. Only intrathecal injection significantly reduces hyperalgesia.

hypotension, possibly because of peripheral vasoconstriction from greater circulating concentrations of clonidine. Other authors reported sustained efficacy for 11 months in a patient with reflex sympathetic dystrophy insensitive to opioids from twice-daily epidural injection (300 μg) or intrathecal injection (150 μg) of clonidine (47). Finally, intrathecal clonidine, 8–17 μg daily, alleviated central neuropathic pain in a patient following spinal cord injury who had not received relief from morphine alone (48).

In summary, α_2-adrenergic agonists often exhibit superior efficacy in clinical reports and trials compared with opioids in patients with neuropathic pain, possibly by suppressing underlying central hyperexcitability. Spinal clonidine can act by at least three different mechanisms to relieve pain in these patients. First, as previously described, α_2-adrenergic agonists reduce nociceptive neurotransmission in the spinal cord dorsal horn by pre- and postsynaptic mechanisms. Second, they decrease sympathetic outflow by an action on spinal preganglionic neurons. Third, they reduce norepinephrine release at peripheral sympathetic nerve endings.

In cancer patients, α_2-adrenergic agonists relieve pain that is unresponsive or poorly responsive to oral or epidural opioids, either because of the nature of the pain (neuropathic) or because of tolerance development to opioids. Eisenach et al., in two studies, demonstrated epidural clonidine is an effective treatment in such cancer patients (49,50). In a pilot study (49), patients with intractable cancer pain responded in a dose-dependent manner to epidural bolus administration of clonidine, 100–900 μg. Analgesia lasted 6 h, and side effects were hemodynamic depression and sedation for doses of 300 μg or more. However, neither pruritus, nausea, and urinary retention (typical side effects from opioids) nor reduction in blood oxygen saturation were observed, and clonidine did not affect cortisol or blood glucose concentrations. In a subsequent, double-blind study (50), 85 patients with pain unresponsive to systemic morphine (100 mg/day) or epidural morphine (20 mg/day), received epidural clonidine (30 μg/h) or placebo for 14 days, through a catheter with tip located at the dermatomal site of their pain. Epidural morphine was allowed as rescue analgesia, and pain scores were evaluated by visual analog scale and McGill pain questionnaire. Clonidine treatment resulted in a 45% success rate (morphine use or pain decreasing without the other variable increasing), compared with 21% with placebo infusion. Even greater was the success rate in patients with neuropathic pain (56% with clonidine compared with 5% with placebo). Overall, clonidine did not affect morphine use, but reduced pain, and pain returned when clonidine was discontinued (Fig. 4). Side effects were similar in the two groups, and only two patients exhibited severe hypotension in the clonidine group. Other authors report efficacy of epidural clonidine alone, 750-μg bolus, producing more than 10-h pain relief, accompanied by hypotension and bradycardia, but not by respiratory depression in patients with Pancoast syndrome (51). They also report sustained analgesia for more than 100 days from lower doses of clonidine (70–170 μg) in combination with local anesthetics and opioids in these patients. There are many case reports and small series of cancer patients who have received intrathecal clonidine for pain unresponsive to opioids. Thus, an intrathecal bolus of 150–300 μg clonidine provides 7–18-h of analgesia, and continuous infusion of 300- to 1500-μg–intrathecal clonidine daily with opioids resulted in sustained efficacy (33,34). Intrathecal administration may be preferable to epidural administration in many cases. In cancer patients, physical factors, such as presence of epidural metastases (not infrequent) or fibrosis around the catheter can limit the diffusion of epidural analgesics. In addition, the intrathecal route can provide greater drug potency, greater dermatomal spread, a longer duration of action, and a smaller injected volume. For these reasons, intrathecal catheters are preferable in some patients, especially because experience has shown that externalized and tunneled intrathecal catheters can be used for a long time without increased complications compared with epidural catheters. A continuous infusion of clonidine, 30 μg daily, combined with opioids and local anesthetics, often is effect in long-term treatment of pain in patients with cancer (52).

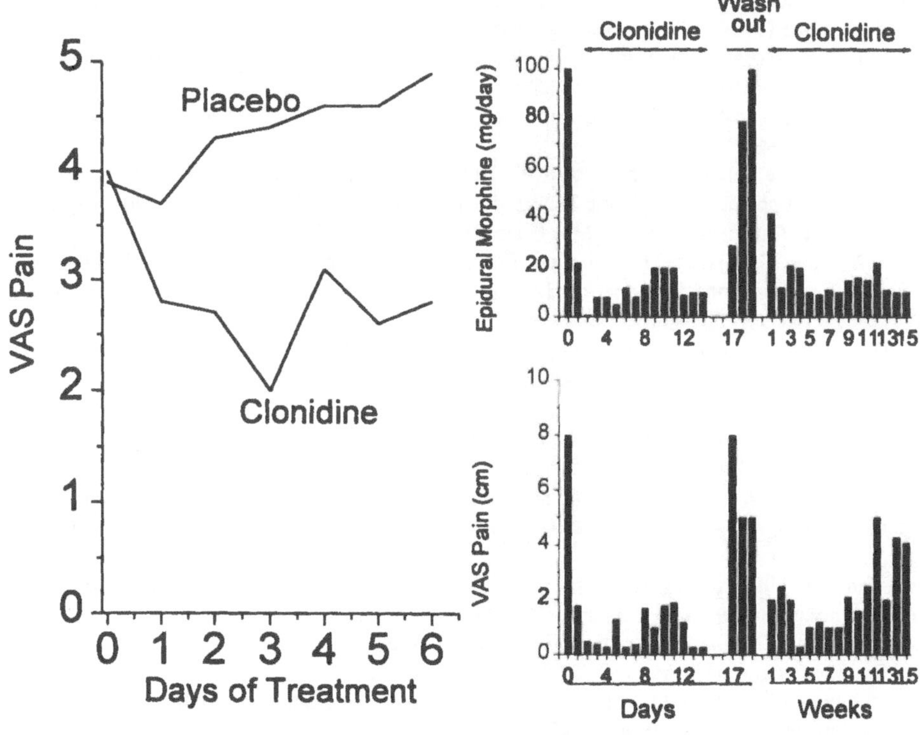

Figure 4 Epidural clonidine versus placebo in patients with intractable cancer pain: Clonidine results in a sustained reduction in pain report (*x*-axis in days), whereas placebo does not (left panel). In a patient with neuropathic pain, epidural morphine use and pain are reduced only during clonidine administration (right panel).

VII. SUMMARY

Spinal clonidine improves cancer pain treatment, especially when a neuropathic or sympathetic component is present, or when tolerance to opioids develops. A retrospective study, taking into account cancer treatments before and after 1990, revealed significant differences, particularly related to a quicker diagnosis of neuropathic pain and to more rational use of drug combinations, such as morphine plus clonidine. Better analgesia, often associated with fewer side effects, can be obtained by combining α_2-adrenergic agonists with opioids and local anesthetics for patients with chronic pain, especially of the neuropathic type.

ACKNOWLEDGMENT

Supported in part by NIH grants GM35523 and GM48085.

REFERENCE

1. Portenoy RK, Foley KM, Inturrisi CE. The nature of opioid responsiveness and its implications for neuropathic pain: new hypotheses derived from studies of opioid infusions. Pain 1990; 43:273–286.

2. Eisenach JC, De Kock M, Klimscha W. α_2-Adrenergic agonists for regional anesthesia—a clinical review of clonidine (1984–1995). Anesthesiology 1996; 85:655–674.
3. Yaksh TL. Pharmacology of spinal adrenergic systems which modulate spinal nociceptive processing. Pharmacol Biochem Behav 1985; 22:845–858.
4. Maze M, Tranquilli W. α-2 Adrenoceptor agonists: defining the role in clinical anesthesia. Anesthesiology 1991; 74:581–605.
5. Smith MS, Schambra UB, Wilson KH, Page SO, Hulette C, Light AR, Schwinn DA. α_2-Adrenergic receptors in human spinal cord: specific localized expression of mRNA encoding α_2-adrenergic receptor subtypes at four distinct levels. Mol Brain Res 1995; 34:109–117.
6. Klimscha W, Tong C, Eisenach JC. Intrathecal α_2-adrenergic agonists stimulate acetylcholine and norepinephrine release from the spinal cord dorsal horn in sheep—an in vivo microdialysis study. Anesthesiology 1997; 87:110–116.
7. Hood DD, Mallak KA, Eisenach JC, Tong CY. Interaction between intrathecal neostigmine and epidural clonidine in human volunteers, Anesthesiology 1996; 85:315–325.
8. Lothe A, Li P, Tong C, Yoon Y, Bouaziz H, Detweiler DJ, Eisenach JC. Spinal cholinergic alpha-2 adrenergic interactions in analgesia and hemodynamic control: role of muscarinic receptor subtypes and nitric oxide. J Pharmacol Exp Ther 1994; 270:1301–1306.
9. Eisenach JC, Hood DD, Tuttle R, Shafer S, Smith T, Tong C. Computer-controlled epidural infusion to targeted cerebrospinal fluid concentrations in humans: clonidine. Anesthesiology 1995; 83:33–47.
10. Valles J, Samso E, Vilar X, Puig MM. Intraoperative requirements of isoflurane after the administration of intramuscular or epidural clonidine. Br J Anaesth 1994; 72:82.
11. Bernard JM, Kick O, Bonnet F. Comparison of intravenous and epidural clonidine for postoperative patient-controlled analgesia. Anesth Analg 1995; 81:706–712.
12. Filos KS, Goudas LC, Patroni O, Polyzou V. Hemodynamic and analgesic profile after intrathecal clonidine in humans: a dose–response study. Anesthesiology 1994; 81:591–601.
13. Mendez R, Eisenach JC, Kashtan K. Epidural clonidine analgesia after cesarean section. Anesthesiology 1990; 73:848–852.
14. Eisenach JC, Tong C. Site of hemodynamic effects of intrathecal α_2-adrenergic agonists. Anesthesiology 1991; 74:766–771.
15. Bailey PL, Sperry RJ, Johnson GK, Eldredge SJ, East KA, East TD, Pace NL, Stanley TH. Respiratory effects of clonidine alone and combined with morphine, in humans. Anesthesiology 1991; 74: 43–48.
16. Muzi M, Goff DR, Kampine JP, Roerig DL, Ebert TJ. Clonidine reduces sympathetic activity but maintains baroreflex responses in normotensive humans. Anesthesiology 1992; 77:864–871.
17. Gentili M, Bonnet F. Spinal clonidine produces less urinary retention than spinal morphine. Br J Anaesth 1996; 76:872–873.
18. Klimscha W, Chiari A, Krafft P, Plattner O, Taslimi R, Mayer N, Weinstabl C, Schneider B, Zimpfer M. Hemodynamic and analgesic effects of clonidine added repetitively to continuous epidural and spinal blocks. Anesth Analg 1995; 80:322–327.
19. Ossipov MH, Harris S, Lloyd P, Messineo E, Lin B–S, Bagley J. Antinociceptive interaction between opioids and medetomidine: systemic additivity and spinal synergy. Anesthesiology 1990; 73:1227–1235.
20. Eisenach JC, D'Angelo R, Taylor C, Hood DD. An isobolographic study of epidural clonidine and fentanyl after cesarean section. Anesth Analg 1994; 79:285–290.
21. Rostaing S, Bonnet F, Levron JC, Vodinh J, Pluskwa F, Saada M. Effect of epidural clonidine on analgesia and pharmacokinetics of epidural fentanyl in postoperative patients. Anesthesiology 1991; 75:420–425.
22. Vercauteren M, Lauwers E, Meert T, De Hert S, Adriaensen H. Comparison of epidural sufentanil plus clonidine with sufentanil alone for postoperative pain relief. Anaesthesia 1990; 45:531–534.
23. Aantaa RE, Kanto JH, Scheinin M, Kallio AMI, Scheinin H. Dexmedetomidine premedication for minor gynecologic surgery. Anesth Analg 1990; 70:407–413.

24. Aho MS, Erkola OA, Scheinin H, Lehtinen A–M, Korttila KT. Effect of intravenously administered dexmedetomidine on pain after laparoscopic tubal ligation. Anesth Analg 1991; 73:112–118.
25. Jaakola M–L, Salonen M, Lehtinen R, Scheinin H. The analgesic action of dexmedetomidine—a novel α_2-adrenoceptor agonist—in healthy volunteers. Pain 1991; 46:281–285.
26. Talke P, Richardson CA, Scheinin M, Fisher DM. Postoperative pharmacokinetics and sympatholytic effects of dexmedetomidine. Anesth Analg 1997; 85:1136–1142.
27. Eisenach JC, Shafer SL, Bucklin BA, Jackson C, Kallio A. Pharmacokinetics and pharmacodynamics of intraspinal dexmedetomidine in sheep. Anesthesiology 1994; 80:1349–1359.
28. Bouaziz H, Hewitt C, Eisenach JC. Subarachnoid neostigmine potentiation of alpha$_2$-adrenergic agonist analgesia. Reg Anesth 1995; 20:121–127.
29. Fukushima K, Nishimi Y, Mori K, Takeda J. Central effect of epidurally administered dexmedetomidine on sympathetic activity and postoperative pain in man. Anesth Analg 1996; 82:S121.
30. Solomon RE, Gebhart GF. Intrathecal morphine and clonidine: antinociceptive tolerance and cross-tolerance and effects on blood pressure. J Pharmacol Exp Ther 1988; 245:444–454.
31. Kalso EA, Sullivan AF, McQuay HJ, Dickenson AH, Roques BP. Cross-tolerance between mu opioid and alpha-$_2$ adrenergic receptors, but not between mu and delta opioid receptors in the spinal cord of the rat. J Pharmacol Exp Ther 1993; 265:551–558.
32. Hayashi Y, Guo TZ, Maze M. Hypnotic and analgesic: effects of the α_2-adrenergic agonist dexmedetomidine in morphine-tolerant rats. Anesth Analg 1996; 83:606–610.
33. Coombs DW, Saunders RL, LaChance D, Savage S, Ragnarsson TS, Jensen LE. Intrathecal morphine tolerance: use of intrathecal clonidine, DADLE, and intraventricular morphine. Anesthesiology 1985; 62:357–363.
34. Coombs DW, Saunders RL, Fratkin JD, Jensen LE, Murphy CA. Continuous intrathecal hydromorphone and clonidine for intractable cancer pain. J Neurosurg 1986; 64:890–894.
35. Yaksh TL, Pogrel JW, Lee YW, and Chaplan SR. Reversal of nerve ligation-induced allodynia by spinal alpha-2 adrenoceptor agonists. J Pharmacol Exp Ther 1995; 272:207–214.
36. Yamamoto T, Yaksh TL. Spinal pharmacology of thermal hyperesthesia induced by incomplete ligation of sciatic nerve: I. Opioid and nonopioid receptors. Anesthesiology 1991; 75:817–826.
37. Puke MJC, Xu X–J, Wiesenfeld–Hallin Z. Intrathecal administration of clonidine suppresses autotomy, a behavioral sign of chronic pain in rats after sciatic nerve section. Neurosci Lett 1991; 133: 199–202.
38. Puke MJC, Wiesenfeld–Hallin Z. The differential effects of morphine and the α_2-adrenoceptor agonists clonidine and dexmedetomidine on the prevention and treatment of experimental neuropathic pain. Anesth Analg 1993; 77:104–109.
39. Yamamoto T, Nozaki–Taguchi N. Clonidine, but not morphine, delays the development of thermal hyperesthesia induced by sciatic nerve constriction injury in the rat. Anesthesiology 1996; 85:835–845.
40. Hao JX, Yu W, Xu XJ, Wiesenfeld–Hallin Z. Effects of intrathecal vs. systemic clonidine in treating chronic allodynia-like response in spinally injured rats. Brain Res 1996; 736:28–34.
41. Eisenach JC, Hood DD, Curry R. Intrathecal, but not IV clonidine reduces pain and hyperalgesia. Anesth Analg 1998; 87:591–596.
42. Glynn C, Dawson D, Sanders R. A double-blind comparison between epidural morphine and epidural clonidine in patients with chronic non-cancer pain. Pain 1988; 34:123–128.
43. Carroll D, Jadad A, King V, Wiffen P, Glynn C, McQuay H. Single-dose, randomized, double-blind, double-dummy cross-over comparison of extradural and i.v. clonidine in chronic pain. Br J Anaesth 1993; 71:665–669.
44. Coventry DM, Todd G. Epidural clonidine in lower limb deafferentation pain. Anesth Analg 1989; 69:424–425.
45. Jahangiri M, Jayatunga AP, Bradley JWP, Dark CH. Prevention of phantom pain after major lower limb amputation by epidural infusion of diamorphine, clonidine and bupivacaine. Ann R Coll Surg Engl 1994; 76:324–326.
46. Rauck RL, Eisenach JC, Jackson K, Young LD, Southern J. Epidural clonidine treatment for refractory reflex sympathetic dystrophy. Anesthesiology 1993; 79:1163–1169.

47. Kabeer AA, Hardy AJ. Long-term use of subarachnoid clonidine for analgesia in refractory reflex sympathetic dystrophy. Reg Anesth 1996; 21:249–252.
48. Siddall PJ, Gray M, Rutkowski S, Cousins MJ. Intrathecal morphine and clonidine in the management of spinal cord injury pain: a case report. Pain 1994; 59:147–148.
49. Eisenach JC, Rauck RL, Buzzanell C, Lysak SZ. Epidural clonidine analgesia for intractable cancer pain: phase I. Anesthesiology 1989; 71:647–652.
50. Eisenach JC, DuPen S, Dubois M, Miguel R, Allin D, Epidural Clonidine Study Group. Epidural clonidine analgesia for intractable cancer pain. Pain 1995; 61:391–399.
51. Ferit PA, Aydinli I, Akra S. Management of cancer pain with epidural clonidine. Reg Anesth 1992; 17(suppl 3S):173–173.
52. Laugner B, Muller A, Theibaut JB, Farcot JM. Analgesie par site implantable pour injections intrathecales iteratives de morphine. Ann Fr Anesth Reanim 1985; 4:511–520.

67

Cellular Implantation for the Treatment of Chronic Pain

Jacqueline Sagen and Mary Eaton
University of Miami School of Medicine, Miami, Florida, U.S.A.

I. INTRODUCTION

Although narcotic analgesics and formulations containing opioids are the most commonly used agents for the treatment of moderate to severe pain, the use of exogenous drug administration on a long-term basis for chronic pain management is often not optimal owing to potentially serious or disturbing side effects, tolerance development, poor pain control, and inconvenience. Over the last two decades, the field of cellular transplantation has exploded as a potential means of providing a local and continually renewable supply of therapeutic molecules. Cell therapy that uses transplants of cells from primary tissue, such as adrenal medullary chromaffin cells, or immortalized, bioengineered cell lines that secrete pain-reducing neuroactive substances into the central nervous system (CNS), offers a feasible alternative in the long-term management of chronic pain. Similar to the more common drug pumps used for opioid delivery, cellular implants permit long-term, low, local dose delivery of antinociceptive agents into the cerebrospinal fluid (CSF), without the side effects associated with large doses or systemic administration. In addition, these biological "cellular minipumps" permit the delivery and utilization of molecules that have biological half-lives that are too short to allow them to be delivered by other means, such as osmotic pumps with intrathecal catheters. With continued viability, cell transplants avoid the problems of catheter-related infections, refilling, and maintenance required with the drug pumps. Although, to date, primary cells have been utilized in initial clinical pain trials, one can envision the possibilities of generating cell lines that can manufacture novel analgesic agents for specific pain indications, or respond to the physiological microenvironment by bioengineering cells to secrete agents only when they are needed, such as with periodic episodes of pain. Some of these pain-reducing neuroactive substances that could be manufactured by the cellular minipumps include opioid peptides (e.g., endorphins and enkephalins) and other peptides such as galanin, neurotensin, somatostatin, and calcitonin; neurotransmitters such as norepinephrine, epinephrine, serotonin, and γ-aminobutyric acid (GABA); neurotrophins such as brain-derived neurotrophic factor (BDNF); cytokines such as interleukin (IL)-10, and numerous other neuroactive molecules, the genes of which can be introduced into bioengineered cell lines.

II. ADRENAL MEDULLARY CHROMAFFIN GRAFTS

A. Chromaffin Cell Sources

Some of the earliest studies describing cell therapy for pain utilized adrenal medullary allografts, containing differentiated chromaffin cells that produce and secrete a variety of antinociceptive molecules, including opioid peptides and catecholamines, as well as a plethora of peptides and neurotrophins able to potentially act at pain-processing sites in the host CNS. This "cocktail" (1) secreted by adrenal chromaffin cell grafts, when transplanted into the subarachnoid space of the spinal cord, is probably responsible for the reversal of pain behaviors reported in a variety of animal models. More recently, xenogeneic sources of chromaffin cells have also been used in pain models, owing partly to the immune-privileged nature of the CNS, as well as the low antigenicity of the neural crest-derived chromaffin cells. Studies in our laboratory have demonstrated minimal rat lymphocytic proliferation in response to isolated bovine chromaffin cells in in vitro lymphocyte proliferation assays (2) and long-term robust survival (at least 1 year) of isolated bovine chromaffin cells in the rat CNS following only a short-term (2–4 weeks) of immunosuppressive treatment (3). Another approach is the use of immunoisolatory devices in which living cells can be encapsulated in semipermeable membranes to allow free passage of nutrients and therapeutic molecules, while hindering passage of cells and host immunoglobulins.

B. Chromaffin Cell Grafts in Preclinical Models

Thus far, adrenal medullary chromaffin cell transplants in the spinal subarachnoid space have demonstrated efficacy in a variety of preclinical rodent pain models, including acute nociceptive assays (4–10), inflammatory pain models (11–15), neuropathic pain models (16–19), and central pain models (20–23). As an example, the effects of isolated bovine chromaffin cell transplants on formalin pain responses are shown in Fig. 1. Chromaffin cells were isolated from bovine adrenal glands as described previously (24), using a series of Percoll gradient separations and differential plating to produce an approximately 95% pure population of chromaffin cells. Adherent bovine adrenal fibroblast cells were left to grow on the plates to serve as control cell implants. For transplantation, cells were resuspended in Hanks' buffered saline solution at a cell density of 50,000s/μL, and 10-μL cell suspensions were implanted by laminectomy and needle puncture at spinal levels L1–L3. Animals were immunosuppressed with cyclosporin beginning 1 day before transplantation for 1 week. The intraplantar injection of formalin (5%, 50 μL, s.c.) resulted in a typical biphasic flinching response in animals implanted with control bovine adrenal fibroblast cells (see Fig. 1), similar to that described by others in normal animals. In contrast, in animals with transplants of bovine chromaffin cells in the spinal subarachnoid space, both phases of the formalin test were markedly attenuated. These findings are similar to those observed in the formalin model following the transplantation of allogeneic adrenal medullary tissue in the spinal subarachnoid space (13). By using tyrosine hydroxylase (TH) immunocytochemistry, healthy clusters of bovine chromaffin cells can be readily identified in the rat spinal subarachnoid space (Fig. 2). These clusters tend to adhere to meningeal surfaces and spinal roots in the region of the cellular implantation sites.

Adrenal medullary transplants also markedly reduce persistent pain symptoms, notably those resulting from peripheral or CNS injury, in rodent models (16–23). In particular, central pain syndromes resulting from spinal cord injury, which are difficult to manage clinically using conventional pain therapies, may be uniquely sensitive to the therapeutic cocktail produced by chromaffin cell transplants. Using three distinct models of spinal cord injury pain, chromaffin cell allografts or xenografts reduce hypersensitivity to mechanical and thermal stimuli (20–23). As an example, an excitotoxic spinal cord injury that results in pathological changes comparable

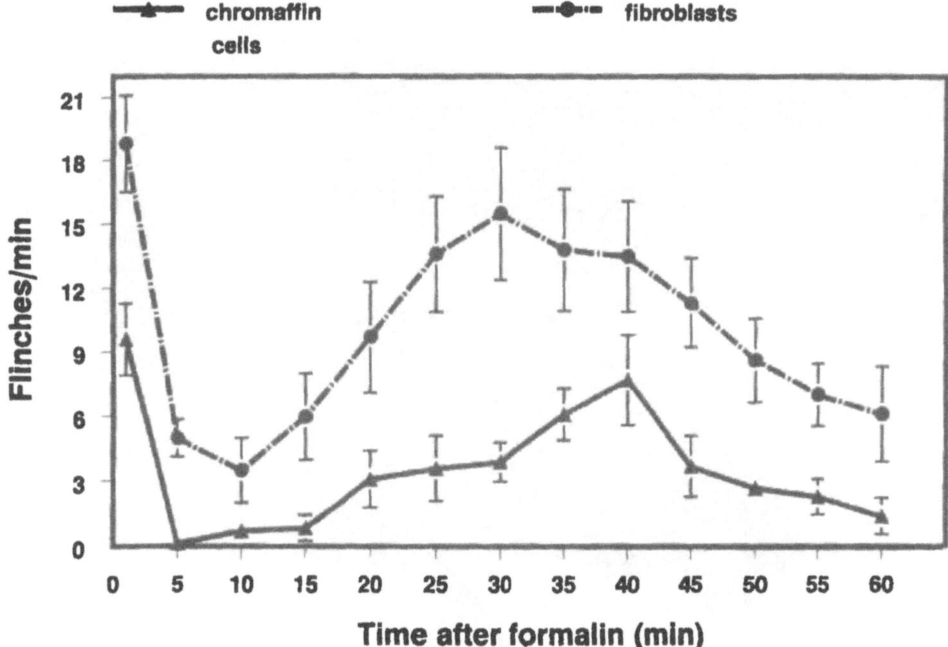

Figure 1 Time course of biphasic flinching response following formalin injection in animals with bovine chromaffin cell transplants or control bovine adrenal medullary fibroblasts in the spinal subarachnoid space: Each point represents the mean ±SEM number of hindpaw flinches observed at 5-min intervals following injection of 5% formalin in the plantar surface of the right hindpaw. $N = 12$ animals per group.

with ischemic and traumatic clinical spinal cord injury can be produced by intraspinal injections of the mixed AMPA/metabotropic receptor agonist quisqualic acid (QUIS) (25). This results in a behavioral syndrome of mechanical and thermal allodynia and excessive grooming at approximately 10–14 days following QUIS injections. At approximately 6 days following the onset of grooming behavior, animals received either adrenal medullary allografts or control skeletal muscle tissue implanted in the spinal subarachnoid space just caudal to the QUIS injection sites. In animals with control transplants, excessive grooming continued to increase in severity over the 25-day posttransplant observation period (Fig. 3). In contrast, in animals with adrenal medullary transplants, this progressive increase in grooming was blocked and, in a couple of cases, skin areas were completely recovered to normal. Both mechanical allodynia, as assessed by von Frey thresholds, and thermal allodynia, as assessed by cold plate test, were also attenuated by adrenal medullary transplants compared with control transplanted animals.

C. Mechanisms of Chromaffin Cell Transplants in Chronic Pain Reduction

These results and those of other groups indicate that transplantation of chromaffin cells into the spinal CSF can markedly reduce symptoms of chronic pain resulting from a variety of etiologies. However, recent studies have suggested that, in addition to opioid peptides and catecholamines released from the transplanted cells, additional mechanisms may be involved in reducing pain symptoms, particularly relative to nonacute pain. Although acute antinociceptive effects of adrenal medullary transplants can be attenuated by opioid or α-adrenergic antagonists (7–9), this

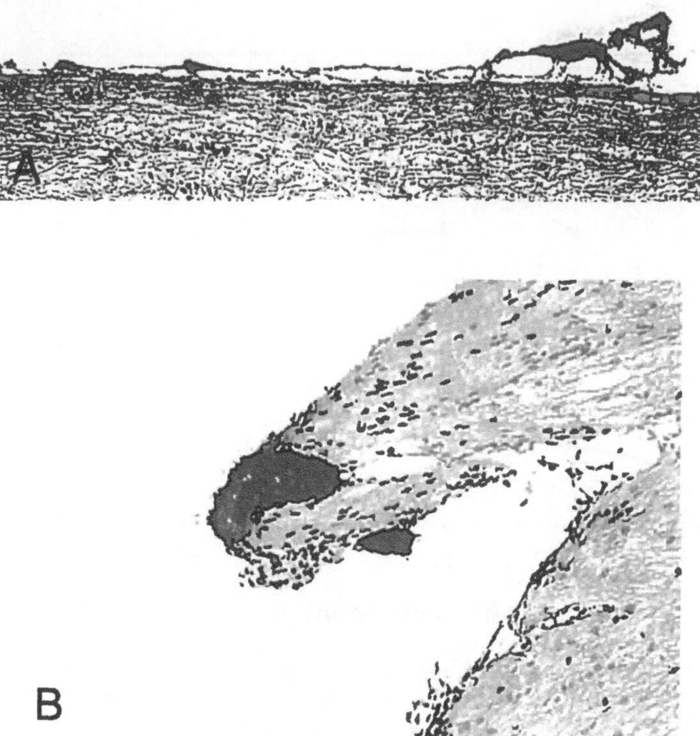

Figure 2 Appearance of bovine chromaffin cell transplants in the rat spinal subarachnoid space: Clusters of chromaffin cells are distributed around the surface of the spinal cord, attached to meninges and roots; (A) several chromaffin cell clusters on the lateral surface of the spinal cord, sectioned longitudinally; (B) a higher magnification of a cluster of chromaffin cells embedded within spinal root fibers. Chromaffin cells have been stained immunocytochemically with tyrosine hydroxylase. Bars: 1.0 mm (A) and 100 μm (B).

does not appear to be a consistent finding in nonacute pain (13,14,22,26). The formalin test is useful as an example because it consists of acute and tonic components that are likely mediated by pharmacologically distinguishable mechanisms. The first phase is thought to be similar to acute noxious stimuli, involving an initial barrage of primary afferent activity. This is followed by a quiescent phase during which a prolonged sensitization and spinal facilitation develop that lead to the second or tonic phase. The tonic phase of the formalin response is thought to be initiated by activation of *N*-methyl-D-aspartate (NMDA) receptors and sustained by a cascade of events including nitric oxide (NO) synthesis (27–31). Using the formalin model in animals with adrenal medullary allografts in the spinal subarachnoid space, both phases of the formalin response were suppressed, as described in the foregoing, for bovine chromaffin cell transplants, in comparison with control striated muscle-transplanted animals. However, pretreatment with the opiate antagonist naloxone (2.0 mg/kg, s.c.) blocked suppression of the phase 1 response in adrenal medullary-transplanted animals, but did not alter the phase 2 suppression (Fig. 4). Similarly, pretreatment with the α-adrenergic antagonist phentolamine significantly attenuated suppression of phase 1 but not phase 2, in adrenal medullary-transplanted animals (13). Since the antinociceptive effects of opiates and α-adrenergic antagonists can block the suppression

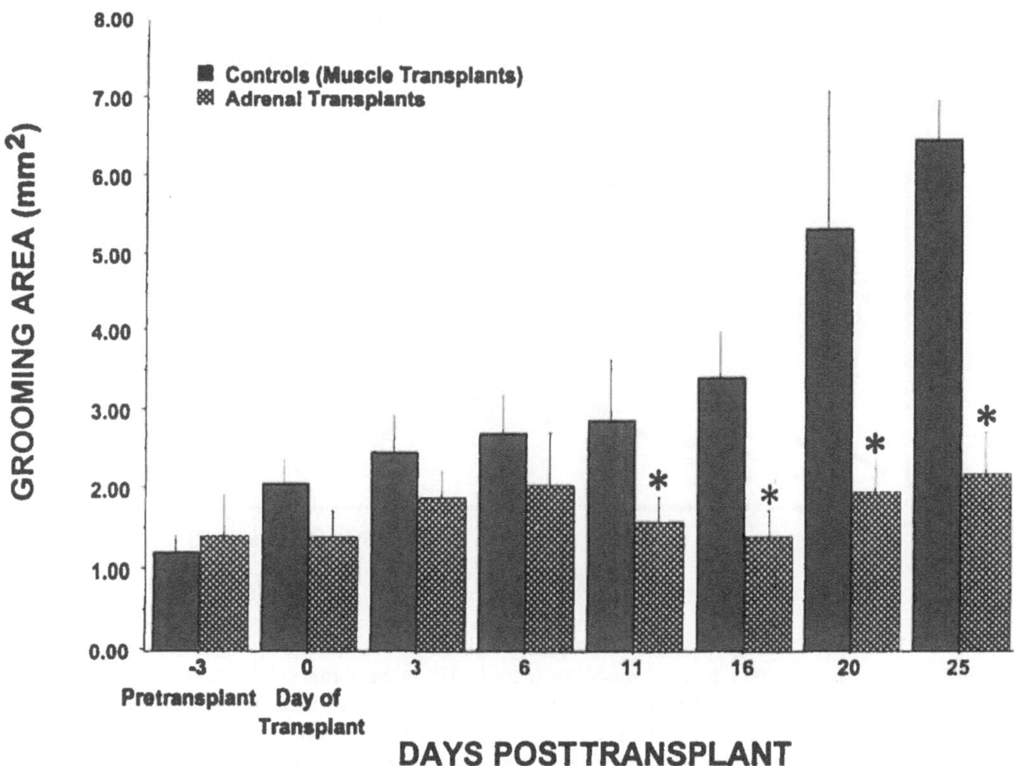

Figure 3 Area of skin targeted for excessive grooming is shown for 25 days following transplantation: Black bars indicate animals receiving transplantation of muscle tissue ($n = 6$); hatched bars show adrenal transplanted animals ($n = 8$). Transplantation was performed an average of 6 days after the onset of grooming behavior and is indicated as time 0. From day 11 through day 25 posttransplant, the area targeted for grooming was significantly smaller for animals receiving adrenal medullary transplants than for those receiving muscle transplants ($p < 0.05$). (From Ref. 20.)

of both formalin phases by their respective agonists (32), these findings suggest the possibility that alternate pharmacological mechanisms are involved in adrenal medullary transplant effects. One possibility is by interaction with the NMDA–NO cascade, for recent findings have revealed that chromaffin cells produce peptides with NMDA antagonist-like activity (33), and adrenal medullary transplants can attenuate exaggerated responses to noxious and innocuous stimuli brought about by direct intrathecal injection of NMDA (26). Finally, the intrathecal administration of adrenal medullary peptide histogranin, which possesses NMDA antagonist activity and attenuates the second, but not the first phase of the formalin test (34), reduces NMDA-mediated nociceptive responses (35), and attenuates pain behaviors following peripheral nerve injury (36). Together, these findings suggest that chromaffin cell transplants may act by direct interaction with spinal NMDA receptors to reduce pain behaviors resulting from central sensitization.

In addition to behavioral findings, neurochemical and morphological evidence indicate that chromaffin cell transplants inhibit spinal hyperexcitability. For example, increases in NO synthase and cGMP following peripheral nerve injury are attenuated by adrenal medullary, but not control transplants in the spinal subarachnoid space (37,38). Activation of the immediate early gene c-*fos* by inflammation in the adjuvant arthritis model or following formalin (39,40) is also markedly reduced in animals with adrenal medullary transplants. Figure 5 shows exam-

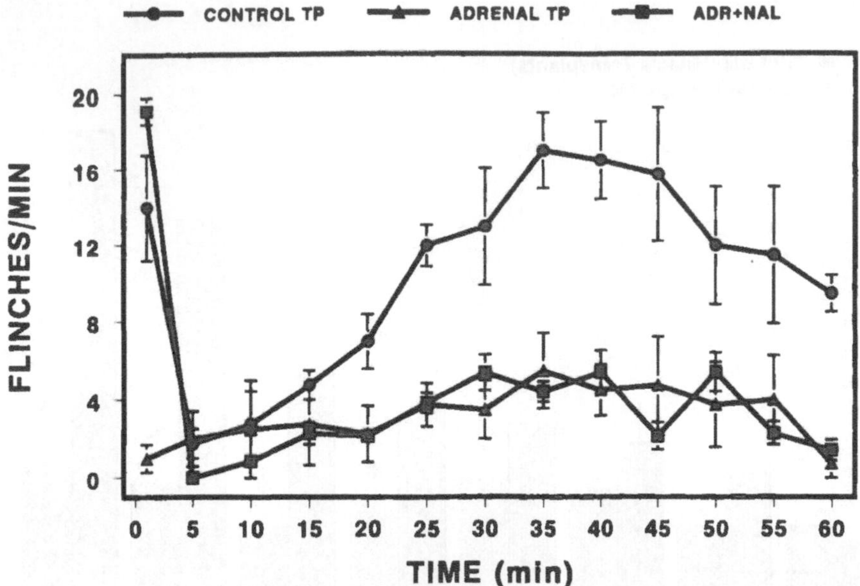

Figure 4 Biphasic flinching response following formalin injection in animals with adrenal medullary (adrenal TP) or control striated muscle transplants (control TP) in the spinal subarachnoid space: An additional group of adrenal medullary-transplanted animals were pretreated with the opiate antagonist naloxone before formalin injection (ADR + NAL). Each point represents the mean ±SEM number of hindpaw flinches observed at 5-min intervals following injection of 5% formalin in the plantar surface of the right hindpaw. $N = 6$–8 animals per group.

ples of c-*fos* activation, using immunocytochemistry for the Fos protein in animals with either control striated muscle transplants or adrenal muscle transplants, 90 min following intraplantar formalin injections.

Adrenal medullary transplants may also provide a degree of neuroprotection as a result of either reducing hyperexcitability or enhancing secretion of neurotrophic factors (1,41). A long-term consequence of persistent noxious activation, such as that resulting from injury to the peripheral or central nervous system, may be a loss of vulnerable inhibitory interneurons which would otherwise serve to limit pain. For example, peripheral nerve injury results in the appearance of hyperchromatic "dark neurons" indicative of transsynaptic degeneration and a loss of inhibitory gabaergic neurons in the superficial spinal dorsal horn (42–45). Both the appearance of dark neurons and the loss of gabaergic neurons are reduced by adrenal medullary transplants (42,43). Thus, adrenal medullary transplants may provide a neuroprotective environment which reduces the long-term detrimental consequences of persistent pain. A model incorporating the potential mechanisms of chronic pain reduction by chromaffin cell transplants in the spinal subarachnoid space is shown in Fig. 6.

D. Chromaffin Cell Transplants in Early Clinical Trials

Initial clinical trials using either human adrenal medullary tissue allografts or encapsulated bovine chromaffin cell implants in patients with cancer pain have been conducted at several centers. At the University of Illinois at Chicago, five patients suffering from severe pain secondary to inoperable cancer received human adrenal medullary implants following enrollment in a University Institutional Review Board-approved study. Adrenal medullary tissue was obtained from

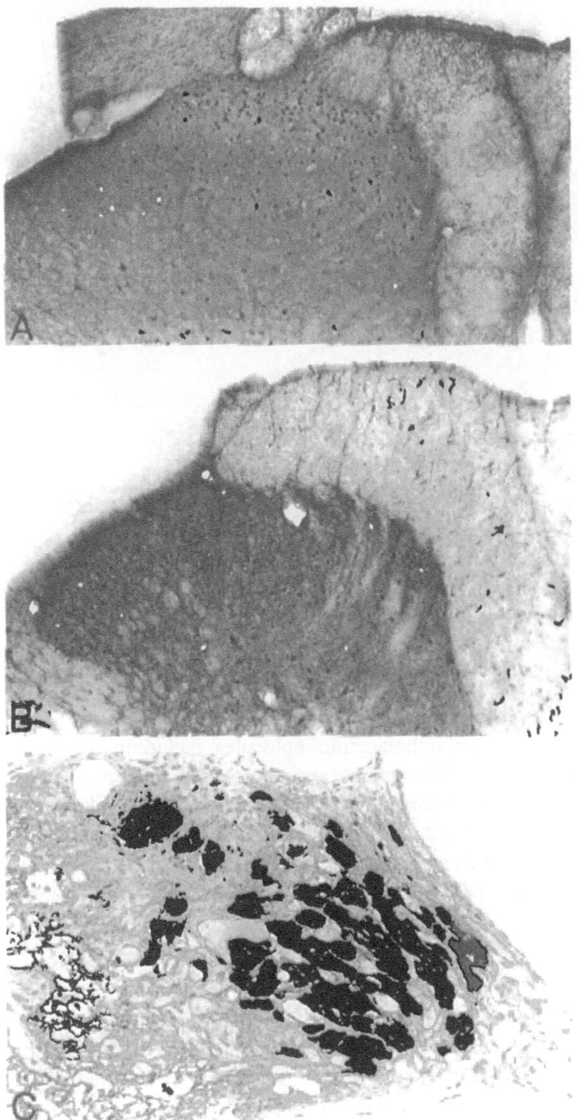

Figure 5 Activation of FOS-IR neurons in the superficial dorsal horn following unilateral injections of formalin (5%) in the plantar hindpaw: (A) from an animal with control striated muscle tissue transplanted in the spinal subarachnoid space; (B) from an animal with adrenal medullary tissue transplanted in the spinal subarachnoid space; (C) the appearance of an adrenal medullary transplant in the rat spinal subarachnoid space, immunocytochemically labeled with tyrosine hydroxylase.

adult glands by the Regional Organ Bank of Illinois following pathogen screening. Adrenal medullary tissue was dissected, cultured, and verified for catecholamine synthesis. Tissue from approximately two adrenal glands was implanted in the subarachnoid space of patients by lumbar puncture using a 14-gauge Touhy needle. Follow-up included visual analog scale (VAS) pain measurements, intake of supplementary pain medications, and daily activity when appropriate. In four of the patients, marked reductions in VAS scores and analgesic consumption was observed within 2–8 weeks following adrenal medullary transplantation. Three of these patients remained free of pain throughout the remainder of their lives, two for approximately 1 year.

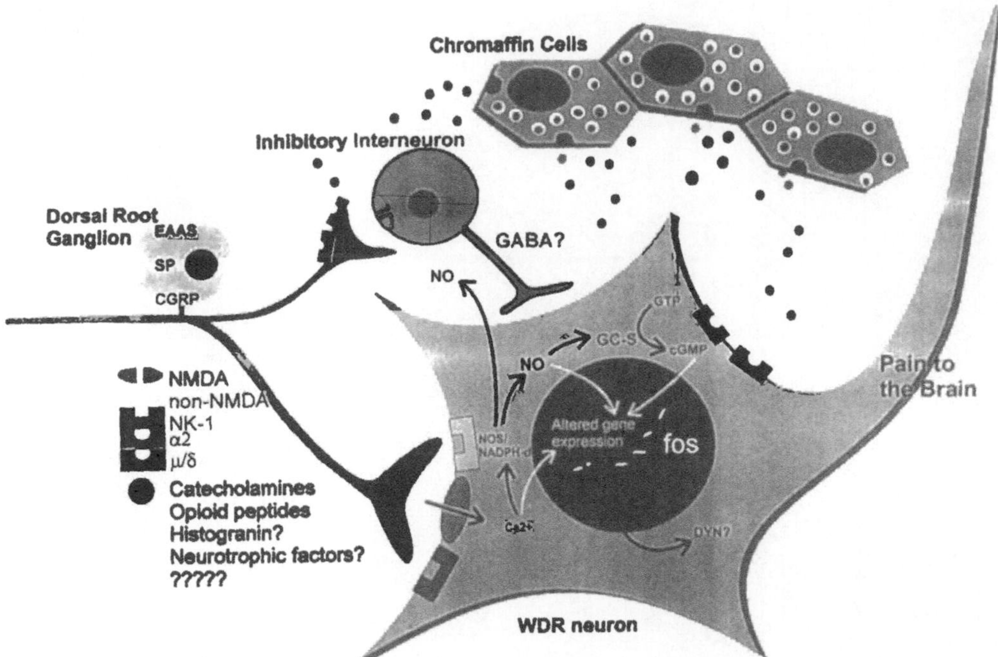

Figure 6 Model for possible routes of intervention in pain transmission by chromaffin cell transplants in the spinal CSF: Chromaffin cells secrete a variety of potential therapeutic molecules, including catecholamines, opioid peptides, putative NMDA antagonist peptide histogranin, and neurotrophic factors. These may interact with host spinal α-adrenergic, μ-, and δ-opioid receptors, NMDA receptors, and others, to reduce activation of spinal pain transmission neurons or excitotoxicity to vulnerable inhibitory interneurons. Previous findings (summarized in the text) have indicated reduced activation of the NMDA–NO cascade and reduced loss of spinal neurons in persistent pain models following adrenal medullary transplantation in the spinal subarachnoid space.

Detailed case histories of the patients can be found in Winnie et al. (46). Using a similar protocol, Lazorthes et al. (47) performed adrenal medullary allogeneic implants in seven patients suffering from intractable pain caused by cancer. A multidisciplinary pain evaluation demonstrated progressively decreased pain scores in six of the patients and opioid analgesic intake was decreased in three of the patients, stabilized in two other patients, and increased in two patients. In addition, CSF met-enkephalin levels were noted to correlate with pain control. Although the results of these studies were promising overall, they must be interpreted cautiously, as a potential placebo effect cannot be ruled out owing to the nature of the study design. This study is ongoing and currently includes 15 patients with similar promising results. A placebo-controlled study is planned for the near future (personal communication).

Two other small studies using human adrenal medullary allografts in patients with cancer pain have been conducted. At Universidad Nacional Autonoma de Mexico, a single patient with intractable pain was implanted with adrenal medullary tissue with "striking results" (Drucker-Colin R, personal communication). In contrast, Vaquero et al. reported a "disappointing outcome" in an end-stage cancer pain patient who experienced only transient pain reduction following adrenal medullary implant (48).

Phase 1 clinical trials have also been conducted at several centers using encapsulated bovine chromaffin cell implants (49–51), and a phase 2 trial is currently in progress in Europe.

Phase 1 clinical trials were conducted to assess safety and preliminary efficacy at the University of Lausanne, Switzerland, in seven patients with severe pain (six with terminal cancer, one with unrelieved neurogenic pain secondary to thoracotomy and scoliosis). Capsules containing approximately 2 million chromaffin cells were implanted by lumbar puncture under local anesthesia. The active portion of the capsule containing the chromaffin cells was placed in the lumbar cistern and held in place by a silicone tether that was sutured to the lumbodorsal fascia and completely covered with skin closure. Except for occasional reports of postdural puncture headaches, no adverse effects from the procedure were noted. Of the seven patients, four who were receiving epidural morphine at the time of the implant were reported to have decreased opioid use following the implant with either a modest improvement or no worsening in pain ratings, and three patients who were not receiving oral or epidural morphine treatment at the time of the implant reported improvement in pain ratings. Histological examination of the spinal cords, when possible, revealed no remarkable pathology, and chromaffin cell viability was confirmed in retrieved capsules by catecholamine release and immunostaining.

A similar phase 1 clinical trial has been conducted in the United States; preliminary results have been reported (51) and detailed findings from this study will be reported shortly (52). This study was conducted under a commercially sponsored Investigational New Drug (IND) application reviewed by the U.S. Food and Drug Administration (FDA). The study included 19 patients with intractable pain secondary to incurable malignancies and with a life expectancy of less than 5 months. Chromaffin–cell-containing devices were provided by Cyto Therapeutics, Inc., Providence, RI. Initially, 15 patients received capsules containing 1×10^6 cells (5.0 cm in length), and an additional 4 patients received capsules containing 3×10^6 cells (7.0 cm in length). Prior to implantation, samples were tested for catecholamine production to ensure chromaffin cell viability. As before, encapsulated chromaffin cell devices were implanted under local anesthesia into the lumbar subarachnoid space through a cannula inserted into the cistern; the silicone tether was secured to the dorsal lumbar fascia; and the skin was sutured closed to completely cover the device tether.

Participants selected for the study were advanced cancer patients with chronic pain inadequately relieved by conventional therapies. In 15 of the patients, aggressive opioid trials had proved ineffective at providing adequate analgesia, whereas in the other 4, opioid use was limited by side effects or individual resistance. As this was primarily a safety trial, patients were carefully monitored for adverse experiences. No serious complications directly attributable to the implant were noted, and routine clinical pathology showed no evidence of adverse reactions. The few mild adverse experiences, including postlumbar puncture headaches (two patients), subcutaneous fluid collections at the implant site (two patients), and subarachnoid–cutaneous fistula (one patient) were easily resolved.

Although assessment of the analgesic efficacy must be evaluated with caution in the absence of appropriate placebo or intervention comparison group, some evidence of analgesic efficacy was suggested by reductions in pain scores in 9 patients, and opiate reduction in 8 of the original 15 patients (51). Mean VAS pain scores showed a gradual decline over time (Fig. 7), with an approximate decline of 39% at 4 weeks postimplant. Of the patients exhibiting improved pain control, most had pain complaints that were localized to body regions innervated by lumbar and sacral nerves. This suggests that diffusion of pain-reducing neuroactive agents to higher levels may be limited. In addition, many of these responsive patients had neuropathic pain caused by local invasion of the lumbar or sacral nerve plexus or nerve roots, which is extremely difficult to manage clinically with opioid analgesics.

In retrieved capsules, catecholamine release assays and histological examination indicated chromaffin cell viability. An example of encapsulated bovine chromaffin cells identified immunocytochemically using a tyrosine hydroxylase antibody is shown in Fig. 8.

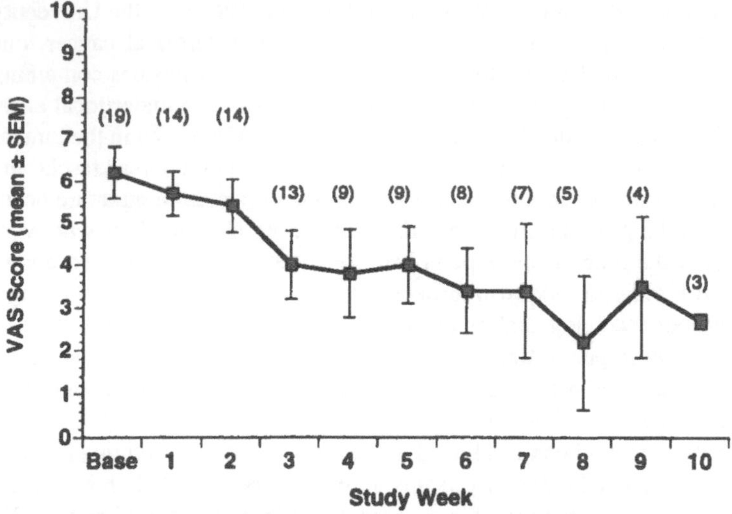

Figure 7 Mean visual analog scores (VAS) of 19 implanted patients in the U.S. phase 1 cancer pain trial: the number of surviving patients at each time point is shown in parentheses.

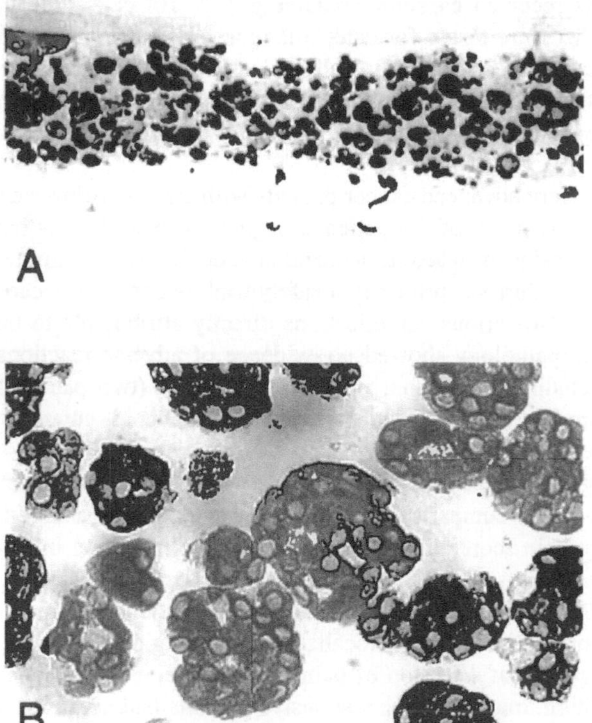

Figure 8 Appearance of bovine chromaffin cell clusters encapsulated in PAN/PVC membranes: (A) a low magnification of chromaffin cell clusters surrounded by the capsule walls; (B) a higher magnification showing numerous viable clusters of chromaffin cells within the capsules. Chromaffin cells are immunocytochemically stained for tyrosine hydroxylase.

Three additional clinical trials to evaluate the safety and efficacy of encapsulated chromaffin cell devices are nearing completion. Two small companion open-label studies in patients with neuropathic pain of various etiologies were initiated in the United States and Switzerland to evaluate the tolerability and retrievability of a modified device. In addition, a large multicenter, placebo-controlled study in patients with cancer-related pain is still ongoing in Switzerland, the Czech Republic, and Poland.

III. BIOENGINEERED CELLS FOR PAIN

A. Tumor Cell Lines

Spontaneously and conditionally immortalized cell lines that could be adapted and genetically engineered for biomedical use are among the most novel of emerging clinical therapies in the treatment of chronic pain in humans. Spontaneous tumor cell lines, such as the adrenal pheochromocytomal PC12 cell line, have been studied extensively as a potential source for grafts in a variety of neurodegenerative diseases, but pheochromocytoma cell lines are inappropriate for therapeutic use owing to the great risk of unrestricted cell division and tumor formation (53–57). Moreover, pheochromocytoma cell lines, such as the rat PC12 line, may not behave as normal mature chromaffin cells, in that they appear to maintain or dedifferentiate to a less mature phenotype. For example, PC12 cells synthesize dopamine and low levels of norepinephrine, but rarely epinephrine, a principal catecholamine in mature chromaffin cells (58). In support for this, these cells also lack detectable levels of phenylethanolamine-*N*-methyltransferase (PNMT) that catalyzes the conversion of norepinephrine to epinephrine (58).

The neuroblastoma line, Neuro2A, which carries the proopiomelanocortin (POMC) gene for β-endorphin secretion has been manipulated to control gene expression as a model "minipump" for pain relief (59). The Neuro2A line and a mouse tumor AtT-20 cell line have been similarly used to secrete β-endorphin and provide analgesia (60–63). When AtT-20 cells were modified to express human enkephalin, analgesia without development of tolerance to the secreted opioids was observed (62,63), suggesting that a combination of biologically manufactured opioids from cells may provide better pain relief and avoid the development of morphine tolerance, compared with pharmacological approaches.

B. Conditionally Immortalized Cell Lines

However, a serious limitation using these approaches is that the immortalized cells generated are oncogenically transformed and continue to divide, creating a risk of tumorigenesis if transplanted into an immune-privileged site, such as the CNS. Conditional immortalization is a means to generate an immortalized cell line that can later be disimmortalized to stop cell division. Several approaches for conditionally immortalizing cell lines have been described in the literature. One approach involving the temperature-sensitive mutant of the SV40 large T antigen (tsTag) (64–67) has been used successfully to conditionally immortalize embryonic CNS neurons (68–71). Using this approach, transfected cells undergo continual cell division under low temperature conditions (e.g., 32–34°C), but differentiate and become postmitotic when the temperature is raised (37–39°C). The host CNS environment to receive these tsTag-immortalized cell lines has a temperature of about 36–39°C, and transplantation allows the cells to cease proliferation and continue differentiation without tumor formation. Thus, conditional immortalization with the tsTag construct incorporates the advantages of cell lines, including the convenience of growing large quantities that can be characterized and safety tested and the ability to genetically engineer additional therapeutic molecules, while reducing the disadvantages of tumor cell lines.

At The Miami Project to Cure Paralysis, we have used conditional immortalization with tsTag to create rodent neuronal cell lines to study the effect of various neurotrophins and agents in vitro to determine how these immortalized neuronal precursors might respond to the transplant CNS environment (72–74). More recently, we have used these immortalized neuronal cell lines bioengineered with novel genes to deliver potentially antinociceptive molecules following grafting into the subarachnoid space (75–76). These cell lines have been transfected with a variety of genes to test the hypothesis that secretion of these agents into the CSF in models of chronic pain can prevent or reverse the hypersensitivity to thermal and tactile stimuli that develops after peripheral nerve or spinal cord injury. The transfected genes tested thus far include brain-derived neurotrophic factor (BDNF); the synthetic enzymes for the neurotransmitters serotonin and GABA; the preproenkephalin gene for met-enkephalin synthesis; and the preprogalanin gene for the peptide galanin synthesis. Examples of the up-regulation of these genes after the cells are differentiated for a week at a nonpermissive temperature (39°C) in vitro are shown in Fig. 9. These conditions stimulate the transplant conditions in the in vivo environment of the spinal subarachnoid space. Expression of GABA or BDNF by the cell grafts 7 weeks after transplantation near the lumber spinal cord is shown in Fig. 10. Cell lines were initially proliferated at

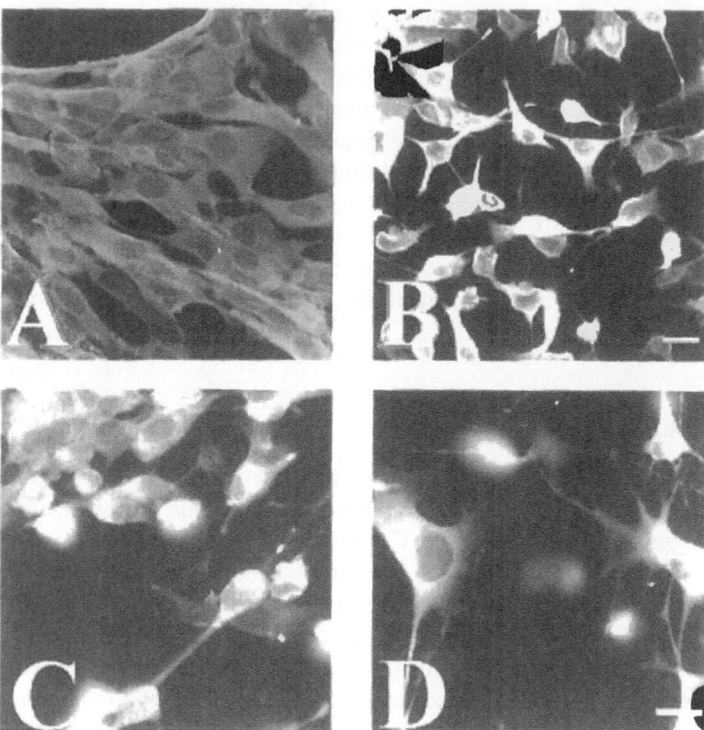

Figure 9 Cell lines in vitro: after proliferation at 33°C in vitro, the (A) 33GAD67.5 cells were stained with an antibody for GABA. After 7 days of differentiation (B) at 39°C in vitro, the 33GAD67.5 cells increase GABA synthesis. Magnification: bar = 150 μm. After proliferation at 33°C in vitro, (C) the 33BDNF.4 cells were stained with an antibody for BDNF. After 7 days of differentiation (D) at 39°C in vitro, the 33BDNF.4 cells increased stain brightly for BDNF-ir. Magnification: bar = 100 μm.

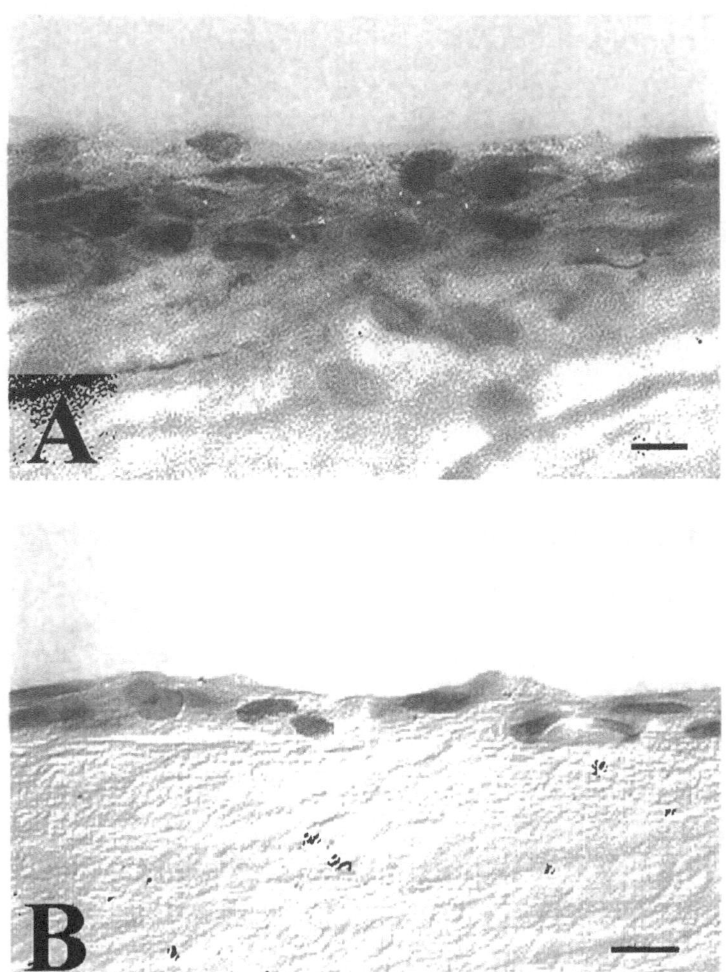

Figure 10 Cell lines in vivo: One week after CCI, the (A) 33GAD67.5 and (B) 33BDNF.4 cell lines were transplanted into the lumbar subarachnoid space. Seven weeks later the cords were sectioned and stained for (A) GABA or (B) BDNF. Each cell line continued to survive and express their relevant genes and synthesize detectable GABA and BDNF. Magnification (A): bar = 75 μm; (B): bar = 100 μm.

permissive temperature (33°C) to expand the cultures for transplantation. One million cells were transplanted at L4–L5 level into the subarachnoid space 1 week following chronic constriction nerve injury (CCI model) (77). As a negative control, cell lines transfected with the vector pCEP4, used to carry the novel gene sequences, were cloned. These vector-only cell lines do not express the novel genes in vitro or in vivo, but survive and differentiate similarly to the antinociceptive cell lines, including after spinal grafting. Both vector-only and bioengineered cell lines cease to proliferate after the temperature-sensitive allele of Tag becomes labile after a few days at 39°C. The presence of grafted cells secreting antinociceptive molecules reversed the behavioral hypersensitivity within 1 week of grafting, and these effects lasted at least throughout the 8-week time course of the study (Fig. 11). In contrast, the control vector-only cell grafts had no effect on the peripheral neuropathic pain.

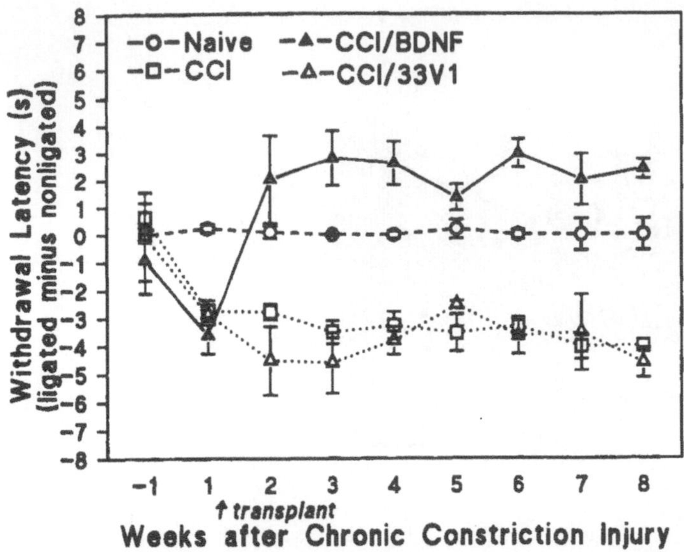

Figure 11 Thermal hyperalgesia after CCI and BDNF cell line transplant. Animals were either left unoperated (open circles), given the CCI (open squares), or transplanted with 33BDNF.4 (filled triangles) or 33V1 cells (open triangles), control cells without the gene for BDNF, 1 week following the CCI, 1 day following behavioral testing. Animals were tested for hindpaw withdrawal once every week for 1 week before and 8 weeks following CCI and before and after transplants. Only animals that demonstrated thermal hyperalgesia 1 week after CCI were transplanted.

C. Conditionally Immortalized Chromaffin Cell Lines

With creation of bioengineered cell lines that secrete specific antinociceptive molecules, the development of the gold standard for cell therapy for pain is the creation of conditionally immortalized chromaffin cell lines. Several attempts have been made to generate immortalized chromaffin cell lines. Birren and Anderson (78) have reported v-*mvc* immortalized sympathoadrenal progenitor cell lines from embryonic rat adrenal glands. Suri et al. (79) have generated adrenal cell lines from tyrosine hydroxylase–SV40 T antigen transgenic mice. However, similar to PC12 cells, in both of these cases, the immortalized cells generated produce dopamine and some norepinephrine, but not epinephrine, and lacked the synthetic enzyme PNMT.

In our laboratory, a recent attempt using the tsTag construct to confer temperature sensitivity has yielded both embryonic rat and neonatal calf chromaffin cell lines (80). Immortalized chromaffin cell lines were chosen by their expression of the catecholamine synthetic enzymes tyrosine hydroxylase (TH), dopamine-β-hydroxylase (DβH), and phenylethanolamine-*N*-methyltransferase (PNMT). Examples of the expression of those enzymes after differentiation for 7 days at nonpermissive temperature in culture are shown in Fig. 12. Expression of these enzymes during proliferation, when the cells are dividing under the control of the Tag protein, is very low. As the Tag protein shuts down during differentiation, enzyme expression increases. These same chromaffin cell lines have recently been grafted in animals with CCI, and appear to behave similar to primary chromaffin grafts, reversing neuropathic pain behaviors for at least 8 weeks following transplantation (81). It may be envisioned that similar conditionally immortalized chromaffin cell lines can be derived from human adrenal chromaffin cultures, providing a virtually unlimited supply for clinical use.

In summary, these studies suggest that cellular transplantation may represent a novel ap-

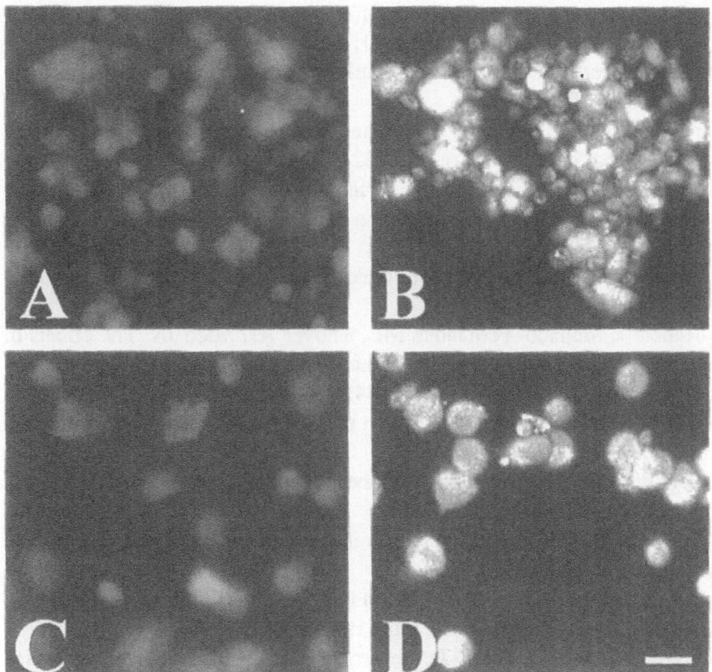

Figure 12 Conditionally immortalized chromaffin cells: (A, C) after proliferation at 33°C and (B, D) differentiation for 7 days at 39°C, the RAD5.2 rat (A, B) and bovine BADA.20 (C, D) chromaffin cells were stained with an antibody for TH. During proliferation, levels of TH-ir are barely detectable, whereas after 7 days of differentiation at 39°C, both the RAD5.2 and BADA.20 cells contained increased TH-ir. Magnification: bar = 70 μm.

proach in the management of chronic pain, particularly for those requiring long-term management or refractory to traditional pharmacological therapies. Although this field is in its infancy, promising preliminary data have already been described, both in the preclinical literature and exploratory clinical trials, and the ability to generate engineered cell lines should lead to improved feasibility and efficacy of this approach.

REFERENCES

1. Unsicker K. The trophic cocktail made by adrenal chromaffin cells. Exp Neurol 1993; 123:167–173.
2. Czech KA, Pollak R, Pappas GD, Sagen J. Bovine chromaffin cells for CNS transplants do not elicit xenogeneic T cell proliferative responses in vitro. Cell Transplant 1996; 5:257–267.
3. Schueler SB, Sagen J, Pappas GD, Kordower JH. Long-term viability of isolated bovine adrenal medullary chromaffin cells following intrastriatal transplantation. Cell Transplant 1995; 4:55–64.
4. Michalewicz P, Laurito CE, Pappas GD, Lu Y, Yeomans DC. Purification of adrenal chromaffin cells increases antinociceptive efficacy of xenotransplants without immunosuppression. Cell Transplant 1999; 8:103–109.
5. Ortega-Alvaro A, Gibert-Rahola J, Chover AJ, Tejedor-Real P, Casas J, Mico JA. Effect of amitriptyline on the analgesia induced by adrenal medullary tissue transplanted in the rat spinal subarachnoid space as measured by an experimental model of acute pain. Exp Neurol 1994; 130: 9–14.

6. Ruz–Franzi JI, Gonzalez–Darder JM. Study of the analgesic effects of the implant of adrenal medullary into the subarachnoid space in rats. Acta Neurochir 1991; 52:39–41.
7. Sagen J, Pappas GD, Perlow MJ. Adrenal medullary tissue transplants in rat spinal cord reduce pain sensitivity. Brain Res 1986; 384:189–194.
8. Sagen J, Pappas GD, Pollard HB. Analgesia induced by isolated bovine chromaffin cells implanted in the rat spinal cord. Proc Natl Acad Sci USA 1986; 83:7522–7526.
9. Sagen J, Wang H, Tresco PA, Aebischer P. Transplants of immunologically isolated xenogeneic chromaffin cells provide a long-term source of pain reducing neuroactive substances. J Neurosci 1993; 13:2415–2423.
10. Wang H, Sagen J. Optimization of adrenal medullary allograft conditions for pain alleviation. J Neural Transplant Plast 1994; 5:49–64.
11. Ortega–Alvaro A, Gibert–Rahola J, Mellado–Fernández ML, Chover AJ, Micó JA. The effects of different monoaminergic antidepressants on the analgesia induced by spinal cord adrenal medullary transplants in the formalin test in rats. Anesth Analg 1997; 84:816–820.
12. Sagen J, Wang H, Pappas GD. Adrenal medullary implants in rat spinal cord reduce nociception in a chronic pain model. Pain 1990; 42:69–79.
13. Siegan JB, Sagen J. Attenuation of formalin pain responses in the rat by adrenal medullary transplants in the spinal subarachnoid space. Pain 1997; 70:279–285.
14. Vaquero J, Arias A, Oya S, Zurita M. Chromaffin allografts into arachnoid of spinal cord reduce basal pain responses in rats. Neuro report 1991; 2:149–151.
15. Wang H, Sagen J. Attenuation of pain-related hyperventilation in adjuvant arthritic rats with adrenal medullary transplants in the spinal subarachnoid space. Pain 1995; 63:313–320.
16. Décosterd I, Buchser E, Gilliard N, Saydoff J, Zurn AD, Aebischer P. Intrathecal implants of bovine chromaffin cells alleviate mechanical allodynia in a rat model of neuropathic pain. Pain 1998; 76: 159–166.
17. Ginzburg R, Seltzer Z. Subarachnoid spinal cord transplantation of adrenal medulla suppresses chronic neuropathic pain behavior in rats. Brain Res 1990; 523:147–150.
18. Hama AT, Sagen J. Reduced pain-related behavior by adrenal medullary transplants in rats with experimental painful peripheral neuropathy. Pain 1993; 52:223–231.
19. Hama AT, Sagen J. Alleviation of neuropathic pain symptoms by xenogeneic chromaffin cell grafts in the spinal subarachnoid space. Brain Res 1994; 651:345–351.
20. Brewer KL, Yezierski RP. Effects of adrenal medullary transplants on pain-related behaviors following excitotoxic spinal cord injury. Brain Res 1998; 798:83–92.
21. Hains BC, Chastain KM, Everhart AW, Hulsebosch CE. Reduction of chronic central pain following spinal cord injury by transplants of adrenal medullary chromaffin cells. Soc Neurosci Abstr 1998; 24:1631.
22. Yu W, Hao J–X, Xu X–J, Saydoff J, Haegerstrand A, Wiesenfeld–Hallin Z. Long-term alleviation of allodynia-like behaviors by intrathecal implantation of bovine chromaffin cells in rats with spinal cord injury. Pain 1998; 74:115–122.
23. Yu W, Hao J–X, Xu X–J, Saydoff J, Haegerstrand A, Wiesenfeld–Hallin Z. Immunoisolating encapsulation of intrathecally implanted bovine chromaffin cells prolongs their survival and produces anti-allodynic effect in spinally injured rats. Eur J Pain 1998; 2:143–151.
24. Schueler SB, Ortega JD, Sagen J, Kordower JH. Robust survival of isolated bovine adrenal chromaffin cells following intrastriatal transplantation: a novel hypothesis of adrenal graft viability. J Neurosci 1993; 13:4496–4510.
25. Yezierski RP, Liu S, Ruenes GL, Kajander KJ, Brewer KL. Behavioral and pathological characteristic of a central pain model following spinal cord injury. Pain 1998; 75:141–155.
26. Siegan JB, Sagen J. Attenuation of NMDA-induced spinal hypersensitivity by adrenal medullary transplants. Brain Res 1995; 680:88–98.
27. Haley JE, Sullivan AF, Dickenson AH. Evidence for spinal *N*-methyl-D-aspartate receptor involvement in prolonged chemical nociception in the rat. Brain Res 1990; 518:218–226.
28. Hunter JC, Singh L. Role of excitatory amino acid receptors in the mediation of the nociceptive response to formalin in the rat. Neurosci Lett 1994; 174:217–221.

29. Malmberg AB, Yaksh TL. Spinal nitric oxide synthesis inhibition blocks NMDA-induced thermal hyperalgesia and produces antinociception in the formalin test in rats. Pain 1993; 54:291–300.
30. Vaccarino AL, Marek P, Kest B, Weber E, Keana JFW, Liebeskind JC. NMDA receptor antagonists, MK-801 and ACEA-1011, prevent the development of tonic pain following subcutaneous formalin. Brain Res 1993; 615:331–334.
31. Yamamoto T, Yaksh TL. Comparison of the antinociceptive effects of pre- and posttreatment with intrathecal morphine and MK801, an NMDA antagonist, on the formalin test in the rat. Anesthesiology 1992; 77:757–763.
32. Malmberg AB, Yaksh TL. Pharmacology of the spinal action of ketorolac, morphine, ST-91, U50488H, and L-PIA on the formalin test and an isobolographic analysis of the NSAID interaction. Anesthesiology 1993; 79:270–281.
33. Lemaire S, Shukla VJ, Rogers C, Ibrahim IH, Lapierre C, Parent P, Dumont M. Isolation and characterization of histogranin, a natural peptide with NMDA receptor antagonist activity. Eur J Pharmacol 1993; 245:247–256.
34. Siegan JB, Sagen J. A natural peptide with NMDA inhibitory activity reduces tonic pain in the formalin model. Neuroreport 1997; 8:1379–1381.
35. Siegan JB, Hama AT, Sagen J. Suppression of neuropathic pain by a naturally-derived peptide with NMDA antagonist activity. Brain Res 1997; 755:331–334.
36. Hama AT, Siegan JB, Herzberg U, Sagen J. NMDA-induced spinal hypersensitivity is reduced by naturally-derived peptide analog [Ser1]histogranin. Pharmacol Biochem Behav 1998; 62:67–74.
37. Hama A, Sagen J. Induction of a spinal NADPH-diaphorase by nerve injury is attenuated by adrenal medullary transplants. Brain Res 1994; 640:345–351.
38. Siegan JB, Hama AT, Sagen J. Alterations in spinal cord cGMP by peripheral nerve injury and adrenal medullary transplantation. Neurosci Lett 1996; 215:49–52.
39. Sagen J, Wang H. Adrenal medullary grafts suppress c-*fos* induction in spinal neurons of arthritic rats. Neurosci Lett 1995; 192:1–4.
40. Siegan JB, Frydel BR, Sagen J. Attenuation of spinal c-*fos* activation in the formalin model by adrenal medullary implants. Am Pain Soc Abstr 1996; 15:A–46.
41. Lachmund A, Gehrke D, Krieglstein K, Unsicker K. Trophic factors from chromaffin granules promote survival of peripheral and central nervous system neurons. Neuroscience 1994; 62:361–370.
42. Hama AT, Pappas GD, Sagen J. Adrenal medullary implants reduce transsynaptic degeneration in the spinal cord of rats following chronic constriction nerve injury. Exp Neurol 1996; 137:81–93.
43. Ibuki T, Hama AT, Wang X–T, Pappas GD, Sagen J. Loss of GABA immunoreactivity in the spinal dorsal horn of rats with peripheral nerve injury and promotion of recovery by adrenal medullary grafts. Neuroscience 1997; 76:845–858.
44. Ralston DD, Coyle DE, Tedesco CS, Milroy AM, Ralston HJ. Long term changes in GABA immunoreactivity (GABA-ir) in a rat model of peripheral mononeuropathy. Soc Neurosci Abstr 1997; 23: 1533.
45. Sugimoto T, Bennett GJ, Kajander KC. Transsynaptic degeneration in the superficial dorsal horn after sciatic nerve injury: effects of chronic constriction injury, transection, and strychnine. Pain 1990; 42:205–213.
46. Winnie AP, Pappas GD, Das Gupta TK, Wang H, Ortega JD, Sagen J. Alleviation of cancer pain by adrenal medullary transplants in the spinal subarachnoid space: a preliminary report. Anesthesiology 1993; 79:644–653.
47. Lazorthes Y, Bès JC, Sagen J, Tafani M, Tkaczuk J, Sallerin B, Nahri I, Verdié JC, Ohayon E, Caratero C, Pappas GD. Transplantation of human chromaffin cells for control of intractable cancer pain. Acta Neurochir 1995; 64:97–100.
48. Vaquero J, Martinez R, Oya S, Coca S, Salazer FG, Colado MI. Transplantation of adrenal medulla into spinal cord for pain relief: disappointing outcome. Lancet 1988; 2:1315.
49. Aebischer P, Buchser E, Joseph JM, Favre J, de Tribolet N, Lysaght M, Rudnick S, Goddard M. Transplantation in humans of encapsulated xenogeneic cells without immunosuppression. Transplantation 1994; 58:1275–1277.

50. Buchser E, Goddard M, Heyd B, Joseph JM, Favre J, Detribolet N, Lysaght M, Aebischer P. Immunoisolated xenogeneic chromaffin cell therapy for chronic pain: initial experience. Anesthesiology 1996; 85:1005–1012.
51. Burgess FW, Goddard M, Savarese D, Wilkinson H. Subarachnoid bovine adrenal chromaffin cell implants for cancer pain management. Am Pain Soc Abstr 1996; 15:A–33.
52. Deleted in proof.
53. Hefti F, Hartikka J, Schlumpf M. Implantation of PC12 cells into the corpus striatum of rats with lesions of the dopaminergic nigrostriatal neurons. Brain Res 1985; 348:283–288.
54. Jaeger CB. Morphological and immunocytochemical characteristics of PC12 cell grafts in rat brain. Ann NY Acad Sci 1987; 495:334–350.
55. Kordower JH, Liu Y, Winn S, Emerich D. Encapsulated PC12 cell transplants into hemiparkinsonian monkeys: a behavioral, neuroanatomical, and neurochemical analysis. Cell Transplant 1995; 4:155–171.
56. Pappas GD, Sagen J. Fine structure of PC 12 cell implants in the rat spinal cord. Neurosci Lett 1986; 70:59–64.
57. Rohrer D, Nilaver G, Nipper V, Machida C. Genetically modified PC12 brain grafts: survivability and inducible nerve growth factor expression. Cell Transplant 1996; 5:57–68.
58. Greene LA, Tischler AS. Establishment of a noradrenergic clonal cell line of rat adrenal pheochromocytoma cells which respond to NGF. Proc Natl Acad Sci USA 1976; 73:2424–2428.
59. Saitoh Y, Eguchi Y, Hagihara Y, Arita N, Watahiki M, Tsujimoto Y, Hayakawa T. Dose-dependent doxycycline-mediated adrenocorticotropic hormone secretion from encapsulated Tet-on proopiomelanocortin Neuro2A cells in the subarachnoid space. Hum Gene Ther 1998; 9:997–1002.
60. Saitoh Y, Taki T, Arita N, Ohnishi T, Hayakawa T. Analgesia induced by transplantation of encapsulated tumor cells secreting β-endorphin. J Neurosurg 1995; 82:630–634.
61. Saitoh Y, Taki T, Arita N, Ohnishi T, Hayakawa T. Cell therapy with encapsulated xenogeneic tumor cells secreting β-endorphin for treatment of peripheral pain. Cell Transplant 1995; 4 (suppl 1):S13–S17.
62. Wu HH, McLoon SC, Wilcox GL. Antinociception following implantation of AtT-20 and genetically modified AtT-20/hENK cells in rat spinal cord. J Neural Transplant Plast 1993; 4:15–26.
63. Wu HH, Wilcox GL, McLoon SC. Implantation of AtT-20 or genetically modified AtT-20–hENK cells in mouse spinal cord induced antinociception and opioid tolerance. J Neurosci 1994; 14:4806–4814.
64. Bredesen DE, Hisanaga MD, Sharp FA. Neural transplantation using temperature sensitive immortalized neural cells: a preliminary report. Ann Neurol 1990; 27:205–207.
65. Giordano M, Takashima H, Herranz A, Poltorak M, Geller HM, Marone M, Freed WJ. Immortalized GAB Aergic cell lines derived from rat striatum using a temperature-sensitive allele of the SV40 large T antigen. Exp Neurol 1993; 124:395–400.
66. Giotta GJ, Heitzmann J, Cohn M. Properties of two temperature-sensitive Rous sarcoma virus transformed cerebellar cell lines. Brain Res 1980; 202:445–458.
67. Jat PS, Sharp PA. Cell lines established by a temperature-sensitive simian virus 40 large T antigen gene are growth restricted at nonpermissive temperature. Mol Cell Biol 1989; 9:1672–1681.
68. Frederiksen K, Jat PS, Valtz N, Levy D, McKay R. Immortalization of precursor cells from the mammalian CNS. Neuron 1988; 1:439–448.
69. Frederiksen K, McKay RDG. Proliferation and differentiation of rat neuroepithelial precursor cells in vivo. J Neurosci 1988; 8:1144–1151.
70. Selmaj K, Raine CS, Farooq M, Norton WT, Brosnan CF. Cytokine cytotoxicity against oligodendrocytes: apoptosis induced by lymphotoxin. J Immunol 1991; 147:1522–1529.
71. Whittemore SR, White LA. Target regulation of neuronal differentiation in a temperature-sensitive cell line derived from medullary raphe. Brain Res 1993; 615:27–40.
72. Eaton MJ, Staley JK, Globus MYT, Whittemore SR. Developmental regulation of early serotonergic neuronal differentiation: the role of brain-derived neurotrophic factor and membrane depolarization. Dev Biol 1995; 170:169–182.

73. Eaton MJ, Whittemore SR. ACTH activation of adenylate cyclase in raphe neurons: multiple regulatory pathways control serotonergic neuronal differentiation. J Neurobiol 1995; 28:465–481.
74. Eaton MJ, Whittemore SR. Autocrine BDNF secretion enhances the survival and serotonergic differentiation of raphe neuronal precursor cells grafted into the adult rat CNS. Exp Neurol 1996; 140: 105–114.
75. Eaton MJ, Dancausse HR, Santiago DI, Whittemore SR. Lumbar transplants of immortalized serotonergic neurons alleviates chronic neuropathic pain. Pain 1997; 72:59–69.
76. Eaton MJ, Plunkett JA, Martinez MA, Lopez T, Karmally S, Cejas P, Whittemore SR. Transplants of neuronal cells bio-engineered to synthesize GABA alleviate chronic neuropathic pain. Cell Transplant 1999; 8:87–101.
77. Bennett GJ, Xie Y–K. A peripheral mononeuropathy in rat that produces disorders of pain sensation like those seen in man. Pain 1988; 33:87–107.
78. Birren SJ, Anderson DJ. A v-*myc*-immortalized sympathoadrenal progenitor cell line in which neuronal differentiation is initiated by FGF not by NGF. Neuron 1990; 4:189–201.
79. Suri C, Fung BP, Tischler AS, Chikaraishi DM. Catecholaminergic cell lines from the brain and adrenal glands of tyrosine hydroxylase–SV40 T antigen transgenic mice. J Neurosci 1993; 13:1280–1291.
80. Frydel B, Eaton MJ, Lopez RF, Nie XT, Sagen J. Generation and characterization of conditionally immortalized chromaffin cell lines. Am Soc Neural Transplant 1999; 6:55.
81. Eaton MJ, Lopez TF, Frydel BR, Martinez MA, Sagen J. Transplants of immortalized chromaffin cells for neuropathic pain. Am Soc Neural Transplant 1999; 6:55.

68

Bone-Seeking Radiopharmaceuticals to Palliate Painful Bone Metastases

Alexander J. B. McEwan
University of Alberta and Cross Cancer Institute, Edmonton, Alberta, Canada

I. INTRODUCTION

Bone-seeking radionuclides have been used to treat painful bone metastases for almost 50 years. Radioisotopes were first used in cancer therapy shortly after the discovery of artificial radioactivity in 1933 (1), and the first report of a potential role in pain palliation was in 1942 in a single patient with prostate cancer who was treated with strontium-89 (^{89}Sr) (2). By 1950, radioisotopes of phosphorus (P) and strontium (Sr) had been reported as bone-seeking radiopharmaceuticals with the potential to contribute to the management of patients with hematological malignancies and solid cancers metastatic to bone (2,3).

Since that initial experience many novel radiolabeled pharmaceuticals have been described as bone-seeking agents, with the potential to deliver targeted doses of radiation to bone metastases (4,5). Few of these have been developed beyond preclinical and pilot clinical studies, and there now remain five in routine clinical use or in clinical development.

Phosphorus-32 (^{32}P) was used extensively in the 1960s and 1970s to palliate pain particularly in patients with cancers of the prostate and breast metastatic to bone. Routine use almost completely stopped because of complexities of administration and perceptions of significant myelosuppression. Despite recent studies supporting a renewal of routine use (6,7) the perceived toxicity remains a significant limitation to reintroduction (8). Of the four other radiopharmaceuticals currently available, ^{89}Sr and samarium-153 ethylenediaminetetramethylene phosphonate ([^{153}Sm]-EDTMP) are licensed for routine use in the United States, and rhenium-186 hydroxyethylidene diphosphonate ([^{186}Re]-HEDP) and tin-117m diethylene triaminepentacetic acid ([^{117m}Sn]-DTPA) are in developmental trials.

Recent data have supported the efficacy and cost effectiveness of this option for treatment, and algorithms have been developed for its routine use in patient care. This chapter will review the principles on which this treatment modality is founded and review the clinical data that support its current role in pain palliation.

II. PRINCIPLES OF RADIONUCLIDE THERAPY

The practice of nuclear medicine requires the targeted delivery of radionuclides to sites of interest to define the presence of disease and to image and quantify pathophysiological processes.

The radionuclide is chemically linked to a pharmaceutical that, when injected intravenously, will be retained or metabolized by a cell, based on a defined biochemical or physiological function or, for example, on a cell membrane receptor. The delivery of a γ-emitting radionuclide allows the derivation of functional images by external detection of the emitted γ-ray. Examples include bone scanning (9), myocardial perfusion scanning (10), and the detection of neuroendocrine tumors with [^{111}In]-octreotide by binding to somatostatin receptors 2, 3, and 5 (11).

In radioisotope therapy, the targeted radionuclide decays with the emission of a β-particle. The short range of the β-particle in tissue delivers a significant radiation dose at the site of interaction and usually within 3–15 mm of the binding site (12). Examples of this form of treatment include radioiodine therapy of thyroid cancer (13), [^{131}I]mIBG therapy of neuroendocrine tumors (14), and palliation of painful bone metastases with bone-seeking radiopharmaceuticals (15).

The basic principles of radioisotope treatment include systemic administration, targeted delivery, radiation delivered at a very low dose rate, and the possibility of repeat administrations. Table 1 summarizes the clinical characteristics of radiopharmaceuticals for palliative treatment of painful bone metastases.

Bone-seeking radiopharmaceuticals have been developed that target bone as a function of osteoblastic activity. At sites of metastatic involvement osteoblastic activity is high, which increases the amount of radionuclide binding to the bone matrix. By specifically targeting these pathophysiological processes with the systemic administration of a bone-seeking radiopharmaceutical, a high therapeutic ratio can be achieved in delivering radiation to metastatic sites. Strontium-89 has a natural affinity for bone and is incorporated into the inorganic bone matrix; ^{32}P, [^{153}Sm]-EDTMP, and [^{186}Re]-HEDP form stable complexes with prolonged retention in the inorganic matrix, and [^{117m}Sn]-DTPA is probably precipitated onto the bone surface at the bone–tumor interface. Phosphorus-32 is also incorporated into the cellular elements of the bone marrow.

Following systemic injection, all bone metastases will be targeted; it follows from the importance of osteoblastic activity for incorporation of the bone-seeking radiopharmaceutical into the bone metastasis that purely lytic neoplasms, such as multiple myeloma, will not respond well to systemic radiopharmaceutical therapy. Theoretical considerations include the possibility that microscopic deposits may also be targeted on the basis of a developing osteoblastic reaction.

The radiation dose that is delivered at the site of localization of the radiopharmaceutical is a function of the amount of radionuclide deposited, the physical half-life of the radionuclide, the biological half-life of the radiopharmaceutical, and the energy of the emitted β-particle. Table 2 provides an overview of the radiopharmaceuticals currently in use (16).

Table 1 Clinical Criteria for Use of Palliative Bone Seeking Radiopharmaceuticals

Preferential uptake at sites of metastases
Low uptake in normal bone
Irradiation of peritumor environment
Reversible myelosuppression
Ability to treat on multiple occasions
No additive toxicity with external-beam irradiation
Ability to administer to patients with extensive prior radiation therapy
Ability to treat recurrent pain in a previously irradiated site
Efficacy comparable with external-beam RT
Toxicity less than hemibody radiotherapy

Table 2 Radiopharmaceuticals for Palliative Therapy

Radionuclide	Pharmaceutical	Half-life (days)	Maximum β-energy (MeV)	Mean β-energy (MeV)	Maximum range in tissue (mm)	γ-Photon keV (%)
^{89}Sr	Chloride	50.5	1.46	0.583	6.7	—
^{32}P	Orthophosphate	14.3	1.71	0.695	8	—
[^{186}Re]-HEDP	HEDP	3.8	1.07	0.349	4.7	137 (9)
[^{153}Sm]-EDTMP	EDTMP	1.95	0.8	0.224	3.4	103 (28)
[^{117m}Sn]-DTPA	DTPA	13.6	(Conversion electrons)	0.129 0.153	0.3	159 (86)

Source: Ref. 16.

The relatively short track length of the particulate radiation emitted by these compounds means that all energy is deposited at or close to the site of binding, with relative sparing of adjacent structures such as bone marrow. This has the theoretical advantage of limiting toxicity by reducing dose delivery to the cellular elements of the bone marrow. The shorter range of the radiation emitted by [^{117m}Sn]-DTPA appears to lead to significant reductions in toxicity. Because these radiopharmaceuticals are incorporated in the inorganic matrix, the complex anatomical relation between tumor and new bone formation means that the irradiation is delivered to the tumor, and also to the peritumor environment, from radionuclide deposited at the bone–tumor interface (17,18), not within tumor cells.

The radiation dose delivered to tumor by systemic radiopharmaceuticals may be cumulatively comparable with that delivered by conventional external-beam radiotherapy techniques. Depending on half-life, the dose may be accumulated over several weeks, although the greatest portion of the dose is deposited within the first one to two effective half-lives. However, the rate at which this dose is delivered is significantly lower—of the order of hundreds of rads a day, rather than a hundred or so rads a minute (19,20). The clinical radiobiology of low-dose–rate therapy has been reviewed (21). The relevant radiobiological factors are defined as the inherent radiosensitivity of the tumor, tumor repair and repopulation rates, cell cycle effects, apoptosis and local pathophysiological conditions within the tumor, and peritumor environment, such as hypoxia and pH.

The palliative effect of bone-seeking radiopharmaceuticals is presumably a function of the absorbed dose deposited in tumor, in bone, and in the peritumor environment by the β-particle emissions. It is interesting that at most administered doses, and for most calculated absorbed doses, there is no clear evidence of a dose–response relations between palliative effect and calculated absorbed dose. This is in contradistinction to response rates to external beam radiation therapy where dose–response relationships have been established for pain palliation and for cytotoxicity (22,23). To what extent the rate at which radiation is delivered by bone-seeking radiopharmaceuticals is a limiting factor in the radiobiological effectiveness of systemic radionuclide therapy remains open to debate; however, published palliative response rates are comparable with those reported for external-beam radiotherapy (22), although no data are available comparing cytotoxicity.

However, the importance of dose rate in palliative treatment at the ranges of very low dose rate (VLDR) therapy has not been tested clinically or in animal models. Calculations of dose administered with any of the five radiopharmaceuticals are less than would be predicted to be effective using the high-dose-rate model of external beam radiotherapy. This may reflect a limited understanding of VLDR radiobiology, also the imprecision of absorbed dose calculations and uncertainty about optimum dosage schedules (24). It may also reflect the target on which the VLDR radiation exerts its effect.

It has been postulated that the primary palliative effect may be related to the dose administered to the peritumor environment, with subsequent reduction in cytokine production and modulation of humoral pain mediators (25–27).

There are some data to support this hypothesis from the literature on the use of low-dose–rate radiotherapy to induce pain relief in patients with arthritides, heterotopic calcification, and the prevention of restenosis after angioplasty (27). Postulated mechanisms of action at these low administered doses include a reduction of nitric oxide production by lowering nitric oxide synthase concentration (28), a reduction in cytokine concentrations (25), induction of early-response genes (29), and activation of intracellular adhesion molecule (ICAM)-1 on endothelial cell surfaces (30). The reduced inflammatory response caused by this cascade of events may be postulated as one of the mechanisms leading to reduction in pain in the days immediately after administration.

In addition, mechanical symptom relief, reduction in hypoxia and periosteal compression, and direct tumor cell cytotoxicity, all are important factors in response to external-beam radiation and may also be important considerations in VLDR therapy (23). These latter mechanisms of relief, however, do not occur immediately after irradiation. It is likely that pain relief is a multifactorial process, perhaps starting with a cytokine or humoral response before proceeding to mechanical and anatomical factors as cumulative dose increases.

To calculate the dose that is delivered to a metastatic deposit, the γ-ray that is emitted by three of the radiopharmaceuticals can be imaged using standard nuclear medicine equipment, and the cumulative activity and retention time can be measured to quantify retained radioactivity and dose delivered using standard MIRD formalism (19,24). Strontium-85 has been used as a tracer to calculate absorbed dose from ^{89}Sr administration (20).

Therefore, the key principles of bone-seeking radiopharmaceutical treatment of bone metastases are systemic distribution, radiation delivered at a low-dose rate, irradiation of tumor by radionuclide distributed at the tumor–bone interface, and limited toxicity. These characteristics have defined the radiopharmaceuticals that are currently in clinical practice and have created the guidelines by which they are used.

III. CLINICAL OVERVIEW

Data have now been accumulated from multicenter trials on the efficacy of these radiopharmaceuticals, and guidelines for practice are being established and accepted by the nuclear medicine and oncology communities. This section will review the currently accepted parameters that guide their use; the data supporting these guidelines will be reviewed in Section IV.

A. Summary of Efficacy

Table 3 summarizes response rates that have been described in the literature for the five radiopharmaceuticals. Overall response rates in terms of efficacy are comparable, and they range from 60–80%. Conventionally, it is said that approximately 20% of patients become pain-free and the remainder have more or less significant pain relief with reduction in analgesic requirements. It is interesting to compare response rates with radiopharmaceutical therapy with those reported for external-beam treatment. Price et al. (31) report a complete response rate of 27% and overall response rate of 85% for patients treated with single fractions and ten fractions; Tong et al. (32) report 53 and 89%, respectively, for 613 patients treated with five to ten fractions. Janjan (22) reports overall response rates in patients with multiple metastases of 40–70% at 2–4 weeks after RT, and in 70–80% at 4–12 weeks. Single and multiple fractions of external beam radiation therapy may be equally as effective in controlling pain, although variations in time to efficacy and in complete response rates may be seen (33). Although pain relief often occurs within 48 h of administration of radiation therapy, the maximum benefit is often not seen until 4 or even 6 weeks after treatment.

Overall response rates of 50–100% and complete response rates of 5–50% are reported in trials of hemibody radiotherapy (34). This population of patients tends to have a greater metastatic burden that is presumably similar in disease extent to that referred for radiopharmaceutical treatment. Care in treatment planning can reduce toxicity, but pneumonitis, thrombocytopenia, and gastrointestinal (GI) symptoms may be severe and are seen in 2–32% of patients in different series (23). The response rates of hemibody radiotherapy are comparable with those seen in appropriately selected patient populations after palliative radiopharmaceutical therapy. The key difference in the two modalities is time to response, which tends to be more rapid with

Table 3 Summary of Responses

	Response rate (%)	Response duration (median)	Response duration/(range)	Time to response (days)	Thrombocytopenia	Flare (%)
[^{186}Re]-HEDP	60–75	1–2	1–4	5–10	Mild–moderate	10
[^{153}Sm]-EDTMP	70–75	2–3	2–6	5–10	Mild–moderate	10
^{32}P	70	2–3	2–6	10–20	Moderate–severe	10–20
^{89}Sr	60–80	3–4	2–12	10–20	Moderate	5–10
[^{117m}Sn]-DTPA	70	2–4	2–6	5–15	None–Mild	<5

Source: Ref. 15

external-beam RT, although as Janjan (22) notes, there is a temporal association with quality of response. The toxicities that are seen with hemibody radiotherapy are not seen following treatment with bone-seeking radiopharmaceuticals.

A flare response, associated with a short-lived increase in pain 24–48 h after administration may be more common than originally believed and may be seen in up to 10% of patients. It may be more common in patients with breast cancer, and it may predict a good response (35).

There is a delay to response with radiopharmaceutical therapy, which is about 10 days following injection. This may be as short as 5 days with those radiopharmaceuticals with shorter half-lives such as [^{186}Re]-HEDP, and up to 15 days following ^{89}Sr administration, which has the longest physical and biological half-life. An increase in the quality of response may be seen for up to 4 weeks after injection.

The duration of response also appears to be directly related to half-life, with median durations of response ranging from 6 weeks to 4 months. Occasionally patients receiving ^{89}Sr may remain pain-free for up to 12 months.

The reported efficacy data and the results of the studies reported by Porter et al. (36) and Quilty et al. (37) provide a rationale for the routine clinical use of these agents. Comparative trial data need to be developed to evaluate efficacy in comparison with that seen in bisphosphonate therapy and to evaluate enhancements of response that may be obtained by the use of cisplatin as a radiosensitizer or possibly in combination with bisphosphonates.

Toxicity is limited to reversible myelosuppression, most often thrombocytopenia. The nadir is seen between 4 and 6 weeks after injection, and recovery is usually complete by 6–10 weeks. The severity of the myelosuppression is related to metastatic burden, and it may be more severe in the longer-lived radiopharmaceuticals and those with more energetic β-particles.

B. Indications

Patient selection is key to the successful and effective use of bone-seeking radiopharmaceuticals in pain palliation. Currently available data support their use in any patient with a positive bone scan with progressive pain, pain requiring increasing levels of analgesics, and recurrent pain in a previously irradiated site (Table 4). Patients with multiple transient sites of pain may achieve the best palliative response. Hospitals that perform large numbers of radiopharmaceutical therapies are tending to move to the model of joint management clinics to ensure appropriate referral and selection.

The data from the adjuvant trial reported by Porter et al. (36) suggest that progression of painful metastases might be significantly reduced in patients with multiple metastases who only

Table 4 Indications for Treatment of Bone Metastases with Bone-Seeking Radiopharmaceuticals

Patient has cancer metastatic to bone
Positive [^{99m}Tc]-MDP bone scan (irrespective of x-ray appearance)
Karnofsky performance score ≥60
Pain requiring narcotic analgesic support
Multiple sites
Diffuse pain
Recurrent pain in a radiotherapy field
Multiple transient pains
Pain requiring radiotherapy to single site with multiple metastases

Source: Ref. 15.

require radiotherapy to a single, painful site. There are, as yet, no convincing data to support the use of radiopharmaceutical therapy in patients with multiple painless metastases, or in those with no bone scan evidence of metastases, but evidence of treatment failure based on a rising PSA. Clinical trials are underway to test this role for both licensed radiopharmaceuticals. Trials are also under consideration to compare the efficacy of bone-seeking radiopharmaceuticals with that of bisphosphonates and to explore the enhancement of efficacy by adjuvant treatment with radiosensitizing chemotherapeutics such as low-dose cisplatin or carboplatin. It is postulated that this enhancement may increase or improve not only palliative efficacy, but that it might lead to increased cytotoxicity and reduction in metastatic burden.

The literature suggests that patients with a low burden of soft-tissue disease do better, and that patients with a superscan may not respond as well. However, the best discriminator may be the Karnofsky Performance Score (38), and this should be one of the key initial screening criteria in patient evaluation.

All the radiopharmaceuticals discussed in this review may be safely used to re-treat patients on multiple occasions—the greatest number of re-treatments reported is nine (35). Requirements for acceptance of patients for subsequent therapies are the same as those for the initial treatment. Most authors, however, indicate that a nonresponder to the first administration is likely to be a nonresponder for subsequent administrations. The minimal time between retreatments is 10–12 weeks for ^{89}Sr and ^{32}P, and 6–10 weeks for the other three radiopharmaceuticals.

Myelosuppression secondary to radiopharmaceutical therapy occurs more slowly than after chemotherapy, and the nadir for ^{89}Sr may not be seen for 4–6 weeks. Recovery is usually complete by 10 weeks. This time scale is shortened for radiopharmaceuticals with shorter half-lives.

C. Contraindications

Even though the radiopharmaceuticals are safe and effective therapies, the practitioner needs to be aware of exclusion criteria before accepting a patient for treatment (Table 5).

Although an absolute platelet count of $60{,}000 \times 10^6$ is the most widely quoted lower level in the literature for administration, the key to the safe use of these radiopharmaceuticals is the relative stability of the counts over the preceding weeks; a stable lower count is more acceptable than a higher count that has fallen rapidly, particularly if there have been no recent therapeutic interventions.

Table 5 Contraindications for Treatment of Bone Metastases with Bone-Seeking Radiopharmaceuticals

Karnofsky performance <50
Extensive soft-tissue metastases
Platelet count $<60{,}000 \times 10^6$
Recent rapid fall in platelet count even if $>60{,}000 \times 10^6$
White cell count $<2.5 \times 10^6$
Disseminated intravascular coagulopathy
Within 1 month of myelosuppressive chemotherapy
Less than 2 months projected survival
Within 2 months of hemibody radiotherapy

Source: Ref. 15.

Two case reports in the literature (39,40) document profound thrombocytopenia in patients with clinical and subclinical disseminated intravascular coagulation (DIC) following administration of ^{89}Sr. DIC is a well-recognized concern of advanced prostate cancer, occurring in up to 16% of patients, and it may often be the terminal event (41,42). In patients with stable counts in the normal range, DIC is probably not a concern. However, in those patients with platelet counts at the lower end of the normal range, or in whom there has been a recent sudden fall in counts, the rate of change of counts is probably more important than the absolute value, and in these patients, it is prudent to screen for DIC before commencing therapy. Our routine practice now is to actively exclude subclinical DIC in patients with advanced and progressive prostate cancer, as judged by bone scan, sequential prostate-specific antigen (PSA) measurements, and sequential blood counts.

The data reported by Schmeler (38) are persuasive on the importance of Karnofsky Performance Scores (KPS) in patient selection. It is now our routine practice not to consider patients for treatment if the KPS is less than 50 and to accept patients on a case-by-case basis at values of 50 and 60.

Impending or actual pathological fractures or cord compression are contraindications to the immediate use of radiopharmaceutical therapy. Those patients require referral for surgical or radiation oncology opinion. Once the acute emergency has been appropriately managed, radiopharmaceuticals may, if otherwise indicated, be safely administered. There is no indication in the literature that radiopharmaceutical therapy leads to a greater incidence of these complications if the patient is appropriately selected, no matter what level of metastatic burden is present.

Unsealed source therapy should not be given before myelosuppressive chemotherapy, as there is anecdotal evidence that myelotoxicity is additive under these conditions. Once recovery from chemotherapy-induced myelosuppression has occurred, treatment may be cautiously administered, possibly at a reduced dose.

Radiopharmaceutical therapy may safely and effectively be given to patients who have previously received hemibody radiotherapy (43). It is our practice to wait for 2 months after completion of the radiation therapy, to avoid enhanced toxicity. Treatment with bone-seeking radiopharmaceuticals is not contraindicated in patients currently receiving local-field radiation therapy; the data of Porter et al. (36) suggest that it may be synergistic.

D. Radiation Safety

The therapeutic administration of radiopharmaceuticals does administer radioactivity to patients; therefore, some precautions have to be put in place to ensure safe practice. Because β-particles are internally absorbed, most patients administered pure β-emitting radionuclides do not become a radiation hazard. Those who emit γ-rays may pose a hazard, and in some national jurisdictions, an overnight stay in an isolation ward may be required. However, with careful patient monitoring risks can be reduced to almost zero.

Most of the administered radioactivity is excreted in urine, and for all the compounds, but especially those with long half-lives, precautions should be taken with urine spills. It is our practice to provide all patients with information sheets on appropriate hygiene practices including double flushing the toilet and, for men, sitting to urinate.

There have also been concerns over exposure to mortuary and crematorium staff should the patient die shortly after treatment. The manufacturers have assessed this and shown no significant risk. To ensure safe practice most centers now follow the practice of Amdur et al. (44) and place a bracelet on the wrist of each patient receiving radiopharmaceutical therapy with a label that states "A Nuclear Medicine Therapy (e.g. Strontium-89) Given: ___/___/___, Questions? Call _____. Keep on for 1 week."

This provides an independent reminder to the patient and the persons with whom he or she comes in contact that a potential hazard may be present.

IV. RADIOPHARMACEUTICALS IN CURRENT PRACTICE

The current indications for the use of bone-seeking radiopharmaceuticals in the management of pain syndromes have been developed from a series of key clinical studies summarized in Table 6. These will be reviewed in the following sections.

A. Strontium-89

Strontium-89 has been used clinically for almost 25 years. However, it is only in the last 10–12 years that multicenter trials have confirmed its role in clinical practice.

It is a pure β-emitting radioisotope of strontium with a maximum β-particle energy of 1.46 MeV; ^{85}Sr has been used as a tracer for ^{89}Sr metabolism in dosimetry studies (20,59).

Biological handling of strontium mimics that of calcium in vivo; strontium is incorporated into the inorganic matrix, with uptake being a function of the degree of osteoblastic activity. Therefore, uptake and retention of ^{89}Sr at sites of metastatic tumor is increased relative to normal bone. ^{85}Sr images are identical with those obtained with ^{99m}Tc MDP. Whole-body retention of ^{89}Sr is proportional to metastatic burden. Excretion is almost entirely by the renal route, the rate of excretion being a complex relation between metastatic burden and renal plasma clearance of

Table 6 Key Studies in the Development of Clinical Protocols for Pain Palliation with Bone-Seeking Radiopharmaceuticals

Author (Ref.)	Radiopharmaceutical	Primary	Trial design
Lewington (46)	^{89}Sr	Prostate	Placebo/crossover
Maxon (47)	[^{186}Re]-HEDP	Mixed	Placebo/crossover
Blake (20)	^{89}Sr	Prostate	Dosimetry
Samaratunga (18)	[^{186}Re]-HEDP	Mixed	Dosimetry
Robinson (35)	^{89}Sr	Mixed	Effectiveness open-label
Porter (36)	^{89}Sr	Prostate	Placebo/adjuvant
Quilty (37)	^{89}Sr	Prostate	Comparison with RT
Sciuto (48)	^{89}Sr	Prostate	Adjuvant chemotherapy
Schmeler (38)	^{89}Sr	Prostate	Patient selection
Serafini (49)	[^{153}Sm]-EDTMP	Mixed	Placebo control
Resche (50)	[^{153}Sm]-EDTMP	Mixed	Dose selection
Collins (51)	[^{153}Sm]-EDTMP	Mixed	Dose escalation
de Klerk (52)	[^{186}Re]-HEDP	Mixed	Dose guidelines
Quirijnen (53)	[^{186}Re]-HEDP	Mixed	Assessment of response
McEwan (54)	^{89}Sr	Prostate	Cost–benefit
Atkins (55)	[^{117m}Sn]-DTPA	Mixed	Proof of principle
Kasalicky (56)	^{89}Sr	Mixed	Repeat treatment
Baziotis (57)	^{89}Sr	Breast	Effectiveness open-label
Tian (58)	[^{153}]Sm EDTMP	Mixed	Effectiveness open-label

Source: Ref. 45.

strontium (60). This may have implications for the use of ^{89}Sr in patients with significant renal impairment, who may require dose modification.

Calculated doses to individual metastases show a wide range and vary between 380 and 2262 rad/mCi, with marrow doses typically being one-tenth of the doses to the metastatic sites (20,61).

The initial clinical experience with ^{89}Sr was in small series of patients, with very different dosing schedules and with, at times, uncertain trial design. McEwan (16) has reviewed these data, which are reproduced in Table 7.

Whereas these contributions may be criticized for unsatisfactory trial design, they do show remarkedly comparable and consistent response rates, and contributed to the early understanding of the potential of palliative treatment with bone-seeking radiopharmaceuticals. Many of the patients in these trials had advanced metastatic cancer, and survival was limited. However, the response rates were comparable with those historically obtained with ^{32}P, and toxicity was reported as being significantly less. It was on the basis of these data that the late Ralph Robinson, M.D. obtained the first U.S. IND at the University of Kansas.

The first dose escalation study of ^{89}Sr was reported by Silberstein and Williams (70), who treated 38 patients with multiple primaries; 45 doses were administered, ranging from 10 μCi/kg (0.4 MBq/kg) to 70 μCi/kg (2.6 MBq/kg). For each decile of dose, no difference was seen in the numbers of patients responding, and no significant myelosuppression was seen. The mean duration of response posttherapy was 1.6 months and the median survival was 4 months. Overall the response rate was 51%.

A second double-blind, placebo-controlled crossover trial was reported by Lewington et al. (46). They evaluated 40 μCi/kg ^{89}Sr compared with the same molar concentration of stable strontium as placebo. Thirty-two patients were evaluated, and there was a crossover option at 6 weeks if no response was seen to the first injection. Patients were evaluated at 6 and 12 weeks after injection. A significant palliative benefit was seen in the active arm at the 6-week evaluation and in those patients who received the second injection and were evaluated at 12 weeks. In addition to confirming an effect of the radiation, it excluded a chemical effect of strontium as the cause of pain relief.

Laing and co-workers (71) also published an open-label dose-escalation study in 83 patients with prostate cancer, using doses of 20, 40, 60, and 80 μCi/kg (0.74, 1.48, 2.22, and 2.96 MBq/kg). An overall response rate of 75% was seen. There was no evidence of a dose–response, although the patient group treated at 20 μCi/kg (0.74 MBq/kg) had a lower overall

Table 7 Review of Strontium-89 as Palliative Therapy for Painful Bone Metastases

Author (Ref.)	Year	Evaluable patients	Patients responding	% responding	Administered activity
Schmidt (62)[a]	1974	10	8	80	10–20 μCi/kg
Firusian (63)[a]	1976	11	8	73	30 μCi/kg
Firusian (64)[a]	1978	43	33	77	15–30 μCi/kg
Kutzner (65)	1978	15	12	80	0.8–2.7 mCi
Hayek (66)	1980	17	7	42	1–2 mCi
Correns (67)	1979	12	8	67	1–2 mCi
Kimmig (68)	1983	12	11	90	3 mCi
Buchali (69)	1983	70	60	86	1 mCi
Total		190	147	77	

[a] Total series includes common patients.
Source: Ref. 16.

response rate than those at the other doses. No clinically significant toxicity was observed, although patients at the highest dose level did show the most, reversible, myelosuppression. Patients with the highest metastatic burden were felt to be those who had the most limited palliation.

The largest published experience of the efficacy of ^{89}Sr derives from the University of Kansas (35). Six hundred and twenty-two patients had been treated; more than 450 had prostate cancer. Patients were treated at two dose levels, 40 and 55 μCi/kg, and some patients were re-treated with doses of 30 μCi/kg. An overall response rate of 81% was reported, with 15% achieving a complete resolution of symptoms and requiring no analgesic support.

Porter et al. (36) reported an adjuvant trial in which patients with pain requiring local-field radiation therapy were randomized to receive either ^{89}Sr or placebo in addition to the standard dose of external-beam radiation. Following injection, patients were followed with standard patterns of care for the balance of their lives. One hundred and twenty-six patients were randomized equally between the two arms of the study. The dose of ^{89}Sr in this study was 10 mCi, larger than the dose currently used in routine practice.

The patients in the arm that received ^{89}Sr in addition to radiation therapy showed significant improvements—at 3 months after injection—in requirements for analgesic support, and in improved quality of life as measured by a visual analog scale. In addition, reduced lifetime requirements for RT were seen in the active group, and there was a reduced rate in the development of new painful bone metastases.

Hematological toxicity was significantly greater in the active arm, but no clinically relevant events were recorded. Reversible thrombocytopenia was the most frequently observed toxicity. No differences in cord compression or pathological fracture were seen between the two arms.

In a second multicenter trial, Quilty and co-workers (37) compared 5.4 mCi of ^{89}Sr with either local-field radiation therapy (148 patients) or wide-field radiation therapy (157 patients). No significant differences in analgesic efficacy were seen in either arm of the two studies. Comparable numbers in all arms of the study showed complete or greater than 50% reductions in pain scores at the index site. In addition, there were significant delays to requirement for additional radiotherapy or other interventions in the ^{89}Sr group in comparison with the local-field radiotherapy group, and there were also significant delays in the development of new pain sites in the ^{89}Sr arm.

Several key elements appear evident from these two trials: (1) analgesic efficacy of ^{89}Sr appears comparable with that of external radiotherapy, although onset may be delayed; (2) significant improvements in quality of life are seen with ^{89}Sr; (3) there is a delay in progression of painful metastases; and (4) there is a reduction in lifetime radiation therapy requirements.

McEwan and co-workers (54) reviewed the data from a single Canadian site, from the study reported by Porter et al. (36), relative to lifetime management costs, evaluating costs of RT, analgesics, hormones, hospitalization, and active support. This cost was Can $5800 lower in the group receiving ^{89}Sr when compared with the placebo group. Cancer Care Ontario has developed a practice guideline for the use of ^{89}Sr in patients with prostate cancer metastatic to bone which will contribute to an enhanced understanding of the most cost-effective practice (72). The America College of Radiology has published guidelines for cost-effective use (73) of radiotherapy, including unsealed sources.

Baziotis and co-workers (57) reported a study in which 64 patients with breast cancer were followed after administration of a standard 4-mCi dose of the radiopharmaceutical for 6 months. Eighty-one percent of patients responded, with 35% appearing to become pain-free. Toxicity was moderate, and in 5 patients it was severe enough to require G-CSF support. These results are comparable with those seen in patients with prostate cancer, and they support the data obtained in patients with breast cancer treated with the other radiopharmaceuticals.

Kasalicky et al. (56) have confirmed the safety and efficacy of multiple administrations of ^{89}Sr in 118 patients with primary cancers of the prostate, breast, or lung, with a maximum of five repeat administrations. This important study shows comparable efficacy among the primary sites and also shows no significant increase in toxicity with succeeding administrations.

Patient selection for administration of ^{89}Sr has been addressed by Schmeler and co-workers (38). Response and survival were correlated with Karnofsky Performance Score (KPS). Limited survival and poor palliative responses were observed in the group with a KPS of 50 or lower. Those patients with a KPS of 70 or higher had a response rate of approximately 75%. A KPS of 60 gave intermediate quality of palliative efficacy, and patient selection in this group should be made on an individual basis. This study should become part of a wider discussion of the most appropriate use of bone-seeking radiopharmaceuticals in the therapeutic armamentarium.

An unexpected finding in the study reported by Porter et al. (36) was a significant fall in PSA levels in the active group. These results should be treated with caution, as this finding was not a secondary endpoint of the study, and data collection was incomplete. However, it may imply that treatment with bone-seeking radiopharmaceuticals may exert a tumoricidal effect, particularly with a radiopharmaceutical, such as ^{89}Sr, with an energetic β-particle.

This concept has been tested by Sciuto and co-workers (48), who compared 4 mCi ^{89}Sr with 4 mCi ^{89}Sr and low-dose carboplatin infusion as radiosensitizer. Fifteen patients were treated in each arm. Not only were the palliative responses significantly better in the arm receiving adjuvant carboplatin as radiosensitizer, but there also appeared to be significant falls in PSA, implying that there was a possible reduction in metastatic burden. These data are preliminary and are being tested in multicenter trials.

B. Samarium-153 EDTMP

The radiopharmaceutical [^{153}Sm]-EDTMP is now licensed for use in the United States for the management of patients with osteoblastic bone metastases. ^{153}Sm is a reactor-produced radioisotope by neutron irradiation of ^{152}Sm. ^{153}Sm has a complex decay scheme, with a principal β_{max} of 0.81 MeV. There is a γ-photon of 103 keV, which can be used for correlative imaging.

The synthesis of ^{153}Sm complexes was first reported by Goeckeler and co-workers (74); EDTMP showed the optimum combination of high bone uptake, rapid blood clearance, and a labeling efficiency of greater than 90%, and was proposed as a potential therapeutic radiopharmaceutical.

Most of the administered dose is localized in the skeleton within 3 hours of injection, and less than 2% is seen in soft tissue. Excretion is almost exclusively renal, and distribution correlates with [^{99m}Tc]-MDP imaging (75). Comparable therapeutic ratios have been demonstrated for [^{153}Sm]-EDTMP as are seen for ^{89}Sr, with bone/soft tissue ratios of up to 10:1 being seen (19,20). The whole-body dose from an injection of [^{153}Sm]-EDTMP has been calculated at 0.44 mGy/mCi. The target organ for toxicity is the marrow.

Metastatic lesion/normal bone ratios and metastatic lesion/soft-tissue ratios have been calculated by Singh and co-workers (76) to be 4.04 and 5.98, respectively. These imply a safe therapeutic ratio for the radiopharmaceutical, and one that will perhaps allow retreatment at an earlier time point than ^{89}Sr.

Several groups have evaluated [^{153}Sm]-EDTMP looking at dose–response and incremental toxicity. Collins and co-workers (51) and Turner et al. (77) have reported incrementally increasing doses up to 4.5 mCi/kg, resulting in total administered doses of up to 300 mCi. There was no convincing evidence of a dose–response, but reversible myelotoxicity was dose-related, and at the highest doses severe. Turner and Claringbold (78) reported safe administration with absorbed dose to marrow of up to 2 Gy. Metastatic burden may also have contributed to toxicity at the highest doses.

Resche et al. (50) have compared two doses of [^{153}Sm]-EDTMP in 114 patients; 55 received 0.5 mCi/kg and 59 received 1.0 mCi/kg, as single administrations. A significant palliative response was seen at the higher-dose level, with patients with breast cancer showing a greater response than patients with prostate and lung cancer. No significant toxicities were seen in either arm. In a second trial, these dose levels of 0.5 and 1.0 mCi/kg were compared with placebo in a double-blind design (49). One hundred and eighteen patients were randomized equally to the three arms. Patients in both active arms fared significantly better than those in the placebo arm, and those at the higher dose had better pain palliation than those treated with 0.5 mCi/kg. Toxicity was greater in the active arms than in the placebo, but was not significantly different between the two active arms. As with the previous study, patients with breast cancer responded better than those with prostate and lung cancer.

A large multicenter trial has also been reported by Tian et al. (58), who treated 105 patients with a variety of primary malignancies with either 0.5 or 1.0 mCi/kg. Effective palliation was observed in 85% of patients, with those in the high-dose group achieving better responses. No clinically significant myelosuppression was observed. Patients with breast cancer tended to do better than the other patient populations.

Overall response rates of 70–80% have been reported at the higher dose of 1.0 mCi/kg. Duration of response may be up to 4–6 months, and time to response is somewhat quicker than that reported for ^{89}Sr (49).

C. Rhenium-186 HEDP

Rhenium-186 HEDP is in routine use in some jurisdictions in Europe to palliate patients with painful bone metastases, but it is not yet available in the United States.

^{186}Re is a group VII metal that decays with the emission of a β-particle of maximum energy 1.07 MeV. A low abundance 137-keV γ-ray is also emitted enabling correlative imaging to be performed.

The synthesis of [^{186}Re]-HEDP was reported in 1986 and, subsequently, a clinical formulation of the product entered clinical trials (79,80). Animal biodistribution studies confirmed high uptake in bone, with 14% of the injected dose remaining in the skeleton 96 h after injection. Up to 43% of the injected dose is excreted in the urine in the first hour. In patient studies, a correlation of uptake and retention with metastatic burden is seen, and up to 38% of the injected dose may be retained in the skeleton 3 h after injection. The percentage of injected dose retained in the skeleton at 4+ days postinjection is less than is seen for [^{153}Sm]-EDTMP and ^{89}Sr, for which up to 90% of the injected dose is retained at 3 months in patients with superscans (81).

Large-scale trials of this radiopharmaceutical have not been reported, although a considerable body of data has been accrued in phase 2 trials showing response rates of up to 80%.

The biodistribution and pharmacokinetics of [^{186}Re]-HEDP have been described (80,82), and dosimetry calculations showed a safe therapeutic ratio with tumor doses of up to 41 rad/mCi and marrow doses of 2.8 rad/mCi. Samaratunga et al. (18) have developed an elegant dosimetry model, which is a Monte Carlo simulation of the microdosimetric environment addressing the questions of heterogeneity of the bone–tumor interface, nonuniform distribution of radiopharmaceutical on bone spicules, and differential energy deposition. This model suggests that, for osteoblastic lesions, standard dosimetric calculations significantly underestimate tumor and marrow dose.

In an initial double-blind, crossover placebo-controlled trial, Maxon et al. (47) compared [^{186}Re]-HEDP with [^{99m}Tc]-MDP as placebo in 13 evaluable patients. The patients were evaluated for response at 4 weeks after injection, and the crossover injection was administered if the patient had failed to respond to the first injection. A statistically significant difference in response was seen with the active administration.

Farhanghi et al. (83) found a lack of a dose–response, associated with dose-related toxicity, in a dose-escalation study, up to 1.0 mCi/kg. They felt that maximum tolerated dose had not been achieved and noted a direct correlation between metastatic burden and retained activity. The response rate was 65% with a duration of response of approximately 4 months.

Dose escalation studies for [^{186}Re]-HEDP have compared incrementally escalating doses from 35 to 95 mCi (53,84,85). There is evidence of a possible dose–response, with significantly more patients at the higher-dose level showing improvements in quality of life and reduction in pain than at the lower-dose levels. de Klerk et al. (52,84) have proposed a dose calculation algorithm using bone scan index and baseline platelet count to individualize the patients' administered dose calculations.

Han et al. (86) have recently performed an open-label, dose-escalation study of [^{186}Re]-HEDP in 30 patients with breast cancer metastatic to bone. Administered doses ranged from 35 to 80 mCi. No dose–response relation was observed, and overall response rates were comparable with those seen in patients with prostate cancer. Dose-related myelosuppression was seen, which apparently recovered more rapidly than with ^{89}Sr.

Responses of up to 75% have been seen in patients with breast cancer (87,88). About one-fifth of patients became pain-free, but the series are small. Schoeneich et al. (89) have reported responses of 60% in 44 patients with prostate cancer treated with 35 mCi [^{186}Re]-HEDP, with a median duration of response of 6 weeks.

Guidelines for dose calculation have also been prepared by Graham et al. (90), recommending doses of up to 80 mCi and suggesting that individual dose calculations be performed. They propose a repetitive-dosing schedule to attain maximum efficacy.

The question of radiosensitization has been addressed by Geldof et al. (91) using [^{186}Re]-HEDP and cisplatin in vitro. Synergy was observed and a proposal for ongoing clinical trials was developed.

D. Tin-117m (4+) DTPA

This innovative radiopharmaceutical is entering phase 2 clinical trials. It is a bone-seeking chelate that shows high bone uptake and very low soft-tissue activity, with rapid renal clearance of the radiopharmaceutical ^{117}Sn is reactor-produced by irradiation of ^{117}Sn. It decays with the emission of low-energy conversion electrons; the short path length of the conversion electron is anticipated to reduce myelotoxicity by reducing the absorbed dose to marrow. A 159-keV photon is emitted, with low abundance, enabling correlative imaging (92). The mechanism of incorporation is believed to be precipitation of the radioactive tin onto the inorganic bone matrix.

Preliminary data show a very high bone dose of up to 300 rad/mCi and lesion/normal tissue ratios of approximately 15:1 (55,93).

A single-dose escalation study of [^{117m}Sn]-DTPA has been performed (93). No toxicity was observed at any level, perhaps reflecting the more limited tissue penetration than is seen with the β-emitting radionuclides. If the efficacy of the radiopharmaceutical can be proved, the limited toxicity may make this an alternative radiopharmaceutical for palliative treatment in an adjuvant setting where multiple administrations are considered.

E. Phosphorus-32

This radiopharmaceutical is included for completeness. Despite the data of Nair (6) and Shah Syed (7), its use is limited. It is, however, less expensive than the other compounds, and additional trials may be developed to evaluate its cost-effectiveness.

Phosphorus-32 decays by β-emission, with a half-life of 14.3 days. Within bone, phosphorus is bound as inorganic phosphorus to the hydroxyapatite matrix with slow turnover. Within soft tissue and in the bone marrow, phosphorus distribution is predominantly intracellular. Excretion is mainly renal (8,94). Uptake is increased at sites of bone metastases relative to normal bone, reflecting increased metabolic turnover in sites of active remodeling.

Published estimates of absorbed dose show a wide range with therapeutic (lesion/bone) ratios of up to 5:1 being reported. The bone marrow receives a higher dose than it does with the other radiopharmaceuticals because of ^{32}P incorporation in bone matrix and in the cellular component of the bone marrow (95,96).

There is an extensive literature of the use of ^{32}P in palliative management that has been reviewed by Silberstein et al. and by Montebello and Hartson–Eaton (8,97). Between 8 and 20 mCi were typically administered, often in fractionated administration schedules of 7–40 days. In addition, treatment with parathormone and testosterone were used to enhance uptake and absorbed dose to metastases.

A wide range of responses were reported—from 20 to 100%—although validated test instruments of efficacy were not available in most of these early trials. Myelosuppression was common and not infrequently severe (98,99).

NOTE IN PROOF

The projected synergistic relationship between low-dose cisplatin and ^{89}Sr has now been validated. Sciuto and co-workers (100) have now published confirmatory data to their preliminary observations (48) that improved palliative efficacy may be achieved. A total of 35 patients treated with 4 mCi ^{89}Sr and cisplatin showed significantly improved pain palliation compared with patients treated with strontium-89 alone.

These data should not only lead to an increase in the routine use of this form of pain palliation but also expand wider research into methods of enhancing radioisotope therapy.

REFERENCES

1. Treadwell AdeG, Low-Beer BVA, Friedell HL, Lawrence JH. Metabolic studies on neoplasm of bone with the aid of radioactive strontium. Am J Med Sci 1942; 204:521–530.
2. Pecher C. Biological investigations with radioactive calcium and strontium: preliminary report on the use of radioactive strontium in the treatment of metastatic bone cancer. Univ Calif Publ Pharmacol 1942; 2:117–149.
3. Lawrence JH, Wasserman LR. Multiple myeloma: a study of 24 patients treated with radioactive isotopes (P^{32} and Sr^{89}). Ann Intern Med 1950; 33:41–55.
4. Hosain F, Spencer RP. Radiopharmaceuticals for palliation of metastatic osseous lesions: biologic and physical background. Semin Nucl Med 1992; 22:1–16.
5. Holmes RA. Radiopharmaceuticals in clinical trials. Semin Oncol 1993; 20(suppl):22–26.
6. Nair N. Relative efficacy of ^{32}P and ^{89}Sr in palliation in skeletal metastases. J Nucl Med 1999; 40: 256–261.
7. Shah Syed GM, Maken RN, Muzzaffar N, Shah MA, Rana F. Effective and economical option for

pain palliation in prostate cancer with skeletal metastases: ^{32}P therapy revisited. Nucl Med Commun 1999; 20:697–702.

8. Silberstein EB, Elgazzar AH, Kapilivsky A. Phosphorus-32 radiopharmaceuticals for the treatment of painful osseous metastases. Semin Nucl Med 1992; 22:17–27.
9. Krasnow AZ, Hellman RS, Timins ME, Collier BD, Anderson T, Isitman AT. Diagnostic bone scanning in oncology. Semin Nucl Med 1997; 27:107–141.
10. Jain D. Technetium-99m labeled myocardial perfusion imaging agents. Semin Nucl Med 1999; 29: 221–236.
11. Olsen JO, Pozderac RV, Hinkle G, Hill T, O'Dorisio TM, Schirmer WJ, Ellison EC, O'Dorisio MS. Somatostatin receptor imaging of neuroendocrine tumors with indium-111 pentetreotide (Octreoscan). Semin Nucl Med 1995; 25:251–261.
12. Sisson JC. Radionuclide therapy for malignancy: influences of physical characteristics of radionuclides and experience with metaiodobenzylguanidine. Clin Oncol 1986; 5:1–21.
13. Reynolds JC, Robbins J. The changing role of radioiodine in the management of differentiated thyroid cancer. Semin Nucl Med 1997; 27:152–164.
14. Hoefnagel CA, Lewington VJ. mIBG therapy. In: Murray IPC, Ell PJ, eds. Nuclear Medicine in Clinical Diagnosis and Treatment. 2nd ed. Edinburgh: Churchill Livingstone, 1998:1067–1081.
15. McEwan AJB. Use of radionuclides for the palliation of bone metastases. Semin Radiat Oncol 2000; 10:103–114.
16. McEwan AJB. Unsealed therapy of painful bone metastases: an update. Semin Nucl Med 1997; 27: 165–182.
17. Ben-Josef E, Lucas DR, Vasan S, Porter AT. Selective accumulation of strontium-89 in metastatic deposits in bone: radio–histological correlation. Nucl Med Commun 1995; 16:457–463.
18. Samaratunga RC, Thomas SR, Hinnefeld JD, Von Kuster LC, Hyams DM, Moulton JS, Sperling MI, Maxon HR III. A Monte Carlo simulation model for radiation dose to metastatic skeletal tumor from rhenium-186(Sn)-HEDP. J Nucl Med 1995; 36:336–350.
19. Logan KW, Volkert WA, Holmes RA. Radiation dose calculations in persons receiving injection of samarium-153 EDTMP. J Nucl Med 1987; 28:505–509.
20. Blake GM, Zivanovic MA, Blaquiere RM, Fine DR, McEwan AJ, Ackery DM. Strontium-89 therapy: measurement of absorbed dose to skeletal metastases. J Nucl Med 1988; 29:549–557.
21. Dale RG, Jones B. The clinical radiobiology of brachytherapy. Br J Radiol 1998; 71:465–483.
22. Janjan NA. Radiation for bone metastases. Conventional techniques and the role of systemic radiopharmaceuticals. Cancer 1997; 80(suppl):1628–1645.
23. Hoskin PJ. Scientific and clinical aspects of radiotherapy in the relief of bone pain. Cancer Surv 1988; 7:69–86.
24. Maxon HR, Thomas SR, Hertzberg VS, Schroder LE, Englaro EE, Samaratunga R, Scher HI, Moulton JS, Deutsch EA, Deutsch KF, Schneider HJ, Williams CC, Ehrhardt GJ. Rhenium-186 hydroxyethylidene diphosphonate for the treatment of painful osseous metastases. Semin Nucl Med 1992; 22:33–40.
25. Dodwell DJ. Malignant bone resorption: cellular and biochemical mechanisms. Ann Oncol 1992; 3: 257–267.
26. Ventafridda V, Sbanotta A, de Conno F. Pain in prostate cancer. Palliat Med 1990; 4:173–184.
27. Trott K–R, Kamprad F. Radiobiological mechanisms of anti-inflammatory radiotherapy. Radiother Oncol 1997; 51:197–203.
28. Hildebrandt G, Seed MP, Freemantle CN, Alam CAS, Colville–Nash PR, Trott KR. Mechanisms of the anti-inflammatory activity of low-dose radiation therapy. Int J Radiat Biol 1998; 74:580–588.
29. Kharbanda S, Yuan ZM, Rubn E, Weichselbaum RR, Kufe D. Activition of SRC-like P56/P53(lyn) tyrosine kinase by ionizing radiation. J Biol Chem 1994; 269:739–743.
30. Eissner G, Lindner H, Behrends U, Kolch W, Hieke A, Klauke I, Bornkamm GW, Holler E. Influence of bacterial endotoxin on radiation-induced activation of human endothelial cells in vitro and in vivo: protective role of IL-10. Transplantation 1996; 62:819–827.
31. Price P, Hoskin PJ, Easton D, Austin A, Palmer SG, Yarnold JR. Prospective randomised trial of

single and multifraction radiotherapy schedules in the treatment of painful bony metastases. Radiother Oncol 1986; 6:247–255.

32. Tong D, Gillick L, Hendrickson FR. The palliation of symptomatic osseous metastases. Final results of the Radiation Therapy Oncology Group. Cancer 1982; 50:893–899.
33. Cole DJ. A randomised trial of a single treatment versus conventional fractionation in the palliative radiotherapy of painful bone metastases. Clin Oncol 1989; 1:59–62.
34. Salazar OM, Rubin P, Hendrickson FR, Komaki R, Poulter C, Newall J, Asbell SO, Mohiuddin M, Van Ess J. Single-dose half-body irradiation for palliation of multiple bone metastases from solid tumors: final Radiation Therapy Oncology Group report. Cancer 1986; 58:29–36.
35. Robinson RG, Preston DF, Schiefelbein M, Baxter KG. Strontium-89 therapy for the palliation of pain due to osseous metastases. JAMA 1995; 274:420–424.
36. Porter AT, McEwan AJB, Powe JE, Reid R, McGowan DG, Lukka H, Sathyanarayana JR, Yakemchuk VN, Thomas GM, Erlich LE, Crook J, Gulenchyn KY, Hong KE, Wesolowski C, Yardley J. Results of a randomized phase-III trial to evaluate the efficacy of strontium-89 adjuvant to local field external beam irradiation in the management of endocrine resistant metastatic prostate cancer. Int J Radiat Oncol Biol Phys 1993; 25:805–813.
37. Quilty PM, Kirk D, Bolger JJ, Dearnaley DP, Lewington VJ, Mason MD, Reed NSE, Russell JM, Yardley J. A comparison of the palliative effects of strontium-89 and external beam radiotherapy in metastatic prostate cancer. Radiother Oncol 1994; 31:33–40.
38. Schmeler K, Bastin K. Strontium-89 for symptomatic metastatic prostate cancer to bone: recommendations for hospice patients. Hosp J 1996; 11:1–10.
39. Cowan RJ, Chilton HM, Cooper MR, Ferree CR, Watson EE, Robinson RG. Hematologic depression following therapy with strontium-89 chloride. Clin Nucl Med 1986; 11:845–846.
40. Leong C, McKenzie MR, Coupland DB, Gascoyne RD. Disseminated intravascular coagulation in a patient with metastatic prostate cancer: fatal outcome following strontium-89 therapy. J Nucl Med 1994; 35:1662–1664.
41. Burgess NA, Hudd C, Rees RWM. Haemostatic pitfalls in advanced prostatic cancer. Br J Urol 1993; 71:231–233.
42. Adamson AS, Witherow RO'N, Francis JL, Snell ME. Coagulopathy in the prostate cancer patient: prevalence and clinical relevance. Ann R Coll Surg Engl 1993; 75:1001–1004.
43. McEwan AJB, Porter AT, Venner PM, Amyotte G. An evaluation of the safety and efficacy of treatment with strontium-89 in patients who have previously received wide field radiotherapy. Antibody Immunoconjugates Radiopharm 1990; 3:91–97.
44. Amdur R, Eaton W, Mitchell S, Leopold K, Filimonov A. The Sr-89 bracelet. Int J Radiat Oncol Biol Physics 1995; 32:897 [correspondence].
45. McEwan AJB. Palliative therapy with bone seeking radiopharmaceuticals. Cancer Biother Radiopharm 1998; 13:413–426.
46. Lewington VJ, McEwan AJ, Ackery DM, Bayly RJ, Keeling DH, Macleod PM, Porter AT, Zivanovic MA. A prospective, randomised double-blind crossover study to examine the efficacy of strontium-89 in pain palliation in patients with advanced prostate cancer metastatic to bone. Eur J Cancer 1991; 27:954–958.
47. Maxon HR, Schroder LE, Hertzberg VS, Thomas SR, Englaro EE, Samaratunga R, Smith H, Moulton JS, Williams CC, Ehrhardt GJ, Schneider HJ. Rhenium-186(Sn)HEDP for treatment of painful osseous metastases: results of a double-blind crossover comparison with placebo. J Nucl Med 1991; 32: 1877–1881.
48. Sciuto R, Maini CL, Tofani A, Fiumara C, Scelsa MG, Broccatelli M. Radiosensitization with low-dose carboplatin enhances pain palliation in radioisotope therapy with strontium-89. Nucl Med Commun 1996; 17:799–804.
49. Serafini AN, Houston SJ, Resche I, Quick DP, Grund FM, Ell PJ, Bertrand A, Ahmann FR, Orihuela E, Reid RH, Lerski RA, Collier BD, McKillop JH, Purnell GL, Pecking AP, Thomas FD, Harrison KA. Palliation of pain associated with metastatic bone cancer using samarium-153 lexidronam: a double-blind placebo-controlled clinical trial. J Clin Oncol 1998; 16:1574–1581.
50. Resche I, Chatal J–F, Pecking A, Ell P, Duchesne G, Rubens R, Fogelman I, Houston S, Fauser A,

Fischer M, Wilkins D. A dose-controlled study of ^{153}Sm-ethylenediaminetetramethylene phosphonate (EDTMP) in the treatment of patients with painful bone metastases. Eur J Cancer 1997; 33:1583–1591.

51. Collins C, Eary JF, Donaldson G, Vernon C, Bush NE, Petersdorf S, Livingston RB, Gordon EE, Chapman CR, Appelbaum FR. Samarium-153-EDTMP in bone metastases of hormone refractory prostate carcinoma: a phase I/II trial. J Nucl Med 1993; 34:1839–1844.
52. de Klerk JMH, van het Schip AD, Zonnenberg BA, van Dijk A, van Rijk PP. Evaluation of thrombocytopenia in patients treated with rhenium-186-HEDP: guidelines for individual dosage recommendations. J Nucl Med 1994; 35:1423–1428.
53. Quirijnen JMSP, Han SH, Zonnenberg BA, de Klerk JMH, van het Schip AD, van Dijk A, ten Kroode HFJ, Blijham GH, van Rijk PP. Efficacy of rhenium-186-etidronate in prostate cancer patients with metastatic bone pain. J Nucl Med 1996; 37:1511–1515.
54. McEwan AJB, Amyotte GA, McGowan DG, MacGillivray JA, Porter AT. A retrospective analysis of the cost effectiveness of treatment with Metastron (^{89}Sr-chloride) in patients with prostate cancer metastatic to bone. Nucl Med Commun 1994; 15:499–504.
55. Atkins HL, Mausner LF, Srivastava SC, Meinken GE, Straub RF, Cabahug CJ, Weber DA, Wong CTC, Sacker DF, Madajewicz S, Park TL, Meek AG. Biodistribution of Sn-117m(4+) DTPA for palliative therapy of painful osseous metastases. Radiology 1993; 186:279–283.
56. Kasalicky J, Krajska V. The effect of repeated strontium-89 chloride therapy on bone pain palliation in patients with skeletal cancer metastases. Eur J Nucl Med 1998; 25:1362–1367.
57. Baziotis N, Yakoumakis E, Zissimopoulos A, Geronicoala–Teapali X, Malamitsi J, Proukakis C. Strontium-89 chloride in the treatment of bone metastases from breast cancer. Oncology 1998; 55: 377–381.
58. Tian JH, Zhang JM, Hou QT, Oyang QH, Wang JM, Luan ZS, Chuan L, He YJ. Multicentre trial on the efficacy and toxicity of single-dose samarium-153-ethylene diamine tetramethylene phosphonate as a palliative treatment for painful skeletal metastases in China. Eur J Nucl Med 1999; 26:2–7.
59. Breen SL, Powe JE, Porter AT. Dose estimation of strontium-89 radiotherapy of metastatic prostatic carcinoma. J Nucl Med, 1992; 33:1316–1323.
60. Blake GM, Wood JF, Wood PJ, Zivanovic MA, Lewington VJ. ^{89}Sr therapy: strontium plasma clearance in disseminated prostatic carcinoma. Eur J Nucl Med 1989; 15:49–54.
61. Blake GM, Gray JM, Zivanovic MA, McEwan AJ, Fleming JS, Ackery DM. Strontium-89 radionuclide therapy: a dosimetric study using impulse response function analysis. Br J Radiol 1987; 60: 685–692.
62. Schmidt CG, Firusian N. 89-Sr for the treatment of incurable pain in patient with neoplastic osseous infiltrations. Int J Clin Pharmacol 1974; 9:199–205.
63. Firusian N, Mellin P, Schmidt CG. Results of ^{89}strontium therapy in patients with carcinoma of the prostate and incurable pain from bone metastases: a preliminary report. J Urol 1976; 16:764–768.
64. Firusian N. Endoossale Isotopen-Therapie maligner Skeleterkrankungen. Z Krebsforsch 1978; 91: 143–156.
65. Kutzner J, Grimm W, Hahn K. Palliative Strahlentherapie mit Strontium-89 bei ausgedehnter Skelettmetastasierung. Strahlentherapie 1978; 154:317–322.
66. Hayek D, Ritschard J, Zwahlen A, Courvoisier B, Donath A. Emploi du strontium-89 dans le traitement antalgique des métastases osseuses. Schweiz Med Wochenschr 1980; 110:1154–1159.
67. Correns H–J, Mebel M, Buchali K, Schnorr D, Seidel C, Mitterlechner E. Strontium 89 therapy of bone metastases of carcinoma of the prostate gland. Eur J Nucl Med 1979; 4:33–35.
68. Kimmig B, Hermann HJ, Kober B. Nuklearmedizinishe Therapie von Knochen metastasen. Röntgenblätter 1983; 36:216–219.
69. Buchali K, Correns HJ, Schnorr D, Schurer M, Sydow K, Lips H. 89-Strontium—therapy of skeletal metastases of prostatic carcinoma. Proceedings of the 1984 Bad Gastein International Radiopharmaceutical Conference. 1984; 151–156.
70. Silberstein EB, Williams C. Strontium-89 therapy for the pain of osseous metastases. J Nucl Med 1985; 26:345–348.
71. Laing AH, Ackery DM, Bayly RJ, Buchanan RB, Lewington VJ, McEwan AJB, Macleod PM, Ziva-

novic MA. Strontium-89 chloride for pain palliation in prostatic skeletal malignancy. Br J Radiol 1991; 64:816–822.

72. Brundage MD, Crook JM, Lukka H, Provincial Genitourinary Cancer Disease Site Group. Use of strontium-89 in endocrine-refractory prostate cancer metastatic to bone. Cancer Prev Control 1998; 2:79–87.
73. Rose CM, Kagan AR. The final report of the expert panel for the Radiation Oncology Bone Metastasis Work Group of the American College of Radiology. Int J Radiat Oncol Biol Phys 1998; 40:1117–1124.
74. Goeckeler WF, Edwards B, Volkert WA, Holmes RA, Simon J, Wilson D. Skeletal localization of samarium-153 chelates: potential therapeutic bone agents. J Nucl Med 1987; 28:495–504.
75. Eary JF, Collins C, Stabin M, Vernon C, Petersdorf S, Baker M, Hartnett S, Ferency S, Addison SJ, Appelbaum F, Gordon EE. Samarium-153-EDTMP biodistribution and dosimetry estimation. J Nucl Med 1993; 34:1031–1036.
76. Singh A, Holmes RA, Farhangi M, Volker WA, Williams A, Stringham LM, Ketring AR. Human pharmacokinetics of samarium-153 EDTMP in metastatic cancer. J Nucl Med 1989; 30:1814–1818.
77. Turner JH, Claringbold PG, Hetherington EL, Sorby P, Martindale AA. A phase I study of samarium-153 ethylenediaminetetramethylene phosphonate therapy for disseminated skeletal metastases. J Clin Oncol 1989; 7:1926–1931.
78. Turner JH, Claringbold PG. A phase II study of treatment of painful multifocal skeletal metastases with single and repeated dose samarium-153 ethylenediaminetetramethylene phosphonate. Eur J Cancer 1991; 27:1084–1086.
79. Deutsch E, Libson K, Vanderheyden JL, Ketring AR, Maxon HR. The chemistry of rhenium and technetium as related to the use of isotopes of these elements in therapeutic and diagnostic nuclear medicine. Int J Nucl Med Biol 1986; 13:465–477.
80. Maxon HR, Deutsch EA, Thomas SR, Libson K, Lukes SJ, Williams CC, Ali S. Re-186(Sn) HEDP for treatment of multiple metastatic foci in bone: human biodistribution and dosimetric studies. Radiology 1988; 166:501–507 (published erratum Radiology 1988; 167:582).
81. Blake GM, Zivanovic MA, McEwan AJ, Ackery DM. Sr-89 therapy: strontium kinetics in disseminated carcinoma of the prostate. Eur J Nucl Med 1986; 12:447–454.
82. de Klerk JMH, van Dijk A, van het Schip AD, Zonnenberg BA, van Rijk PP. Pharmacokinetics of rhenium-186 after administration of rhenium-186-HEDP to patients with bone metastases. J Nucl Med 1992; 33:646–651.
83. Farhanghi M, Holmes RA, Volkert WA, Logan KW, Singh A. Samarium-153-EDTMP: pharmacokinetic, toxicity and pain response using an escalating dose schedule in treatment of metastatic bone cancer. J Nucl Med 1992; 33:1451–1458.
84. de Klerk JMH, Zonnenberg BA, van het Schip AD, van Dijk A, Han SH, Quirijnen JMSP, Blijham GH, van Rijk PP. Dose escalation study of rhenium-186 hydroxyethylidene diphosphonate in patients with metastatic prostate cancer. Eur J Nucl Med 1994; 21:1114–1120.
85. Zonnenberg BA, de Klerk JMH, van Rijk PP, Quirijnen JMSP, van het Schip AD, van Dijk A, ten Kroode NFJ. Re-186-HEDP for treatment of painful bone metastases in patients with metastatic prostate or breast cancer. Preliminary results (abstr). J Nucl Med 1991; 32:1082.
86. Han SH, Zonnenberg BA, de Klerk JM, Quirijnen JM, van het Schip AD, van Dijk A, Blijham GH, van Rijk PP. ^{186}Re-etidronate in breast cancer patients with metastatic bone pain. J Nucl Med 1999; 40:639–642.
87. Guerra UP, Englaro E, Cattaruzzi E. Palliative therapy with rhenium-186-HEDP for bone metastases of breast cancer. Tumori 1997; 83:560–562.
88. Limouris GS, Shukla SK, Condi–Paphiti A, Gennatas C, Kouvaris I, Vitoratos N, Manetou A, Dardoufas C, Rigas V, Vlahos L. Palliative therapy using rhenium-186-HEDP in painful breast osseous metastases. Anticancer Res 1997; 17:1767–1772.
89. Schoeneich G, Palmedo H, Dierke–Dzierzon C, Muller SC, Biersack HJ. Rhenium-186 HEDP: palliative radionuclide therapy of painful bone metastases. Preliminary results. Scand J Urol Nephrol 1997; 31:445–448.

90. Graham MC, Scher HI, Liu GB, Yeh SD, Curley T, Daghighian F, Goldsmith SJ, Larson SM. Rhenium-186-labeled hydroxyethylidene diphosphonate dosimetry and dosing guidelines for the palliation of skeletal metastases from androgen-independent prostate cancer. Clin Cancer Res 1999; 5: 1307–1318.
91. Geldof AA, de Rooij L, Versteegh RT, Newling DW, Teule GJ. Combination ^{186}Re-HEDP and cisplatin supra-additive treatment effects in prostate cancer cells. J Nucl Med 1999; 40:667–671.
92. Yano Y, Chu P, Anger HO. Tin-117m: production, chemistry and evaluation as a bone-scanning agent. Int J Appl Radiat Isot 1973; 24:319–325.
93. Srivastava SC. Treatment of metastatic bone pain with tin-117m stannic diethylenetriaminepentaacetic acid: a phase I/II clinical study. Clin Cancer Res 1998; 4:61–68.
94. Wilkinson R. Absorption of calcium, phosphorus and magnesium. In: Nordin BEC, ed. Calcium, Phosphate and Magnesium Metabolism. New York: Churchill Livingstone, 1976; 36–113.
95. Potsaid MS, Irwin RJ Jr, Castronovo FP, Prout GR Jr, Harvey WJ, Francis MD, Tofe AJ, Zamenhof RG. [^{32}P]Diphosphonate dose determination in patients with bone metastases from prostatic carcinoma. J Nucl Med 1978; 19:98–104.
96. Spiers FW, Beddoe AH, King SD. The absorbed dose of bone marrow in the treatment of polycythemia by ^{32}P. Br J Radiol 1976; 49:133–140.
97. Montebello JF, Hartson–Eaton M. The palliation of osseous metastasis with ^{32}P or ^{89}Sr compared with external beam and hemibody irradiation: a historical perspective. Cancer Invest 1989; 7:139–160.
98. Cheung A, Driedger AA. Evaluation of radiophosphorus in the palliation of metastatic bone lesions from carcinoma of the breast and prostate. Radiology 1980; 134:209–212.
99. Storaasli JP, King RL, Krieger H, Abbott WE, Friedell HL. Palliation of osseous metastases from breast carcinoma with radioactive phosphorus alone and in combination with adrenalectomy. Radiology 1961; 76:422–429.
100. Sciuto R, Festa A, Rea S, Pasqualoni R, Bergomi S, Petrilli G, Maini CL. Effects of low-dose cisplatin on ^{89}Sr therapy for painful bone metastases from prostate cancer: a randomized clinical trial. J Nucl Med 2002; 43:79–86.

Appendix I: Currently Marketed Analgesics (U.S.A.; 1998–2001) (compiled by William K. Schmidt)

OPIOID AND NON-OPIOID COMBINATION ANALGESICS (ORAL USE)

TRADE NAME	COMPOSITION	DISTRIBUTOR	REGULATORY STATUS
Anexsia	hydrocodone + APAP	Mallinckrodt	C-III
Damason-P	hydrocodone + aspirin	Mason	C-III
Darvocet-N	propoxyphene + APAP	Lilly	C-IV
Darvon Cmpd-65	propoxyphene, aspirin, caffeine	Lilly	C-IV
DHCplus	dihydrocodeine, aspirin, caffeine	Purdue Frederick	C-III
Endocet	oxycodone + APAP	Endo	C-II
Endodan	oxycodone + aspirin	Endo	C-II
Fioricet w/codeine	codeine, butalbital, caffeine, APAP	Novartis	C-III
Fiorinal w/codeine	codeine, butalbital, caffeine, aspirin	Novartis	C-III
Hydrocet	hydrocodone + APAP	Carnrick	C-III
Lorcet	hydrocodone + APAP	Forest	C-III
Lortab	hydrocodone + APAP	UCB	C-III
Lortab ASA	hydrocodone + aspirin	UCB	C-III
Maxidone	hydrocodone + APAP	Watson	C-III
Norco	hydrocodone + APAP	Watson	C-III
Phenaphen w/codeine	codeine + APAP	A. H. Robins	C-III
Percocet	oxycodone + APAP	Endo	C-II
Percodan	oxycodone + aspirin	Endo	C-II
Roxicet	oxycodone + APAP	Roxane	C-II
Roxilox	oxycodone + APAP	Roxane	C-II
Roxiprin	oxycodone + aspirin	Roxane	C-II
Synalgos-DC	dihydrocodeine, aspirin, caffeine	Wyeth-Ayerst	C-III
Talacen	pentazocine + APAP	Sanofi-Synthelabo	C-IV
Talwin Compound	pentazocine + aspirin	Sanofi-Synthelabo	C-IV
Tylenol w/codeine	codeine + APAP	Ortho-McNeil	C-III
Tylox	oxycodone + APAP	Ortho-McNeil	C-II
Ultracet	tramadol + APAP	Ortho-McNeil	Non-Narcotic ℞
Vicodin	hydrocodone + APAP	Knoll	C-III
Vicoprofen	hydrocodone + ibuprofen	Knoll	C-III
Wygesic	propoxyphene + APAP	Wyeth-Ayerst	C-IV
Zydone	hydrocodone + APAP	Endo	C-III

APAP = acetaminophen; ℞ = Prescription

• New Products ('97–'01): Vicoprofen (hydromorphone + ibuprofen), Ultracet (tramadol + APAP)

Note: codeine, hydrocodone, and dihydrocodeine combinations sold as cough suppressants or which are combined with sedatives, anxiolytics, decongestants, muscle relaxants, expectorants, or other products are not shown. Aspirin + APAP combinations are not shown. Generics are not shown. C-II, C-III, C-IV, and C-V designate narcotics regulated under the U.S. Controlled Substances Act.

SINGLE-ENTITY ANALGESICS, MODERATE-SEVERE PAIN

A. ORAL PRODUCTS

TRADE NAME	COMPOSITION	DISTRIBUTOR	REGULATORY STATUS
Darvon, Darvon-N	propoxyphene	Lilly	C-IV
Demerol	meperidine (pethidine)	Sanofi-Synthelabo	C-II
Dilaudid	hydromorphone	Knoll	C-II
Dolophine	methadone	Roxane	C-II
Duract*	bromfenac sodium	Wyeth-Ayerst	Non-Narcotic ℞ (NSAID)
Kadian	morphine (controlled rel.)	Faulding	C-II
Levo-Dromoran	levorphanol	ICN	C-II
MS Contin	morphine (controlled rel.)	Purdue Frederick	C-II
MSIR	morphine	Purdue Frederick	C-II
Oramorph SR	morphine (controlled rel.)	Roxane	C-II
OxyContin	oxycodone (controlled rel.)	Purdue Pharma	C-II
OxyFast	oxycodone	Purdue Pharma	C-II
OxylR	oxycodone	Purdue Pharma	C-II
Percalone	oxycodone	Endo	C-II
Rescudose	morphine	Roxane	C-II
Roxanol	morphine	Roxane	C-II
Roxicodone	oxycodone	Roxane	C-II
Talwin Nx	pentazocine + naloxone	Sanofi-Synthelabo	C-IV
Toradol	ketorolac	Syntex	Non-Narcotic ℞ (NSAID)
Ultram	tramadol	Ortho-McNeil	Non-Narcotic ℞†

† Ultram (tramadol) is metabolized to a weak mu agonist with narcotic analgesic properties

• New products ('95–'01): OxylR (immediate release oxycodone), OxyContin (12-hr controlled release oxycodone), Kadian (24-hr controlled release morphine), Duract (bromfenac).

* Discontinued: Duract (bromfenac).

Note: Generics are not shown. C-II, C-III, C-IV, and C-V designate narcotics regulated under the U.S. Controlled Substances Act. "Non-narcotic" designates higher efficacy non-controlled prescription products.

Note (2): hydromorphone (Dilaudid) and oxycodone (Numorphan) are also available in rectal suppositories.

SINGLE-ENTITY ANALGESICS, MODERATE-SEVERE PAIN

B. INJECTABLE PRODUCTS

TRADE NAME	COMPOSITION	DISTRIBUTOR	REGULATORY STATUS
Alfenta	alfentanil	Janssen	C-II
Astramorph	morphine	AstraZeneca	C-II
Buprenex	buprenorphine	Reckitt Benckiser	C-V
Dalgan	dezocine	AstraZeneca	Non-Narcotic ℞
Demerol	meperidine (pethidine)	Sanofi-Synthelabo	C-II
Dilaudid	hydromorphone	Knoll	C-II
Dolophine	methadone	Roxane	C-II
Duramorph	morphine	Elkins-Sinn	C-II
Infumorph	morphine	Elkins-Sinn	C-II
Levo-Dromoran	levorphanol	ICN	C-II
Levoprome	methotrimeprazine	Immunex	Non-Narcotic ℞
Mepergan	meperidine (pethidine) + promethazine	Wyeth-Ayerst	C-II
Nubain	nalbuphine	Endo	Non-Narcotic ℞
Numorphan	oxymorphone	Endo	C-II
Stadol†	butorphanol	Bristol-Myers Squibb	C-IV
Sublimaze	fentanyl	Taylor	C-II
Sufenta	sufentanil	Janssen	C-II
Talwin	pentazocine	Sanofi-Synthelabo	C-IV
Toradol	ketorolac	Syntex	Non-Narcotic ℞ (NSAID)

† Stadol is also available as an intranasal formulation (Stadol NS)

Note: Generics are not shown. C-II, C-III, C-IV, and C-V designate narcotics regulated under the U.S. Controlled Substances Act. "Non-narcotic" designates higher efficacy non-controlled prescription products.

MILD-MODERATE PAIN, ARTHRITIS, INFLAMMATION, FEVER: ANTI-INFLAMMATORY/ANTIPYRETIC ANALGESICS (NSAID; ORAL)

TRADE NAME	COMPOSITION	DISTRIBUTOR	REGULATORY STATUS
Actron	ketoprofen	Bayer	OTC
Advil	ibuprofen	Whitehall-Robins	OTC
Aleve	naproxen	Bayer	OTC
Anaprox	naproxen sodium	Roche	℞
Ansaid	flurbiprofen	Pharmacia & Upjohn	℞
Arthrotec	diclofenac + misoprostel	Searle	℞
Bayer aspirin	aspirin	Bayer	OTC
Cataflam	diclofenac potassium	Novartis	℞
Celebrex*	celecoxib	Searle-Pharmacia	℞
Clinoril	sulindac	Merck	℞
Daypro	oxaprozin	Searle	℞
Disalcid	salsalate	3M	℞
Dolobid	diflunisal	Merck	℞
Feldene	piroxicam	Pfizer	℞
Indocin	indomethacin	Merck	℞
Lodine	etodolac	Wyeth-Ayerst	℞
Mobic	meloxicam	Boehringer Ingelheim	℞
Motrin	ibuprofen	McNeil	OTC, ℞
Nalfon	fenoprofen	Dista	℞
Naprelan	naproxen (controlled rel.)	Wyeth-Ayerst	℞
Naprosyn	naproxen	Roche	℞
Nuprin	ibuprofen	Bristol-Myers	OTC
Orudis	ketoprofen	Wyeth-Ayerst	OTC, ℞
Oruvail	ketoprofen (controlled rel.)	Wyeth-Ayerst	℞
Ponstel	mefenamic acid	Parke-Davis	℞
Relafen	nabumetone	GlaxoSmithKline	℞
Tolectin	tolmetin sodium	Ortho-McNeil	℞
Trilisate	choline magnesium trisalicylate	Purdue Frederick	℞
Tylenol	acetaminophen	Ortho-McNeil	OTC
Vioxx*	rofecoxib	Merck	℞
Voltaren	diclofenac sodium	Novartis	℞

OTC = over-the-counter (non-prescription); ℞ = Prescription

* COX-2 selective

• New products ('95–'01): Naprelan (24-hr controlled release naproxen), Arthrotec (diclofenac + misoprostel), Celebrex (celecoxib), Vioxx (rofecoxib), Mobic (meloxicam).

Discontinued: Meclomen (meclofenamate, Parke-Davis); may still be available as generic

Note: Generics, multiple brand names of aspirin, acetaminophen, ibuprofen, and OTC combination products with other analgesics, sedatives, anxiolytics, caffeine, muscle relaxants, or other products are not shown. Acetaminophen (a non-NSAID) lacks anti-inflammatory activity.

MIGRAINE PAIN (ORAL UNLESS OTHERWISE INDICATED):

TRADE NAME	COMPOSITION	DISTRIBUTOR	REGULATORY STATUS
Amerge	naratriptan	Glaxo Wellcome	℞
Blockadren	timolol	Merck	℞
Cafergot	ergotamine + caffeine (oral, suppository)	Novartis	℞
Depakote	divalproex sodium	Abbott	℞
D.H.E.	dihydroergotamine (inj.)	Novartis	℞
Ergomar	ergotamine (sublingual)	Lotus	℞
Excedrin Migraine	aspirin, APAP, caffeine	Bristol-Myers	OTC
Inderal	propranolol (oral, inj.)	Wyeth-Ayerst	℞
Imitrex	sumitriptan (oral, inj., nasal)	Glaxo Wellcome	℞
Maxalt	rizatriptan	Merck	℞
Midrin	isometheptene, dichloralphenazone, APAP	Carnrick	℞
Migranal	dihydroergotamine (nasal)	Novartis	℞
Motrin migraine	ibuprofen	McNeil Consumer	OTC
Sansert	methysergide	Novartis	℞
Wigraine	ergotamine + caffeine	Organon	℞
Zomig	zolmitriptan	AstraZeneca	℞

OTC = over-the-counter (non-prescription); ℞ = Prescription

APAP = acetaminophen

• New Products ('97–'98): Amerge (naratriptan), Migranal (nasal dihydroergotamine), Imitrex-nasal (sumitriptan), Zomig (zolmitriptan), Maxalt (rizatriptan)

Note: Beta blockers and divalproex (valproic acid) are intended only for prophylaxis. Ergotamine and methysergide are intended for prophylaxis or treatment. Other products are indicated only for treatment.

SPECIAL USE ANALGESICS

TRADE NAME	COMPOSITION	DISTRIBUTOR	REGULATORY STATUS
Actiq	fentanyl, oral transmucosal Use limited to break-through cancer pain in combination with opioids	Anesta	C-II
Duraclon	clonidine, epidural Use limited to cancer pain in combination with opioids	Roxane	℞
Duragesic	fentanyl, transdermal Use limited to chronic pain & cancer pain	Janssen	C-II
Elmiron	pentosan polysulfate interstitial cystitis; bladder pain	Alza	℞
Fentanyl Oralet	fentanyl, transmucosal pediatric and adult preanesthestic; "monitored anesthesia care"	Abbott	C-II
Hyalgan	sodium hyaluronate intra-articular joint lubricant for osteoarthritis of the knee (5 weekly injections)	Sanofi-Synthelabo	℞
Lidoderm Patch	lidocaine (5%) dermal patch Use limited to post-herpetic neuralgia	Endo	℞
Metastron	Strontium-89 chloride Radionuclide for metastatic bone cancer	Amersham	℞
Naropin	ropivacaine anesthetic-analgesic (spinal, epidural, local)	AstraZeneca	℞
Quadramet	Samarium 153-EDTMP Radionuclide for metastatic bone cancer	DuPont Merck	℞
Synvisc	hylan A + hylan B intra-articular joint lubricant for osteoarthritis of the knee (3 weekly injections)	Wyeth-Ayerst	℞
Ultiva	remifentanil Ultra-short acting mu agonist analgesic-anesthetic	GlaxoSmithKline	C-II

℞ = Prescription.

• New products ('95–'01): Duraclon (epidural clonidine), Elmiron (pentosan polysulfate), Hyalgan (hyaluronate), Lidoderm (lidocaine patch), Naropin (ropivacaine), Quadramet (Sm 153-EDTMP), Synvisc (hylan), Ultiva (remifentanil)

General use local anesthetics are not shown.

Appendix II: 21–Year Survey of Analgesics in Development for Treatment of Acute or Chronic Pain

Ref.: Pharmaprojects (updated to 2/02) used with permission; Scrip, corporate, literature & patent references
"Status" is international drug development or regulatory status and may not indicate status in USA
Sponsor: Original company name is retained if product is discontinued or inactive after merger, acquisition, company name change, etc.
Users of this table are encouraged to independently verify the status, activity, and mechanism of action of drugs of interest

GENERIC / TRADE NAME	STATUS	SPONSOR (S)	MECHANISM OF ACTION	REF. UPDATE
SORTED BY MECHANISM OF ACTION / THERAPEUTIC ACTIVITY				
ADENOSINE / ANTAGONISTS				
SEP-89068 / SEP-42960	Discontinued	Sepracor (US)	Adenosine A2A / A3 antags.	Jun-00
L-249313	Discontinued	Merck & Co (US)	Adenosine A3 antagonist (inflam.)	Sep-99
UP-202-32	Discontinued	Bristol-Myers Squibb / UPSA	Adenosine agonist	Mar-97
5'd-5IT	Discontinued	Abbott (US)	Adenosine kinase inhibitor	Oct-99
GP-1-515	Discontinued	Metabasis Therapeutics	Adenosine regulating agent (ARA)	Feb-02
GR-79236	Discontinued (ph. I)	Glaxo Wellcome (UK)	Adenosine A1 agonist	1998
GP-04012	Inactive	Metabasis Therapeutics	Adenosine A1 agonist/antag.	Feb-02
Pharmaprojects No. 3775	Preclinical	Novo-Nordisk (Denmark)	Adenosine A1 antagonist	Nov-93
ADRENERGICS				
Pharmaprojects No. 5623	Discontinued	Johnson & Johnson (US)	Alpha-2 agonist	Jun-99
RWJ-52807	Discontinued	Johnson & Johnson (US)	Alpha-2 agonist	Feb-02
Alpha-2 agonists	Discontinued	Synaptic (US)	Alpha-2a, 2b, 2c agonists	May-99
Pharmaprojects No. 4931	Discontinued	Allergan (US)	Alpha-2a+2b+2c agonist	1997
Clonidine, intrathecal	Discontinued	Orphan Medical / Medtronic	Clonidine intrathecal	May-98
FG-5530	Discontinued	Kabi Pharmacia (Sweden)	Clonidine-like neurolep.	Mar-89
Azepexole	Discontinued (ph. II)	Boehringer Ingelheim (Ger)	Alpha-2 agonist	1983
Chinoin-150 (JATE-1023)	Discontinued (ph. II)	Chinoin (Hungary)	Beta-1 adrenergic antagonist	Jun-86
CP-18534-1	Inactive	Pfizer (US)	Alpha-2 agonist	1986
RWJ-52353	Inactive	Johnson & Johnson (US)	Alpha-2 agonist	Feb-02
U-47,476A	Inactive	Upjohn (US)	Alpha-2 agonist	1985
MPV-2426	Inactive	Orion Pharma (Finland)	Alpha-2(a+b+c) agonist (spinal)	Feb-02
Dexmedetomidine (spinal)	LAUNCHED	Orion (Finland) / Abbott (US)	Alpha-2 agonist sedative-analgesic	Dec-99
Clonidine (DURACLON™ epidural)	LAUNCHED	Roxane (US) / Fujisawa	Formulation, epidural; cancer	Jan-97
Pharmaprojects No. 5761	Preclinical	Synaptic (US) / Gruenenthal (Ger)	Alpha-2 agonist	Mar-98
2-amino imidazole derivatives	Preclinical	Allergan (US)	Alpha-2 agonist / peripheral	Sep-95
ANALGESIC COMBINATIONS				
oxycodone + naloxone, Purdue	CLINICAL	Purdue Pharma (US)	Analgesic combination	Feb-02
ROBAXACET®	CLINICAL	Wyeth-Ayerst (US)	Methocarbamol + APAP	May-93
Etodolac + dextromethorphan	CLINICAL (I)	Algos (US)	Etodolac + dextromethorphan	May-97
HydrocoDex	CLINICAL (II)	Endo / Algos (US)	Hydrocodone + dextromethorphan	Feb-02
Ibuprofen + dextromethorphan	CLINICAL (II)	Algos (US) / J&J (US)	Ibuprofen + dextromethorphan	May-97
PTI-501 (morphine + naloxone)	CLINICAL (II)	Pain Therapeutics (US)	morphine + ultra low dose antag.	Feb-02
PTI-555 (morphine + naltrexone)	CLINICAL (II)	Pain Therapeutics (US)	morphine + ultra low dose antag.	Feb-02
hydromorphone combination	CLINICAL (II)	Pain Therapeutics (US)	Opioid + low dose antagonist	Feb-02
OxycoDex® combination	CLINICAL (II)	Endo / Algos (US)	Oxycodone + dextromethorphan	Jun-00
PTI-801 (oxycodone + naltrexone)	CLINICAL (II)	Pain Therapeutics (US)	oxycodone + ultra low dose antag.	Feb-02
amitriptyline+ketamine,Epitome	CLINICAL (II)	EpiCept (US) / Epitome (Canada)	Topical; neuropathy, surg. pain	Feb-02
MorphiDex® combination	CLINICAL (III)	Endo / Algos (US)	Morphine + dextromethorphan	Feb-02
Acetaminophen + dextromethorphan	CLINICAL (III)	Algos (US) / J&J (US)	OTC: APAP + dextromethorphan	May-97
Dextromethorphan comb.	Discontinued	Whitby Pharmaceut. (US)	Dextr.+ antacids + antiflat.	1984
Ibuprofen + codeine	Discontinued	Alza (US)	Ibuprofen + opioid	Mar-89
Nalbuphine combinations	Discontinued	DuPont Merck (US)	Indomethacin combination	Sep-84
Ibuprofen + dihydrocodeine	Discontinued (ph. II)	IVX BioSciences (US)	Formulation, oral	Sep-96
oxycodone + paracetamol, Barr	Inactive	Barr Laboratories (US)	Analgesic combination	Feb-02
ibuprofen (CR) + codeine, Napp	LAUNCHED	Napp (UK)	Analgesic combination	Feb-02
feprazone+paracetamol+guaifen	LAUNCHED	Schwarz (Ger)	Analgesic combination	Feb-02
trimebutine + ruscogenines	LAUNCHED	Pfizer (US)	Analgesic combination	Feb-02
paracetamol+dihydrocodeine	LAUNCHED	Napp (UK)	Analgesic combination	Feb-02
Diclofenac + misoprostol (Arthrotec®)	LAUNCHED	Searle/Monsanto (US)	Cytoprotective formulation	Nov-96
Ibuprofen combination	LAUNCHED	Adcock Ingram (RSA)	Ibuprofen + APAP + codeine	Apr-92
Ibuprofen + codeine	LAUNCHED	Boots (UK)	Ibuprofen + opioid (low dose)	1995
VISCERALGINE FORTE®	LAUNCHED	Akzo (Netherlands)	Muscarinic + anti-inflam.	Dec-91
Ibuprofen+hydrocodone (VICOPROFEN®)	LAUNCHED	Knoll (Germany) / Abbott (US)	Oral combination analgesic	Apr-98
Lidocaine + Dex. (LidoDex-NS®)	Preclinical	Algos (US) / Interneuron (US)	Lidocaine + dextromethorphan	Feb-97
oxycodone + ibuprofen, BTG	PRE-REGISTRATION	Forest (US) / BTG	Analgesic combination	Feb-02
ibuprofen + codeine,bioMerieux	PRE-REGISTRATION	bioMerieux-Pierre Fabre (France)	Formulation, oral combination	Feb-02

Ref.: Pharmaprojects (updated to 2/02) used with permission; Scrip, corporate, literature & patent references
"Status" is international drug development or regulatory status and may not indicate status in USA
Sponsor: Original company name is retained if product is discontinued or inactive after merger, acquisition, company name change, etc.
Users of this table are encouraged to independently verify the status, activity, and mechanism of action of drugs of interest

GENERIC / TRADE NAME	STATUS	SPONSOR (S)	MECHANISM OF ACTION	REF. UPDATE
Ibuprofen + oxycodone	PRE-REGISTRATION	Forest Laboratories (US)	Ibuprofen + opioid	Feb-02
ANTI-INFLAMMATORY / ANTIARTHRITIC (PGSI, COX, 5-LO, TNF, MMP, etc.)				
LAS-33826	CLINICAL	Almirall-Prodesfarma (Spain)	Antiarthritic	Feb-02
Bindarit	CLINICAL	Angelini (Italy)	Anti-inflammatory	Jun-93
GP-03	CLINICAL (I)	BioPhausia (Sweden)	Antiarthritic	Feb-02
IRA-378	CLINICAL (I)	Kyorin	Antiarthritic	Feb-02
ONO-4817	CLINICAL (I)	Ono (Japan)	Antiarthritic	Feb-02
Ro-320-1195	CLINICAL (I)	Roche (Switz)	Antiarthritic	Feb-02
SMP-114	CLINICAL (I)	Sumitomo (Japan)	Antiarthritic	Feb-02
SCIO-469	CLINICAL (I)	Scios (US)	Antiarthritic	Feb-02
RWJ-67657	CLINICAL (I)	Johnson & Johnson (US)	Antiarthritic	Feb-02
BIRB-796	CLINICAL (I)	Boehringer Ingelheim (Ger)	Antiarthritic	Feb-02
SB-273005	CLINICAL (I)	GlaxoSmithKline (UK)	Antiarthritic	Feb-02
ABT-963	CLINICAL (I)	Abbott (US)	Antiarthritic	Feb-02
SVT-2016	CLINICAL (I)	SALVAT	Antiarthritic	Feb-02
NGD-2000-1	CLINICAL (I)	Neurogen (US)	Antiinflammatory	Feb-02
E-6087	CLINICAL (I)	Esteve (Spain)	Antiinflammatory	Feb-02
IC-485	CLINICAL (I)	ICOS (US)	Antiinflammatory	Feb-02
IPL-512602	CLINICAL (I)	Inflazyme (US)	Antiinflammatory	Feb-02
IPL-550260	CLINICAL (I)	Inflazyme (US)	Antiinflammatory	Feb-02
L-791456	CLINICAL (I)	Merck & Co (US)	COX-2 inhibitor	Sep-99
Dextromethorphan, IriSys	CLINICAL (I)	Avanir (US) / IriSys (US)	Dextrometh. + P450/2D6 inhib.	Jun-99
D-5410	CLINICAL (I)	Chiroscience (UK)	MMP / TNF convertase inhibitor	Mar-97
D-1927	CLINICAL (I)	Celltech (UK)	MMP inhibitor / antiinflammatory	Feb-02
dersalazine	CLINICAL (I)	Uriach (Spain)	NSAID	Feb-02
ketoprofen, NexACT	CLINICAL (I)	NexMed	NSAID	Feb-02
2-ethoxybenzoic acid	CLINICAL (I)	Pfleger	NSAID	Feb-02
GW-406381	CLINICAL (I)	GlaxoSmithKline (UK)	NSAID	Feb-02
Piroxicam, Anesta	CLINICAL (I)	Cephalon (US)	NSAID	Jun-00
NCX-701	CLINICAL (I)	NicOx (France)	NSAID + NO releaser	Feb-02
Bay 12-9566	CLINICAL (I)	Bayer (Germany)	Stromelysin inhibitor; OA	Jun-97
SelCID	CLINICAL (I)	Celgene (US)	TNF-alpha inhibitor	Dec-97
DPC-333	CLINICAL (II)	Bristol-Myers Squibb (US)	Antiarthritic	Feb-02
THC:CBD broad ratio, GW Pharm	CLINICAL (II)	GW Pharmaceuticals (UK)	Antiarthritic	Feb-02
S-2474	CLINICAL (II)	Shionogi (Japan)	Antiarthritic	Feb-02
BMS-347070	CLINICAL (II)	Bristol-Myers Squibb (US)	Antiinflammatory	Feb-02
S-3013	CLINICAL (II)	Shionogi (Japan)	Antiinflammatory	Feb-02
JTE-607	CLINICAL (II)	Japan Tobacco (Japan)	Antiinflammatory	Feb-02
PBI-1101	CLINICAL (II)	ProMetic LifeSciences	Antiinflammatory	Feb-02
CNI-1493	CLINICAL (II)	Cytokine PharmaSciences	Antiinflammatory	Feb-02
IPR-6001	CLINICAL (II)	Inst. Pharm Research (Switz)	Antiinflammatory / chronic pain	Feb-97
TAK-603	CLINICAL (II)	Takeda (Japan)	Bone formation stimulant	Jun-96
5G1.1-SC	CLINICAL (II)	Alexion (US)	C5a complement inhibitor	Oct-97
CI-1004	CLINICAL (II)	Warner-Lambert (US)	COX-2 / 5-LO inhibitor; OA/RA	Apr-98
CS-502	CLINICAL (II)	Sankyo (Japan)	COX-2 inhibitor	Feb-02
JTE-522	CLINICAL (II)	Japan Tobacco / J&J (US)	COX-2 inhibitor (RA, OA)	Dec-97
CBF-BS2	CLINICAL (II)	KS Biomedix (UK)	G6PDH inhib. (glucose 6-PO4 DH)	Dec-96
Superoxide dismutase (PC-SOD)	CLINICAL (II)	Seikagaku Kogyo (Japan)	Lecithinized superoxide dismutase	Jun-99
FK-011	CLINICAL (II)	Fujisawa (Japan)	Leukotriene antagonist	Jul-97
Ro-1130830	CLINICAL (II)	Roche (Switz)	Metalloproteinase inhibitor	Jun-00
Pharmaprojects No. 5179	CLINICAL (II)	Bayer (Germany)	MMP (Metalloproteinase inhibitor)	Nov-96
Cizolirtine citrate (E-4018)	CLINICAL (II)	Esteve (Spain)	NSAID	Mar-98
Eltenac	CLINICAL (II)	Byk Gulden (Ger) / Sankyo (Jp)	NSAID	Apr-98
(R)-ketoprofen, Sepracor	CLINICAL (II)	Sepracor (US)	NSAID (single isomer)	Feb-02
HCT-3012	CLINICAL (II)	NicOx (France)	NSAID + NO releaser	Feb-02
P-07	CLINICAL (II)	Novogen (Australia)	Phytoestrogen form. (mastalgia)	Jul-98
PEGsTHFr1	CLINICAL (II)	Amgen (US)	TNF receptor antagonist / RA	Nov-99
TRK-530	CLINICAL (II)	Toray (Japan)	Unidentified antiarthritic	Jun-00
CDP-870	CLINICAL (II)	Celltech (UK)	Unidentified anti-inflammatory	Feb-99
NC-503 (Fibrillex)	CLINICAL (III)	Neurochem (Canada)	Amyloid deposit inhibitor (arthritis)	Mar-00
ST-1482	CLINICAL (III)	Sigma-Tau (Italy)	Antiarthritic	Feb-02
ML-3000	CLINICAL (III)	Merckle (Germany)	COX + 5-LO inhibitor	Feb-02

Ref.: Pharmaprojects (updated to 2/02) used with permission; Scrip, corporate, literature & patent references
"Status" is international drug development or regulatory status and may not indicate status in USA
Sponsor: Original company name is retained if product is discontinued or inactive after merger, acquisition, company name change, etc.
Users of this table are encouraged to independently verify the status, activity, and mechanism of action of drugs of interest

GENERIC / TRADE NAME	STATUS	SPONSOR (S)	MECHANISM OF ACTION	REF. UPDATE
COX-189	CLINICAL (III)	Novartis (Switz.)	COX-2 inhibitor	Feb-02
MK-663	CLINICAL (III)	Merck & Co (US)	COX-2 inhibitor (RA, OA, pain)	Jan-00
Pelubiprofen (CS-670)	CLINICAL (III)	Sankyo (Japan)	T cell stimulant, anti-inflam.	Mar-98
Pharmaprojects No. 4702	Discontinued	Wyeth-Ayerst (US)	5-Lipoxygenase (5-LO) inhib.	May-98
Pharmaprojects No. 4710	Discontinued	Servier (France)	5-Lipoxygenase (5-LO) inhib.	May-99
CGS-25997	Discontinued	Novartis (Switz.)	5-Lipoxygenase (5-LO) inhibitor	Sep-98
CGS-26529	Discontinued	Novartis (Switz.)	5-Lipoxygenase (5-LO) inhibitor	May-98
ER-34122	Discontinued	Eisai (Japan)	5-LO / COX inhibitor	Jun-99
eprovafen	Discontinued	Aventis (France)	5-LO inhibitor	Feb-02
ICI-211965 (ICI-216800)	Discontinued	Zeneca (UK)	5-LO inhibitor	Aug-92
Pharmaprojects No. 3444	Discontinued	Lilly (US)	5-LO inhibitor	Nov-94
Pharmaprojects No. 4890	Discontinued	Searle/Monsanto (US)	5-LO inhibitor	Dec-97
R-85355	Discontinued	Janssen / J&J (US)	5-LO inhibitor	Dec-94
RWJ-63556	Discontinued	Johnson & Johnson (US)	5-LO inhibitor; anti-inflam.	Mar-99
Pharmaprojects No. 5999	Discontinued	Procter & Gamble (US)	5-LO/COX-2 inhibitor; RA, OA	Jun-00
Methotrexate analogs	Discontinued	SRI International (US)	60 MTX analogs / RA	Mar-99
Pharmaprojects No. 5262	Discontinued	Bayer (Germany)	Acetylsalicyclic acid + NO	Sep-98
Pharmaprojects No. 3553	Discontinued	Novartis (Switz.)	Antiarthritic	May-98
aminothiophenols	Discontinued	ISIS Innovation	Antiarthritic	Feb-02
ATSA	Discontinued	Pharmacia (US)	Antiarthritic	Feb-02
clobuzarit	Discontinued	AstraZeneca (UK)	Antiarthritic	Feb-02
collagen antagonists, Xoma	Discontinued	Xoma (US)	Antiarthritic	Feb-02
EN-780	Discontinued	Bristol-Myers Squibb (US)	Antiarthritic	Feb-02
GP-44	Discontinued	Protherics	Antiarthritic	Feb-02
GYKI-44688	Discontinued	ICN (US)	Antiarthritic	Feb-02
honey bee venom	Discontinued	Pharmacia (US)	Antiarthritic	Feb-02
HYC-141	Discontinued	Fidia (Italy)	Antiarthritic	Feb-02
ICI-115432	Discontinued	AstraZeneca (UK)	Antiarthritic	Feb-02
lotifazole	Discontinued	bioMerieux-Pierre Fabre (France)	Antiarthritic	Feb-02
neutrophil elastase inhib, Imm	Discontinued	Texas Biotechnology	Antiarthritic	Feb-02
nicocortonide	Discontinued	Yamanouchi (Japan)	Antiarthritic	Feb-02
NPC-17923	Discontinued	Scios (US)	Antiarthritic	Feb-02
oxindanac	Discontinued	Novartis (Switz.)	Antiarthritic	Feb-02
Pharmaprojects No. 1261	Discontinued	Aventis (France)	Antiarthritic	Feb-02
Pharmaprojects No. 2015	Discontinued	Bristol-Myers Squibb (US)	Antiarthritic	Feb-02
Pharmaprojects No. 2029	Discontinued	American Home Products (US)	Antiarthritic	Feb-02
Pharmaprojects No. 2193	Discontinued	Abbott (US)	Antiarthritic	Feb-02
Pharmaprojects No. 2850	Discontinued	Kureha Chemical	Antiarthritic	Feb-02
Pharmaprojects No. 3240	Discontinued	Boehringer Ingelheim (Ger)	Antiarthritic	Feb-02
Pharmaprojects No. 3282	Discontinued	Biofor (US)	Antiarthritic	Feb-02
Pharmaprojects No. 3647	Discontinued	Abbott (US)	Antiarthritic	Feb-02
Pharmaprojects No. 4079	Discontinued	Bristol-Myers Squibb (US)	Antiarthritic	Feb-02
PKH152	Discontinued	CytRx (US)	Antiarthritic	Feb-02
Ro-31-9790	Discontinued	Roche (Switz)	Antiarthritic	Feb-02
S-16276-1	Discontinued	Servier (France)	Antiarthritic	Feb-02
SC-106	Discontinued	Scotia (UK)	Antiarthritic	Feb-02
SKF-104351	Discontinued	GlaxoSmithKline (UK)	Antiarthritic	Feb-02
SKF-36914	Discontinued	GlaxoSmithKline (UK)	Antiarthritic	Feb-02
spirogermanium, Unimed	Discontinued	Solvay (Netherlands)	Antiarthritic	Feb-02
ST-875	Discontinued	bioMerieux-Pierre Fabre (France)	Antiarthritic	Feb-02
TMC-851	Discontinued	Taiyo Pharmaceutical	Antiarthritic	Feb-02
TSC-5	Discontinued	Takeda (Japan)	Antiarthritic	Feb-02
U-24522	Discontinued	AstraZeneca (UK)	Antiarthritic	Feb-02
BB-2983	Discontinued	British Biotech (UK)	Antiarthritic	Feb-02
CH-138	Discontinued	Celltech (UK)	Antiarthritic	Feb-02
Pharmaprojects No. 2434	Discontinued	Novartis Consumer (Switz.)	Antiarthritic	Feb-02
superoxide dismutase, QLT	Discontinued	QLT	Antiarthritic	Feb-02
superoxide dismutase, Takeda	Discontinued	Takeda (Japan)	Antiarthritic	Feb-02
Wy-45368	Discontinued	American Home Products (US)	Antiarthritic	Feb-02
tiflamizole	Discontinued	Bristol-Myers Squibb (US)	Antiarthritic	Feb-02
AI-202	Discontinued	AutoImmune (US)	Antiarthritic	Feb-02
Pharmaprojects No. 919	Discontinued	American Home Products (US)	Antiarthritic	Feb-02
Pharmaprojects No. 3582	Discontinued	Pharmacia (US)	Antiarthritic	Feb-02

Ref.: Pharmaprojects (updated to 2/02) used with permission; Scrip, corporate, literature & patent references
"Status" is international drug development or regulatory status and may not indicate status in USA
Sponsor: Original company name is retained if product is discontinued or inactive after merger, acquisition, company name change, etc.
Users of this table are encouraged to independently verify the status, activity, and mechanism of action of drugs of interest

GENERIC / TRADE NAME	STATUS	SPONSOR (S)	MECHANISM OF ACTION	REF. UPDATE
ß-elemonic acid	Discontinued	Aventis (France)	Antiarthritic	Feb-02
BB-1101	Discontinued	British Biotech (UK)	Antiarthritic	Feb-02
dexindoprofen	Discontinued	Pharmacia (US)	Antiarthritic	Feb-02
DuP-697	Discontinued	Bristol-Myers Squibb (US)	Antiarthritic	Feb-02
flosulide	Discontinued	Schering AG (Germany)	Antiarthritic	Feb-02
tiopinac	Discontinued	Roche (Switz)	Antiarthritic	Feb-02
lodelaben	Discontinued	Pharmacia (US)	Antiarthritic	Feb-02
ZD-2138	Discontinued	AstraZeneca (UK)	Antiarthritic	Feb-02
tepoxalin	Discontinued	Johnson & Johnson (US)	Antiarthritic	Feb-02
leucotriene analogues, ResCo	Discontinued	Research Corp. Tech. (US)	Antiarthritic	Feb-02
Pharmaprojects No. 5152	Discontinued	Merck (US) / CollaGenex (US)	Antiarthritic (unknown)	Jul-98
Mesoporphyrin	Discontinued	Taiho (Japan)	Antiarthritic T-cell inhibitor	Feb-98
MMP inhibitors, NIH	Discontinued	NIH (US)	Antibodies; type IV collagenase	Nov-98
A-162-ester	Discontinued	Alpharma (US)	Antiinflammatory	Feb-02
A-52795	Discontinued	Abbott (US)	Antiinflammatory	Feb-02
AH-7170	Discontinued	GlaxoSmithKline (UK)	Antiinflammatory	Feb-02
AMA-60	Discontinued	Kureha Chemical	Antiinflammatory	Feb-02
anti-inflammatories, Karo	Discontinued	Karo Bio (Sweden)	Antiinflammatory	Feb-02
ANW-82	Discontinued	Boehringer Ingelheim (Ger)	Antiinflammatory	Feb-02
AY-24873	Discontinued	American Home Products (US)	Antiinflammatory	Feb-02
AZER	Discontinued	Pliva	Antiinflammatory	Feb-02
bendazac meglumine	Discontinued	Therapicon (Italy)	Antiinflammatory	Feb-02
BI-L-93BS	Discontinued	Boehringer Ingelheim (Ger)	Antiinflammatory	Feb-02
BN-50370	Discontinued	Beaufour-Ipsen (France)	Antiinflammatory	Feb-02
BR-703	Discontinued	Italfarmaco (Italy)	Antiinflammatory	Feb-02
BW-70C	Discontinued	GlaxoSmithKline (UK)	Antiinflammatory	Feb-02
BW-755C	Discontinued	GlaxoSmithKline (UK)	Antiinflammatory	Feb-02
calcineurin inhibitors, Ag	Discontinued	Pfizer (US)	Antiinflammatory	Feb-02
carbazomycin B	Discontinued	Bristol-Myers Squibb (US)	Antiinflammatory	Feb-02
CBS-1108	Discontinued	Bausch & Lomb (US)	Antiinflammatory	Feb-02
CGP-25157	Discontinued	Novartis (Switz.)	Antiinflammatory	Feb-02
CGP-47900	Discontinued	Novartis (Switz.)	Antiinflammatory	Feb-02
CGS-22745	Discontinued	Novartis (Switz.)	Antiinflammatory	Feb-02
CGS-23885	Discontinued	Novartis (Switz.)	Antiinflammatory	Feb-02
CHF-1021	Discontinued	Chiesi (Italy)	Antiinflammatory	Feb-02
CHF-1909	Discontinued	Chiesi (Italy)	Antiinflammatory	Feb-02
cicloprofen	Discontinued	Bristol-Myers Squibb (US)	Antiinflammatory	Feb-02
clopirac	Discontinued	Pharmacia (US)	Antiinflammatory	Feb-02
CP-0364	Discontinued	Cortech (US)	Antiinflammatory	Feb-02
CT-737	Discontinued	American Home Products (US)	Antiinflammatory	Feb-02
D-10242	Discontinued	Asta Medica (Germany)	Antiinflammatory	Feb-02
ENA	Discontinued	Mediolanum	Antiinflammatory	Feb-02
ethanoarachidonic acids, ResCo	Discontinued	Research Corp. Tech. (US)	Antiinflammatory	Feb-02
etodolac meglumine	Discontinued	Therapicon (Italy)	Antiinflammatory	Feb-02
evandamine	Discontinued	Aventis (France)	Antiinflammatory	Feb-02
flazalone	Discontinued	3M (US)	Antiinflammatory	Feb-02
fluquazone	Discontinued	Merck & Co (US)	Antiinflammatory	Feb-02
foliaspongin	Discontinued	Fujisawa (Japan)	Antiinflammatory	Feb-02
folipastatin	Discontinued	Sankyo (Japan)	Antiinflammatory	Feb-02
furaprofen	Discontinued	3M (US)	Antiinflammatory	Feb-02
furcloprofen	Discontinued	Roche (Switz)	Antiinflammatory	Feb-02
GP-53633	Discontinued	Novartis (Switz.)	Antiinflammatory	Feb-02
GYKI-66114	Discontinued	Gedeon Richter	Antiinflammatory	Feb-02
hexaprofen	Discontinued	Uriach (Spain)	Antiinflammatory	Feb-02
IND-9	Discontinued	Alter	Antiinflammatory	Feb-02
intrazole	Discontinued	Bristol-Myers Squibb (US)	Antiinflammatory	Feb-02
KF-17515	Discontinued	Kyowa Hakko (Japan)	Antiinflammatory	Feb-02
KF-18280	Discontinued	Kyowa Hakko (Japan)	Antiinflammatory	Feb-02
L-8322	Discontinued	Aventis (France)	Antiinflammatory	Feb-02
LC-546	Discontinued	Alcon (US)	Antiinflammatory	Feb-02
leucotriene antags, Aventis	Discontinued	Aventis (France)	Antiinflammatory	Feb-02
LS-4249	Discontinued	BTG (UK)	Antiinflammatory	Feb-02
LU-20884	Discontinued	Abbott (US)	Antiinflammatory	Feb-02

Ref.: Pharmaprojects (updated to 2/02) used with permission; Scrip, corporate, literature & patent references
"Status" is international drug development or regulatory status and may not indicate status in USA
Sponsor: Original company name is retained if product is discontinued or inactive after merger, acquisition, company name change, etc.
Users of this table are encouraged to independently verify the status, activity, and mechanism of action of drugs of interest

GENERIC / TRADE NAME	STATUS	SPONSOR (S)	MECHANISM OF ACTION	REF. UPDATE
LY-280810	Discontinued	Lilly (US)	Antiinflammatory	Feb-02
metbufen	Discontinued	American Home Products (US)	Antiinflammatory	Feb-02
morniflumate	Discontinued	Aventis (France)	Antiinflammatory	Feb-02
MS-731	Discontinued	Schering AG (Germany)	Antiinflammatory	Feb-02
NE 1704	Discontinued	Neose Technologies	Antiinflammatory	Feb-02
nitrosoxacin-A	Discontinued	Bristol-Myers Squibb (US)	Antiinflammatory	Feb-02
odalprofen	Discontinued	Chiesi (Italy)	Antiinflammatory	Feb-02
ONO-5349	Discontinued	Ono (Japan)	Antiinflammatory	Feb-02
oxaprozin meglumine	Discontinued	Therapicon (Italy)	Antiinflammatory	Feb-02
Pharmaprojects No. 1001	Discontinued	Bristol-Myers Squibb (US)	Antiinflammatory	Feb-02
Pharmaprojects No. 12059	Discontinued	Abbott (US)	Antiinflammatory	Feb-02
Pharmaprojects No. 1302	Discontinued	Bristol-Myers Squibb (US)	Antiinflammatory	Feb-02
Pharmaprojects No. 1524	Discontinued	American Home Products (US)	Antiinflammatory	Feb-02
Pharmaprojects No. 1657	Discontinued	Schering AG (Germany)	Antiinflammatory	Feb-02
Pharmaprojects No. 1660	Discontinued	Roche (Switz)	Antiinflammatory	Feb-02
Pharmaprojects No. 1749	Discontinued	GlaxoSmithKline (UK)	Antiinflammatory	Feb-02
Pharmaprojects No. 1763	Discontinued	Kayaku	Antiinflammatory	Feb-02
Pharmaprojects No. 1860	Discontinued	Schering Plough (US)	Antiinflammatory	Feb-02
Pharmaprojects No. 1967	Discontinued	Schering Plough (US)	Antiinflammatory	Feb-02
Pharmaprojects No. 1970	Discontinued	AstraZeneca (UK)	Antiinflammatory	Feb-02
Pharmaprojects No. 2157	Discontinued	Pharmacia (US)	Antiinflammatory	Feb-02
Pharmaprojects No. 2167	Discontinued	Toa Eiyo	Antiinflammatory	Feb-02
Pharmaprojects No. 2332	Discontinued	Roche (Switz)	Antiinflammatory	Feb-02
Pharmaprojects No. 2503	Discontinued	Kaken (Japan)	Antiinflammatory	Feb-02
Pharmaprojects No. 2541	Discontinued	Mitsubishi Pharma (Japan)	Antiinflammatory	Feb-02
Pharmaprojects No. 2553	Discontinued	Abbott (US)	Antiinflammatory	Feb-02
Pharmaprojects No. 2660	Discontinued	Dainippon (Japan)	Antiinflammatory	Feb-02
Pharmaprojects No. 2662	Discontinued	Sanofi-Synthelabo (France)	Antiinflammatory	Feb-02
Pharmaprojects No. 2794	Discontinued	Aventis (France)	Antiinflammatory	Feb-02
Pharmaprojects No. 3169	Discontinued	Oxford GlycoSciences (UK)	Antiinflammatory	Feb-02
Pharmaprojects No. 3258	Discontinued	Sanofi-Synthelabo (France)	Antiinflammatory	Feb-02
Pharmaprojects No. 3863	Discontinued	Peptech (Australia)	Antiinflammatory	Feb-02
Pharmaprojects No. 4107	Discontinued	GlaxoSmithKline (UK)	Antiinflammatory	Feb-02
Pharmaprojects No. 4234	Discontinued	Menarini (Italy)	Antiinflammatory	Feb-02
Pharmaprojects No. 647	Discontinued	Sanofi-Synthelabo (France)	Antiinflammatory	Feb-02
Pharmaprojects No. 929	Discontinued	American Home Products (US)	Antiinflammatory	Feb-02
phospholipase A2 inhib, La Jol	Discontinued	La Jolla Pharmaceutical	Antiinflammatory	Feb-02
phospholipase C inhibitor, Bri	Discontinued	British Biotech (UK)	Antiinflammatory	Feb-02
phospholipase C inhibitor, Med	Discontinued	Mediolanum	Antiinflammatory	Feb-02
phospholipase inhibitors, Poli	Discontinued	Polifarma (Italy)	Antiinflammatory	Feb-02
prenafen	Discontinued	Ferrer (Spain)	Antiinflammatory	Feb-02
pyrroben	Discontinued	Spofa	Antiinflammatory	Feb-02
Rev-5367	Discontinued	Aventis (France)	Antiinflammatory	Feb-02
Ro-1-9564	Discontinued	Roche (Switz)	Antiinflammatory	Feb-02
Ro-3-1314	Discontinued	Roche (Switz)	Antiinflammatory	Feb-02
robinosole	Discontinued	Inflazyme (US)	Antiinflammatory	Feb-02
RP 66364	Discontinued	Aventis (France)	Antiinflammatory	Feb-02
SDZ-210-610	Discontinued	Novartis (Switz.)	Antiinflammatory	Feb-02
SKF-104493	Discontinued	GlaxoSmithKline (UK)	Antiinflammatory	Feb-02
sudoxicam	Discontinued	Pfizer (US)	Antiinflammatory	Feb-02
TAI-764	Discontinued	Takeda (Japan)	Antiinflammatory	Feb-02
THC-1102	Discontinued	Therapicon (Italy)	Antiinflammatory	Feb-02
THC-1104	Discontinued	Therapicon (Italy)	Antiinflammatory	Feb-02
THC-1105	Discontinued	Therapicon (Italy)	Antiinflammatory	Feb-02
THC-1108	Discontinued	Therapicon (Italy)	Antiinflammatory	Feb-02
THC-1110	Discontinued	Therapicon (Italy)	Antiinflammatory	Feb-02
THC-1112	Discontinued	Therapicon (Italy)	Antiinflammatory	Feb-02
thielavins	Discontinued	Sankyo (Japan)	Antiinflammatory	Feb-02
tianafac	Discontinued	Sanofi-Synthelabo (France)	Antiinflammatory	Feb-02
tolmetin glycine amide	Discontinued	Johnson & Johnson (US)	Antiinflammatory	Feb-02
TY-10214	Discontinued	Toa Eiyo	Antiinflammatory	Feb-02
Wy-23205	Discontinued	American Home Products (US)	Antiinflammatory	Feb-02
ZG-1494Alpha	Discontinued	Novo Nordisk (Denmark)	Antiinflammatory	Feb-02

Ref.: Pharmaprojects (updated to 2/02) used with permission; Scrip, corporate, literature & patent references
"Status" is international drug development or regulatory status and may not indicate status in USA
Sponsor: Original company name is retained if product is discontinued or inactive after merger, acquisition, company name change, etc.
Users of this table are encouraged to independently verify the status, activity, and mechanism of action of drugs of interest

GENERIC / TRADE NAME	STATUS	SPONSOR (S)	MECHANISM OF ACTION	REF. UPDATE
ICI-10652	Discontinued	AstraZeneca (UK)	Antiinflammatory	Feb-02
CGP-47969A	Discontinued	Novartis (Switz.)	Antiinflammatory	Feb-02
GR-80907	Discontinued	GlaxoSmithKline (UK)	Antiinflammatory	Feb-02
anti-inflammatories, ResCo	Discontinued	Research Corp. Tech. (US)	Antiinflammatory	Feb-02
Sch-12223	Discontinued	Schering Plough (US)	Antiinflammatory	Feb-02
Pharmaprojects No. 1741	Discontinued	American Home Products (US)	Antiinflammatory	Feb-02
LN-1520	Discontinued	Roche (Switz)	Antiinflammatory	Feb-02
furofenac	Discontinued	Alfa Wassermann	Antiinflammatory	Feb-02
phospholipase inhibitor, Scios	Discontinued	Scios (US)	Antiinflammatory	Feb-02
Pharmaprojects No. 1673	Discontinued	Aventis (France)	Antiinflammatory	Feb-02
ER-3826	Discontinued	Eisai (Japan)	Antiinflammatory	Feb-02
superoxide dismutase, Tosoh	Discontinued	Tosoh Corporation	Antiinflammatory	Feb-02
Corleukin compounds	Discontinued	Corvas	Antiinflammatory	Feb-02
Pharmaprojects No. 1707	Discontinued	Novartis (Switz.)	Antiinflammatory	Feb-02
Pharmaprojects No. 3337	Discontinued	Manchester Innovation	Antiinflammatory	Feb-02
TAN-1515	Discontinued	Takeda (Japan)	Antiinflammatory	Feb-02
MDL-9563	Discontinued	Aventis (France)	Antiinflammatory	Feb-02
KC-8973	Discontinued	Kaken (Japan)	Antiinflammatory	Feb-02
ACP	Discontinued	Kureha Chemical	Antiinflammatory	Feb-02
collismycin A	Discontinued	Kirin Brewery	Antiinflammatory	Feb-02
SC-41661A	Discontinued	Pharmacia (US)	Antiinflammatory	Feb-02
GM7-050	Discontinued	Ligand (US)	Antiinflammatory	Feb-02
Pharmaprojects No. 3973	Discontinued	Schering Plough (US)	Antiinflammatory	Feb-02
Wy-28342	Discontinued	American Home Products (US)	Antiinflammatory	Feb-02
Pharmaprojects No. 2857	Discontinued	Vinas (Spain)	Antiinflammatory	Feb-02
pyrrolostatin	Discontinued	Kirin Brewery	Antiinflammatory	Feb-02
TR-35	Discontinued	Mitsubishi Pharma (Japan)	Antiinflammatory	Feb-02
seclazone	Discontinued	Wallace Pharmaceuticals	Antiinflammatory	Feb-02
EGIS-2829	Discontinued	Servier (France)	Antiinflammatory	Feb-02
prodolic acid	Discontinued	American Home Products (US)	Antiinflammatory	Feb-02
AD-1491	Discontinued	Dainippon (Japan)	Antiinflammatory	Feb-02
AFP-802	Discontinued	Recordati	Antiinflammatory	Feb-02
amfenac resinate	Discontinued	Meiji Seika (Japan)	Antiinflammatory	Feb-02
bermoprofen	Discontinued	Dainippon (Japan)	Antiinflammatory	Feb-02
CHF-2003	Discontinued	Chiesi (Italy)	Antiinflammatory	Feb-02
clofurac	Discontinued	Novartis (Switz.)	Antiinflammatory	Feb-02
CPP, Eisai	Discontinued	Eisai (Japan)	Antiinflammatory	Feb-02
F-1044	Discontinued	Procter & Gamble (US)	Antiinflammatory	Feb-02
F-2329	Discontinued	Faes (Spain)	Antiinflammatory	Feb-02
GP-650	Discontinued	Grelan	Antiinflammatory	Feb-02
H-88	Discontinued	Hisamitsu	Antiinflammatory	Feb-02
HAI-105	Discontinued	Hisamitsu	Antiinflammatory	Feb-02
HN-1857	Discontinued	Hisamitsu	Antiinflammatory	Feb-02
HN-2836	Discontinued	Hisamitsu	Antiinflammatory	Feb-02
IG-243-Na	Discontinued	Taiho (Japan)	Antiinflammatory	Feb-02
isofezolac	Discontinued	Aventis (France)	Antiinflammatory	Feb-02
KB-1043	Discontinued	Akzo Nobel (Netherlands)	Antiinflammatory	Feb-02
M-75168	Discontinued	Aventis (France)	Antiinflammatory	Feb-02
MG-18311	Discontinued	Sanofi-Synthelabo (France)	Antiinflammatory	Feb-02
MG-18755	Discontinued	Sanofi-Synthelabo (France)	Antiinflammatory	Feb-02
miroprofen	Discontinued	Mitsubishi Pharma (Japan)	Antiinflammatory	Feb-02
MR-653	Discontinued	Recordati	Antiinflammatory	Feb-02
MR-654	Discontinued	Recordati	Antiinflammatory	Feb-02
nitraquazone	Discontinued	Bayer (Germany)	Antiinflammatory	Feb-02
NS-398	Discontinued	Taisho (Japan)	Antiinflammatory	Feb-02
Pharmaprojects No. 1018	Discontinued	Novartis (Switz.)	Antiinflammatory	Feb-02
Pharmaprojects No. 1084	Discontinued	Mediolanum	Antiinflammatory	Feb-02
Pharmaprojects No. 1653	Discontinued	Recordati	Antiinflammatory	Feb-02
Pharmaprojects No. 1756	Discontinued	Alpharma (US)	Antiinflammatory	Feb-02
Pharmaprojects No. 1910	Discontinued	Abbott (US)	Antiinflammatory	Feb-02
Pharmaprojects No. 4717	Discontinued	GlaxoSmithKline (UK)	Antiinflammatory	Feb-02
Pharmaprojects No. 943	Discontinued	Bristol-Myers Squibb (US)	Antiinflammatory	Feb-02
PR-8	Discontinued	Dainippon (Japan)	Antiinflammatory	Feb-02

Ref.: Pharmaprojects (updated to 2/02) used with permission; Scrip, corporate, literature & patent references
"Status" is international drug development or regulatory status and may not indicate status in USA
Sponsor: Original company name is retained if product is discontinued or inactive after merger, acquisition, company name change, etc.
Users of this table are encouraged to independently verify the status, activity, and mechanism of action of drugs of interest

GENERIC / TRADE NAME	STATUS	SPONSOR (S)	MECHANISM OF ACTION	REF. UPDATE
SX-1032	Discontinued	SSP (Japan)	Antiinflammatory	Feb-02
tazeprofen	Discontinued	Merck KGaA (Germany)	Antiinflammatory	Feb-02
TY-10246	Discontinued	Toa Eiyo	Antiinflammatory	Feb-02
TY-10474	Discontinued	Toa Eiyo	Antiinflammatory	Feb-02
TZI-615	Discontinued	Teikoku Hormone	Antiinflammatory	Feb-02
YM-09561	Discontinued	Yamanouchi (Japan)	Antiinflammatory	Feb-02
YM-13162	Discontinued	Yamanouchi (Japan)	Antiinflammatory	Feb-02
AHR-6293	Discontinued	American Home Products (US)	Antiinflammatory	Feb-02
xenyhexenic acid	Discontinued	Aventis (France)	Antiinflammatory	Feb-02
Z-4003	Discontinued	Zambon	Antiinflammatory	Feb-02
AF/AI-1	Discontinued	Recordati	Antiinflammatory	Feb-02
CP-331	Discontinued	Zeria	Antiinflammatory	Feb-02
Wy-41770	Discontinued	American Home Products (US)	Antiinflammatory	Feb-02
AFP-860	Discontinued	Recordati	Antiinflammatory	Feb-02
SKF-86002	Discontinued	GlaxoSmithKline (UK)	Antiinflammatory	Feb-02
L-776967	Discontinued	Merck & Co (US)	Antiinflammatory	Feb-02
RP 67580	Discontinued	Aventis (France)	Antiinflammatory	Feb-02
Wy-19735	Discontinued	American Home Products (US)	Antiinflammatory	Feb-02
CGS-21595	Discontinued	Novartis (Switz.)	Antiinflammatory	Feb-02
epocarbazolin-A	Discontinued	Bristol-Myers Squibb (US)	Antiinflammatory	Feb-02
D-20682	Discontinued	Asta Medica (Germany)	Antiinflammatory	Feb-02
Pharmaprojects No. 2119	Discontinued	Roche (Switz)	Antiinflammatory	Feb-02
Pharmaprojects No. 4350	Discontinued	Abbott (US)	Antiinflammatory	Feb-02
Anti-inflammatories, Wyeth	Discontinued	Wyeth-Ayerst / Panlabs (US)	Anti-inflammatory	Dec-94
BIO-1006	Discontinued	Biogen (US)	Anti-inflammatory	Feb-98
Tetrandrine	Discontinued	Inst. Med. Res. (Australia)	Anti-inflammatory	Jun-94
Pharmaprojects No. 4206	Discontinued	Proteus Molecular Design (UK)	Antiinflammatory (unidentified)	May-98
Pharmaprojects No. 4809	Discontinued	Watson (US)	Antiinflammatory (unidentified)	Jun-00
Pharmaprojects No. 5036	Discontinued	Fujisawa (Japan)	Antiinflammatory (unidentified)	Jun-00
Pharmaprojects No. 4670	Discontinued	Servier (France)	Antiinflammatory (unspecified)	Jan-99
Pharmaprojects No. 5620	Discontinued	AstraZeneca (UK)	Antiinflammatory (unspecified)	Jun-99
Pharmaprojects No. 3505	Discontinued	Procter & Gamble (US)	Antiinflammatory / antiarthritic	May-98
BI-L-45XX	Discontinued	Boehringer Ingelheim (Ger.)	Antiinflammatory analgesic	Feb-87
MTDQ-DS	Discontinued	Human Inst. Serobac. Res. (Hung.)	Antiinflammatory, antioxidant	1990
hIAP-1 inhibitor	Discontinued	Human Genome Sciences (US)	Apoptosis hIAP-1 inhibitor	Sep-98
Pharmaprojects No. 3858	Discontinued	Peptech (Australia)	Arachidonic acid antagonist	Jun-00
LA-351	Discontinued	Lacer (Spain)	Benzopyran antiinflammatory	May-97
Pharmaprojects No. 5016	Discontinued	Takeda (Japan)	Bone formation stimulant	Feb-98
Pharmaprojects No. 5180	Discontinued	Bayer (Germany)	Bone formation stimulant	Jul-98
collagenase inhibitors, ResC	Discontinued	Research Corp. Tech. (US)	Collagenase inhibitors	Feb-02
collagenase IX inhibitor	Discontinued	BioCryst (US)	Collagenase inhibitors	Feb-02
BB-2827	Discontinued	British Biotech (UK)	Collagenase-specific MMP inhib.	Nov-99
TK9C	Discontinued	Avant Immunother. (US)	Complement factor inhibitor	May-98
Diflumidone (BA-4164-8)	Discontinued	3M (US)	COX inhibitor	Feb-81
BW-540C	Discontinued	Glaxo Wellcome (UK)	COX/5-LO inhibitor	Mar-87
PD-136005	Discontinued	Warner-Lambert (US)	COX/5-LO inhibitor	Aug-95
Pharmaprojects No. 4214	Discontinued	Glaxo Wellcome (UK)	COX/5-LO inhibitor	Jan-97
Pharmaprojects No. 2523	Discontinued	Merck & Co (US)	COX/LTB4 inhibitor	Apr-92
A-183827.0	Discontinued	Abbott (US)	COX-2 inhibitor	Mar-99
CS-179	Discontinued	Searle/Monsanto (US)	COX-2 inhibitor	Nov-98
L-768277	Discontinued	Merck & Co (US)	COX-2 inhibitor	Feb-99
L-804600, L-818571	Discontinued	Merck & Co (US)	COX-2 inhibitor	Dec-99
Pharmaprojects No. 4540	Discontinued	Merck & Co (US)	COX-2 inhibitor	May-99
Pharmaprojects No. 4720	Discontinued	Searle/Monsanto (US)	COX-2 inhibitor	May-99
Pharmaprojects No. 5135	Discontinued	Glaxo Wellcome (UK)	COX-2 inhibitor	1997
Pharmaprojects No. 5318	Discontinued	Merck & Co (US)	COX-2 inhibitor	Nov-98
Pharmaprojects No. 5606	Discontinued	Chugai (Japan)	COX-2 inhibitor	Apr-99
Pharmaprojects No. 5633	Discontinued	Sankyo (Japan)	COX-2 inhibitor	Jun-99
Pharmaprojects No. 5661	Discontinued	UPSA / Bristol-Myers Squibb (US)	COX-2 inhibitor	May-99
RS-113472	Discontinued	Roche (Switz)	COX-2 inhibitor	Jun-00
Pharmaprojects No. 5124	Discontinued	Servier (France)	COX-LO inhibitor	Jun-00
GR-373	Discontinued	Merck & Co (US)	Cysteine protease inhib; arthritis	Nov-99
Pharmaprojects No. 742	Discontinued	Roche (Switz)	Delta-5 lipoxygenase inhibitor	1982

Ref.: Pharmaprojects (updated to 2/02) used with permission; Scrip, corporate, literature & patent references
"Status" is international drug development or regulatory status and may not indicate status in USA
Sponsor: Original company name is retained if product is discontinued or inactive after merger, acquisition, company name change, etc.
Users of this table are encouraged to independently verify the status, activity, and mechanism of action of drugs of interest

GENERIC / TRADE NAME	STATUS	SPONSOR (S)	MECHANISM OF ACTION	REF. UPDATE
ISIS-4730	Discontinued	ISIS Pharmaceuticals (US)	ELAM-1 antisense; antiinflam.	Aug-99
Elastase inhibitor, Biopharm	Discontinued	Merck KGaA (Ger)/Biopharm (Can)	Elastase inhib / RA	May-98
Pharmaprojects No. 4549	Discontinued	Taiho (Japan)	Elastase inhibitor	Mar-97
SLPI fragments	Discontinued	Teijin (Japan)	Elastase inhibitor	Jun-00
Cell adhesion inhibitors	Discontinued	Warner-Lambert (US)	E-selectin / ICAM-1 antag.	May-97
Pharmaprojects No. 4822	Discontinued	Yamanouchi (Japan) / Tularik (US)	Gene expression inhibitor	May-98
Glycosidase inhibitors	Discontinued	Oxford GlycoSciences (UK)	Glycosidase inhib. / RA	Dec-98
PD-144795	Discontinued	Warner-Lambert (US)	ICAM 1 antagonist	May-97
SDZ-224-015	Discontinued	Novartis (Switz.)	ICE (IL-1beta conv. enzyme) inhib.	Sep-98
RSD-931	Discontinued	Nortran (Canada)	Ion channel modulator	Jun-00
Pharmaprojects No. 5409	Discontinued	Tularik (US)	IRAK: IL-1 recep.-assoc. kinase inhib.	Jun-00
Anirolac (RS-37326)	Discontinued	Syntex/Roche (Switz)	Ketorolac analog	Jun-90
Pharmaprojects No. 6071	Discontinued	Boehringer Ingelheim (Ger)	Leucotriene B4 antag.	Jun-00
LM-1376	Discontinued	Menarini (Italy)	Leukotriene D4 antagonist	May-98
Pharmaprojects No. 5933	Discontinued	Santen (Japan)	Leukotriene LTA4 antagonist	Jun-00
Pharmaprojects No. 5977	Discontinued	Bioproject / INSERM (France)	Leukotriene LTA4 antagonist	Jun-00
LY-210073	Discontinued	Lilly (US)	Leukotriene LTB4 antagonist	Jan-95
Pharmaprojects No. 3492	Discontinued	Roche (Switz)	Leukotriene LTB4 antagonist	Dec-94
SB-201146	Discontinued	SmithKline Beecham (UK)	Leukotriene LTB4 antagonist	May-96
SC-411930	Discontinued	Searle/Monsanto (US)	Leukotriene LTB4 antagonist	May-94
SC-51146	Discontinued	Searle/Monsanto (US)	Leukotriene LTB4 antagonist	May-94
Forsythiaside	Discontinued	Ehime Univ. (Japan)	Lipoxygenase (5-LO) inhibitor	1987
BAY-o-8276	Discontinued	Bayer (Germany)	Lipoxygenase inhibitor	Oct-89
anti-L-selectin oligo, Gilead	Discontinued	NeXstar / Gilead (US)	L-selectin inhibitor; anti-inflam.	Nov-98
RP-66364 (RP-60532; RP-69929)	Discontinued	Rhone-Poulenc Rorer (France)	LTB4 / CO antagonist	Nov-94
CVX	Discontinued	Bayer (Ger) / CV Ther (US)	Macrophage inhib.; anti-inflam.	Jun-99
PD-98059	Discontinued	Warner-Lambert (US)	MAP kinase inhibitor	Jun-00
TEI-8535	Discontinued	Teijin (Japan)	MCP-1 antagonist /PGE-1 agonist	Jul-98
Pharmaprojects No. 5433	Discontinued	Trega Biosciences (US)	Melanocortin MC-1 agonist	Jun-00
Pharmaprojects No. 4032	Discontinued	Novartis (Switz.)	Metalloproteinase inhib.	May-98
MMP inhibitors, Synt:em	Discontinued	Syntem (France)	Metalloproteinase inhibitor	Dec-98
Pharmaprojects No. 5687	Discontinued	Pharmacia & Upjohn (UK)	Metalloproteinase inhibitors	May-99
Pharmaprojects No. 3802	Discontinued	Roche (Switz)	Microbial collagenase inhibitor	May-98
RPR-122818 derivatives	Discontinued	Aventis (France)	MMP / PDE-IV inhibitor	Jun-00
CMTs (Chemically Mod. Tetracyclines)	Discontinued	CollaGenex (US) / Boehringer Man.	MMP inhib.; tetracycline analogs	Sep-99
XR-168	Discontinued	Xenova (US)	MMP inhibitor (collagenase inhib.)	Nov-96
Pharmaprojects No. 6067	Discontinued	DuPont (US)	MMP inhibitor / arthritis	Jun-00
PGE-2946979 (PGE-5747401)	Discontinued	Procter & Gamble (US)	MMP inhibitor / OA	Jun-00
PS-508	Discontinued	ProScript (US)	MMP-3 inhibitor / RA	May-99
Pharmaprojects No. 5573	Discontinued	Warner-Lambert (US)	MMP-3, MMP-2 inhibitors	Mar-99
RS-130830	Discontinued	Roche (Switz)	Neutrophil collagenase inhib./OA	Jun-00
MDL-104238 (MDL-101286)	Discontinued	Hoechst Marion Roussel (Ger)	Neutrophil elastase inhibitor	Sep-97
tenoxicam meglumine	Discontinued	Therapicon (Italy)	NSAID	Feb-02
isoprofen	Discontinued	Bristol-Myers Squibb (US)	NSAID	Feb-02
naproxen meglumine	Discontinued	Therapicon (Italy)	NSAID	Feb-02
piridoxiprofen	Discontinued	Crinos	NSAID	Feb-02
AY-30068	Discontinued	American Home Products (US)	NSAID	Feb-02
CGP-37861A	Discontinued	Novartis (Switz.)	NSAID	Feb-02
dizatrifone	Discontinued	bioMerieux-Pierre Fabre (France)	NSAID	Feb-02
F-2341	Discontinued	bioMerieux-Pierre Fabre (France)	NSAID	Feb-02
FX-205-754	Discontinued	Novartis (Switz.)	NSAID	Feb-02
MG-8681	Discontinued	Sanofi-Synthelabo (France)	NSAID	Feb-02
moxifadol	Discontinued	Byk Gulden (Ger)	NSAID	Feb-02
Pharmaprojects No. 2520	Discontinued	Roche (Switz)	NSAID	Feb-02
Pharmaprojects No. 3484	Discontinued	AstraZeneca (UK)	NSAID	Feb-02
S-01	Discontinued	Sanwa Kagaku Kenkyusho	NSAID	Feb-02
S-1528	Discontinued	Sanofi-Synthelabo (France)	NSAID	Feb-02
SM-9064	Discontinued	Sumitomo (Japan)	NSAID	Feb-02
THC-1301	Discontinued	Therapicon (Italy)	NSAID	Feb-02
ST-793	Discontinued	bioMerieux-Pierre Fabre (France)	NSAID	Feb-02
A-45474	Discontinued	Abbott (US)	NSAID	Feb-02
araprofen	Discontinued	Sanofi-Synthelabo (France)	NSAID	Feb-02
CO-893	Discontinued	Boehringer Ingelheim (Ger)	NSAID	Feb-02

Ref.: Pharmaprojects (updated to 2/02) used with permission; Scrip, corporate, literature & patent references
"Status" is international drug development or regulatory status and may not indicate status in USA
Sponsor: Original company name is retained if product is discontinued or inactive after merger, acquisition, company name change, etc.
Users of this table are encouraged to independently verify the status, activity, and mechanism of action of drugs of interest

GENERIC / TRADE NAME	STATUS	SPONSOR (S)	MECHANISM OF ACTION	REF. UPDATE
fendosal	Discontinued	Aventis (France)	NSAID	Feb-02
fluproquazone	Discontinued	Novartis (Switz.)	NSAID	Feb-02
MR-714	Discontinued	Recordati	NSAID	Feb-02
Pharmaprojects No. 2354	Discontinued	Grunenthal (Germany)	NSAID	Feb-02
Pharmaprojects No. 965	Discontinued	bioMerieux-Pierre Fabre (France)	NSAID	Feb-02
RUB-265	Discontinued	Sankyo (Japan)	NSAID	Feb-02
tifurac	Discontinued	Roche (Switz)	NSAID	Feb-02
TY-10222	Discontinued	Toa Eiyo	NSAID	Feb-02
Y-20003	Discontinued	Mitsubishi Pharma (Japan)	NSAID	Feb-02
EM-405	Discontinued	Grunenthal (Germany)	NSAID	Feb-02
AY-31633	Discontinued	Wyeth-Ayerst (US)	NSAID	Mar-88
CGP-25449	Discontinued	Novartis (Switz.)	NSAID	May-92
Cloximate (DU-22599)	Discontinued	Solvay (Netherlands)	NSAID	Jul-83
Flubichin (VUFB-12950; VUFB-15950)	Discontinued	VUFB (Czech Republic)	NSAID	Mar-94
Pharmaprojects No. 5129	Discontinued	Univ. Thessalonika (Greece)	NSAID	Jul-98
RMM-318	Discontinued	Roemmers	NSAID	Jun-00
Rhodanine derivatives	Discontinued	Univ. L'viv (Ukraine)	NSAID	Jun-00
HCT-2035	Discontinued	NicOx (France)	NSAID + NO releaser	Jun-99
dexflurbiprofen	Discontinued	Abbott (US)	NSAID, single isomer	Feb-02
(R)-Ketorolac	Discontinued	Sepracor (US)	NSAID, single isomer	Mar-99
SC-XX906	Discontinued	Pharmacia (US)	P38 kinase inhibitor	Jun-00
Pharmaprojects No. 4596	Discontinued	Japan Energy (Japan)	PAF antagonist / anti-inflam.	Dec-98
ABT-491 (A-13791)	Discontinued	Abbott (US)	PAF antagonist; inflamm. dis.	Nov-98
Pharmaprojects No. 6012	Discontinued	SSP (Japan)	PDE-IV / TNF-α inhibitor	Jun-00
CP-353164	Discontinued	Pfizer (US)	PDE-IV inhibitor	Dec-98
RPR-132294	Discontinued	Aventis (France)	PDE-IV inhibitor	Jun-00
ONO-NT-012	Discontinued	Ono (Japan)	PGE1/E3 prostanoid agonist	Nov-96
Benzodiazepine-piperidines	Discontinued	Hoechst (Ger)	PGSI	Feb-87
DU-608	Discontinued	Dainippon (Japan)	PGSI	1979
ER-10103	Discontinued	Euroresearch (Italy)	PGSI	Apr-88
Pidocetamol	Discontinued	Pan Medica (France)	PGSI	Jan-92
PR-870-714A	Discontinued	Fisons (UK)	PGSI	Dec-93
RO 11-4337	Discontinued	Roche (Switz)	PGSI	Mar-84
RO 12-9150	Discontinued	Roche (Switz)	PGSI	Nov-85
Sch-30497	Discontinued	Schering Plough (US)	PGSI	Sep-86
Veradoline	Discontinued	Fisons (UK)	PGSI	Aug-82
Verilopam	Discontinued	Fisons (UK)	PGSI	Feb-80
RS-17597	Discontinued	Syntex / Roche (Switz)	Phosphodiesterase (PDE-IV) inhib.	May-98
GW-3600	Discontinued	Glaxo Wellcome (UK)	Phosphodiesterase IV inhib.	Sep-97
AGN-190383	Discontinued	Allergan (US)	Phospholipase PLA2 inhibitor	Nov-92
Duramycin B (Duramycin C)	Discontinued	Novartis (Switz.)	Phospholipase PLA2 inhibitor	May-92
Pharmaprojects No. 4404	Discontinued	Merckle (Germany)	Phospholipase PLA2 inhibitor	Jun-00
Ro-23-9358	Discontinued	Roche (Switz)	Phospholipase PLA2 inhibitor	Mar-95
Thielocin	Discontinued	Shionogi (Japan)	Phospholipase PLA2 inhibitor	Dec-92
WAY-121520 (WAY-122220)	Discontinued	Wyeth-Ayerst (US)	Phospholipase PLA2 inhibitor	Apr-95
YM-26734	Discontinued	Yamanouchi (Japan)	Phospholipase PLA2 inhibitor	May-98
Pharmaprojects No. 2540	Discontinued	Genetics Institute	PLA2 inhibitor	Jun-00
WA-8242B	Discontinued	Fujisawa (Japan)	PLA2 inhibitor; inflam., allergy	Jun-00
Ro-31-8425 (Ro-32-0432)	Discontinued	Roche (Switz)	Protein kinase PKC inhibitor	Nov-95
cysteine protease inhibs,Celer	Discontinued	Celera Genomics	RA, OA, osteoporosis	Feb-02
Cysteine protease inhibs.	Discontinued	AxyS (US)	RA, OA, osteoporosis	May-98
Pharmaprojects No. 5488	Discontinued	Novartis (Switz.)	Selectin antag.; anti-inflam.	Jun-00
Selectin inhibitors	Discontinued	Nisshin Oil Mills (Japan)	Selectin antag.; anti-inflam.	Jun-00
GM-1986	Discontinued	Glycomed / Ligand (US)	Selectin antagonist	Feb-97
Pharmaprojects No. 4784	Discontinued	Kanebo (Japan)	Selectin blocker; anti-inflam.	Nov-98
Anti-inflammatories	Discontinued	Affymax (Glaxo Wellcome-UK)	Selectin inhibitor	May-98
GM-1998 (Celadin)	Discontinued	Ligand (US)	Selectin inhibitor; anti-inflam.	Mar-00
KPI-022	Discontinued	Scios (US)	Serine protease inhibitor (inflam.)	Nov-99
LEX analogues	Discontinued	SuperGen (US)	Serine protease inhibitor (inflam.)	Sep-99
L-758354	Discontinued	Merck & Co (US)	Stromelysin-1 (MMP-3) inhibitor	Jun-99
AQ-588	Discontinued	Avant (US) / ArQule (US)	T-cell inhib.; immunosuppressant	Nov-99
D-21151	Discontinued	Asta Medica (Germany)	Thromboxane B2 antagonist	Mar-97
F-2349	Discontinued	Pierre Fabre (France)	Thromboxane synthase inhibitor	Mar-88

Ref.: Pharmaprojects (updated to 2/02) used with permission; Scrip, corporate, literature & patent references
"Status" is international drug development or regulatory status and may not indicate status in USA
Sponsor: Original company name is retained if product is discontinued or inactive after merger, acquisition, company name change, etc.
Users of this table are encouraged to independently verify the status, activity, and mechanism of action of drugs of interest

GENERIC / TRADE NAME	STATUS	SPONSOR (S)	MECHANISM OF ACTION	REF. UPDATE
CV-6504	Discontinued	Takeda (Japan)	Thromboxane TXA2/5-LO inhib.	Aug-95
CI-987	Discontinued	Warner-Lambert (US)	Thromboxane TXB2 release inhib.	May-94
Pharmaprojects No. 5913	Discontinued	Novo Nordisk (Denmark)	TNF / cytokine inhib.; arthritis	Jun-00
Pharmaprojects No. 6069	Discontinued	DuPont (US)	TNF convertase inhib. / RA	Jun-00
Pharmaprojects No. 5679	Discontinued	Sumitomo (Japan)	TNF-α inhibitor	Jun-99
Xyloadenosine	Discontinued	Amgen (US)	TNF-alpha inhibitor	Dec-97
CB-28	Discontinued	KS Biomedix (UK)	Unident. muscle elasticity enhanc.	Sep-99
Pharmaprojects No. 4282	Discontinued	Proteus Molecular Design (UK)	Unidentified	Jan-97
EN-08	Discontinued	Essential Nutrition (UK)	Unidentified (arthritis pain)	1998
TRK-240	Discontinued	Toray (Japan)	Unidentified / anti-inflammatory	May-99
Dazidamine (AF-2322)	Discontinued	Angelini (Italy)	Unidentified anti-inflammatory	Mar-87
VLA-4 antagonist	Discontinued	Hoechst Marion Roussel (Ger)	VLA-4 inhibitor; RA	Jun-00
Talmetacin	Discontinued (Clin)	Resfar (Italy) / Bago (Argen)	Cyclooxygenase inhibitor	May-98
HB-328	Discontinued (Clin.)	Synthelabo (France)	Antiinflamatory 5-ASA prodrug	Nov-91
Fenclorac (WHR-539)	Discontinued (Clin.)	Rhone-Poulenc Rorer (France)	COX inhibitor	Dec-82
HP-573	Discontinued (Clin.)	Hoechst Marion Roussel (Ger)	NSAID	Jul-84
Orpanoxin (F-776)	Discontinued (Clin.)	Procter & Gamble (US)	NSAID	Jun-86
RU-29693	Discontinued (Clin.)	Hoechst Marion Roussel (Ger)	NSAID	1983
Delmetacin (UR-2301)	Discontinued (Clin.)	Uriach (Spain)	NSAID / indomethacin analog	Mar-84
Niacinamide (vitamin B3)	Discontinued (Clin.)	NIH (US)	Unidentified (osteoarthritis)	Jul-98
CRE-109	Discontinued (Clin.)	Cermol (Switz.)	Unidentified anti-inflammatory	Jun-94
SQ-11579	Discontinued (Clin.)	Bristol-Myers Squibb (US)	Unidentified anti-inflammatory	Jul-80
Oxapadol (MD-720111)	Discontinued (Clin.)	Synthelabo (France)	Unidentified antiinflammatory analg.	Feb-83
Suprofen	Discontinued (LNCHD)	Johnson & Johnson (US)	PGSI inhibitor	1989
BF-389 (Biofor 389)	Discontinued (ph. I)	Biofor (US)	5-LO / COX inhibitor	Nov-95
A-78773	Discontinued (ph. I)	Abbott (US)	5-LO inhibitor	May-95
Diaveridine, EGIS (EGIS-5645)	Discontinued (ph. I)	EGIS (Hungary)	Anti-inflammatory	Nov-91
· Manoalide (luffariellolide)	Discontinued (ph. I)	Allergan (US) / Scripps Inst.	Anti-inflammatory	May-92
FPL-62064	Discontinued (ph. I)	Fisons (RPR; Ger.)	COX + lipoxygenase inhibitor	Jun-94
Ro-12-9150	Discontinued (ph. I)	Roche (Switz)	COX inhibitor	Nov-85
SQ-20650	Discontinued (ph. I)	Bristol-Myers Squibb (US)	COX inhibitor	Jan-80
BF-389 (Biofor 389)	Discontinued (ph. I)	Biofor (US)	COX/5-LO inhibitor	Nov-97
CBS-1114	Discontinued (ph. I)	Chauvin (France)	COX/5-LO inhibitor	Oct-85
L-652343	Discontinued (ph. I)	Merck & Co (US)	COX/5-LO inhibitor	1986
SKF-105809 (SK&F-105561)	Discontinued (ph. I)	SmithKline Beecham (UK)	COX/5-LO inhibitor	Jan-93
D-1367	Discontinued (ph. I)	Chiroscience (UK)	COX-2 inhibitor	May-98
SC-57666	Discontinued (ph. I)	Searle/Monsanto (US)	COX-2 inhibitor	May-99
GI-245402 / BB-2983	Discontinued (ph. I)	Glaxo Wellcome / British Biotech	MMP / TNF inhibitor (arthritis)	Oct-97
IQB-821	Discontinued (ph. I)	IQB (Spain)	Nefopam analog	Jan-86
AU-8001	Discontinued (ph. I)	Aldo-Union (Spain)	NSAID	Oct-91
CGP-17829	Discontinued (ph. I)	Novartis (Switz.)	NSAID	Jan-90
CGP-19416	Discontinued (ph. I)	Novartis (Switz.)	NSAID	Apr-90
CGP-28237 / ZK-34228	Discontinued (ph. I)	Novartis / Schering AG (Ger)	NSAID	May-89
CGP-31081	Discontinued (ph. I)	Novartis (Switz.)	NSAID	May-94
EP-322 (EP-323)	Discontinued (ph. I)	Edmond Pharma (Italy)	NSAID	Nov-91
Isoprazone (DL-809-IT)	Discontinued (ph. I)	Hoechst Marion Roussel (Ger)	NSAID	1983
LCB-1892	Discontinued (ph. I)	Merck KGaA (Germany)	NSAID	Mar-96
Pemedolac (AY-30715)	Discontinued (ph. I)	Wyeth-Ayerst (US)	NSAID	May-96
Pimetacin	Discontinued (ph. I)	Rhone-Poulenc Rorer (France)	NSAID	Feb-90
SaH-46-798	Discontinued (ph. I)	Novartis (Switz.)	NSAID	Feb-83
Fluorometacin (FA-401)	Discontinued (ph. I)	Yoshitomi (Japan)	NSAID (ph. Indomethacin derivative)	Sep-89
Chinoin-127	Discontinued (ph. I)	Chinon (Hungary)	NSAID (rimazolium analog)	Mar-88
Ibuproxam-beta-cyclodextrin	Discontinued (ph. I)	Lex Pharma. (Slovenia)	NSAID, solubilized ibuproxam	Mar-91
ZK-31945 (SH-405)	Discontinued (ph. I)	Schering AG (Germany)	NSAID; Clidanac isomer	Apr-84
V-2	Discontinued (ph. I)	Prodesfarma (Spain)	PGSI / peripheral analgesic	Jul-95
ITF-2357	Discontinued (ph. I)	Italfarmaco (Italy)	TNF-alpha, IL-1b synthesis inhib.	Feb-02
ICI-95527	Discontinued (ph. I)	Zeneca (UK)	Unidentified anti-inflammatory	Apr-90
Ro-21-5521	Discontinued (ph. I)	Roche (Switz)	Unidentified anti-inflammatory	Feb-85
Xenipentone (RP-48-482)	Discontinued (ph. I)	Novartis (Switz.)	Unidentified anti-inflammatory	Feb-85
AA-2379	Discontinued (ph. II)	Takeda (Japan)	Ant-inflammatory/antipyretic	May-92
TZI-41078	Discontinued (ph. II)	Teikoku Hormone (Japan)	COX + lipoxygenase inhibitor	May-90
Curcumin	Discontinued (ph. II)	Central Drug Research (India)	COX inhibitor / 12-HETE	May-98
KME-4	Discontinued (ph. II)	Kaneka (Japan)	COX/5-LO inhibitor	Jul-91

Ref.: Pharmaprojects (updated to 2/02) used with permission; Scrip, corporate, literature & patent references
"Status" is international drug development or regulatory status and may not indicate status in USA
Sponsor: Original company name is retained if product is discontinued or inactive after merger, acquisition, company name change, etc.
Users of this table are encouraged to independently verify the status, activity, and mechanism of action of drugs of interest

GENERIC / TRADE NAME	STATUS	SPONSOR (S)	MECHANISM OF ACTION	REF. UPDATE
Darbufelone mesylate (CI-1004)	Discontinued (ph. II)	Warner-Lambert (US)	COX-2 / 5-LO inhibitor; OA/RA	Feb-02
L-783003	Discontinued (ph. II)	Merck & Co (US)	COX-2 inhibitor	Sep-98
SC-106	Discontinued (ph. II)	Scotia (UK)	γ-linolenic acid combo (RA, OA)	Jan-99
TA-60	Discontinued (ph. II)	Taisho (Japan)	Ibuprofen analog	1985
Lobuprofen (frabuprofen)	Discontinued (ph. II)	Juste (Spain)	Ibuprofen ester	May-93
CGS-25019C	Discontinued (ph. II)	Ciba-Geigy (Switz)	LTB4 antagonist	Feb-96
Ontazolast (BI-RM-270)	Discontinued (ph. II)	Boehringer Ingelheim (Ger)	LTB4 synthesis inhibitor	May-97
Mipragoside (AGF-44, FISER-A503)	Discontinued (ph. II)	Fidia (Italy)	Membrane perm. inhib./anti-inflam.	May-99
CGP-16789A	Discontinued (ph. II)	Novartis (Switz.)	NSAID	Apr-90
E-5110	Discontinued (ph. II)	Eisai (Japan)	NSAID	Jun-91
FK-3311	Discontinued (ph. II)	Fujisawa (Japan)	NSAID	Dec-94
Florifenine (FI-2500; FI-2522)	Discontinued (ph. II)	Ferrer (Spain)	NSAID	Oct-97
Flunixin (Banamine; Sch-14714)	Discontinued (ph. II)	Schering Plough (US)	NSAID	Mar-84
FS-205-397	Discontinued (ph. II)	Novartis (Switz.)	NSAID	Jan-97
S-14080	Discontinued (ph. II)	Servier (France)	NSAID	Sep-93
SY-6001	Discontinued (ph. II)	SSP (Japan)	NSAID	Mar-93
Tebufelone (NE-11740)	Discontinued (ph. II)	Procter & Gamble (US)	NSAID	May-94
V-144	Discontinued (ph. II)	Vita-Invest (Spain)	NSAID	Apr-85
Apyramide	Discontinued (ph. II)	Laboratoires Richard (France)	NSAID (ph. Indomethacin+APAP ester)	Feb-92
Sumacetamol	Discontinued (ph. II)	Eastman Kodak (US)	PGSI	1985
Peptide T	Discontinued (ph. II)	Peptech (Australia) / NIH	TNF-alpha inhibitor / HIV	Mar-97
CL-225385	Discontinued (ph. II)	Lederle / Am. Home Prod. (US)	Unidentified anti-inflammatory	Nov-84
JI-36 (TCA)	Discontinued (ph. II)	Otsuka (Japan)	Unidentified anti-inflammatory	Apr-93
Niflangel	Discontinued (ph. II)	Yoshitomi (Japan)	Unidentified anti-inflammatory	Nov-87
T-3788	Discontinued (ph. II)	Toyama (Japan)	Unidentified antiinflammatory analg.	Apr-98
CB-2431	Discontinued (ph. II)	KS Biomedix (UK)	Unknown (drug combo)	Feb-02
Sfericase (A1-794; Ponase)	Discontinued (ph. III)	Meiji Seika (Japan)	Antiinflammatory/expectorant	Feb-89
Superoxide dismutase, OXIS	Discontinued (ph. III)	OXIS (US) / Grunenthal (Ger)	Bovine SOD (osteoarthritis)	Mar-97
Fopirtoline (D-1126)	Discontinued (ph. III)	Asta Medica (Germany)	COX inhibitor	Feb-84
Fenflumizole (A-214)	Discontinued (ph. III)	Alpharma (US)	COX/5-LO inhibitor	Jan-86
Timegadine (SR-1368)	Discontinued (ph. III)	Leo (Denmark)	COX/5-LO inhibitor	Mar-88
EF-5 (SC-106)	Discontinued (ph. III)	Scotia (UK)	γ-linolenic acid combo (RA, OA)	Feb-02
Trocade (Ro-32-3555)	Discontinued (ph. III)	Roche (Switz.)	MMP inhibitor / RA	Feb-02
Chlorotenoxicam	Discontinued (ph. III)	Nycomed Amersham (Norway)	NSAID	Jan-94
Ibuprofen aluminum (U-18573G)	Discontinued (ph. III)	Pharmacia & Upjohn (UK)	NSAID	1980
Lofemizole	Discontinued (ph. III)	Farmatis (Italy)	NSAID	Sep-82
Nerbacadol (HWA-272)	Discontinued (ph. III)	Hoechst Marion Roussel (Ger.)	NSAID	May-90
ONO-3144 (AI-3144)	Discontinued (ph. III)	Ono (Japan)	NSAID	Sep-87
Prinomide (CGS-10787B)	Discontinued (ph. III)	Novartis (Switz.)	NSAID	Feb-90
Tinoprofen arbamel (Y-23023)	Discontinued (ph. III)	Yoshitomi/Japan Tobacco (Japan)	NSAID	May-99
Zoliprofen (156-S)	Discontinued (ph. III)	Shionogi (Japan)	NSAID	May-89
Fenclozine (S-1429)	Discontinued (ph. III)	Synthelabo (France)	NSAID / anxiolytic	May-92
Icodulinium HCl	Discontinued (ph. III)	Chauvin (France)	Ophthalmic anti-inflam. (COX+LO)	Nov-94
Oxepinac (DD-3314)	Discontinued (ph. III)	Daiichi (Japan)	Prostaglandin synthase inhib.	1980s
Tenidap	Discontinued (PRE-REG)	Pfizer (US)	COX / 5-LO inhib. (LTB4/IL1)	May-98
Flurbiprofen meglumine (THC-1103)	Discontinued (PRE-REG)	Therapicon (Italy)	NSAID	May-99
Salmisteine (EP-321)	Discontinued (PRE-REG)	Edmond Pharma (Italy)	NSAID	May-93
Zidometacin (P-74180)	Discontinued (PRE-REG)	Pharmacia & Upjohn (UK)	NSAID / indomethacin analog	Apr-88
filenadol	Discontinued (PRE-REG)	Ferrer (Spain)	PGSI	Feb-02
Parcetasal	Discontinued (PRE-REG)	Medea Research (Italy)	PGSI	1997
Pirazolac (MY-309, SH-376)	Discontinued (REGIS.)	Schering AG (Germany)	NSAID	May-99
GV-3658 (Diflusol)	Discontinued (REGIS.)	Edmond Pharma (It) / Resfar	NSAID / diflunisal derivative	Feb-99
GV-3659	Discontinued (REGIS.)	Edmond Pharma (It) / Resfar	NSAID / diflunisal derivative	Feb-99
atliprofen methyl ester	Inactive	IDPL	Antiarthritic	Feb-02
CP-850	Inactive	Pharmacia (US)	Antiarthritic	Feb-02
disalazine	Inactive	VUFB (Czech Republic)	Antiarthritic	Feb-02
GR-129574A	Inactive	GlaxoSmithKline (UK)	Antiarthritic	Feb-02
LY-289415	Inactive	Lilly (US)	Antiarthritic	Feb-02
MCI-426	Inactive	Mitsubishi Pharma (Japan)	Antiarthritic	Feb-02
MDL-201331	Inactive	Aventis (France)	Antiarthritic	Feb-02
methylprednisolone prodrug	Inactive	Pharmacia (US)	Antiarthritic	Feb-02
moxilubant maleate	Inactive	Novartis (Switz.)	Antiarthritic	Feb-02
PD-057081	Inactive	Pfizer (US)	Antiarthritic	Feb-02

Ref.: Pharmaprojects (updated to 2/02) used with permission; Scrip, corporate, literature & patent references
"Status" is international drug development or regulatory status and may not indicate status in USA
Sponsor: Original company name is retained if product is discontinued or inactive after merger, acquisition, company name change, etc.
Users of this table are encouraged to independently verify the status, activity, and mechanism of action of drugs of interest

GENERIC / TRADE NAME	STATUS	SPONSOR (S)	MECHANISM OF ACTION	REF. UPDATE
Pharmaprojects No. 1573	Inactive	Pharmacia (US)	Antiarthritic	Feb-02
Pharmaprojects No. 2016	Inactive	Toyobo	Antiarthritic	Feb-02
Pharmaprojects No. 2755	Inactive	American Home Products (US)	Antiarthritic	Feb-02
Pharmaprojects No. 2969	Inactive	GlaxoSmithKline (UK)	Antiarthritic	Feb-02
Pharmaprojects No. 3722	Inactive	Japan Tobacco (Japan)	Antiarthritic	Feb-02
Pharmaprojects No. 4850	Inactive	Pfizer (US)	Antiarthritic	Feb-02
Pharmaprojects No. 653	Inactive	Roche (Switz)	Antiarthritic	Feb-02
Pharmaprojects No. 883	Inactive	Roche (Switz)	Antiarthritic	Feb-02
Ro-31-4724	Inactive	Roche (Switz)	Antiarthritic	Feb-02
RS-113-080	Inactive	Roche (Switz)	Antiarthritic	Feb-02
RU-43526	Inactive	Aventis (France)	Antiarthritic	Feb-02
SAM-PFH	Inactive	Gibipharma	Antiarthritic	Feb-02
SR-26831	Inactive	Sanofi-Synthelabo (France)	Antiarthritic	Feb-02
TA-383	Inactive	Tanabe Seiyaku (Japan)	Antiarthritic	Feb-02
U-81581	Inactive	Pharmacia (US)	Antiarthritic	Feb-02
NPC-15670	Inactive	Scios (US)	Antiarthritic	Feb-02
Pharmaprojects No. 3253	Inactive	Ligand (US)	Antiarthritic	Feb-02
holmium hydroxyapatite	Inactive	Mallinckrodt (US)	Antiarthritic	Feb-02
DGI	Inactive	Innogenetics	Antiarthritic	Feb-02
PD-172084	Inactive	Millennium (US)	Antiarthritic	Feb-02
GI-155704A	Inactive	GlaxoSmithKline (UK)	Antiarthritic	Feb-02
Pharmaprojects No. 3056	Inactive	Ariad	Antiarthritic	Feb-02
phospholipase D inhibitors, Sp	Inactive	Lilly (US)	Antiarthritic	Feb-02
Pharmaprojects No. 3694	Inactive	Aventis (France)	Antiarthritic	Feb-02
Pharmaprojects No. 874	Inactive	Fujisawa (Japan)	Antiarthritic	Feb-02
Pharmaprojects No. 6318	Inactive	Pfizer (US)	Antiarthritic	Feb-02
Pharmaprojects No. 6319	Inactive	Pfizer (US)	Antiarthritic	Feb-02
Pharmaprojects No. 6417	Inactive	Procter & Gamble (US)	Antiarthritic	Feb-02
itrocinonide	Inactive	AstraZeneca (UK)	Antiarthritic	Feb-02
Pharmaprojects No. 3395	Inactive	Pharmacia (US)	Antiarthritic	Feb-02
Pharmaprojects No. 4388	Inactive	Pharmacia (US)	Antiarthritic	Feb-02
holy basil oil, Delhi	Inactive	Non-industrial source	Antiarthritic	Feb-02
Pharmaprojects No. 2968	Inactive	GlaxoSmithKline (UK)	Antiarthritic	Feb-02
SC-107	Inactive	Scotia (UK)	Antiarthritic	Feb-02
Pharmaprojects No. 6408	Inactive	Pan Pacific	Antiarthritic	Feb-02
Pharmaprojects No. 5073	Inactive	Phytera	Antiarthritic	Feb-02
A-121798	Inactive	Abbott (US)	Antiarthritic	Feb-02
Pharmaprojects No. 2456	Inactive	Novartis (Switz.)	Antiarthritic	Feb-02
ZM-216800	Inactive	AstraZeneca (UK)	Antiarthritic	Feb-02
hyaluronic acid, Kyowa Hakko	Inactive	Kyowa Hakko (Japan)	Antiarthritic	Feb-02
Pharmaprojects No. 3274	Inactive	Novartis (Switz.)	Antiarthritic	Feb-02
CVT-857 (CVT-710)	Inactive	CV Therapeutics (US)	Antiinflamatory protease inhib.	Oct-98
hyaluronidase, BioPhausia	Inactive	BioPhausia (Sweden)	Antiinflamatory; interstitial edema	Feb-02
A-80263	Inactive	Abbott (US)	Antiinflammatory	Feb-02
anti-collagenase	Inactive	Chiron (US)	Antiinflammatory	Feb-02
anti-inflammatories, Affymax	Inactive	GlaxoSmithKline (UK)	Antiinflammatory	Feb-02
anti-inflammatories, Ankara	Inactive	Non-industrial source	Antiinflammatory	Feb-02
anti-inflammatories, Ligand	Inactive	Ligand (US)	Antiinflammatory	Feb-02
anti-inflammatories, Praxis	Inactive	Praxis (Austr.)	Antiinflammatory	Feb-02
BL-016	Inactive	Theracel	Antiinflammatory	Feb-02
BMS-192066	Inactive	Bristol-Myers Squibb (US)	Antiinflammatory	Feb-02
borjatriol	Inactive	Non-industrial source	Antiinflammatory	Feb-02
BPC-15	Inactive	Pfizer (US)	Antiinflammatory	Feb-02
C5a antagonist, Abbott	Inactive	Abbott (US)	Antiinflammatory	Feb-02
CD11b/CD18 antags, Selectide	Inactive	Aventis (France)	Antiinflammatory	Feb-02
cell adhesion inhibitors, Park	Inactive	Pfizer (US)	Antiinflammatory	Feb-02
cinfenoac	Inactive	Biorex Labs	Antiinflammatory	Feb-02
CO-1827	Inactive	Aventis (France)	Antiinflammatory	Feb-02
CPR-2001	Inactive	Clarion (US)	Antiinflammatory	Feb-02
dendalone 3-hydroxybutyrate	Inactive	Roche (Switz)	Antiinflammatory	Feb-02
dibenzosuberone	Inactive	Pfizer (US)	Antiinflammatory	Feb-02
EN-07	Inactive	Essential Nutrition (UK)	Antiinflammatory	Feb-02
EN-105	Inactive	Mitsubishi Pharma (Japan)	Antiinflammatory	Feb-02

Ref.: Pharmaprojects (updated to 2/02) used with permission; Scrip, corporate, literature & patent references
"Status" is international drug development or regulatory status and may not indicate status in USA
Sponsor: Original company name is retained if product is discontinued or inactive after merger, acquisition, company name change, etc.
Users of this table are encouraged to independently verify the status, activity, and mechanism of action of drugs of interest

GENERIC / TRADE NAME	STATUS	SPONSOR (S)	MECHANISM OF ACTION	REF. UPDATE
flumazole	Inactive	Lilly (US)	Antiinflammatory	Feb-02
FPP-028	Inactive	Non-industrial source	Antiinflammatory	Feb-02
GF-109203X	Inactive	Pfizer (US)	Antiinflammatory	Feb-02
ICAM antagonists, Genentech	Inactive	Genentech	Antiinflammatory	Feb-02
ICF-650	Inactive	Non-industrial source	Antiinflammatory	Feb-02
inhibitor B	Inactive	Merck & Co (US)	Antiinflammatory	Feb-02
K562 factor, INSERM	Inactive	Non-industrial source	Antiinflammatory	Feb-02
kallikrein inhibitors, Celera	Inactive	Celera Genomics	Antiinflammatory	Feb-02
kallolide-A	Inactive	Non-industrial source	Antiinflammatory	Feb-02
L-695499	Inactive	Merck & Co (US)	Antiinflammatory	Feb-02
L-709049	Inactive	Merck & Co (US)	Antiinflammatory	Feb-02
L-804600	Inactive	Merck & Co (US)	Antiinflammatory	Feb-02
leumedins, Scios	Inactive	Scios (US)	Antiinflammatory	Feb-02
LY-112101	Inactive	Lilly (US)	Antiinflammatory	Feb-02
LY-233569	Inactive	Lilly (US)	Antiinflammatory	Feb-02
LY-243062	Inactive	Lilly (US)	Antiinflammatory	Feb-02
M-5	Inactive	Fujisawa (Japan)	Antiinflammatory	Feb-02
MAFP, Merck	Inactive	Merck & Co (US)	Antiinflammatory	Feb-02
manoalogue	Inactive	Lilly (US)	Antiinflammatory	Feb-02
MB-432	Inactive	Non-industrial source	Antiinflammatory	Feb-02
MDL-19301D	Inactive	Aventis (France)	Antiinflammatory	Feb-02
NACAS	Inactive	Non-industrial source	Antiinflammatory	Feb-02
NADPH inhibitors, Selectide	Inactive	Aventis (France)	Antiinflammatory	Feb-02
Org-7258	Inactive	Akzo Nobel (Netherlands)	Antiinflammatory	Feb-02
p-benzyloxyphenol	Inactive	Pfizer (US)	Antiinflammatory	Feb-02
PD-127443	Inactive	Pfizer (US)	Antiinflammatory	Feb-02
PD-145246	Inactive	Pfizer (US)	Antiinflammatory	Feb-02
Pharmaprojects No. 1141	Inactive	Merck & Co (US)	Antiinflammatory	Feb-02
Pharmaprojects No. 1247	Inactive	Non-industrial source	Antiinflammatory	Feb-02
Pharmaprojects No. 1251	Inactive	Aventis (France)	Antiinflammatory	Feb-02
Pharmaprojects No. 1311	Inactive	Non-industrial source	Antiinflammatory	Feb-02
Pharmaprojects No. 1550	Inactive	Merck & Co (US)	Antiinflammatory	Feb-02
Pharmaprojects No. 1805	Inactive	Abbott (US)	Antiinflammatory	Feb-02
Pharmaprojects No. 1894	Inactive	AstraZeneca (UK)	Antiinflammatory	Feb-02
Pharmaprojects No. 1903	Inactive	Fujisawa (Japan)	Antiinflammatory	Feb-02
Pharmaprojects No. 2010	Inactive	Yamanouchi (Japan)	Antiinflammatory	Feb-02
Pharmaprojects No. 2264	Inactive	Bayer (Germany)	Antiinflammatory	Feb-02
Pharmaprojects No. 2505	Inactive	Schering Plough (US)	Antiinflammatory	Feb-02
Pharmaprojects No. 2515	Inactive	American Home Products (US)	Antiinflammatory	Feb-02
Pharmaprojects No. 2516	Inactive	American Home Products (US)	Antiinflammatory	Feb-02
Pharmaprojects No. 2671	Inactive	Kuraray	Antiinflammatory	Feb-02
Pharmaprojects No. 2707	Inactive	Pfizer (US)	Antiinflammatory	Feb-02
Pharmaprojects No. 2800	Inactive	Pfizer (US)	Antiinflammatory	Feb-02
Pharmaprojects No. 2848	Inactive	American Home Products (US)	Antiinflammatory	Feb-02
Pharmaprojects No. 2871	Inactive	Aventis (France)	Antiinflammatory	Feb-02
Pharmaprojects No. 2943	Inactive	Pfizer (US)	Antiinflammatory	Feb-02
Pharmaprojects No. 3197	Inactive	ISIS Pharmaceuticals (US)	Antiinflammatory	Feb-02
Pharmaprojects No. 3217	Inactive	Millennium (US)	Antiinflammatory	Feb-02
Pharmaprojects No. 3259	Inactive	Lilly (US)	Antiinflammatory	Feb-02
Pharmaprojects No. 3268	Inactive	Lilly (US)	Antiinflammatory	Feb-02
Pharmaprojects No. 3335	Inactive	Pfizer (US)	Antiinflammatory	Feb-02
Pharmaprojects No. 3350	Inactive	Pharmacia (US)	Antiinflammatory	Feb-02
Pharmaprojects No. 3355	Inactive	Bayer (Germany)	Antiinflammatory	Feb-02
Pharmaprojects No. 3357	Inactive	Merck & Co (US)	Antiinflammatory	Feb-02
Pharmaprojects No. 3435	Inactive	Abbott (US)	Antiinflammatory	Feb-02
Pharmaprojects No. 3490	Inactive	Johnson & Johnson (US)	Antiinflammatory	Feb-02
Pharmaprojects No. 3503	Inactive	Procter & Gamble (US)	Antiinflammatory	Feb-02
Pharmaprojects No. 3532	Inactive	Pharmacia (US)	Antiinflammatory	Feb-02
Pharmaprojects No. 3957	Inactive	Telik (US)	Antiinflammatory	Feb-02
Pharmaprojects No. 4373	Inactive	Pharmacia (US)	Antiinflammatory	Feb-02
Pharmaprojects No. 4521	Inactive	Johnson & Johnson (US)	Antiinflammatory	Feb-02
Pharmaprojects No. 4527	Inactive	Toyobo	Antiinflammatory	Feb-02
Pharmaprojects No. 4580	Inactive	Bristol-Myers Squibb (US)	Antiinflammatory	Feb-02

Ref.: Pharmaprojects (updated to 2/02) used with permission; Scrip, corporate, literature & patent references
"Status" is international drug development or regulatory status and may not indicate status in USA
Sponsor: Original company name is retained if product is discontinued or inactive after merger, acquisition, company name change, etc.
Users of this table are encouraged to independently verify the status, activity, and mechanism of action of drugs of interest

GENERIC / TRADE NAME	STATUS	SPONSOR (S)	MECHANISM OF ACTION	REF. UPDATE
Pharmaprojects No. 4603	Inactive	Allergan (US)	Antiinflammatory	Feb-02
Pharmaprojects No. 4619	Inactive	GlaxoSmithKline (UK)	Antiinflammatory	Feb-02
Pharmaprojects No. 4648	Inactive	AstraZeneca (UK)	Antiinflammatory	Feb-02
Pharmaprojects No. 4828	Inactive	Sanofi-Synthelabo (France)	Antiinflammatory	Feb-02
Pharmaprojects No. 4916	Inactive	Johnson & Johnson (US)	Antiinflammatory	Feb-02
Pharmaprojects No. 4975	Inactive	Amgen (US)	Antiinflammatory	Feb-02
Pharmaprojects No. 5679	Inactive	Sumitomo (Japan)	Antiinflammatory	Feb-02
Pharmaprojects No. 6425	Inactive	Italfarmaco (Italy)	Antiinflammatory	Feb-02
Pharmaprojects No. 6438	Inactive	Arachnova	Antiinflammatory	Feb-02
Pharmaprojects No. 799	Inactive	Abbott (US)	Antiinflammatory	Feb-02
podoverine A	Inactive	Aventis (France)	Antiinflammatory	Feb-02
QZ-16	Inactive	Non-industrial source	Antiinflammatory	Feb-02
R-62230	Inactive	Non-industrial source	Antiinflammatory	Feb-02
Ro-31-8830	Inactive	Roche (Switz)	Antiinflammatory	Feb-02
S-19812	Inactive	Servier (France)	Antiinflammatory	Feb-02
SC-299	Inactive	Pharmacia (US)	Antiinflammatory	Feb-02
SC-53228	Inactive	Pharmacia (US)	Antiinflammatory	Feb-02
SP-123	Inactive	UCM-Difme	Antiinflammatory	Feb-02
ß-glucan receptor antagonists	Inactive	Alpha-Beta Technology	Antiinflammatory	Feb-02
T-0757	Inactive	Tanabe Seiyaku (Japan)	Antiinflammatory	Feb-02
TA-668	Inactive	Taisho (Japan)	Antiinflammatory	Feb-02
TEI-1338	Inactive	Teijin (Japan)	Antiinflammatory	Feb-02
TEI-1345	Inactive	Teijin (Japan)	Antiinflammatory	Feb-02
TMK-919	Inactive	Terumo	Antiinflammatory	Feb-02
TR-9109	Inactive	Tanabe Seiyaku (Japan)	Antiinflammatory	Feb-02
Win-72052	Inactive	Sanofi-Synthelabo (France)	Antiinflammatory	Feb-02
Wy-48489	Inactive	American Home Products (US)	Antiinflammatory	Feb-02
Wy-49422	Inactive	American Home Products (US)	Antiinflammatory	Feb-02
YM-26567-1	Inactive	Yamanouchi (Japan)	Antiinflammatory	Feb-02
ZK-90695	Inactive	Schering AG (Germany)	Antiinflammatory	Feb-02
naphterpin	Inactive	Non-industrial source	Antiinflammatory	Feb-02
Pharmaprojects No. 1369	Inactive	Maruzen Seiyaku	Antiinflammatory	Feb-02
Pharmaprojects No. 3443	Inactive	Aventis (France)	Antiinflammatory	Feb-02
Pharmaprojects No. 1996	Inactive	Chiesi (Italy)	Antiinflammatory	Feb-02
Pharmaprojects No. 3232	Inactive	Eisai (Japan)	Antiinflammatory	Feb-02
disogluside	Inactive	Non-industrial source	Antiinflammatory	Feb-02
LEX-028	Inactive	SuperGen (US)	Antiinflammatory	Feb-02
PEG-catalase, Sterling	Inactive	Sanofi-Synthelabo (France)	Antiinflammatory	Feb-02
Pharmaprojects No. 3089	Inactive	MacroNex	Antiinflammatory	Feb-02
catalase, Enzon	Inactive	Enzon	Antiinflammatory	Feb-02
U-78517	Inactive	Pharmacia (US)	Antiinflammatory	Feb-02
Pharmaprojects No. 4876	Inactive	GlaxoSmithKline (UK)	Antiinflammatory	Feb-02
Pharmaprojects No. 1878	Inactive	Akzo Nobel (Netherlands)	Antiinflammatory	Feb-02
Pharmaprojects No. 4542	Inactive	Bristol-Myers Squibb (US)	Antiinflammatory	Feb-02
benzydamine, Angelini	Inactive	Angelini (Italy)	Antiinflammatory	Feb-02
glucocorticoids, Aventis	Inactive	Aventis (France)	Antiinflammatory	Feb-02
Pharmaprojects No. 4295	Inactive	Aventis (France)	Antiinflammatory	Feb-02
Pharmaprojects No. 4322	Inactive	Roche (Switz)	Antiinflammatory	Feb-02
Pharmaprojects No. 4488	Inactive	Aventis (France)	Antiinflammatory	Feb-02
sialophorin, LSB	Inactive	Large Scale Biology	Antiinflammatory	Feb-02
TMC-86A	Inactive	Tanabe Seiyaku (Japan)	Antiinflammatory	Feb-02
cell adhesion inhibitors, Tana	Inactive	Tanabe Seiyaku (Japan)	Antiinflammatory	Feb-02
Pharmaprojects No. 640	Inactive	GlaxoSmithKline (UK)	Antiinflammatory	Feb-02
TMC-95A	Inactive	Tanabe Seiyaku (Japan)	Antiinflammatory	Feb-02
CY-9652	Inactive	Epimmune	Antiinflammatory	Feb-02
WF-11605	Inactive	Fujisawa (Japan)	Antiinflammatory	Feb-02
Pharmaprojects No. 3359	Inactive	Lilly (US)	Antiinflammatory	Feb-02
Pharmaprojects No. 4566	Inactive	Pfizer (US)	Antiinflammatory	Feb-02
MCP enzyme inhibitors,Cephalon	Inactive	Cephalon (US)	Antiinflammatory	Feb-02
Pharmaprojects No. 4490	Inactive	Merck & Co (US)	Antiinflammatory	Feb-02
Pharmaprojects No. 1688	Inactive	Sanofi-Synthelabo (France)	Antiinflammatory	Feb-02
EN-03	Inactive	Essential Nutrition (UK)	Antiinflammatory	Feb-02
M-7074	Inactive	Mochida	Antiinflammatory	Feb-02

Ref.: Pharmaprojects (updated to 2/02) used with permission; Scrip, corporate, literature & patent references
"Status" is international drug development or regulatory status and may not indicate status in USA
Sponsor: Original company name is retained if product is discontinued or inactive after merger, acquisition, company name change, etc.
Users of this table are encouraged to independently verify the status, activity, and mechanism of action of drugs of interest

GENERIC / TRADE NAME	STATUS	SPONSOR (S)	MECHANISM OF ACTION	REF. UPDATE
Pharmaprojects No. 3898	Inactive	Pharmacia (US)	Antiinflammatory	Feb-02
CAM inhibitors, Syntex	Inactive	Roche (Switz)	Antiinflammatory	Feb-02
FI-302	Inactive	Taisho (Japan)	Antiinflammatory	Feb-02
HG/3	Inactive	UCM-Difme	Antiinflammatory	Feb-02
oxanthinecarboxylic acid	Inactive	Takeda (Japan)	Antiinflammatory	Feb-02
Pharmaprojects No. 1079	Inactive	Boehringer Ingelheim (Ger)	Antiinflammatory	Feb-02
Pharmaprojects No. 1472	Inactive	Sanofi-Synthelabo (France)	Antiinflammatory	Feb-02
Pharmaprojects No. 2139	Inactive	Merck & Co (US)	Antiinflammatory	Feb-02
Pharmaprojects No. 4088	Inactive	Pfizer (US)	Antiinflammatory	Feb-02
Pharmaprojects No. 475	Inactive	GlaxoSmithKline (UK)	Antiinflammatory	Feb-02
Pharmaprojects No. 4920	Inactive	Pharmacia (US)	Antiinflammatory	Feb-02
Pharmaprojects No. 760	Inactive	GlaxoSmithKline (UK)	Antiinflammatory	Feb-02
Pharmaprojects No. 900	Inactive	GlaxoSmithKline (UK)	Antiinflammatory	Feb-02
Pharmaprojects No. 981	Inactive	Takeda (Japan)	Antiinflammatory	Feb-02
PV-108	Inactive	Resfar (Italy)	Antiinflammatory	Feb-02
pyrimidant	Inactive	Non-industrial source	Antiinflammatory	Feb-02
RU-42738	Inactive	Aventis (France)	Antiinflammatory	Feb-02
salicylamide esters	Inactive	Merck & Co (US)	Antiinflammatory	Feb-02
TB-219	Inactive	Teikoku Chemical	Antiinflammatory	Feb-02
YS-134	Inactive	Medea Research (Italy)	Antiinflammatory	Feb-02
zoanthamine	Inactive	Non-industrial source	Antiinflammatory	Feb-02
YS-1033	Inactive	Asahi Kasei (Japan)	Antiinflammatory	Feb-02
BGI	Inactive	Non-industrial source	Antiinflammatory	Feb-02
talosalate	Inactive	Bago	Antiinflammatory	Feb-02
Pharmaprojects No. 2054	Inactive	Mitsubishi Pharma (Japan)	Antiinflammatory	Feb-02
HN-3392	Inactive	Hisamitsu	Antiinflammatory	Feb-02
Pharmaprojects No. 2462	Inactive	Novartis (Switz.)	Antiinflammatory	Feb-02
RU-48057	Inactive	Aventis (France)	Antiinflammatory	Feb-02
Pharmaprojects No. 4877	Inactive	Bristol-Myers Squibb (US)	Antiinflammatory	Feb-02
Pharmaprojects No. 4099	Inactive	Merck & Co (US)	Antiinflammatory	Feb-02
Pharmaprojects No. 4421	Inactive	Merck & Co (US)	Antiinflammatory	Feb-02
LY-178002	Inactive	Lilly (US)	Antiinflammatory	Feb-02
SPI-42	Inactive	Johnson & Johnson (US)	Antiinflammatory	Feb-02
MDL-100948A	Inactive	Aventis (France)	Antiinflammatory	Feb-02
KCN-TEI-6172	Inactive	Teijin (Japan)	Antiinflammatory	Feb-02
Pharmaprojects No. 4029	Inactive	Celltech (UK)	Antiinflammatory	Feb-02
Pharmaprojects No. 6492	Inactive	Cytopia	Antiinflammatory	Feb-02
phospholipase A2 inhibs, Sphin	Inactive	Lilly (US)	Antiinflammatory	Feb-02
A-69412	Inactive	Abbott (US)	Antiinflammatory	Feb-02
BI-L-357	Inactive	Boehringer Ingelheim (Ger)	Antiinflammatory	Feb-02
Pharmaprojects No. 3360	Inactive	Novartis (Switz.)	Antiinflammatory	Feb-02
MM-7002	Inactive	Meiji Milk (Japan)	Antiinflammatory	Feb-02
Pharmaprojects No. 3193	Inactive	Pharmagenesis	Antiinflammatory	Feb-02
Fanetizole	Inactive	Pfizer (US)	Anti-inflammatory	Unk.
NCX-099	Inactive	NicOx (France)	Antiinflammatory (unspecified)	Feb-02
Pharmaprojects No. 5356	Inactive	DuPont Merck (US)	Chemotactic mod.; anti-inflam.	Feb-02
collagenase, Yakult Honsha	Inactive	Yakult Honsha	Collagenase inhibitors	Feb-02
BCX-1170	Inactive	BioCryst (US)	Complement factor D inhib.	Nov-98
COX-2 inhibitor, Roche	Inactive	Roche (Switz)	COX-2 inhibitor	Feb-02
COX-2 inhibitors, Almirall-Pro	Inactive	Almirall-Prodesfarma (Spain)	COX-2 inhibitor	Feb-02
NMI-346 (diclofenac-SNO)	Inactive	NitroMed (US) / J&J (US)	Diclofenac w/nitric oxide donor	Jun-00
NMI-377	Inactive	NitroMed (US)	Diclofenac w/nitric oxide donor	Aug-99
NMI-172 (ibuprofen-SNO)	Inactive	NitroMed (US) / J&J (US)	Ibuprofen w/nitric oxide donor	Apr-00
Pharmaprojects No. 6007	Inactive	Idun (US)	ICE (IL-1beta conv. enzyme) inhib.	Feb-02
NMI-267 (indomethacin-SNO)	Inactive	NitroMed (US) / J&J (US)	Indomethacin w/nitric oxide donor	Nov-99
Pharmaprojects No. 6080	Inactive	Merck & Co (US)	iNOS inhibitor / anti-inflam.	Feb-02
NMI-246 (ketoprofen-SNO)	Inactive	NitroMed (US) / J&J (US)	Ketoprofen w/nitric oxide donor	Nov-99
elastase inhibitors, Servier	Inactive	Servier (France)	Leucocyte elastase inhib. /inflam.	Feb-02
KB-R7785	Inactive	Akzo Nobel / Kanebo (Japan)	Metalloproteinase, TNF, FasL inhib.	Feb-02
Pharmaprojects No. 5441	Inactive	DuPont Merck (US)	Metalloproteinase-3 inhib.	Sep-97
CH-5902	Inactive	Celltech / Chiroscience (UK)	MMP inhibitor / anti-inflam.	Feb-02
Orazipone (OR-1384)	Inactive	Orion Pharma (Finland)	Neutrophil superoxide antag.	Mar-99
EU-11300	Inactive	Euroresearch	NSAID	Feb-02

Ref.: Pharmaprojects (updated to 2/02) used with permission; Scrip, corporate, literature & patent references
"Status" is international drug development or regulatory status and may not indicate status in USA
Sponsor: Original company name is retained if product is discontinued or inactive after merger, acquisition, company name change, etc.
Users of this table are encouraged to independently verify the status, activity, and mechanism of action of drugs of interest

GENERIC / TRADE NAME	STATUS	SPONSOR (S)	MECHANISM OF ACTION	REF. UPDATE
AHR-10037	Inactive	American Home Products (US)	NSAID	Feb-02
BRL-37959	Inactive	GlaxoSmithKline (UK)	NSAID	Feb-02
LY-108964	Inactive	Lilly (US)	NSAID	Feb-02
Pharmaprojects No. 886	Inactive	GlaxoSmithKline (UK)	NSAID	Feb-02
SC-56567	Inactive	Pharmacia (US)	NSAID	Feb-02
tazadolene	Inactive	Pharmacia (US)	NSAID	Feb-02
anthrotainin	Inactive	Sanofi-Synthelabo (France)	NSAID	Feb-02
dexibuprofen lysine	Inactive	Merck & Co (US)	NSAID	Feb-02
FZ	Inactive	Nippon Zoki (Japan)	NSAID	Feb-02
Pharmaprojects No. 1379	Inactive	Sankyo (Japan)	NSAID	Feb-02
Pharmaprojects No. 1618	Inactive	Non-industrial source	NSAID	Feb-02
Pharmaprojects No. 2145	Inactive	Biosearch Italia (Italy)	NSAID	Feb-02
Pharmaprojects No. 2368	Inactive	Aventis (France)	NSAID	Feb-02
Pharmaprojects No. 514	Inactive	American Home Products (US)	NSAID	Feb-02
Pharmaprojects No. 1738	Inactive	GlaxoSmithKline (UK)	NSAID	Feb-02
piroxicam olamine	Inactive	Pfizer (US)	NSAID	Feb-02
NCX-284	Inactive	NicOx (France)	NSAID + NO releaser	Feb-02
CPR-3016	Inactive	Clarion (US)	PAF antag.; anti-inflam./asthma	Feb-02
NCS-700	Inactive	CNRS (France)	PDE-IV + TNF-α inhibitor	Jul-99
Pharmaprojects No. 6141	Inactive	Rhone-Poulenc Rorer (France)	PDE-IV inhibitor / inflam.	Feb-02
Praxiterol	Inactive	Kyowa Hakko (Japan)	PGSI	Mar-92
RU-49289	Inactive	Roussel-Uclaf (France)	PGSI	1988
TAI-998	Inactive	Takeda (Japan)	PGSI	1985
Tolpadol	Inactive	Univ. Complutense (Spain)	PGSI	1983
ML-3176	Inactive	Merckle (Germany)	Phospholipase PLA2 inhibitor	Jul-99
Pharmaprojects No. 5712	Inactive	AstraZeneca (UK)	Pink tarantula venom extract	Feb-02
Cysteine protease inhibitors	Inactive	British Biotech (UK) / SynPhar	RA, OA, osteoporosis	Feb-02
Pharmaprojects No. 5341	Inactive	Pharmos (US)	Steroid analogs; anti-inflam.	Feb-02
CLX-1100 / CLX-1200	Inactive	Calyx Therapeutics (US)	TNF-α antagonist; plant extract	Jun-00
Melanin analogs	Inactive	Biosource Technologies (US)	TNF-alpha inhibitor; anti-inflam.	Aug-97
TSK-204 (KF-20444)	Inactive	Taisho / Kyowa Hakko (Japan)	Unidentified (RA)	Feb-02
Pharmaprojects No. 5552	Inactive	CombiChem (US) / Sumitomo	Unidentified (RA, OA)	Feb-02
CMI-546	Inactive	CytoMed / Millennium (US)	Unidentified anti-inflammatory	Feb-02
Pharmaprojects No. 5431	Inactive	LeukoSite (US)	Unidentified; RA, MS, psoriasis	Feb-02
auranofin	LAUNCHED	GlaxoSmithKline (UK)	Antiarthritic	Feb-02
glucametacin	LAUNCHED	Farmades	Antiarthritic	Feb-02
halopredone	LAUNCHED	Dainippon (Japan)	Antiarthritic	Feb-02
hyaluronic acid, Fidia	LAUNCHED	Fidia (Italy)	Antiarthritic	Feb-02
hyaluronic acid, Seikagaku	LAUNCHED	Seikagaku Kogyo (Japan)	Antiarthritic	Feb-02
hylans	LAUNCHED	Genzyme (US)	Antiarthritic	Feb-02
meclofenamate sodium	LAUNCHED	Pfizer (US)	Antiarthritic	Feb-02
copper complexes, Arkansas	LAUNCHED	Non-industrial source	Antiarthritic	Feb-02
piproxen	LAUNCHED	Aventis (France)	Antiarthritic	Feb-02
loxoprofen	LAUNCHED	Sankyo (Japan)	Antiarthritic	Feb-02
tiaprofenic acid	LAUNCHED	Aventis (France)	Antiarthritic	Feb-02
tropine indometacinate, Spofa	LAUNCHED	VUFB (Czech Republic)	Antiarthritic	Feb-02
cloprednol	LAUNCHED	Roche (Switz)	Antiarthritic	Feb-02
Mofezolac	LAUNCHED	Pasteur Merieux (Fr) / Taiho	Antiinflamatory/analgesic	Nov-95
amfenac sodium	LAUNCHED	American Home Products (US)	Antiinflammatory	Feb-02
bufexamac	LAUNCHED	Pharmacia (US)	Antiinflammatory	Feb-02
chondroitin sulfate	LAUNCHED	American Home Products (US)	Antiinflammatory	Feb-02
clidanac	LAUNCHED	Bristol-Myers Squibb (US)	Antiinflammatory	Feb-02
difenpyramide	LAUNCHED	GlaxoSmithKline (UK)	Antiinflammatory	Feb-02
droxicam	LAUNCHED	Esteve (Spain)	Antiinflammatory	Feb-02
enfenamic acid	LAUNCHED	Unichem	Antiinflammatory	Feb-02
epirizole	LAUNCHED	Daiichi (Japan)	Antiinflammatory	Feb-02
feprazone	LAUNCHED	Boehringer Ingelheim (Ger)	Antiinflammatory	Feb-02
flurbiprofen	LAUNCHED	Abbott (US)	Antiinflammatory	Feb-02
lonazolac calcium	LAUNCHED	Byk Gulden (Ger)	Antiinflammatory	Feb-02
mabuprofen	LAUNCHED	Aldo-Union	Antiinflammatory	Feb-02
oxametacin	LAUNCHED	ABC	Antiinflammatory	Feb-02
protizinic acid	LAUNCHED	Aventis (France)	Antiinflammatory	Feb-02
sulindac	LAUNCHED	Merck & Co (US)	Antiinflammatory	Feb-02

Ref.: Pharmaprojects (updated to 2/02) used with permission; Scrip, corporate, literature & patent references
"Status" is international drug development or regulatory status and may not indicate status in USA
Sponsor: Original company name is retained if product is discontinued or inactive after merger, acquisition, company name change, etc.
Users of this table are encouraged to independently verify the status, activity, and mechanism of action of drugs of interest

GENERIC / TRADE NAME	STATUS	SPONSOR (S)	MECHANISM OF ACTION	REF. UPDATE
superoxide dismutase, Sidus	LAUNCHED	Sidus	Antiinflammatory	Feb-02
thiazolinobutazone	LAUNCHED	Almirall-Prodesfarma (Spain)	Antiinflammatory	Feb-02
tolfenamic acid	LAUNCHED	Bristol-Myers Squibb (US)	Antiinflammatory	Feb-02
tolmetin sodium	LAUNCHED	Johnson & Johnson (US)	Antiinflammatory	Feb-02
venoglobulin-1H	LAUNCHED	Mitsubishi Pharma (Japan)	Antiinflammatory	Feb-02
etersalate	LAUNCHED	Alter	Antiinflammatory	Feb-02
superoxide dismutase, Cantacuz	LAUNCHED	Non-industrial source	Antiinflammatory	Feb-02
carprofen	LAUNCHED	Roche (Switz)	Antiinflammatory	Feb-02
azapropazone	LAUNCHED	Siegfried	Antiinflammatory	Feb-02
acemetacin	LAUNCHED	Bayer (Germany)	Antiinflammatory	Feb-02
AF-2259	LAUNCHED	Angelini (Italy)	Antiinflammatory	Feb-02
cinmetacin	LAUNCHED	Chiesi (Italy)	Antiinflammatory	Feb-02
emorfazone	LAUNCHED	Aventis (France)	Antiinflammatory	Feb-02
fentiazac	LAUNCHED	American Home Products (US)	Antiinflammatory	Feb-02
imidazole salicylate	LAUNCHED	Italfarmaco (Italy)	Antiinflammatory	Feb-02
nimesulide	LAUNCHED	Helsinn	Antiinflammatory	Feb-02
perisoxal citrate	LAUNCHED	Shionogi (Japan)	Antiinflammatory	Feb-02
proglumetacin	LAUNCHED	Rotta (Italy)	Antiinflammatory	Feb-02
proquazone	LAUNCHED	Novartis (Switz.)	Antiinflammatory	Feb-02
talniflumate	LAUNCHED	Bago	Antiinflammatory	Feb-02
zaltoprofen	LAUNCHED	Nippon Chemiphar	Antiinflammatory	Feb-02
butibufen	LAUNCHED	Juste (Spain)	Antiinflammatory	Feb-02
persalmide	LAUNCHED	Sanofi-Synthelabo (France)	Antiinflammatory	Feb-02
diclofenac potassium	LAUNCHED	Novartis (Switz.)	Antiinflammatory	Feb-02
guaimesal	LAUNCHED	GlaxoSmithKline (UK)	Antiinflammatory	Feb-02
superoxide dismutase, Isnardi	LAUNCHED	Sanofi-Synthelabo (France)	Antiinflammatory	Feb-02
Diacerein (ARTRODAR; FISIODAR)	LAUNCHED	Proter (Italy)	Arthritis; chelator; IL-1, TNFα antag.	Mar-96
Naproxen betinate	LAUNCHED	Applied Pharma Res. (Switz.)	Combination naproxen + betaine	Jun-98
Meloxicam (MOBIC®)	LAUNCHED	Boehringer Ingelheim (Ger)	COX 1-2 inhibitor, 1x daily	Dec-96
Celecoxib (CELEBRA, CELEBREX)	LAUNCHED	Pharmacia (US)	COX-2 inhibitor	May-00
Rofecoxib (VIOXX, MK-966)	LAUNCHED	Merck & Co (US)	COX-2 inhibitor / RA-OA	Jun-99
TJ-114	LAUNCHED	Tsumura (Jp)	Herbal med. (induces IL-1ra)	Aug-95
NRD-101	Launched	Aventis (France)	Hyaluronic acid (inj.); arthritis	Feb-02
Hylan (SYNVISC®)	LAUNCHED	Wyeth-Ayerst (US) / Biomatrix	Hylan A + B (joint lubricant, inj)	Jul-96
alclofenac	LAUNCHED	Pharmacia (US)	NSAID	Feb-02
ampiroxicam	LAUNCHED	Pfizer (US)	NSAID	Feb-02
ibuproxam	LAUNCHED	GlaxoSmithKline (UK)	NSAID	Feb-02
ketoprofen	LAUNCHED	Aventis (France)	NSAID	Feb-02
indometacin farnesil	LAUNCHED	Eisai (Japan)	NSAID	Feb-02
nabumetone	LAUNCHED	GlaxoSmithKline (UK)	NSAID	Feb-02
pranoprofen	LAUNCHED	Mitsubishi Pharma (Japan)	NSAID	Feb-02
fenbufen	LAUNCHED	American Home Products (US)	NSAID	Feb-02
flunoxaprofen	LAUNCHED	Abbott (US)	NSAID	Feb-02
piroxicam	LAUNCHED	Pfizer (US)	NSAID	Feb-02
floctafenine	LAUNCHED	Aventis (France)	NSAID	Feb-02
ketorolac	LAUNCHED	Roche (Switz)	NSAID	Feb-02
lysine salicylate	LAUNCHED	Polytechna	NSAID	Feb-02
nefopam	LAUNCHED	3M (US)	NSAID	Feb-02
denaverine hydrochloride	LAUNCHED	Apogepha	NSAID	Feb-02
alminoprofen	LAUNCHED	Recordati	NSAID	Feb-02
diflunisal	LAUNCHED	Merck & Co (US)	NSAID	Feb-02
isonixin	LAUNCHED	Hermes	NSAID	Feb-02
lysine clonixinate	LAUNCHED	Laplex	NSAID	Feb-02
rimazolium metilsulfate	LAUNCHED	Chinoin (Hungary)	NSAID	Feb-02
lornoxicam	LAUNCHED	Nycomed Pharma (Norway)	NSAID	Feb-02
fosfosal	LAUNCHED	Uriach (Spain)	NSAID	Feb-02
dexibuprofen	LAUNCHED	PAZ Pharma (Ger)	NSAID	Feb-02
Aceclofenac (Airtal, Barcan)	LAUNCHED	BMS / Almirall-Prodesfarma	NSAID	Aug-98
Etodolac (LODINE®)	LAUNCHED	P&G (US) / Am Home Prod	NSAID	May-96
Piroxicam cinnamate	LAUNCHED	SPA (Italy)	NSAID	Aug-96
Tenoxicam	LAUNCHED	HMR (Ger) / Roche (Switz)	NSAID	Oct-94
Lornoxicam (LORCAM, XEFO)	LAUNCHED	Nycomed Pharma (Norway)	NSAID (oral, suppository)	Jan-00
Oxaprozin (DAYPRO®)	LAUNCHED	Searle (US)/Am Home Prod	NSAID, 1x daily	Mar-96

Ref.: Pharmaprojects (updated to 2/02) used with permission; Scrip, corporate, literature & patent references
"Status" is international drug development or regulatory status and may not indicate status in USA
Sponsor: Original company name is retained if product is discontinued or inactive after merger, acquisition, company name change, etc.
Users of this table are encouraged to independently verify the status, activity, and mechanism of action of drugs of interest

GENERIC / TRADE NAME	STATUS	SPONSOR (S)	MECHANISM OF ACTION	REF. UPDATE
Carbasalte calcium	LAUNCHED	Bristol-Myers Squibb (US)	NSAID, non-ulcerogenic	Jan-96
bromfenac, ophthalmic	LAUNCHED	Senju (Japan)	NSAID: COX + peroxidase inhib.	Feb-02
(S)-Ibuprofen, PAZ	LAUNCHED	PAZ Pharma (Ger)	NSAID; single isomer	Jul-96
Amtolmetin guacil (Eufans)	LAUNCHED	Sigma-Tau (Italy)	NSAID; tolmetin prodrug	Dec-98
Fepramol	LAUNCHED	Schwarz (Ger)	PGSI	Dec-91
Piroxicam betadex (BREXECAM)	LAUNCHED	Chiesi (Italy)	Piroxicam beta-cyclodextrin	May-99
Hyaluronic acid (HYALGAN®)	LAUNCHED	Sanofi (France) / Fidia (Italy)	Purified hyaluronic acid for OA	Nov-97
Dexketoprofen [(S)-ketoprofen]	LAUNCHED	Menarini / Chiroscience (UK)	Single isomer formulation	Jul-96
Glucosamine sulfate	LAUNCHED	Rotta (Italy)	Superoxide free radical antag.	Jan-96
etanercept (ENBREL™)	LAUNCHED	Immunex (US) / Wyeth-Ayerst	TNF receptor fusion protein (RA)	Nov-98
Infliximab (REMICADE)	LAUNCHED	Centocor (US)	TNF-alpha antibody, RA	Feb-02
Biphenyl-acetohydroxamic acids	Preclinical	Wellcome (UK)	5-LO / COX inhibitor	Jan-95
Aggrecanase inhibitors	Preclinical	Zeneca (UK)/Celltech (UK)	Aggrecanase inhibitors	Mar-97
arthritis therapy, LGCI	Preclinical	LG Chem Investment	Antiarthritic	Feb-02
AZD-8309	Preclinical	AstraZeneca (UK)	Antiarthritic	Feb-02
AZD-9056	Preclinical	AstraZeneca (UK)	Antiarthritic	Feb-02
KSB-306	Preclinical	KS Biomedix	Antiarthritic	Feb-02
MITO-2227	Preclinical	MitoKor	Antiarthritic	Feb-02
MPYS-333 ligands	Preclinical	Myriad Genetics	Antiarthritic	Feb-02
MX-1094	Preclinical	Medinox (US)	Antiarthritic	Feb-02
OA-5025	Preclinical	Genzyme (US)	Antiarthritic	Feb-02
osteoarthritis therapy, Incyt	Preclinical	Incyte Genomics	Antiarthritic	Feb-02
PGE-4304887	Preclinical	Procter & Gamble (US)	Antiarthritic	Feb-02
SP-057	Preclinical	Bristol-Myers Squibb (US)	Antiarthritic	Feb-02
TST-500	Preclinical	Twinstrand Therapeutics	Antiarthritic	Feb-02
viscoelastic collagen, Collage	Preclinical	Collagenesis	Antiarthritic	Feb-02
SB-380732	Preclinical	GlaxoSmithKline (UK)	Antiarthritic	Feb-02
C24	Preclinical	GlaxoSmithKline (UK)	Antiarthritic	Feb-02
SP-600125	Preclinical	Celgene (US)	Antiarthritic	Feb-02
Pharmaprojects No. 6625	Preclinical	Sunesis	Antiarthritic	Feb-02
TNF-Alpha antagonists, Dynavax	Preclinical	Dynavax Technologies	Antiarthritic	Feb-02
Vapill	Preclinical	BioTie Therapies	Antiarthritic	Feb-02
CPI-1714	Preclinical	Centaur	Antiarthritic	Feb-02
E-6259	Preclinical	Esteve (Spain)	Antiarthritic	Feb-02
AP-1 inhibitors, Toyama	Preclinical	Toyama (Japan)	Antiarthritic	Feb-02
bradykinin antags, Drug Discov	Preclinical	Drug Discovery	Antiarthritic	Feb-02
A-155918	Preclinical	Abbott (US)	Antiinflammatory	Feb-02
A-293507	Preclinical	Abbott (US)	Antiinflammatory	Feb-02
Alpha-D modulator, ICOS	Preclinical	ICOS (US)	Antiinflammatory	Feb-02
anti-inflammatory, GeneMax	Preclinical	GeneMax	Antiinflammatory	Feb-02
BIO-2421	Preclinical	Biogen (US)	Antiinflammatory	Feb-02
CR-3294	Preclinical	Rotta (Italy)	Antiinflammatory	Feb-02
GW-4459	Preclinical	GlaxoSmithKline (UK)	Antiinflammatory	Feb-02
ICAM-1 antagonists, Abbott	Preclinical	Abbott (US)	Antiinflammatory	Feb-02
IDN-6126	Preclinical	Idun (US)	Antiinflammatory	Feb-02
M3, Xenova	Preclinical	Xenova (US)	Antiinflammatory	Feb-02
metalloenzyme inhibitors, Sero	Preclinical	Serono	Antiinflammatory	Feb-02
NF-AT decoy, Corgentech	Preclinical	Corgentech	Antiinflammatory	Feb-02
NF-kappaB decoy, Corgentech	Preclinical	Corgentech	Antiinflammatory	Feb-02
P61	Preclinical	Phytopharm (UK)	Antiinflammatory	Feb-02
Pharmaprojects No. 4915	Preclinical	Avanir (US)	Antiinflammatory	Feb-02
Pharmaprojects No. 5270	Preclinical	Pharmacopeia (US)	Antiinflammatory	Feb-02
Pharmaprojects No. 6263	Preclinical	OXiGENE	Antiinflammatory	Feb-02
Pharmaprojects No. 6325	Preclinical	Structural Bioinformatics	Antiinflammatory	Feb-02
Pharmaprojects No. 6624	Preclinical	AtheroGenics	Antiinflammatory	Feb-02
RDP-58, 2nd-generation	Preclinical	SangStat (US)	Antiinflammatory	Feb-02
RS-635	Preclinical	Abbott (US)	Antiinflammatory	Feb-02
TNF-Alpha inhibitors, Message	Preclinical	Message Pharmaceuticals (US)	Antiinflammatory	Feb-02
VLA-4 antagonist, Merck	Preclinical	Merck & Co (US)	Antiinflammatory	Feb-02
VLA-4 antagonists, Biogen	Preclinical	Biogen (US)	Antiinflammatory	Feb-02
VT-224	Preclinical	Viron Therapeutics (Canada)	Antiinflammatory	Feb-02
VT-239	Preclinical	Viron Therapeutics (Canada)	Antiinflammatory	Feb-02
VT-346	Preclinical	Viron Therapeutics (Canada)	Antiinflammatory	Feb-02

Ref.: Pharmaprojects (updated to 2/02) used with permission; Scrip, corporate, literature & patent references
"Status" is international drug development or regulatory status and may not indicate status in USA
Sponsor: Original company name is retained if product is discontinued or inactive after merger, acquisition, company name change, etc.
Users of this table are encouraged to independently verify the status, activity, and mechanism of action of drugs of interest

GENERIC / TRADE NAME	STATUS	SPONSOR (S)	MECHANISM OF ACTION	REF. UPDATE
VT-900	Preclinical	Viron Therapeutics (Canada)	Antiinflammatory	Feb-02
KP-364	Preclinical	Kinetek	Antiinflammatory	Feb-02
chemokine ligands, Dompe	Preclinical	Dompe	Antiinflammatory	Feb-02
SB-265610	Preclinical	GlaxoSmithKline (UK)	Antiinflammatory	Feb-02
MASP inhibitors, Natimmune	Preclinical	Natimmune	Antiinflammatory	Feb-02
PT-17	Preclinical	Palatin Technologies	Antiinflammatory	Feb-02
VX-702	Preclinical	Vertex Pharmaceuticals (US)	Antiinflammatory	Feb-02
VX-765	Preclinical	Vertex Pharmaceuticals (US)	Antiinflammatory	Feb-02
AS-602801	Preclinical	Serono	Antiinflammatory	Feb-02
Pharmaprojects No. 6558	Preclinical	Kowa	Antiinflammatory	Feb-02
CXCR2 antagonists, Celltech	Preclinical	Celltech (UK)	Antiinflammatory	Feb-02
anti-inflammatories, Icagen	Preclinical	Icagen	Antiinflammatory	Feb-02
haem oxygenase agonist, SangSt	Preclinical	SangStat (US)	Antiinflammatory	Feb-02
G-protein inhibitors, ICOS	Preclinical	ICOS (US)	Antiinflammatory	Feb-02
Pharmaprojects No. 6661	Preclinical	CombinatoRx	Antiinflammatory	Feb-02
MC1 agonists, Melacure	Preclinical	Melacure Therapeutics	Antiinflammatory	Feb-02
NF-kB inhibitors, Aventis	Preclinical	Aventis (France)	Antiinflammatory	Feb-02
Pharmaprojects No. 6570	Preclinical	Cephalon (US)	Antiinflammatory	Feb-02
Pharmaprojects No. 6612	Preclinical	Celgene (US)	Antiinflammatory	Feb-02
p38 MAP kinase inhibs, Uriach	Preclinical	Uriach (Spain)	Antiinflammatory	Feb-02
LV-216	Preclinical	Vinas (Spain)	Antiinflammatory	Feb-02
UR-8880	Preclinical	Uriach (Spain)	Antiinflammatory	Feb-02
PLR-14	Preclinical	Pliva	Antiinflammatory	Feb-02
PPI-3088	Preclinical	Praecis Pharmaceuticals	Antiinflammatory	Feb-02
SPC-839	Preclinical	Serono	Antiinflammatory	Feb-02
chemokine antags, Neurocrine	Preclinical	Neurocrine Biosciences (US)	Antiinflammatory	Feb-02
DRF-4848	Preclinical	Dr Reddy's	Antiinflammatory	Feb-02
HGP-12	Preclinical	HG Pars (US)	Antiinflammatory	Feb-02
NK2 antagonists, Schering-Plou	Preclinical	Schering Plough (US)	Antiinflammatory	Feb-02
DP-103	Preclinical	D-Pharm (Israel)	Antiinflammatory	Feb-02
AntiPARP-1, Octamer	Preclinical	Octamer	Antiinflammatory	Feb-02
cell adhesion inhibs, Kaken	Preclinical	Kaken (Japan)	Antiinflammatory	Feb-02
PLR-13	Preclinical	Pliva	Antiinflammatory	Feb-02
T25	Preclinical	Manchester Innovation	Antiinflammatory	Feb-02
tryptase inhibitors, Array	Preclinical	Array BioPharma	Antiinflammatory	Feb-02
cathepsin F inhibitors, Celera	Preclinical	Celera Genomics	Antiinflammatory	Feb-02
Yissum P-1025	Preclinical	Yissum (Israel)	Antiinflammatory / Antioxidant	Apr-98
Cathepsin S Inhibitors	Preclinical	Rhone-Poulenc Rorer/AxyS (US)	Cathepsin S inhib. / anti-inflam.	Feb-99
Chemokine binding proteins	Preclinical	Viron Therapeutics (Canada)	Chemokine receptor antag	Aug-99
Collagenase inhibitors	Preclinical	SmithKline Beecham (UK)	Collagenase inhibitors	Mar-97
Complement inhibitors	Preclinical	AdProTech (UK)	Complement factor inhib. / arthritis	Apr-99
APT-070	Preclinical	AdProTech (UK)	Complement inhibitor; arthritis	Jun-99
GR-253035	Preclinical	Glaxo Wellcome (UK)	COX-2 inhibitor	Jan-97
Pharmaprojects No. 4539	Preclinical	DuPont Merck (US)	COX-2 inhibitor	Mar-97
Pharmaprojects No. 5899	Preclinical	Laboratorios SALVAT (Spain)	COX-2 inhibitor	Jul-98
Pharmaprojects No. 6089	Preclinical	Kotobuki (Japan)	COX-2 inhibitor	Oct-98
S-33516	Preclinical	Servier (France)	COX-2 inhibitor	Jun-00
Elastase inhibitors	Preclinical	Cortech (US)	Elastase inhibition	Mar-97
Elastase inhibitors, Cortech	Preclinical	Ono (Japan) / Cortech (US)	Elastase inhibitor, oral: RA	Jun-99
Pharmaprojects No. 5480	Preclinical	Tularik (US) / Roche (Switz)	Gene regulation anti-inflam.	Sep-97
Core-2 GLcNAc-T inhibitors	Preclinical	GlycoDesign (Canada)	Glycosyl transferase inhib. / inflam.	Jan-99
A-252444.0	Preclinical	Abbott (US)	ICAM-1 & E-selectin antagonists	Sep-99
GW-273629, GW-27415	Preclinical	Glaxo Wellcome (UK)	iNOS inhibitor; inflammation	Sep-99
IPL 423 (bispan)	Preclinical	Inflazyme (US)	Kinase activator (anti-inflam.)	Feb-98
Pharmaprojects No. 5594	Preclinical	Kissei (Japan) / Vertex (US)	MAP kinase inhibitor; anti-inflam.	Dec-97
VX-475	Preclinical	Vertex (US) / Kissei (Japan)	MAP kinase inhibitor; RA	Oct-98
HGP-3	Preclinical	HG Pars (US)	Menabitan progrug (anti-inflam.)	Jan-96
MMP inhibitors	Preclinical	DuPont (US)	Metalloproteinase + TNF-α inhib.	Sep-99
ZD-2315	Preclinical	Zeneca (UK)	MHCII antagonist (RA)	Jan-98
D-2163	Preclinical	Chiroscience (UK)	MMP inhibitor / antiinflammatory	Mar-97
Pharmaprojects No. 5610	Preclinical	Shionogi (Japan)	MMP inhibitor; anti-inflam.	Dec-97
NSAID prodrugs, Medinox	Preclinical	Medinox (US)	NSAID	Feb-02
ABT-702	Preclinical	Abbott (US)	NSAID	Feb-02

Ref.: Pharmaprojects (updated to 2/02) used with permission; Scrip, corporate, literature & patent references
"Status" is international drug development or regulatory status and may not indicate status in USA
Sponsor: Original company name is retained if product is discontinued or inactive after merger, acquisition, company name change, etc.
Users of this table are encouraged to independently verify the status, activity, and mechanism of action of drugs of interest

GENERIC / TRADE NAME	STATUS	SPONSOR (S)	MECHANISM OF ACTION	REF. UPDATE
DRF-4367	Preclinical	Dr Reddy's	NSAID	Feb-02
L-745337	Preclinical	Merck & Co (US)	NSAID	Feb-02
Pharmaprojects No. 8653	Preclinical	Biofrontera	NSAID	Feb-02
HCT-8015	Preclinical	NicOx (France)	NSAID + NO releaser	Feb-02
NO-NSAIDS	Preclinical	NitroMed (US) / J&J (US)	NSAID + NO releaser	Jul-97
NO-NSAIDS, NicOx	Preclinical	NicOx (France)	NSAID + NO releaser	Feb-02
UPA-780	Preclinical	NAS (Ukraine)	PGSI / Leukotriene inhib.	Oct-95
PDE-IV inhibitors	Preclinical	ICOS (US)	Phosphodiesterase IV inhib.	May-99
Acylpyrrole-alkanoic acids	Preclinical	Merckle (Germany)	PLA1 inhibitor	Jul-95
Lactacystin analogs	Preclinical	ProScript (US)	Proteasome inhib.; anti-inflam.	Dec-97
PS-519 (lactacystin analog)	Preclinical	ProScript (US)	Proteasome inhib.; anti-inflam.	May-98
Pharmaprojects No. 5488	Preclinical	Novartis (Switz.)	Selectin antag.; anti-inflam.	Sep-97
Kunitz protease inhibitor	Preclinical	Scios (US)	Serine protease inhib; APP	Jun-97
M-40403	Preclinical	Metaphore (US)	Superoxide dismutase inhibitor	Dec-99
Pharmaprojects No. 5463	Preclinical	Searle/Monsanto (US)	Superoxide dismutase stim.	Sep-97
Pharmaprojects No. 4581	Preclinical	Takeda (Japan)	T-cell suppression	Mar-97
ISIS-104838	Preclinical	ISIS Pharmaceuticals (US)	TNF-a antagonist; RA, Crohn's	Jan-00
TACE antagnoists	Preclinical	Immunex (US) / Wyeth-Ayerst	TNF-α converting enzyme antag.	Feb-97
Pharmaprojects No. 6181	Preclinical	Peptor / Teva (Israel)	TNF-alpha inhib. / RA-Crohn's	Mar-99
Pharmaprojects No. 5537	Preclinical	Oxford GlycoSciences (UK)	Unidentified (RA)	Oct-97
Anti-inflammatories	Preclinical	Praxis (Austr.)	Unidentified anti-inflammatory	Feb-00
Pharmaprojects No. 6035	Preclinical	Active Biotech (Sweden)	Unidentified anti-inflammatory	Sep-98
TBC-3342	Preclinical	Texas Biotechnology (US)	VLA-4 inhibitor; RA	May-98
Reumacon	PRE-REGISTRATION	Conpharm (Sweden) / Pharmacia	Amyloid deposit inhibitor (arthritis)	Jun-00
oxaprozin potassium	PRE-REGISTRATION	Pharmacia (US)	Antiarthritic	Feb-02
Parecoxib	PRE-REGISTRATION	Pharmacia (US)	COX-2 antagonist (inj.)	Feb-02
Hyaluronic acid (ORTHOVISC®)	PRE-REGISTRATION	Anika Therapeutics (US)	Purified hyaluronic acid for OA	Jan-98
etoricoxib	REGISTERED	Merck & Co (US)	Antiarthritic	Feb-02
Rimexolone	REGISTERED	Alcon (US) / Akzo Nobel (NE)	Corticosteroid (topical, intra-articular)	Mar-96
Valdecoxib	REGISTERED	Pharmacia / Pfizer (US)	COX-2 inhibitor, 2nd generation	Feb-02
Arthrovas (AE-941)	Suspended	Aterna Labs (Canada)	Shark cartilage extract / RA-OA	Jan-99
POL-647	Suspended	Polifarma (Italy)	TNF-alpha antag.; anti-inflam.	Nov-98
VX-745	Suspended (ph. II)	Vertex (US) / Kissei (Japan)	MAP kinase inhib. / anti-inflam.	Feb-02
diftalone	WITHDRAWN	Biosearch Italia (Italy)	Antiinflammatory	Feb-02
Indoprofen	WITHDRAWN	Pharmacia (US)	Antiinflammatory	Feb-02
Bromfenac, Biovail	WITHDRAWN	Biovail (Canada)	Controlled-release (1x/day)	Aug-98
antrafenine	WITHDRAWN	Sanofi-Synthelabo (France)	COX inhibitor	Feb-02
isoxicam	WITHDRAWN	Pfizer (US)	NSAID	Feb-02
Pirprofen (RENGASIL)	WITHDRAWN	Novartis (Switz.)	NSAID	1990
Benoxaprofen (ORAFLEX, OPREN)	WITHDRAWN	Lilly (US)	NSAID / photosensitivity tox.	1982
Bromfenac (DURACT™)	WITHDRAWN	Wyeth-Ayerst (US)	NSAID: COX + peroxidase inhib.	Aug-98
Glafenine, Sopar	WITHDRAWN (LNCHD)	Rhone-Poulenc Rorer (France)	Unidentified (NSAID); fatalities	Apr-91
ANTIDEPRESSANT ANALGESICS; SEROTONERGICS; 5-HT/NE UPTAKE INHIBITORS; MAO INHIBITORS				
E-5296	CLINICAL (I)	Devp (UK) / Esteve (Spain)	5-HT uptake inhib; sigma antag.	Feb-02
P16CM	Discontinued	Florida A&M Univ. (US)	16-substituted prednisolone der.	May-97
FR-64822	Discontinued	Fujisawa (Japan)	5-HT agonist	Jan-92
Pyranopyrazolones	Discontinued	Dainippon (Japan)	5-HT uptake inhibitor	Apr-86
B-777-81	Discontinued	Byk Gulden (Ger)	Antidepressant analgesic	Mar-87
MD-260185	Discontinued	Synthelabo (France)	NE uptake inhib.	1984
Esflurbiprofen (BTS-24332)	Discontinued (Clin.)	Knoll (Ger.) / Nichiiko (Japan)	(S)-flurbiprofen isomer	Mar-89
SP-186	Discontinued (ph. I)	Serotonin Pharma. (US)	5-HT agonist	May-93
Ro-15-8081	Discontinued (ph. I)	Roche (Switz.)	5-HT/NE uptake inhibitor	May-92
Anpirtoline (D-16949)	Discontinued (ph. I)	Asta Medica (Germany)	5-HT1 agonist; antidepressant	May-93
Fluradoline (HP-494)	Discontinued (ph. I)	Hoechst Marion Roussel (Ger)	Antidepressant analgesic	Feb-87
UP-26-91	Discontinued (ph. II)	UPSA / Bristol-Myers Squibb (US)	5-HT neuromodulator	Mar-97
CPR-2015	Inactive	Clarion (US)	5-ASA analog; anti-inflam./asthma	Feb-02
Nonane / Decane derv.	Inactive	Procter & Gamble (US)	5-HT agonist	Unk.
LY-214281	Inactive	Lilly (US)	5-HT uptake inhibitor	1989
DuP-631	Inactive	Endo Pharmaceuticals (US)	5-HT/NE uptake inhib.	Feb-02
Indolylimidazolones	Inactive	King George's Med. College	MAO inhibitor	1987
Nefazodone	LAUNCHED	Bristol-Myers Squibb (US)	5-HT uptake inhib.; 5-HT2 antag.	Apr-96
Tramadol (TRAMAL®, ULTRAM®)	LAUNCHED	Gruenthal (Ger); J&J (US)	5-HT/NE uptake inhib.	Apr-95

Ref.: Pharmaprojects (updated to 2/02) used with permission; Scrip, corporate, literature & patent references
"Status" is international drug development or regulatory status and may not indicate status in USA
Sponsor: Original company name is retained if product is discontinued or inactive after merger, acquisition, company name change, etc.
Users of this table are encouraged to independently verify the status, activity, and mechanism of action of drugs of interest

GENERIC / TRADE NAME	STATUS	SPONSOR (S)	MECHANISM OF ACTION	REF. UPDATE
Paroxetine (PAXIL®)	LAUNCHED	Novo-Nordisk (Denmark)	Antidepress; 5-HT uptake inh.	Mar-97
Piperadinyl-cyclohexanols	Preclinical	Bristol-Myers Squibb (US)	5-HT1a antagonists	Jul-93
BENZODIAZEPINES / ANXIOLYTICS (ANALGESIC ADJUNCTS)				
SEN-215	Discontinued	Kyowa Hakko (Japan)	Unk. / Benzodiazepine	Jul-84
Midazolam	LAUNCHED	Roche (Switz)	Benzodiazepine	Feb-92
BRADYKININ ANTAGONISTS				
CP-0126 / CP-0499 heterodimers	Discontinued	Cortech (US)	B2 + NK1/NK2 antag; B2 + μ ag.	Mar-97
Pharmaprojects No. 3856	Discontinued	Scios Nova (US)	BK antagonist, 2nd generation	1997
B-4148	Discontinued	Scios Nova (US)	Bradykinin antagonist	Nov-88
NPC-349	Discontinued	Scios Nova (US)	Bradykinin antagonist	Feb-92
NPC-567	Discontinued	Scios Nova (US)	Bradykinin antagonist	Feb-92
Pharmaprojects No. 5518	Discontinued	Sanofi-Synthelabo (France)	Bradykinin B1 antagonist	Feb-02
Pharmaprojects No. 5220	Discontinued	Pharmacopeia (US)	Bradykinin B1/B2 antagonist	Jun-00
FR-173657	Discontinued	Fujisawa (Japan)	Bradykinin B2 antagonist	Feb-00
NPC-18545 (NPC-18608)	Discontinued	Scios (US)	Bradykinin B2 antagonist	Oct-97
Pharmaprojects No. 2936	Discontinued	DuPont (US)	Kallikrein antagonist	Sep-93
CP-0840 (CP-0880)	Discontinued	Cortech (US)	Peripheral B2 antag. + μ agonist	Feb-99
FR-193517	Inactive	Fujisawa (Japan)	B2 bradykinin antag., non-peptide	Feb-02
LF-521	Inactive	Fournier (France)	Bradykinin B1 antagonist	Feb-02
Pharmaprojects No. 5665	Inactive	Aventis (France)	Bradykinin B2 antagonist	Feb-02
NPC-17731	Preclinical	Scios Nova (US)	B2 antagonist	Oct-93
Win-64338	Preclinical	Eastman Kodak (US)	B2 antagonist	Nov-93
NPC-16731	Preclinical	Scios Nova (US)	Bradykinin antagonist	May-91
NPC-17730	Preclinical	Novo-Nordisk (Denmark)	Bradykinin antagonist	Jan-92
Pharmaprojects No. 5503	Preclinical	Fournier (France)	Bradykinin B2 antagonist	Oct-97
CP-0880	Preclinical	Cortech (US)	Peripheral B2 antag. + μ agonist	Mar-97
CP-0127 (BRADYCOR®)	Suspended (ph. II)	Cortech (US)	B2 antagonist	Jan-97
CALCITONIN AGONISTS				
ACT-15	Discontinued	Asahi Glass (Jp) / Chugai (Jp)	Calcitonin stimulant	May-97
Elcatonin, intrathecal	Discontinued	Innapharma (US)	Eel calcitonin (intrathecal)	Aug-99
Elcatonin	LAUNCHED	Asahi Chemical (Japan)	Modified eel calcitonin	Oct-93
CANNABINOIDS				
CT3 (DMH-11C)	CLINICAL (I)	Atlantic Tech. Ventures (US)	THC analog; non-psychoactive	Feb-02
high THC cannabis deriv, GW	CLINICAL (III)	GW Pharmaceuticals (UK)	Cannabinoid	Feb-02
Nabitan	Discontinued	HG Pars (US)	Cannabinoid	Mar-92
Nantradol	Discontinued	Pfizer (US)	Cannabinoid	1979
Levonantradol (CP-50556-1)	Discontinued (ph. II)	Pfizer (US)	Cannabinoid	1984
Pravadoline (Win-48098)	Discontinued (ph. II)	Sanofi (France)	Cannabinoid / PGSI	May-93
CP-47497	Inactive	Pfizer (US)	Cannabinoid	1984
CP-55244	Inactive	Pfizer (US)	Cannabinoid	1983
Aminoalkylindoles	Preclinical	Eastman Kodak (US)	Cannabinoid	Sep-92
cannabinoid agonist, Bayer-2	Preclinical	Bayer (Germany)	Cannabinoid	Feb-02
cannabinoid agonists, AMRAD	Preclinical	AMRAD (Australia)	Cannabinoid	Feb-02
AM-512	Preclinical	AMRAD (Australia)	CB1 cannabinoid agonist	May-99
Cannabis (THC)	Preclinical	GW Pharmaceuticals (UK)	MS, spinal injuries, phantom limb	Aug-98
cannabinoid agonists, Adolor	Preclinical	Adolor (US)	Peripheral analgesic	Feb-02
Anandamide	REGISTERED	Yissum (Israel)	Cannabinoid agonist	Oct-95
CCK ANALOGS / ANTAGONISTS				
Devacade	CLINICAL (II)	ML Laboratories / Panos (UK)	CCK-A antagonist; analgesic pot.	Feb-02
Colykade	CLINICAL (II)	ML Laboratories / Panos (UK)	CCK-B antagonist; analgesic pot.	Apr-99
CCK(27-32)	Discontinued	Kanebo (Japan)	CCK fragment	Mar-93
CCK(27-32), Akzo Nobel	Discontinued	Akzo Nobel (Netherlands)	CCK fragment	Feb-02
PD-122263	Inactive	Warner-Lambert (US)	CCK analogs	Jul-92
Ceruletide diethylamine	LAUNCHED	Pharmacia / Erbamont (Italy)	CCK peptide analog	Dec-91
Neuroactive peptides	Preclinical	NeuroSearch (Denmark)	CCK analogs	Jan-93
Tetronothiodin	Preclinical	Roche (Switz)	CCK-B antagonist	Feb-93
CHOLINERGICS / CHOLINESTERASE INHIBITORS				

Ref.: Pharmaprojects (updated to 2/02) used with permission; Scrip, corporate, literature & patent references
"Status" is international drug development or regulatory status and may not indicate status in USA
Sponsor: Original company name is retained if product is discontinued or inactive after merger, acquisition, company name change, etc.
Users of this table are encouraged to independently verify the status, activity, and mechanism of action of drugs of interest

GENERIC / TRADE NAME	STATUS	SPONSOR (S)	MECHANISM OF ACTION	REF. UPDATE
ABT-594	CLINICAL (II)	Abbott (US)	Nicotonic α4/β2 agonist	Jun-99
FID-072021	Discontinued	Fidia (Italy)	ACh release stimulant	Oct-96
Eseroline (MCV-4481; NIH-10398)	Discontinued	Univ. Florence (Italy)	Cholinesterase inhibitor	1984
LY-297802 / NNC-11-1053	Discontinued (ph. II)	Lilly (US) / Novo Nordisk (Den)	Muscarinic M1 agonist	May-99
Pharmaprojects No. 4616	Discontinued (ph. II)	Lilly (US)	Muscarinic M4 agonist	May-99
RU-35963	Inactive	Roussel-Uclaf (France)	Cholinergic agonist	1990
L-689660	Inactive	Merck & Co (US)	Cholinomimetic (M1 ag.)	Nov-92
CMI-980	Inactive	CytoMed / Millennium (US)	Muscarinic agonist	Feb-02
epibatidine analogues, Bayer	Preclinical	Bayer (Germany)	Nicotinic agonist	Feb-02
DOPAMINERGICS / NEUROLEPTICS				
CY-208-243	Discontinued	Sandoz (Switz)	D1/D2 partial agonist	1988
Pharmaprojects No. 4632	Discontinued	Takeda (Japan)	Dopamine D1 antag. / D2 ag.	1997
HP-818	Discontinued	Hoechst (Ger)	Neuroleptic analgesic	Sep-91
Tetrahydroisoquinolines	Preclinical	Boots (UK)	D1/D2 antagonists	Sep-93
EXCITATORY AMINO ACID ANTAGONISTS (Glutamate, Kainate, NMDA, Glycine)				
Memantine	CLINICAL (II)	Merz / Neurobiological Tech. (US)	NMDA antag. / neuropathic pain	Apr-98
NPS-846	Discontinued	NPS Pharmaceuticals (US)	Glutamate antagonist (Aradn)	1997
SYM-2192	Discontinued	Symphony (US)	Kainate/glutamate partial ag.	Nov-96
FPL-15609	Discontinued	Astra/Fisons (Sweden)	NMDA antagonist / non-compet.	1997
GV-196771	Discontinued (ph. II)	GlaxoSmithKline (UK)	Glycine antag. / neuropathic	Feb-02
CPP	Discontinued (ph. II)	Sandoz (Switz)	NMDA antagonist (neuroprotec)	Nov-95
LY-189709	Inactive	Lilly (US)	NMDA antagonist	1986
Lamotrigine (LAMICTAL®)	LAUNCHED	Wellcome (UK)	Glutamate inhib. / anticonvul.	May-93
NMDA antagonist, Vernalis	Preclinical	Vernalis (UK)	Centrally-acting analgesic	Feb-02
NPC-12626	Preclinical	Scios Nova (US)	Excitatory amino acid antag.	Jan-92
Pharmaprojects No. 4171	Preclinical	Astra (Sweden)	Excitatory amino acid antag.	Nov-94
Quinoxalinediones	Preclinical	Sumitomo (Japan)	Glutamate antagonist	May-93
BW-524C79	Preclinical	Wellcome (UK)	Glutamate release inhibitor	May-93
ZD-9379	Preclinical	Zeneca (UK)	Glycine antag. / neuropathic pain	Jan-98
GlyT-1 inhibitors	Preclinical	Gliatech (US)	Glycine reuptake inhibitor (GlyT2)	Feb-99
SYM-2007	Preclinical	Symphony (US)	Kainate/glutamate partial ag.	Apr-95
SYM-2081	Preclinical	Symphony (US)	Kainate/glutamate partial ag.	Sep-95
mGLUR antagonists	Preclinical	Novartis (Switz.) / Merck (US)	mGLUR (glutamate) antag.	Oct-99
Indoylpropenoic acids	Preclinical	Marion Merrell Dow (US)	NMDA antagonist	Jan-95
FPL-15765	Preclinical	Astra/Fisons (Sweden)	NMDA antagonist / non-compet.	Apr-95
Kappagems / glystasins	Preclinical	CoCensys (US)	NMDA associated	Feb-93
FOLK MEDICINES				
P54	CLINICAL (II)	Phytopharm (UK)	OA, IBS: phytomedicine; NSAID	May-98
Epibatidine	Discontinued	Merck & Co (US)	Nicotinic agonist	Jun-95
alpha-Viniferin	Inactive	Chung-Ang Univ. (Japan)	Korean folk medicine	1990
FORMULATIONS / DELIVERY SYSTEMS				
Paracetamol formulation	CLINICAL	Himedics (US)	APAP formulation	1991
Buprenorphine, transmucosal	CLINICAL	3M (US)	Buccal release patch	Mar-95
Dermatan sulfate	CLINICAL	CytRx (US)	Dermatan topical form.	Feb-93
morphine, Dainippon-2	CLINICAL	Dainippon (Japan)	Formulation	Feb-02
Morphine formulation	CLINICAL	Eurand (Italy)	Sustained-release MS	Mar-91
capsaicin, NeurogesX	CLINICAL	NeurogesX (US)	Topical capsaicin	Feb-02
Pharmaprojects No. 5689	CLINICAL	Core Technologies (UK)	Unidentified (vulvar vestibulitis)	Jan-98
fentanyl, Latitude	CLINICAL (I)	3M (US)	Formulation	Feb-02
morphine, Generex	CLINICAL (I)	Generex	Formulation	Feb-02
Tramadol, Labopharm	CLINICAL (I)	Labopharm	Formulation	Feb-02
morphine, Premaire	CLINICAL (I)	Sheffield Pharmaceuticals (US)	Inhalation formulation	Jul-99
Naproxen, injectable (NANOX®)	CLINICAL (I)	Mimetix (US)	Injectable naproxen	Apr-97
Pharmaprojects No. 5976	CLINICAL (I)	Elan (Ireland) / Sheffield (US)	Pulmonary delivery, MSI technol.	Jun-99
Morphine	CLINICAL (I)	West Pharmaceutical (US)	Transnasal formulation	Jan-00
lidocaine, EpiCept-2	CLINICAL (II)	EpiCept (US)	Dermal formulation	Feb-02
lidocaine, EpiCept-3	CLINICAL (II)	EpiCept (US)	Dermal formulation	Feb-02
Morphine, DepoMorphine (D-0401)	CLINICAL (II)	DepoTech (US)	Epidural sustained rel. morphine	Dec-98
ibuprofen, SEPA	CLINICAL (II)	MacroChem (US)	Formulation	Feb-02

Ref.: Pharmaprojects (updated to 2/02) used with permission; Scrip, corporate, literature & patent references
"Status" is international drug development or regulatory status and may not indicate status in USA
Sponsor: Original company name is retained if product is discontinued or inactive after merger, acquisition, company name change, etc.
Users of this table are encouraged to independently verify the status, activity, and mechanism of action of drugs of interest

GENERIC / TRADE NAME	STATUS	SPONSOR (S)	MECHANISM OF ACTION	REF. UPDATE
buprenorphine, Toyobo	CLINICAL (II)	Toyobo	Formulation	Feb-02
fentanyl, Watson	CLINICAL (II)	Watson (US)	Formulation	Feb-02
morphine, West	CLINICAL (II)	West Pharmaceutical (US)	Formulation	Feb-02
etomidate, Anesta	CLINICAL (II)	Cephalon (US)	Formulation	Feb-02
AERx Morphine pulmonary system	CLINICAL (II)	SmithKline Beecham / Aradigm (US)	Formulation, pulmonary	Jun-98
Buprenorphine, transdermal	CLINICAL (II)	Ethical (UK)	Formulation, transdermal	Mar-95
Ibuprofen + SEPA enhancers	CLINICAL (II)	MacroChem (US)	Formulation, transdermal	Nov-96
BL-1834	CLINICAL (II)	Bioglan Laboratories (UK)	Intranasal doxepin; severe pain	May-00
Morphine (TNK-951)	CLINICAL (II)	Nippon Kayaku (Japan)	Morphine formulation	Feb-99
Diclofenac gel (ORALEASE)	CLINICAL (II)	SkyePharma (UK)	Oral gel formulation; mouth ulcers	Feb-02
morphine, AERx	CLINICAL (II)	Aradigm	Pulmonary delivery	Feb-02
capsaicin cream, Maruishi	CLINICAL (II)	Maruishi Pharmaceutical	Topical capsaicin	Feb-02
Ibuprofen gel, topical	CLINICAL (II)	Macrochem (US)	Topical gel formulation	Apr-99
Loperamide (ADL 2-1294)	CLINICAL (II)	Adolor (US) / Santen	Topical, ophthalmic formulations	May-00
PTI-801 (naltrexone + tramadol)	CLINICAL (II)	Pain Therapeutics (US)	Tramadol + ultra low dose antag.	Feb-02
Oxycodone, Mundipharma	CLINICAL (III)	Shionogi (Jp) / Mundipharma	Controlled release	Nov-97
Tramadol, Biovail	CLINICAL (III)	Biovail (Canada)	Controlled-release (1x/day)	Feb-02
oxymorphone, TIMERx	CLINICAL (III)	Endo Pharmaceuticals (US)	Controlled-release formulation	Feb-02
Lidocaine, PowderJect	CLINICAL (III)	Chiroscience / PowderJect (UK)	Dermal, oral formulations	Jun-99
lidocaine, Vyteris	CLINICAL (III)	Vyteris	Formulation	Feb-02
BL-1832	CLINICAL (III)	Bioglan Laboratories	Formulation	Feb-02
morphine, DepoFoam	CLINICAL (III)	SkyePharma (UK)	Formulation	Feb-02
sufentanil, DUROS	CLINICAL (III)	Durect	Formulation	Feb-02
Morphine, Gacel	CLINICAL (III)	Gacell (Sweden)	Formulation, oral 24 hr morphine	Nov-96
Panoderm hydromorphone	CLINICAL (III)	Elan (Ireland)	Formulation, transdermal	Jul-96
morphine, Multipor	CLINICAL (III)	Amarin (UK)	Oral 1x daily morphine	Feb-02
Diclofenac spray	CLINICAL (III)	Dr Kade (Germany)	Topical spray	Nov-99
Fentanyl, E-TRANS	CLINICAL (III)	Johnson & Johnson / Alza (US)	Transdermal formulations	Feb-02
TSN-09 (Buprenorphine)	CLINICAL (III)	Teijin (Japan)	Transdermal tape formulation	Feb-99
Morphine formulation	Discontinued	Forest Laboratories (US)	Buccal formulation	Feb-88
Buprenorphine, 3M	Discontinued	3M (US)	Buccal patch	Sep-99
Pharmaprojects No. 5817	Discontinued	BioChem Pharma (Canada)	Central μ ag. + NMDA antag.	Jun-00
Paracetamol + codeine	Discontinued	Alza (US)	Controlled release	Mar-89
Paracetamol formulation	Discontinued	Alza (US)	Controlled release	Mar-90
Yissum P-0558	Discontinued	Yissum (Israel)	Controlled release system	Feb-93
Paracetamol formulation	Discontinued	Scios Nova (US)	Edible whip APAP	Mar-91
ibuprofen topical, bioMerieux	Discontinued	bioMerieux-Pierre Fabre (France)	Formulation	Feb-02
ketorolac, TheraTech	Discontinued	Watson (US)	Formulation	Feb-02
Anchor drug delivery	Discontinued	Redcell (Canada)	Formulation, site-specific	Mar-99
THIP	Discontinued	Lundbeck (Denmark)	GABA agonist	1985
Nalbuphine, nasal	Discontinued	Nastech (US)	Intranasal formulation	Jul-99
analgesics, Vestar	Discontinued	Vestar (US)	Liposomal formulations	Sep-91
Ketoprofen, CEFORM	Discontinued	Biovail (Canada)	Oral formulation	Oct-99
Naproxen, CEFORM	Discontinued	Biovail (Canada)	Oral formulation	Oct-99
Fentanyl formulation	Discontinued	Hercon (US)	Transdermal fentanyl	Feb-90
Ketorolac, TCPI	Discontinued	Technical Chemicals (US)	Transdermal formulation	Dec-98
Capsaicin	Discontinued (Clin)	Andromaco (Argentina)	Topical capsaicin; OA, RA	Mar-98
flurbiprofen, microCRYSTAL	Discontinued (Clin.)	Pharma-Logic (US)	Lecithin-coated formulation	Feb-02
Diclofenac, Pharmos	Discontinued (ph. I)	Pharmos (US)	Formulation, diclofenac	May-99
Dexmedetomidine, Cygnus	Discontinued (ph. I)	Cygnus (US)	Formulation, transdermal	Dec-94
Diclofenac, FOAM-SYS	Discontinued (ph. I)	Poli (Italy)	Local / topical formulation	Sep-99
Buprenorphine, nasal	Discontinued (ph. I)	Nastech (US)	Opioid agonist/antagonist	Feb-02
Buprenorphine, transdermal	Discontinued (ph. I)	Pierre Fabre (France)	Transdermal buprenorphine	May-97
Fentanyl, iontophoretic (TS-36)	Discontinued (ph. II)	Fournier (France)	Electronic iontophoretic transderm.	Nov-97
Buprenorphine, transmucosal	Discontinued (ph. II)	Watson (US)	Formulation, buccal release	May-99
Buprenorphine, transdermal	Discontinued (ph. II)	Ethical (UK)	Formulation, transdermal	May-99
Piroxicam meglumine	Discontinued (ph. II)	Therapicon (ph. Italy)	Hydrolysable salt of piroxicam	Apr-95
SR-206 (ph. Ibuprofen 1x/day)	Discontinued (ph. II)	SSP (Japan)	Ibuprofen formulation	Oct-96
Fentanyl, inhaler	Discontinued (ph. II)	3M (US)	Metered dose inhaler	May-97
Lidocaine, E-TRANS	Discontinued (ph. II)	Alza (US)	Topical lidocaine	Mar-00
Dihydrocodeine (S-8115)	Discontinued (ph. III)	Shionogi / Mundipharma (Switz)	Controlled release formulation	Oct-98
Hyaluronic formul. (Hyanalgese-D™)	Discontinued (ph. III)	Hyal Pharmaceutical (Canada)	Diclofenac + hyaluronic acid (ph. lv)	Dec-97
Panoderm calcitonin	Discontinued (ph. III)	Elan (Ireland)	Iontophoretic transdermal opioids	Jun-99

Ref.: Pharmaprojects (updated to 2/02) used with permission; Scrip, corporate, literature & patent references
"Status" is international drug development or regulatory status and may not indicate status in USA
Sponsor: Original company name is retained if product is discontinued or inactive after merger, acquisition, company name change, etc.
Users of this table are encouraged to independently verify the status, activity, and mechanism of action of drugs of interest

GENERIC / TRADE NAME	STATUS	SPONSOR (S)	MECHANISM OF ACTION	REF. UPDATE
Fentanyl, transdermal	Discontinued (ph. III)	Cygnus (US)	Transdermal 24 hr patch	Feb-97
Morphine, Repro-Dose	Discontinued (PRE-REG)	Nycomed Amersham (Norway)	Formulation, 1-2x daily oral	May-99
Ibuprofen gel, topical	Discontinued (PRE-REG)	Pierre Fabre (France)	Topical gel formulation	Apr-99
paracetamol, Elan PharmaZome	Inactive	Elan (Ireland)	APAP formulation	Feb-02
dyclonine HCl, BEMA, Atrix	Inactive	Atrix (US)	Buccal film / canker sores	Feb-02
LM-001	Inactive	American Home Products (US)	Formulation	Feb-02
ibuprofen, CEFORM	Inactive	Biovail (Canada)	Formulation	Feb-02
ketoprofen, Poli	Inactive	Poli (Italy)	Formulation	Feb-02
SK-982	Inactive	Sanwa Kagaku Kenkyusho	Formulation	Feb-02
analgesics, Endo	Inactive	Endo Pharmaceuticals (US)	Formulation	Feb-02
buprenorphine, Elan	Inactive	Elan (Ireland)	Formulation	Feb-02
Piroxicam, granular	Inactive	Applied Pharma Res. (Switz.)	Formulation, oral fast-acting	Jun-99
diclofenac-2, Applied	Inactive	Applied Pharma Res. (Switz.)	Oral formulation #2	Feb-02
Orolip E	Inactive	EpiCept (US)	Oral sustained-rel. enkephalins	Feb-02
ketorolac tromethamine, Pharme	Inactive	Technical Chemicals (US)	Patch formulation, 1x daily	Feb-02
Morphine (INFUSETTE®)	Inactive	Advanced Medical (Canada)	Rectal controlled release	Nov-91
Orolip DP	Inactive	EpiCapt (US)	Timed-release neuropeptides	Feb-02
CPR-2006	Inactive	Clarion (US)	Topical; menthol conjugate	Feb-02
Paracetamol suppositories	LAUNCHED	SS Pharmaceutical (Japan)	APAP formulation	Dec-91
paracetamol, EFVDAS	LAUNCHED	Elan (Ireland)	APAP formulation	Feb-02
Capsaicin (ZOSTRIX®)	LAUNCHED	Knoll (US) / GenDerm (US)	Capsaicin /anesthetic formul.	Jun-96
Capsaicin	LAUNCHED	Vinas (Spain)	Capsicum oleoresin	Mar-94
Dextropropoxyphene form.	LAUNCHED	Hafslund Nycomed (Norway)	Controlled release	Aug-91
Dihydrocodeine formulation	LAUNCHED	Biovail (Canada)	Controlled release DHC	Dec-91
Morphine formulation	LAUNCHED	Karo Bio (Sweden)	Epidural morphine	Mar-92
Morphine formulation	LAUNCHED	Wyeth-Ayerst (US)	Epidural morphine	Dec-91
Fentanyl citrate (ORALET, ACTIQ)	LAUNCHED	Abbott (US) / Anesta (US)	Fentanyl oral transmucusal	Jun-99
naproxen, AW	LAUNCHED	Alfa Wassermann	Formulation	Feb-02
flurbiprofen transdermal, Lead	LAUNCHED	Mikasa Seiyaku	Formulation	Feb-02
tetracine, percutaneous	LAUNCHED	Smith & Nephew	Formulation	Feb-02
ibuprofen, Flash Dose	LAUNCHED	Biovail (Canada)	Formulation	Feb-02
diclofenac once-daily, SSP	LAUNCHED	SSP (Japan)	Formulation	Feb-02
fentanyl, Alza	LAUNCHED	Johnson & Johnson (US)	Formulation	Feb-02
hydromorphone, Napp	LAUNCHED	Napp (UK)	Formulation	Feb-02
morphine, Ethypharm	LAUNCHED	Ethypharm	Formulation	Feb-02
morphine, Nycomed Amersham	LAUNCHED	Nycomed Pharma (Norway)	Formulation	Feb-02
buprenorphine, Gruenenthal	LAUNCHED	Grunenthal (Germany)	Formulation	Feb-02
Hydrocodone + APAP (NORCO™)	LAUNCHED	Watson (US)	Formulation, high dose HC	Feb-97
Oxycodone (OXYCONTIN®)	LAUNCHED	Purdue Pharma (US)	Formulation, oral 12 hr oxycodone	Apr-98
Ibuprofen, EFVDAS (IBUSCENT)	LAUNCHED	Searle (US) / Elan (Ireland)	Formulation, oral fast-acting	Jun-99
morphine, Rhotard	LAUNCHED	Amarin (UK)	Formulation, oral morphine	Feb-02
Paracetamol + dihydrocodeine	LAUNCHED	Napp (UK)	Formulation, paracetamol + DHC	Mar-96
Ametop	LAUNCHED	Mylan (US) / Smith&Nephew (UK)	Formulation, topical amethocaine	Jun-96
Propacetamol (PRO-DAFALGAN)	LAUNCHED	UPSA (France)	Injectable paracetamol	May-93
Carbamazepine (CARBATROL)	LAUNCHED	Shire (UK) / Elan (Ireland)	Na+ channel antag.; Microtrol b.i.d.	Jun-99
Naproxen, cont. rel. (NAPRELAN®)	LAUNCHED	Wyeth-Ayerst (US) / Elan	Naproxen, 1x/day formulation	Mar-97
Buprenorphine	LAUNCHED	Reckitt & Colman (UK)	Opioid agonist/antagonist	Jun-91
Butorphanol, nasal (STADOL® NS)	LAUNCHED	Bristol-Myers Squibb (US)	Opioid agonist/antagonist	Oct-92
Morphine (KADIAN®, KAPINOL®)	LAUNCHED	Faulding (Austr)	Oral 24 hr formulation	May-99
Diclofenac, Applied	LAUNCHED	Novartis / Applied Pharma (Switz.)	Oral formulation	Nov-99
Hydromorphone (HYDROMORPH CONTIN®)	LAUNCHED	Napp (UK)	Oral sustained release	Apr-98
Benzocaine, Vinas (DENTISPRAY)	LAUNCHED	Vinas (Spain)	OTC 5% benzocaine; dental	Jun-99
Diclofenac (Arthrex Duo)	LAUNCHED	Klinge (Germany)	Quick/Slow pellets in capsule	Mar-99
Diclofenac, topical	LAUNCHED	Mika Pharma (Germany)	Topical liposome spray-gel	Apr-00
Prednisolone farnesil	LAUNCHED	Taiho / Kuraray (Japan)	Topical steroid; OA + RA	Nov-98
Tramadol + acetaminophen (ULTREX)	LAUNCHED	Johnson & Johnson (US)	Tramadol + APAP formulation	Feb-02
Lidocaine patch (LIDODERM)	LAUNCHED	Endo (US) / Elan (IR) / Hind (US)	Transdermal formulation; PHN	May-00
Fentanyl (DURAGESIC®)	LAUNCHED	J&J / Alza (US)	Transdermal narcotic	Apr-97
Lidocaine (DentiPatch)	LAUNCHED	Noven Pharma (US)	Transoral mucosal anesthetic	Feb-99
Lidocaine, Noven	LAUNCHED	Noven Pharmaceuticals (US)	Transoral mucosal delivery	Jun-97
BL-1828	Preclinical	Bioglan Laboratories (UK)	Aerosal opioid antagonist	May-00
Lidocaine, LIDOMER MICROSPHERES	Preclinical	Guilford (US)	Biodegradable microspheres (inj.)	Apr-00
Fentanyl citrate	Preclinical	Samchundang (S. Korea)	Fentanyl formulation (unspec.)	Apr-00

Ref.: Pharmaprojects (updated to 2/02) used with permission; Scrip, corporate, literature & patent references
"Status" is international drug development or regulatory status and may not indicate status in USA
Sponsor: Original company name is retained if product is discontinued or inactive after merger, acquisition, company name change, etc.
Users of this table are encouraged to independently verify the status, activity, and mechanism of action of drugs of interest

GENERIC / TRADE NAME	STATUS	SPONSOR (S)	MECHANISM OF ACTION	REF. UPDATE
lidocaine ring, Enhance	Preclinical	Enhance Pharmaceuticals	Formulation	Feb-02
analgesic, Nobex	Preclinical	Nobex	Formulation	Feb-02
fentanyl citrate, Samchundang	Preclinical	Samchundang (S. Korea)	Formulation	Feb-02
fentanyl, BEMA film	Preclinical	Atrix (US)	Formulation	Feb-02
fentanyl, Generex	Preclinical	Generex	Formulation	Feb-02
hydromorphone, DUROS	Preclinical	Durect	Formulation	Feb-02
IP-01	Preclinical	Ionix Pharmaceuticals	Formulation	Feb-02
morphine, TDS	Preclinical	TransDermal Technologies	Formulation	Feb-02
neuropathic pain ther, ProVec	Preclinical	GlaxoSmithKline (UK)	Formulation	Feb-02
oxycodone, Bentley	Preclinical	Bentley	Formulation	Feb-02
pain therapies, Arakis	Preclinical	Arakis	Formulation	Feb-02
sufentanil, S BioSystems	Preclinical	Durect	Formulation	Feb-02
buprenorphine, Mundipharma	Preclinical	Mundipharma	Formulation	Feb-02
PJ2204	Preclinical	Powderject (UK)	Formulation, antimigraine	Dec-97
OT-Piroxicam	Preclinical	Anesta (US)	Oral transmucosal formulation	Mar-99
Bupivacaine (DepoBupivacaine)	Preclinical	DepoTech (US)	Sustained release formulation	Dec-98
Lipocaine	Preclinical	Deprenyl Research (Canada)	Topical lidocaine formula	Jul-93
Analgesics, Endo	Preclinical	Endo (US) / Lavipharm (Greece)	Transdermal analgesic (unspec.)	Dec-99
Eptazocine formulation	Preclinical	TheraTech (US)	Transdermal eptazocine	Oct-92
Buprenorphine, transdermal	Preclinical	Cygnus Research (US)	Transdermal formulation	Mar-93
Narcotic analgesic patch	Preclinical	Amarin (UK)	Transdermal narcotic patch	Aug-99
narcotic analgesic patch, Elan	Preclinical	Elan (Ireland)	Transdermal narcotic patch	Feb-02
fentanyl, buccal, 3M	Preclinical	3M (US)	Transdermal, transmusocal forms.	Feb-02
Ibuprofen, Ceform	PRE-REGISTRATION	Fuisz Technologies	"Flash Dose" oral delivery	Jul-98
Tramadol, Purdue	PRE-REGISTRATION	Purdue Pharma (US)	Controlled release formulation	Jun-00
Acetaminophen (FEVERALL EXT. REL.)	PRE-REGISTRATION	Ascent Pediatrics (US)	Extended release, pediatric	Jan-98
Diclofenac formulation	PRE-REGISTRATION	Applied Pharma Res. (Switz.)	Fast/slow controlled release	Jun-98
Diclofenac (1x/day formulation)	PRE-REGISTRATION	SSP (Japan)	Formulation	May-98
Morphine (MORAXEN)	PRE-REGISTRATION	CeNeS (UK) / BTG (UK)	Hydrogel morphine suppository	Apr-00
hydromorphone, OROS	PRE-REGISTRATION	Johnson & Johnson (US)	Oral 24hr hydromorphone	Feb-02
Morphine, rectal	PRE-REGISTRATION	Core Technologies (UK)	Suppository gel, 12-24 hr activity	Apr-97
Diclofenac (PENNSAID™)	PRE-REGISTRATION	Dimethaid Research (Canada)	Topical formulation	Mar-98
diclofenac + HA topical, Skye	PRE-REGISTRATION	SkyePharma (UK)	Topical formulation	Feb-02
ph-913 (LidoPain®)	PRE-REGISTRATION	EpiCept (US)	Transdermal patch; unknown opioid	Feb-98
Morphine (MORPHELAN)	REGISTERED	Ligand (US) / Elan (Ireland)	Controlled rel. 1x/day SODAS	Feb-02
Ibuprofen, APR	REGISTERED	Applied Pharma Res. (Switz.)	Fast/slow controlled release	Jun-98
Morphine, Takeda, MH-100	REGISTERED	Takeda (Japan)	Formulation, inj. high-concentr.	Feb-02
diclofenac, OSAT	Suspended	CeNeS (UK)	Oral sustained release	Feb-02
Analgesic aerosol (BL-1827)	Suspended	CeNeS (UK) / Bioglan Labs (UK)	Sublingual opioid	Feb-00
ph-921A	Suspended	pharmed (Ger)	Transdermal opioids	Jun-92
morphine, OSAT	Suspended (ph. I)	CeNeS (UK)	Oral sustained release	Feb-02
ibuprofen, OSAT	Suspended (REGIS)	CeNeS (UK)	Oral sustained release	Feb-02
GABA AGONISTS / ANTAGONISTS				
R-baclofen, Paladin Labs	CLINICAL (II)	Pharmascience (Canada)	GABA antagonist	Feb-02
Pregabalin	CLINICAL (II/III)	Warner-Lambert (US)	Neuropathic pain, epilepsy	Apr-98
thiocolchicoside	Discontinued	Sanofi-Synthelabo (France)	GABA antagonist; analg., anti-inflam.	Feb-02
Pharmaprojects No. 5261	Discontinued	Novo Nordisk (Denmark)	GABA uptake inhibitor (GAT-4)	1997
Pharmaprojects No. 5065	Discontinued	Lundbeck (Denmark)	GABA uptake inhibitors	Mar-98
Gaboxadol (Lu2-030; THIP)	Discontinued (ph. II)	Lundbeck (Denmark)	GABA agonist; muscimol analog	Mar-85
Gabapentin (US Phase IV Pain)	LAUNCHED	Warner-Lambert (US)	GABA releaser / antiepileptic	Apr-96
IL-1 / CYTOKINE ANTAGONISTS / IMMUNOMODULATORS				
anti-inflammatory peptide, BTG	CLINICAL	BTG (UK)	Cytokine antag.; inflam., RA	Feb-02
HP-228	CLINICAL (II)	LION bioscience (US)	Cytokine antagonist	Feb-02
VX-740 (HMR-3480)	CLINICAL (II)	Aventis (France)	IL-1beta conv. enzyme inhib./RA	Jun-00
T-614	CLINICAL (III)	Eisai / Toyama (Japan)	IL-1b, IL-6, IL-8 antag./ RA	Dec-98
Pharmaprojects No. 5758	Discontinued	RepliGen (US) / GW (UK)	Cytokine (glyceptor) anti-inflam.	Mar-98
Pharmaprojects No. 2817	Discontinued	Boron Biologicals (US)	IL-1 antagonist, TNF-a antagonist	Jun-00
Pharmaprojects No. 4332	Discontinued	BioResearch (Ireland)	IL-1 antagonist, TNF-α antagonist	Sep-98
Pharmaprojects No. 5905	Discontinued	Servier (France)	IL-1 beta antagonist; non-peptide	Jun-00
E-5090	Discontinued	Eisai (Japan)	IL-1 inhibitor	Jan-92
EI-1507-1	Discontinued	Kyowa Hakko (Japan)	IL-1b converting enz. Inhib.	Sep-99

Ref.: Pharmaprojects (updated to 2/02) used with permission; Scrip, corporate, literature & patent references
"Status" is international drug development or regulatory status and may not indicate status in USA
Sponsor: Original company name is retained if product is discontinued or inactive after merger, acquisition, company name change, etc.
Users of this table are encouraged to independently verify the status, activity, and mechanism of action of drugs of interest

GENERIC / TRADE NAME	STATUS	SPONSOR (S)	MECHANISM OF ACTION	REF. UPDATE
ICE inhibitors	Discontinued	Ono (Japan)	IL-1beta conv. enzyme inhib.	Jan-99
ICE inhibitors (PD-163594)	Discontinued	Warner-Lambert (US)	IL-1beta conv. enzyme inhib.	Jan-00
Pharmaprojects No. 5094	Discontinued	Pharmacopeia / Regeneron (US)	IL-6, IFN-γ, EPO, G-CSF inhibitors	Jun-00
Pharmaprojects No. 5568	Discontinued	SmithKline Beecham (UK)	IL-8 receptor B antagonist	Jun-00
CBX-10913 / CBX-12266	Inactive	Ciblex (US)	Cytokine release inhibitor; RA	Jan-00
LK-423	Inactive	Fujimoto (Japan)	IL-10 agonist; Interferon-γ antag.	Jun-99
IL-8 antagonists, Pharmacopeia	Inactive	Pharmacopeia (US)	IL-8 receptor antagonist (inflam.)	Feb-02
Anakinra (KINERET®)	LAUNCHED	Amgen (US)	IL-1 receptor antagonist / RA	Feb-02
Anticytokines	Preclinical	Sigma-Tau (Italy)	Cytokine antagonist; RA	Jul-99
IL-1Hy1	Preclinical	Hyseq (US)	IL-1 receptor antagonist	Aug-99
Caspase 1 / ICE inhibs	Preclinical	Vertex Pharmaceuticals (US)	IL-1β converting enz. Inhib.	Jan-00
IL-8 antagonists	Preclinical	Pharmacopeia (US) / Organon	IL-8 receptor antagonist (inflam.)	Jan-00
Adamantylamide dipeptide	Preclinical	Leciva (Czechoslovakia)	Immunostimulant	Feb-92
RWJ-68354	Preclinical	Johnson & Johnson (US)	Inhib. p38 kinase, TNF-α, IL-1b/RA	Jan-99
ION CHANNEL ANTAGONISTS (Na+, Ca++ antagonists)				
RSD-921 / Nociblockers	CLINICAL (I)	Nortran (Canada)	Ion channel antagonist (iv)	May-97
AM-336	CLINICAL (II)	Xenome / AMRAD (Austr.)	Conotoxins, Ca++ channel antag.	Feb-02
Omega-conotoxin GVIA	Discontinued	Biomolecular Res. Inst. (Austr.)	Ca++ antagonist; cone shell toxin	Feb-02
Gabapentin analogues	Discontinued	Warner-Lambert (US)	Ca++ antagonist; pain + epilepsy	Jan-00
NS-649 (NS-626)	Discontinued	NeuroSearch (Denmark)	Ca++ channel antag., N-type	Feb-96
Pharmaprojects No. 4499	Discontinued	NPS Pharmaceuticals (US)	Ca++ channel antag., receptor-type	Sep-95
(S)-mexiletine	Discontinued	Celgene (US)	Na+ Channel antag.; neuropathic	Mar-00
Imidazopyrazoles	Discontinued	Roussel-Uclaf (France)	Na+ channel antagonist	Mar-89
Isoquinolines	Discontinued	Richter (Hungary)	Na+ channel antagonist	Apr-86
Lodaxaprine	Discontinued	Sanofi (France)	Na+ channel antagonist	Mar-92
GW-286103	Discontinued	Glaxo Wellcome (UK)	Na+ channel inhib.	Feb-02
Pharmaprojects No. 5595	Discontinued	Roche (Switz)	Sodium channel antag.; neuropathy	Mar-99
4030W92	Discontinued (ph. II)	Glaxo Wellcome (UK)	Na+ Channel antag.; chronic pain	Jul-99
LTA	Discontinued (ph. II)	AstraZeneca (UK)	Na+ channel antagonist, topical	Feb-02
SNX-239	Inactive	Elan (Ireland)	Ca++ channel antag., N-type	Feb-02
SNX-185	Inactive	Elan (Ireland)	Conotoxin; N-type Ca++ antag.	Feb-02
Pharmaprojects No. 5565	Inactive	NPS Pharmaceuticals (US)	Ion channel blocker; neuropathy	Feb-02
Benzofuropyridines	Inactive	Hoechst (Ger)	Na+ channel antagonist	Unk.
Lomerizine (TERANAS; MIGSIS)	LAUNCHED	Akzo Nobel (Netherlands)	Ca++ antagonist; migraine	Jul-99
Conus toxins, AMRAD	Preclinical	AMRAD (Australia)	Ca++ channel antagonist	May-98
contulakin-G	Preclinical	Cognetix	Calcium channel antagonist	Feb-02
N-calcium channel blockers	Preclinical	NeuroMed Technologies	Centrally-acting analgesic	Feb-02
ion channel blockers, NeuroS	Preclinical	NeuroSearch (Denmark)	ion channel blockers	Feb-02
Co-102862	Preclinical	CoCensys (US) / U. Saskatchewan	Na+ channel antagonist	Dec-97
Contulakin-G (CGX-1160)	Preclinical	Elan (Ireland) / Cognetix (US)	Neurotensin agonist; conopeptide	Feb-00
Ziconotide (SNX-111, intrathecal)	PRE-REGISTRATION	Elan (Ireland) / Neurex (US)	Ca++ channel antag. / intrathecal	Jun-00
CNS-5161	Suspended (ph. II)	CeNeS / Cambridge Neurosci.	NMDA ion chan. antag.; neuropathy	Feb-02
MIGRAINE (Serotonin 5-HT1d agonists, 5-HT antagonists, etc.)				
PNU-142633	CLINICAL	Pharmacia & Upjohn (UK)	5-HT1d agonist; migraine	Jun-99
F-12640	CLINICAL (I)	Pierre Fabre (France)	5-HT1b/1d agonist; migraine	Mar-00
MT-500 (RS-127445)	CLINICAL (I)	POZEN (US) / Roche (Switz)	5-HT2b antagonist (migraine)	Feb-02
donitriptan mesylate	CLINICAL (I)	bioMerieux-Pierre Fabre (France)	Antimigraine	Feb-02
ALX-0646	CLINICAL (I)	NPS / Allelix (Canada)	serotonin agonist (selective)	Apr-98
(S)-Fluoxetine	CLINICAL (II)	Sepracor (US)	5-HT uptake inhibitor	Feb-97
(R)-Fluoxetine	CLINICAL (II)	Lilly / Sepracor (US)	5-HT uptake inhibitor / migraine	Feb-99
BIBN-4096	CLINICAL (II)	Boehringer Ingelheim (Ger)	CGRP antagonist (migraine)	Jul-98
Ganaxolone (CCD-1042)	CLINICAL (II)	CoCensys (US)	Epalon neurosteroid (migraine)	Dec-97
GR-205171	CLINICAL (II)	Glaxo Wellcome (UK)	NK-1 antagonist / antiemetic	Feb-97
Tonabersat (SB-220453)	CLINICAL (II)	SmithKline Beecham (UK)	Unidentified (antimigraine)	May-99
Pharmaprojects No. 1943	Discontinued	Servier (France)	5-HT antagonist	Apr-90
Pharmaprojects No. 2657	Discontinued	SmithKline Beecham (UK)	5-HT antagonist	Aug-92
S-2441	Discontinued	Pharmacia & Upjohn (UK) /Kabi	5-HT antagonist / NK antagonist	Apr-91
GR-127607	Discontinued	Glaxo Wellcome (UK)	5-HT1 agonist	Nov-93
GR-40370	Discontinued	Glaxo Wellcome (UK)	5-HT1 agonist	Feb-92
GR-57426	Discontinued	Glaxo Wellcome (UK)	5-HT1 agonist	Jun-90
GR-69354	Discontinued	Glaxo Wellcome (UK)	5-HT1 agonist	Jun-89

Ref.: Pharmaprojects (updated to 2/02) used with permission; Scrip, corporate, literature & patent references
"Status" is international drug development or regulatory status and may not indicate status in USA
Sponsor: Original company name is retained if product is discontinued or inactive after merger, acquisition, company name change, etc.
Users of this table are encouraged to independently verify the status, activity, and mechanism of action of drugs of interest

GENERIC / TRADE NAME	STATUS	SPONSOR (S)	MECHANISM OF ACTION	REF. UPDATE
Pharmaprojects No. 3976	Discontinued	Glaxo Wellcome (UK)	5-HT1 agonist	1997
Pharmaprojects No. 4044	Discontinued	SmithKline Beecham (UK)	5-HT1 agonist	Feb-96
Pharmaprojects No. 3893	Discontinued	Merck & Co (US)	5-HT1a/2c agonist	Oct-95
CP-93129	Discontinued	Pfizer (US)	5-HT1b agonist	Aug-94
L-694247	Discontinued	Merck & Co (US)	5-HT1d agonist	Oct-95
PNU-109291	Discontinued	Pharmacia & Upjohn (UK)	5-HT1d agonist; migraine	Jun-00
ALX-1323	Discontinued	NPS / Allelix (Canada)	5-HT1d antagonist	1997
LY-39	Discontinued	Univ. Upsala (Sweden)	5-HT1d/D2 agonist	Jan-96
VS-395	Discontinued	Vita-Invest (Spain)	5-HT1d-alpha/beta agonist	Jun-98
Pharmaprojects No. 5037	Discontinued	Bristol-Myers Squibb (US)	5-HT2 antagonist	Feb-98
EGIS-7625	Discontinued	Servier (France)	5-HT2b+sigma-1 antag.; migraine	Mar-00
AH-25086B	Discontinued	GlaxoSmithKline (UK)	Antimigraine	Feb-02
L-782097	Discontinued	Merck & Co (US)	Antimigraine	Feb-02
Org-GC94	Discontinued	Akzo Nobel (Netherlands)	Antimigraine	Feb-02
tropanserin	Discontinued	Aventis (France)	Antimigraine	Feb-02
bemesetron	Discontinued	Biosearch Italia (Italy)	Antimigraine	Feb-02
taclamine	Discontinued	American Home Products (US)	Antimigraine	Feb-02
ICI-118551	Discontinued	AstraZeneca (UK)	Antimigraine	Feb-02
Pharmaprojects No. 5328	Discontinued	Glaxo Wellcome (UK)	Migraine: 5-HT1a modulator	Jun-99
CGRP antagonists	Discontinued	SmithKline Beecham (UK)	Migraine; inflammation, pain	Oct-99
324C91	Discontinued	Glaxo Wellcome (UK)	Unidentified (antimigraine)	Dec-94
NM-105	Discontinued	GeriatRx (Canada)	Unidentified (antimigraine)	Oct-96
Pharmaprojects No. 4620	Discontinued	Spectra / Glaxo Wellcome (UK)	Unidentified (antimigraine)	Feb-96
Pharmaprojects No. 2519	Discontinued	Vita-Invest (Spain)	Unidentified (antimigraine)	Mar-96
Tolnapersine	Discontinued (ph. I)	Novartis (Switz.)	5-HT antagonist	Apr-92
BMS-181885	Discontinued (ph. I)	Bristol-Myers Squibb (US)	5-HT1d antagonist	Jul-97
SB-216842	Discontinued (ph. I)	GlaxoSmithKline (UK)	Antimigraine	Feb-02
CP-122288	Discontinued (ph. II)	Pfizer (US)	5-HT1B/5-HT1D antag. / migr.	Jan-99
Alniditan	Discontinued (ph. II)	Johnson & Johnson (US)	5-HT1d-alpha/beta agonist	1997
LY-334370	Discontinued (ph. II)	Synaptic (US) / Lilly (US)	5-HT1f agonist; antimigraine	May-99
Emopamil	Discontinued (ph. II)	Knoll (Ger)	5-HT2 / Ca++ antagonist	Aug-93
LY-053857	Discontinued (ph. II)	Lilly (US)	5-HT2 antagonist	Oct-94
Sergolexole	Discontinued (ph. II)	Lilly (US)	5-HT2 antagonist	Aug-96
4991W93	Discontinued (ph. II)	Glaxo Wellcome (UK)	Unidentified (antimigraine)	Sep-98
Pharmaprojects No. 3449	Discontinued (ph. II)	Phytopharm (UK)	Unidentified (antimigraine)	Apr-95
aldinitan (PASMIGREN®)	Discontinued (ph. III)	Janssen (Belgium)	5-HT1d agonist	Mar-98
Avitriptan	Discontinued (ph. III)	Bristol-Myers Squibb (US)	5-HT1d agonist / migraine	Sep-96
Tenosal	Discontinued (PRE-REG)	Medea Research (Italy)	COX inhibitor / Ca++ antag. / migraine	Feb-97
dotarizine	Discontinued (PRE-REG.)	Ferrer (Spain)	5-HT2 antagonist / Ca++ antag.	Feb-02
feverfew	Inactive	Non-industrial source	Antimigraine	Feb-02
Pharmaprojects No. 1257	Inactive	Aventis (France)	Antimigraine	Feb-02
Pharmaprojects No. 439	Inactive	Roche (Switz)	Antimigraine	Feb-02
Tropoxin	Inactive	Non-industrial source	Antimigraine	Feb-02
Pharmaprojects No. 568	Inactive	Aventis (France)	Antimigraine	Feb-02
leucotriene inhibitors, Glaxo	Inactive	GlaxoSmithKline (UK)	Antimigraine	Feb-02
pipethiadene	Inactive	Spofa	Antimigraine	Feb-02
AIT-297	Inactive	NeoTherapeutics (US)	Unidentified; anti-migraine	Feb-02
Rizatriptan benzoate (MAXALT®)	LAUNCHED	Merck & Co (US)	5-HT1b/1d agonist	Oct-98
Sumitriptan (IMIGRAN®/IMITREX®)	LAUNCHED	Glaxo Wellcome (UK)	5-HT1d agonist	Jan-97
Sumitriptan, nasal (IMITREX®)	LAUNCHED	Glaxo Wellcome (UK)	5-HT1d agonist (migraine)	Nov-97
Almotriptan (LAS-31416)	LAUNCHED	Almirall-Prodesfarma (Spain)	5-HT1d agonist; migraine	Feb-02
Eletriptan (Relpax)	LAUNCHED	Pfizer (US)	5-HT1d partial agonist	Feb-02
Naratriptan (NARAMIG®; AMERGE™)	LAUNCHED	Glaxo Wellcome (UK)	5-HT1d/1b agonist	Apr-98
Zolmitriptan (ZOMIG®; 311C90)	LAUNCHED	Zeneca (UK)	5-HT1d/1b agonist	Apr-98
alpiropride	LAUNCHED	Sanofi-Synthelabo (France)	Antimigraine	Feb-02
oxetorone	LAUNCHED	Sanofi-Synthelabo (France)	Antimigraine	Feb-02
pizotifen	LAUNCHED	Novartis (Switz.)	Antimigraine	Feb-02
flunarizine	LAUNCHED	Johnson & Johnson (US)	Antimigraine	Feb-02
gepefrine	LAUNCHED	Aventis (France)	Antimigraine	Feb-02
Alpha-dihydroergocryptine	LAUNCHED	Poli (Italy)	Ergot alkaloid; antimigraine	May-98
L-0076	Preclinical	Pierre Fabre (France)	5-HT1d agonist	May-96
Pharmaprojects No. 4318	Preclinical	Allelix (Canada)	5-HT1d agonist	May-96
L-747201	Preclinical	Merck & Co (US)	5-HT1d-alpha agonist	Nov-97

Ref.: Pharmaprojects (updated to 2/02) used with permission; Scrip, corporate, literature & patent references
"Status" is international drug development or regulatory status and may not indicate status in USA
Sponsor: Original company name is retained if product is discontinued or inactive after merger, acquisition, company name change, etc.
Users of this table are encouraged to independently verify the status, activity, and mechanism of action of drugs of interest

GENERIC / TRADE NAME	STATUS	SPONSOR (S)	MECHANISM OF ACTION	REF. UPDATE
Pharmaprojects No. 4924	Preclinical	Merck & Co (US)	5-HT1d-alpha agonist	Aug-96
LY-344864	Preclinical	Synaptic (US)	5-HT1f agonist	Oct-98
Pharmaprojects No. 4731	Preclinical	Servier (France)	5-HT2c antagonist	Feb-96
antimigraine, First Horizon	Preclinical	First Horizon (US)	Antimigraine	Feb-02
migraine prophylaxis, Biofront	Preclinical	Biofrontera	Antimigraine	Feb-02
migraine ther, BMS	Preclinical	Bristol-Myers Squibb (US)	Antimigraine	Feb-02
migraine therapy, NeuroMed	Preclinical	NeuroMed Technologies	Antimigraine	Feb-02
S-19014	Preclinical	Servier (France)	Antimigraine	Feb-02
Frovatriptan (VML-251; SB-209505)	REGISTERED	Vernalis (UK)	5-HT1d/1b partial agonist; migraine	Feb-02
IS-159	Suspended (ph. II)	Medicines Company (US)	5-HT1d agonist / migraine	Feb-02
NEUROPEPTIDE Y (NPY) ANTAGONISTS				
BMS-192548	Discontinued	Bristol-Myers Squibb (US)	NPY antagonist (Y1+Y2)	Aug-96
Alpha-trinositol (PP-56)	Discontinued (ph. II)	Perstorp (Sweden)	NPY antagonist	Feb-99
NEUROTENSIN ANALOGS				
ADA-KPYIL	Discontinued	DuPont Merck (US)	Neurotensin analog	Mar-93
neurotensin, Merck	Inactive	Merck & Co (US)	Neurotensin & analogs	1982
NITRIC OXIDE (NO) SYNTHASE INHIBITORS				
Nitric oxide blockers	Discontinued	NeuroSearch (Denmark)	Nitric oxide receptor antag.	Sep-96
NOX-200	Discontinued	Medinox (US)	Nitric oxide scavenger; arthritis	Feb-00
Pharmaprojects No. 4715	Discontinued	Glaxo Wellcome (UK)	Nitric oxide synthase inhibitor	1997
BN-52296	Discontinued	Beaufour-Ipsen (France)	NO synthetase inhib.; migraine	Nov-98
Pharmaprojects No. 5681	Inactive	AstraZeneca (UK)	Nitric oxide synthase inhibitor	Feb-02
L-NAME	Preclinical	King's College, London	Nitric oxide synthase inhibitor	Jan-93
OPIOID ANALGESICS: MU AGONISTS / AGONIST-ANTAGONISTS / NARCOTICS				
morphine-6-glucuronide, CeNeS	CLINICAL (II)	CeNeS (UK)	Morphine metabolite	Feb-02
morphine-6-glucuronide, UFC	CLINICAL (II)	UFC Pharma	Morphine metabolite	Feb-02
frakefamide (BCH-3963, LEF-576)	CLINICAL (II)	Shire (UK)	Mu agonist peptide	Feb-02
Xorphanol	CLINICAL (II)	HG Pars (US)	Opioid agonist/antagonist	Mar-92
morphine gluconate, Nastech	CLINICAL (II)	Nastech (US)	Opioid mu agonist	Feb-02
Morphine-6-glucuronide (M6G)	CLINICAL (II)	ML Laboratories (UK)	Opioid mu agonist; nebulized	Apr-98
ADL 2-1294	CLINICAL (II)	Adolor (US)	Topical; peripheral mu opioid	Feb-98
Propiram fumarate	CLINICAL (III)	Shire (UK) / Bayer (Ger)	Opioid agonist/antagonist	Apr-98
Pharmaprojects No. 2790	Discontinued	Faes (Spain)	Fentanyl analog	Aug-95
Pharmaprojects No. 2876	Discontinued	Warner-Lambert (US)	Fentanyl analog, short acting	May-94
ICI-120518	Discontinued	Zeneca (US)	Narcotic analgesic	Feb-82
A-3622	Discontinued	Baxter / Ohmeda (US)	Opioid agonist	Apr-91
Azabicycloheptanes	Discontinued	Pfizer (US)	Opioid agonist	1982
MG-8958	Discontinued	Eastman Kodak (US)	Opioid agonist	Mar-81
Morphinan derivative	Discontinued	Daiichi (Japan)	Opioid agonist	Mar-87
Morphinan derivative	Discontinued	Univ. Innsbruck (Austria)	Opioid agonist	1984
Opioid peptides	Discontinued	Unigene (US)	Opioid agonist	Mar-87
Opioid peptides	Discontinued	Univ. Arizona (US)	Opioid agonist	Sep-98
R-18936	Discontinued	Johnson & Johnson (US)	Opioid agonist	Jul-81
R-26800	Discontinued	Johnson & Johnson (US)	Opioid agonist	Jul-81
R-34994	Discontinued	Johnson & Johnson (US)	Opioid agonist	Jul-81
R-4066	Discontinued	Johnson & Johnson (US)	Opioid agonist	Jul-81
TR-5385	Discontinued	Bayer (Germany)	Opioid agonist	Mar-91
VUFB-13757	Discontinued	VUFB (Czech Republic)	Opioid agonist	Dec-92
Wy-42320	Discontinued	Wyeth-Ayerst (US)	Opioid agonist	Feb-82
HP-736	Discontinued	Hoechst (Ger)	Opioid agonist (mu ag.)	Apr-89
NAGA	Discontinued	Asahi Brewery (Japan)	Opioid agonist tetrapeptide	1986
Pharmaprojects No. 5143	Discontinued	Astra (Sweden) / Agouron (US)	Opioid agonist, novel	May-99
Acylmorphinans	Discontinued	Roche (Switz)	Opioid agonist/antagonist	1985
AD-1211	Discontinued	Dainippon (Japan)	Opioid agonist/antagonist	Apr-86
Bremazocine	Discontinued	Sandoz (Switz)	Opioid agonist/antagonist	Feb-83
CM-32113	Discontinued	Sanofi (France)	Opioid agonist/antagonist	Mar-87
Cyclazocine	Discontinued	Eastman Kodak (US)	Opioid agonist/antagonist	Mar-84
J-8970	Discontinued	DuPont Merck (US)	Opioid agonist/antagonist	Mar-92
KT-90	Discontinued	Chugai (Japan)	Opioid agonist/antagonist	Aug-91

Ref.: Pharmaprojects (updated to 2/02) used with permission; Scrip, corporate, literature & patent references
"Status" is international drug development or regulatory status and may not indicate status in USA
Sponsor: Original company name is retained if product is discontinued or inactive after merger, acquisition, company name change, etc.
Users of this table are encouraged to independently verify the status, activity, and mechanism of action of drugs of interest

GENERIC / TRADE NAME	STATUS	SPONSOR (S)	MECHANISM OF ACTION	REF. UPDATE
Morphinan derivative	Discontinued	SRI Int'l (US)	Opioid agonist/antagonist	Apr-86
MR-1268	Discontinued	Boehringer Ingelheim (Ger)	Opioid agonist/antagonist	1983
Pharmaprojects No. 2446	Discontinued	SRI Int'l (US)	Opioid agonist/antagonist	Apr-95
Proxorphan tartrate (BL-5572)	Discontinued	Bristol-Myers Squibb (US)	Opioid agonist/antagonist	Feb-84
Win-42610	Discontinued	Eastman Kodak (US)	Opioid agonist/antagonist	Feb-85
MT-45	Discontinued	Dainippon (Japan)	Opioid analgesic	1985
Pharmaprojects No. 5474	Discontinued	Nycomed Amersham (Norway)	Opioid mu agonist; morph. der.	May-99
SEP-130551 / SEP-130169	Discontinued	Sepracor (US)	Opioid mu/kappa agonist	Jun-00
Oxymorphonazine	Discontinued	Scios Nova (US)	Opioid mu-1 agonist	Nov-88
KF-24705	Discontinued	Kyowa Hakko (Japan)	Opioid mu2 agonist	Feb-00
Bromadoline (U-47931E)	Discontinued (Clin.)	Upjohn (US)	Opioid agonist	1986
S-20682	Discontinued (Clin.)	Shionogi (Japan)	Opioid agonist / narcotic	May-84
Cyclic opioid peptides	Discontinued (Clin.)	Astra (Sweden) / P. Schiller	Opioid mu agonist	Oct-95
Brifentanil (A-3331)	Discontinued (ph. I)	Ohmeda (US)	Fentanyl analog, short acting	Aug-91
Butinazocine	Discontinued (ph. I)	Brocacef / Novartis (Switz)	Opioid agonist/antagonist	Apr-85
Ocfentanil	Discontinued (ph. II)	Ohmeda (US)	Fentanyl analog	Jun-91
Conorphone (HGP-10)	Discontinued (ph. II)	HG Pars (US)	Opioid agonist/antagonist	Nov-93
Moxazocine (BL-4566)	Discontinued (ph. II)	Bristol-Myers Squibb (US)	Opioid agonist/antagonist	Mar-83
Tonazocine (Win-421562)	Discontinued (ph. II)	Sanofi (France)	Opioid agonist/antagonist	May-94
Lofentanil (R-34995)	Discontinued (ph. II)	Janssen / J&J (US)	Opioid mu agonist (long acting)	1987
Mirfentanil (A-3508)	Discontinued (ph. II)	Baxter / Ohmeda (US)	Opioid mu/delta agonist	May-97
Trefentanil	Discontinued (ph. II)	Ohmeda (US)	Ultra-short acting mu opioid	May-97
Metkephamide (LY-127623)	Discontinued (ph. III)	Lilly (US)	Enkephalin analog	Feb-88
Picenadol (LY-136595)	Discontinued (ph. III)	Lilly (US)	Opioid agonist/antagonist	May-94
Pentamorphone (A-4492; RX-77989)	Discontinued (ph. III)	Baxter / Ohmeda (US)	Opioid mu agonist	Jul-91
Ciramadol (Wy-15705)	Discontinued (PRE-REG)	Wyeth-Ayerst (US)	Opioid agonist/antagonist	Jan-87
DuP-769	Inactive	Endo Pharmaceuticals (US)	nalbuphine N-oxide prodrug	Feb-02
A-3443	Inactive	Baxter / Ohmeda (US)	Opioid agonist	Feb-90
Benzotricycloundecanes	Inactive	Merck & Co (US)	Opioid agonist	Unk.
CP-42096	Inactive	Pfizer (US)	Opioid agonist	1985
Doxpicomine	Inactive	Lilly (US)	Opioid agonist	1982
Ethenomorphinan der.	Inactive	Univ. California (US)	Opioid agonist	1985
Hexahydrobenzazocines	Inactive	Research Corp. Tech. (US)	Opioid agonist	1987
Morphinan derivative	Inactive	Roche (Switz)	Opioid agonist	1984
benzomorphan derivatives, Mada	Inactive	Madaus (Ger)	Opioid agonist (weak)	Jun-91
Isoquinolinylphenols	Inactive	Lilly (US)	Opioid agonist/antagonist	1988
Pentazocine, nasal	Inactive	Nastech (US)	Opioid agonist/antagonist	Oct-84
Phenylmorpholines	Inactive	Wyeth-Ayerst (US)	Opioid agonist/antagonist	Apr-83
Zenazocine mesilate	Inactive	Eastman Kodak (US)	Opioid agonist/antagonist	1981
KK3	Inactive	Nagasaki Univ. (Japan)	Opioid analgesic	1990
NIH-10494	Inactive	NIH (US)	Opioid analgesic	1989
P-7521	Inactive	Shankai Inst. Materia Med.	Opioid analgesic	1987
Benzodiazocines	Inactive	Roussel-Uclaf (France)	Opioid mu agonist	1990
Morphiceptin analog	Inactive	Wellcome (UK)	Opioid mu agonist	Sep-84
B.TEHM	Inactive	Takeda (Japan)	Opioids	1984
Piperidinepropanoic acids	Inactive	Warner-Lambert (US)	Ultra-short acting opioid	Aug-91
Remifentanil (ULTIVA™)	LAUNCHED	Glaxo Wellcome (UK)	Mu opioid: ultra-short anesthesia	Mar-98
Butorphanol (STADOL®)	LAUNCHED	Bristol-Myers Squibb (US)	Opioid agonist/antagonist	Feb-92
Dezocine	LAUNCHED	Wyeth-Ayerst (US)	Opioid agonist/antagonist	Mar-91
Eptazocine	LAUNCHED	Nichiiko (Japan)	Opioid agonist/antagonist	Dec-94
Meptazinol	LAUNCHED	Wyeth-Ayerst (US)	Opioid agonist/antagonist	Dec-91
Nalbuphine (NUBAIN®)	LAUNCHED	DuPont Merck (US)	Opioid agonist/antagonist	Feb-92
Alfentanil	LAUNCHED	Johnson & Johnson (US)	Opioid analgesic	Feb-92
Sufentanil (SUFENTA®)	LAUNCHED	Johnson & Johnson (US)	Opioid mu agonist	Jan-95
Hydroisoquinolines	Preclinical	SmithKline Beecham (UK)	Agonist/antagonist opioid	Mar-95
Morphine-6-glucuronide analog	Preclinical	BTG (UK)	Chronic pain	Apr-96
HGP-14	Preclinical	HG Pars (US)	Narcotic analgesic	Apr-99
HGP-15	Preclinical	HG Pars (US)	Narcotic analgesic	Apr-99
HGP-16	Preclinical	HG Pars (US)	Narcotic analgesic	Apr-99
Ketorfanol	Preclinical	HG Pars (US)	Narcotic analgesic	Nov-95
HGP-17	Preclinical	HG Pars (US)	Opioid agonist/antagonist	Nov-95
HGP-18	Preclinical	HG Pars (US)	Opioid agonist/antagonist	Nov-95
Ketorfanol (HGP-13)	Preclinical	HG Pars (US)	Opioid agonist/antagonist	Apr-99

Ref.: Pharmaprojects (updated to 2/02) used with permission; Scrip, corporate, literature & patent references
"Status" is international drug development or regulatory status and may not indicate status in USA
Sponsor: Original company name is retained if product is discontinued or inactive after merger, acquisition, company name change, etc.
Users of this table are encouraged to independently verify the status, activity, and mechanism of action of drugs of interest

GENERIC / TRADE NAME	STATUS	SPONSOR (S)	MECHANISM OF ACTION	REF. UPDATE
N-a-Me-CPM-normorphine	Preclinical	SRI Int'l (US)	Opioid agonist/antagonist	Jul-91
4-Aminopiperidines	Preclinical	E. Merck (Ger)	Opioid mu agonist	Sep-93
Cyclic opioid peptides	Preclinical	Astra (Sweden)	Opioid mu agonist	Aug-92
Fentanyl analogues	Preclinical	Faes (Spain)	Opioid mu agonist	May-92
OPIOID ANALGESICS: ENKEPHALINASE INHIBITORS				
D-Phe-AHPA	Discontinued	Meiji Seika (Japan)	Enk'ase inhibitor	Mar-87
Enkephalin Convertase Inhib.	Discontinued	Scios Nova (US)	Enk'ase inhibitor	Mar-91
Enkephalinase Inhibitors	Discontinued	Dainippon (Japan)	Enk'ase inhibitor	Aug-93
Propioxatin-A	Discontinued	Sankyo (Japan)	Enk'ase inhibitor	Dec-86
SQ-28133	Discontinued	Bristol-Myers Squibb (US)	Enk'ase inhibitor	Oct-85
APHA	Discontinued	Meiji Seika (Japan)	Enk'ase Inhibitors	Jan-89
Thiorphan	Discontinued (ph. I)	Bioproject / INSERM (France)	Enk'ase inhibitor	Feb-94
Sch-32615	Discontinued (ph. II)	Schering Plough (US)	Enk'ase inhibitor; phase II	Mar-93
Sch-34826	Discontinued (ph. II)	Schering Plough (US)	Enk'ase inhibitor; phase II	Mar-93
UK-69578	Discontinued (ph. II)	Pfizer (US)	Enk'ase inhibitor; phase II	1990
ONO-9902	Discontinued (ph. II)	Ono (Japan)	Enkephalinase inhibitor, oral	Feb-96
Enkastatin ID	Inactive	Hoechst (Ger)	Enk'ase inhibitor	1989
Kelatorphan	Inactive	INSERM (France)	Enk'ase inhibitor	1985
Leucine derivative	Inactive	Univ. Rouen (France)	Enk'ase inhibitor	1983
MDL-100250	Inactive	Marion Merrell Dow (US)	Enk'ase inhibitor	Jan-93
RB-38B	Inactive	Univ. Cadiz (Spain)	Enk'ase inhibitor	1990
RU-42827	Inactive	Roussel-Uclaf (France)	Enk'ase inhibitor	1986
RU-44004	Inactive	Roussel-Uclaf (France)	Enk'ase inhibitor	Sep-92
Mercaptoacetylamide azepines	Preclinical	Hoechst Marion Roussel (Ger)	Enk'ase inhibitor	Sep-95
OPIOID DELTA AGONISTS				
DPI-3290	CLINICAL (II)	Ardent Pharmaceuticals	Delta-mu agonist analgesic	Feb-02
SNC-80	Discontinued	GlaxoSmithKline (UK)	Delta agonist	Feb-02
Pharmaprojects No. 3389	Discontinued	Searle/Monsanto (US)	Delta agonist peptide	Mar-94
TIPP-NH2	Discontinued	Astra / Clin. Res. Inst. (Canada)	Delta opioid peptide	Sep-97
Pharmaprojects No. 4445	Discontinued	NIH (US)	Delta opioid peptides	Feb-97
LSZ-1025	Discontinued	Univ. Arizona (US)	Glycopeptide δ antagonist	Apr-97
BW-373U86	Discontinued	Burroughs Wellcome (UK)	Opioid delta agonists (non-peptide)	Mar-97
SB-237596	Discontinued	SmithKline Beecham (UK)	Opioid delta agonists (non-peptide)	Jun-00
BW-2378W92	Discontinued	Delta / Glaxo Wellcome (US)	Opioid delta-mu agonist	Feb-98
OHM-3295	Discontinued	Ohmeda (US)	Fentanyl analog	May-96
Peptidomimetic	Inactive	Univ. Arizona (US)	Delta agonist	1989
Pharmaprojects No. 5468	Inactive	SmithKline Beecham (UK)	Delta receptor agonist/antag.	Sep-97
Delta agonists	Preclinical	Searle/Monsanto (US)	Delta agonist	Mar-93
Di-, Tri-, cyclic peptides	Preclinical	NIH (US)	Delta agonist	Aug-95
Diarylmethylpiperazines	Preclinical	Glaxo Wellcome (UK)	Mu + delta agonist	Mar-95
Tan-67	Preclinical	Hoshi Univ. (Japan)	Non-peptide delta agonist	Oct-96
DPI-3338	Preclinical	Delta Pharmaceuticals (US)	Opioid delta ag. / narcotic combo.	Feb-98
DPI-584	Preclinical	Delta Pharmaceuticals (US)	Opioid delta ag. / urinary incontinence	Feb-98
Pharmaprojects No. 4680	Preclinical	Astra (Sweden)	Opioid delta agonist (non-peptide)	Dec-97
Delta agonists, Astra	Preclinical	Astra (Sweden)	Opioid delta agonists (non-peptide)	Feb-98
OPIOID KAPPA AGONISTS				
ADL 10-0116	CLINICAL (I)	Adolor (US)	Peripheral kappa agonist	Feb-02
Asimadoline (EMD-61753)	CLINICAL (II)	Merck KGaA (Germany)	Kappa agonist (peripheral)	Jun-97
TRK-820	CLINICAL (II)	Toray (Japan) / Daiichi (Japan)	Kappa agonist analgesic	Sep-97
ADL 10-0101	CLINICAL (II)	Adolor (US)	Peripheral kappa agonist	Feb-02
EMD-60400	Discontinued	Merck KGaA (Germany)	Kappa agonist	May-94
GR-45809	Discontinued	Glaxo (UK)	Kappa agonist	Nov-93
GR-94839	Discontinued	Glaxo Wellcome (UK)	Kappa agonist	Oct-96
HZ-2	Discontinued	Grunenthal (Germany)	Kappa agonist	Feb-02
ICI-199441	Discontinued	Zeneca (US)	Kappa agonist	Mar-89
ICI-204448	Discontinued	Zeneca (US)	Kappa agonist	Feb-90
PD-117302	Discontinued	Warner-Lambert (US)	Kappa agonist	Mar-94
Pharmaprojects No. 5139	Discontinued	Pfizer (US)	Kappa agonist	Jul-98
Pyrrolidinylethylacetamides	Discontinued	Zeneca (US)	Kappa agonist	Mar-92
R-84760	Discontinued	Sankyo (Japan)	Kappa agonist	Apr-97

Ref.: Pharmaprojects (updated to 2/02) used with permission; Scrip, corporate, literature & patent references
"Status" is international drug development or regulatory status and may not indicate status in USA
Sponsor: Original company name is retained if product is discontinued or inactive after merger, acquisition, company name change, etc.
Users of this table are encouraged to independently verify the status, activity, and mechanism of action of drugs of interest

GENERIC / TRADE NAME	STATUS	SPONSOR (S)	MECHANISM OF ACTION	REF. UPDATE
Tetrahydroisoquinolines	Discontinued	SmithKline Beecham (UK)	Kappa agonist	Nov-92
Thienylacetamides	Discontinued	Boehringer Mannheim (Ger)	Kappa agonist	1990
Tifluadom	Discontinued	Solvay (Netherlands)	Kappa agonist	Jul-91
XB375, XE440	Discontinued	DuPont Merck (US)	Kappa agonist	Jun-93
ZT-52656A	Discontinued (ph. I)	SmithKline Beecham (UK)	Kappa agonist	Jan-93
HN-11608 (HN-11600)	Discontinued (ph. I?)	Hafslund Nycomed (Norway)	Kappa agonist	May-95
Dynorphin A	Discontinued (ph. II)	Neurobiological Technologies	Dynorphin A (1-13) peptide	Feb-02
E-2078	Discontinued (ph. II)	Eisai (Japan)	Dynorphin analog, kappa agon.	Aug-93
Apadoline (RP 60180)	Discontinued (ph. II)	Rhone-Poulenc Rorer (France)	Kappa agonist	Jun-99
Spiradoline (U-62066E)	Discontinued (ph. II)	Pharmacia & Upjohn (UK)	Kappa agonist	Dec-93
Niravoline (RU 51599)	Discontinued (ph. II)	Hoechst Marion Roussel (Ger)	Kappa agonist "aquaretic"	Aug-96
Enadoline	Discontinued (ph. II)	Warner-Lambert (US)	Kappa agonist / head injuries	May-97
AK-235	Inactive	Univ. Arizona (US)	Dynorphin A analog	1989
DuP-747	Inactive	Endo Pharmaceuticals (US)	Kappa agonist	Feb-02
GR-103545	Inactive	Glaxo (UK)	Kappa agonist	Jan-92
PD-129290	Inactive	Warner-Lambert (US)	Kappa agonist	Aug-91
U-50,488H	Inactive	Upjohn (US)	Kappa agonist	1989
Cyclopropylmethylmorphinan	Preclinical	SRI Int'l (US)	Kappa agonist	Nov-93
Opioid analgesics, Adolor	Preclinical	Adolor (US)	Kappa agonists, peripheral	Jun-99
Pharmaprojects No. 5821	Preclinical	Adolor (US)	Peripheral kappa agonist	Jun-98
TAN-684	Preclinical	Toray (Japan)	Peripheral kappa agonist	Jun-00
OPIOID PEPTIDES / ENDORPHINS / ENKEPHALINS				
BCH-2687 (LEF-553)	Discontinued	Shire / BioChem Pharma	Dermorphin tetrapeptide	May-97
β-endorphin	Discontinued	Amgen (US)	Endorphin	Mar-85
β-endorphin	Discontinued	Cambridge Biotech (US)	Endorphin	Dec-84
Org-5878	Discontinued	Akzo (Netherlands)	Endorphin	Apr-91
BW-831C	Discontinued	Wellcome (UK)	Enkephalin analog	Mar-88
DN-1504	Discontinued	Daiichi (Japan)	Enkephalin analog	Dec-84
EK-399	Discontinued	Takeda (Japan)	Enkephalin analog	Jul-89
Lipoenkephalins	Discontinued	Merck & Co (US)	Enkephalin analog	Jan-84
Nifalatide	Discontinued	Wellcome (UK)	Enkephalin analog	Mar-87
RX-783006	Discontinued	Reckitt & Colman (UK)	Enkephalin analog	Feb-84
RX-783016	Discontinued	Reckitt & Colman (UK)	Enkephalin analog	Feb-84
SC-34871	Discontinued	Searle/Monsanto (US)	Enkephalin analog	Jul-89
SC-39566	Discontinued	Searle/Monsanto (US)	Enkephalin analog	Nov-90
SD-41	Discontinued	Dainippon (Japan)	Enkephalin analog	Jan-92
Syndyphalin (SD-33)	Discontinued	Otsuka (Japan)	Enkephalin analog	1983
CDRI-82-205	Discontinued	Central Drug Research (India)	Met-enkephalin analog	May-97
Pharmaprojects No. 4974	Discontinued	Chiron (US)	Opioid ligands (peptidomimetic)	1997
Leumorphin	Discontinued	Mitsubishi Kasei (Japan)	Opioid peptide	1984
Yissum P-0883	Discontinued	Yissum (Israel)	Peripheral opioid inducer	Mar-97
BW-180C	Discontinued (ph. II)	Glaxo Wellcome (UK)	Enkephalin analog	Mar-87
BW-443C81	Discontinued (ph. II)	Wellcome (UK)	Enkephalin analog	Oct-91
Ocitide (Hoe-825)	Discontinued (ph. II)	Hoechst Marion Roussel (Ger)	Enkephalin analog	Oct-88
FK-33-824 (DAMME)	Discontinued (ph. II)	Novartis (Switz.)	Met-enkephalin analog	1979
443C81	Discontinued (ph. II)	Glaxo Wellcome (UK)	Peripherally-acting enkephalin	Nov-91
β-endorphin	Inactive	Mitsubishi Kasei (Japan)	Endorphin	Unk.
Endorphin, pancreatic	Inactive	Endorphin Inc. (US)	Endorphin	Feb-85
alpha-Neoendorphin	Inactive	Suntory (Japan)	Endorphin (synthetic)	Dec-81
Met-enkephalin	Inactive	TNI (US)	Enkephalin	1988
Biphalin	Inactive	Univ. Arizona (US)	Enkephalin analog	May-92
DALECK	Inactive	Hungarian Acad. Sciences	Enkephalin analog	Unk.
EK-209	Inactive	Takeda (Japan)	Enkephalin analog	Unk.
LY-281217	Inactive	Lilly (US)	Enkephalin analog	Nov-91
LY-97292	Inactive	Lilly (US)	Enkephalin analog	1984
Wy-42186	Inactive	Wyeth-Ayerst (US)	Enkephalin analog	1983
Enkephalins	Inactive	Peptide Technology (Austr)	Enkephalins	Mar-86
PL-030	Inactive	Peninsula Laboratories (US)	Morphiceptin analog	1983
Metorphamide	Inactive	Stanford Univ. (US)	Opioid octapeptide	Unk.
Wheat-derived peptide	Inactive	Nisshin Flour (Japan)	Opioid peptide	Jul-91
BCH-150	Preclinical	BioChem Pharma (Canada)	Dermorphin analog	1992
UA 621/859	Preclinical	Univ. Arizona (US)	Opioid endorphins	Apr-97

Ref.: Pharmaprojects (updated to 2/02) used with permission; Scrip, corporate, literature & patent references
"Status" is international drug development or regulatory status and may not indicate status in USA
Sponsor: Original company name is retained if product is discontinued or inactive after merger, acquisition, company name change, etc.
Users of this table are encouraged to independently verify the status, activity, and mechanism of action of drugs of interest

GENERIC / TRADE NAME	STATUS	SPONSOR (S)	MECHANISM OF ACTION	REF. UPDATE
Pharmaprojects No. 4724	Preclinical	Astra (Sweden)/BioChem Pharma	Opioid peptide μ ag. / δ antag.	Jun-96
OPIOID, OTHER / UNSPECIFIED				
Nociceptin	Discontinued	Euroscreen (Belgium)	Opioid ORL-1 agonist	Aug-99
CAP, Nycomed Amersham	Discontinued (ph. II)	Nycomed (Norway)	Unknown	Feb-02
Analgesic gene therapy	Inactive	NIH (US)	β-endorphin gene (adenovirus)	Sep-99
opioid analgesics, BTG	Inactive	BTG (UK)	Opioid analgesic	Feb-02
Pharmaprojects No. 4137	Inactive	Trega Biosciences (US)	Opioid mu antagonist (peripheral)	Feb-02
Nociceptin/orphanin antags.	Inactive	CoCensys (US)	Opioid orphan receptor antag.	Jun-99
Flupirtine	LAUNCHED	Carter Wallace / Asta Medica	Weak opioid / NMDA antag.	Jun-96
ORL-1 antagonists, Adolor	Preclinical	Adolor (US)	Central opioid analgesic	Feb-02
opioid agonists, Molecumetics	Preclinical	Molecumetics	Opioid analgesic	Feb-02
VAN project	Preclinical	Vita-Invest (Spain)	Opioid analgesic (unidentified)	Jun-98
Nociceptive	Preclinical	Merck (US) / Banyu (Japan)	Opioid ORL-1 antagonist	Jan-00
Pain gene therapy	Preclinical	Univ. South Carolina (US)	Preproenkephalin gene (HSV vector)	Jun-99
PROSTAGLANDIN RECEPTOR ANTAGONISTS				
ONO-8711	CLINICAL (I)	Ono (Japan)	Prostaglandin EP1 antagonist	Apr-00
ZD-6416	Discontinued	AstraZeneca (UK)	EP1 prostaglandin antagonist	Feb-02
Pharmaprojects No. 3651	Discontinued	Searle/Monsanto (US)	PGE2 receptor antagonist	Mar-94
Pharmaprojects No. 4217	Discontinued	Searle/Monsanto (US)	PGE2 receptor antagonist	May-98
S- 19220 / Dibenzoxazepines	Discontinued	Searle/Monsanto (US)	PGE2 receptor antagonist	Sep-93
M-5011	Discontinued	Maruho (Japan)	PGF1a antagonist	Apr-98
Tomoxiprole (MDL-035)	Discontinued (Clin.)	Hoechst Marion Roussel (Ger)	PGE2 / PGF1-alpha antag.	Mar-87
ZD-4953	Discontinued (ph. II)	AstraZeneca (UK)	EP1 prostaglandin antagonist	Jun-00
SC-42867	Discontinued (ph. II)	Searle/Monsanto (US)	Prostaglandin antagonist	Apr-93
NXTHIO	Discontinued (PRE-REG)	Applied Pharma Res. (Switz)	Naproxen + mucolytic	Jun-98
ZD-6804	Preclinical	Zeneca (UK)	EP1 prostaglandin antagonist	Jan-98
SC 51089 / Dibenzoxazepines	Preclinical	Searle/Monsanto (US)	PGE2 receptor antagonist	1993
Thiazepines	Preclinical	Searle/Monsanto (US)	PGE2 receptor antagonist	Feb-95
RADIONUCLIDES				
117m-Sn-DTPA	CLINICAL (II)	Schering AG (Germany)	Radionuclide, Tin-117 isotope	Feb-02
Rhenium-HEDP	Discontinued (PRE-REG)	Mallinckrodt (US)	Radionuclutide; bone cancer pain	Jun-96
Sm153 lexidronam (QUADRAMET®)	LAUNCHED	DuPont Merck / Cytogen (US)	Radionuclide / bone cancer pain	Apr-98
Strontium-89 Chloride	LAUNCHED	Amersham (US)	Radionuclide, Sr-89 isotope	1994
OR-1384	Preclinical	Orion Pharma (Finland)	Polymorph. neutrophil inhib.	Oct-98
SEROTONIN / NOREPINEPHRINE ANTAGONISTS				
Dimethylethylamines	Discontinued	Hoechst (Ger)	5-HT antagonist	Unk.
ADR-882	Discontinued	Erbamont (Italy)	5-HT3 antagonist	Jun-93
Lappaconitine	Discontinued	Mercian (Japan)	NE/5-HT antagonist	Jul-94
CGP-29030A	Discontinued (ph. II)	Ciba-Geigy (Switz)	5-HT2 / A1 antagonist	Mar-94
TMS-ethoxymethylimidazoles	Inactive	Pfizer (US)	5-HT3 antagonists	1990
Pharmaprojects No. 3905	Preclinical	Almirall (Spain)	5-HT3 antagonist	Apr-94
SOMATOSTATIN / ANALOGS				
Somatostatin	LAUNCHED	6 University Study	I.C.V./Intrathecal/Epidural	1984
Octreotide (SANDOSTATIN®)	LAUNCHED	Sandoz (Switz)	Somatostatin analog (I.th.)	1993
SPINAL / EPIDURAL / INTRATHECAL / LOCAL ANESTHETICS				
Levobupivacaine (CHIROCAINE®)	CLINICAL (III)	Zeneca (UK) / Chiroscience (UK)	Local anesthetic / (S)-isomer	May-96
Sameridine	Discontinued (ph. II)	Astra (Sweden)	Local anesthetic (spinal)	Jan-98
Ropivacaine (NAROPIN™)	LAUNCHED	Pharmacia & Upjohn / Astra	Local anesthetic (epidural/spinal)	May-96
STEROIDS				
FP16CM	Discontinued	Florida A&M Univ. (US)	Antiinflammatory steroid	Nov-98
Lipocortin, Shionogi	Discontinued	Shionogi (Japan)	Corticoid	Feb-02
Pharmaprojects No. 4042	Discontinued	Rhone-Poulenc Rorer (France)	Glucocorticoid antag. steroid	Feb-96
Pharmaprojects No. 4091	Discontinued	Rhone-Poulenc Rorer (France)	Glucocorticoid antag. steroid	Mar-96
SEP-119249	Discontinued	Sepracor (US)	Glucocorticoid; anti-inflam.	Jun-00
NM-135	Discontinued	Nissin Food Products (Japan)	Prodrug steriod; anti-inflam.	Feb-02
Lipocortin	Inactive	Biogen (US)	Corticoid	May-85

Ref.: Pharmaprojects (updated to 2/02) used with permission; Scrip, corporate, literature & patent references
"Status" is international drug development or regulatory status and may not indicate status in USA
Sponsor: Original company name is retained if product is discontinued or inactive after merger, acquisition, company name change, etc.
Users of this table are encouraged to independently verify the status, activity, and mechanism of action of drugs of interest

GENERIC / TRADE NAME	STATUS	SPONSOR (S)	MECHANISM OF ACTION	REF. UPDATE
Antevate, TO-186	PRE-REGISTRATION	Mitsubishi Kasei (Japan)	Dermatological steroid	Sep-93
SUBSTANCE P ANTAGONISTS / NEUROKININ ANTAGONISTS / CAPSAICIN				
Nolpitantium chloride (SR-140333)	CLINICAL (I)	Sanofi (France)	NK-1 antag.; inflam. & migraine	Aug-98
SR-48968	CLINICAL (II)	Sanofi (France)	NK-2 antagonist	Dec-97
DA-5018 (KR-25018)	CLINICAL (II)	Dong-A (Korea)	Synthetic capsanoid	Feb-02
N-vanillylnonamide analogues	Discontinued	Procter & Gamble (US)	Capsaicin analogues	Apr-85
Capsazepine	Discontinued	Novartis (Switz.)	Capsaicin antagonist	Oct-93
SDZ-249-482	Discontinued	Novartis (Switz.)	Capsaicin derivatives	Jan-99
Win-64821	Discontinued	Sanofi (France)	NK1 + NK2 antagonist	Dec-95
L-732138	Discontinued	Merck & Co (US)	NK-1 antagonist	Nov-96
L-733060	Discontinued	Merck & Co (US)	NK-1 antagonist	May-98
NKT-343 (SDZ-NKT-343)	Discontinued	Novartis (Switz.)	NK-1 antagonist	May-99
TAN-1612	Discontinued	Takeda (Japan)	NK-1 antagonist	May-98
L-740141	Discontinued	Merck & Co (US)	NK-1 antagonist	Feb-99
S-18523	Discontinued	Servier (France)	NK-1 antagonist (pseudopept.)	May-99
GR-82334	Discontinued	Glaxo Wellcome (UK)	NK-1 antagonist peptide	Jan-97
OT-7100	Discontinued	Otsuka (Japan)	NK-1 receptor antag.	Jan-99
CP-99994	Discontinued	Pfizer (US)	NK1/Substance P antag., 2nd gen.	May-99
Pharmaprojects No. 3347	Discontinued	Merck & Co (US)	Substance P antagnoist	1997
Pharmaprojects No. 3879	Discontinued	Takeda (Japan)	Substance P antagonist	Aug-95
Pharmaprojects No. 5533	Discontinued	Johnson & Johnson (US)	Substance P antagonist	Feb-99
RP-67580	Discontinued	Rhone-Poulenc Rorer (France)	Substance P antagonist	Mar-93
Tachykinin analogues	Discontinued	Yissum (Israel)	Substance P antagonist	Feb-93
Pharmaprojects No. 4006	Discontinued	Rhone-Poulenc Rorer (France)	Substance P antagonist (migraine)	Jan-96
Resiniferatoxin, NIH	Discontinued	NIH (US)	Substance P depletor	Jul-98
Pharmaprojects No. 3818	Discontinued	Merck & Co (US)	Tachykinin antagonist	Jan-94
RPR-100893	Discontinued (ph. II)	Rhone-Poulenc Rorer (France)	NK-1 antagonist	Oct-96
Lanepitant (LY-303870)	Discontinued (ph. II)	Lilly (US)	NK-1 antagonist (oral)	Sep-97
Olvanil	Inactive	Procter & Gamble (US)	Capsaicin analogue	Jul-91
GR-71251	Inactive	Glaxo (UK)	NK-1 antagonist (peptide)	Jul-91
L-659837	Inactive	Merck & Co (US)	NK-2 antagonist	1991
L-659877	Inactive	Merck & Co (US)	NK-2 antagonist	Nov-92
MEN-10207	Inactive	Menarini (Italy)	NK-A Antagonist	Oct-93
Pharmaprojects No. 6051	Inactive	Lilly (US)	Substance P / glutamate antag.	Feb-02
Heptapeptides	Inactive	Ferring (Sweden)	Substance P antagonist	Unk.
SPA-58	Inactive	Takeda (Japan)	Substance P antagonist	1983
tachykinin antagonists, Lilly	Inactive	Lilly (US)	Substance P antagonist	Feb-02
N-1103	Preclinical	GenDerm (US)	Capsanoid	Nov-92
6b-I, NIH	Preclinical	NIH (US)	NK-1 antagonist	Sep-99
CP-96345 / CP-96344	Preclinical	Pfizer (US)	NK-1 antagonist	Dec-99
BL-1872	Preclinical	Bioglan Laboratories (UK)	NK-1 antagonist; capsanoid	May-00
Morpholines, Thiomorpholines	Preclinical	Merck & Co (US)	Substance P antag / depletor	Oct-95
Pharmaprojects No. 6015	Preclinical	Merck & Co (US)	Substance P antag.; pain, inflam.	Sep-98
Diphenylpropanes	Preclinical	Merck & Co (US)	Substance P antagonist	Feb-93
Substance P-neurotoxin compound	Preclinical	Univ. Minnesota (US)	Substance P cell toxin (I.th.)	Oct-97
MISCELLANEOUS / OTHER / UNKNOWN				
D-6428	CLINICAL (I)	Celltech (UK)	Centrally-acting analgesic	Feb-02
VAN-H36	CLINICAL (I)	Vita-Invest (Spain)	Centrally-acting analgesic	Feb-02
GPI-5693	CLINICAL (I)	Guilford (US)	Centrally-acting analgesic	Feb-02
BCX-1470	CLINICAL (I)	BioCryst (US)	Factor D serine protease inhib.	Jun-98
MX-68	CLINICAL (I)	Chugai (Japan)	Methotrexate analog; DHFR antag.	Feb-00
Prosaptide TX14(A)	CLINICAL (I)	Myelos Neurosciences (US)	Neuropathic pain	Mar-98
NNC-05-1869	CLINICAL (I)	Novo Nordisk (Denmark)	Unknown / diabetic neuropathy	Apr-97
CJC-1008	CLINICAL (II)	ConjuChem (US)	Centrally-acting analgesic	Feb-02
JTC-801	CLINICAL (II)	Japan Tobacco (Japan)	Centrally-acting analgesic	Feb-02
CPC-111	CLINICAL (II)	Cypros (US)	Cytoprotective (sickle cell pain)	Nov-97
LeukoVax	CLINICAL (II)	Viragen / Inflammatics (US)	Immunomod. cell prep; RA	Nov-98
Bicifadine (CL-220075)	CLINICAL (II)	Dov (US) / Wyeth-Ayerst (US)	NSAID	Jul-97
hCG (LDI-200), Milkhaus	CLINICAL (III)	Milkhaus (US)	Antileukemic; ph. I cancer pain	Feb-98
Esterom	CLINICAL (III)	Entropin	Cocaine hydrolysis esters; topical	Feb-02
Small peptides, Centocor	Discontinued	Centocor (US)	Adhesion molecule antag. / RA	Dec-94

Ref.: Pharmaprojects (updated to 2/02) used with permission; Scrip, corporate, literature & patent references
"Status" is international drug development or regulatory status and may not indicate status in USA
Sponsor: Original company name is retained if product is discontinued or inactive after merger, acquisition, company name change, etc.
Users of this table are encouraged to independently verify the status, activity, and mechanism of action of drugs of interest

GENERIC / TRADE NAME	STATUS	SPONSOR (S)	MECHANISM OF ACTION	REF. UPDATE
butinazocine	Discontinued	Brocacef	Centrally-acting analgesic	Feb-02
Latranal	Discontinued	Praecis Pharmaceuticals	Centrally-acting analgesic	Feb-02
Pharmaprojects No. 1205	Discontinued	SRI International	Centrally-acting analgesic	Feb-02
Pharmaprojects No. 1248	Discontinued	Dainippon (Japan)	Centrally-acting analgesic	Feb-02
Pharmaprojects No. 1421	Discontinued	Non-industrial source	Centrally-acting analgesic	Feb-02
Pharmaprojects No. 1446	Discontinued	Aventis (France)	Centrally-acting analgesic	Feb-02
Pharmaprojects No. 1490	Discontinued	Aventis (France)	Centrally-acting analgesic	Feb-02
Pharmaprojects No. 1687	Discontinued	Roche (Switz)	Centrally-acting analgesic	Feb-02
Pharmaprojects No. 1874	Discontinued	Daiichi (Japan)	Centrally-acting analgesic	Feb-02
Pharmaprojects No. 2120	Discontinued	Fresenius	Centrally-acting analgesic	Feb-02
Pharmaprojects No. 2737	Discontinued	Aventis (France)	Centrally-acting analgesic	Feb-02
Pharmaprojects No. 2782	Discontinued	GlaxoSmithKline (UK)	Centrally-acting analgesic	Feb-02
Pharmaprojects No. 2840	Discontinued	Shionogi (Japan)	Centrally-acting analgesic	Feb-02
Pharmaprojects No. 2853	Discontinued	AstraZeneca (UK)	Centrally-acting analgesic	Feb-02
Pharmaprojects No. 711	Discontinued	American Home Products (US)	Centrally-acting analgesic	Feb-02
Pharmaprojects No. 962	Discontinued	BTG (UK)	Centrally-acting analgesic	Feb-02
pidocetamol	Discontinued	Pan Medica (France)	Centrally-acting analgesic	Feb-02
Ro-11-4337	Discontinued	Roche (Switz)	Centrally-acting analgesic	Feb-02
Sch-32615	Discontinued	Schering Plough (US)	Centrally-acting analgesic	Feb-02
D-19050	Discontinued	Asta Medica (Germany)	CNS + peripheral action	Oct-91
D-16120	Discontinued	Asta Medica (Germany)	CNS action	Jul-87
Peptidomimetic	Discontinued	Yissum (Israel)	Cyclic peptide	Jan-93
FY95-0006	Discontinued	UAB Research Foundation (US)	Disacharides; selectin inhibition	Sep-98
Protease Inhibitors	Discontinued	Unigene (US)	Endothelin antagonist	Aug-92
NRT-115	Discontinued	Centaur (US)	Free radical scavenger; arthritis	Dec-99
TSG-6 inhibitors	Discontinued	NYU Medical Center (US)	Inflammatory protein	Jun-00
Pharmaprojects No. 3877	Discontinued	Medarex (US)	Intract. pain: destroys periph. nerves	Apr-96
Benzenemethanamine	Discontinued	Hoechst (Ger)	Non-opioid	Unk.
RU-54808	Discontinued	Hoechst Marion Roussel (Ger)	Peripheral analgesic	Feb-97
NB1 (Nociblocker)	Discontinued	Nortran (Canada)	Peripheral analgesic (unidentified)	Dec-99
PDE inhibitors, Bayer	Discontinued	Bayer (Germany)	Phosphodiesterase inhibitor	Mar-98
SKF-10049	Discontinued	SmithKline Beecham (UK)	Sigma agonist	Mar-81
Pharmaprojects No. 5459	Discontinued	Searle/Monsanto (US)	Steroid nitrite ester / inflam.	Jan-99
OF-743	Discontinued	Moscow State Univ. (Russia)	Unidentified	Mar-97
Pharmaprojects No. 5742	Discontinued	Toray (Japan)	Unidentified (cancer pain)	Jun-00
Pharmaprojects No. 4963	Discontinued	Roche (Switz.) / Agouron (US)	Unidentified / pain	May-99
Pharmaprojects No. 4423	Discontinued	Dong Wha (S. Korea)	Unidentified analgesic	Mar-98
Pharmaprojects No. 6187	Discontinued	Roche (Switz) / AxyS (US)	Unidentified genomic technology	Feb-02
Pharmaprojects No. 5458	Discontinued	Novo Nordisk (Denmark)	Unidentified; analg., anti-inflam.	Jun-00
RMM-295	Discontinued	Roemmers	Unk. (non-narcotic)	Jun-00
ATBO	Discontinued	Univ. Seville (Spain)	Unknown	1997
Benzopyranopyridimines	Discontinued	Ciba-Geigy (Switz)	Unknown	Jun-85
Hoe-302	Discontinued	Hoechst (Ger)	Unknown	Feb-87
Hoe-S-2922	Discontinued	Hoechst (Ger)	Unknown	Mar-89
Lorcinadol	Discontinued	Johnson & Johnson (US)	Unknown	Mar-89
McN-5195	Discontinued	Johnson & Johnson (US)	Unknown	1987
Oxadiazolylarylmethanones	Discontinued	Hoechst (Ger)	Unknown	Mar-88
Pharmaprojects No. 4734	Discontinued	Servier (France)	Unknown	1997
SD-46	Discontinued	Dainippon (Japan)	Unknown	Aug-85
SD-62	Discontinued	Dainippon (Japan)	Unknown	Feb-89
Tetrahydrothiopyraneindoles	Discontinued	Shionogi (Japan)	Unknown	Mar-93
Tropanes / Benzomorphans	Discontinued	BTG (UK)	Unknown	Nov-91
Pharmaprojects No. 3420	Discontinued	Servier (France)	Unknown (non-opioid)	Mar-95
F-9004T	Discontinued	Faes (Spain)	Unknown (oral non-narcotic)	Feb-94
Pharmaprojects No. 3953	Discontinued	Boehringer Ingelheim (Ger)	Unknown / indazolone	Mar-96
S-1490 (S-1491)	Discontinued (Clin.)	Synthelabo (France)	Unidentified analgesic	Mar-85
SKF-10047 (NANM)	Discontinued (ph. I)	SmithKline Beecham (UK)	Sigma receptor agonist	Dec-92
Pinadoline (SC-25469)	Discontinued (ph. I)	Searle/Monsanto (US)	Unidentified analgesic	1984
CereCRIB	Discontinued (ph. I/II)	Astra (Swed.) / CytoTherapeutics	Encapsulated cells (ph. I.th. implant)	Mar-97
GW-275919	Discontinued (ph. II)	Glaxo Wellcome (UK)	Back pain (unspec. Mechanism)	Feb-02
UP-5222-04	Discontinued (ph. II)	UPSA (France)	Central non-opioid analgesic	Mar-91
HGP-4	Discontinued (ph. II)	HG Pars (US)	Centrally-acting analgesic	Feb-02
NIK-264	Discontinued (ph. II)	Nikken Chemical (Japan)	Unidentified (cancer pain)	Feb-02

Ref.: Pharmaprojects (updated to 2/02) used with permission; Scrip, corporate, literature & patent references
"Status" is international drug development or regulatory status and may not indicate status in USA
Sponsor: Original company name is retained if product is discontinued or inactive after merger, acquisition, company name change, etc.
Users of this table are encouraged to independently verify the status, activity, and mechanism of action of drugs of interest

GENERIC / TRADE NAME	STATUS	SPONSOR (S)	MECHANISM OF ACTION	REF. UPDATE
P-1230	Discontinued (ph. II)	Poli (Italy)	Unidentified analgesic	Jul-87
AI-200	Discontinued (ph. III)	AutoImmune (US)	Collagen, type II; RA	Sep-99
CKD-303	Discontinued (ph. III)	Chong Kun Dang (S. Korea)	Unidentified (analgesic)	Feb-00
Peltazone	Discontinued (ph. III)	Takeda (Japan)	Unidentified analgesic	Feb-95
AM-543	Inactive	AMRAD (Australia)	Centrally-acting analgesic	Feb-02
Pharmaprojects No. 1135	Inactive	Merck & Co (US)	Centrally-acting analgesic	Feb-02
Pharmaprojects No. 1376	Inactive	Roche (Switz)	Centrally-acting analgesic	Feb-02
Pharmaprojects No. 1586	Inactive	Pharmacia (US)	Centrally-acting analgesic	Feb-02
Pharmaprojects No. 1587	Inactive	Non-industrial source	Centrally-acting analgesic	Feb-02
Pharmaprojects No. 1863	Inactive	Pfizer (US)	Centrally-acting analgesic	Feb-02
Pharmaprojects No. 1928	Inactive	Research Corp. Tech. (US)	Centrally-acting analgesic	Feb-02
Pharmaprojects No. 2008	Inactive	Nycomed Pharma (Norway)	Centrally-acting analgesic	Feb-02
Pharmaprojects No. 2096	Inactive	Procter & Gamble (US)	Centrally-acting analgesic	Feb-02
Pharmaprojects No. 2356	Inactive	Lilly (US)	Centrally-acting analgesic	Feb-02
Pharmaprojects No. 2552	Inactive	Non-industrial source	Centrally-acting analgesic	Feb-02
Pharmaprojects No. 2744	Inactive	Sanofi-Synthelabo (France)	Centrally-acting analgesic	Feb-02
Pharmaprojects No. 2866	Inactive	Nisshin Flour (Japan)	Centrally-acting analgesic	Feb-02
Pharmaprojects No. 3680	Inactive	Merck KGaA (Germany)	Centrally-acting analgesic	Feb-02
Pharmaprojects No. 6293	Inactive	ICN (US)	Centrally-acting analgesic	Feb-02
Pharmaprojects No. 6321	Inactive	Merck & Co (US)	Centrally-acting analgesic	Feb-02
Pharmaprojects No. 6327	Inactive	NIH (US)	Centrally-acting analgesic	Feb-02
Pharmaprojects No. 6448	Inactive	AstraZeneca (UK)	Centrally-acting analgesic	Feb-02
Pharmaprojects No. 780	Inactive	Roche (Switz)	Centrally-acting analgesic	Feb-02
Pharmaprojects No. 916	Inactive	Non-industrial source	Centrally-acting analgesic	Feb-02
Pharmaprojects No. 932	Inactive	Abbott (US)	Centrally-acting analgesic	Feb-02
PN1 antagonists, Allelix	Inactive	NPS Pharmaceuticals (US)	Centrally-acting analgesic	Feb-02
RP 63494	Inactive	Aventis (France)	Centrally-acting analgesic	Feb-02
RWJ-314313	Inactive	Johnson & Johnson (US)	Centrally-acting analgesic	Feb-02
S-18920	Inactive	Servier (France)	Centrally-acting analgesic	Feb-02
Pharmaprojects No. 4507	Inactive	Aventis (France)	Centrally-acting analgesic	Feb-02
Pharmaprojects No. 931	Inactive	American Home Products (US)	Centrally-acting analgesic	Feb-02
Pharmaprojects No. 5399	Inactive	Southern Research Institute	Centrally-acting analgesic	Feb-02
Pharmaprojects No. 835	Inactive	Aventis (France)	Centrally-acting analgesic	Feb-02
Pharmaprojects No. 2362	Inactive	Non-industrial source	Centrally-acting analgesic	Feb-02
Pharmaprojects No. 6375	Inactive	Elan (Ireland)	Centrally-acting analgesic	Feb-02
Pharmaprojects No. 2886	Inactive	Aventis (France)	Centrally-acting analgesic	Feb-02
BDP-3	Inactive	Non-industrial source	Centrally-acting analgesic	Feb-02
Pyrrolidones	Inactive	Hoechst (Ger)	Cognition / analgesia	Aug-91
GEMM-1 antagonists	Inactive	GEMMA Biotechnology	GEMM-1 antagonist; arthritis	Feb-02
BOP-3	Inactive	Klinikum der Univerl. (Ger)	Imaging agent	1986
Methotrexate	Inactive	Dartmouth College (US)	Low back pain (intrathecal)	Feb-00
TRIM	Inactive	Non-industrial source	Neural nitric oxide synthase inhib.	Feb-02
Oxazepines	Inactive	Knoll (Ger)	Oxidoreductase	Apr-85
D-20450	Inactive	Asta Medica (Germany)	Peripheral site action	Apr-92
Pharmaprojects No. 5218	Inactive	Origene Technologies (US)	Snake venom gene product	Feb-02
Pharmaprojects No. 5504	Inactive	Glaxo Wellcome (UK)	Uniden. (androstane deriv./inflam)	Feb-02
Pharmaprojects No. 5425	Inactive	Roche (Switz) / Clontech (US)	Unidentified; analg., anti-inflam.	Feb-02
Pharmaprojects No. 2502	Inactive	Pharmol Pacific (Austral)	Unk. / centrally-acting	1988
Yissum P-0873	Inactive	Yissum (Israel)	Unk. / peripheral	Feb-02
2-Halopyridines	Inactive	Lacer (Spain)	Unknown	May-92
Alkynamides	Inactive	Procter & Gamble (US)	Unknown	Unk.
Biphenylacetic acid der.	Inactive	Upjohn (US)	Unknown	Unk.
Cyclohexadienes	Inactive	Roche (Switz)	Unknown	Unk.
Diaminocyclohexanes	Inactive	Upjohn (US)	Unknown	Unk.
Diaminocyclohexylamides	Inactive	Warner-Lambert (US)	Unknown	Unk.
Dibenzthiepines	Inactive	Hoechst (Ger)	Unknown	1982
MR-549	Inactive	Medea Research (Italy)	Unknown	Nov-85
NE-21610	Inactive	Procter & Gamble (US)	Unknown	1989
Phenyliminoimidazolines	Inactive	Hafslund Nycomed (Norway)	Unknown	Unk.
Win-52114-2	Inactive	Eastman Kodak (US)	Unknown	1988
Icilin	Inactive	Canada Packers (Canada)	Unknown; "Feels cold"	1984
Neurotropin	LAUNCHED	Nippon Zoki (Japan)	Inflam. rabbit skin extract	Jan-92
Evening Primrose Oil	LAUNCHED	Efamol (UK)	Linoleic acid (PMS pain)	Sep-93

Ref.: Pharmaprojects (updated to 2/02) used with permission; Scrip, corporate, literature & patent references
"Status" is international drug development or regulatory status and may not indicate status in USA
Sponsor: Original company name is retained if product is discontinued or inactive after merger, acquisition, company name change, etc.
Users of this table are encouraged to independently verify the status, activity, and mechanism of action of drugs of interest

GENERIC / TRADE NAME	STATUS	SPONSOR (S)	MECHANISM OF ACTION	REF. UPDATE
Guacetisal	LAUNCHED	Bayer (Germany)	Mucin antagonist	Dec-91
clodronate disodium, Abiogen	LAUNCHED	Merck & Co (US)	Osteoporosis / bone pain	Feb-02
Pharmaprojects No. 5150	Preclinical	Novo Nordisk (Denmark)	Amylin / CGRP release inhibitor	Jan-97
Pharmaprojects No. 4571	Preclinical	Innapharma (US)	Cancer pain; IND	Oct-95
Pharmaprojects No. 3945	Preclinical	Theracel / Titan (US)	Cells / CNS implant	May-94
analgesic, Sigyn	Preclinical	Sigyn Pharmaceuticals	Centrally-acting analgesic	Feb-02
analgesic, TIMERx	Preclinical	Sanofi-Synthelabo (France)	Centrally-acting analgesic	Feb-02
analgesics, Icagen	Preclinical	Icagen	Centrally-acting analgesic	Feb-02
analgesics, Ionix	Preclinical	Ionix Pharmaceuticals	Centrally-acting analgesic	Feb-02
AR-M390	Preclinical	Roche (Switz)	Centrally-acting analgesic	Feb-02
AZD-4282	Preclinical	AstraZeneca (UK)	Centrally-acting analgesic	Feb-02
calcium channel blockers, Ono	Preclinical	Ono (Japan)	Centrally-acting analgesic	Feb-02
CGX-1002	Preclinical	Cognetix	Centrally-acting analgesic	Feb-02
DD-161515	Preclinical	DiverDrugs	Centrally-acting analgesic	Feb-02
FE200 665	Preclinical	Ferring (Sweden)	Centrally-acting analgesic	Feb-02
GAT-3/4 inhibitors, BTG	Preclinical	BTG (UK)	Centrally-acting analgesic	Feb-02
GT-094	Preclinical	GoBang Therapeutics	Centrally-acting analgesic	Feb-02
HGP-18	Preclinical	HG Pars (US)	Centrally-acting analgesic	Feb-02
IP-02	Preclinical	Ionix Pharmaceuticals	Centrally-acting analgesic	Feb-02
IP-03	Preclinical	Ionix Pharmaceuticals	Centrally-acting analgesic	Feb-02
J-113397	Preclinical	Merck & Co (US)	Centrally-acting analgesic	Feb-02
NaN, TransMolecular	Preclinical	TransMolecular	Centrally-acting analgesic	Feb-02
NW-1029	Preclinical	Newron	Centrally-acting analgesic	Feb-02
ONO-2921	Preclinical	Ono (Japan)	Centrally-acting analgesic	Feb-02
Org-25543	Preclinical	Akzo Nobel (Netherlands)	Centrally-acting analgesic	Feb-02
Pharmaprojects No. 6636	Preclinical	Juvantia	Centrally-acting analgesic	Feb-02
RWJ-37210	Preclinical	Johnson & Johnson (US)	Centrally-acting analgesic	Feb-02
TKA-731	Preclinical	Novartis (Switz.)	Centrally-acting analgesic	Feb-02
Xen-001	Preclinical	Xenome	Centrally-acting analgesic	Feb-02
vanilloid receptor antag,Neuro	Preclinical	Neurogen (US)	Centrally-acting analgesic	Feb-02
A-286501	Preclinical	Abbott (US)	Centrally-acting analgesic	Feb-02
MET-157	Preclinical	NicOx (France)	Centrally-acting analgesic	Feb-02
NCX-285	Preclinical	NicOx (France)	Centrally-acting analgesic	Feb-02
GRI-2	Preclinical	NPS Pharmaceuticals (US)	Centrally-acting analgesic	Feb-02
Pharmaprojects No. 6592	Preclinical	Abbott (US)	Centrally-acting analgesic	Feb-02
BP-2.94	Preclinical	Bioproject (France)	H3-receptor agonist analgesic	Jun-98
CEE-04-420; CEE-04-421	Preclinical	CeNeS (UK) / BTG (UK)	Lys-D-Pro-Thr; neuropathic pain	Jun-99
NGX.231	Preclinical	NeurogesX (US)	Neuropathic pain / antiinflammatory	Feb-02
Oligopeptides	Preclinical	SPA (Italy)	Oral lysozyme metabolites	May-96
Pharmaprojects No. 6101	Preclinical	Molecumetics / BMS (US)	Transcription factor inhib.	Nov-98
PDE-IV inhibitors	Preclinical	Syntex/Roche (Switzerland)	Type IV Phosphodiesterase inhib.	Apr-95
NC-164	Preclinical	CAMR (UK)	Unidentified (botulinum frag.)	Jan-99
Pharmaprojects No. 6152	Preclinical	CAMR (UK)	Unidentified (botulinum frag.)	Jan-99
SPA-S-646	Preclinical	SPA (Italy)	Unidentified analgesic	Feb-02
Anchoring protein modulators	Preclinical	ICOS (US)	Unidentified anti-inflammatory	Jul-97
AGN-197075	Preclinical	ACADIA (US) / Allergan (US)	Unidentified G-protein receptor agon.	Feb-02
Osteoarthritis therapy	Preclinical	Genzyme (US)	Unidentified mech. (osteoarthritis)	Nov-99
Pharmaprojects No. 3063	Preclinical	Adcock Ingram (RSA)	Unk. / non-narcotic	Apr-92
Pharmaprojects No. 3873	Preclinical	Telor Ophthalmic (US)	Unk. / ocular pain	Mar-94
Menabitan	Preclinical	HG Pars (US)	Unknown	Mar-92
Non-narcotic plant derivative	Preclinical	Dong Wha (Korea)	Unknown	Jul-95
Pharmaprojects No. 3874	Preclinical	Regeneron / Glaxo (US)	Unknown	Mar-94
SNX-236	Preclinical	Neurex (US)	Unknown	Feb-93
Lysozyme metabolites	Suspended	SPA (Italy)	Oligopeptides	Mar-99

SORTED ALPHABETICALLY BY DRUG NAME

(R)-Fluoxetine	CLINICAL (II)	Lilly / Sepracor (US)	5-HT uptake inhibitor / migraine	Feb-99
(R)-ketoprofen, Sepracor	CLINICAL (II)	Sepracor (US)	NSAID (single isomer)	Feb-02
(R)-Ketorolac	Discontinued	Sepracor (US)	NSAID, single isomer	Mar-99

Ref.: Pharmaprojects (updated to 2/02) used with permission; Scrip, corporate, literature & patent references
"Status" is international drug development or regulatory status and may not indicate status in USA
Sponsor: Original company name is retained if product is discontinued or inactive after merger, acquisition, company name change, etc.
Users of this table are encouraged to independently verify the status, activity, and mechanism of action of drugs of interest

GENERIC / TRADE NAME	STATUS	SPONSOR (S)	MECHANISM OF ACTION	REF. UPDATE
(S)-Fluoxetine	CLINICAL (II)	Sepracor (US)	5-HT uptake inhibitor	Feb-97
(S)-Ibuprofen, PAZ	LAUNCHED	PAZ Pharma (Ger)	NSAID; single isomer	Jul-96
(S)-mexiletine	Discontinued	Celgene (US)	Na+ Channel antag.; neuropathic	Mar-00
117m-Sn-DTPA	CLINICAL (II)	Schering AG (Germany)	Radionuclide, Tin-117 isotope	Feb-02
2-amino imidazole derivatives	Preclinical	Allergan (US)	Alpha-2 agonist / peripheral	Sep-95
2-ethoxybenzoic acid	CLINICAL (I)	Pfleger	NSAID	Feb-02
2-Halopyridines	Inactive	Lacer (Spain)	Unknown	May-92
324C91	Discontinued	Glaxo Wellcome (UK)	Unidentified (antimigraine)	Dec-94
4030W92	Discontinued (ph. II)	Glaxo Wellcome (UK)	Na+ Channel antag.; chronic pain	Jul-99
443C81	Discontinued (ph. II)	Glaxo Wellcome (UK)	Peripherally-acting enkephalin	Nov-91
4991W93	Discontinued (ph. II)	Glaxo Wellcome (UK)	Unidentified (antimigraine)	Sep-98
4-Aminopiperidines	Preclinical	E. Merck (Ger)	Opioid mu agonist	Sep-93
5'd-5IT	Discontinued	Abbott (US)	Adenosine kinase inhibitor	Oct-99
5G1.1-SC	CLINICAL (II)	Alexion (US)	C5a complement inhibitor	Oct-97
6b-I, NIH	Preclinical	NIH (US)	NK-1 antagonist	Sep-99
A-121798	Inactive	Abbott (US)	Antiarthritic	Feb-02
A-156918	Preclinical	Abbott (US)	Antiinflammatory	Feb-02
A-162-ester	Discontinued	Alpharma (US)	Antiinflammatory	Feb-02
A-183827.0	Discontinued	Abbott (US)	COX-2 inhibitor	Mar-99
A-252444.0	Preclinical	Abbott (US)	ICAM-1 & E-selectin antagonists	Sep-99
A-286501	Preclinical	Abbott (US)	Centrally-acting analgesic	Feb-02
A-293507	Preclinical	Abbott (US)	Antiinflammatory	Feb-02
A-3443	Inactive	Baxter / Ohmeda (US)	Opioid agonist	Feb-90
A-3622	Discontinued	Baxter / Ohmeda (US)	Opioid agonist	Apr-91
A-45474	Discontinued	Abbott (US)	NSAID	Feb-02
A-52795	Discontinued	Abbott (US)	Antiinflammatory	Feb-02
A-69412	Inactive	Abbott (US)	Antiinflammatory	Feb-02
A-78773	Discontinued (ph. I)	Abbott (US)	5-LO inhibitor	May-95
A-80263	Inactive	Abbott (US)	Antiinflammatory	Feb-02
AA-2379	Discontinued (ph. II)	Takeda (Japan)	Ant-inflammatory/antipyretic	May-92
ABT-491 (A-13791)	Discontinued	Abbott (US)	PAF antagonist; inflamm. dis.	Nov-98
ABT-594	CLINICAL (II)	Abbott (US)	Nicotonic α4/β2 agonist	Jun-99
ABT-702	Preclinical	Abbott (US)	NSAID	Feb-02
ABT-963	CLINICAL (I)	Abbott (US)	Antiarthritic	Feb-02
Aceclofenac (Airtal, Barcan)	LAUNCHED	BMS / Almirall-Prodesfarma	NSAID	Aug-98
acemetacin	LAUNCHED	Bayer (Germany)	Antiinflammatory	Feb-02
Acetaminophen (FEVERALL EXT. REL.)	PRE-REGISTRATION	Ascent Pediatrics (US)	Extended release, pediatric	Jan-98
Acetaminophen + dextromethorphan	CLINICAL (III)	Algos (US) / J&J (US)	OTC: APAP + dextromethorphan	May-97
ACP	Discontinued	Kureha Chemical	Antiinflammatory	Feb-02
ACT-15	Discontinued	Asahi Glass (Jp) / Chugai (Jp)	Calcitonin stimulant	May-97
Acylmorphinans	Discontinued	Roche (Switz)	Opioid agonist/antagonist	1985
Acylpyrrole-alkanoic acids	Preclinical	Merckle (Germany)	PLA1 inhibitor	Jul-95
AD-1211	Discontinued	Dainippon (Japan)	Opioid agonist/antagonist	Apr-86
AD-1491	Discontinued	Dainippon (Japan)	Antiinflammatory	Feb-02
ADA-KPYIL	Discontinued	DuPont Merck (US)	Neurotensin analog	Mar-93
Adamantylamide dipeptide	Preclinical	Lachema (Czechoslovakia)	Immunostimulant	Feb-92
ADL 10-0101	CLINICAL (II)	Adolor (US)	Peripheral kappa agonist	Feb-02
ADL 10-0116	CLINICAL (I)	Adolor (US)	Peripheral kappa agonist	Feb-02
ADL 2-1294	CLINICAL (II)	Adolor (US)	Topical; peripheral mu opioid	Feb-98
ADR-882	Discontinued	Erbamont (Italy)	5-HT3 antagonist	Jun-93
AERx Morphine pulmonary system	CLINICAL (II)	SmithKline Beecham / Aradigm (US)	Formulation, pulmonary	Jun-98
AF/AI-1	Discontinued	Recordati	Antiinflammatory	Feb-02
AF-2259	LAUNCHED	Angelini (Italy)	Antiinflammatory	Feb-02
AFP-802	Discontinued	Recordati	Antiinflammatory	Feb-02
AFP-860	Discontinued	Recordati	Antiinflammatory	Feb-02
Aggrecanase inhibitors	Preclinical	Zeneca (UK)/Celltech (UK)	Aggrecanase inhibitors	Mar-97
AGN-190383	Discontinued	Allergan (US)	Phospholipase PLA2 inhibitor	Nov-92
AGN-197075	Preclinical	ACADIA (US) / Allergan (US)	Unidentified G-protein receptor agon.	Feb-02
AH-25086B	Discontinued	GlaxoSmithKline (UK)	Antimigraine	Feb-02
AH-7170	Discontinued	GlaxoSmithKline (UK)	Antiinflammatory	Feb-02
AHR-10037	Inactive	American Home Products (US)	NSAID	Feb-02
AHR-6293	Discontinued	American Home Products (US)	Antiinflammatory	Feb-02
AI-200	Discontinued (ph. III)	AutoImmune (US)	Collagen, type II; RA	Sep-99

Ref.: Pharmaprojects (updated to 2/02) used with permission; Scrip, corporate, literature & patent references
"Status" is international drug development or regulatory status and may not indicate status in USA
Sponsor: Original company name is retained if product is discontinued or inactive after merger, acquisition, company name change, etc.
Users of this table are encouraged to independently verify the status, activity, and mechanism of action of drugs of interest

GENERIC / TRADE NAME	STATUS	SPONSOR (S)	MECHANISM OF ACTION	REF. UPDATE
AI-202	Discontinued	AutoImmune (US)	Antiarthritic	Feb-02
AIT-297	Inactive	NeoTherapeutics (US)	Unidentified; anti-migraine	Feb-02
AK-235	Inactive	Univ. Arizona (US)	Dynorphin A analog	1989
Aklynamides	Inactive	Procter & Gamble (US)	Unknown	Unk.
alclofenac	LAUNCHED	Pharmacia (US)	NSAID	Feb-02
aldinitan (PASMIGREN®)	Discontinued (ph. III)	Janssen (Belgium)	5-HT1d agonist	Mar-98
Alfentanil	LAUNCHED	Johnson & Johnson (US)	Opioid analgesic	Feb-92
alminoprofen	LAUNCHED	Recordati	NSAID	Feb-02
Almotriptan (LAS-31416)	LAUNCHED	Almirall-Prodesfarma (Spain)	5-HT1d agonist; migraine	Feb-02
Alniditan	Discontinued (ph. II)	Johnson & Johnson (US)	5-HT1d-alpha/beta agonist	1997
Alpha-2 agonists	Discontinued	Synaptic (US)	Alpha-2a, 2b, 2c agonists	May-99
Alpha-D modulator, ICOS	Preclinical	ICOS (US)	Antiinflammatory	Feb-02
Alpha-dihydroergocryptine	LAUNCHED	Poli (Italy)	Ergot alkaloid; antimigraine	May-98
alpha-Neoendorphin	Inactive	Suntory (Japan)	Endorphin (synthetic)	Dec-81
Alpha-trinositol (PP-56)	Discontinued (ph. II)	Perstorp (Sweden)	NPY antagonist	Feb-99
alpha-Viniferin	Inactive	Chung-Ang Univ. (Japan)	Korean folk medicine	1990
alpiropride	LAUNCHED	Sanofi-Synthelabo (France)	Antimigraine	Feb-02
ALX-0646	CLINICAL (I)	NPS / Allelix (Canada)	serotonin agonist (selective)	Apr-98
ALX-1323	Discontinued	NPS / Allelix (Canada)	5-HT1d antagonist	1997
AM-336	CLINICAL (II)	Xenome / AMRAD (Austr.)	Conotoxins, Ca++ channel antag.	Feb-02
AM-512	Preclinical	AMRAD (Australia)	CB1 cannabinoid agonist	May-99
AM-543	Inactive	AMRAD (Australia)	Centrally-acting analgesic	Feb-02
AMA-60	Discontinued	Kureha Chemical	Antiinflammatory	Feb-02
Ametop	LAUNCHED	Mylan (US) / Smith&Nephew (UK)	Formulation, topical amethocaine	Jun-96
amfenac resinate	Discontinued	Meiji Seika (Japan)	Antiinflammatory	Feb-02
amfenac sodium	LAUNCHED	American Home Products (US)	Antiinflammatory	Feb-02
Aminoalkylindoles	Preclinical	Eastman Kodak (US)	Cannabinoid	Sep-92
aminothiophenols	Discontinued	ISIS Innovation	Antiarthritic	Feb-02
amitriptyline+ketamine,Epitome	CLINICAL (II)	EpiCept (US) / Epitome (Canada)	Topical; neuropathy, surg. pain	Feb-02
ampiroxicam	LAUNCHED	Pfizer (US)	NSAID	Feb-02
Amtolmetin guacil (Eufans)	LAUNCHED	Sigma-Tau (Italy)	NSAID; tolmetin prodrug	Dec-98
Anakinra (KINERET®)	LAUNCHED	Amgen (US)	IL-1 receptor antagonist / RA	Feb-02
Analgesic aerosol (BL-1827)	Suspended	CeNeS (UK) / Bioglan Labs (UK)	Sublingual opioid	Feb-00
Analgesic gene therapy	Inactive	NIH (US)	β-endorphin gene (adenovirus)	Sep-99
analgesic, Nobex	Preclinical	Nobex	Formulation	Feb-02
analgesic, Sigyn	Preclinical	Sigyn Pharmaceuticals	Centrally-acting analgesic	Feb-02
analgesic, TIMERx	Preclinical	Sanofi-Synthelabo (France)	Centrally-acting analgesic	Feb-02
analgesics, Endo	Inactive	Endo Pharmaceuticals (US)	Formulation	Feb-02
Analgesics, Endo	Preclinical	Endo (US) / Lavipharm (Greece)	Transdermal analgesic (unspec.)	Dec-99
analgesics, Icagen	Preclinical	Icagen	Centrally-acting analgesic	Feb-02
analgesics, Ionix	Preclinical	Ionix Pharmaceuticals	Centrally-acting analgesic	Feb-02
analgesics, Vestar	Discontinued	Vestar (US)	Liposomal formulations	Sep-91
Anandamide	REGISTERED	Yissum (Israel)	Cannabinoid agonist	Oct-95
Anchor drug delivery	Discontinued	Redcell (Canada)	Formulation, site-specific	Mar-99
Anchoring protein modulators	Preclinical	ICOS (US)	Unidentified anti-inflammatory	Jul-97
Anirolac (RS-37326)	Discontinued	Syntex/Roche (Switz)	Ketorolac analog	Jun-90
Anpirtoline (D-16949)	Discontinued (ph. I)	Asta Medica (Germany)	5-HT1 agonist; antidepressant	May-93
Antevate, TO-186	PRE-REGISTRATION	Mitsubishi Kasei (Japan)	Dermatological steroid	Sep-93
anthrotainin	Inactive	Sanofi-Synthelabo (France)	NSAID	Feb-02
anti-collagenase	Inactive	Chiron (US)	Antiinflammatory	Feb-02
Anticytokines	Preclinical	Sigma-Tau (Italy)	Cytokine antagonist; RA	Jul-99
Anti-inflammatories	Discontinued	Affymax (Glaxo Wellcome-UK)	Selectin inhibitor	May-98
Anti-inflammatories	Preclinical	Praxis (Austr.)	Unidentified anti-inflammatory	Feb-00
anti-inflammatories, Affymax	Inactive	GlaxoSmithKline (UK)	Antiinflammatory	Feb-02
anti-inflammatories, Ankara	Inactive	Non-industrial source	Antiinflammatory	Feb-02
anti-inflammatories, Icagen	Preclinical	Icagen	Antiinflammatory	Feb-02
anti-inflammatories, Karo	Discontinued	Karo Bio (Sweden)	Antiinflammatory	Feb-02
anti-inflammatories, Ligand	Inactive	Ligand (US)	Antiinflammatory	Feb-02
anti-inflammatories, Praxis	Inactive	Praxis (Austr.)	Antiinflammatory	Feb-02
anti-inflammatories, ResCo	Discontinued	Research Corp. Tech. (US)	Antiinflammatory	Feb-02
Anti-inflammatories, Wyeth	Discontinued	Wyeth-Ayerst / Panlabs (US)	Anti-inflammatory	Dec-94
anti-inflammatory peptide, BTG	CLINICAL	BTG (UK)	Cytokine antag.; inflam., RA	Feb-02
anti-inflammatory, GeneMax	Preclinical	GeneMax	Antiinflammatory	Feb-02

Ref.: Pharmaprojects (updated to 2/02) used with permission; Scrip, corporate, literature & patent references
"Status" is international drug development or regulatory status and may not indicate status in USA
Sponsor: Original company name is retained if product is discontinued or inactive after merger, acquisition, company name change, etc.
Users of this table are encouraged to independently verify the status, activity, and mechanism of action of drugs of interest

GENERIC / TRADE NAME	STATUS	SPONSOR (S)	MECHANISM OF ACTION	REF. UPDATE
anti-L-selectin oligo, Gilead	Discontinued	NeXstar / Gilead (US)	L-selectin inhibitor; anti-inflam.	Nov-98
antimigraine, First Horizon	Preclinical	First Horizon (US)	Antimigraine	Feb-02
AntiPARP-1, Octamer	Preclinical	Octamer	Antiinflammatory	Feb-02
antrafenine	WITHDRAWN	Sanofi-Synthelabo (France)	COX inhibitor	Feb-02
ANW-82	Discontinued	Boehringer Ingelheim (Ger)	Antiinflammatory	Feb-02
AP-1 inhibitors, Toyama	Preclinical	Toyama (Japan)	Antiarthritic	Feb-02
Apadoline (RP 60180)	Discontinued (ph. II)	Rhone-Poulenc Rorer (France)	Kappa agonist	Jun-99
APHA	Discontinued	Meiji Seika (Japan)	Enk'ase Inhibitors	Jan-89
APT-070	Preclinical	AdProTech (UK)	Complement inhibitor; arthritis	Jun-99
Apyramide	Discontinued (ph. II)	Laboratoires Richard (France)	NSAID (ph. Indomethacin+APAP ester)	Feb-92
AQ-588	Discontinued	Avant (US) / ArQule (US)	T-cell inhib.; immunosuppressant	Nov-99
araprofen	Discontinued	Sanofi-Synthelabo (France)	NSAID	Feb-02
AR-M390	Preclinical	Roche (Switz)	Centrally-acting analgesic	Feb-02
arthritis therapy, LGCI	Preclinical	LG Chem Investment	Antiarthritic	Feb-02
Arthrovas (AE-941)	Suspended	Aterna Labs (Canada)	Shark cartilage extract / RA-OA	Jan-99
AS-602801	Preclinical	Serono	Antiinflammatory	Feb-02
Asimadoline (EMD-61753)	CLINICAL (II)	Merck KGaA (Germany)	Kappa agonist (peripheral)	Jun-97
ATBO	Discontinued	Univ. Seville (Spain)	Unknown	1997
atliprofen methyl ester	Inactive	IDPL	Antiarthritic	Feb-02
ATSA	Discontinued	Pharmacia (US)	Antiarthritic	Feb-02
AU-8001	Discontinued (ph. I)	Aldo-Union (Spain)	NSAID	Oct-91
auranofin	LAUNCHED	GlaxoSmithKline (UK)	Antiarthritic	Feb-02
Avitriptan	Discontinued (ph. III)	Bristol-Myers Squibb (US)	5-HT1d agonist / migraine	Sep-96
AY-24873	Discontinued	American Home Products (US)	Antiinflammatory	Feb-02
AY-30068	Discontinued	American Home Products (US)	NSAID	Feb-02
AY-31633	Discontinued	Wyeth-Ayerst (US)	NSAID	Mar-88
Azabicycloheptanes	Discontinued	Pfizer (US)	Opioid agonist	1982
azapropazone	LAUNCHED	Siegfried	Antiinflammatory	Feb-02
AZD-4282	Preclinical	AstraZeneca (UK)	Centrally-acting analgesic	Feb-02
AZD-8309	Preclinical	AstraZeneca (UK)	Antiarthritic	Feb-02
AZD-9056	Preclinical	AstraZeneca (UK)	Antiarthritic	Feb-02
Azepexole	Discontinued (ph. II)	Boehringer Ingelheim (Ger)	Alpha-2 agonist	1983
AZER	Discontinued	Pliva	Antiinflammatory	Feb-02
B.TEHM	Inactive	Takeda (Japan)	Opioids	1984
B-4148	Discontinued	Scios Nova (US)	Bradykinin antagonist	Nov-88
B-777-81	Discontinued	Byk Gulden (Ger)	Antidepressant analgesic	Mar-87
Bay 12-9566	CLINICAL (I)	Bayer (Germany)	Stromelysin inhibitor; OA	Jun-97
BAY-o-8276	Discontinued	Bayer (Germany)	Lipoxygenase inhibitor	Oct-89
BB-1101	Discontinued	British Biotech (UK)	Antiarthritic	Feb-02
BB-2827	Discontinued	British Biotech (UK)	Collagenase-specific MMP inhib.	Nov-99
BB-2983	Discontinued	British Biotech (UK)	Antiarthritic	Feb-02
BCH-150	Preclinical	BioChem Pharma (Canada)	Dermorphin analog	1992
BCH-2687 (LEF-553)	Discontinued	Shire / BioChem Pharma	Dermorphin tetrapeptide	May-97
BCX-1170	Inactive	BioCryst (US)	Complement factor D inhib.	Nov-98
BCX-1470	CLINICAL (I)	BioCryst (US)	Factor D serine protease inhib.	Jun-98
BDP-3	Inactive	Non-industrial source	Centrally-acting analgesic	Feb-02
bemesetron	Discontinued	Biosearch Italia (Italy)	Antimigraine	Feb-02
bendazac meglumine	Discontinued	Therapicon (Italy)	Antiinflammatory	Feb-02
β-endorphin	Discontinued	Amgen (US)	Endorphin	Mar-85
β-endorphin	Discontinued	Cambridge Biotech (US)	Endorphin	Dec-84
β-endorphin	Inactive	Mitsubishi Kasei (Japan)	Endorphin	Unk.
Benoxaprofen (ORAFLEX, OPREN)	WITHDRAWN	Lilly (US)	NSAID / photosensitivity tox.	1982
Benzenemethanamine	Discontinued	Hoechst (Ger)	Non-opioid	Unk.
Benzocaine, Vinas (DENTISPRAY)	LAUNCHED	Vinas (Spain)	OTC 5% benzocaine; dental	Jun-99
Benzodiazepine-piperidines	Discontinued	Hoechst (Ger)	PGSI	Feb-87
Benzodiazocines	Inactive	Roussel-Uclaf (France)	Opioid mu agonist	1990
Benzofuropyridines	Inactive	Hoechst (Ger)	Na+ channel antagonist	Unk.
benzomorphan derivatives, Mada	Inactive	Madaus (Ger)	Opioid agonist (weak)	Jun-91
Benzopyranopyridimines	Discontinued	Ciba-Geigy (Switz)	Unknown	Jun-85
Benzotricycloundecanes	Inactive	Merck & Co (US)	Opioid agonist	Unk.
benzydamine, Angelini	Inactive	Angelini (Italy)	Antiinflammatory	Feb-02
bermoprofen	Discontinued	Dainippon (Japan)	Antiinflammatory	Feb-02
BF-389 (Biofor 389)	Discontinued (ph. I)	Biofor (US)	5-LO / COX inhibitor	Nov-95

Ref.: Pharmaprojects (updated to 2/02) used with permission; Scrip, corporate, literature & patent references
"Status" is international drug development or regulatory status and may not indicate status in USA
Sponsor: Original company name is retained if product is discontinued or inactive after merger, acquisition, company name change, etc.
Users of this table are encouraged to independently verify the status, activity, and mechanism of action of drugs of interest

GENERIC / TRADE NAME	STATUS	SPONSOR (S)	MECHANISM OF ACTION	REF. UPDATE
BF-389 (Biofor 389)	Discontinued (ph. I)	Biofor (US)	COX/5-LO inhibitor	Nov-97
BGI	Inactive	Non-industrial source	Antiinflammatory	Feb-02
BIBN-4096	CLINICAL (II)	Boehringer Ingelheim (Ger)	CGRP antagonist (migraine)	Jul-98
Bicifadine (CL-220075)	CLINICAL (II)	Dov (US) / Wyeth-Ayerst (US)	NSAID	Jul-97
BI-L-357	Inactive	Boehringer Ingelheim (Ger)	Antiinflammatory	Feb-02
BI-L-45XX	Discontinued	Boehringer Ingelheim (Ger.)	Antiinflammatory analgesic	Feb-87
BI-L-93BS	Discontinued	Boehringer Ingelheim (Ger)	Antiinflammatory	Feb-02
Bindarit	CLINICAL	Angelini (Italy)	Anti-inflammatory	Jun-93
BIO-1006	Discontinued	Biogen (US)	Anti-inflammatory	Feb-98
BIO-2421	Preclinical	Biogen (US)	Antiinflammatory	Feb-02
Biphalin	Inactive	Univ. Arizona (US)	Enkephalin analog	May-92
Biphenylacetic acid der.	Inactive	Upjohn (US)	Unknown	Unk.
Biphenyl-acetohydroxamic acids	Preclinical	Wellcome (UK)	5-LO / COX inhibitor	Jan-95
BIRB-796	CLINICAL (I)	Boehringer Ingelheim (Ger)	Antiarthritic	Feb-02
BL-016	Inactive	Theracel	Antiinflammatory	Feb-02
BL-1828	Preclinical	Bioglan Laboratories (UK)	Aerosal opioid antagonist	May-00
BL-1832	CLINICAL (III)	Bioglan Laboratories	Formulation	Feb-02
BL-1834	CLINICAL (II)	Bioglan Laboratories (UK)	Intranasal doxepin; severe pain	May-00
BL-1872	Preclinical	Bioglan Laboratories (UK)	NK-1 antagonist; capsanoid	May-00
BMS-181885	Discontinued (ph. I)	Bristol-Myers Squibb (US)	5-HT1d antagonist	Jul-97
BMS-192066	Inactive	Bristol-Myers Squibb (US)	Antiinflammatory	Feb-02
BMS-192548	Discontinued	Bristol-Myers Squibb (US)	NPY antagonist (Y1+Y2)	Aug-96
BMS-347070	CLINICAL (II)	Bristol-Myers Squibb (US)	Antiinflammatory	Feb-02
BN-50370	Discontinued	Beaufour-Ipsen (France)	Antiinflammatory	Feb-02
BN-52296	Discontinued	Beaufour-Ipsen (France)	NO synthetase inhib.; migraine	Nov-98
BOP-3	Inactive	Klinikum der Univeri. (Ger)	Imaging agent	1986
borjatriol	Inactive	Non-industrial source	Antiinflammatory	Feb-02
BP-2.94	Preclinical	Bioproject (France)	H3-receptor agonist analgesic	Jun-98
BPC-15	Inactive	Pfizer (US)	Antiinflammatory	Feb-02
BR-703	Discontinued	Italfarmaco (Italy)	Antiinflammatory	Feb-02
bradykinin antags, Drug Discov	Preclinical	Drug Discovery	Antiarthritic	Feb-02
Bremazocine	Discontinued	Sandoz (Switz)	Opioid agonist/antagonist	Feb-83
Brifentanil (A-3331)	Discontinued (ph. I)	Ohmeda (US)	Fentanyl analog, short acting	Aug-91
BRL-37959	Inactive	GlaxoSmithKline (UK)	NSAID	Feb-02
Bromadoline (U-47931E)	Discontinued (Clin.)	Upjohn (US)	Opioid agonist	1986
Bromfenac (DURACT™)	WITHDRAWN	Wyeth-Ayerst (US)	NSAID: COX + peroxidase inhib.	Aug-98
Bromfenac, Biovail	WITHDRAWN	Biovail (Canada)	Controlled-release (1x/day)	Aug-98
bromfenac, ophthalmic	LAUNCHED	Senju (Japan)	NSAID: COX + peroxidase inhib.	Feb-02
bufexamac	LAUNCHED	Pharmacia (US)	Antiinflammatory	Feb-02
Bupivacaine (DepoBupivacaine)	Preclinical	DepoTech (US)	Sustained release formulation	Dec-98
Buprenorphine	LAUNCHED	Reckitt & Colman (UK)	Opioid agonist/antagonist	Jun-91
Buprenorphine, 3M	Discontinued	3M (US)	Buccal patch	Sep-99
buprenorphine, Elan	Inactive	Elan (Ireland)	Formulation	Feb-02
buprenorphine, Gruenenthal	LAUNCHED	Grunenthal (Germany)	Formulation	Feb-02
buprenorphine, Mundipharma	Preclinical	Mundipharma	Formulation	Feb-02
Buprenorphine, nasal	Discontinued (ph. I)	Nastech (US)	Opioid agonist/antagonist	Feb-02
buprenorphine, Toyobo	CLINICAL (II)	Toyobo	Formulation	Feb-02
Buprenorphine, transdermal	CLINICAL (II)	Ethical (UK)	Formulation, transdermal	Mar-95
Buprenorphine, transdermal	Discontinued (ph. II)	Ethical (UK)	Formulation, transdermal	May-99
Buprenorphine, transdermal	Discontinued (ph. I)	Pierra Fabre (France)	Transdermal buprenorphine	May-97
Buprenorphine, transdermal	Preclinical	Cygnus Research (US)	Transdermal formulation	Mar-93
Buprenorphine, transmucosal	CLINICAL	3M (US)	Buccal release patch	Mar-95
Buprenorphine, transmucosal	Discontinued (ph. II)	Watson (US)	Formulation, buccal release	May-99
butibufen	LAUNCHED	Juste (Spain)	Antiinflammatory	Feb-02
butinazocine	Discontinued	Brocacef	Centrally-acting analgesic	Feb-02
Butinazocine	Discontinued (ph. I)	Brocacef / Novartis (Switz)	Opioid agonist/antagonist	Apr-85
Butorphanol (STADOL®)	LAUNCHED	Bristol-Myers Squibb (US)	Opioid agonist/antagonist	Feb-92
Butorphanol, nasal (STADOL® NS)	LAUNCHED	Bristol-Myers Squibb (US)	Opioid agonist/antagonist	Oct-92
BW-180C	Discontinued (ph. II)	Glaxo Wellcome (UK)	Enkephalin analog	Mar-87
BW-2378W92	Discontinued	Delta / Glaxo Wellcome (US)	Opioid delta-mu agonist	Feb-98
BW-373U86	Discontinued	Burroughs Wellcome (UK)	Opioid delta agonists (non-peptide)	Mar-97
BW-443C81	Discontinued (ph. II)	Wellcome (UK)	Enkephalin analog	Oct-91
BW-524C79	Preclinical	Wellcome (UK)	Glutamate release inhibitor	May-93

Ref.: Pharmaprojects (updated to 2/02) used with permission; Scrip, corporate, literature & patent references
"Status" is international drug development or regulatory status and may not indicate status in USA
Sponsor: Original company name is retained if product is discontinued or inactive after merger, acquisition, company name change, etc.
Users of this table are encouraged to independently verify the status, activity, and mechanism of action of drugs of interest

GENERIC / TRADE NAME	STATUS	SPONSOR (S)	MECHANISM OF ACTION	REF. UPDATE
BW-540C	Discontinued	Glaxo Wellcome (UK)	COX/5-LO inhibitor	Mar-87
BW-70C	Discontinued	GlaxoSmithKline (UK)	Antiinflammatory	Feb-02
BW-755C	Discontinued	GlaxoSmithKline (UK)	Antiinflammatory	Feb-02
BW-831C	Discontinued	Wellcome (UK)	Enkephalin analog	Mar-88
C24	Preclinical	GlaxoSmithKline (UK)	Antiarthritic	Feb-02
C5a antagonist, Abbott	Inactive	Abbott (US)	Antiinflammatory	Feb-02
calcineurin inhibitors, Ag	Discontinued	Pfizer (US)	Antiinflammatory	Feb-02
calcium channel blockers, Ono	Preclinical	Ono (Japan)	Centrally-acting analgesic	Feb-02
CAM inhibitors, Syntex	Inactive	Roche (Switz)	Antiinflammatory	Feb-02
cannabinoid agonist, Bayer-2	Preclinical	Bayer (Germany)	Cannabinoid	Feb-02
cannabinoid agonists, Adolor	Preclinical	Adolor (US)	Peripheral analgesic	Feb-02
cannabinoid agonists, AMRAD	Preclinical	AMRAD (Australia)	Cannabinoid	Feb-02
Cannabis (THC)	Preclinical	GW Pharmaceuticals (UK)	MS, spinal injuries, phantom limb	Aug-98
CAP, Nycomed Amersham	Discontinued (ph. II)	Nycomed (Norway)	Unknown	Feb-02
Capsaicin	LAUNCHED	Vinas (Spain)	Capsicum oleoresin	Mar-94
Capsaicin	Discontinued (Clin)	Andromaco (Argentina)	Topical capsaicin; OA, RA	Mar-98
Capsaicin (ZOSTRIX®)	LAUNCHED	Knoll (US) / GenDerm (US)	Capsaicin /anesthetic formul.	Jun-96
capsaicin cream, Maruishi	CLINICAL (II)	Maruishi Pharmaceutical	Topical capsaicin	Feb-02
capsaicin, NeurogesX	CLINICAL	NeurogesX (US)	Topical capsaicin	Feb-02
Capsazepine	Discontinued	Novartis (Switz.)	Capsaicin antagonist	Oct-93
Carbamazepine (CARBATROL)	LAUNCHED	Shire (UK) / Elan (Ireland)	Na+ channel antag.; Microtrol b.i.d.	Jun-99
Carbasalte calcium	LAUNCHED	Bristol-Myers Squibb (US)	NSAID, non-ulcerogenic	Jan-96
carbazomycin B	Discontinued	Bristol-Myers Squibb (US)	Antiinflammatory	Feb-02
carprofen	LAUNCHED	Roche (Switz)	Antiinflammatory	Feb-02
Caspase 1 / ICE inhibs	Preclinical	Vertex Pharmaceuticals (US)	IL-1β converting enz. Inhib.	Jan-00
catalase, Enzon	Inactive	Enzon	Antiinflammatory	Feb-02
cathepsin F inhibitors, Celera	Preclinical	Celera Genomics	Antiinflammatory	Feb-02
Cathepsin S Inhibitors	Preclinical	Rhone-Poulenc Rorer/AxyS (US)	Cathepsin S inhib. / anti-inflam.	Feb-99
CB-2431	Discontinued (ph. II)	KS Biomedix (UK)	Unknown (drug combo)	Feb-02
CB-28	Discontinued	KS Biomedix (UK)	Unident. muscle elasticity enhanc.	Sep-99
CBF-BS2	CLINICAL (II)	KS Biomedix (UK)	G6PDH inhib. (glucose 6-PO4 DH)	Dec-96
CBS-1108	Discontinued	Bausch & Lomb (US)	Antiinflammatory	Feb-02
CBS-1114	Discontinued (ph. I)	Chauvin (France)	COX/5-LO inhibitor	Oct-85
CBX-10913 / CBX-12266	Inactive	Cibiex (US)	Cytokine release inhibitor; RA	Jan-00
CCK(27-32)	Discontinued	Kanebo (Japan)	CCK fragment	Mar-93
CCK(27-32), Akzo Nobel	Discontinued	Akzo Nobel (Netherlands)	CCK fragment	Feb-02
CD11b/CD18 antags, Selectide	Inactive	Aventis (France)	Antiinflammatory	Feb-02
CDP-870	CLINICAL (II)	Celltech (UK)	Unidentified anti-inflammatory	Feb-99
CDRI-82-205	Discontinued	Central Drug Research (India)	Met-enkephalin analog	May-97
CEE-04-420; CEE-04-421	Preclinical	CeNeS (UK) / BTG (UK)	Lys-D-Pro-Thr; neuropathic pain	Jun-99
Celecoxib (CELEBRA, CELEBREX)	LAUNCHED	Pharmacia (US)	COX-2 inhibitor	May-00
Cell adhesion inhibitors	Discontinued	Warner-Lambert (US)	E-selectin / ICAM-1 antag.	May-97
cell adhesion inhibitors, Park	Inactive	Pfizer (US)	Antiinflammatory	Feb-02
cell adhesion inhibitors, Tana	Inactive	Tanabe Seiyaku (Japan)	Antiinflammatory	Feb-02
cell adhesion inhibs, Kaken	Preclinical	Kaken (Japan)	Antiinflammatory	Feb-02
CereCRIB	Discontinued (ph. I/II)	Astra (Swed.) / CytoTherapeutics	Encapsulated cells (ph. I.th. implant)	Mar-97
Ceruletide diethylamine	LAUNCHED	Pharmacia / Erbamont (Italy)	CCK peptide analog	Dec-91
CGP-16789A	Discontinued (ph. II)	Novartis (Switz.)	NSAID	Apr-90
CGP-17829	Discontinued (ph. I)	Novartis (Switz.)	NSAID	Jan-90
CGP-19416	Discontinued (ph. I)	Novartis (Switz.)	NSAID	Apr-90
CGP-25157	Discontinued	Novartis (Switz.)	Antiinflammatory	Feb-02
CGP-25449	Discontinued	Novartis (Switz.)	NSAID	May-92
CGP-28237 / ZK-34228	Discontinued (ph. I)	Novartis / Schering AG (Ger)	NSAID	May-89
CGP-29030A	Discontinued (ph. II)	Ciba-Geigy (Switz)	5-HT2 / A1 antagonist	Mar-94
CGP-31081	Discontinued (ph. I)	Novartis (Switz.)	NSAID	May-94
CGP-37861A	Discontinued	Novartis (Switz.)	NSAID	Feb-02
CGP-47900	Discontinued	Novartis (Switz.)	Antiinflammatory	Feb-02
CGP-47969A	Discontinued	Novartis (Switz.)	Antiinflammatory	Feb-02
CGRP antagonists	Discontinued	SmithKline Beecham (UK)	Migraine; inflammation, pain	Oct-99
CGS-21595	Discontinued	Novartis (Switz.)	Antiinflammatory	Feb-02
CGS-22745	Discontinued	Novartis (Switz.)	Antiinflammatory	Feb-02
CGS-23885	Discontinued	Novartis (Switz.)	Antiinflammatory	Feb-02
CGS-25019C	Discontinued (ph. II)	Ciba-Geigy (Switz)	LTB4 antagonist	Feb-96

Ref.: Pharmaprojects (updated to 2/02) used with permission; Scrip, corporate, literature & patent references
"Status" is international drug development or regulatory status and may not indicate status in USA
Sponsor: Original company name is retained if product is discontinued or inactive after merger, acquisition, company name change, etc.
Users of this table are encouraged to independently verify the status, activity, and mechanism of action of drugs of interest

GENERIC / TRADE NAME	STATUS	SPONSOR (S)	MECHANISM OF ACTION	REF. UPDATE
CGS-25997	Discontinued	Novartis (Switz.)	5-Lipoxygenase (5-LO) inhibitor	Sep-98
CGS-26529	Discontinued	Novartis (Switz.)	5-Lipoxygenase (5-LO) inhibitor	May-98
CGX-1002	Preclinical	Cognetix	Centrally-acting analgesic	Feb-02
CH-138	Discontinued	Celltech (UK)	Antiarthritic	Feb-02
CH-5902	Inactive	Celltech / Chiroscience (UK)	MMP inhibitor / anti-inflam.	Feb-02
chemokine antags, Neurocrine	Preclinical	Neurocrine Biosciences (US)	Antiinflammatory	Feb-02
Chemokine binding proteins	Preclinical	Viron Therapeutics (Canada)	Chemokine receptor antag	Aug-99
chemokine ligands, Dompe	Preclinical	Dompe	Antiinflammatory	Feb-02
CHF-1021	Discontinued	Chiesi (Italy)	Antiinflammatory	Feb-02
CHF-1909	Discontinued	Chiesi (Italy)	Antiinflammatory	Feb-02
CHF-2003	Discontinued	Chiesi (Italy)	Antiinflammatory	Feb-02
Chinoin-127	Discontinued (ph. I)	Chinon (Hungary)	NSAID (rimazolium analog)	Mar-88
Chinoin-150 (JATE-1023)	Discontinued (ph. II)	Chinoin (Hungary)	Beta-1 adrenergic antagonist	Jun-86
Chlorotenoxicam	Discontinued (ph. III)	Nycomed Amersham (Norway)	NSAID	Jan-94
chondroitin sulfate	LAUNCHED	American Home Products (US)	Antiinflammatory	Feb-02
CI-1004	CLINICAL (II)	Warner-Lambert (US)	COX-2 / 5-LO inhibitor; OA/RA	Apr-98
CI-987	Discontinued	Warner-Lambert (US)	Thromboxane TXB2 release inhib.	May-94
cicloprofen	Discontinued	Bristol-Myers Squibb (US)	Antiinflammatory	Feb-02
cinfenoac	Inactive	Biorex Labs	Antiinflammatory	Feb-02
cinmetacin	LAUNCHED	Chiesi (Italy)	Antiinflammatory	Feb-02
Ciramadol (Wy-15705)	Discontinued (PRE-REG)	Wyeth-Ayerst (US)	Opioid agonist/antagonist	Jan-87
Cizolirtine citrate (E-4018)	CLINICAL (II)	Esteve (Spain)	NSAID	Mar-98
CJC-1008	CLINICAL (II)	ConjuChem (US)	Centrally-acting analgesic	Feb-02
CKD-303	Discontinued (ph. III)	Chong Kun Dang (S. Korea)	Unidentified (analgesic)	Feb-00
CL-225385	Discontinued (ph. II)	Lederle / Am. Home Prod. (US)	Unidentified anti-inflammatory	Nov-84
clidanac	LAUNCHED	Bristol-Myers Squibb (US)	Antiinflammatory	Feb-02
clobuzarit	Discontinued	AstraZeneca (UK)	Antiarthritic	Feb-02
clodronate disodium, Abiogen	LAUNCHED	Merck & Co (US)	Osteoporosis / bone pain	Feb-02
clofurac	Discontinued	Novartis (Switz.)	Antiinflammatory	Feb-02
Clonidine (DURACLON™ epidural)	LAUNCHED	Roxane (US) / Fujisawa	Formulation, epidural; cancer	Jan-97
Clonidine, intrathecal	Discontinued	Orphan Medical / Medtronic	Clonidine intrathecal	May-98
clopirac	Discontinued	Pharmacia (US)	Antiinflammatory	Feb-02
cloprednol	LAUNCHED	Roche (Switz)	Antiarthritic	Feb-02
Cloximate (DU-22599)	Discontinued	Solvay (Netherlands)	NSAID	Jul-83
CLX-1100 / CLX-1200	Inactive	Calyx Therapeutics (US)	TNF-α antagonist; plant extract	Jun-00
CM-32113	Discontinued	Sanofi (France)	Opioid agonist/antagonist	Mar-87
CMI-546	Inactive	CytoMed / Millennium (US)	Unidentified anti-inflammatory	Feb-02
CMI-980	Inactive	CytoMed / Millennium (US)	Muscarinic agonist	Feb-02
CMTs (Chemically Mod. Tetracyclines)	Discontinued	CollaGenex (US) / Boehringer Man.	MMP inhib.; tetracycline analogs	Sep-99
CNI-1493	CLINICAL (II)	Cytokine PharmaSciences	Antiinflammatory	Feb-02
CNS-5161	Suspended (ph. II)	CeNeS / Cambridge Neurosci.	NMDA ion chan. antag.; neuropathy	Feb-02
Co-102862	Preclinical	CoCensys (US) / U. Saskatchewan	Na+ channel antagonist	Dec-97
CO-1827	Inactive	Aventis (France)	Antiinflammatory	Feb-02
CO-893	Discontinued	Boehringer Ingelheim (Ger)	NSAID	Feb-02
collagen antagonists, Xoma	Discontinued	Xoma (US)	Antiarthritic	Feb-02
Collagenase inhibitors	Preclinical	SmithKline Beecham (UK)	Collagenase inhibitors	Mar-97
collagenase inhibitors, ResC	Discontinued	Research Corp. Tech. (US)	Collagenase inhibitors	Feb-02
collagenase IX inhibitor	Discontinued	BioCryst (US)	Collagenase inhibitors	Feb-02
collagenase, Yakult Honsha	Inactive	Yakult Honsha	Collagenase inhibitors	Feb-02
collismycin A	Discontinued	Kirin Brewery	Antiinflammatory	Feb-02
Colykade	CLINICAL (II)	ML Laboratories / Panos (UK)	CCK-B antagonist; analgesic pot.	Apr-99
Complement inhibitors	Preclinical	AdProTech (UK)	Complement factor inhib. / arthritis	Apr-99
Conorphone (HGP-10)	Discontinued (ph. II)	HG Pars (US)	Opioid agonist/antagonist	Nov-93
contulakin-G	Preclinical	Cognetix	Calcium channel antagonist	Feb-02
Contulakin-G (CGX-1160)	Preclinical	Elan (Ireland) / Cognetix (US)	Neurotensin agonist; conopeptide	Feb-00
Conus toxins, AMRAD	Preclinical	AMRAD (Australia)	Ca++ channel antagonist	May-98
copper complexes, Arkansas	LAUNCHED	Non-industrial source	Antiarthritic	Feb-02
Core-2 GlcNAc-T inhibitors	Preclinical	GlycoDesign (Canada)	Glycosyl transferase inhib. / inflam.	Jan-99
Corleukin compounds	Discontinued	Corvas	Antiinflammatory	Feb-02
COX-189	CLINICAL (III)	Novartis (Switz.)	COX-2 inhibitor	Feb-02
COX-2 inhibitor, Roche	Inactive	Roche (Switz)	COX-2 inhibitor	Feb-02
COX-2 inhibitors, Almirall-Pro	Inactive	Almirall-Prodesfarma (Spain)	COX-2 inhibitor	Feb-02
CP-0126 / CP-0499 heterodimers	Discontinued	Cortech (US)	B2 + NK1/NK2 antag; B2 + μ ag.	Mar-97

Ref.: Pharmaprojects (updated to 2/02) used with permission; Scrip, corporate, literature & patent references
"Status" is international drug development or regulatory status and may not indicate status in USA
Sponsor: Original company name is retained if product is discontinued or inactive after merger, acquisition, company name change, etc.
Users of this table are encouraged to independently verify the status, activity, and mechanism of action of drugs of interest

GENERIC / TRADE NAME	STATUS	SPONSOR (S)	MECHANISM OF ACTION	REF. UPDATE
CP-0127 (BRADYCOR®)	Suspended (ph. II)	Cortech (US)	B2 antagonist	Jan-97
CP-0364	Discontinued	Cortech (US)	Antiinflammatory	Feb-02
CP-0840 (CP-0880)	Discontinued	Cortech (US)	Peripheral B2 antag. + µ agonist	Feb-99
CP-0880	Preclinical	Cortech (US)	Peripheral B2 antag. + µ agonist	Mar-97
CP-122288	Discontinued (ph. II)	Pfizer (US)	5-HT1B/5-HT1D antag. / migr.	Jan-99
CP-18534-1	Inactive	Pfizer (US)	Alpha-2 agonist	1986
CP-331	Discontinued	Zeria	Antiinflammatory	Feb-02
CP-353164	Discontinued	Pfizer (US)	PDE-IV inhibitor	Dec-98
CP-42096	Inactive	Pfizer (US)	Opioid agonist	1985
CP-47497	Inactive	Pfizer (US)	Cannabinoid	1984
CP-55244	Inactive	Pfizer (US)	Cannabinoid	1983
CP-850	Inactive	Pharmacia (US)	Antiarthritic	Feb-02
CP-93129	Discontinued	Pfizer (US)	5-HT1b agonist	Aug-94
CP-96345 / CP-96344	Preclinical	Pfizer (US)	NK-1 antagonist	Dec-99
CP-99994	Discontinued	Pfizer (US)	NK1/Substance P antag., 2nd gen.	May-99
CPC-111	CLINICAL (II)	Cypros (US)	Cytoprotective (sickle cell pain)	Nov-97
CPI-1714	Preclinical	Centaur	Antiarthritic	Feb-02
CPP	Discontinued (ph. II)	Sandoz (Switz)	NMDA antagonist (neuroprotec)	Nov-95
CPP, Eisai	Discontinued	Eisai (Japan)	Antiinflammatory	Feb-02
CPR-2001	Inactive	Clarion (US)	Antiinflammatory	Feb-02
CPR-2006	Inactive	Clarion (US)	Topical; menthol conjugate	Feb-02
CPR-2015	Inactive	Clarion (US)	5-ASA analog; anti-inflam./asthma	Feb-02
CPR-3016	Inactive	Clarion (US)	PAF antag.; anti-inflam./asthma	Feb-02
CR-3294	Preclinical	Rotta (Italy)	Antiinflammatory	Feb-02
CRE-109	Discontinued (Clin.)	Cermol (Switz.)	Unidentified anti-inflammatory	Jun-94
CS-179	Discontinued	Searle/Monsanto (US)	COX-2 inhibitor	Nov-98
CS-502	CLINICAL (II)	Sankyo (Japan)	COX-2 inhibitor	Feb-02
CT3 (DMH-11C)	CLINICAL (I)	Atlantic Tech. Ventures (US)	THC analog; non-psychoactive	Feb-02
CT-737	Discontinued	American Home Products (US)	Antiinflammatory	Feb-02
Curcumin	Discontinued (ph. II)	Central Drug Research (India)	COX inhibitor / 12-HETE	May-98
CV-6504	Discontinued	Takeda (Japan)	Thromboxane TXA2/5-LO inhib.	Aug-95
CVT-857 (CVT-710)	Inactive	CV Therapeutics (US)	Antiinflamatory protease inhib.	Oct-98
CVX	Discontinued	Bayer (Ger) / CV Ther (US)	Macrophage inhib.; anti-inflam.	Jun-99
CXCR2 antagonists, Celltech	Preclinical	Celltech (UK)	Antiinflammatory	Feb-02
CY-208-243	Discontinued	Sandoz (Switz)	D1/D2 partial agonist	1988
CY-9652	Inactive	Epimmune	Antiinflammatory	Feb-02
Cyclazocine	Discontinued	Eastman Kodak (US)	Opioid agonist/antagonist	Mar-84
Cyclic opioid peptides	Preclinical	Astra (Sweden)	Opioid mu agonist	Aug-92
Cyclic opioid peptides	Discontinued (Clin.)	Astra (Sweden) / P. Schiller	Opioid mu agonist	Oct-95
Cyclohexadienes	Inactive	Roche (Switz)	Unknown	Unk.
Cyclopropylmethylmorphinan	Preclinical	SRI Int'l (US)	Kappa agonist	Nov-93
Cysteine protease inhibitors	Inactive	British Biotech (UK) / SynPhar	RA, OA, osteoporosis	Feb-02
cysteine protease inhibs,Celer	Discontinued	Celera Genomics	RA, OA, osteoporosis	Feb-02
Cysteine protease inhibs.	Discontinued	AxyS (US)	RA, OA, osteoporosis	May-98
D-10242	Discontinued	Asta Medica (Germany)	Antiinflammatory	Feb-02
D-1367	Discontinued (ph. I)	Chiroscience (UK)	COX-2 inhibitor	May-98
D-16120	Discontinued	Asta Medica (Germany)	CNS action	Jul-87
D-19050	Discontinued	Asta Medica (Germany)	CNS + peripheral action	Oct-91
D-1927	CLINICAL (I)	Celltech (UK)	MMP inhibitor / antiinflammatory	Feb-02
D-20450	Inactive	Asta Medica (Germany)	Peripheral site action	Apr-92
D-20882	Discontinued	Asta Medica (Germany)	Antiinflammatory	Feb-02
D-21151	Discontinued	Asta Medica (Germany)	Thromboxane B2 antagonist	Mar-97
D-2163	Preclinical	Chiroscience (UK)	MMP inhibitor / antiinflammatory	Mar-97
D-5410	CLINICAL (I)	Chiroscience (UK)	MMP / TNF convertase inhibitor	Mar-97
D-6428	CLINICAL (I)	Celltech (UK)	Centrally-acting analgesic	Feb-02
DA-5018 (KR-25018)	CLINICAL (II)	Dong-A (Korea)	Synthetic capsanoid	Feb-02
DALECK	Inactive	Hungarian Acad. Sciences	Enkephalin analog	Unk.
Darbufelone mesylate (CI-1004)	Discontinued (ph. II)	Warner-Lambert (US)	COX-2 / 5-LO inhibitor; OA/RA	Feb-02
Dazidamine (AF-2322)	Discontinued	Angelini (Italy)	Unidentified anti-inflammatory	Mar-87
DD-161515	Preclinical	DiverDrugs	Centrally-acting analgesic	Feb-02
Delmetacin (UR-2301)	Discontinued (Clin.)	Uriach (Spain)	NSAID / indomethacin analog	Mar-84
Delta agonists	Preclinical	Searle/Monsanto (US)	Delta agonist	Mar-93
Delta agonists, Astra	Preclinical	Astra (Sweden)	Opioid delta agonists (non-peptide)	Feb-98

Ref.: Pharmaprojects (updated to 2/02) used with permission; Scrip, corporate, literature & patent references
"Status" is international drug development or regulatory status and may not indicate status in USA
Sponsor: Original company name is retained if product is discontinued or inactive after merger, acquisition, company name change, etc.
Users of this table are encouraged to independently verify the status, activity, and mechanism of action of drugs of interest

GENERIC / TRADE NAME	STATUS	SPONSOR (S)	MECHANISM OF ACTION	REF. UPDATE
denaverine hydrochloride	LAUNCHED	Apogepha	NSAID	Feb-02
dendalone 3-hydroxybutyrate	Inactive	Roche (Switz)	Antiinflammatory	Feb-02
Dermatan sulfate	CLINICAL	CytRx (US)	Dermatan topical form.	Feb-93
dersalazine	CLINICAL (I)	Uriach (Spain)	NSAID	Feb-02
Devacade	CLINICAL (II)	ML Laboratories / Panos (UK)	CCK-A antagonist; analgesic pot.	Feb-02
dexflurbiprofen	Discontinued	Abbott (US)	NSAID, single isomer	Feb-02
dexibuprofen	LAUNCHED	PAZ Pharma (Ger)	NSAID	Feb-02
dexibuprofen lysine	Inactive	Merck & Co (US)	NSAID	Feb-02
dexindoprofen	Discontinued	Pharmacia (US)	Antiarthritic	Feb-02
Dexketoprofen [(S)-ketoprofen]	LAUNCHED	Menarini / Chiroscience (UK)	Single isomer formulation	Jul-96
Dexmedetomidine (spinal)	LAUNCHED	Orion (Finland) / Abbott (US)	Alpha-2 agonist sedative-analgesic	Dec-99
Dexmedetomidine, Cygnus	Discontinued (ph. I)	Cygnus (US)	Formulation, transdermal	Dec-94
Dextromethorphan comb.	Discontinued	Whitby Pharmaceut. (US)	Dextr.+ antacids + antiflat.	1984
Dextromethorphan, IriSys	CLINICAL (I)	Avanir (US) / IriSys (US)	Dextrometh. + P450/2D6 inhib.	Jun-99
Dextropropoxyphene form.	LAUNCHED	Hafslund Nycomed (Norway)	Controlled release	Aug-91
Dezocine	LAUNCHED	Wyeth-Ayerst (US)	Opioid agonist/antagonist	Mar-91
DGI	Inactive	Innogenetics	Antiarthritic	Feb-02
Di-, Tri-, cyclic peptides	Preclinical	NIH (US)	Delta agonist	Aug-95
Diacerein (ARTRODAR; FISIODAR)	LAUNCHED	Proter (Italy)	Arthritis; chelator; IL-1, TNFα antag.	Mar-96
Diaminocyclohexanes	Inactive	Upjohn (US)	Unknown	Unk.
Diaminocyclohexylamides	Inactive	Warner-Lambert (US)	Unknown	Unk.
Diarylmethylpiperazines	Preclinical	Glaxo Wellcome (UK)	Mu + delta agonist	Mar-95
Diaveridine, EGIS (EGIS-5645)	Discontinued (ph. I)	EGIS (Hungary)	Anti-inflammatory	Nov-91
dibenzosuberone	Inactive	Pfizer (US)	Antiinflammatory	Feb-02
Dibenzthiepines	Inactive	Hoechst (Ger)	Unknown	1982
Diclofenac (1x/day formulation)	PRE-REGISTRATION	SSP (Japan)	Formulation	May-98
Diclofenac (Arthrex Duo)	LAUNCHED	Klinge (Germany)	Quick/Slow pellets in capsule	Mar-99
Diclofenac (PENNSAID™)	PRE-REGISTRATION	Dimethaid Research (Canada)	Topical formulation	Mar-98
diclofenac + HA topical, Skye	PRE-REGISTRATION	SkyePharma (UK)	Topical formulation	Feb-02
Diclofenac + misoprostol (Arthrotec®)	LAUNCHED	Searle/Monsanto (US)	Cytoprotective formulation	Nov-96
Diclofenac formulation	PRE-REGISTRATION	Applied Pharma Res. (Switz.)	Fast/slow controlled release	Jun-98
Diclofenac gel (ORALEASE)	CLINICAL (II)	SkyePharma (UK)	Oral gel formulation; mouth ulcers	Feb-02
diclofenac once-daily, SSP	LAUNCHED	SSP (Japan)	Formulation	Feb-02
diclofenac potassium	LAUNCHED	Novartis (Switz.)	Antiinflammatory	Feb-02
Diclofenac spray	CLINICAL (III)	Dr Kade (Germany)	Topical spray	Nov-99
Diclofenac, Applied	LAUNCHED	Novartis / Applied Pharma (Switz.)	Oral formulation	Nov-99
Diclofenac, FOAM-SYS	Discontinued (ph. I)	Poli (Italy)	Local / topical formulation	Sep-99
diclofenac, OSAT	Suspended	CeNeS (UK)	Oral sustained release	Feb-02
Diclofenac, Pharmos	Discontinued (ph. I)	Pharmos (US)	Formulation, diclofenac	May-99
Diclofenac, topical	LAUNCHED	Mika Pharma (Germany)	Topical liposome spray-gel	Apr-00
diclofenac-2, Applied	Inactive	Applied Pharma Res. (Switz.)	Oral formulation #2	Feb-02
difenpyramide	LAUNCHED	GlaxoSmithKline (UK)	Antiinflammatory	Feb-02
Diflumidone (BA-4164-8)	Discontinued	3M (US)	COX inhibitor	Feb-81
diflunisal	LAUNCHED	Merck & Co (US)	NSAID	Feb-02
diftalone	WITHDRAWN	Bioesearch Italia (Italy)	Antiinflammatory	Feb-02
Dihydrocodeine (S-8115)	Discontinued (ph. III)	Shionogi / Mundipharma (Switz)	Controlled release formulation	Oct-98
Dihydrocodeine formulation	LAUNCHED	Biovail (Canada)	Controlled release DHC	Dec-91
Dimethylethylamines	Discontinued	Hoechst (Ger)	5-HT antagonist	Unk.
Diphenylpropanes	Preclinical	Merck & Co (US)	Substance P antagonist	Feb-93
disalazine	Inactive	VUFB (Czech Republic)	Antiarthritic	Feb-02
disogluside	Inactive	Non-industrial source	Antiinflammatory	Feb-02
dizatrifone	Discontinued	bioMerieux-Pierre Fabre (France)	NSAID	Feb-02
DN-1504	Discontinued	Daiichi (Japan)	Enkephalin analog	Dec-84
donitriptan mesylate	CLINICAL (I)	bioMerieux-Pierre Fabre (France)	Antimigraine	Feb-02
dotarizine	Discontinued (PRE-REG.)	Ferrer (Spain)	5-HT2 antagonist / Ca++ antag.	Feb-02
Doxpicomine	Inactive	Lilly (US)	Opioid agonist	1982
DP-103	Preclinical	D-Pharm (Israel)	Antiinflammatory	Feb-02
DPC-333	CLINICAL (II)	Bristol-Myers Squibb (US)	Antiarthritic	Feb-02
D-Phe-AHPA	Discontinued	Meiji Seika (Japan)	Enk'ase inhibitor	Mar-87
DPI-3290	CLINICAL (II)	Ardent Pharmaceuticals	Delta-mu agonist analgesic	Feb-02
DPI-3338	Preclinical	Delta Pharmaceuticals (US)	Opioid delta ag. / narcotic combo.	Feb-98
DPI-584	Preclinical	Delta Pharmaceuticals (US)	Opioid delta ag. / urinary incontinence	Feb-98
DRF-4367	Preclinical	Dr Reddy's	NSAID	Feb-02

Ref.: Pharmaprojects (updated to 2/02) used with permission; Scrip, corporate, literature & patent references
"Status" is international drug development or regulatory status and may not indicate status in USA
Sponsor: Original company name is retained if product is discontinued or inactive after merger, acquisition, company name change, etc.
Users of this table are encouraged to independently verify the status, activity, and mechanism of action of drugs of interest

GENERIC / TRADE NAME	STATUS	SPONSOR (S)	MECHANISM OF ACTION	REF. UPDATE
DRF-4848	Preclinical	Dr Reddy's	Antiinflammatory	Feb-02
droxicam	LAUNCHED	Esteve (Spain)	Antiinflammatory	Feb-02
DU-608	Discontinued	Dainippon (Japan)	PGSI	1979
DuP-631	Inactive	Endo Pharmaceuticals (US)	5-HT/NE uptake inhib.	Feb-02
DuP-697	Discontinued	Bristol-Myers Squibb (US)	Antiarthritic	Feb-02
DuP-747	Inactive	Endo Pharmaceuticals (US)	Kappa agonist	Feb-02
DuP-769	Inactive	Endo Pharmaceuticals (US)	nalbuphine N-oxide prodrug	Feb-02
Duramycin B (Duramycin C)	Discontinued	Novartis (Switz.)	Phospholipase PLA2 inhibitor	May-92
dyclonine HCl, BEMA, Atrix	Inactive	Atrix (US)	Buccal film / canker sores	Feb-02
Dynorphin A	Discontinued (ph. II)	Neurobiological Technologies	Dynorphin A (1-13) peptide	Feb-02
E-2078	Discontinued (ph. II)	Eisai (Japan)	Dynorphin analog, kappa agon.	Aug-93
E-5090	Discontinued	Eisai (Japan)	IL-1 inhibitor	Jan-92
E-5110	Discontinued (ph. II)	Eisai (Japan)	NSAID	Jun-91
E-5296	CLINICAL (I)	Devp (UK) / Esteve (Spain)	5-HT uptake inhib; sigma antag.	Feb-02
E-6087	CLINICAL (I)	Esteve (Spain)	Antiinflammatory	Feb-02
E-6259	Preclinical	Esteve (Spain)	Antiarthritic	Feb-02
EF-5 (SC-106)	Discontinued (ph. III)	Scotia (UK)	γ-linolenic acid combo (RA, OA)	Feb-02
EGIS-2829	Discontinued	Servier (France)	Antiinflammatory	Feb-02
EGIS-7625	Discontinued	Servier (France)	5-HT2b+sigma-1 antag.; migraine	Mar-00
EI-1507-1	Discontinued	Kyowa Hakko (Japan)	IL-1b converting enz. Inhib.	Sep-99
EK-209	Inactive	Takeda (Japan)	Enkephalin analog	Unk.
EK-399	Discontinued	Takeda (Japan)	Enkephalin analog	Jul-89
Elastase inhibitor, Biopharm	Discontinued	Merck KGaA (Ger)/Biopharm (Can)	Elastase inhib / RA	May-98
Elastase inhibitors	Preclinical	Cortech (US)	Elastase inhibition	Mar-97
Elastase inhibitors, Cortech	Preclinical	Ono (Japan) / Cortech (US)	Elastase inhibitor, oral: RA	Jun-99
elastase inhibitors, Servier	Inactive	Servier (France)	Leucocyte elastase inhib. /inflam.	Feb-02
Elcatonin	LAUNCHED	Asahi Chemical (Japan)	Modified eel calcitonin	Oct-93
Elcatonin, intrathecal	Discontinued	Innapharma (US)	Eel calcitonin (intrathecal)	Aug-99
Eletriptan (Relpax)	LAUNCHED	Pfizer (US)	5-HT1d partial agonist	Feb-02
Eltenac	CLINICAL (II)	Byk Gulden (Ger) / Sankyo (Jp)	NSAID	Apr-98
EM-405	Discontinued	Grunenthal (Germany)	NSAID	Feb-02
EMD-60400	Discontinued	Merck KGaA (Germany)	Kappa agonist	May-94
Emopamil	Discontinued (ph. II)	Knoll (Ger)	5-HT2 / Ca++ antagonist	Aug-93
emorfazone	LAUNCHED	Aventis (France)	Antiinflammatory	Feb-02
EN-03	Inactive	Essential Nutrition (UK)	Antiinflammatory	Feb-02
EN-07	Inactive	Essential Nutrition (UK)	Antiinflammatory	Feb-02
EN-08	Discontinued	Essential Nutrition (UK)	Unidentified (arthritis pain)	1998
EN-105	Inactive	Mitsubishi Pharma (Japan)	Antiinflammatory	Feb-02
EN-760	Discontinued	Bristol-Myers Squibb (US)	Antiarthritic	Feb-02
ENA	Discontinued	Mediolanum	Antiinflammatory	Feb-02
Enadoline	Discontinued (ph. II)	Warner-Lambert (US)	Kappa agonist / head injuries	May-97
Endorphin, pancreatic	Inactive	Endorphin Inc. (US)	Endorphin	Feb-85
enfenamic acid	LAUNCHED	Unichem	Antiinflammatory	Feb-02
Enkastatin ID	Inactive	Hoechst (Ger)	Enk'ase inhibitor	1989
Enkephalin Convertase Inhib.	Discontinued	Scios Nova (US)	Enk'ase inhibitor	Mar-91
Enkephalinase Inhibitors	Discontinued	Dainippon (Japan)	Enk'ase inhibitor	Aug-93
Enkephalins	Inactive	Peptide Technology (Austr)	Enkephalins	Mar-86
EP-322 (EP-323)	Discontinued (ph. I)	Edmond Pharma (Italy)	NSAID	Nov-91
Epibatidine	Discontinued	Merck & Co (US)	Nicotinic agonist	Jun-95
epibatidine analogues, Bayer	Preclinical	Bayer (Germany)	Nicotinic agonist	Feb-02
epirizole	LAUNCHED	Daiichi (Japan)	Antiinflammatory	Feb-02
epocarbazolin-A	Discontinued	Bristol-Myers Squibb (US)	Antiinflammatory	Feb-02
eprovafen	Discontinued	Aventis (France)	5-LO inhibitor	Feb-02
Eptazocine	LAUNCHED	Nichiiko (Japan)	Opioid agonist/antagonist	Dec-94
Eptazocine formulation	Preclinical	TheraTech (US)	Transdermal eptazocine	Oct-92
ER-10103	Discontinued	Euroresearch (Italy)	PGSI	Apr-88
ER-34122	Discontinued	Eisai (Japan)	5-LO / COX inhibitor	Jun-99
ER-3826	Discontinued	Eisai (Japan)	Antiinflammatory	Feb-02
Eseroline (MCV-4481; NIH-10398)	Discontinued	Univ. Florence (Italy)	Cholinesterase inhibitor	1984
Esflurbiprofen (BTS-24332)	Discontinued (Clin.)	Knoll (Ger.) / Nichiiko (Japan)	(S)-flurbiprofen isomer	Mar-89
Esterom	CLINICAL (III)	Entropin	Cocaine hydrolysis esters; topical	Feb-02
etanercept (ENBREL™)	LAUNCHED	Immunex (US) / Wyeth-Ayerst	TNF receptor fusion protein (RA)	Nov-98
etersalate	LAUNCHED	Alter	Antiinflammatory	Feb-02

Ref.: Pharmaprojects (updated to 2/02) used with permission; Scrip, corporate, literature & patent references
"Status" is international drug development or regulatory status and may not indicate status in USA
Sponsor: Original company name is retained if product is discontinued or inactive after merger, acquisition, company name change, etc.
Users of this table are encouraged to independently verify the status, activity, and mechanism of action of drugs of interest

GENERIC / TRADE NAME	STATUS	SPONSOR (S)	MECHANISM OF ACTION	REF. UPDATE
ethenoarachidonic acids, ResCo	Discontinued	Research Corp. Tech. (US)	Antiinflammatory	Feb-02
Ethenomorphinan der.	Inactive	Univ. California (US)	Opioid agonist	1985
Etodolac (LODINE®)	LAUNCHED	P&G (US) / Am Home Prod	NSAID	May-96
Etodolac + dextromethorphan	CLINICAL (I)	Algos (US)	Etodolac + dextromethorphan	May-97
etodolac meglumine	Discontinued	Therapicon (Italy)	Antiinflammatory	Feb-02
etomidate, Anesta	CLINICAL (II)	Cephalon (US)	Formulation	Feb-02
etoricoxib	REGISTERED	Merck & Co (US)	Antiarthritic	Feb-02
EU-11300	Inactive	Euroresearch	NSAID	Feb-02
evandamine	Discontinued	Aventis (France)	Antiinflammatory	Feb-02
Evening Primrose Oil	LAUNCHED	Efamol (UK)	Linoleic acid (PMS pain)	Sep-93
F-1044	Discontinued	Procter & Gamble (US)	Antiinflammatory	Feb-02
F-12640	CLINICAL (I)	Pierre Fabre (France)	5-HT1b/1d agonist; migraine	Mar-00
F-2329	Discontinued	Faes (Spain)	Antiinflammatory	Feb-02
F-2341	Discontinued	bioMerieux-Pierre Fabre (France)	NSAID	Feb-02
F-2349	Discontinued	Pierre Fabre (France)	Thromboxane synthase inhibitor	Mar-88
F-9004T	Discontinued	Faes (Spain)	Unknown (oral non-narcotic)	Feb-94
Fanetizole	Inactive	Pfizer (US)	Anti-inflammatory	Unk.
FE200 665	Preclinical	Ferring (Sweden)	Centrally-acting analgesic	Feb-02
fenbufen	LAUNCHED	American Home Products (US)	NSAID	Feb-02
Fenclorac (WHR-539)	Discontinued (Clin.)	Rhone-Poulenc Rorer (France)	COX inhibitor	Dec-82
Fenclozine (S-1429)	Discontinued (ph. III)	Synthelabo (France)	NSAID / anxiolytic	May-92
fendosal	Discontinued	Aventis (France)	NSAID	Feb-02
Fenflumizole (A-214)	Discontinued (ph. III)	Alpharma (US)	COX/5-LO inhibitor	Jan-86
Fentanyl (DURAGESIC®)	LAUNCHED	J&J / Alza (US)	Transdermal narcotic	Apr-97
Fentanyl analogues	Preclinical	Faes (Spain)	Opioid mu agonist	May-92
Fentanyl citrate	Preclinical	Samchundang (S. Korea)	Fentanyl formulation (unspec.)	Apr-00
Fentanyl citrate (ORALET, ACTIQ)	LAUNCHED	Abbott (US) / Anesta (US)	Fentanyl oral transmucusal	Jun-99
fentanyl citrate, Samchundang	Preclinical	Samchundang (S. Korea)	Formulation	Feb-02
Fentanyl formulation	Discontinued	Hercon (US)	Transdermal fentanyl	Feb-90
fentanyl, Alza	LAUNCHED	Johnson & Johnson (US)	Formulation	Feb-02
fentanyl, BEMA film	Preclinical	Atrix (US)	Formulation	Feb-02
fentanyl, buccal, 3M	Preclinical	3M (US)	Transdermal, transmusocal forms.	Feb-02
Fentanyl, E-TRANS	CLINICAL (III)	Johnson & Johnson / Alza (US)	Transdermal formulations	Feb-02
fentanyl, Generex	Preclinical	Generex	Formulation	Feb-02
Fentanyl, inhaler	Discontinued (ph. II)	3M (US)	Metered dose inhaler	May-97
Fentanyl, iontophoretic (TS-36)	Discontinued (ph. II)	Fournier (France)	Electronic iontophoretic transderm.	Nov-97
fentanyl, Latitude	CLINICAL (I)	3M (US)	Formulation	Feb-02
Fentanyl, transdermal	Discontinued (ph. III)	Cygnus (US)	Transdermal 24 hr patch	Feb-97
fentanyl, Watson	CLINICAL (II)	Watson (US)	Formulation	Feb-02
fentiazac	LAUNCHED	American Home Products (US)	Antiinflammatory	Feb-02
Fepramol	LAUNCHED	Schwarz (Ger)	PGSI	Dec-91
feprazone	LAUNCHED	Boehringer Ingelheim (Ger)	Antiinflammatory	Feb-02
feprazone+paracetamol+guaifen	LAUNCHED	Schwarz (Ger)	Analgesic combination	Feb-02
feverfew	Inactive	Non-industrial source	Antimigraine	Feb-02
FG-5530	Discontinued	Kabi Pharmacia (Sweden)	Clonidine-like neurolep.	Mar-89
FI-302	Inactive	Taisho (Japan)	Antiinflammatory	Feb-02
FID-072021	Discontinued	Fidia (Italy)	ACh release stimulant	Oct-96
filenadol	Discontinued (PRE-REG)	Ferrer (Spain)	PGSI	Feb-02
FK-011	CLINICAL (II)	Fujisawa (Japan)	Leukotriene antagonist	Jul-97
FK-3311	Discontinued (ph. II)	Fujisawa (Japan)	NSAID	Dec-94
FK-33-824 (DAMME)	Discontinued (ph. II)	Novartis (Switz.)	Met-enkephalin analog	1979
flazalone	Discontinued	3M (US)	Antiinflammatory	Feb-02
floctafenine	LAUNCHED	Aventis (France)	NSAID	Feb-02
Florifenine (FI-2500; FI-2522)	Discontinued (ph. II)	Ferrer (Spain)	NSAID	Oct-97
flosulide	Discontinued	Schering AG (Germany)	Antiarthritic	Feb-02
Flubichin (VUFB-12950; VUFB-15950)	Discontinued	VUFB (Czech Republic)	NSAID	Mar-94
flumazole	Inactive	Lilly (US)	Antiinflammatory	Feb-02
flunarizine	LAUNCHED	Johnson & Johnson (US)	Antimigraine	Feb-02
Flunixin (Banamine; Sch-14714)	Discontinued (ph. II)	Schering Plough (US)	NSAID	Mar-84
flunoxaprofen	LAUNCHED	Abbott (US)	NSAID	Feb-02
Fluorometacin (FA-401)	Discontinued (ph. I)	Yoshitomi (Japan)	NSAID (ph. Indomethacin derivative)	Sep-89
Flupirtine	LAUNCHED	Carter Wallace / Asta Medica	Weak opioid / NMDA antag.	Jun-96
fluproquazone	Discontinued	Novartis (Switz.)	NSAID	Feb-02

Ref.: Pharmaprojects (updated to 2/02) used with permission; Scrip, corporate, literature & patent references
"Status" is international drug development or regulatory status and may not indicate status in USA
Sponsor: Original company name is retained if product is discontinued or inactive after merger, acquisition, company name change, etc.
Users of this table are encouraged to independently verify the status, activity, and mechanism of action of drugs of interest

GENERIC / TRADE NAME	STATUS	SPONSOR (S)	MECHANISM OF ACTION	REF. UPDATE
fluquazone	Discontinued	Merck & Co (US)	Antiinflammatory	Feb-02
Fluradoline (HP-494)	Discontinued (ph. I)	Hoechst Marion Roussel (Ger)	Antidepressant analgesic	Feb-87
flurbiprofen	LAUNCHED	Abbott (US)	Antiinflammatory	Feb-02
Flurbiprofen meglumine (THC-1103)	Discontinued (PRE-REG)	Therapicon (Italy)	NSAID	May-99
flurbiprofen transdermal, Lead	LAUNCHED	Mikasa Seiyaku	Formulation	Feb-02
flurbiprofen, microCRYSTAL	Discontinued (Clin.)	Pharma-Logic (US)	Lecithin-coated formulation	Feb-02
foliaspongin	Discontinued	Fujisawa (Japan)	Antiinflammatory	Feb-02
folipastatin	Discontinued	Sankyo (Japan)	Antiinflammatory	Feb-02
Fopirtoline (D-1126)	Discontinued (ph. III)	Asta Medica (Germany)	COX inhibitor	Feb-84
Forsythiaside	Discontinued	Ehime Univ. (Japan)	Lipoxygenase (5-LO) inhibitor	1987
fosfosal	LAUNCHED	Uriach (Spain)	NSAID	Feb-02
FP16CM	Discontinued	Florida A&M Univ. (US)	Antiinflammatory steroid	Nov-98
FPL-15609	Discontinued	Astra/Fisons (Sweden)	NMDA antagonist / non-compet.	1997
FPL-15765	Preclinical	Astra/Fisons (Sweden)	NMDA antagonist / non-compet.	Apr-95
FPL-62064	Discontinued (ph. I)	Fisons (RPR; Ger.)	COX + lipoxygenase inhibitor	Jun-94
FPP-028	Inactive	Non-industrial source	Antiinflammatory	Feb-02
FR-173657	Discontinued	Fujisawa (Japan)	Bradykinin B2 antagonist	Feb-00
FR-193517	Inactive	Fujisawa (Japan)	B2 bradykinin antag., non-peptide	Feb-02
FR-64822	Discontinued	Fujisawa (Japan)	5-HT agonist	Jan-92
frakefamide (BCH-3963, LEF-576)	CLINICAL (II)	Shire (UK)	Mu agonist peptide	Feb-02
Frovatriptan (VML-251; SB-209505)	REGISTERED	Vernalis (UK)	5-HT1d/1b partial agonist; migraine	Feb-02
FS-205-397	Discontinued (ph. II)	Novartis (Switz.)	NSAID	Jan-97
furaprofen	Discontinued	3M (US)	Antiinflammatory	Feb-02
furcloprofen	Discontinued	Roche (Switz)	Antiinflammatory	Feb-02
furofenac	Discontinued	Alfa Wassermann	Antiinflammatory	Feb-02
FX-205-754	Discontinued	Novartis (Switz.)	NSAID	Feb-02
FY95-0006	Discontinued	UAB Research Foundation (US)	Disacharides; selectin inhibition	Sep-98
FZ	Inactive	Nippon Zoki (Japan)	NSAID	Feb-02
Gabapentin (US Phase IV Pain)	LAUNCHED	Warner-Lambert (US)	GABA releaser / antiepileptic	Apr-96
Gabapentin analogues	Discontinued	Warner-Lambert (US)	Ca++ antagonist; pain + epilepsy	Jan-00
Gaboxadol (Lu2-030; THIP)	Discontinued (ph. II)	Lundbeck (Denmark)	GABA agonist; muscimol analog	Mar-85
Ganaxolone (CCD-1042)	CLINICAL (II)	CoCensys (US)	Epalon neurosteroid (migraine)	Dec-97
GAT-3/4 inhibitors, BTG	Preclinical	BTG (UK)	Centrally-acting analgesic	Feb-02
GEMM-1 antagonists	Inactive	GEMMA Biotechnology	GEMM-1 antagonist; arthritis	Feb-02
gepefrine	LAUNCHED	Aventis (France)	Antimigraine	Feb-02
GF-109203X	Inactive	Pfizer (US)	Antiinflammatory	Feb-02
GI-156704A	Inactive	GlaxoSmithKline (UK)	Antiarthritic	Feb-02
GI-245402 / BB-2983	Discontinued (ph. I)	Glaxo Wellcome / British Biotech	MMP / TNF inhibitor (arthritis)	Oct-97
Glafenine, Sopar	WITHDRAWN (LNCHD)	Rhone-Poulenc Rorer (France)	Unidentified (NSAID); fatalities	Apr-91
glucametacin	LAUNCHED	Farmades	Antiarthritic	Feb-02
glucocorticoids, Aventis	Inactive	Aventis (France)	Antiinflammatory	Feb-02
Glucosamine sulfate	LAUNCHED	Rotta (Italy)	Superoxide free radical antag.	Jan-96
Glycosidase inhibitors	Discontinued	Oxford GlycoSciences (UK)	Glycosidase inhib. / RA	Dec-98
GlyT-1 inhibitors	Preclinical	Gliatech (US)	Glycine reuptake inhibitor (GlyT2)	Feb-99
GM-1986	Discontinued	Glycomed / Ligand (US)	Selectin antagonist	Feb-97
GM-1998 (Celadin)	Discontinued	Ligand (US)	Selectin inhibitor; anti-inflam.	Mar-00
GM7-050	Discontinued	Ligand (US)	Antiinflammatory	Feb-02
GP-03	CLINICAL (I)	BioPhausia (Sweden)	Antiarthritic	Feb-02
GP-04012	Inactive	Metabasis Therapeutics	Adenosine A1 agonist/antag.	Feb-02
GP-1-515	Discontinued	Metabasis Therapeutics	Adenosine regulating agent (ARA)	Feb-02
GP-44	Discontinued	Protherics	Antiarthritic	Feb-02
GP-53633	Discontinued	Novartis (Switz.)	Antiinflammatory	Feb-02
GP-650	Discontinued	Greian	Antiinflammatory	Feb-02
GPI-5693	CLINICAL (I)	Guilford (US)	Centrally-acting analgesic	Feb-02
G-protein inhibitors, ICOS	Preclinical	ICOS (US)	Antiinflammatory	Feb-02
GR-103545	Inactive	Glaxo (UK)	Kappa agonist	Jan-92
GR-127607	Discontinued	Glaxo Wellcome (UK)	5-HT1 agonist	Nov-93
GR-129574A	Inactive	GlaxoSmithKline (UK)	Antiarthritic	Feb-02
GR-205171	CLINICAL (II)	Glaxo Wellcome (UK)	NK-1 antagonist / antiemetic	Feb-97
GR-253035	Preclinical	Glaxo Wellcome (UK)	COX-2 inhibitor	Jan-97
GR-373	Discontinued	Merck & Co (US)	Cysteine protease inhib; arthritis	Nov-99
GR-40370	Discontinued	Glaxo Wellcome (UK)	5-HT1 agonist	Feb-92
GR-45809	Discontinued	Glaxo (UK)	Kappa agonist	Nov-93

Ref.: Pharmaprojects (updated to 2/02) used with permission; Scrip, corporate, literature & patent references
"Status" is international drug development or regulatory status and may not indicate status in USA
Sponsor: Original company name is retained if product is discontinued or inactive after merger, acquisition, company name change, etc.
Users of this table are encouraged to independently verify the status, activity, and mechanism of action of drugs of interest

GENERIC / TRADE NAME	STATUS	SPONSOR (S)	MECHANISM OF ACTION	REF. UPDATE
GR-57426	Discontinued	Glaxo Wellcome (UK)	5-HT1 agonist	Jun-90
GR-69354	Discontinued	Glaxo Wellcome (UK)	5-HT1 agonist	Jun-89
GR-71251	Inactive	Glaxo (UK)	NK-1 antagonist (peptide)	Jul-91
GR-79236	Discontinued (ph. I)	Glaxo Wellcome (UK)	Adenosine A1 agonist	1998
GR-80907	Discontinued	GlaxoSmithKline (UK)	Antiinflammatory	Feb-02
GR-82334	Discontinued	Glaxo Wellcome (UK)	NK-1 antagonist peptide	Jan-97
GR-94839	Discontinued	Glaxo Wellcome (UK)	Kappa agonist	Oct-96
GRI-2	Preclinical	NPS Pharmaceuticals (US)	Centrally-acting analgesic	Feb-02
GT-094	Preclinical	GoBang Therapeutics	Centrally-acting analgesic	Feb-02
Guacetisal	LAUNCHED	Bayer (Germany)	Mucin antagonist	Dec-91
guaimesal	LAUNCHED	GlaxoSmithKline (UK)	Antiinflammatory	Feb-02
GV-196771	Discontinued (ph. II)	GlaxoSmithKline (UK)	Glycine antag. / neuropathic	Feb-02
GV-3658 (Diflusol)	Discontinued (REGIS.)	Edmond Pharma (It) / Resfar	NSAID / diflunisal derivative	Feb-99
GV-3659	Discontinued (REGIS.)	Edmond Pharma (It) / Resfar	NSAID / diflunisal derivative	Feb-99
GW-273629, GW-27415	Preclinical	Glaxo Wellcome (UK)	iNOS inhibitor; inflammation	Sep-99
GW-275919	Discontinued (ph. II)	Glaxo Wellcome (UK)	Back pain (unspec. Mechanism)	Feb-02
GW-286103	Discontinued	Glaxo Wellcome (UK)	Na+ channel inhib.	Feb-02
GW-3600	Discontinued	Glaxo Wellcome (UK)	Phosphodiesterase IV inhib.	Sep-97
GW-406381	CLINICAL (I)	GlaxoSmithKline (UK)	NSAID	Feb-02
GW-4459	Preclinical	GlaxoSmithKline (UK)	Antiinflammatory	Feb-02
GYKI-44688	Discontinued	ICN (US)	Antiarthritic	Feb-02
GYKI-86114	Discontinued	Gedeon Richter	Antiinflammatory	Feb-02
H-88	Discontinued	Hisamitsu	Antiinflammatory	Feb-02
haem oxygenase agonist, SangSt	Preclinical	SangStat (US)	Antiinflammatory	Feb-02
HAI-105	Discontinued	Hisamitsu	Antiinflammatory	Feb-02
halopredone	LAUNCHED	Dainippon (Japan)	Antiarthritic	Feb-02
HB-328	Discontinued (Clin.)	Synthelabo (France)	Antiinflamatory 5-ASA prodrug	Nov-91
hCG (LDI-200), Milkhaus	CLINICAL (III)	Milkhaus (US)	Antileukemic; ph. I cancer pain	Feb-98
HCT-2035	Discontinued	NicOx (France)	NSAID + NO releaser	Jun-99
HCT-3012	CLINICAL (II)	NicOx (France)	NSAID + NO releaser	Feb-02
HCT-6015	Preclinical	NicOx (France)	NSAID + NO releaser	Feb-02
Heptapeptides	Inactive	Ferring (Sweden)	Substance P antagonist	Unk.
Hexahydrobenzazocines	Inactive	Research Corp. Tech. (US)	Opioid agonist	1987
hexaprofen	Discontinued	Uriach (Spain)	Antiinflammatory	Feb-02
HG/3	Inactive	UCM-Difme	Antiinflammatory	Feb-02
HGP-12	Preclinical	HG Pars (US)	Antiinflammatory	Feb-02
HGP-14	Preclinical	HG Pars (US)	Narcotic analgesic	Apr-99
HGP-15	Preclinical	HG Pars (US)	Narcotic analgesic	Apr-99
HGP-16	Preclinical	HG Pars (US)	Narcotic analgesic	Apr-99
HGP-17	Preclinical	HG Pars (US)	Opioid agonist/antagonist	Nov-95
HGP-18	Preclinical	HG Pars (US)	Centrally-acting analgesic	Feb-02
HGP-18	Preclinical	HG Pars (US)	Opioid agonist/antagonist	Nov-95
HGP-3	Preclinical	HG Pars (US)	Menabitan progrug (anti-inflam.)	Jan-96
HGP-4	Discontinued (ph. II)	HG Pars (US)	Centrally-acting analgesic	Feb-02
hIAP-1 inhibitor	Discontinued	Human Genome Sciences (US)	Apoptosis hIAP-1 inhibitor	Sep-98
high THC cannabis deriv, GW	CLINICAL (III)	GW Pharmaceuticals (UK)	Cannabinoid	Feb-02
HN-11608 (HN-11600)	Discontinued (ph. I?)	Hafslund Nycomed (Norway)	Kappa agonist	May-95
HN-1657	Discontinued	Hisamitsu	Antiinflammatory	Feb-02
HN-2836	Discontinued	Hisamitsu	Antiinflammatory	Feb-02
HN-3392	Inactive	Hisamitsu	Antiinflammatory	Feb-02
Hoe-302	Discontinued	Hoechst (Ger)	Unknown	Feb-87
Hoe-S-2922	Discontinued	Hoechst (Ger)	Unknown	Mar-89
holmium hydroxyapatite	Inactive	Mallinckrodt (US)	Antiarthritic	Feb-02
holy basil oil, Delhi	Inactive	Non-industrial source	Antiarthritic	Feb-02
honey bee venom	Discontinued	Pharmacia (US)	Antiarthritic	Feb-02
HP-228	CLINICAL (II)	LION bioscience (US)	Cytokine antagonist	Feb-02
HP-573	Discontinued (Clin.)	Hoechst Marion Roussel (Ger)	NSAID	Jul-84
HP-736	Discontinued	Hoechst (Ger)	Opioid agonist (mu ag.)	Apr-89
HP-818	Discontinued	Hoechst (Ger)	Neuroleptic analgesic	Sep-91
Hyaluronic acid (HYALGAN®)	LAUNCHED	Sanofi (France) / Fidia (Italy)	Purified hyaluronic acid for OA	Nov-97
Hyaluronic acid (ORTHOVISC®)	PRE-REGISTRATION	Anika Therapeutics (US)	Purified hyaluronic acid for OA	Jan-98
hyaluronic acid, Fidia	LAUNCHED	Fidia (Italy)	Antiarthritic	Feb-02
hyaluronic acid, Kyowa Hakko	Inactive	Kyowa Hakko (Japan)	Antiarthritic	Feb-02

Ref.: Pharmaprojects (updated to 2/02) used with permission; Scrip, corporate, literature & patent references
"Status" is international drug development or regulatory status and may not indicate status in USA
Sponsor: Original company name is retained if product is discontinued or inactive after merger, acquisition, company name change, etc.
Users of this table are encouraged to independently verify the status, activity, and mechanism of action of drugs of interest

GENERIC / TRADE NAME	STATUS	SPONSOR (S)	MECHANISM OF ACTION	REF. UPDATE
hyaluronic acid, Seikagaku	LAUNCHED	Seikagaku Kogyo (Japan)	Antiarthritic	Feb-02
Hyaluronic formul. (Hyanalgese-D™)	Discontinued (ph. III)	Hyal Pharmaceutical (Canada)	Diclofenac + hyaluronic acid (ph. IV)	Dec-97
hyaluronidase, BioPhausia	Inactive	BioPhausia (Sweden)	Antiinflamatory; interstitial edema	Feb-02
HYC-141	Discontinued	Fidia (Italy)	Antiarthritic	Feb-02
HydrocoDex	CLINICAL (II)	Endo / Algos (US)	Hydrocodone + dextromethorphan	Feb-02
Hydrocodone + APAP (NORCO™)	LAUNCHED	Watson (US)	Formulation, high dose HC	Feb-97
Hydroisoquinolines	Preclinical	SmithKline Beecham (UK)	Agonist/antagonist opioid	Mar-95
Hydromorphone (HYDROMORPH CONTIN®)	LAUNCHED	Napp (UK)	Oral sustained release	Apr-98
hydromorphone combination	CLINICAL (II)	Pain Therapeutics (US)	Opioid + low dose antagonist	Feb-02
hydromorphone, DUROS	Preclinical	Durect	Formulation	Feb-02
hydromorphone, Napp	LAUNCHED	Napp (UK)	Formulation	Feb-02
hydromorphone, OROS	PRE-REGISTRATION	Johnson & Johnson (US)	Oral 24hr hydromorphone	Feb-02
Hylan (SYNVISC®)	LAUNCHED	Wyeth-Ayerst (US) / Biomatrix	Hylan A + B (joint lubricant, inj)	Jul-96
hylans	LAUNCHED	Genzyme (US)	Antiarthritic	Feb-02
HZ-2	Discontinued	Grunenthal (Germany)	Kappa agonist	Feb-02
ibuprofen (CR) + codeine, Napp	LAUNCHED	Napp (UK)	Analgesic combination	Feb-02
Ibuprofen + codeine	Discontinued	Alza (US)	Ibuprofen + opioid	Mar-89
Ibuprofen + codeine	LAUNCHED	Boots (UK)	Ibuprofen + opioid (low dose)	1995
ibuprofen + codeine,bioMerieux	PRE-REGISTRATION	bioMerieux-Pierre Fabre (France)	Formulation, oral combination	Feb-02
Ibuprofen + dextromethorphan	CLINICAL (II)	Algos (US) / J&J (US)	Ibuprofen + dextromethorphan	May-97
Ibuprofen + dihydrocodeine	Discontinued (ph. II)	IVX BioSciences (US)	Formulation, oral	Sep-96
Ibuprofen + oxycodone	PRE-REGISTRATION	Forest Laboratories (US)	Ibuprofen + opioid	Feb-02
Ibuprofen + SEPA enhancers	CLINICAL (II)	MacroChem (US)	Formulation, transdermal	Nov-96
Ibuprofen aluminum (U-18573G)	Discontinued (ph. III)	Pharmacia & Upjohn (UK)	NSAID	1980
Ibuprofen combination	LAUNCHED	Adcock Ingram (RSA)	Ibuprofen + APAP + codeine	Apr-92
Ibuprofen gel, topical	CLINICAL (II)	Macrochem (US)	Topical gel formulation	Apr-99
Ibuprofen gel, topical	Discontinued (PRE-REG)	Pierre Fabre (France)	Topical gel formulation	Apr-99
ibuprofen topical, bioMerieux	Discontinued	bioMerieux-Pierre Fabre (France)	Formulation	Feb-02
Ibuprofen, APR	REGISTERED	Applied Pharma Res. (Switz.)	Fast/slow controlled release	Jun-98
Ibuprofen, Ceform	PRE-REGISTRATION	Fuisz Technologies	"Flash Dose" oral delivery	Jul-98
ibuprofen, CEFORM	Inactive	Biovail (Canada)	Formulation	Feb-02
Ibuprofen, EFVDAS (IBUSCENT)	LAUNCHED	Searle (US) / Elan (Ireland)	Formulation, oral fast-acting	Jun-99
ibuprofen, Flash Dose	LAUNCHED	Biovail (Canada)	Formulation	Feb-02
ibuprofen, OSAT	Suspended (REGIS)	CeNeS (UK)	Oral sustained release	Feb-02
ibuprofen, SEPA	CLINICAL (II)	MacroChem (US)	Formulation	Feb-02
Ibuprofen+hydrocodone (VICOPROFEN®)	LAUNCHED	Knoll (Germany) / Abbott (US)	Oral combination analgesic	Apr-98
ibuproxam	LAUNCHED	GlaxoSmithKline (UK)	NSAID	Feb-02
Ibuproxam-beta-cyclodextrin	Discontinued (ph. I)	Lex Pharma. (Slovenia)	NSAID, solubilized ibuproxam	Mar-91
IC-485	CLINICAL (I)	ICOS (US)	Antiinflammatory	Feb-02
ICAM antagonists, Genentech	Inactive	Genentech	Antiinflammatory	Feb-02
ICAM-1 antagonists, Abbott	Preclinical	Abbott (US)	Antiinflammatory	Feb-02
ICE inhibitors	Discontinued	Ono (Japan)	IL-1beta conv. enzyme inhib.	Jan-99
ICE inhibitors (PD-163594)	Discontinued	Warner-Lambert (US)	IL-1beta conv. enzyme inhib.	Jan-00
ICF-650	Inactive	Non-industrial source	Antiinflammatory	Feb-02
ICI-10552	Discontinued	AstraZeneca (UK)	Antiinflammatory	Feb-02
ICI-115432	Discontinued	AstraZeneca (UK)	Antiarthritic	Feb-02
ICI-118551	Discontinued	AstraZeneca (UK)	Antimigraine	Feb-02
ICI-120518	Discontinued	Zeneca (US)	Narcotic analgesic	Feb-82
ICI-199441	Discontinued	Zeneca (US)	Kappa agonist	Mar-89
ICI-204448	Discontinued	Zeneca (US)	Kappa agonist	Feb-90
ICI-211965 (ICI-216800)	Discontinued	Zeneca (UK)	5-LO inhibitor	Aug-92
ICI-95527	Discontinued (ph. I)	Zeneca (UK)	Unidentified anti-inflammatory	Apr-90
Icilin	Inactive	Canada Packers (Canada)	Unknown; "Feels cold"	1984
Icodulinium HCl	Discontinued (ph. III)	Chauvin (France)	Ophthalmic anti-inflam. (COX+LO)	Nov-94
IDN-8128	Preclinical	Idun (US)	Antiinflammatory	Feb-02
IG-243-Na	Discontinued	Taiho (Japan)	Antiinflammatory	Feb-02
IL-1Hy1	Preclinical	Hyseq (US)	IL-1 receptor antagonist	Aug-99
IL-8 antagonists	Preclinical	Pharmacopeia (US) / Organon	IL-8 receptor antagonist (inflam.)	Jan-00
IL-8 antagonists, Pharmacopeia	Inactive	Pharmacopeia (US)	IL-8 receptor antagonist (inflam.)	Feb-02
imidazole salicylate	LAUNCHED	Italfarmaco (Italy)	Antiinflammatory	Feb-02
Imidazopyrazoles	Discontinued	Roussel-Uclaf (France)	Na+ channel antagonist	Mar-89
IND-9	Discontinued	Alter	Antiinflammatory	Feb-02
Indolylimidazolones	Inactive	King George's Med. College	MAO inhibitor	1987

Ref.: Pharmaprojects (updated to 2/02) used with permission; Scrip, corporate, literature & patent references
"Status" is international drug development or regulatory status and may not indicate status in USA
Sponsor: Original company name is retained if product is discontinued or inactive after merger, acquisition, company name change, etc.
Users of this table are encouraged to independently verify the status, activity, and mechanism of action of drugs of interest

GENERIC / TRADE NAME	STATUS	SPONSOR (S)	MECHANISM OF ACTION	REF. UPDATE
indometacin farnesil	LAUNCHED	Eisai (Japan)	NSAID	Feb-02
indoprofen	WITHDRAWN	Pharmacia (US)	Antiinflammatory	Feb-02
Indoylpropenoic acids	Preclinical	Marion Merrell Dow (US)	NMDA antagonist	Jan-95
Infliximab (REMICADE)	LAUNCHED	Centocor (US)	TNF-alpha antibody, RA	Feb-02
inhibitor B	Inactive	Merck & Co (US)	Antiinflammatory	Feb-02
intrazole	Discontinued	Bristol-Myers Squibb (US)	Antiinflammatory	Feb-02
ion channel blockers, NeuroS	Preclinical	NeuroSearch (Denmark)	Ion channel blockers	Feb-02
IP-01	Preclinical	Ionix Pharmaceuticals	Formulation	Feb-02
IP-02	Preclinical	Ionix Pharmaceuticals	Centrally-acting analgesic	Feb-02
IP-03	Preclinical	Ionix Pharmaceuticals	Centrally-acting analgesic	Feb-02
IPL 423 (bispan)	Preclinical	Inflazyme (US)	Kinase activator (anti-inflam.)	Feb-98
IPL-512602	CLINICAL (I)	Inflazyme (US)	Antiinflammatory	Feb-02
IPL-550260	CLINICAL (I)	Inflazyme (US)	Antiinflammatory	Feb-02
IPR-6001	CLINICAL (II)	Inst. Pharm Research (Switz)	Antiinflammatory / chronic pain	Feb-97
IQB-821	Discontinued (ph. I)	IQB (Spain)	Nefopam analog	Jan-86
IRA-378	CLINICAL (I)	Kyorin	Antiarthritic	Feb-02
IS-159	Suspended (ph. II)	Medicines Company (US)	5-HT1d agonist / migraine	Feb-02
ISIS-104838	Preclinical	ISIS Pharmaceuticals (US)	TNF-a antagonist; RA, Crohn's	Jan-00
ISIS-4730	Discontinued	ISIS Pharmaceuticals (US)	ELAM-1 antisense; antiinflam.	Aug-99
isofezolac	Discontinued	Aventis (France)	Antiinflammatory	Feb-02
isonixin	LAUNCHED	Hermes	NSAID	Feb-02
Isoprazone (DL-809-IT)	Discontinued (ph. I)	Hoechst Marion Roussel (Ger)	NSAID	1983
isoprofen	Discontinued	Bristol-Myers Squibb (US)	NSAID	Feb-02
Isoquinolines	Discontinued	Richter (Hungary)	Na+ channel antagonist	Apr-86
Isoquinolinylphenols	Inactive	Lilly (US)	Opioid agonist/antagonist	1988
isoxicam	WITHDRAWN	Pfizer (US)	NSAID	Feb-02
ITF-2357	Discontinued (ph. I)	Italfarmaco (Italy)	TNF-alpha, IL-1b synthesis inhib.	Feb-02
itrocinonide	Inactive	AstraZeneca (UK)	Antiarthritic	Feb-02
J-113397	Preclinical	Merck & Co (US)	Centrally-acting analgesic	Feb-02
J-8970	Discontinued	DuPont Merck (US)	Opioid agonist/antagonist	Mar-92
JI-36 (TCA)	Discontinued (ph. II)	Otsuka (Japan)	Unidentified anti-inflammatory	Apr-93
JTC-801	CLINICAL (II)	Japan Tobacco (Japan)	Centrally-acting analgesic	Feb-02
JTE-522	CLINICAL (II)	Japan Tobacco / J&J (US)	COX-2 inhibitor (RA, OA)	Dec-97
JTE-607	CLINICAL (II)	Japan Tobacco (Japan)	Antiinflammatory	Feb-02
K562 factor, INSERM	Inactive	Non-industrial source	Antiinflammatory	Feb-02
kallikrein inhibitors, Celera	Inactive	Celera Genomics	Antiinflammatory	Feb-02
kallolide-A	Inactive	Non-industrial source	Antiinflammatory	Feb-02
Kappagems / glystasins	Preclinical	CoCensys (US)	NMDA associated	Feb-93
KB-1043	Discontinued	Akzo Nobel (Netherlands)	Antiinflammatory	Feb-02
KB-R7785	Inactive	Akzo Nobel / Kanebo (Japan)	Metalloproteinase, TNF, FasL inhib.	Feb-02
KC-8973	Discontinued	Kaken (Japan)	Antiinflammatory	Feb-02
KCN-TEI-6172	Inactive	Teijin (Japan)	Antiinflammatory	Feb-02
Kelatorphan	Inactive	INSERM (France)	Enk'ase inhibitor	1985
ketoprofen	LAUNCHED	Aventis (France)	NSAID	Feb-02
Ketoprofen, CEFORM	Discontinued	Biovail (Canada)	Oral formulation	Oct-99
ketoprofen, NexACT	CLINICAL (I)	NexMed	NSAID	Feb-02
ketoprofen, Poli	Inactive	Poli (Italy)	Formulation	Feb-02
Ketorfanol	Preclinical	HG Pars (US)	Narcotic analgesic	Nov-95
Ketorfanol (HGP-13)	Preclinical	HG Pars (US)	Opioid agonist/antagonist	Apr-99
ketorolac	LAUNCHED	Roche (Switz)	NSAID	Feb-02
ketorolac tromethamine, Pharme	Inactive	Technical Chemicals (US)	Patch formulation, 1x daily	Feb-02
Ketorolac, TCPI	Discontinued	Technical Chemicals (US)	Transdermal formulation	Dec-98
ketorolac, TheraTech	Discontinued	Watson (US)	Formulation	Feb-02
KF-17515	Discontinued	Kyowa Hakko (Japan)	Antiinflammatory	Feb-02
KF-18280	Discontinued	Kyowa Hakko (Japan)	Antiinflammatory	Feb-02
KF-24705	Discontinued	Kyowa Hakko (Japan)	Opioid mu2 agonist	Feb-00
KK3	Inactive	Nagasaki Univ. (Japan)	Opioid analgesic	1990
KME-4	Discontinued (ph. II)	Kaneka (Japan)	COX/5-LO inhibitor	Jul-91
KP-354	Preclinical	Kinetek	Antiinflammatory	Feb-02
KPI-022	Discontinued	Scios (US)	Serine protease inhibitor (inflam.)	Nov-99
KSB-308	Preclinical	KS Biomedix	Antiarthritic	Feb-02
KT-90	Discontinued	Chugai (Japan)	Opioid agonist/antagonist	Aug-91
Kunitz protease inhibitor	Preclinical	Scios (US)	Serine protease inhib; APP	Jun-97

Ref.: Pharmaprojects (updated to 2/02) used with permission; Scrip, corporate, literature & patent references
"Status" is international drug development or regulatory status and may not indicate status in USA
Sponsor: Original company name is retained if product is discontinued or inactive after merger, acquisition, company name change, etc.
Users of this table are encouraged to independently verify the status, activity, and mechanism of action of drugs of interest

GENERIC / TRADE NAME	STATUS	SPONSOR (S)	MECHANISM OF ACTION	REF. UPDATE
L-0076	Preclinical	Pierre Fabre (France)	5-HT1d agonist	May-96
L-249313	Discontinued	Merck & Co (US)	Adenosine A3 antagonist (inflam.)	Sep-99
L-652343	Discontinued (ph. I)	Merck & Co (US)	COX/5-LO inhibitor	1986
L-659837	Inactive	Merck & Co (US)	NK-2 antagonist	1991
L-659877	Inactive	Merck & Co (US)	NK-2 antagonist	Nov-92
L-689660	Inactive	Merck & Co (US)	Cholinomimetic (M1 ag.)	Nov-92
L-694247	Discontinued	Merck & Co (US)	5-HT1d agonist	Oct-95
L-695499	Inactive	Merck & Co (US)	Antiinflammatory	Feb-02
L-709049	Inactive	Merck & Co (US)	Antiinflammatory	Feb-02
L-732138	Discontinued	Merck & Co (US)	NK-1 antagonist	Nov-96
L-733060	Discontinued	Merck & Co (US)	NK-1 antagonist	May-98
L-740141	Discontinued	Merck & Co (US)	NK-1 antagonist	Feb-99
L-745337	Preclinical	Merck & Co (US)	NSAID	Feb-02
L-747201	Preclinical	Merck & Co (US)	5-HT1d-alpha agonist	Nov-97
L-758354	Discontinued	Merck & Co (US)	Stromelysin-1 (MMP-3) inhibitor	Jun-99
L-768277	Discontinued	Merck & Co (US)	COX-2 inhibitor	Feb-99
L-776967	Discontinued	Merck & Co (US)	Antiinflammatory	Feb-02
L-782097	Discontinued	Merck & Co (US)	Antimigraine	Feb-02
L-783003	Discontinued (ph. II)	Merck & Co (US)	COX-2 inhibitor	Sep-98
L-791456	CLINICAL (I)	Merck & Co (US)	COX-2 inhibitor	Sep-99
L-804600	Inactive	Merck & Co (US)	Antiinflammatory	Feb-02
L-804600, L-818571	Discontinued	Merck & Co (US)	COX-2 inhibitor	Dec-99
L-8322	Discontinued	Aventis (France)	Antiinflammatory	Feb-02
LA-351	Discontinued	Lacer (Spain)	Benzopyran antiinflammatory	May-97
Lactacystin analogs	Preclinical	ProScript (US)	Proteasome inhib.; anti-inflam.	Dec-97
Lamotrigine (LAMICTAL®)	LAUNCHED	Wellcome (UK)	Glutamate inhib. / anticonvul.	May-93
Lanepitant (LY-303870)	Discontinued (ph. II)	Lilly (US)	NK-1 antagonist (oral)	Sep-97
Lappaconitine	Discontinued	Mercian (Japan)	NE/5-HT antagonist	Jul-94
LAS-33826	CLINICAL	Almirall-Prodesfarma (Spain)	Antiarthritic	Feb-02
Latranal	Discontinued	Praecis Pharmaceuticals	Centrally-acting analgesic	Feb-02
LC-546	Discontinued	Alcon (US)	Antiinflammatory	Feb-02
LCB-1892	Discontinued (ph. I)	Merck KGaA (Germany)	NSAID	Mar-96
Leucine derivative	Inactive	Univ. Rouen (France)	Enk'ase inhibitor	1983
leucotriene analogues, ResCo	Discontinued	Research Corp. Tech. (US)	Antiarthritic	Feb-02
leucotriene antags, Aventis	Discontinued	Aventis (France)	Antiinflammatory	Feb-02
leucotriene inhibitors, Glaxo	Inactive	GlaxoSmithKline (UK)	Antimigraine	Feb-02
LeukoVax	CLINICAL (II)	Viragen / Inflammatics (US)	Immunomod. cell prep; RA	Nov-98
leumedins, Scios	Inactive	Scios (US)	Antiinflammatory	Feb-02
Leumorphin	Discontinued	Mitsubishi Kasei (Japan)	Opioid peptide	1984
Levobupivacaine (CHIROCAINE®)	CLINICAL (III)	Zeneca (UK) / Chiroscience (UK)	Local anesthetic / (S)-isomer	May-96
Levonantradol (CP-50556-1)	Discontinued (ph. II)	Pfizer (US)	Cannabinoid	1984
LEX analogues	Discontinued	SuperGen (US)	Serine protease inhibitor (inflam.)	Sep-99
LEX-028	Inactive	SuperGen (US)	Antiinflammatory	Feb-02
LF-521	Inactive	Fournier (France)	Bradykinin B1 antagonist	Feb-02
Lidocaine (DentiPatch)	LAUNCHED	Noven Pharma (US)	Transoral mucosal anesthetic	Feb-99
Lidocaine + Dex. (LidoDex-NS®)	Preclinical	Algos (US) / Interneuron (US)	Lidocaine + dextromethorphan	Feb-97
Lidocaine patch (LIDODERM)	LAUNCHED	Endo (US) / Elan (IR) / Hind (US)	Transdermal formulation; PHN	May-00
lidocaine ring, Enhance	Preclinical	Enhance Pharmaceuticals	Formulation	Feb-02
lidocaine, EpiCept-2	CLINICAL (II)	EpiCept (US)	Dermal formulation	Feb-02
lidocaine, EpiCept-3	CLINICAL (II)	EpiCept (US)	Dermal formulation	Feb-02
Lidocaine, E-TRANS	Discontinued (ph. II)	Alza (US)	Topical lidocaine	Mar-00
Lidocaine, LIDOMER MICROSPHERES	Preclinical	Guilford (US)	Biodegradable microspheres (inj.)	Apr-00
Lidocaine, Noven	LAUNCHED	Noven Pharmaceuticals (US)	Transoral mucosal delivery	Jun-97
Lidocaine, PowderJect	CLINICAL (III)	Chiroscience / PowderJect (UK)	Dermal, oral formulations	Jun-99
lidocaine, Vyteris	CLINICAL (III)	Vyteris	Formulation	Feb-02
Lipocaine	Preclinical	Deprenyl Research (Canada)	Topical lidocaine formula	Jul-93
Lipocortin	Inactive	Biogen (US)	Corticoid	May-85
Lipocortin, Shionogi	Discontinued	Shionogi (Japan)	Corticoid	Feb-02
Lipoenkephalins	Discontinued	Merck & Co (US)	Enkephalin analog	Jan-84
LK-423	Inactive	Fujimoto (Japan)	IL-10 agonist; Interferon-γ antag.	Jun-99
LM-001	Inactive	American Home Products (US)	Formulation	Feb-02
LM-1376	Discontinued	Menarini (Italy)	Leukotriene D4 antagonist	May-98
LN-1520	Discontinued	Roche (Switz)	Antiinflammatory	Feb-02

Ref.: Pharmaprojects (updated to 2/02) used with permission; Scrip, corporate, literature & patent references
"Status" is international drug development or regulatory status and may not indicate status in USA
Sponsor: Original company name is retained if product is discontinued or inactive after merger, acquisition, company name change, etc.
Users of this table are encouraged to independently verify the status, activity, and mechanism of action of drugs of interest

GENERIC / TRADE NAME	STATUS	SPONSOR (S)	MECHANISM OF ACTION	REF. UPDATE
L-NAME	Preclinical	King's College, London	Nitric oxide synthase inhibitor	Jan-93
Lobuprofen (frabuprofen)	Discontinued (ph. II)	Juste (Spain)	Ibuprofen ester	May-93
Lodaxaprine	Discontinued	Sanofi (France)	Na+ channel antagonist	Mar-92
lodelaben	Discontinued	Pharmacia (US)	Antiarthritic	Feb-02
Lofemizole	Discontinued (ph. III)	Farmatis (Italy)	NSAID	Sep-82
Lofentanil (R-34995)	Discontinued (ph. II)	Janssen / J&J (US)	Opioid mu agonist (long acting)	1987
Lomerizine (TERANAS; MIGSIS)	LAUNCHED	Akzo Nobel (Netherlands)	Ca++ antagonist; migraine	Jul-99
lonazolac calcium	LAUNCHED	Byk Gulden (Ger)	Antiinflammatory	Feb-02
Loperamide (ADL 2-1294)	CLINICAL (II)	Adolor (US) / Santen	Topical, ophthalmic formulations	May-00
Lorcinadol	Discontinued	Johnson & Johnson (US)	Unknown	Mar-89
lornoxicam	LAUNCHED	Nycomed Pharma (Norway)	NSAID	Feb-02
Lornoxicam (LORCAM, XEFO)	LAUNCHED	Nycomed Pharma (Norway)	NSAID (oral, suppository)	Jan-00
lotifazole	Discontinued	bioMerieux-Pierre Fabre (France)	Antiarthritic	Feb-02
loxoprofen	LAUNCHED	Sankyo (Japan)	Antiarthritic	Feb-02
LS-4249	Discontinued	BTG (UK)	Antiinflammatory	Feb-02
LSZ-1025	Discontinued	Univ. Arizona (US)	Glycopeptide δ antagonist	Apr-97
LTA	Discontinued (ph. II)	AstraZeneca (UK)	Na+ channel antagonist, topical	Feb-02
LU-20884	Discontinued	Abbott (US)	Antiinflammatory	Feb-02
LV-216	Preclinical	Vinas (Spain)	Antiinflammatory	Feb-02
LY-053857	Discontinued (ph. II)	Lilly (US)	5-HT2 antagonist	Oct-94
LY-108964	Inactive	Lilly (US)	NSAID	Feb-02
LY-112101	Inactive	Lilly (US)	Antiinflammatory	Feb-02
LY-178002	Inactive	Lilly (US)	Antiinflammatory	Feb-02
LY-189709	Inactive	Lilly (US)	NMDA antagonist	1986
LY-210073	Discontinued	Lilly (US)	Leukotriene LTB4 antagonist	Jan-95
LY-214281	Inactive	Lilly (US)	5-HT uptake inhibitor	1989
LY-233569	Inactive	Lilly (US)	Antiinflammatory	Feb-02
LY-243062	Inactive	Lilly (US)	Antiinflammatory	Feb-02
LY-269415	Inactive	Lilly (US)	Antiarthritic	Feb-02
LY-280810	Discontinued	Lilly (US)	Antiinflammatory	Feb-02
LY-281217	Inactive	Lilly (US)	Enkephalin analog	Nov-91
LY-297802 / NNC-11-1053	Discontinued (ph. II)	Lilly (US) / Novo Nordisk (Den)	Muscarinic M1 agonist	May-99
LY-334370	Discontinued (ph. II)	Synaptic (US) / Lilly (US)	5-HT1f agonist; antimigraine	May-99
LY-344864	Preclinical	Synaptic (US)	5-HT1f agonist	Oct-98
LY-39	Discontinued	Univ. Upsala (Sweden)	5-HT1d/D2 agonist	Jan-96
LY-97292	Inactive	Lilly (US)	Enkephalin analog	1984
lysine clonixinate	LAUNCHED	Laplex	NSAID	Feb-02
lysine salicylate	LAUNCHED	Polytechna	NSAID	Feb-02
Lysozyme metabolites	Suspended	SPA (Italy)	Oligopeptides	Mar-99
M3, Xenova	Preclinical	Xenova (US)	Antiinflammatory	Feb-02
M-40403	Preclinical	Metaphore (US)	Superoxide dismutase inhibitor	Dec-99
M-5	Inactive	Fujisawa (Japan)	Antiinflammatory	Feb-02
M-5011	Discontinued	Maruho (Japan)	PGF1a antagonist	Apr-98
M-7074	Inactive	Mochida	Antiinflammatory	Feb-02
M-75168	Discontinued	Aventis (France)	Antiinflammatory	Feb-02
mabuprofen	LAUNCHED	Aldo-Union	Antiinflammatory	Feb-02
MAFP, Merck	Inactive	Merck & Co (US)	Antiinflammatory	Feb-02
Manoalide (luffariellolide)	Discontinued (ph. I)	Allergan (US) / Scripps Inst.	Anti-inflammatory	May-92
manoalogue	Inactive	Lilly (US)	Antiinflammatory	Feb-02
MASP inhibitors, Natimmune	Preclinical	Natimmune	Antiinflammatory	Feb-02
MB-432	Inactive	Non-industrial source	Antiinflammatory	Feb-02
MC1 agonists, Melacure	Preclinical	Melacure Therapeutics	Antiinflammatory	Feb-02
MCI-426	Inactive	Mitsubishi Pharma (Japan)	Antiarthritic	Feb-02
McN-5195	Discontinued	Johnson & Johnson (US)	Unknown	1987
MCP enzyme inhibitors,Cephalon	Inactive	Cephalon (US)	Antiinflammatory	Feb-02
MD-260185	Discontinued	Synthelabo (France)	NE uptake inhib.	1984
MDL-100250	Inactive	Marion Merrell Dow (US)	Enk'ase inhibitor	Jan-93
MDL-100948A	Inactive	Aventis (France)	Antiinflammatory	Feb-02
MDL-104238 (MDL-101286)	Discontinued	Hoechst Marion Roussel (Ger)	Neutrophil elastase inhibitor	Sep-97
MDL-19301D	Inactive	Aventis (France)	Antiinflammatory	Feb-02
MDL-201331	Inactive	Aventis (France)	Antiarthritic	Feb-02
MDL-9563	Discontinued	Aventis (France)	Antiinflammatory	Feb-02
meclofenamate sodium	LAUNCHED	Pfizer (US)	Antiarthritic	Feb-02

Ref.: Pharmaprojects (updated to 2/02) used with permission; Scrip, corporate, literature & patent references
"Status" is international drug development or regulatory status and may not indicate status in USA
Sponsor: Original company name is retained if product is discontinued or inactive after merger, acquisition, company name change, etc.
Users of this table are encouraged to independently verify the status, activity, and mechanism of action of drugs of interest

GENERIC / TRADE NAME	STATUS	SPONSOR (S)	MECHANISM OF ACTION	REF. UPDATE
Melanin analogs	Inactive	Biosource Technologies (US)	TNF-alpha inhibitor; anti-inflam.	Aug-97
Meloxicam (MOBIC®)	LAUNCHED	Boehringer Ingelheim (Ger)	COX 1-2 inhibitor, 1x daily	Dec-96
Memantine	CLINICAL (II)	Merz / Neurobiological Tech. (US)	NMDA antag. / neuropathic pain	Apr-98
MEN-10207	Inactive	Menarini (Italy)	NK-A Antagonist	Oct-93
Menabitan	Preclinical	HG Pars (US)	Unknown	Mar-92
Meptazinol	LAUNCHED	Wyeth-Ayerst (US)	Opioid agonist/antagonist	Dec-91
Mercaptoacetylamide azepines	Preclinical	Hoechst Marion Roussel (Ger)	Enk'ase inhibitor	Sep-95
Mesoporphyrin	Discontinued	Taiho (Japan)	Antiarthritic T-cell inhibitor	Feb-98
MET-157	Preclinical	NicOx (France)	Centrally-acting analgesic	Feb-02
metalloenzyme inhibitors, Sero	Preclinical	Serono	Antiinflammatory	Feb-02
metbufen	Discontinued	American Home Products (US)	Antiinflammatory	Feb-02
Met-enkephalin	Inactive	TNI (US)	Enkephalin	1988
Methotrexate	Inactive	Dartmouth College (US)	Low back pain (intrathecal)	Feb-00
Methotrexate analogs	Discontinued	SRI International (US)	60 MTX analogs / RA	Mar-99
methylprednisolone prodrug	Inactive	Pharmacia (US)	Antiarthritic	Feb-02
Metkephamide (LY-127623)	Discontinued (ph. III)	Lilly (US)	Enkephalin analog	Feb-88
Metorphamide	Inactive	Stanford Univ. (US)	Opioid octapeptide	Unk.
MG-18311	Discontinued	Sanofi-Synthelabo (France)	Antiinflammatory	Feb-02
MG-18755	Discontinued	Sanofi-Synthelabo (France)	Antiinflammatory	Feb-02
MG-6881	Discontinued	Sanofi-Synthelabo (France)	NSAID	Feb-02
MG-8958	Discontinued	Eastman Kodak (US)	Opioid agonist	Mar-81
mGLUR antagonists	Preclinical	Novartis (Switz.) / Merck (US)	mGLUR (glutamate) antag.	Oct-99
Midazolam	LAUNCHED	Roche (Switz)	Benzodiazepine	Feb-92
migraine prophylaxis, Biofront	Preclinical	Biofrontera	Antimigraine	Feb-02
migraine ther, BMS	Preclinical	Bristol-Myers Squibb (US)	Antimigraine	Feb-02
migraine therapy, NeuroMed	Preclinical	NeuroMed Technologies	Antimigraine	Feb-02
Mipragoside (AGF-44, FISER-A503)	Discontinued (ph. II)	Fidia (Italy)	Membrane perm. inhib./anti-inflam.	May-99
Mirfentanil (A-3508)	Discontinued (ph. II)	Baxter / Ohmeda (US)	Opioid mu/delta agonist	May-97
miroprofen	Discontinued	Mitsubishi Pharma (Japan)	Antiinflammatory	Feb-02
MITO-2227	Preclinical	MitoKor	Antiarthritic	Feb-02
MK-663	CLINICAL (III)	Merck & Co (US)	COX-2 inhibitor (RA, OA, pain)	Jan-00
ML-3000	CLINICAL (III)	Merckle (Germany)	COX + 5-LO inhibitor	Feb-02
ML-3176	Inactive	Merckle (Germany)	Phospholipase PLA2 inhibitor	Jul-99
MM-7002	Inactive	Meiji Milk (Japan)	Antiinflammatory	Feb-02
MMP inhibitors	Preclinical	DuPont (US)	Metalloproteinase + TNF-α inhib.	Sep-99
MMP inhibitors, NIH	Discontinued	NIH (US)	Antibodies; type IV collagenase	Nov-98
MMP inhibitors, Synt:em	Discontinued	Syntem (France)	Metalloproteinase inhibitor	Dec-98
Mofezolac	LAUNCHED	Pasteur Merieux (Fr) / Taiho	Antiinflamatory/analgesic	Nov-95
morniflumate	Discontinued	Aventis (France)	Antiinflammatory	Feb-02
Morphiceptin analog	Inactive	Wellcome (UK)	Opioid mu agonist	Sep-84
MorphiDex® combination	CLINICAL (III)	Endo / Algos (US)	Morphine + dextromethorphan	Feb-02
Morphinan derivative	Discontinued	Daiichi (Japan)	Opioid agonist	Mar-87
Morphinan derivative	Inactive	Roche (Switz)	Opioid agonist	1984
Morphinan derivative	Discontinued	Univ. Innsbruck (Austria)	Opioid agonist	1984
Morphinan derivative	Discontinued	SRI Int'l (US)	Opioid agonist/antagonist	Apr-86
Morphine	CLINICAL (I)	West Pharmaceutical (US)	Transnasal formulation	Jan-00
Morphine (INFUSETTE®)	Inactive	Advanced Medical (Canada)	Rectal controlled release	Nov-91
Morphine (KADIAN®, KAPINOL®)	LAUNCHED	Faulding (Austr)	Oral 24 hr formulation	May-99
Morphine (MORAXEN)	PRE-REGISTRATION	CeNeS (UK) / BTG (UK)	Hydrogel morphine suppository	Apr-00
Morphine (MORPHELAN)	REGISTERED	Ligand (US) / Elan (Ireland)	Controlled rel. 1x/day SODAS	Feb-02
Morphine (TNK-951)	CLINICAL (II)	Nippon Kayaku (Japan)	Morphine formulation	Feb-99
Morphine formulation	Discontinued	Forest Laboratories (US)	Buccal formulation	Feb-88
Morphine formulation	LAUNCHED	Karo Bio (Sweden)	Epidural morphine	Mar-92
Morphine formulation	LAUNCHED	Wyeth-Ayerst (US)	Epidural morphine	Dec-91
Morphine formulation	CLINICAL	Eurand (Italy)	Sustained-release MS	Mar-91
morphine gluconate, Nastech	CLINICAL (II)	Nastech (US)	Opioid mu agonist	Feb-02
morphine, AERx	CLINICAL (II)	Aradigm	Pulmonary delivery	Feb-02
morphine, Dainippon-2	CLINICAL	Dainippon (Japan)	Formulation	Feb-02
morphine, DepoFoam	CLINICAL (III)	SkyePharma (UK)	Formulation	Feb-02
Morphine, DepoMorphine (D-0401)	CLINICAL (II)	DepoTech (US)	Epidural sustained rel. morphine	Dec-98
morphine, Ethypharm	LAUNCHED	Ethypharm	Formulation	Feb-02
Morphine, Gacel	CLINICAL (III)	Gacell (Sweden)	Formulation, oral 24 hr morphine	Nov-96
morphine, Generex	CLINICAL (I)	Generex	Formulation	Feb-02

Ref.: Pharmaprojects (updated to 2/02) used with permission; Scrip, corporate, literature & patent references
"Status" is international drug development or regulatory status and may not indicate status in USA
Sponsor: Original company name is retained if product is discontinued or inactive after merger, acquisition, company name change, etc.
Users of this table are encouraged to independently verify the status, activity, and mechanism of action of drugs of interest

GENERIC / TRADE NAME	STATUS	SPONSOR (S)	MECHANISM OF ACTION	REF. UPDATE
morphine, Multipor	CLINICAL (III)	Amarin (UK)	Oral 1x daily morphine	Feb-02
morphine, Nycomed Amersham	LAUNCHED	Nycomed Pharma (Norway)	Formulation	Feb-02
morphine, OSAT	Suspended (ph. I)	CeNeS (UK)	Oral sustained release	Feb-02
morphine, Premaire	CLINICAL (I)	Sheffield Pharmaceuticals (US)	Inhalation formulation	Jul-99
Morphine, rectal	PRE-REGISTRATION	Core Technologies (UK)	Suppository gel, 12-24 hr activity	Apr-97
Morphine, Repro-Dose	Discontinued (PRE-REG)	Nycomed Amersham (Norway)	Formulation, 1-2x daily oral	May-99
morphine, Rhotard	LAUNCHED	Amarin (UK)	Formulation, oral morphine	Feb-02
Morphine, Takeda, MH-100	REGISTERED	Takeda (Japan)	Formulation, inj. high-concentr.	Feb-02
morphine, TDS	Preclinical	TransDermal Technologies	Formulation	Feb-02
morphine, West	CLINICAL (II)	West Pharmaceutical (US)	Formulation	Feb-02
Morphine-6-glucuronide (M6G)	CLINICAL (II)	ML Laboratories (UK)	Opioid mu agonist; nebulized	Apr-98
Morphine-6-glucuronide analog	Preclinical	BTG (UK)	Chronic pain	Apr-96
morphine-6-glucuronide, CeNeS	CLINICAL (II)	CeNeS (UK)	Morphine metabolite	Feb-02
morphine-6-glucuronide, UFC	CLINICAL (II)	UFC Pharma	Morphine metabolite	Feb-02
Morpholines, Thiomorpholines	Preclinical	Merck & Co (US)	Substance P antag / depletor	Oct-95
Moxazocine (BL-4566)	Discontinued (ph. II)	Bristol-Myers Squibb (US)	Opioid agonist/antagonist	Mar-83
moxifadol	Discontinued	Byk Gulden (Ger)	NSAID	Feb-02
moxilubant maleate	Inactive	Novartis (Switz.)	Antiarthritic	Feb-02
MPV-2426	Inactive	Orion Pharma (Finland)	Alpha-2(a+b+c) agonist (spinal)	Feb-02
MPYS-333 ligands	Preclinical	Myriad Genetics	Antiarthritic	Feb-02
MR-1268	Discontinued	Boehringer Ingelheim (Ger)	Opioid agonist/antagonist	1983
MR-549	Inactive	Medea Research (Italy)	Unknown	Nov-85
MR-853	Discontinued	Recordati	Antiinflammatory	Feb-02
MR-854	Discontinued	Recordati	Antiinflammatory	Feb-02
MR-714	Discontinued	Recordati	NSAID	Feb-02
MS-731	Discontinued	Schering AG (Germany)	Antiinflammatory	Feb-02
MT-45	Discontinued	Dainippon (Japan)	Opioid analgesic	1985
MT-500 (RS-127445)	CLINICAL (I)	POZEN (US) / Roche (Switz)	5-HT2b antagonist (migraine)	Feb-02
MTDQ-DS	Discontinued	Human Inst. Serobac. Res. (Hung.)	Antiinflammatory, antioxidant	1990
MX-1094	Preclinical	Medinox (US)	Antiarthritic	Feb-02
MX-68	CLINICAL (I)	Chugai (Japan)	Methotrexate analog; DHFR antag.	Feb-00
N-1103	Preclinical	GenDerm (US)	Capsanoid	Nov-92
Nabitan	Discontinued	HG Pars (US)	Cannabinoid	Mar-92
nabumetone	LAUNCHED	GlaxoSmithKline (UK)	NSAID	Feb-02
NACAS	Inactive	Non-industrial source	Antiinflammatory	Feb-02
NADPH inhibitors, Selectide	Inactive	Aventis (France)	Antiinflammatory	Feb-02
NAGA	Discontinued	Asahi Brewery (Japan)	Opioid agonist tetrapeptide	1986
Nalbuphine (NUBAIN®)	LAUNCHED	DuPont Merck (US)	Opioid agonist/antagonist	Feb-92
Nalbuphine combinations	Discontinued	DuPont Merck (US)	Indomethacin combination	Sep-84
Nalbuphine, nasal	Discontinued	Nastech (US)	Intranasal formulation	Jul-99
N-a-Me-CPM-normorphine	Preclinical	SRI Int'l (US)	Opioid agonist/antagonist	Jul-91
NaN, TransMolecular	Preclinical	TransMolecular	Centrally-acting analgesic	Feb-02
Nantradol	Discontinued	Pfizer (US)	Cannabinoid	1979
naphlerpin	Inactive	Non-industrial source	Antiinflammatory	Feb-02
Naproxen betinate	LAUNCHED	Applied Pharma Res. (Switz.)	Combination naproxen + betaine	Jun-98
naproxen meglumine	Discontinued	Therapicon (Italy)	NSAID	Feb-02
naproxen, AW	LAUNCHED	Alfa Wassermann	Formulation	Feb-02
Naproxen, CEFORM	Discontinued	Biovail (Canada)	Oral formulation	Oct-99
Naproxen, cont. rel. (NAPRELAN®)	LAUNCHED	Wyeth-Ayerst (US) / Elan	Naproxen, 1x/day formulation	Mar-97
Naproxen, injectable (NANOX®)	CLINICAL (I)	Mimetix (US)	Injectable naproxen	Apr-97
Naratriptan (NARAMIG®; AMERGE™)	LAUNCHED	Glaxo Wellcome (UK)	5-HT1d/1b agonist	Apr-98
Narcotic analgesic patch	Preclinical	Amarin (UK)	Transdermal narcotic patch	Aug-99
narcotic analgesic patch, Elan	Preclinical	Elan (Ireland)	Transdermal narcotic patch	Feb-02
NB1 (Nociblocker)	Discontinued	Nortran (Canada)	Peripheral analgesic (unidentified)	Dec-99
NC-164	Preclinical	CAMR (UK)	Unidentified (botulinum frag.)	Jan-99
NC-503 (Fibrillex)	CLINICAL (III)	Neurochem (Canada)	Amyloid deposit inhibitor (arthritis)	Mar-00
N-calcium channel blockers	Preclinical	NeuroMed Technologies	Centrally-acting analgesic	Feb-02
NCS-700	Inactive	CNRS (France)	PDE-IV + TNF-α inhibitor	Jul-99
NCX-099	Inactive	NicOx (France)	Antiinflammatory (unspecified)	Feb-02
NCX-284	Inactive	NicOx (France)	NSAID + NO releaser	Feb-02
NCX-285	Preclinical	NicOx (France)	Centrally-acting analgesic	Feb-02
NCX-701	CLINICAL (I)	NicOx (France)	NSAID + NO releaser	Feb-02
NE 1704	Discontinued	Neose Technologies	Antiinflammatory	Feb-02

Ref.: Pharmaprojects (updated to 2/02) used with permission; Scrip, corporate, literature & patent references
"Status" is international drug development or regulatory status and may not indicate status in USA
Sponsor: Original company name is retained if product is discontinued or inactive after merger, acquisition, company name change, etc.
Users of this table are encouraged to independently verify the status, activity, and mechanism of action of drugs of interest

GENERIC / TRADE NAME	STATUS	SPONSOR (S)	MECHANISM OF ACTION	REF. UPDATE
NE-21610	Inactive	Procter & Gamble (US)	Unknown	1989
Nefazodone	LAUNCHED	Bristol-Myers Squibb (US)	5-HT uptake inhib.; 5-HT2 antag.	Apr-96
nefopam	LAUNCHED	3M (US)	NSAID	Feb-02
Nerbacadol (HWA-272)	Discontinued (ph. III)	Hoechst Marion Roussel (Ger.)	NSAID	May-90
Neuroactive peptides	Preclinical	NeuroSearch (Denmark)	CCK analogs	Jan-93
neuropathic pain ther, ProVec	Preclinical	GlaxoSmithKline (UK)	Formulation	Feb-02
neurotensin, Merck	Inactive	Merck & Co (US)	Neurotensin & analogs	1982
Neurotropin	LAUNCHED	Nippon Zoki (Japan)	Inflam. rabbit skin extract	Jan-92
neutrophil elastase inhib, Imm	Discontinued	Texas Biotechnology	Antiarthritic	Feb-02
NF-AT decoy, Corgentech	Preclinical	Corgentech	Antiinflammatory	Feb-02
NF-kappaB decoy, Corgentech	Preclinical	Corgentech	Antiinflammatory	Feb-02
NF-kB inhibitors, Aventis	Preclinical	Aventis (France)	Antiinflammatory	Feb-02
NGD-2000-1	CLINICAL (I)	Neurogen (US)	Antiinflammatory	Feb-02
NGX.231	Preclinical	NeurogesX (US)	Neuropathic pain / antiinflammatory	Feb-02
Niacinamide (vitamin B3)	Discontinued (Clin.)	NIH (US)	Unidentified (osteoarthritis)	Jul-98
nicocortonide	Discontinued	Yamanouchi (Japan)	Antiarthritic	Feb-02
Nifalatide	Discontinued	Wellcome (UK)	Enkephalin analog	Mar-87
Niflangel	Discontinued (ph. II)	Yoshitomi (Japan)	Unidentified anti-inflammatory	Nov-87
NIH-10494	Inactive	NIH (US)	Opioid analgesic	1989
NIK-264	Discontinued (ph. II)	Nikken Chemical (Japan)	Unidentified (cancer pain)	Feb-02
nimesulide	LAUNCHED	Helsinn	Antiinflammatory	Feb-02
Niravoline (RU 51599)	Discontinued (ph. II)	Hoechst Marion Roussel (Ger)	Kappa agonist "aquaretic"	Aug-96
nitraquazone	Discontinued	Bayer (Germany)	Antiinflammatory	Feb-02
Nitric oxide blockers	Discontinued	NeuroSearch (Denmark)	Nitric oxide receptor antag.	Sep-96
nitrosoxacin-A	Discontinued	Bristol-Myers Squibb (US)	Antiinflammatory	Feb-02
NK2 antagonists, Schering-Plou	Preclinical	Schering Plough (US)	Antiinflammatory	Feb-02
NKT-343 (SDZ-NKT-343)	Discontinued	Novartis (Switz.)	NK-1 antagonist	May-99
NM-105	Discontinued	GeriatRx (Canada)	Unidentified (antimigraine)	Oct-96
NM-135	Discontinued	Nissin Food Products (Japan)	Prodrug steriod; anti-inflam.	Feb-02
NMDA antagonist, Vernalis	Preclinical	Vernalis (UK)	Centrally-acting analgesic	Feb-02
NMI-172 (ibuprofen-SNO)	Inactive	NitroMed (US) / J&J (US)	Ibuprofen w/nitric oxide donor	Apr-00
NMI-246 (ketoprofen-SNO)	Inactive	NitroMed (US) / J&J (US)	Ketoprofen w/nitric oxide donor	Nov-99
NMI-267 (indomethacin-SNO)	Inactive	NitroMed (US) / J&J (US)	Indomethacin w/nitric oxide donor	Nov-99
NMI-346 (diclofenac-SNO)	Inactive	NitroMed (US) / J&J (US)	Diclofenac w/nitric oxide donor	Jun-00
NMI-377	Inactive	NitroMed (US)	Diclofenac w/nitric oxide donor	Aug-99
NNC-05-1869	CLINICAL (I)	Novo Nordisk (Denmark)	Unknown / diabetic neuropathy	Apr-97
Nociceptin	Discontinued	Euroscreen (Belgium)	Opioid ORL-1 agonist	Aug-99
Nociceptin/orphanin antags.	Inactive	CoCensys (US)	Opioid orphan receptor antag.	Jun-99
Nociceptive	Preclinical	Merck (US) / Banyu (Japan)	Opioid ORL-1 antagonist	Jan-00
Nolpitantium chloride (SR-140333)	CLINICAL (I)	Sanofi (France)	NK-1 antag.; inflam. & migraine	Aug-98
Nonane / Decane derv.	Inactive	Procter & Gamble (US)	5-HT agonist	Unk.
Non-narcotic plant derivative	Preclinical	Dong Wha (Korea)	Unknown	Jul-95
NO-NSAIDS	Preclinical	NitroMed (US) / J&J (US)	NSAID + NO releaser	Jul-97
NO-NSAIDS, NicOx	Preclinical	NicOx (France)	NSAID + NO releaser	Feb-02
NOX-200	Discontinued	Medinox (US)	Nitric oxide scavenger; arthritis	Feb-00
NPC-12626	Preclinical	Scios Nova (US)	Excitatory amino acid antag.	Jan-92
NPC-15670	Inactive	Scios (US)	Antiarthritic	Feb-02
NPC-16731	Preclinical	Scios Nova (US)	Bradykinin antagonist	May-91
NPC-17730	Preclinical	Novo-Nordisk (Denmark)	Bradykinin antagonist	Jan-92
NPC-17731	Preclinical	Scios Nova (US)	B2 antagonist	Oct-93
NPC-17923	Discontinued	Scios (US)	Antiarthritic	Feb-02
NPC-18545 (NPC-18608)	Discontinued	Scios (US)	Bradykinin B2 antagonist	Oct-97
NPC-349	Discontinued	Scios Nova (US)	Bradykinin antagonist	Feb-92
NPC-567	Discontinued	Scios Nova (US)	Bradykinin antagonist	Feb-92
NPS-846	Discontinued	NPS Pharmaceuticals (US)	Glutamate antagonist (Araxin)	1997
NRD-101	Launched	Aventis (France)	Hyaluronic acid (inj.); arthritis	Feb-02
NRT-115	Discontinued	Centaur (US)	Free radical scavenger; arthritis	Dec-99
NS-398	Discontinued	Taisho (Japan)	Antiinflammatory	Feb-02
NS-649 (NS-626)	Discontinued	NeuroSearch (Denmark)	Ca++ channel antag., N-type	Feb-96
NSAID prodrugs, Medinox	Preclinical	Medinox (US)	NSAID	Feb-02
N-vanillylnonamide analogues	Discontinued	Procter & Gamble (US)	Capsaicin analogues	Apr-85
NW-1029	Preclinical	Newron	Centrally-acting analgesic	Feb-02
NXTHIO	Discontinued (PRE-REG)	Applied Pharma Res. (Switz)	Naproxen + mucolytic	Jun-98

Ref.: Pharmaprojects (updated to 2/02) used with permission; Scrip, corporate, literature & patent references
"Status" is international drug development or regulatory status and may not indicate status in USA
Sponsor: Original company name is retained if product is discontinued or inactive after merger, acquisition, company name change, etc.
Users of this table are encouraged to independently verify the status, activity, and mechanism of action of drugs of interest

GENERIC / TRADE NAME	STATUS	SPONSOR (S)	MECHANISM OF ACTION	REF. UPDATE
OA-6025	Preclinical	Genzyme (US)	Antiarthritic	Feb-02
Ocfentanil	Discontinued (ph. II)	Ohmeda (US)	Fentanyl analog	Jun-91
Ociltide (Hoe-825)	Discontinued (ph. II)	Hoechst Marion Roussel (Ger)	Enkephalin analog	Oct-88
Octreotide (SANDOSTATIN®)	LAUNCHED	Sandoz (Switz)	Somatostatin analog (i.th.)	1993
odalprofen	Discontinued	Chiesi (Italy)	Antiinflammatory	Feb-02
OF-743	Discontinued	Moscow State Univ. (Russia)	Unidentified	Mar-97
OHM-3295	Discontinued	Ohmeda (US)	Fentanyl analog	May-96
Oligopeptides	Preclinical	SPA (Italy)	Oral lysozyme metabolites	May-96
Olvanil	Inactive	Procter & Gamble (US)	Capsaicin analogue	Jul-91
Omega-conotoxin GVIA	Discontinued	Biomolecular Res. Inst. (Austr.)	Ca++ antagonist; cone shell toxin	Feb-02
ONO-2921	Preclinical	Ono (Japan)	Centrally-acting analgesic	Feb-02
ONO-3144 (AI-3144)	Discontinued (ph. III)	Ono (Japan)	NSAID	Sep-87
ONO-4817	CLINICAL (I)	Ono (Japan)	Antiarthritic	Feb-02
ONO-5349	Discontinued	Ono (Japan)	Antiinflammatory	Feb-02
ONO-8711	CLINICAL (I)	Ono (Japan)	Prostaglandin EP1 antagonist	Apr-00
ONO-9902	Discontinued (ph. II)	Ono (Japan)	Enkephalinase inhibitor, oral	Feb-96
ONO-NT-012	Discontinued	Ono (Japan)	PGE1/E3 prostanoid agonist	Nov-96
Ontazolast (BI-RM-270)	Discontinued (ph. II)	Boehringer Ingelheim (Ger)	LTB4 synthesis inhibitor	May-97
opioid agonists, Molecumetics	Preclinical	Molecumetics	Opioid analgesic	Feb-02
Opioid analgesics, Adolor	Preclinical	Adolor (US)	Kappa agonists, peripheral	Jun-99
opioid analgesics, BTG	Inactive	BTG (UK)	Opioid analgesic	Feb-02
Opioid peptides	Discontinued	Unigene (US)	Opioid agonist	Mar-87
Opioid peptides	Discontinued	Univ. Arizona (US)	Opioid agonist	Sep-98
OR-1384	Preclinical	Orion Pharma (Finland)	Polymorph. neutrophil inhib.	Oct-98
Orazipone (OR-1384)	Inactive	Orion Pharma (Finland)	Neutrophil superoxide antag.	Mar-99
Org-25543	Preclinical	Akzo Nobel (Netherlands)	Centrally-acting analgesic	Feb-02
Org-5878	Discontinued	Akzo (Netherlands)	Endorphin	Apr-91
Org-7258	Inactive	Akzo Nobel (Netherlands)	Antiinflammatory	Feb-02
Org-GC94	Discontinued	Akzo Nobel (Netherlands)	Antimigraine	Feb-02
ORL-1 antagonists, Adolor	Preclinical	Adolor (US)	Central opioid analgesic	Feb-02
Orolip DP	Inactive	EpiCept (US)	Timed-release neuropeptides	Feb-02
Orolip E	Inactive	EpiCept (US)	Oral sustained-rel. enkephalins	Feb-02
Orpanoxin (F-776)	Discontinued (Clin.)	Procter & Gamble (US)	NSAID	Jun-86
Osteoarthritis therapy	Preclinical	Genzyme (US)	Unidentified mech. (osteoarthritis)	Nov-99
osteoarthritis therapy, Incyt	Preclinical	Incyte Genomics	Antiarthritic	Feb-02
OT-7100	Discontinued	Otsuka (Japan)	NK-1 receptor antag.	Jan-99
OT-Piroxicam	Preclinical	Anesta (US)	Oral transmucosal formulation	Mar-99
Oxadiazolylarylmethanones	Discontinued	Hoechst (Ger)	Unknown	Mar-88
oxametacin	LAUNCHED	ABC	Antiinflammatory	Feb-02
oxanthinecarboxylic acid	Inactive	Takeda (Japan)	Antiinflammatory	Feb-02
Oxapadol (MD-720111)	Discontinued (Clin.)	Synthelabo (France)	Unidentified antiinflammatory analg.	Feb-83
Oxaprozin (DAYPRO®)	LAUNCHED	Searle (US)/Am Home Prod	NSAID, 1x daily	Mar-96
oxaprozin meglumine	Discontinued	Therapicon (Italy)	Antiinflammatory	Feb-02
oxaprozin potassium	PRE-REGISTRATION	Pharmacia (US)	Antiarthritic	Feb-02
Oxazepines	Inactive	Knoll (Ger)	Oxidoreductase	Apr-85
Oxepinac (DD-3314)	Discontinued (ph. III)	Daiichi (Japan)	Prostaglandin synthase inhib.	1980s
oxetorone	LAUNCHED	Sanofi-Synthelabo (France)	Antimigraine	Feb-02
oxindanac	Discontinued	Novartis (Switz.)	Antiarthritic	Feb-02
OxycoDex® combination	CLINICAL (II)	Endo / Algos (US)	Oxycodone + dextromethorphan	Jun-00
Oxycodone (OXYCONTIN®)	LAUNCHED	Purdue Pharma (US)	Formulation, oral 12 hr oxycodone	Apr-98
oxycodone + ibuprofen, BTG	PRE-REGISTRATION	Forest (US) / BTG	Analgesic combination	Feb-02
oxycodone + naloxone, Purdue	CLINICAL	Purdue Pharma (US)	Analgesic combination	Feb-02
oxycodone + paracetamol, Barr	Inactive	Barr Laboratories (US)	Analgesic combination	Feb-02
oxycodone, Bentley	Preclinical	Bentley	Formulation	Feb-02
Oxycodone, Mundipharma	CLINICAL (III)	Shionogi (Jp) / Mundipharma	Controlled release	Nov-97
Oxymorphonazine	Discontinued	Scios Nova (US)	Opioid mu-1 agonist	Nov-88
oxymorphone, TIMERx	CLINICAL (III)	Endo Pharmaceuticals (US)	Controlled-release formulation	Feb-02
P-07	CLINICAL (II)	Novogen (Australia)	Phytoestrogen form. (mastalgia)	Jul-98
P-1230	Discontinued (ph. II)	Poli (Italy)	Unidentified analgesic	Jul-87
P16CM	Discontinued	Florida A&M Univ. (US)	16-substituted prednisolone der.	May-97
p38 MAP kinase inhibs, Uriach	Preclinical	Uriach (Spain)	Antiinflammatory	Feb-02
P54	CLINICAL (II)	Phytopharm (UK)	OA, IBS: phytomedicine; NSAID	May-98
P61	Preclinical	Phytopharm (UK)	Antiinflammatory	Feb-02

Ref.: Pharmaprojects (updated to 2/02) used with permission; Scrip, corporate, literature & patent references
"Status" is international drug development or regulatory status and may not indicate status in USA
Sponsor: Original company name is retained if product is discontinued or inactive after merger, acquisition, company name change, etc.
Users of this table are encouraged to independently verify the status, activity, and mechanism of action of drugs of interest

GENERIC / TRADE NAME	STATUS	SPONSOR (S)	MECHANISM OF ACTION	REF. UPDATE
P-7521	Inactive	Shenkai Inst. Materia Med.	Opioid analgesic	1987
Pain gene therapy	Preclinical	Univ. South Carolina (US)	Preproenkephalin gene (HSV vector)	Jun-99
pain therapies, Arakis	Preclinical	Arakis	Formulation	Feb-02
Panoderm calcitonin	Discontinued (ph. III)	Elan (Ireland)	Iontophoretic transdermal opioids	Jun-99
Panoderm hydromorphone	CLINICAL (III)	Elan (Ireland)	Formulation, transdermal	Jul-96
Paracetamol + codeine	Discontinued	Alza (US)	Controlled release	Mar-89
Paracetamol + dihydrocodeine	LAUNCHED	Napp (UK)	Formulation, paracetamol + DHC	Mar-96
Paracetamol formulation	CLINICAL	Himedics (US)	APAP formulation	1991
Paracetamol formulation	Discontinued	Alza (US)	Controlled release	Mar-90
Paracetamol formulation	Discontinued	Scios Nova (US)	Edible whip APAP	Mar-91
Paracetamol suppositories	LAUNCHED	SS Pharmaceutical (Japan)	APAP formulation	Dec-91
paracetamol, EFVDAS	LAUNCHED	Elan (Ireland)	APAP formulation	Feb-02
paracetamol, Elan PharmaZome	Inactive	Elan (Ireland)	APAP formulation	Feb-02
paracetamol+dihydrocodeine	LAUNCHED	Napp (UK)	Analgesic combination	Feb-02
Parcetasal	Discontinued (PRE-REG)	Medea Research (Italy)	PGSI	1997
Parecoxib	PRE-REGISTRATION	Pharmacia (US)	COX-2 antagonist (inj.)	Feb-02
Paroxetine (PAXIL®)	LAUNCHED	Novo-Nordisk (Denmark)	Antidepress; 5-HT uptake inh.	Mar-97
parsalmide	LAUNCHED	Sanofi-Synthelabo (France)	Antiinflammatory	Feb-02
p-benzyloxyphenol	Inactive	Pfizer (US)	Antiinflammatory	Feb-02
PBI-1101	CLINICAL (II)	ProMetic LifeSciences	Antiinflammatory	Feb-02
PD-057081	Inactive	Pfizer (US)	Antiarthritic	Feb-02
PD-117302	Discontinued	Warner-Lambert (US)	Kappa agonist	Mar-94
PD-122263	Inactive	Warner-Lambert (US)	CCK analogs	Jul-92
PD-127443	Inactive	Pfizer (US)	Antiinflammatory	Feb-02
PD-129290	Inactive	Warner-Lambert (US)	Kappa agonist	Aug-91
PD-136005	Discontinued	Warner-Lambert (US)	COX/5-LO inhibitor	Aug-95
PD-144795	Discontinued	Warner-Lambert (US)	ICAM 1 antagonist	May-97
PD-145246	Inactive	Pfizer (US)	Antiinflammatory	Feb-02
PD-172084	Inactive	Millennium (US)	Antiarthritic	Feb-02
PD-98059	Discontinued	Warner-Lambert (US)	MAP kinase inhibitor	Jun-00
PDE inhibitors, Bayer	Discontinued	Bayer (Germany)	Phosphodiesterase inhibitor	Mar-98
PDE-IV inhibitors	Preclinical	ICOS (US)	Phosphodiesterase IV inhib.	May-99
PDE-IV inhibitors	Preclinical	Syntex/Roche (Switzerland)	Type IV Phosphodiesterase inhib.	Apr-95
PEG-catalase, Sterling	Inactive	Sanofi-Synthelabo (France)	Antiinflammatory	Feb-02
PEGsTHFr1	CLINICAL (II)	Amgen (US)	TNF receptor antagonist / RA	Nov-99
Peltazone	Discontinued (ph. III)	Takeda (Japan)	Unidentified analgesic	Feb-95
Pelubiprofen (CS-670)	CLINICAL (III)	Sankyo (Japan)	T cell stimulant, anti-inflam.	Mar-98
Pemedolac (AY-30715)	Discontinued (ph. I)	Wyeth-Ayerst (US)	NSAID	May-96
Pentamorphone (A-4492; RX-77989)	Discontinued (ph. III)	Baxter / Ohmeda (US)	Opioid mu agonist	Jul-91
Pentazocine, nasal	Inactive	Nastech (US)	Opioid agonist/antagonist	Oct-84
Peptide T	Discontinued (ph. II)	Peptech (Australia) / NIH	TNF-alpha inhibitor / HIV	Mar-97
Peptidomimetic	Discontinued	Yissum (Israel)	Cyclic peptide	Jan-93
Peptidomimetic	Inactive	Univ. Arizona (US)	Delta agonist	1989
perisoxal citrate	LAUNCHED	Shionogi (Japan)	Antiinflammatory	Feb-02
PGE-2946979 (PGE-5747401)	Discontinued	Procter & Gamble (US)	MMP inhibitor / OA	Jun-00
PGE-4304887	Preclinical	Procter & Gamble (US)	Antiarthritic	Feb-02
ph-913 (LidoPain®)	PRE-REGISTRATION	EpiCept (US)	Transdermal patch; unknown opioid	Feb-98
ph-921A	Suspended	pharmed (Ger)	Transdermal opioids	Jun-92
Pharmaprojects No. 1001	Discontinued	Bristol-Myers Squibb (US)	Antiinflammatory	Feb-02
Pharmaprojects No. 1018	Discontinued	Novartis (Switz.)	Antiinflammatory	Feb-02
Pharmaprojects No. 1079	Inactive	Boehringer Ingelheim (Ger)	Antiinflammatory	Feb-02
Pharmaprojects No. 1084	Discontinued	Mediolanum	Antiinflammatory	Feb-02
Pharmaprojects No. 1135	Inactive	Merck & Co (US)	Centrally-acting analgesic	Feb-02
Pharmaprojects No. 1141	Inactive	Merck & Co (US)	Antiinflammatory	Feb-02
Pharmaprojects No. 1205	Discontinued	SRI International	Centrally-acting analgesic	Feb-02
Pharmaprojects No. 12059	Discontinued	Abbott (US)	Antiinflammatory	Feb-02
Pharmaprojects No. 1247	Inactive	Non-industrial source	Antiinflammatory	Feb-02
Pharmaprojects No. 1248	Discontinued	Dainippon (Japan)	Centrally-acting analgesic	Feb-02
Pharmaprojects No. 1251	Inactive	Aventis (France)	Antiinflammatory	Feb-02
Pharmaprojects No. 1257	Inactive	Aventis (France)	Antimigraine	Feb-02
Pharmaprojects No. 1261	Discontinued	Aventis (France)	Antiarthritic	Feb-02
Pharmaprojects No. 1302	Discontinued	Bristol-Myers Squibb (US)	Antiinflammatory	Feb-02
Pharmaprojects No. 1311	Inactive	Non-industrial source	Antiinflammatory	Feb-02

Ref.: Pharmaprojects (updated to 2/02) used with permission; Scrip, corporate, literature & patent references
"Status" is international drug development or regulatory status and may not indicate status in USA
Sponsor: Original company name is retained if product is discontinued or inactive after merger, acquisition, company name change, etc.
Users of this table are encouraged to independently verify the status, activity, and mechanism of action of drugs of interest

GENERIC / TRADE NAME	STATUS	SPONSOR (S)	MECHANISM OF ACTION	REF. UPDATE
Pharmaprojects No. 1369	Inactive	Maruzen Seiyaku	Antiinflammatory	Feb-02
Pharmaprojects No. 1376	Inactive	Roche (Switz)	Centrally-acting analgesic	Feb-02
Pharmaprojects No. 1379	Inactive	Sankyo (Japan)	NSAID	Feb-02
Pharmaprojects No. 1421	Discontinued	Non-industrial source	Centrally-acting analgesic	Feb-02
Pharmaprojects No. 1446	Discontinued	Aventis (France)	Centrally-acting analgesic	Feb-02
Pharmaprojects No. 1472	Inactive	Sanofi-Synthelabo (France)	Antiinflammatory	Feb-02
Pharmaprojects No. 1490	Discontinued	Aventis (France)	Centrally-acting analgesic	Feb-02
Pharmaprojects No. 1524	Discontinued	American Home Products (US)	Antiinflammatory	Feb-02
Pharmaprojects No. 1550	Inactive	Merck & Co (US)	Antiinflammatory	Feb-02
Pharmaprojects No. 1573	Inactive	Pharmacia (US)	Antiarthritic	Feb-02
Pharmaprojects No. 1586	Inactive	Pharmacia (US)	Centrally-acting analgesic	Feb-02
Pharmaprojects No. 1587	Inactive	Non-industrial source	Centrally-acting analgesic	Feb-02
Pharmaprojects No. 1618	Inactive	Non-industrial source	NSAID	Feb-02
Pharmaprojects No. 1653	Discontinued	Recordati	Antiinflammatory	Feb-02
Pharmaprojects No. 1657	Discontinued	Schering AG (Germany)	Antiinflammatory	Feb-02
Pharmaprojects No. 1660	Discontinued	Roche (Switz)	Antiinflammatory	Feb-02
Pharmaprojects No. 1673	Discontinued	Aventis (France)	Antiinflammatory	Feb-02
Pharmaprojects No. 1687	Discontinued	Roche (Switz)	Centrally-acting analgesic	Feb-02
Pharmaprojects No. 1688	Inactive	Sanofi-Synthelabo (France)	Antiinflammatory	Feb-02
Pharmaprojects No. 1707	Discontinued	Novartis (Switz.)	Antiinflammatory	Feb-02
Pharmaprojects No. 1738	Inactive	GlaxoSmithKline (UK)	NSAID	Feb-02
Pharmaprojects No. 1741	Discontinued	American Home Products (US)	Antiinflammatory	Feb-02
Pharmaprojects No. 1749	Discontinued	GlaxoSmithKline (UK)	Antiinflammatory	Feb-02
Pharmaprojects No. 1756	Discontinued	Alpharma (US)	Antiinflammatory	Feb-02
Pharmaprojects No. 1763	Discontinued	Kayaku	Antiinflammatory	Feb-02
Pharmaprojects No. 1805	Inactive	Abbott (US)	Antiinflammatory	Feb-02
Pharmaprojects No. 1860	Discontinued	Schering Plough (US)	Antiinflammatory	Feb-02
Pharmaprojects No. 1863	Inactive	Pfizer (US)	Centrally-acting analgesic	Feb-02
Pharmaprojects No. 1874	Discontinued	Daiichi (Japan)	Centrally-acting analgesic	Feb-02
Pharmaprojects No. 1878	Inactive	Akzo Nobel (Netherlands)	Antiinflammatory	Feb-02
Pharmaprojects No. 1894	Inactive	AstraZeneca (UK)	Antiinflammatory	Feb-02
Pharmaprojects No. 1903	Inactive	Fujisawa (Japan)	Antiinflammatory	Feb-02
Pharmaprojects No. 1910	Discontinued	Abbott (US)	Antiinflammatory	Feb-02
Pharmaprojects No. 1928	Inactive	Research Corp. Tech. (US)	Centrally-acting analgesic	Feb-02
Pharmaprojects No. 1943	Discontinued	Servier (France)	5-HT antagonist	Apr-90
Pharmaprojects No. 1967	Discontinued	Schering Plough (US)	Antiinflammatory	Feb-02
Pharmaprojects No. 1970	Discontinued	AstraZeneca (UK)	Antiinflammatory	Feb-02
Pharmaprojects No. 1998	Inactive	Chiesi (Italy)	Antiinflammatory	Feb-02
Pharmaprojects No. 2008	Inactive	Nycomed Pharma (Norway)	Centrally-acting analgesic	Feb-02
Pharmaprojects No. 2010	Inactive	Yamanouchi (Japan)	Antiinflammatory	Feb-02
Pharmaprojects No. 2015	Discontinued	Bristol-Myers Squibb (US)	Antiarthritic	Feb-02
Pharmaprojects No. 2016	Inactive	Toyobo	Antiarthritic	Feb-02
Pharmaprojects No. 2029	Discontinued	American Home Products (US)	Antiarthritic	Feb-02
Pharmaprojects No. 2054	Inactive	Mitsubishi Pharma (Japan)	Antiinflammatory	Feb-02
Pharmaprojects No. 2096	Inactive	Procter & Gamble (US)	Centrally-acting analgesic	Feb-02
Pharmaprojects No. 2119	Discontinued	Roche (Switz)	Antiinflammatory	Feb-02
Pharmaprojects No. 2120	Discontinued	Fresenius	Centrally-acting analgesic	Feb-02
Pharmaprojects No. 2139	Inactive	Merck & Co (US)	Antiinflammatory	Feb-02
Pharmaprojects No. 2145	Inactive	Biosearch Italia (Italy)	NSAID	Feb-02
Pharmaprojects No. 2157	Discontinued	Pharmacia (US)	Antiinflammatory	Feb-02
Pharmaprojects No. 2167	Discontinued	Toa Eiyo	Antiinflammatory	Feb-02
Pharmaprojects No. 2193	Discontinued	Abbott (US)	Antiarthritic	Feb-02
Pharmaprojects No. 2264	Inactive	Bayer (Germany)	Antiinflammatory	Feb-02
Pharmaprojects No. 2332	Discontinued	Roche (Switz)	Antiinflammatory	Feb-02
Pharmaprojects No. 2354	Discontinued	Grunenthal (Germany)	NSAID	Feb-02
Pharmaprojects No. 2356	Inactive	Lilly (US)	Centrally-acting analgesic	Feb-02
Pharmaprojects No. 2362	Inactive	Non-industrial source	Centrally-acting analgesic	Feb-02
Pharmaprojects No. 2368	Inactive	Aventis (France)	NSAID	Feb-02
Pharmaprojects No. 2434	Discontinued	Novartis Consumer (Switz.)	Antiarthritic	Feb-02
Pharmaprojects No. 2446	Discontinued	SRI Int'l (US)	Opioid agonist/antagonist	Apr-95
Pharmaprojects No. 2456	Inactive	Novartis (Switz.)	Antiarthritic	Feb-02
Pharmaprojects No. 2462	Inactive	Novartis (Switz.)	Antiinflammatory	Feb-02
Pharmaprojects No. 2502	Inactive	Pharmol Pacific (Austral)	Unk. / centrally-acting	1988

Ref.: Pharmaprojects (updated to 2/02) used with permission; Scrip, corporate, literature & patent references
"Status" is international drug development or regulatory status and may not indicate status in USA
Sponsor: Original company name is retained if product is discontinued or inactive after merger, acquisition, company name change, etc.
Users of this table are encouraged to independently verify the status, activity, and mechanism of action of drugs of interest

GENERIC / TRADE NAME	STATUS	SPONSOR (S)	MECHANISM OF ACTION	REF. UPDATE
Pharmaprojects No. 2503	Discontinued	Kaken (Japan)	Antiinflammatory	Feb-02
Pharmaprojects No. 2506	Inactive	Schering Plough (US)	Antiinflammatory	Feb-02
Pharmaprojects No. 2515	Inactive	American Home Products (US)	Antiinflammatory	Feb-02
Pharmaprojects No. 2516	Inactive	American Home Products (US)	Antiinflammatory	Feb-02
Pharmaprojects No. 2519	Discontinued	Vita-Invest (Spain)	Unidentified (antimigraine)	Mar-96
Pharmaprojects No. 2520	Discontinued	Roche (Switz)	NSAID	Feb-02
Pharmaprojects No. 2523	Discontinued	Merck & Co (US)	COX/LTB4 inhibitor	Apr-92
Pharmaprojects No. 2540	Discontinued	Genetics Institute	PLA2 inhibitor	Jun-00
Pharmaprojects No. 2541	Discontinued	Mitsubishi Pharma (Japan)	Antiinflammatory	Feb-02
Pharmaprojects No. 2552	Inactive	Non-industrial source	Centrally-acting analgesic	Feb-02
Pharmaprojects No. 2553	Discontinued	Abbott (US)	Antiinflammatory	Feb-02
Pharmaprojects No. 2657	Discontinued	SmithKline Beecham (UK)	5-HT antagonist	Aug-92
Pharmaprojects No. 2660	Discontinued	Dainippon (Japan)	Antiinflammatory	Feb-02
Pharmaprojects No. 2662	Discontinued	Sanofi-Synthelabo (France)	Antiinflammatory	Feb-02
Pharmaprojects No. 2671	Inactive	Kuraray	Antiinflammatory	Feb-02
Pharmaprojects No. 2707	Inactive	Pfizer (US)	Antiinflammatory	Feb-02
Pharmaprojects No. 2737	Discontinued	Aventis (France)	Centrally-acting analgesic	Feb-02
Pharmaprojects No. 2744	Inactive	Sanofi-Synthelabo (France)	Centrally-acting analgesic	Feb-02
Pharmaprojects No. 2755	Inactive	American Home Products (US)	Antiarthritic	Feb-02
Pharmaprojects No. 2782	Discontinued	GlaxoSmithKline (UK)	Centrally-acting analgesic	Feb-02
Pharmaprojects No. 2790	Discontinued	Faes (Spain)	Fentanyl analog	Aug-95
Pharmaprojects No. 2794	Discontinued	Aventis (France)	Antiinflammatory	Feb-02
Pharmaprojects No. 2800	Inactive	Pfizer (US)	Antiinflammatory	Feb-02
Pharmaprojects No. 2817	Discontinued	Boron Biologicals (US)	IL-1 antagonist, TNF-a antagonist	Jun-00
Pharmaprojects No. 2840	Discontinued	Shionogi (Japan)	Centrally-acting analgesic	Feb-02
Pharmaprojects No. 2848	Inactive	American Home Products (US)	Antiinflammatory	Feb-02
Pharmaprojects No. 2850	Discontinued	Kureha Chemical	Antiarthritic	Feb-02
Pharmaprojects No. 2853	Discontinued	AstraZeneca (UK)	Centrally-acting analgesic	Feb-02
Pharmaprojects No. 2857	Discontinued	Vinas (Spain)	Antiinflammatory	Feb-02
Pharmaprojects No. 2866	Inactive	Nisshin Flour (Japan)	Centrally-acting analgesic	Feb-02
Pharmaprojects No. 2871	Inactive	Aventis (France)	Antiinflammatory	Feb-02
Pharmaprojects No. 2876	Discontinued	Warner-Lambert (US)	Fentanyl analog, short acting	May-94
Pharmaprojects No. 2886	Inactive	Aventis (France)	Centrally-acting analgesic	Feb-02
Pharmaprojects No. 2936	Discontinued	DuPont (US)	Kallikrein antagonist	Sep-93
Pharmaprojects No. 2943	Inactive	Pfizer (US)	Antiinflammatory	Feb-02
Pharmaprojects No. 2968	Inactive	GlaxoSmithKline (UK)	Antiarthritic	Feb-02
Pharmaprojects No. 2969	Inactive	GlaxoSmithKline (UK)	Antiarthritic	Feb-02
Pharmaprojects No. 3056	Inactive	Ariad	Antiarthritic	Feb-02
Pharmaprojects No. 3063	Preclinical	Adcock Ingram (RSA)	Unk. / non-narcotic	Apr-92
Pharmaprojects No. 3089	Inactive	MacroNex	Antiinflammatory	Feb-02
Pharmaprojects No. 3169	Discontinued	Oxford GlycoSciences (UK)	Antiinflammatory	Feb-02
Pharmaprojects No. 3193	Inactive	Pharmagenesis	Antiinflammatory	Feb-02
Pharmaprojects No. 3197	Inactive	ISIS Pharmaceuticals (US)	Antiinflammatory	Feb-02
Pharmaprojects No. 3217	Inactive	Millennium (US)	Antiinflammatory	Feb-02
Pharmaprojects No. 3232	Inactive	Eisai (Japan)	Antiinflammatory	Feb-02
Pharmaprojects No. 3240	Discontinued	Boehringer Ingelheim (Ger)	Antiarthritic	Feb-02
Pharmaprojects No. 3253	Inactive	Ligand (US)	Antiarthritic	Feb-02
Pharmaprojects No. 3258	Discontinued	Sanofi-Synthelabo (France)	Antiinflammatory	Feb-02
Pharmaprojects No. 3259	Inactive	Lilly (US)	Antiinflammatory	Feb-02
Pharmaprojects No. 3268	Inactive	Lilly (US)	Antiinflammatory	Feb-02
Pharmaprojects No. 3274	Inactive	Novartis (Switz.)	Antiarthritic	Feb-02
Pharmaprojects No. 3282	Discontinued	Biofor (US)	Antiarthritic	Feb-02
Pharmaprojects No. 3335	Inactive	Pfizer (US)	Antiinflammatory	Feb-02
Pharmaprojects No. 3337	Discontinued	Manchester Innovation	Antiinflammatory	Feb-02
Pharmaprojects No. 3347	Discontinued	Merck & Co (US)	Substance P antagnoist	1997
Pharmaprojects No. 3350	Inactive	Pharmacia (US)	Antiinflammatory	Feb-02
Pharmaprojects No. 3355	Inactive	Bayer (Germany)	Antiinflammatory	Feb-02
Pharmaprojects No. 3357	Inactive	Merck & Co (US)	Antiinflammatory	Feb-02
Pharmaprojects No. 3359	Inactive	Lilly (US)	Antiinflammatory	Feb-02
Pharmaprojects No. 3360	Inactive	Novartis (Switz.)	Antiinflammatory	Feb-02
Pharmaprojects No. 3389	Discontinued	Searle/Monsanto (US)	Delta agonist peptide	Mar-94
Pharmaprojects No. 3395	Inactive	Pharmacia (US)	Antiarthritic	Feb-02
Pharmaprojects No. 3420	Discontinued	Servier (France)	Unknown (non-opioid)	Mar-95

Ref.: Pharmaprojects (updated to 2/02) used with permission; Scrip, corporate, literature & patent references
"Status" is international drug development or regulatory status and may not indicate status in USA
Sponsor: Original company name is retained if product is discontinued or inactive after merger, acquisition, company name change, etc.
Users of this table are encouraged to independently verify the status, activity, and mechanism of action of drugs of interest

GENERIC / TRADE NAME	STATUS	SPONSOR (S)	MECHANISM OF ACTION	REF. UPDATE
Pharmaprojects No. 3435	Inactive	Abbott (US)	Antiinflammatory	Feb-02
Pharmaprojects No. 3443	Inactive	Aventis (France)	Antiinflammatory	Feb-02
Pharmaprojects No. 3444	Discontinued	Lilly (US)	5-LO inhibitor	Nov-94
Pharmaprojects No. 3449	Discontinued (ph. II)	Phytopharm (UK)	Unidentified (antimigraine)	Apr-95
Pharmaprojects No. 3484	Discontinued	AstraZeneca (UK)	NSAID	Feb-02
Pharmaprojects No. 3490	Inactive	Johnson & Johnson (US)	Antiinflammatory	Feb-02
Pharmaprojects No. 3492	Discontinued	Roche (Switz)	Leukotriene LTB4 antagonist	Dec-94
Pharmaprojects No. 3503	Inactive	Procter & Gamble (US)	Antiinflammatory	Feb-02
Pharmaprojects No. 3505	Discontinued	Procter & Gamble (US)	Antiinflammatory / antiarthritic	May-98
Pharmaprojects No. 3532	Inactive	Pharmacia (US)	Antiinflammatory	Feb-02
Pharmaprojects No. 3553	Discontinued	Novartis (Switz.)	Antiarthritic	May-98
Pharmaprojects No. 3582	Discontinued	Pharmacia (US)	Antiarthritic	Feb-02
Pharmaprojects No. 3647	Discontinued	Abbott (US)	Antiarthritic	Feb-02
Pharmaprojects No. 3651	Discontinued	Searle/Monsanto (US)	PGE2 receptor antagonist	Mar-94
Pharmaprojects No. 3680	Inactive	Merck KGaA (Germany)	Centrally-acting analgesic	Feb-02
Pharmaprojects No. 3694	Inactive	Aventis (France)	Antiarthritic	Feb-02
Pharmaprojects No. 3722	Inactive	Japan Tobacco (Japan)	Antiarthritic	Feb-02
Pharmaprojects No. 3775	Preclinical	Novo-Nordisk (Denmark)	Adenosine A1 antagonist	Nov-93
Pharmaprojects No. 3802	Discontinued	Roche (Switz)	Microbial collagenase inhibitor	May-98
Pharmaprojects No. 3818	Discontinued	Merck & Co (US)	Tachykinin antagonist	Jan-94
Pharmaprojects No. 3856	Discontinued	Scios Nova (US)	BK antagonist, 2nd generation	1997
Pharmaprojects No. 3858	Discontinued	Peptech (Australia)	Arachidonic acid antagonist	Jun-00
Pharmaprojects No. 3863	Discontinued	Peptech (Australia)	Antiinflammatory	Feb-02
Pharmaprojects No. 3873	Preclinical	Telor Ophthalmic (US)	Unk. / ocular pain	Mar-94
Pharmaprojects No. 3874	Preclinical	Regeneron / Glaxo (US)	Unknown	Mar-94
Pharmaprojects No. 3877	Discontinued	Medarex (US)	Intract. pain: destroys periph. nerves	Apr-96
Pharmaprojects No. 3879	Discontinued	Takeda (Japan)	Substance P antagonist	Aug-95
Pharmaprojects No. 3893	Discontinued	Merck & Co (US)	5-HT1a/2c agonist	Oct-95
Pharmaprojects No. 3896	Inactive	Pharmacia (US)	Antiinflammatory	Feb-02
Pharmaprojects No. 3905	Preclinical	Almirall (Spain)	5-HT3 antagonist	Apr-94
Pharmaprojects No. 3945	Preclinical	Theracel / Titan (US)	Cells / CNS implant	May-94
Pharmaprojects No. 3953	Discontinued	Boehringer Ingelheim (Ger)	Unknown / indazolone	Mar-96
Pharmaprojects No. 3957	Inactive	Telik (US)	Antiinflammatory	Feb-02
Pharmaprojects No. 3973	Discontinued	Schering Plough (US)	Antiinflammatory	Feb-02
Pharmaprojects No. 3976	Discontinued	Glaxo Wellcome (UK)	5-HT1 agonist	1997
Pharmaprojects No. 4006	Discontinued	Rhone-Poulenc Rorer (France)	Substance P antagonist (migraine)	Jan-96
Pharmaprojects No. 4029	Inactive	Celltech (UK)	Antiinflammatory	Feb-02
Pharmaprojects No. 4032	Discontinued	Novartis (Switz.)	Metalloproteinase inhib.	May-98
Pharmaprojects No. 4042	Discontinued	Rhone-Poulenc Rorer (France)	Glucocorticoid antag. steroid	Feb-96
Pharmaprojects No. 4044	Discontinued	SmithKline Beecham (UK)	5-HT1 agonist	Feb-96
Pharmaprojects No. 4079	Discontinued	Bristol-Myers Squibb (US)	Antiarthritic	Feb-02
Pharmaprojects No. 4088	Inactive	Pfizer (US)	Antiinflammatory	Feb-02
Pharmaprojects No. 4091	Discontinued	Rhone-Poulenc Rorer (France)	Glucocorticoid antag. steroid	Mar-96
Pharmaprojects No. 4099	Inactive	Merck & Co (US)	Antiinflammatory	Feb-02
Pharmaprojects No. 4107	Discontinued	GlaxoSmithKline (UK)	Antiinflammatory	Feb-02
Pharmaprojects No. 4137	Inactive	Trega Biosciences (US)	Opioid mu antagonist (peripheral)	Feb-02
Pharmaprojects No. 4171	Preclinical	Astra (Sweden)	Excitatory amino acid antag.	Nov-94
Pharmaprojects No. 4206	Discontinued	Proteus Molecular Design (UK)	Antiinflammatory (unidentified)	May-98
Pharmaprojects No. 4214	Discontinued	Glaxo Wellcome (UK)	COX/5-LO inhibitor	Jan-97
Pharmaprojects No. 4217	Discontinued	Searle/Monsanto (US)	PGE2 receptor antagonist	May-98
Pharmaprojects No. 4234	Discontinued	Menarini (Italy)	Antiinflammatory	Feb-02
Pharmaprojects No. 4282	Discontinued	Proteus Molecular Design (UK)	Unidentified	Jan-97
Pharmaprojects No. 4295	Inactive	Aventis (France)	Antiinflammatory	Feb-02
Pharmaprojects No. 4318	Preclinical	Allelix (Canada)	5-HT1d agonist	May-96
Pharmaprojects No. 4322	Inactive	Roche (Switz)	Antiinflammatory	Feb-02
Pharmaprojects No. 4332	Discontinued	BioResearch (Ireland)	IL-1 antagonist, TNF-α antagonist	Sep-98
Pharmaprojects No. 4350	Discontinued	Abbott (US)	Antiinflammatory	Feb-02
Pharmaprojects No. 4373	Inactive	Pharmacia (US)	Antiinflammatory	Feb-02
Pharmaprojects No. 4388	Inactive	Pharmacia (US)	Antiarthritic	Feb-02
Pharmaprojects No. 439	Inactive	Roche (Switz)	Antimigraine	Feb-02
Pharmaprojects No. 4404	Discontinued	Merckle (Germany)	Phospholipase PLA2 inhibitor	Jun-00
Pharmaprojects No. 4421	Inactive	Merck & Co (US)	Antiinflammatory	Feb-02
Pharmaprojects No. 4423	Discontinued	Dong Wha (S. Korea)	Unidentified analgesic	Mar-98

Ref.: Pharmaprojects (updated to 2/02) used with permission; Scrip, corporate, literature & patent references
"Status" is international drug development or regulatory status and may not indicate status in USA
Sponsor: Original company name is retained if product is discontinued or inactive after merger, acquisition, company name change, etc.
Users of this table are encouraged to independently verify the status, activity, and mechanism of action of drugs of interest

GENERIC / TRADE NAME	STATUS	SPONSOR (S)	MECHANISM OF ACTION	REF. UPDATE
Pharmaprojects No. 4445	Discontinued	NIH (US)	Delta opioid peptides	Feb-97
Pharmaprojects No. 4488	Inactive	Aventis (France)	Antiinflammatory	Feb-02
Pharmaprojects No. 4490	Inactive	Merck & Co (US)	Antiinflammatory	Feb-02
Pharmaprojects No. 4499	Discontinued	NPS Pharmaceuticals (US)	Ca++ channel antag., receptor-type	Sep-95
Pharmaprojects No. 4507	Inactive	Aventis (France)	Centrally-acting analgesic	Feb-02
Pharmaprojects No. 4521	Inactive	Johnson & Johnson (US)	Antiinflammatory	Feb-02
Pharmaprojects No. 4527	Inactive	Toyobo	Antiinflammatory	Feb-02
Pharmaprojects No. 4539	Preclinical	DuPont Merck (US)	COX-2 inhibitor	Mar-97
Pharmaprojects No. 4540	Discontinued	Merck & Co (US)	COX-2 inhibitor	May-99
Pharmaprojects No. 4542	Inactive	Bristol-Myers Squibb (US)	Antiinflammatory	Feb-02
Pharmaprojects No. 4549	Discontinued	Taiho (Japan)	Elastase inhibitor	Mar-97
Pharmaprojects No. 4568	Inactive	Pfizer (US)	Antiinflammatory	Feb-02
Pharmaprojects No. 4571	Preclinical	Innapharma (US)	Cancer pain; IND	Oct-95
Pharmaprojects No. 4580	Inactive	Bristol-Myers Squibb (US)	Antiinflammatory	Feb-02
Pharmaprojects No. 4581	Preclinical	Takeda (Japan)	T-cell suppression	Mar-97
Pharmaprojects No. 4596	Discontinued	Japan Energy (Japan)	PAF antagonist / anti-inflam.	Dec-98
Pharmaprojects No. 4603	Inactive	Allergan (US)	Antiinflammatory	Feb-02
Pharmaprojects No. 4616	Discontinued (ph. II)	Lilly (US)	Muscarinic M4 agonist	May-99
Pharmaprojects No. 4619	Inactive	GlaxoSmithKline (UK)	Antiinflammatory	Feb-02
Pharmaprojects No. 4620	Discontinued	Spectra / Glaxo Wellcome (UK)	Unidentified (antimigraine)	Feb-96
Pharmaprojects No. 4632	Discontinued	Takeda (Japan)	Dopamine D1 antag. / D2 ag.	1997
Pharmaprojects No. 4648	Inactive	AstraZeneca (UK)	Antiinflammatory	Feb-02
Pharmaprojects No. 4670	Discontinued	Servier (France)	Antiinflammatory (unspecified)	Jan-99
Pharmaprojects No. 4680	Preclinical	Astra (Sweden)	Opioid delta agonist (non-peptide)	Dec-97
Pharmaprojects No. 4702	Discontinued	Wyeth-Ayerst (US)	5-Lipoxygenase (5-LO) inhib.	May-98
Pharmaprojects No. 4710	Discontinued	Servier (France)	5-Lipoxygenase (5-LO) inhib.	May-99
Pharmaprojects No. 4715	Discontinued	Glaxo Wellcome (UK)	Nitric oxide synthase inhibitor	1997
Pharmaprojects No. 4717	Discontinued	GlaxoSmithKline (UK)	Antiinflammatory	Feb-02
Pharmaprojects No. 4720	Discontinued	Searle/Monsanto (US)	COX-2 inhibitor	May-99
Pharmaprojects No. 4724	Preclinical	Astra (Sweden)/BioChem Pharma	Opioid peptide μ ag. / δ antag.	Jun-96
Pharmaprojects No. 4731	Preclinical	Servier (France)	5-HT2c antagonist	Feb-96
Pharmaprojects No. 4734	Discontinued	Servier (France)	Unknown	1997
Pharmaprojects No. 475	Inactive	GlaxoSmithKline (UK)	Antiinflammatory	Feb-02
Pharmaprojects No. 4784	Discontinued	Kanebo (Japan)	Selectin blocker; anti-inflam.	Nov-98
Pharmaprojects No. 4809	Discontinued	Watson (US)	Antiinflammatory (unidentified)	Jun-00
Pharmaprojects No. 4822	Discontinued	Yamanouchi (Japan) / Tularik (US)	Gene expression inhibitor	May-98
Pharmaprojects No. 4828	Inactive	Sanofi-Synthelabo (France)	Antiinflammatory	Feb-02
Pharmaprojects No. 4850	Inactive	Pfizer (US)	Antiarthritic	Feb-02
Pharmaprojects No. 4876	Inactive	GlaxoSmithKline (UK)	Antiinflammatory	Feb-02
Pharmaprojects No. 4877	Inactive	Bristol-Myers Squibb (US)	Antiinflammatory	Feb-02
Pharmaprojects No. 4890	Discontinued	Searle/Monsanto (US)	5-LO inhibitor	Dec-97
Pharmaprojects No. 4915	Preclinical	Avanir (US)	Antiinflammatory	Feb-02
Pharmaprojects No. 4916	Inactive	Johnson & Johnson (US)	Antiinflammatory	Feb-02
Pharmaprojects No. 4920	Inactive	Pharmacia (US)	Antiinflammatory	Feb-02
Pharmaprojects No. 4924	Preclinical	Merck & Co (US)	5-HT1d-alpha agonist	Aug-96
Pharmaprojects No. 4931	Discontinued	Allergan (US)	Alpha-2a+2b+2c agonist	1997
Pharmaprojects No. 4963	Discontinued	Roche (Switz.) / Agouron (US)	Unidentified / pain	May-99
Pharmaprojects No. 4974	Discontinued	Chiron (US)	Opioid ligands (peptidomimetic)	1997
Pharmaprojects No. 4975	Inactive	Amgen (US)	Antiinflammatory	Feb-02
Pharmaprojects No. 5016	Discontinued	Takeda (Japan)	Bone formation stimulant	Feb-98
Pharmaprojects No. 5036	Discontinued	Fujisawa (Japan)	Antiinflammatory (unidentified)	Jun-00
Pharmaprojects No. 5037	Discontinued	Bristol-Myers Squibb (US)	5-HT2 antagonist	Feb-98
Pharmaprojects No. 5065	Discontinued	Lundbeck (Denmark)	GABA uptake inhibitors	Mar-98
Pharmaprojects No. 5073	Inactive	Phytera	Antiarthritic	Feb-02
Pharmaprojects No. 5094	Discontinued	Pharmacopeia / Regeneron (US)	IL-6, IFN-γ, EPO, G-CSF inhibitors	Jun-00
Pharmaprojects No. 5124	Discontinued	Servier (France)	COX-LO inhibitor	Jun-00
Pharmaprojects No. 5129	Discontinued	Univ. Thessalonika (Greece)	NSAID	Jul-98
Pharmaprojects No. 5135	Discontinued	Glaxo Wellcome (UK)	COX-2 inhibitor	1997
Pharmaprojects No. 5139	Discontinued	Pfizer (US)	Kappa agonist	Jul-98
Pharmaprojects No. 514	Inactive	American Home Products (US)	NSAID	Feb-02
Pharmaprojects No. 5143	Discontinued	Astra (Sweden) / Agouron (US)	Opioid agonist, novel	May-99
Pharmaprojects No. 5150	Preclinical	Novo Nordisk (Denmark)	Amylin / CGRP release inhibitor	Jan-97
Pharmaprojects No. 5152	Discontinued	Merck (US) / CollaGenex (US)	Antiarthritic (unknown)	Jul-98

Ref.: Pharmaprojects (updated to 2/02) used with permission; Scrip, corporate, literature & patent references
"Status" is international drug development or regulatory status and may not indicate status in USA
Sponsor: Original company name is retained if product is discontinued or inactive after merger, acquisition, company name change, etc.
Users of this table are encouraged to independently verify the status, activity, and mechanism of action of drugs of interest

GENERIC / TRADE NAME	STATUS	SPONSOR (S)	MECHANISM OF ACTION	REF. UPDATE
Pharmaprojects No. 5179	CLINICAL (II)	Bayer (Germany)	MMP (Metalloproteinase inhibitor)	Nov-96
Pharmaprojects No. 5180	Discontinued	Bayer (Germany)	Bone formation stimulant	Jul-98
Pharmaprojects No. 5218	Inactive	Origene Technologies (US)	Snake venom gene product	Feb-02
Pharmaprojects No. 5220	Discontinued	Pharmacopeia (US)	Bradykinin B1/B2 antagonist	Jun-00
Pharmaprojects No. 5261	Discontinued	Novo Nordisk (Denmark)	GABA uptake inhibitor (GAT-4)	1997
Pharmaprojects No. 5262	Discontinued	Bayer (Germany)	Acetylsalicyclic acid + NO	Sep-98
Pharmaprojects No. 5270	Preclinical	Pharmacopeia (US)	Antiinflammatory	Feb-02
Pharmaprojects No. 5318	Discontinued	Merck & Co (US)	COX-2 inhibitor	Nov-98
Pharmaprojects No. 5328	Discontinued	Glaxo Wellcome (UK)	Migraine: 5-HT1a modulator	Jun-99
Pharmaprojects No. 5341	Inactive	Pharmos (US)	Steroid analogs; anti-inflam.	Feb-02
Pharmaprojects No. 5356	Inactive	DuPont Merck (US)	Chemotactic mod.; anti-inflam.	Feb-02
Pharmaprojects No. 5399	Inactive	Southern Research Institute	Centrally-acting analgesic	Feb-02
Pharmaprojects No. 5409	Discontinued	Tularik (US)	IRAK: IL-1 recep.-assoc. kinase inhib.	Jun-00
Pharmaprojects No. 5425	Inactive	Roche (Switz) / Clontech (US)	Unidentified; analg., anti-inflam.	Feb-02
Pharmaprojects No. 5431	Inactive	LeukoSite (US)	Unidentified; RA, MS, psoriasis	Feb-02
Pharmaprojects No. 5433	Discontinued	Trega Biosciences (US)	Melanocortin MC-1 agonist	Jun-00
Pharmaprojects No. 5441	Inactive	DuPont Merck (US)	Metalloproteinase-3 inhib.	Sep-97
Pharmaprojects No. 5458	Discontinued	Novo Nordisk (Denmark)	Unidentified; analg., anti-inflam.	Jun-00
Pharmaprojects No. 5459	Discontinued	Searle/Monsanto (US)	Steroid nitrite ester / inflam.	Jan-99
Pharmaprojects No. 5463	Preclinical	Searle/Monsanto (US)	Superoxide dismutase stim.	Sep-97
Pharmaprojects No. 5468	Inactive	SmithKline Beecham (UK)	Delta receptor agonist/antag.	Sep-97
Pharmaprojects No. 5474	Discontinued	Nycomed Amersham (Norway)	Opioid mu agonist; morph. der.	May-99
Pharmaprojects No. 5480	Preclinical	Tularik (US) / Roche (Switz)	Gene regulation anti-inflam.	Sep-97
Pharmaprojects No. 5488	Preclinical	Novartis (Switz.)	Selectin antag.; anti-inflam.	Sep-97
Pharmaprojects No. 5488	Discontinued	Novartis (Switz.)	Selectin antag.; anti-inflam.	Jun-00
Pharmaprojects No. 5503	Preclinical	Fournier (France)	Bradykinin B2 antagonist	Oct-97
Pharmaprojects No. 5504	Inactive	Glaxo Wellcome (UK)	Uniden. (androstane deriv./inflam)	Feb-02
Pharmaprojects No. 5518	Discontinued	Sanofi-Synthelabo (France)	Bradykinin B1 antagonist	Feb-02
Pharmaprojects No. 5533	Discontinued	Johnson & Johnson (US)	Substance P antagonist	Feb-99
Pharmaprojects No. 5537	Preclinical	Oxford GlycoSciences (UK)	Unidentified (RA)	Oct-97
Pharmaprojects No. 5552	Inactive	CombiChem (US) / Sumitomo	Unidentified (RA, OA)	Feb-02
Pharmaprojects No. 5565	Inactive	NPS Pharmaceuticals (US)	Ion channel blocker; neuropathy	Feb-02
Pharmaprojects No. 5568	Discontinued	SmithKline Beecham (UK)	IL-8 receptor B antagonist	Jun-00
Pharmaprojects No. 5573	Discontinued	Warner-Lambert (US)	MMP-3, MMP-2 inhibitors	Mar-99
Pharmaprojects No. 5594	Preclinical	Kissei (Japan) / Vertex (US)	MAP kinase inhibitor; anti-inflam.	Dec-97
Pharmaprojects No. 5595	Discontinued	Roche (Switz)	Sodium channel antag.; neuropathy	Mar-99
Pharmaprojects No. 5606	Discontinued	Chugai (Japan)	COX-2 inhibitor	Apr-99
Pharmaprojects No. 5610	Preclinical	Shionogi (Japan)	MMP inhibitor; anti-inflam.	Dec-97
Pharmaprojects No. 5620	Discontinued	AstraZeneca (UK)	Antiinflammatory (unspecified)	Jun-99
Pharmaprojects No. 5623	Discontinued	Johnson & Johnson (US)	Alpha-2 agonist	Jun-99
Pharmaprojects No. 5633	Discontinued	Sankyo (Japan)	COX-2 inhibitor	Jun-99
Pharmaprojects No. 5661	Discontinued	UPSA / Bristol-Myers Squibb (US)	COX-2 inhibitor	May-99
Pharmaprojects No. 5665	Inactive	Aventis (France)	Bradykinin B2 antagonist	Feb-02
Pharmaprojects No. 5679	Inactive	Sumitomo (Japan)	Antiinflammatory	Feb-02
Pharmaprojects No. 5679	Discontinued	Sumitomo (Japan)	TNF-α inhibitor	Jun-99
Pharmaprojects No. 568	Inactive	Aventis (France)	Antimigraine	Feb-02
Pharmaprojects No. 5681	Inactive	AstraZeneca (UK)	Nitric oxide synthase inhibitor	Feb-02
Pharmaprojects No. 5687	Discontinued	Pharmacia & Upjohn (UK)	Metalloproteinase inhibitors	May-99
Pharmaprojects No. 5689	CLINICAL	Core Technologies (UK)	Unidentified (vulvar vestibulitis)	Jan-98
Pharmaprojects No. 5712	Inactive	AstraZeneca (UK)	Pink tarantula venom extract	Feb-02
Pharmaprojects No. 5742	Discontinued	Toray (Japan)	Unidentified (cancer pain)	Jun-00
Pharmaprojects No. 5758	Discontinued	RepliGen (US) / GW (UK)	Cytokine (glyceptor) anti-inflam.	Mar-98
Pharmaprojects No. 5761	Preclinical	Synaptic (US) / Gruenenthal (Ger)	Alpha-2 agonist	Mar-98
Pharmaprojects No. 5817	Discontinued	BioChem Pharma (Canada)	Central μ ag. + NMDA antag.	Jun-00
Pharmaprojects No. 5821	Preclinical	Adolor (US)	Peripheral kappa agonist	Jun-98
Pharmaprojects No. 5899	Preclinical	Laboratorios SALVAT (Spain)	COX-2 inhibitor	Jul-98
Pharmaprojects No. 5905	Discontinued	Servier (France)	IL-1 beta antagonist; non-peptide	Jun-00
Pharmaprojects No. 5913	Discontinued	Novo Nordisk (Denmark)	TNF / cytokine inhib.; arthritis	Jun-00
Pharmaprojects No. 5933	Discontinued	Santen (Japan)	Leukotriene LTA4 antagonist	Jun-00
Pharmaprojects No. 5976	CLINICAL (I)	Elan (Ireland) / Sheffield (US)	Pulmonary delivery, MSI technol.	Jun-99
Pharmaprojects No. 5977	Discontinued	Bioproject / INSERM (France)	Leukotriene LTA4 antagonist	Jun-00
Pharmaprojects No. 5999	Discontinued	Procter & Gamble (US)	5-LO/COX-2 inhibitor; RA, OA	Jun-00
Pharmaprojects No. 6007	Inactive	Idun (US)	ICE (IL-1beta conv. enzyme) inhib.	Feb-02

Ref.: Pharmaprojects (updated to 2/02) used with permission; Scrip, corporate, literature & patent references
"Status" is international drug development or regulatory status and may not indicate status in USA
Sponsor: Original company name is retained if product is discontinued or inactive after merger, acquisition, company name change, etc.
Users of this table are encouraged to independently verify the status, activity, and mechanism of action of drugs of interest

GENERIC / TRADE NAME	STATUS	SPONSOR (S)	MECHANISM OF ACTION	REF. UPDATE
Pharmaprojects No. 6012	Discontinued	SSP (Japan)	PDE-IV / TNF-α inhibitor	Jun-00
Pharmaprojects No. 6015	Preclinical	Merck & Co (US)	Substance P antag.; pain, inflam.	Sep-98
Pharmaprojects No. 6035	Preclinical	Active Biotech (Sweden)	Unidentified anti-inflammatory	Sep-98
Pharmaprojects No. 6051	Inactive	Lilly (US)	Substance P / glutamate antag.	Feb-02
Pharmaprojects No. 6067	Discontinued	DuPont (US)	MMP inhibitor / arthritis	Jun-00
Pharmaprojects No. 6069	Discontinued	DuPont (US)	TNF convertase inhib. / RA	Jun-00
Pharmaprojects No. 6071	Discontinued	Boehringer Ingelheim (Ger)	Leucotriene B4 antag.	Jun-00
Pharmaprojects No. 6080	Inactive	Merck & Co (US)	iNOS inhibitor / anti-inflam.	Feb-02
Pharmaprojects No. 6089	Preclinical	Kotobuki (Japan)	COX-2 inhibitor	Oct-98
Pharmaprojects No. 6101	Preclinical	Molecumetics / BMS (US)	Transcription factor inhib.	Nov-98
Pharmaprojects No. 6141	Inactive	Rhone-Poulenc Rorer (France)	PDE-IV inhibitor / inflam.	Feb-02
Pharmaprojects No. 6152	Preclinical	CAMR (UK)	Unidentified (botulinum frag.)	Jan-99
Pharmaprojects No. 6181	Preclinical	Peptor / Teva (Israel)	TNF-alpha inhib. / RA-Crohn's	Mar-99
Pharmaprojects No. 6187	Discontinued	Roche (Switz) / AxyS (US)	Unidentified genomic technology	Feb-02
Pharmaprojects No. 6283	Preclinical	OXIGENE	Antiinflammatory	Feb-02
Pharmaprojects No. 6293	Inactive	ICN (US)	Centrally-acting analgesic	Feb-02
Pharmaprojects No. 6318	Inactive	Pfizer (US)	Antiarthritic	Feb-02
Pharmaprojects No. 6319	Inactive	Pfizer (US)	Antiarthritic	Feb-02
Pharmaprojects No. 6321	Inactive	Merck & Co (US)	Centrally-acting analgesic	Feb-02
Pharmaprojects No. 6325	Preclinical	Structural Bioinformatics	Antiinflammatory	Feb-02
Pharmaprojects No. 6327	Inactive	NIH (US)	Centrally-acting analgesic	Feb-02
Pharmaprojects No. 6375	Inactive	Elan (Ireland)	Centrally-acting analgesic	Feb-02
Pharmaprojects No. 640	Inactive	GlaxoSmithKline (UK)	Antiinflammatory	Feb-02
Pharmaprojects No. 6408	Inactive	Pan Pacific	Antiarthritic	Feb-02
Pharmaprojects No. 6417	Inactive	Procter & Gamble (US)	Antiarthritic	Feb-02
Pharmaprojects No. 6425	Inactive	Italfarmaco (Italy)	Antiinflammatory	Feb-02
Pharmaprojects No. 6438	Inactive	Arachnova	Antiinflammatory	Feb-02
Pharmaprojects No. 6448	Inactive	AstraZeneca (UK)	Centrally-acting analgesic	Feb-02
Pharmaprojects No. 647	Discontinued	Sanofi-Synthelabo (France)	Antiinflammatory	Feb-02
Pharmaprojects No. 6492	Inactive	Cytopia	Antiinflammatory	Feb-02
Pharmaprojects No. 653	Inactive	Roche (Switz)	Antiarthritic	Feb-02
Pharmaprojects No. 6558	Preclinical	Kowa	Antiinflammatory	Feb-02
Pharmaprojects No. 6570	Preclinical	Cephalon (US)	Antiinflammatory	Feb-02
Pharmaprojects No. 6592	Preclinical	Abbott (US)	Centrally-acting analgesic	Feb-02
Pharmaprojects No. 6612	Preclinical	Celgene (US)	Antiinflammatory	Feb-02
Pharmaprojects No. 6624	Preclinical	AtheroGenics	Antiinflammatory	Feb-02
Pharmaprojects No. 6625	Preclinical	Sunesis	Antiarthritic	Feb-02
Pharmaprojects No. 6636	Preclinical	Juvantia	Centrally-acting analgesic	Feb-02
Pharmaprojects No. 6653	Preclinical	Biofrontera	NSAID	Feb-02
Pharmaprojects No. 6661	Preclinical	CombinatoRx	Antiinflammatory	Feb-02
Pharmaprojects No. 711	Discontinued	American Home Products (US)	Centrally-acting analgesic	Feb-02
Pharmaprojects No. 742	Discontinued	Roche (Switz)	Delta-5 lipoxygenase inhibitor	1982
Pharmaprojects No. 760	Inactive	GlaxoSmithKline (UK)	Antiinflammatory	Feb-02
Pharmaprojects No. 780	Inactive	Roche (Switz)	Centrally-acting analgesic	Feb-02
Pharmaprojects No. 799	Inactive	Abbott (US)	Antiinflammatory	Feb-02
Pharmaprojects No. 835	Inactive	Aventis (France)	Centrally-acting analgesic	Feb-02
Pharmaprojects No. 874	Inactive	Fujisawa (Japan)	Antiarthritic	Feb-02
Pharmaprojects No. 883	Inactive	Roche (Switz)	Antiarthritic	Feb-02
Pharmaprojects No. 886	Inactive	GlaxoSmithKline (UK)	NSAID	Feb-02
Pharmaprojects No. 900	Inactive	GlaxoSmithKline (UK)	Antiinflammatory	Feb-02
Pharmaprojects No. 916	Inactive	Non-industrial source	Centrally-acting analgesic	Feb-02
Pharmaprojects No. 919	Discontinued	American Home Products (US)	Antiarthritic	Feb-02
Pharmaprojects No. 929	Discontinued	American Home Products (US)	Antiinflammatory	Feb-02
Pharmaprojects No. 931	Inactive	American Home Products (US)	Centrally-acting analgesic	Feb-02
Pharmaprojects No. 932	Inactive	Abbott (US)	Centrally-acting analgesic	Feb-02
Pharmaprojects No. 943	Discontinued	Bristol-Myers Squibb (US)	Antiinflammatory	Feb-02
Pharmaprojects No. 962	Discontinued	BTG (UK)	Centrally-acting analgesic	Feb-02
Pharmaprojects No. 965	Discontinued	bioMerieux-Pierre Fabre (France)	NSAID	Feb-02
Pharmaprojects No. 981	Inactive	Takeda (Japan)	Antiinflammatory	Feb-02
Phenyliminoimidazolines	Inactive	Hafslund Nycomed (Norway)	Unknown	Unk.
Phenylmorpholines	Inactive	Wyeth-Ayerst (US)	Opioid agonist/antagonist	Apr-83
phospholipase A2 inhib, La Jol	Discontinued	La Jolla Pharmaceutical	Antiinflammatory	Feb-02
phospholipase A2 inhibs, Sphin	Inactive	Lilly (US)	Antiinflammatory	Feb-02

Ref.: Pharmaprojects (updated to 2/02) used with permission; Scrip, corporate, literature & patent references
"Status" is international drug development or regulatory status and may not indicate status in USA
Sponsor: Original company name is retained if product is discontinued or inactive after merger, acquisition, company name change, etc.
Users of this table are encouraged to independently verify the status, activity, and mechanism of action of drugs of interest

GENERIC / TRADE NAME	STATUS	SPONSOR (S)	MECHANISM OF ACTION	REF. UPDATE
phospholipase C inhibitor, Bri	Discontinued	British Biotech (UK)	Antiinflammatory	Feb-02
phospholipase C inhibitor, Med	Discontinued	Mediolanum	Antiinflammatory	Feb-02
phospholipase D inhibitors, Sp	Inactive	Lilly (US)	Antiarthritic	Feb-02
phospholipase inhibitor, Scios	Discontinued	Scios (US)	Antiinflammatory	Feb-02
phospholipase inhibitors, Poli	Discontinued	Polifarma (Italy)	Antiinflammatory	Feb-02
Picenadol (LY-136595)	Discontinued (ph. III)	Lilly (US)	Opioid agonist/antagonist	May-94
Pidocetamol	Discontinued	Pan Medica (France)	PGSI	Jan-92
pidocetamol	Discontinued	Pan Medica (France)	Centrally-acting analgesic	Feb-02
Pimetacin	Discontinued (ph. I)	Rhone-Poulenc Rorer (France)	NSAID	Feb-90
Pinadoline (SC-25469)	Discontinued (ph. I)	Searle/Monsanto (US)	Unidentified analgesic	1984
Piperadinyl-cyclohexanols	Preclinical	Bristol-Myers Squibb (US)	5-HT1a antagonists	Jul-93
Piperidinepropanoic acids	Inactive	Warner-Lambert (US)	Ultra-short acting opioid	Aug-91
pipethiadene	Inactive	Spofa	Antimigraine	Feb-02
piproxen	LAUNCHED	Aventis (France)	Antiarthritic	Feb-02
Pirazolac (MY-309, SH-376)	Discontinued (REGIS.)	Schering AG (Germany)	NSAID	May-99
piridoxiprofen	Discontinued	Crinos	NSAID	Feb-02
piroxicam	LAUNCHED	Pfizer (US)	NSAID	Feb-02
Piroxicam betadex (BREXECAM)	LAUNCHED	Chiesi (Italy)	Piroxicam beta-cyclodextrin	May-99
Piroxicam cinnamate	LAUNCHED	SPA (Italy)	NSAID	Aug-96
Piroxicam meglumine	Discontinued (ph. II)	Therapicon (ph. Italy)	Hydrolysable salt of piroxicam	Apr-95
piroxicam olamine	Inactive	Pfizer (US)	NSAID	Feb-02
Piroxicam, Anesta	CLINICAL (I)	Cephalon (US)	NSAID	Jun-00
Piroxicam, granular	Inactive	Applied Pharma Res. (Switz.)	Formulation, oral fast-acting	Jun-99
Pirprofen (RENGASIL)	WITHDRAWN	Novartis (Switz.)	NSAID	1990
pizotifen	LAUNCHED	Novartis (Switz.)	Antimigraine	Feb-02
PJ2204	Preclinical	PowderJect (UK)	Formulation, antimigraine	Dec-97
PKH152	Discontinued	CytRx (US)	Antiarthritic	Feb-02
PL-030	Inactive	Peninsula Laboratories (US)	Morphiceptin analog	1983
PLR-13	Preclinical	Pliva	Antiinflammatory	Feb-02
PLR-14	Preclinical	Pliva	Antiinflammatory	Feb-02
PN1 antagonists, Allelix	Inactive	NPS Pharmaceuticals (US)	Centrally-acting analgesic	Feb-02
PNU-109291	Discontinued	Pharmacia & Upjohn (UK)	5-HT1d agonist; migraine	Jun-00
PNU-142633	CLINICAL	Pharmacia & Upjohn (UK)	5-HT1d agonist; migraine	Jun-99
podoverine A	Inactive	Aventis (France)	Antiinflammatory	Feb-02
POL-647	Suspended	Polifarma (Italy)	TNF-alpha antag.; anti-inflam.	Nov-98
PPI-3088	Preclinical	Praecis Pharmaceuticals	Antiinflammatory	Feb-02
PR-870-714A	Discontinued	Fisons (UK)	PGSI	Dec-93
pranoprofen	LAUNCHED	Mitsubishi Pharma (Japan)	NSAID	Feb-02
Pravadoline (Win-48098)	Discontinued (ph. II)	Sanofi (France)	Cannabinoid / PGSI	May-93
Praxiterol	Inactive	Kyowa Hakko (Japan)	PGSI	Mar-92
PR-B	Discontinued	Dainippon (Japan)	Antiinflammatory	Feb-02
Prednisolone farnesil	LAUNCHED	Taiho / Kuraray (Japan)	Topical steroid; OA + RA	Nov-98
Pregabalin	CLINICAL (II/III)	Warner-Lambert (US)	Neuropathic pain, epilepsy	Apr-98
prenafen	Discontinued	Ferrer (Spain)	Antiinflammatory	Feb-02
Prinomide (CGS-10787B)	Discontinued (ph. III)	Novartis (Switz.)	NSAID	Feb-90
prodolic acid	Discontinued	American Home Products (US)	Antiinflammatory	Feb-02
proglumetacin	LAUNCHED	Rotta (Italy)	Antiinflammatory	Feb-02
Propacetamol (PRO-DAFALGAN)	LAUNCHED	UPSA (France)	Injectable paracetamol	May-93
Propioxatin-A	Discontinued	Sankyo (Japan)	Enk'ase inhibitor	Dec-86
Propiram fumarate	CLINICAL (III)	Shire (UK) / Bayer (Ger)	Opioid agonist/antagonist	Apr-98
proquazone	LAUNCHED	Novartis (Switz.)	Antiinflammatory	Feb-02
Prosaptide TX14(A)	CLINICAL (I)	Myelos Neurosciences (US)	Neuropathic pain	Mar-98
Protease Inhibitors	Discontinued	Unigene (US)	Endothelin antagonist	Aug-92
protizinic acid	LAUNCHED	Aventis (France)	Antiinflammatory	Feb-02
Proxorphan tartrate (BL-5572)	Discontinued	Bristol-Myers Squibb (US)	Opioid agonist/antagonist	Feb-84
PS-508	Discontinued	ProScript (US)	MMP-3 inhibitor / RA	May-99
PS-519 (lactacystin analog)	Preclinical	ProScript (US)	Proteasome inhib.; anti-inflam.	May-98
PT-17	Preclinical	Palatin Technologies	Antiinflammatory	Feb-02
PTI-501 (morphine + naloxone)	CLINICAL (II)	Pain Therapeutics (US)	morphine + ultra low dose antag.	Feb-02
PTI-555 (morphine + naltrexone)	CLINICAL (II)	Pain Therapeutics (US)	morphine + ultra low dose antag.	Feb-02
PTI-601 (naltrexone + tramadol)	CLINICAL (II)	Pain Therapeutics (US)	Tramadol + ultra low dose antag.	Feb-02
PTI-801 (oxycodone + naltrexone)	CLINICAL (II)	Pain Therapeutics (US)	oxycodone + ultra low dose antag.	Feb-02
PV-108	Inactive	Resfar (Italy)	Antiinflammatory	Feb-02

Ref.: Pharmaprojects (updated to 2/02) used with permission; Scrip, corporate, literature & patent references
"Status" is international drug development or regulatory status and may not indicate status in USA
Sponsor: Original company name is retained if product is discontinued or inactive after merger, acquisition, company name change, etc.
Users of this table are encouraged to independently verify the status, activity, and mechanism of action of drugs of interest

GENERIC / TRADE NAME	STATUS	SPONSOR (S)	MECHANISM OF ACTION	REF. UPDATE
Pyranopyrazolones	Discontinued	Dainippon (Japan)	5-HT uptake inhibitor	Apr-86
pyrimidant	Inactive	Non-industrial source	Antiinflammatory	Feb-02
pyrroben	Discontinued	Spofa	Antiinflammatory	Feb-02
Pyrrolidinylethylacetamides	Discontinued	Zeneca (US)	Kappa agonist	Mar-92
Pyrrolidones	Inactive	Hoechst (Ger)	Cognition / analgesia	Aug-91
pyrrolostatin	Discontinued	Kirin Brewery	Antiinflammatory	Feb-02
Quinoxalinediones	Preclinical	Sumitomo (Japan)	Glutamate antagonist	May-93
QZ-16	Inactive	Non-industrial source	Antiinflammatory	Feb-02
R-18936	Discontinued	Johnson & Johnson (US)	Opioid agonist	Jul-81
R-26800	Discontinued	Johnson & Johnson (US)	Opioid agonist	Jul-81
R-34994	Discontinued	Johnson & Johnson (US)	Opioid agonist	Jul-81
R-4066	Discontinued	Johnson & Johnson (US)	Opioid agonist	Jul-81
R-62230	Inactive	Non-industrial source	Antiinflammatory	Feb-02
R-84760	Discontinued	Sankyo (Japan)	Kappa agonist	Apr-97
R-85355	Discontinued	Janssen / J&J (US)	5-LO inhibitor	Dec-94
RB-38B	Inactive	Univ. Cadiz (Spain)	Enk'ase inhibitor	1990
R-baclofen, Paladin Labs	CLINICAL (II)	Pharmascience (Canada)	GABA antagonist	Feb-02
RDP-58, 2nd-generation	Preclinical	SangStat (US)	Antiinflammatory	Feb-02
Remifentanil (ULTIVA™)	LAUNCHED	Glaxo Wellcome (UK)	Mu opioid: ultra-short anesthesia	Mar-98
Resiniferatoxin, NIH	Discontinued	NIH (US)	Substance P depletor	Jul-98
Reumacon	PRE-REGISTRATION	Conpharm (Sweden) / Pharmacia	Amyloid deposit inhibitor (arthritis)	Jun-00
Rev-5367	Discontinued	Aventis (France)	Antiinflammatory	Feb-02
Rhenium-HEDP	Discontinued (PRE-REG)	Mallinckrodt (US)	Radionuclutide; bone cancer pain	Jun-96
Rhodanine derivatives	Discontinued	Univ. L'viv (Ukraine)	NSAID	Jun-00
rimazolium metilsulfate	LAUNCHED	Chinoin (Hungary)	NSAID	Feb-02
Rimexolone	REGISTERED	Alcon (US) / Akzo Nobel (NE)	Corticosteroid (topical, intra-articular)	Mar-96
Rizatriptan benzoate (MAXALT®)	LAUNCHED	Merck & Co (US)	5-HT1b/1d agonist	Oct-98
RMM-295	Discontinued	Roemmers	Unk. (non-narcotic)	Jun-00
RMM-318	Discontinued	Roemmers	NSAID	Jun-00
RO 11-4337	Discontinued	Roche (Switz)	PGSI	Mar-84
RO 12-9150	Discontinued	Roche (Switz)	PGSI	Nov-85
Ro-1130830	CLINICAL (II)	Roche (Switz)	Metalloproteinase inhibitor	Jun-00
Ro-11-4337	Discontinued	Roche (Switz)	Centrally-acting analgesic	Feb-02
Ro-12-9150	Discontinued (ph. I)	Roche (Switz)	COX inhibitor	Nov-85
Ro-15-8081	Discontinued (ph. I)	Roche (Switz.)	5-HT/NE uptake inhibitor	May-92
Ro-1-9564	Discontinued	Roche (Switz)	Antiinflammatory	Feb-02
Ro-21-5521	Discontinued (ph. I)	Roche (Switz)	Unidentified anti-inflammatory	Feb-85
Ro-23-9358	Discontinued	Roche (Switz)	Phospholipase PLA2 inhibitor	Mar-95
Ro-3-1314	Discontinued	Roche (Switz)	Antiinflammatory	Feb-02
Ro-31-4724	Inactive	Roche (Switz)	Antiarthritic	Feb-02
Ro-31-8425 (Ro-32-0432)	Discontinued	Roche (Switz)	Protein kinase PKC inhibitor	Nov-95
Ro-31-8830	Inactive	Roche (Switz)	Antiinflammatory	Feb-02
Ro-31-9790	Discontinued	Roche (Switz)	Antiarthritic	Feb-02
Ro-320-1195	CLINICAL (I)	Roche (Switz)	Antiarthritic	Feb-02
ROBAXACET®	CLINICAL	Wyeth-Ayerst (US)	Methocarbamol + APAP	May-93
robinoeole	Discontinued	Inflazyme (US)	Antiinflammatory	Feb-02
Rofecoxib (VIOXX, MK-966)	LAUNCHED	Merck & Co (US)	COX-2 inhibitor / RA-OA	Jun-99
Ropivacaine (NAROPIN™)	LAUNCHED	Pharmacia & Upjohn / Astra	Local anesthetic (epidural/spinal)	May-96
RP 63494	Inactive	Aventis (France)	Centrally-acting analgesic	Feb-02
RP 66364	Discontinued	Aventis (France)	Antiinflammatory	Feb-02
RP 67580	Discontinued	Aventis (France)	Antiinflammatory	Feb-02
RP-66364 (RP-60532; RP-69929)	Discontinued	Rhone-Poulenc Rorer (France)	LTB4 / CO antagonist	Nov-94
RP-67580	Discontinued	Rhone-Poulenc Rorer (France)	Substance P antagonist	Mar-93
RPR-100893	Discontinued (ph. II)	Rhone-Poulenc Rorer (France)	NK-1 antagonist	Oct-96
RPR-122818 derivatives	Discontinued	Aventis (France)	MMP / PDE-IV inhibitor	Jun-00
RPR-132294	Discontinued	Aventis (France)	PDE-IV inhibitor	Jun-00
RS-113-080	Inactive	Roche (Switz)	Antiarthritic	Feb-02
RS-113472	Discontinued	Roche (Switz)	COX-2 inhibitor	Jun-00
RS-130830	Discontinued	Roche (Switz)	Neutrophil collagenase inhib./OA	Jun-00
RS-17597	Discontinued	Syntex / Roche (Switz)	Phosphodiesterase (PDE-IV) inhib.	May-98
RS-635	Preclinical	Abbott (US)	Antiinflammatory	Feb-02
RSD-921 / Nociblockers	CLINICAL (I)	Nortran (Canada)	Ion channel antagonist (iv)	May-97
RSD-931	Discontinued	Nortran (Canada)	Ion channel modulator	Jun-00

Ref.: Pharmaprojects (updated to 2/02) used with permission; Scrip, corporate, literature & patent references
"Status" is international drug development or regulatory status and may not indicate status in USA
Sponsor: Original company name is retained if product is discontinued or inactive after merger, acquisition, company name change, etc.
Users of this table are encouraged to independently verify the status, activity, and mechanism of action of drugs of interest

GENERIC / TRADE NAME	STATUS	SPONSOR (S)	MECHANISM OF ACTION	REF. UPDATE
RU-29693	Discontinued (Clin.)	Hoechst Marion Roussel (Ger)	NSAID	1983
RU-35963	Inactive	Roussel-Uclaf (France)	Cholinergic agonist	1990
RU-42738	Inactive	Aventis (France)	Antiinflammatory	Feb-02
RU-42827	Inactive	Roussel-Uclaf (France)	Enk'ase inhibitor	1986
RU-43526	Inactive	Aventis (France)	Antiarthritic	Feb-02
RU-44004	Inactive	Roussel-Uclaf (France)	Enk'ase inhibitor	Sep-92
RU-46057	Inactive	Aventis (France)	Antiinflammatory	Feb-02
RU-49289	Inactive	Roussel-Uclaf (France)	PGSI	1988
RU-54808	Discontinued	Hoechst Marion Roussel (Ger)	Peripheral analgesic	Feb-97
RUB-265	Discontinued	Sankyo (Japan)	NSAID	Feb-02
RWJ-314313	Inactive	Johnson & Johnson (US)	Centrally-acting analgesic	Feb-02
RWJ-37210	Preclinical	Johnson & Johnson (US)	Centrally-acting analgesic	Feb-02
RWJ-52353	Inactive	Johnson & Johnson (US)	Alpha-2 agonist	Feb-02
RWJ-52807	Discontinued	Johnson & Johnson (US)	Alpha-2 agonist	Feb-02
RWJ-63556	Discontinued	Johnson & Johnson (US)	5-LO inhibitor; anti-inflam.	Mar-99
RWJ-67657	CLINICAL (I)	Johnson & Johnson (US)	Antiarthritic	Feb-02
RWJ-68354	Preclinical	Johnson & Johnson (US)	Inhib. p38 kinase, TNF-α, IL-1b/RA	Jan-99
RX-783006	Discontinued	Reckitt & Colman (UK)	Enkephalin analog	Feb-84
RX-783016	Discontinued	Reckitt & Colman (UK)	Enkephalin analog	Feb-84
S- 19220 / Dibenzoxazepines	Discontinued	Searle/Monsanto (US)	PGE2 receptor antagonist	Sep-93
S-01	Discontinued	Sanwa Kagaku Kenkyusho	NSAID	Feb-02
S-14080	Discontinued (ph. II)	Servier (France)	NSAID	Sep-93
S-1490 (S-1491)	Discontinued (Clin.)	Synthelabo (France)	Unidentified analgesic	Mar-85
S-1528	Discontinued	Sanofi-Synthelabo (France)	NSAID	Feb-02
S-16276-1	Discontinued	Servier (France)	Antiarthritic	Feb-02
S-18523	Discontinued	Servier (France)	NK-1 antagonist (pseudopept.)	May-99
S-18920	Inactive	Servier (France)	Centrally-acting analgesic	Feb-02
S-19014	Preclinical	Servier (France)	Antimigraine	Feb-02
S-19812	Inactive	Servier (France)	Antiinflammatory	Feb-02
S-20682	Discontinued (Clin.)	Shionogi (Japan)	Opioid agonist / narcotic	May-84
S-2441	Discontinued	Pharmacia & Upjohn (UK) /Kabi	5-HT antagonist / NK antagonist	Apr-91
S-2474	CLINICAL (II)	Shionogi (Japan)	Antiarthritic	Feb-02
S-3013	CLINICAL (II)	Shionogi (Japan)	Antiinflammatory	Feb-02
S-33516	Preclinical	Servier (France)	COX-2 inhibitor	Jun-00
SaH-46-798	Discontinued (ph. I)	Novartis (Switz.)	NSAID	Feb-83
salicylamide esters	Inactive	Merck & Co (US)	Antiinflammatory	Feb-02
Salmisteine (EP-321)	Discontinued (PRE-REG)	Edmond Pharma (Italy)	NSAID	May-93
Sameridine	Discontinued (ph. II)	Astra (Sweden)	Local anesthetic (spinal)	Jan-98
SAM-PFH	Inactive	Gibipharma	Antiarthritic	Feb-02
SB-201146	Discontinued	SmithKline Beecham (UK)	Leukotriene LTB4 antagonist	May-96
SB-218842	Discontinued (ph. I)	GlaxoSmithKline (UK)	Antimigraine	Feb-02
SB-237596	Discontinued	SmithKline Beecham (UK)	Opioid delta agonists (non-peptide)	Jun-00
SB-265610	Preclinical	GlaxoSmithKline (UK)	Antiinflammatory	Feb-02
SB-273005	CLINICAL (I)	GlaxoSmithKline (UK)	Antiarthritic	Feb-02
SB-380732	Preclinical	GlaxoSmithKline (UK)	Antiarthritic	Feb-02
SC 51089 / Dibenzoxazepines	Preclinical	Searle/Monsanto (US)	PGE2 receptor antagonist	1993
SC-105	Discontinued	Scotia (UK)	Antiarthritic	Feb-02
SC-106	Discontinued (ph. II)	Scotia (UK)	γ-linolenic acid combo (RA, OA)	Jan-99
SC-107	Inactive	Scotia (UK)	Antiarthritic	Feb-02
SC-299	Inactive	Pharmacia (US)	Antiinflammatory	Feb-02
SC-34871	Discontinued	Searle/Monsanto (US)	Enkephalin analog	Jul-89
SC-39566	Discontinued	Searle/Monsanto (US)	Enkephalin analog	Nov-90
SC-411930	Discontinued	Searle/Monsanto (US)	Leukotriene LTB4 antagonist	May-94
SC-41661A	Discontinued	Pharmacia (US)	Antiinflammatory	Feb-02
SC-42867	Discontinued (ph. II)	Searle/Monsanto (US)	Prostaglandin antagonist	Apr-93
SC-51146	Discontinued	Searle/Monsanto (US)	Leukotriene LTB4 antagonist	May-94
SC-53228	Inactive	Pharmacia (US)	Antiinflammatory	Feb-02
SC-56557	Inactive	Pharmacia (US)	NSAID	Feb-02
SC-57666	Discontinued (ph. I)	Searle/Monsanto (US)	COX-2 inhibitor	May-99
Sch-12223	Discontinued	Schering Plough (US)	Antiinflammatory	Feb-02
Sch-30497	Discontinued	Schering Plough (US)	PGSI	Sep-86
Sch-32615	Discontinued	Schering Plough (US)	Centrally-acting analgesic	Feb-02
Sch-32615	Discontinued (ph. II)	Schering Plough (US)	Enk'ase inhibitor; phase II	Mar-93

Ref.: Pharmaprojects (updated to 2/02) used with permission; Scrip, corporate, literature & patent references
"Status" is international drug development or regulatory status and may not indicate status in USA
Sponsor: Original company name is retained if product is discontinued or inactive after merger, acquisition, company name change, etc.
Users of this table are encouraged to independently verify the status, activity, and mechanism of action of drugs of interest

GENERIC / TRADE NAME	STATUS	SPONSOR (S)	MECHANISM OF ACTION	REF. UPDATE
Sch-34826	Discontinued (ph. II)	Schering Plough (US)	Enk'ase inhibitor; phase II	Mar-93
SCIO-469	CLINICAL (I)	Scios (US)	Antiarthritic	Feb-02
SC-XX906	Discontinued	Pharmacia (US)	P38 kinase inhibitor	Jun-00
SD-41	Discontinued	Dainippon (Japan)	Enkephalin analog	Jan-92
SD-46	Discontinued	Dainippon (Japan)	Unknown	Aug-85
SD-62	Discontinued	Dainippon (Japan)	Unknown	Feb-89
SDZ-210-610	Discontinued	Novartis (Switz.)	Antiinflammatory	Feb-02
SDZ-224-015	Discontinued	Novartis (Switz.)	ICE (IL-1beta conv. enzyme) inhib.	Sep-98
SDZ-249-482	Discontinued	Novartis (Switz.)	Capsaicin derivatives	Jan-99
seclazone	Discontinued	Wallace Pharmaceuticals	Antiinflammatory	Feb-02
SelCID	CLINICAL (I)	Celgene (US)	TNF-alpha inhibitor	Dec-97
Selectin inhibitors	Discontinued	Nisshin Oil Mills (Japan)	Selectin antag.; anti-inflam.	Jun-00
SEN-215	Discontinued	Kyowa Hakko (Japan)	Unk. / Benzodiazepine	Jul-84
SEP-119249	Discontinued	Sepracor (US)	Glucocorticoid; anti-inflam.	Jun-00
SEP-130551 / SEP-130169	Discontinued	Sepracor (US)	Opioid mu/kappa agonist	Jun-00
SEP-89068 / SEP-42960	Discontinued	Sepracor (US)	Adenosine A2A / A3 antags.	Jun-00
Sergolexole	Discontinued (ph. II)	Lilly (US)	5-HT2 antagonist	Aug-96
Sfericase (A1-794; Ponase)	Discontinued (ph. III)	Meiji Seika (Japan)	Antiinflammatory/expectorant	Feb-89
sialophorin, LSB	Inactive	Large Scale Biology	Antiinflammatory	Feb-02
SK-962	Inactive	Sanwa Kagaku Kenkyusho	Formulation	Feb-02
SKF-10047 (NANM)	Discontinued (ph. I)	SmithKline Beecham (UK)	Sigma receptor agonist	Dec-92
SKF-10049	Discontinued	SmithKline Beecham (UK)	Sigma agonist	Mar-81
SKF-104351	Discontinued	GlaxoSmithKline (UK)	Antiarthritic	Feb-02
SKF-104493	Discontinued	GlaxoSmithKline (UK)	Antiinflammatory	Feb-02
SKF-105809 (SK&F-105561)	Discontinued (ph. I)	SmithKline Beecham (UK)	COX/5-LO inhibitor	Jan-93
SKF-36914	Discontinued	GlaxoSmithKline (UK)	Antiarthritic	Feb-02
SKF-86002	Discontinued	GlaxoSmithKline (UK)	Antiinflammatory	Feb-02
SLPI fragments	Discontinued	Teijin (Japan)	Elastase inhibitor	Jun-00
Sm153 lexidronam (QUADRAMET®)	LAUNCHED	DuPont Merck / Cytogen (US)	Radionuclide / bone cancer pain	Apr-98
SM-9064	Discontinued	Sumitomo (Japan)	NSAID	Feb-02
Small peptides, Centocor	Discontinued	Centocor (US)	Adhesion molecule antag. / RA	Dec-94
SMP-114	CLINICAL (I)	Sumitomo (Japan)	Antiarthritic	Feb-02
SNC-80	Discontinued	GlaxoSmithKline (UK)	Delta agonist	Feb-02
SNX-185	Inactive	Elan (Ireland)	Conotoxin; N-type Ca++ antag.	Feb-02
SNX-236	Preclinical	Neurex (US)	Unknown	Feb-93
SNX-239	Inactive	Elan (Ireland)	Ca++ channel antag., N-type	Feb-02
Somatostatin	LAUNCHED	6 University Study	I.C.V./Intrathecal/Epidural	1984
SP-057	Preclinical	Bristol-Myers Squibb (US)	Antiarthritic	Feb-02
SP-123	Inactive	UCM-Difme	Antiinflammatory	Feb-02
SP-186	Discontinued (ph. I)	Serotonin Pharma. (US)	5-HT agonist	May-93
SP-600125	Preclinical	Celgene (US)	Antiarthritic	Feb-02
SPA-58	Inactive	Takeda (Japan)	Substance P antagonist	1983
SPA-S-646	Preclinical	SPA (Italy)	Unidentified analgesic	Feb-02
SPC-839	Preclinical	Serono	Antiinflammatory	Feb-02
SPI-42	Inactive	Johnson & Johnson (US)	Antiinflammatory	Feb-02
Spiradoline (U-62066E)	Discontinued (ph. II)	Pharmacia & Upjohn (UK)	Kappa agonist	Dec-93
spirogermanium, Unimed	Discontinued	Solvay (Netherlands)	Antiarthritic	Feb-02
SQ-11579	Discontinued (Clin.)	Bristol-Myers Squibb (US)	Unidentified anti-inflammatory	Jul-80
SQ-20650	Discontinued (ph. I)	Bristol-Myers Squibb (US)	COX inhibitor	Jan-80
SQ-28133	Discontinued	Bristol-Myers Squibb (US)	Enk'ase inhibitor	Oct-85
SR-206 (ph. Ibuprofen 1x/day)	Discontinued (ph. II)	SSP (Japan)	Ibuprofen formulation	Oct-96
SR-26831	Inactive	Sanofi-Synthelabo (France)	Antiarthritic	Feb-02
SR-48968	CLINICAL (II)	Sanofi (France)	NK-2 antagonist	Dec-97
ß-elemonic acid	Discontinued	Aventis (France)	Antiarthritic	Feb-02
ß-glucan receptor antagonists	Inactive	Alpha-Beta Technology	Antiinflammatory	Feb-02
ST-1482	CLINICAL (III)	Sigma-Tau (Italy)	Antiarthritic	Feb-02
ST-793	Discontinued	bioMerieux-Pierre Fabre (France)	NSAID	Feb-02
ST-875	Discontinued	bioMerieux-Pierre Fabre (France)	Antiarthritic	Feb-02
Strontium-89 Chloride	LAUNCHED	Amersham (US)	Radionuclide, Sr-89 isotope	1994
Substance P-neurotoxin compound	Preclinical	Univ. Minnesota (US)	Substance P cell toxin (I.th.)	Oct-97
sudoxicam	Discontinued	Pfizer (US)	Antiinflammatory	Feb-02
Sufentanil (SUFENTA®)	LAUNCHED	Johnson & Johnson (US)	Opioid mu agonist	Jan-95
sufentanil, DUROS	CLINICAL (III)	Durect	Formulation	Feb-02

Ref.: Pharmaprojects (updated to 2/02) used with permission; Scrip, corporate, literature & patent references
"Status" is international drug development or regulatory status and may not indicate status in USA
Sponsor: Original company name is retained if product is discontinued or inactive after merger, acquisition, company name change, etc.
Users of this table are encouraged to independently verify the status, activity, and mechanism of action of drugs of interest

GENERIC / TRADE NAME	STATUS	SPONSOR (S)	MECHANISM OF ACTION	REF. UPDATE
sufentanil, S BioSystems	Preclinical	Durect	Formulation	Feb-02
sulindac	LAUNCHED	Merck & Co (US)	Antiinflammatory	Feb-02
Sumacetamol	Discontinued (ph. II)	Eastman Kodak (US)	PGSI	1985
Sumitriptan (IMIGRAN®/IMITREX®)	LAUNCHED	Glaxo Wellcome (UK)	5-HT1d agonist	Jan-97
Sumitriptan, nasal (IMITREX®)	LAUNCHED	Glaxo Wellcome (UK)	5-HT1d agonist (migraine)	Nov-97
Superoxide dismutase (PC-SOD)	CLINICAL (II)	Seikagaku Kogyo (Japan)	Lecithinized superoxide dismutase	Jun-99
superoxide dismutase, Cantacuz	LAUNCHED	Non-industrial source	Antiinflammatory	Feb-02
superoxide dismutase, Isnardi	LAUNCHED	Sanofi-Synthelabo (France)	Antiinflammatory	Feb-02
Superoxide dismutase, OXIS	Discontinued (ph. III)	OXIS (US) / Grunenthal (Ger)	Bovine SOD (osteoarthritis)	Mar-97
superoxide dismutase, QLT	Discontinued	QLT	Antiarthritic	Feb-02
superoxide dismutase, Sidus	LAUNCHED	Sidus	Antiinflammatory	Feb-02
superoxide dismutase, Takeda^	Discontinued	Takeda (Japan)	Antiarthritic	Feb-02
superoxide dismutase, Tosoh	Discontinued	Tosoh Corporation	Antiinflammatory	Feb-02
Suprofen	Discontinued (LNCHD)	Johnson & Johnson (US)	PGSI inhibitor	1989
SVT-2016	CLINICAL (I)	SALVAT	Antiarthritic	Feb-02
SX-1032	Discontinued	SSP (Japan)	Antiinflammatory	Feb-02
SY-6001	Discontinued (ph. II)	SSP (Japan)	NSAID	Mar-93
SYM-2007	Preclinical	Symphony (US)	Kainate/glutamate partial ag.	Apr-95
SYM-2081	Preclinical	Symphony (US)	Kainate/glutamate partial ag.	Sep-95
SYM-2192	Discontinued	Symphony (US)	Kainate/glutamate partial ag.	Nov-96
Syndyphalin (SD-33)	Discontinued	Otsuka (Japan)	Enkephalin analog	1983
T-0757	Inactive	Tanabe Seiyaku (Japan)	Antiinflammatory	Feb-02
T25	Preclinical	Manchester Innovation	Antiinflammatory	Feb-02
T-3788	Discontinued (ph. II)	Toyama (Japan)	Unidentified antiinflammatory analg.	Apr-98
T-614	CLINICAL (III)	Eisai / Toyama (Japan)	IL-1b, IL-6, IL-8 antag./ RA	Dec-98
TA-383	Inactive	Tanabe Seiyaku (Japan)	Antiarthritic	Feb-02
TA-60	Discontinued (ph. II)	Taisho (Japan)	Ibuprofen analog	1985
TA-668	Inactive	Taisho (Japan)	Antiinflammatory	Feb-02
TACE antagnoists	Preclinical	Immunex (US) / Wyeth-Ayerst	TNF-α converting enzyme antag.	Feb-97
Tachykinin analogues	Discontinued	Yissum (Israel)	Substance P antagonist	Feb-93
tachykinin antagonists, Lilly	Inactive	Lilly (US)	Substance P antagonist	Feb-02
taclamine	Discontinued	American Home Products (US)	Antimigraine	Feb-02
TAI-764	Discontinued	Takeda (Japan)	Antiinflammatory	Feb-02
TAI-998	Inactive	Takeda (Japan)	PGSI	1985
TAK-603	CLINICAL (II)	Takeda (Japan)	Bone formation stimulant	Jun-96
Talmetacin	Discontinued (Clin)	Resfar (Italy) / Bago (Argen)	Cyclooxygenase inhibitor	May-98
talniflumate	LAUNCHED	Bago	Antiinflammatory	Feb-02
talosalate	Inactive	Bago	Antiinflammatory	Feb-02
TAN-1515	Discontinued	Takeda (Japan)	Antiinflammatory	Feb-02
TAN-1612	Discontinued	Takeda (Japan)	NK-1 antagonist	May-98
Tan-67	Preclinical	Hoshi Univ. (Japan)	Non-peptide delta agonist	Oct-96
TAN-684	Preclinical	Toray (Japan)	Peripheral kappa agonist	Jun-00
tazadolene	Inactive	Pharmacia (US)	NSAID	Feb-02
tazaprofen	Discontinued	Merck KGaA (Germany)	Antiinflammatory	Feb-02
TB-219	Inactive	Teikoku Chemical	Antiinflammatory	Feb-02
TBC-3342	Preclinical	Texas Biotechnology (US)	VLA-4 inhibitor; RA	May-98
Tebufelone (NE-11740)	Discontinued (ph. II)	Procter & Gamble (US)	NSAID	May-94
TEI-1338	Inactive	Teijin (Japan)	Antiinflammatory	Feb-02
TEI-1345	Inactive	Teijin (Japan)	Antiinflammatory	Feb-02
TEI-8535	Discontinued	Teijin (Japan)	MCP-1 antagonist /PGE-1 agonist	Jul-98
Tenidap	Discontinued (PRE-REG)	Pfizer (US)	COX / 5-LO inhib. (LTB4/IL1)	May-98
Tenosal	Discontinued (PRE-REG)	Medea Research (Italy)	COX inhibitor / Ca++ antag. / migraine	Feb-97
Tenoxicam	LAUNCHED	HMR (Ger) / Roche (Switz)	NSAID	Oct-94
tenoxicam meglumine	Discontinued	Therapicon (Italy)	NSAID	Feb-02
tepoxalin	Discontinued	Johnson & Johnson (US)	Antiarthritic	Feb-02
tetracine, percutaneous	LAUNCHED	Smith & Nephew	Formulation	Feb-02
Tetrahydroisoquinolines	Preclinical	Boots (UK)	D1/D2 antagonists	Sep-93
Tetrahydroisoquinolines	Discontinued	SmithKline Beecham (UK)	Kappa agonist	Nov-92
Tetrahydrothiopyraneindoles	Discontinued	Shionogi (Japan)	Unknown	Mar-93
Tetrandrine	Discontinued	Inst. Med. Res. (Australia)	Anti-inflammatory	Jun-94
Tetronothiodin	Preclinical	Roche (Switz)	CCK-B antagonist	Feb-93
THC:CBD broad ratio, GW Pharm	CLINICAL (II)	GW Pharmaceuticals (UK)	Antiarthritic	Feb-02
THC-1102	Discontinued	Therapicon (Italy)	Antiinflammatory	Feb-02

Ref.: Pharmaprojects (updated to 2/02) used with permission; Scrip, corporate, literature & patent references
"Status" is international drug development or regulatory status and may not indicate status in USA
Sponsor: Original company name is retained if product is discontinued or inactive after merger, acquisition, company name change, etc.
Users of this table are encouraged to independently verify the status, activity, and mechanism of action of drugs of interest

GENERIC / TRADE NAME	STATUS	SPONSOR (S)	MECHANISM OF ACTION	REF. UPDATE
THC-1104	Discontinued	Therapicon (Italy)	Antiinflammatory	Feb-02
THC-1105	Discontinued	Therapicon (Italy)	Antiinflammatory	Feb-02
THC-1108	Discontinued	Therapicon (Italy)	Antiinflammatory	Feb-02
THC-1110	Discontinued	Therapicon (Italy)	Antiinflammatory	Feb-02
THC-1112	Discontinued	Therapicon (Italy)	Antiinflammatory	Feb-02
THC-1301	Discontinued	Therapicon (Italy)	NSAID	Feb-02
Thiazepines	Preclinical	Searle/Monsanto (US)	PGE2 receptor antagonist	Feb-95
thiazolinobutazone	LAUNCHED	Almirall-Prodesfarma (Spain)	Antiinflammatory	Feb-02
thielavins	Discontinued	Sankyo (Japan)	Antiinflammatory	Feb-02
Thielocin	Discontinued	Shionogi (Japan)	Phospholipase PLA2 inhibitor	Dec-92
Thienylacetamides	Discontinued	Boehringer Mannheim (Ger)	Kappa agonist	1990
thiocolchicoside	Discontinued	Sanofi-Synthelabo (France)	GABA antagonist; analg., anti-inflam.	Feb-02
Thiorphan	Discontinued (ph. I)	Bioproject / INSERM (France)	Enk'ase inhibitor	Feb-94
THIP	Discontinued	Lundbeck (Denmark)	GABA agonist	1985
tianafac	Discontinued	Sanofi-Synthelabo (France)	Antiinflammatory	Feb-02
tiaprofenic acid	LAUNCHED	Aventis (France)	Antiarthritic	Feb-02
tiflamizole	Discontinued	Bristol-Myers Squibb (US)	Antiarthritic	Feb-02
Tifluadom	Discontinued	Solvay (Netherlands)	Kappa agonist	Jul-91
tifurac	Discontinued	Roche (Switz)	NSAID	Feb-02
Tilnoprofen arbamel (Y-23023)	Discontinued (ph. III)	Yoshitomi/Japan Tobacco (Japan)	NSAID	May-99
Timegadine (SR-1368)	Discontinued (ph. III)	Leo (Denmark)	COX/5-LO inhibitor	Mar-88
tiopinac	Discontinued	Roche (Switz)	Antiarthritic	Feb-02
TIPP-NH2	Discontinued	Astra / Clin. Res. Inst. (Canada)	Delta opioid peptide	Sep-97
TJ-114	LAUNCHED	Tsumura (Jp)	Herbal med. (induces IL-1ra)	Aug-95
TK9C	Discontinued	Avant Immunother. (US)	Complement factor inhibitor	May-98
TKA-731	Preclinical	Novartis (Switz.)	Centrally-acting analgesic	Feb-02
TMC-851	Discontinued	Taiyo Pharmaceutical	Antiarthritic	Feb-02
TMC-86A	Inactive	Tanabe Seiyaku (Japan)	Antiinflammatory	Feb-02
TMC-95A	Inactive	Tanabe Seiyaku (Japan)	Antiinflammatory	Feb-02
TMK-919	Inactive	Terumo	Antiinflammatory	Feb-02
TMS-ethoxymethylimidazoles	Inactive	Pfizer (US)	5-HT3 antagonists	1990
TNF-Alpha antagonists, Dynavax	Preclinical	Dynavax Technologies	Antiarthritic	Feb-02
TNF-Alpha inhibitors, Message	Preclinical	Message Pharmaceuticals (US)	Antiinflammatory	Feb-02
tolfenamic acid	LAUNCHED	Bristol-Myers Squibb (US)	Antiinflammatory	Feb-02
tolmetin glycine amide	Discontinued	Johnson & Johnson (US)	Antiinflammatory	Feb-02
tolmetin sodium	LAUNCHED	Johnson & Johnson (US)	Antiinflammatory	Feb-02
Tolnapersine	Discontinued (ph. I)	Novartis (Switz.)	5-HT antagonist	Apr-92
Tolpadol	Inactive	Univ. Complutense (Spain)	PGSI	1983
Tomoxiprole (MDL-035)	Discontinued (Clin.)	Hoechst Marion Roussel (Ger)	PGE2 / PGF1-alpha antag.	Mar-87
Tonabersat (SB-220453)	CLINICAL (II)	SmithKline Beecham (UK)	Unidentified (antimigraine)	May-99
Tonazocine (Win-421562)	Discontinued (ph. II)	Sanofi (France)	Opioid agonist/antagonist	May-94
TR-35	Discontinued	Mitsubishi Pharma (Japan)	Antiinflammatory	Feb-02
TR-5385	Discontinued	Bayer (Germany)	Opioid agonist	Mar-91
TR-9109	Inactive	Tanabe Seiyaku (Japan)	Antiinflammatory	Feb-02
Tramadol (TRAMAL®, ULTRAM®)	LAUNCHED	Gruenthal (Ger); J&J (US)	5-HT/NE uptake inhib.	Apr-95
Tramadol + acetaminophen (ULTREX)	LAUNCHED	Johnson & Johnson (US)	Tramadol + APAP formulation	Feb-02
Tramadol, Biovail	CLINICAL (III)	Biovail (Canada)	Controlled-release (1x/day)	Feb-02
Tramadol, Labopharm	CLINICAL (I)	Labopharm	Formulation	Feb-02
Tramadol, Purdue	PRE-REGISTRATION	Purdue Pharma (US)	Controlled release formulation	Jun-00
Trefentanil	Discontinued (ph. II)	Ohmeda (US)	Ultra-short acting mu opioid	May-97
TRIM	Inactive	Non-industrial source	Neural nitric oxide synthase inhib.	Feb-02
trimebutine + ruscogenines	LAUNCHED	Pfizer (US)	Analgesic combination	Feb-02
TRK-240	Discontinued	Toray (Japan)	Unidentified / anti-inflammatory	May-99
TRK-530	CLINICAL (II)	Toray (Japan)	Unidentified antiarthritic	Jun-00
TRK-820	CLINICAL (II)	Toray (Japan) / Daiichi (Japan)	Kappa agonist analgesic	Sep-97
Trocade (Ro-32-3555)	Discontinued (ph. III)	Roche (Switz.)	MMP inhibitor / RA	Feb-02
Tropanes / Benzomorphans	Discontinued	BTG (UK)	Unknown	Nov-91
tropanserin	Discontinued	Aventis (France)	Antimigraine	Feb-02
tropine indometacinate, Spofa	LAUNCHED	VUFB (Czech Republic)	Antiarthritic	Feb-02
Tropoxin	Inactive	Non-industrial source	Antimigraine	Feb-02
tryptase inhibitors, Array	Preclinical	Array BioPharma	Antiinflammatory	Feb-02
TSC-5	Discontinued	Takeda (Japan)	Antiarthritic	Feb-02
TSG-6 inhibitors	Discontinued	NYU Medical Center (US)	Inflammatory protein	Jun-00

Ref.: Pharmaprojects (updated to 2/02) used with permission; Scrip, corporate, literature & patent references
"Status" is international drug development or regulatory status and may not indicate status in USA
Sponsor: Original company name is retained if product is discontinued or inactive after merger, acquisition, company name change, etc.
Users of this table are encouraged to independently verify the status, activity, and mechanism of action of drugs of interest

GENERIC / TRADE NAME	STATUS	SPONSOR (S)	MECHANISM OF ACTION	REF. UPDATE
TSK-204 (KF-20444)	Inactive	Taisho / Kyowa Hakko (Japan)	Unidentified (RA)	Feb-02
TSN-09 (Buprenorphine)	CLINICAL (III)	Teijin (Japan)	Transdermal tape formulation	Feb-99
TST-500	Preclinical	Twinstrand Therapeutics	Antiarthritic	Feb-02
TY-10214	Discontinued	Toa Eiyo	Antiinflammatory	Feb-02
TY-10222	Discontinued	Toa Eiyo	NSAID	Feb-02
TY-10246	Discontinued	Toa Eiyo	Antiinflammatory	Feb-02
TY-10474	Discontinued	Toa Eiyo	Antiinflammatory	Feb-02
TZI-41078	Discontinued (ph. II)	Teikoku Hormone (Japan)	COX + lipoxygenase inhibitor	May-90
TZI-615	Discontinued	Teikoku Hormone	Antiinflammatory	Feb-02
U-24522	Discontinued	AstraZeneca (UK)	Antiarthritic	Feb-02
U-47,476A	Inactive	Upjohn (US)	Alpha-2 agonist	1985
U-50,488H	Inactive	Upjohn (US)	Kappa agonist	1989
U-78517	Inactive	Pharmacia (US)	Antiinflammatory	Feb-02
U-81581	Inactive	Pharmacia (US)	Antiarthritic	Feb-02
UA 621/859	Preclinical	Univ. Arizona (US)	Opioid endorphins	Apr-97
UK-69578	Discontinued (ph. II)	Pfizer (US)	Enk'ase inhibitor; phase II	1990
UP-202-32	Discontinued	Bristol-Myers Squibb / UPSA	Adenosine agonist	Mar-97
UP-26-91	Discontinued (ph. II)	UPSA / Bristol-Myers Squibb (US)	5-HT neuromodulator	Mar-97
UP-5222-04	Discontinued (ph. II)	UPSA (France)	Central non-opioid analgesic	Mar-91
UPA-780	Preclinical	NAS (Ukraine)	PGSI / Leukotriene inhib.	Oct-95
UR-8880	Preclinical	Uriach (Spain)	Antiinflammatory	Feb-02
V-144	Discontinued (ph. II)	Vita-Invest (Spain)	NSAID	Apr-85
V-2	Discontinued (ph. I)	Prodesfarma (Spain)	PGSI / peripheral analgesic	Jul-95
Valdecoxib	REGISTERED	Pharmacia / Pfizer (US)	COX-2 inhibitor, 2nd generation	Feb-02
VAN project	Preclinical	Vita-Invest (Spain)	Opioid analgesic (unidentified)	Jun-98
VAN-H36	CLINICAL (I)	Vita-Invest (Spain)	Centrally-acting analgesic	Feb-02
vanilloid receptor antag,Neuro	Preclinical	Neurogen (US)	Centrally-acting analgesic	Feb-02
Vapill	Preclinical	BioTie Therapies	Antiarthritic	Feb-02
venoglobulin-1H	LAUNCHED	Mitsubishi Pharma (Japan)	Antiinflammatory	Feb-02
Veradoline	Discontinued	Fisons (UK)	PGSI	Aug-82
Verilopam	Discontinued	Fisons (UK)	PGSI	Feb-80
VISCERALGINE FORTE®	LAUNCHED	Akzo (Netherlands)	Muscarinic + anti-inflam.	Dec-91
viscoelastic collagen, Collage	Preclinical	Collagenesis	Antiarthritic	Feb-02
VLA-4 antagonist	Discontinued	Hoechst Marion Roussel (Ger)	VLA-4 inhibitor; RA	Jun-00
VLA-4 antagonist, Merck	Preclinical	Merck & Co (US)	Antiinflammatory	Feb-02
VLA-4 antagonists, Biogen	Preclinical	Biogen (US)	Antiinflammatory	Feb-02
VS-395	Discontinued	Vita-Invest (Spain)	5-HT1d-alpha/beta agonist	Jun-98
VT-224	Preclinical	Viron Therapeutics (Canada)	Antiinflammatory	Feb-02
VT-239	Preclinical	Viron Therapeutics (Canada)	Antiinflammatory	Feb-02
VT-346	Preclinical	Viron Therapeutics (Canada)	Antiinflammatory	Feb-02
VT-900	Preclinical	Viron Therapeutics (Canada)	Antiinflammatory	Feb-02
VUFB-13757	Discontinued	VUFB (Czech Republic)	Opioid agonist	Dec-92
VX-475	Preclinical	Vertex (US) / Kissei (Japan)	MAP kinase inhibitor; RA	Oct-98
VX-702	Preclinical	Vertex Pharmaceuticals (US)	Antiinflammatory	Feb-02
VX-740 (HMR-3480)	CLINICAL (II)	Aventis (France)	IL-1beta conv. enzyme inhib./RA	Jun-00
VX-745	Suspended (ph. II)	Vertex (US) / Kissei (Japan)	MAP kinase inhib. / anti-inflam.	Feb-02
VX-765	Preclinical	Vertex Pharmaceuticals (US)	Antiinflammatory	Feb-02
WA-8242B	Discontinued	Fujisawa (Japan)	PLA2 inhibitor; inflam., allergy	Jun-00
WAY-121520 (WAY-122220)	Discontinued	Wyeth-Ayerst (US)	Phospholipase PLA2 inhibitor	Apr-95
WF-11605	Inactive	Fujisawa (Japan)	Antiinflammatory	Feb-02
Wheat-derived peptide	Inactive	Nisshin Flour (Japan)	Opioid peptide	Jul-91
Win-42610	Discontinued	Eastman Kodak (US)	Opioid agonist/antagonist	Feb-85
Win-52114-2	Inactive	Eastman Kodak (US)	Unknown	1988
Win-64338	Preclinical	Eastman Kodak (US)	B2 antagonist	Nov-93
Win-64821	Discontinued	Sanofi (France)	NK1 + NK2 antagonist	Dec-95
Win-72052	Inactive	Sanofi-Synthelabo (France)	Antiinflammatory	Feb-02
Wy-19735	Discontinued	American Home Products (US)	Antiinflammatory	Feb-02
Wy-23205	Discontinued	American Home Products (US)	Antiinflammatory	Feb-02
Wy-28342	Discontinued	American Home Products (US)	Antiinflammatory	Feb-02
Wy-41770	Discontinued	American Home Products (US)	Antiinflammatory	Feb-02
Wy-42186	Inactive	Wyeth-Ayerst (US)	Enkephalin analog	1983
Wy-42320	Discontinued	Wyeth-Ayerst (US)	Opioid agonist	Feb-82
Wy-45368	Discontinued	American Home Products (US)	Antiarthritic	Feb-02

Ref.: Pharmaprojects (updated to 2/02) used with permission; Scrip, corporate, literature & patent references
"Status" is international drug development or regulatory status and may not indicate status in USA
Sponsor: Original company name is retained if product is discontinued or inactive after merger, acquisition, company name change, etc.
Users of this table are encouraged to independently verify the status, activity, and mechanism of action of drugs of interest

GENERIC / TRADE NAME	STATUS	SPONSOR (S)	MECHANISM OF ACTION	REF. UPDATE
Wy-48489	Inactive	American Home Products (US)	Antiinflammatory	Feb-02
Wy-49422	Inactive	American Home Products (US)	Antiinflammatory	Feb-02
XB375, XE440	Discontinued	DuPont Merck (US)	Kappa agonist	Jun-93
Xen-001	Preclinical	Xenome	Centrally-acting analgesic	Feb-02
Xenipentone (RP-48-482)	Discontinued (ph. I)	Novartis (Switz.)	Unidentified anti-inflammatory	Feb-85
xenyhexenic acid	Discontinued	Aventis (France)	Antiinflammatory	Feb-02
Xorphanol	CLINICAL (II)	HG Pars (US)	Opioid agonist/antagonist	Mar-92
XR-168	Discontinued	Xenova (US)	MMP inhibitor (collagenase inhib.)	Nov-96
Xyloadenosine	Discontinued	Amgen (US)	TNF-alpha inhibitor	Dec-97
Y-20003	Discontinued	Mitsubishi Pharma (Japan)	NSAID	Feb-02
Yissum P-0558	Discontinued	Yissum (Israel)	Controlled release system	Feb-93
Yissum P-0873	Inactive	Yissum (Israel)	Unk. / peripheral	Feb-02
Yissum P-0883	Discontinued	Yissum (Israel)	Peripheral opioid inducer	Mar-97
Yissum P-1025	Preclinical	Yissum (Israel)	Antiinflammatory / Antioxidant	Apr-98
YM-09561	Discontinued	Yamanouchi (Japan)	Antiinflammatory	Feb-02
YM-13162	Discontinued	Yamanouchi (Japan)	Antiinflammatory	Feb-02
YM-26567-1	Inactive	Yamanouchi (Japan)	Antiinflammatory	Feb-02
YM-26734	Discontinued	Yamanouchi (Japan)	Phospholipase PLA2 inhibitor	May-98
YS-1033	Inactive	Asahi Kasei (Japan)	Antiinflammatory	Feb-02
YS-134	Inactive	Medea Research (Italy)	Antiinflammatory	Feb-02
Z-4003	Discontinued	Zambon	Antiinflammatory	Feb-02
zaltoprofen	LAUNCHED	Nippon Chemiphar	Antiinflammatory	Feb-02
ZD-2138	Discontinued	AstraZeneca (UK)	Antiarthritic	Feb-02
ZD-2315	Preclinical	Zeneca (UK)	MHCII antagonist (RA)	Jan-98
ZD-4953	Discontinued (ph. II)	AstraZeneca (UK)	EP1 prostaglandin antagonist	Jun-00
ZD-6416	Discontinued	AstraZeneca (UK)	EP1 prostaglandin antagonist	Feb-02
ZD-6804	Preclinical	Zeneca (UK)	EP1 prostaglandin antagonist	Jan-98
ZD-9379	Preclinical	Zeneca (UK)	Glycine antag. / neuropathic pain	Jan-98
Zenazocine mesilate	Inactive	Eastman Kodak (US)	Opioid agonist/antagonist	1981
ZG-1494Alpha	Discontinued	Novo Nordisk (Denmark)	Antiinflammatory	Feb-02
Ziconotide (SNX-111, intrathecal)	PRE-REGISTRATION	Elan (Ireland) / Neurex (US)	Ca++ channel antag. / intrathecal	Jun-00
Zidometacin (P-74180)	Discontinued (PRE-REG)	Pharmacia & Upjohn (UK)	NSAID / indomethacin analog	Apr-88
ZK-31945 (SH-405)	Discontinued (ph. I)	Schering AG (Germany)	NSAID; Clidanac isomer	Apr-84
ZK-90695	Inactive	Schering AG (Germany)	Antiinflammatory	Feb-02
ZM-216800	Inactive	AstraZeneca (UK)	Antiarthritic	Feb-02
zoanthamine	Inactive	Non-industrial source	Antiinflammatory	Feb-02
Zoliprofen (156-S)	Discontinued (ph. III)	Shionogi (Japan)	NSAID	May-89
Zolmitriptan (ZOMIG®; 311C90)	LAUNCHED	Zeneca (UK)	5-HT1d/1b agonist	Apr-98
ZT-52656A	Discontinued (ph. I)	SmithKline Beecham (UK)	Kappa agonist	Jan-93

Further Readings

SECTION 1: BASIC ASPECTS

1. Mechanism-Based Classifications of Pain and Analgesic Drug Discovery

Samad TA, Sapirstein A, Woolf CJ. (2002) Prostanoids and pain: unraveling mechanisms and revealing therapeutic targets. Trends Mol Med 8(8):390–396.

2. Sites of Analgesic Action

Whiteside GT, Munglani R. (2001) Cell death in the superficial dorsal horn in a model of neuropathic pain. J Neurosci Res 64(2):168–173.

3. From Acute to Chronic Pain: Peripheral and Central Mechanisms

Cervero F. (2000) Visceral pain—central sensitisation. Gut 47(Suppl 4):56–57.
Cervero F. (2000) Visceral hyperalgesia revisited. Lancet 356(9236):1127–1128.

4. Central and Peripheral Components of Neuropathic Pain

Hashizume H, DeLeo JA, Colburn RW, Weinstein JN. (2000) Spinal glial activation and cytokine expression after lumbar root injury in the rat. Spine 25(10):1206–1217.

5. A New Perspective on Signal Transduction in Neuropathic Pain: The Emerging Role of the G Protein by βγ Dimer in Transducing and Modulating Opioid Signaling

McCormack K, Kidd BL, Morris V. (2000) Assay of topically administered ibuprofen using a model of post-injury hypersensitivity—A randomised, double-blind, placebo-controlled study. Eur J Clin Pharm 56(6-7):459–462.

6. Pain and the Somatosensory Cortex

Lenz FA, Treede RD. (2002) Attention, novelty, and pain. Pain 99(1-2):1–3.
Baumgartner U, Magerl W, Klein T, Hopf HC, Treede RD. (2002) Neurogenic hyperalgesia versus painful hypoalgesia: two distinct mechanisms of neuropathic pain. Pain 96(1–2):141–51.

Treede RD, Apkarian AV, Bromm B, Greenspan JD, Lenz FA. (2000) Cortical representation of pain: functional characterization of nociceptive areas near the lateral sulcus. Pain 87(2):113–119.

7. Descending Pathways in Spinal Cord Stimulation and Pain Control

Baba H, Shimoji K, Yoshimura M. (2000) Norepinephrine facilitates inhibitory transmission in substantia gelatinosa of adult rat spinal cord (part 1): effects on axon terminals of GABAergic and glycinergic neurons. Anesth 92(2):473–484.

Baba H, Goldstein PA, Okamoto M, Kohno T, Ataka T, Yoshimura M, Shimoji K. (2000) Norepinephrine facilitates inhibitory transmission in substantia gelatinosa of adult rat spinal cord (part 2): effects on somatodendritic sites of GABAergic neurons. Anesth 92(2):485–492.

8. Local Neuroimmune Interactions in Visceral Hyperalgesia: Bradykinin, Neurotrophins, and Cannabinoids

Rice AS, Farquhar-Smith WP, Nagy I. (2002) Endocannabinoids and pain: spinal and peripheral analgesia in inflammation and neuropathy. Prostaglandins Leukot Essent Fatty Acids 66(2–3):243–256.

Farquhar-Smith WP, Jaggar SI, Rice AS. (2002) Attenuation of nerve growth factor-induced visceral hyperalgesia via cannabinoid CB(1) and CB(2)-like receptors. Pain 97(1–2):11–21.

Bridges D, Thompson SW, Rice AS. (2001) Mechanisms of neuropathic Pain Br J Anaesth 87(1):12–26.

9. Pain Processing in the Periphery: Development of Analgesics

Lembo PMC, Grazzini E, Groblewski T, O'Donnell D, Roy MO, Zhang J, Hoffert C, Cao J, Schmidt R, Pelletier M, Labarre M, Gosselin M, Fortin Y, Banville D, Shen SH, Strom P, Payza K, Dray A, Walker P, Ahmad S. (2002) Proenkephalin A gene products activate a new family of sensory neuron-specific GPCRs. Nat Neuro 5(3):201–209.

SECTION 2: CLINICAL ASPECTS

10. Neuroimaging of Pain: Possibilities of Objective Measurements of Analgesic Actions in Human Subjects

DaSilva AFM, Becerra L, Makris N, Strassman AM, Gonzalez RG, Geatrakis N, Borsook D. (2002) Somatotopic activation in the human trigeminal pain pathway. J Neurosci 22(18):8183–8192.

Becerra L, Breiter HC, Wise R, Gonzalez RG, Borsook D. (2001) Reward circuitry activation by noxious thermal stimuli. Neuron 32(5):927–946.

Tracey I, Becerra L, Chang I, Breiter H, Jenkins L, Borsook D, Gonzalez RG. (2000) Noxious hot and cold stimulation produce common patterns of brain activation in humans: a functional magnetic resonance imaging study. Neurosci Lett 288(2):159–162.

11. Surrogate Models of Pain

Baumgartner U, Magerl W, Klein T, Hopf HC, Treede RD. (2002) Neurogenic hyperalgesia versus painful hypoalgesia: two distinct mechanisms of neuropathic pain. Pain 96(1–2):141–151.

12. Acute Trauma and Postoperative Pain

Cooper JA, Bromley LM, Baranowski AP, Barker SGE. (2000) Evaluation of a needle-free injection system for local anaesthesia prior to venous cannulation. Anaesth 55(3):247–250.

13. Effectiveness of Needling Techniques with Special Reference to Myofascial Pain Syndromes

Irnich D, Behrens N, Gleditsch JM, Stor W, Schreiber MA, Schops P, Vickers AJ, Beyer A. (2002) Immediate effects of dry needling and acupuncture at distant points in chronic neck pain: results of a randomized, double-blind, sham-controlled crossover trial. Pain 99(1–2):83–89.

14. Advances in the Management of Spinal Pain and Radiofrequency Techniques

Whitworth LA, Feler CA. (2002) Application of spinal ablative techniques for the treatment of benign chronic painful conditions: history, methods, and outcomes. Spine 27(22):2607–2612.

Geurts JW, van Wijk RM, Stolker RJ, Groen GJ. (2001) Efficacy of radiofrequency procedures for the treatment of spinal pain: a systematic review of randomized clinical trials. Reg Anesth Pain Med 26(5): 394–400.

Leclaire R, Fortin L, Lambert R, Bergeron YM, Rossignol M. (2001) Radiofrequency facet joint denervation in the treatment of low back pain: a placebo-controlled clinical trial to assess efficacy. Spine 26(13): 1411–1416.

15. Pulsed Radiofrequency Treatment of Chronic Neck, Back, Sympathetic, and Peripheral Neuroma-Derived Pain

Forouzanfar T, van Kleef M, Weber WE. (2000) Radiofrequency lesions of the stellate ganglion in chronic pain syndromes: retrospective analysis of clinical efficacy in 86 patients. Clin J Pain 16(2):164–168.

16. Spinal Cord Stimulation

North RB, Wetzel FT. (2002) Spinal cord stimulation for chronic pain of spinal origin: a valuable long-term solution. Spine 27(22):2584–2591.

Oakley JC, Prager JP. (2002) Spinal cord stimulation: mechanisms of action. Spine 27(22):2574–2583.

17. Spinal Endoscopy: Its Current Status and Role in Lumbosacral Radiculopathy

Geurts JW, Kallewaard JW, Richardson J, Groen GJ. (2002) Targeted methylprednisolone acetate/hyaluronidase/clonidine injection after diagnostic epiduroscopy for chronic sciatica: a prospective, 1-year follow-up study. Reg Anesth Pain Med 27(4):343–352.

Richardson J, McGurgan P, Cheema S, Prasad R, Gupta S. (2001) Spinal endoscopy in chronic low back pain with radiculopathy. A prospective case series. Anaesth 56(5):454–460.

18. Cancer Pain Treatment

Meier DE. (2002) United States: overview of cancer pain and palliative care. J Pain Symp Man 24(2): 265–269. [NB: See other country-by-country reviews in this special journal issue].

19. Inflammatory Joint Disease and Pain

Isaacs JD, Greer S, Sharma S, Symmons D, Smith M, Johnston J, Waldmann H, Hale G, Hazleman BL. (2001) Morbidity and mortality in rheumatoid arthritis patients with prolonged and profound therapy-induced lymphopenia. Arthritis & Rheum 44(9):1998–2008.

20. Chronic Nonmalignant Visceral Pain Syndromes of the Abdomen, Pelvis, and Bladder and Chronic Urogenital and Rectal Pain

Wesselmann U. (2001) Neurogenic inflammation and chronic pelvic pain. World J Urology 19(3):180–185.

Wesselmann U. (2001) Interstitial cystitis: A chronic visceral pain syndrome. Urology 57(6A Suppl S): 32–39.

Ali Z, Raja SN, Wesselmann U, Fuchs PN, Meyer RA, Campbell JN. (2000) Intradermal injection of norepinephrine evokes pain in patients with sympathetically maintained pain. Pain 88(2):161–168.

21. Nerve Injury Pain

Khodorova A, Fareed MU, Gokin A, Strichartz GR, Davar G. (2002) Local injection of a selective endothelin-B receptor agonist inhibits endothelin-1-induced pain-like behavior and excitation of nociceptors in a naloxone-sensitive manner. J Neurosci 22(17):7788–7796.

Zhou ZR, Davar G, Strichartz G. (2002) Endothelin-1 (ET-1) selectively enhances the activation gating of slowly inactivating tetrodotoxin-resistant sodium currents in rat sensory neurons: A mechanism for the pain-inducing actions of ET-1. J Neurosci 22(15):6325–6330.

Zhou QL, Strichartz G, Davar G. (2001) Endothelin-1 activates ETA receptors to increase intracellular calcium in model sensory neurons. NeuroReport 12(17):3853–3857.

22. Sympathetically Maintained Pain

Wasner G, Schattschneider J, Baron R. (2002) Skin temperature side differences–a diagnostic tool for CRPS? Pain 98(1–2):19–26.

Baron R, Raja SN. (2002) Role of adrenergic transmitters and receptors in nerve and tissue injury related pain. MECHANISMS AND MEDIATORS OF NEUROPATHIC PAIN. pp. 153–174.

Wasner G, Brechot A, Schattschneider J, Allardt A, Binder A, Jensen TS, Baron R. (2002) Effect of sympathetic muscle vasoconstrictor activity on capsaicin-induced muscle pain. Musc & Nerve 26(1): 113–121.

23. Headache: Basic Anatomy and Physiology of the Trigeminovascular System

Goadsby PJ, Lance J, Ferrari M, Dahlof C, Watson D, Mathew N, Diener HC, Goldstein J, Salonen R, Messina E, Rapaport A, O'Sullivan E, Saxena PR, Dowson A. (2001) Imigran: Ten years of improving the lives of migraine patients–Rome, 24 March 2000–Questions from the audience. Cephal 21(Suppl 1):39–41.

24. Psychological Factors in Measurement of Pain

Koutantji M, Pearce S, Harrold E. (2000) Psychological aspects of vasculitis. Rheumatol 39(11):1173–1179.

Koutantji M, Pearce SA, Oskley DA. (2000) Cognitive processing of pain-related words and psychological adjustment in high and low pain frequency participants. Br J Health Psychol 5(Part 3):275–288.

25. Challenges and Pitfalls of Clinical Trials: Evaluating Novel Analgesics for Neuropathic Pain

Sang CN. (2000) NMDA-receptor antagonists in neuropathic pain: experimental methods to clinical trials. J Pain Symp Man 19(1 Suppl):S21–S25.

SECTION 3: NOVEL APPROACHES TO DRUG DISCOVERY

26. Molecular Approaches to the Study of Pain

Lawson SN. (2002) Phenotype and function of somatic primary afferent nociceptive neurones with C-, Adelta- or Aalpha/beta-fibres. Exp Physiol 87(2):239–244.

Newton RA, Bingham S, Davey PD, Medhurst AD, Piercy V, Raval P, Parsons AA, Sanger GJ, Case CP, Lawson SN. (2000) Identification of differentially expressed genes in dorsal root ganglia following partial sciatic nerve injury. Neurosci 95(4):1111–1120.

27. Molecular Validation of Pain Targets

Decosterd I, Ji RR, Abdi S, Tate S, Woolf CJ. (2002) The pattern of expression of the voltage-gated sodium channels Na(v)1.8 and Na(v)1.9 does not change in uninjured primary sensory neurons in experimental neuropathic pain models. Pain 96(3):269–277.

Bucknill AT, Coward K, Plumpton C, Tate S, Bountra C, Birch R, Sandison A, Hughes SPF, Anand P. (2002) Nerve fibers in lumbar spine structures and injured spinal roots express the sensory neuron-specific sodium channels SNS/PN3 and NaN/SNS2. Spine 27(2):135–140.

Shembalkar PK, Till S, Boettger MK, Terenghi G, Tate S, Bountra C, Anand P. (2001) Increased sodium channel SNS/PN3 immunoreactivity in a causalgic finger. Eur J Pain 5(3):319–323.

Benn SC, Costigan M, Tate S, Fitzgerald M, Woolf CJ. (2001) Developmental expression of the TTX-resistant voltage-gated sodium channels Na(v)1.8 (SNS) and Na(v)1.9 (SNS2) in primary sensory neurons. J Neurosci 21(16):6077–6085.

Coward K, Mosahebi A, Plumpton C, Facer P, Birch R, Tate S, Bountra C, Terenghi G, Anand P. (2001) Immunolocalisation of sodium channel NaG in the intact and injured human peripheral nervous system. J Anat 198(Part 2):175–180.

Coward K, Jowett A, Plumpton C, Powell A, Birch R, Tate S, Bountra C, Anand P. (2001) Sodium channel beta 1 and beta 2 subunits parallel SNS/PN3 alpha-subunit changes in injured human sensory neurons. NeuroReport 12(3):483–488.

28. Genetics of Pain

Duckworth DM, Sanseau P. (2002) In silico identification of novel therapeutic targets. Drug Disc Today 7(11 Suppl S):S64–S69.

Sanseau P. (2001) Transgenic gene knockouts: a functional platform for the industry. Drug Disc Today 6(15):770–771.

Sanseau P. (2001) Impact of human genome sequencing for in silico target discovery. Drug Disc Today 6(6):316–323.

Delany NS, Hurle M, Facer P, Alnadaf T, Plumpton C, Kinghorn I, See CG, Costigan M, Anand P, Woolf CJ, Crowther D, Sanseau P, Tate SN. (2001) Identification and characterization of a novel human vanilloid receptor-like protein, VRL-2. Physio Gen 4(3):165–174.

29. Animal Models of Pain

Drew GM, Siddall PJ, Duggan AW. (2001) Responses of spinal neurones to cutaneous and dorsal root stimuli in rats with mechanical allodynia after contusive spinal cord injury. Brain Res 893(1–2):59–69.

Siddall PJ, Molloy AR, Walker S, Mather LE, Rutkowski SB, Cousins MJ. (2000) The efficacy of intrathecal morphine and clonidine in the treatment of pain after spinal cord injury. Anesth Analg 91(6):1493–1498.

SECTION 4: NEW and EMERGING THERAPIES

30. An Overview of Current and Investigational Drugs for the Treatment of Acute and Chronic Pain

Furst DE, Manning DC. (2001) Future directions in pain management. Clin Exp Rheumatol 19(6 Suppl 25):S71–S76.

31. Novel Mu, Delta, and Kappa Agonists: Potential for Development of Novel Analgesic Agent

Gardell LR, Burgess SE, Dogrul A, Ossipov MH, Malan TP, Lai J, Porreca F. (2002) Pronociceptive effects of spinal dynorphin promote cannabinoid-induced pain and antinociceptive tolerance. Pain 98(1–2):79–88.

Gardell LR, Wang RZ, Burgess SE, Ossipov MH, Vanderah TW, Malan TP, Lai J, Porreca F. (2002) Sustained morphine exposure induces a spinal dynorphin-dependent enhancement of excitatory transmitter release from primary afferent fibers. J Neurosci 22(15):6747–6755.

Porreca F, Ossipov MH, Gebhart GF. (2002) Chronic pain and medullary descending facilitation. Trends in Neurosci 25(6):319–325.

Hruby VJ. (2001) Design in topographical space of peptide and peptidomimetic ligands that affect behavior. A chemist's glimpse at the mind—body problem. Acc Chem Res 34(5):389–397.

32. Delta-Receptor, Nonpeptide Agonists: The Development of Safe, Strong Analgesics with a Novel Mechanism of Action

Dondio G. (2000) Development of novel pain relief agents acting through the selective activation of the delta-opioid receptor. Farmaco 55(3):178–180.

33. Peripheral Opioid Analgesia: Neuroimmune Interactions and Therapeutic Implications

Machelska H, Stein C. (2002) Immune mechanisms in pain control. Anesth Analg 95(4):1002–1008.

Machelska H, Mousa SA, Brack A, Schopohl JK, Rittner HL, Schafer M, Stein C. (2002) Opioid control of inflammatory pain regulated by intercellular adhesion molecule-1. J Neurosci 22(13):5588–5596.

Mousa SA, Machelska H, Schafer M, Stein C. (2002) Immunohistochemical localization of endomorphin-1 and endomorphin-2 in immune cells and spinal cord in a model of inflammatory pain. J Neuroimmunology 126(1–2):5–15.

Stein C, Machelska H, Schafer A. (2001) Peripheral analgesic and antiinflammatory effects of opioids. Zeitschrift fur Rheumatologie 60(6):416.

Rittner HL, Brack A, Machelska H, Mousa SA, Bauer M, Schafer M, Stein C. (2001) Opioid peptide-expressing leukocytes–Identification, recruitment, and simultaneously increasing inhibition of inflammatory pain. Anesth 95(2):500–508.

Binder W, Machelska H, Mousa S, Schmitt T, Riviere PJM, Junien JL, Stein C, Schafer M. (2001) Analgesic and antiinflammatory effects of two novel kappa-opioid peptides. Anesth 94(6):1034–1044.

34. Profile of ADL 2-1294, an Opioid Antihyperalgesic Agent with Selectivity for Peripheral Mu- Opiate Receptors

DeHaven-Hudkins DL, Cowan A, Cortes Burgos L, Daubert JD, Cassel JA, DeHaven RN, Kehner GB, Kumar V. (2002) Antipruritic and antihyperalgesic actions of loperamide and analogs. Life Sci 71(23): 2787–2796.

Sandner-Kiesling A, Pan HL, Chen SR, James RL, DeHaven-Hudkins DL, Dewan DM, Eisenach JC. (2002) Effect of kappa opioid agonists on visceral nociception induced by uterine cervical distension in rats. Pain 96(1–2):13–22.

35. Controlled-Release Opioids

Simpson KH. (2002) Individual choice of opioids and formulations: strategies to achieve the optimum for the patient. Rheumatol 21 Suppl 1:S5–S8.

Sinatra RS, Torres J, Bustos AM. (2002) Pain management after major orthopaedic surg•y: current strategies and new concepts. J Am Acad Orthop Surg 10(2):117–129.

Reder RF. (2001) Opioid formulations: tailoring to the needs in chronic pain. Eur J Pain 5 Suppl A:109–111.

Cherny N. (2000) New strategies in opioid therapy for cancer pain. J Oncol Manag 9(1):8–15.

36. NMDA-Receptor Antagonists as Enhancers of Analgesic Activity: The MorphiDex™ Morphine–Dextromethorphan Combination

Weinbroum AA, Gorodetzky A, Nirkin A, Kollender Y, Bickels J, Marouani N, Rudick V, Meller I. (2002) Dextromethorphan for the reduction of immediate and late postoperative pain and morphine consumption in orthopedic oncology patients: a randomized, placebo-controlled, double-blind study. Cancer 95(5):1164–1170.

Weinbroum AA. (2002) Dextromethorphan reduces immediate and late postoperative analgesic requirements and improves patients' subjective scorings after epidural lidocaine and general anesthesia. Anesth Analg 94(6):1547–1552.

Heiskanen T, Hartel B, Dahl ML, Seppala T, Kalso E. (2002) Analgesic effects of dextromethorphan and morphine in patients with chronic pain. Pain 96(3):261–267.

Goldblum R. (2000) Long-term safety of MorphiDex. J Pain Symp Man 19(1 Suppl):S50–S56.

Price DD, Mayer DJ, Mao J, Caruso FS. (2000) NMDA-receptor antagonists and opioid receptor interactions as related to analgesia and tolerance. J Pain Symp Man 19(1 Suppl):S7–S11.

37. CCK Antagonist Potentiation of Opioid Analgesia

Coudore-Civiale MA, Courteix C, Fialip J, Boucher M, Eschalier A. (2000) Spinal effect of the cholecystokinin-B receptor antagonist CI-988 on hyperalgesia, allodynia and morphine-induced analgesia in diabetic and mononeuropathic rats. Pain 88(1):15–22.

Wiesenfeld-Hallin Z, de Arauja Lucas G, Alster P, Xu XJ, Hokfelt T. (1999) Cholecystokinin/opioid interactions. Brain Res 848(1–2):78–89.

38. Profile of NSAID + Opioid Combination Analgesics

Olson NZ, Otero AM, Marrero I, Tirado S, Cooper S, Doyle G, Jayawardena S, Sunshine A. (2001) Onset of analgesia for liquigel ibuprofen 400 mg, acetaminophen 1000 mg, ketoprofen 25 mg, and placebo in the treatment of postoperative dental pain. J Clin Pharm 41(11):1238–1247.

Sunshine A, Laska E, Meisner M. (2000) Oral aspirin in post-operative pain: a quantitative, systematic review. Edwards et al., PAIN 81 (1999) 289-297. Pain 88(3):309–310.

Sunshine A. (2000) A comparison of the newer COX-2 drugs and older nonnarcotic oral analgesics. J Pain 1(3 Suppl 1):10–13.

39. NSAIDs and COX-2 Inhibitors

Sonnenblick EH. (2002) Differences between COX-2-specific inhibitors: clinical and economic implications. Am J Manag Care 8(15 Suppl):S428–S430.

Howes LG, Krum H. (2002) Selective cyclo-oxygenase-2 inhibitors and myocardial infarction: how strong is the link? Drug Saf 25(12):829–835.

Katz N. The impact of pain management on quality of life. J Pain Symp Man 24(1 Suppl):S38-47, 2002.

Sinatra R. (2002) Role of COX-2 inhibitors in the evolution of acute pain management. J Pain Symp Man 24(1 Suppl):S18–S27.

Staats PS. (2002) Pain management and beyond: evolving concepts and treatments involving cyclooxygenase inhibition. J Pain Symp Man 24(1 Suppl):S4–S9.

Lin DT, Subbaramaiah K, Shah JP, Dannenberg AJ, Boyle JO. (2002) Cyclooxygenase-2: a novel molecular target for the prevention and treatment of head and neck cancer. Head Neck 24(8):792–799.

Moore RA. (2002) The hidden costs of arthritis treatment and the cost of new therapy—the burden of non-steroidal anti-inflammatory drug gastropathy. Rheumatol (Oxford) 41 Suppl:7–15.

40. COX-2–Specific Inhibitors: Celecoxib and Second-Generation Agents

Bensen WG. (2000) Antiinflammatory and analgesic efficacy of COX-2 specific inhibition: from investigational trials to clinical experience. J Rheumatol Suppl 60:17–24.

Bensen WG, Zhao SZ, Burke TA, Zabinski RA, Makuch RW, Maurath CJ, Agrawal NM, Geis GS. (2000) Upper gastrointestinal tolerability of celecoxib, a COX-2 specific inhibitor, compared to naproxen and placebo. J Rheumatol 27(8):1876–1883.

41. NK_1 Receptor Antagonists: Potential Analgesics?

Smith D, Hill RG, Edvinsson L, Longmore J. (2002) An immunocytochemical investigation of human trigeminal nucleus caudalis: CGRP, substance P and 5-HT1D-receptor immunoreactivities are expressed by trigeminal sensory fibres. Cephal 22(6):424–431.

Fields HL, Hill RG. (2001) Neuropathic pain: The near and far horizon. NEUROPATHIC PAIN: PATHOPHYSIOLOGY AND TREATMENT. pp. 251–264.

Hill RG. (2002) Substance P, opioid, and catecholamine systems in the mouse central nervous system (CNS). Proc Natl Acad Sci USA 99(2):549–551.

42. Vanilloids

Nagy I, Rang H. (2000) Comparison of currents activated by noxious heat in rat and chicken primary sensory neurons. Reg Peptides 96(1—2 Special Issue SI):3–6.

43. The Development of Bradykinin Antagonists as Therapeutic Agents

Dziadulewicz EK, Ritchie TJ, Hallett A, Snell CR, Davies JW, Wrigglesworth R, Dunstan AR, Bloomfield GC, Drake GS, McIntyre P, Brown MC, Burgess GM, Lee W, Davis C, Yaqoob M, Phagoo SB, Phillips E, Perkins MN, Campbell EA, Davis AJ, Rang HP. (2002) Nonpeptide bradykinin B2 receptor antagonists: conversion of rodent-selective bradyzide analogues into potent, orally-active human bradykinin B2 receptor antagonists. J Med Chem 45(11):2160–2172.

Burgess GM, Perkins MN, Rang HP, Campbell EA, Brown MC, McIntyre P, Urban L, Dziadulewicz EK, Ritchie TJ, Hallett A, Snell CR, Wrigglesworth R, Lee W, Davis C, Phagoo SB, Davis AJ, Phillips E, Drake GS, Hughes GA, Dunstan A, Bloomfield GC. (2000) Bradyzide, a potent non-peptide B(2) bradykinin receptor antagonist with long-lasting oral activity in animal models of inflammatory hyperalgesia. Br J Pharmacol 129(1):77–86.

44. The Treatment of Neuropathic Pain: Anticonvulsants, Antidepressants, Na Channel Blockers, NMDA Receptor Blockers and Capsaicin

Bowsher D. (2002) Human 'autotomy'. Pain 95(1–2):187–189.

Bowsher D. (2001) Stroke and central poststroke pain in an elderly population. J Pain 2(5):258–261.

Bowsher D. (2001) Painful stimulation. J Neuro, Neurosurg & Psych 71(3):416.
Bowsher D. (2001) Postherpetic neuralgia–Findings differ from earlier results. Br Med J 322(7290):859–860.
Bowsher D. (2000) The important time parameter is missing. Comment on Sindrup and Jensen, PAIN 83 (1999) 389–400. Pain 88(3):313.

45. *N*-Methyl-D-Aspartate (NMDA) Receptors as a Target for Pain Therapy

Chizh BA. (2002) Novel approaches to targeting glutamate receptors for the treatment of chronic pain: Review article. Amino Acids 23(1–3):169–176.
Chizh BA, Headley PM, Tzschentke TM. (2001) NMDA receptor antagonists as analgesics: focus on the NR2B subtype. Trends in Pharmacol Sci 22(12):636–642.
Chizh BA, Reissmuller E, Schlutz H, Scheede M, Haase G, Englberger W. (2001) Supraspinal vs spinal sites of the antinociceptive action of the subtype-selective NMDA antagonist ifenprodil. Neuropharm 40(2):212–220.
Chizh BA, Schlutz H, Scheede M, Englberger W. (2000) The N-methyl-D-aspartate antagonistic and opioid components of d-methadone antinociception in the rat spinal cord. Neurosci Lett 296(2–3):117–120.

46. Profile of Ketamine, CPP, Dextromethorphan, and Memantine

Duncan MA, Spiller JA. (2002) Analgesia with ketamine in a patient with perioperative opioid tolerance. J Pain Symp Man 24(1):8–11.
Mitchell AC, Fallon MT. (2002) A single infusion of intravenous ketamine improves pain relief in patients with critical limb ischaemia: results of a double blind randomised controlled trial. Pain 97(3):275–281.
Hewitt DJ. (2000) The use of NMDA-receptor antagonists in the treatment of chronic pain. Clin J Pain 16(2 Suppl):S73–S79.

47. GV 196771A, a New Glycine Site Antagonist of the NMDA Receptor with Potent Antihyperalgesic Activity

Quartaroli M, Fasdelli N, Bettelini L, Maraia G, Corsi M. (2001) GV196771A, an NMDA receptor/glycine site antagonist, attenuates mechanical allodynia in neuropathic rats and reduces tolerance induced by morphine in mice. Eur J Pharma 430(2–3):219–227.
Bordi F, Quartaroli M. (2000) Modulation of nociceptive transmission by NMDA/glycine site receptor in the ventroposterolateral nucleus of the thalamus. Pain 84(2–3):213–224.

48. Voltage-Gated Sodium Channels and Pain: Recent Advances

Decosterd I, Ji RR, Abdi S, Tate S, Woolf CJ. (2002) The pattern of expression of the voltage-gated sodium channels Na(v)1.8 and Na(v)1.9 does not change in uninjured primary sensory neurons in experimental neuropathic pain models. Pain 96(3):269–277.
Bucknill AT, Coward K, Plumpton C, Tate S, Bountra C, Birch R, Sandison A, Hughes SP, Anand P. (2002) Nerve fibers in lumbar spine structures and injured spinal roots express the sensory neuron-specific sodium channels SNS/PN3 and NaN/SNS2. Spine 27(2):135–140.
Benn SC, Costigan M, Tate S, Fitzgerald M, Woolf CJ. (2001) Developmental expression of the TTX-resistant voltage-gated sodium channels Nav1.8 (SNS) and Nav1.9 (SNS2) in primary sensory neurons. J Neurosci 21(16):6077–6085.
Coward K, Mosahebi A, Plumpton C, Facer P, Birch R, Tate S, Bountra C, Terenghi G, Anand P. (2001) Immunolocalisation of sodium channel NaG in the intact and injured human peripheral nervous system. J Anat 198(Pt 2):175–180.

Clare JJ, Tate SN, Nobbs M, Romanos MA. (2000) Voltage-gated sodium channels as therapeutic targets. Drug Discov Today 5(11):506–520.

49. Calcium Channel Antagonists and the Control of Pain

Chapman V, Dickenson AH. (2002) Pharmacological plasticity associated with neuropathic pain states. MECHANISMS AND MEDIATORS OF NEUROPATHIC PAIN. pp. 79–87.

Suzuki R, Dickenson AH. (2002) The pharmacology of central sensitization. J Musc Pain 10(1–2):35–43.

Dickenson AH. (2002) Gate Control Theory of pain stands the test of time. Br J Anaesth 88(6):755–757A.

Matthews EA, Dickenson AH. (2001) Effects of spinally delivered N- and P-type voltage-dependent calcium channel antagonists on dorsal horn neuronal responses in a rat model of neuropathy. Pain 92(1–2):235–246.

Dickenson AH, Matthews EA, Suzuki R. (2001) Central nervous system mechanisms of pain in peripheral neuropathy. NEUROPATHIC PAIN: PATHOPHYSIOLOGY AND TREATMENT. pp. 85–106.

50. Profile of Ziconotide (SNX-111): A Neuronal N-Type Voltage-Sensitive Calcium Channel Blocker

Jain KK. (2000) An evaluation of intrathecal ziconotide for the treatment of chronic pain. Expert Opin Investig Drugs 9(10):2403–2410.

Cox B. (2000) Calcium channel blockers and pain therapy. Curr Rev Pain 4(6):488–498.

Atanassoff PG, Hartmannsgruber MW, Thrasher J, Wermeling D, Longton W, Gaeta R, Singh T, Mayo M, McGuire D, Luther RR. (2000) Ziconotide, a new N-type calcium channel blocker, administered intrathecally for acute postoperative pain. Reg Anesth Pain Med 25(3):274–278.

Wang YX, Gao D, Pettus M, Phillips C, Bowersox SS. (2000) Interactions of intrathecally administered ziconotide, a selective blocker of neuronal N-type voltage-sensitive calcium channels, with morphine on nociception in rats. Pain 84(2–3):271–281.

51. Nitric Oxide Synthase Inhibitors and the Role of Nitric Oxide in Nociception

Blantz RC, Munger K. (2002) Role of nitric oxide in inflammatory conditions. Nephron 90(4):373–378.

Salerno L, Sorrenti V, Di Giacomo C, Romeo G, Siracusa MA. (2002) Progress in the development of selective nitric oxide synthase (NOS) inhibitors. Curr Pharm Des (3):177–200.

52. Adenosine and Pain

Burnstock G. (2002) Potential therapeutic targets in the rapidly expanding field of purinergic signalling. Clin Med 2(1):45–53.

McGaraughty S, Cowart M, Jarvis MF. (2001) Recent developments in the discovery of novel adenosine kinase inhibitors: mechanism of action and therapeutic potential. CNS Drug Rev 7(4):415–432.

Keeling SE, Albinson FD, Ayres BE, Butchers PR, Chambers CL, Cherry PC, Ellis F, Ewan GB, Gregson M, Knight J, Mills K, Ravenscroft P, Reynolds LH, Sanjar S, Sheehan MJ. (2000) The discovery and synthesis of highly potent, A2a receptor agonists. Bioorg Med Chem Lett 10(4):403–406.

53. Adenosine Kinase Inhibition as a Therapeutic Approach to Analgesia

Jarvis MF, Mikusa J, Chu KL, Wismer CT, Honore P, Kowaluk EA, McGaraughty S. (2002) Comparison of the ability of adenosine kinase inhibitors and adenosine receptor agonists to attenuate thermal hyperalgesia and reduce motor performance in rats. Pharm Biochem Behav 73(3):573–581.

Gomtsyan A, Didomenico S, Lee CH, Matulenko MA, Kim K, Kowaluk EA, Wismer CT, Mikusa J, Yu HX, Kohlhaas K, Jarvis MF. Bhagwat SS. (2002) Design, synthesis, and structure-activity relationship of 6-alkynylpyrimidines as potent adenosine kinase inhibitors. J Med Chem 45(17):3639–3648.

Jarvis MF, Yu HX, McGaraughty S, Wismer CT, Mikusa J, Zhu C, Chu K, Kohlhaas K, Cowart M, Lee CH, Stewart AO, Cox BF, Polakowski J, Kowaluk EA. (2002) Analgesic and anti-inflammatory effects of A-286501, a novel orally active adenosine kinase inhibitor. Pain 96(1–2):107–118.

Zheng GZ, Lee CH, Pratt JK, Perner RJ, Jiang MQ, Gomtsyan A, Matulenko MA, Mao Y, Koenig JR, Kim KH, Muchmore S, Yu HX, Kohlhaas K, Alexander KM, McGaraughty S, Chu KL, Wismer CT, Mikusa J, Jarvis MF, Marsh K, Kowaluk EA, Bhagwat SS. Stewart AO. (2001) Pyridopyrimidine analogues as novel adenosine kinase inhibitors. Bioorg Med Chem Lett 11(16):2071–2074.

Zhu CZ, Mikusa J, Chu KL, Cowart M, Kowaluk EA, Jarvis MF, McGaraughty S. (2001) A-134974: a novel adenosine kinase inhibitor, relieves tactile allodynia via spinal sites of action in peripheral nerve injured rats. Brain Res 905(1–2):104–110.

Lee CH, Jiang MQ, Cowart M, Gfesser G, Perner R, Kim KH, Gu YG, Williams M, Jarvis MF, Kowaluk EA, Stewart AO, Bhagwat SS. (2001) Discovery of 4-amino-5-(3-bromophenyl)-7-(6-morpholino-pyridin-3-yl)pyrido[2,3-d]pyrimidine, an orally active, non-nucleoside adenosine kinase inhibitor. J Med Chem 44(13):2133–2138.

54. P2X Purinergic Receptors for ATP in Nociception

Hibell AD, Thompson KM, Simon J, Xing M, Humphrey PP, Michel AD. (2001) Species- and agonist-dependent differences in the deactivation-kinetics of P2X7 receptors. Naunyn Schmiedebergs Arch Pharmacol 363(6):639–648.

Hibell AD, Kidd EJ, Chessell IP, Humphrey PP, Michel AD. (2000) Apparent species differences in the kinetic properties of P2X(7) receptors. Br J Pharmacol 130(1):167–173.

Jones CA, Chessell IP, Simon J, Barnard EA, Miller KJ, Michel AD, Humphrey PP. (2000) Functional characterization of the P2X(4) receptor orthologues. Br J Pharmacol 129(2):388–394.

Bland-Ward PA, Humphrey PPA. (2000) P2X receptors mediate ATP-induced primary nociceptive neurone activation. J Autonom Nerv Sys 81(1–3):146–151.

55. Somatostatin Receptors in Analgesia

Abdu F, Hicks GA, Hennig G, Allen JP, Grundy D. (2002) Somatostatin sst(2) receptors inhibit peristalsis in the rat and mouse jejunum. Am J Physiol–Gastro Liver Physiol 282(4):G624–G633.

Booth CE, Kirkup AJ, Hicks GA, Humphrey PPA, Grundy D. (2001) Somatostatin sst(2) receptor-mediated inhibition of mesenteric afferent nerves of the jejunum in the anesthetized rat. Gastroent 121(2):358–369.

Selmer I, Schindler M, Allen JP, Humphrey PP, Emson PC. (2000) Advances in understanding neuronal somatostatin receptors. Regul Pept 90(1–3):1–18.

56. Cannabinoids

Gauldie SD, McQueen DS, Pertwee R, Chessell IP. (2001) Anandamide activates peripheral nociceptors in normal and arthritic rat knee joints. Br J Pharm 132(3):617–621.

Pertwee R. (2000) Marijuana and medicine. Assessing the science base. 95(2):291–292.

57. Antinociceptive Effects of Centrally Administered Neurotrophic Factors

MacQueen GM, Ramakrishnan K, Croll SD, Siuciak JA, Yu GH, Young LT, Fahnestock M. (2001) Performance of heterozygous brain-derived neurotrophic factor knockout mice on behavioral analogues of anxiety, nociception, and depression. Behav Neurosci 115(5):1145–1153.

58. Peripheral Neurotrophic Factors and Pain

Arvanian VL, Mendell LM. (2001) Acute modulation of synaptic transmission to motoneurons by BDNF in the neonatal rat spinal cord. Eur J Neurosci 14(11):1800–1808.

Shu X, Mendell LM. (2001) Acute sensitization by NGF of the response of small-diameter sensory neurons to capsaicin. J Neurophys 86(6):2931–2938.

Arvanian VL, Mendell LM. (2001) Removal of NMDA receptor Mg2+ block extends the action of NT-3 on synaptic transmission in neonatal rat motoneurons. J Neurophys 86(1):123–129.

Mendell LM, Munson JB, Arvanian VL. (2001) Neurotrophins and synaptic plasticity in the mammalian spinal cord. J Physiol–London 533(1):91–97.

59. Profile of Tramadol and Tramadol Analogues

Wu WN, McKown LA, Codd EE, Raffa RB. (2002) In vitro metabolism of the analgesic agent, tramadol-N-oxide, in mouse, rat, and human. Eur J Drug Metab Pharmacokinet 27(3):193–197.

Tzschentke TM, Bruckmann W, Friderichs E. (2002) Lack of sensitization during place conditioning in rats is consistent with the low abuse potential of tramadol. Neurosci Lettt 329(1):25–28.

Tao Q, Stone DJ, Borenstein MR, Codd EE, Coogan TP, Desai-Krieger D, Liao S, Raffa RB. (2002) Differential tramadol and O-desmethyl metabolite levels in brain vs. plasma of mice and rats administered tramadol hydrochloride orally. J Clin Pharm Ther 27(2):99–106.

Raffa RB. (2001) Pharmacology of oral combination analgesics: rational therapy for pain. J Clin Pharm Ther 26(4):257–264.

60. Sumatriptan and Related 5-HT$_{1B/1D}$ Receptor Agonists: Novel Treatments for Migraine

Palmer JB, Salonen R. (2002) Triptan medications to treat acute migraine. Lancet 359(9312):1151.

Salonen R, Scott A. (2002) Triptans: do they differ? Curr Pain Headache Rep 6(2):133–139.

Connor HE. (2001) Building on the sumatriptan experience: the development of naratriptan. Cephal 21 Suppl 1:32–34.

Salonen R. (2001) The sumatriptan difference. Cephal 21 Suppl 1:18–20.

Humphrey PP. (2001) How it started. Cephal 21 Suppl 1:2–5.

Storer RJ, Akerman S, Connor HE, Goadsby PJ. (2001) 4991W93, a potent blocker of neurogenic plasma protein extravasation, inhibits trigeminal neurons at 5-hydroxytryptamine (5-HT1B/1D) agonist doses. Neuropharm 40(7):911–917.

Salonen R. (2000) Drug comparisons: why are they so difficult? Cephal 20 Suppl 2:25–32.

61. Cholinergic Approaches to Pain Therapy

Schroder H, Schutz U, Burghaus L, Lindstrom J, Kuryatov A, Monteggia L, DeVos RAI, van Noort G, Wevers A, Nowacki S, Happich E, Moser N, Arneric SP, Maelicke A. (2001) Expression of the alpha 4 isoform of the nicotinic acetylcholine receptor in the fetal human cerebral cortex. Devel Brain Res 132(1):33–45.

Lin NH, Li YH, He Y, Holladay MW, Kuntzweiler T, Anderson DJ, Campbell JE, Arneric SP. (2001) Synthesis and structure-activity relationships of 5-substituted pyridine analogues of 3-[2-((S)-pyrrolidinyl)methoxyl pyridine, A-84543: A potent nicotinic receptor ligand. Bioorg Med Chem Lett 11(5): 631–633.

62. Analgesic Effects of Vedaclidine, a Mixed Agonist–Antagonist at Muscarinic Receptor Subtypes

Shannon HE, Jones CK, Li DL, Peters SC, Simmons RMA, Iyengar S. (2001) Antihyperalgesic effects of the muscarinic receptor ligand vedaclidine in models involving central sensitization in rats. Pain 93(3):221–227.

Rasmussen T, Fink-Jensen A, Sauerberg P, Swedberg MDB, Thomsen C, Sheardown MJ, Jeppesen L, Calligaro DO, DeLapp NW, Whitesitt C, Ward JS, Shannon HE, Bymaster FP. (2001) The muscarinic receptor agonist BuTAC, a novel potential antipsychotic, does not impair learning and memory in mouse passive avoidance. Schizo Res 49(1-2):193–201.

Bymaster FP, Carter PA, Zhang L, Falcone JF, Stengel PW, Cohen ML, Shannon HE, Gomeza J, Wess J, Felder CC. (2001) Investigations into the physiological role of muscarinic M-2 and M-4 muscarinic and M-4 receptor subtypes using receptor knockout mice. Life Sci 68(22–23):2473–2479.

Perry KW, Nisenbaum LK, George CA, Shannon HE, Felder CC, Bymaster FP. (2001) The muscarinic agonist xanomeline increases monoamine release and immediate early gene expression in the rat prefrontal cortex. Bio Psych 49(8):716–725.

63. Gabapentin and Related Compounds

Field MJ, Gonzalez MI, Tallarida RJ, Singh L. (2002) Gabapentin and the neurokinin(1) receptor antagonist CI-1021 act synergistically in two rat models of neuropathic pain. J Pharmacol Exp Ther 303(2):730–735.

Andrews N, Loomis S, Blake R, Ferrigan L, Singh L, McKnight AT. (2001) Effect of gabapentin-like compounds on development and maintenance of morphine-induced conditioned place preference. Psychopharmacology (Berl) 157(4):381–387.

Field MJ, Hughes J, Singh L. (2000) Further evidence for the role of the alpha(2)delta subunit of voltage dependent calcium channels in models of neuropathic pain. Br J Pharmacol 131(2):282–286.

64. The Role of Gabapentin in the Management of Neuropathic Pain

Backonja MM. (2002) Use of anticonvulsants for treatment of neuropathic pain. Neurol 59(5 Suppl 2): S14–S17.

Wheeler G. (2002) Gabapentin. Pfizer. Curr Opin Investig Drugs 3(3):470–477.

Rose MA, Kam PC. (2002) Gabapentin: pharmacology and its use in pain management. Anaesth 57(5): 451–462.

Jensen TS. (2002) Anticonvulsants in neuropathic pain: rationale and clinical evidence. Eur J Pain 2002; 6 Suppl A:61–A68.

Mellegers MA, Furlan AD, Mailis A. (2001) Gabapentin for neuropathic pain: systematic review of controlled and uncontrolled literature. Clin J Pain 17(4):284–295.

65. New Local Anesthetic Analgesics

Stocks GM, Hallworth SP, Fernando R, England AJ, Columb MO, Lyons G. (2001) Minimum local analgesic dose of intrathecal bupivacaine in labor and the effect of intrathecal fentanyl. Anesth 94(4):593–598.

Robinson AP, Lyons GR, Wilson RC, Gorton HJ, Columb MO. (2001) Levobupivacaine for epidural analgesia in labor: the sparing effect of epidural fentanyl. Anesth Analg 92(2):410–414.

66. Spinal α_2-Adrenergic Agonists for Intractable Cancer Pain

Docquier MA, Lavand'homme P, Collet V. De Kock M. (2002) Spinal alpha(2)-adrenoceptors are involved in the MACbar-sparing effect of systemic clonidine in rats. Anesth Analg 95(4):935–939.

Lavand'homme PM, Ma W, De Kock M, Eisenach JC. (2002) Perineural alpha(2A)-adrenoceptor activation inhibits spinal cord neuroplasticity and tactile allodynia after nerve injury. Anesth 97(4):972–980.

Duflo F, Li X, Bantel C, Pancaro C, Vincler M, Eisenach JC. (2002) Peripheral nerve injury alters the alpha2 adrenoceptor subtype activated by clonidine for analgesia. Anesth 97(3):636–641.

Paqueron X, Li X, Bantel C, Tobin JR, Voytko ML, Eisenach JC. (2001) An obligatory role for spinal cholinergic neurons in the antiallodynic effects of clonidine after peripheral nerve injury. Anesth 94(6): 1074–1081.

De Kock M, Gautier P, Fanard L, Hody JL, Lavand'homme P. (2001) Intrathecal ropivacaine and clonidine for ambulatory knee arthroscopy—A dose-response study. Anesth 94(4):574–578.

67. Cellular Implantation for the Treatment of Chronic Pain

Siegan JB, Herzberg U, Frydel BR, Sagen J. (2002) Adrenal medullary transplants reduce formalin-evoked c-fos expression in the rat spinal cord. Brain Res 944(1–2):174-183.

Eaton MJ, Herman JP, Jullien N, Lopez TL, Martinez M, Huang J. (2002) Immortalized chromaffin cells disimmortalized with Cre/lox site-directed recombination for use in cell therapy for pain after partial nerve injury. Exp Neurol 175(1):49–60.

Castellanos DA, Tsoulfas P, Frydel BR, Gajavelli S, Bes JC, Sagen J. (2002) TrkC overexpression enhances survival and migration of neural stem cell transplants in the rat spinal cord. Cell Trans 11(3):297–307.

Hama A, Sagen J. (2002) Selective antihyperalgesic effect of [Ser(1)] histogranin on complete Freund's adjuvant-induced hyperalgesia in rats. Pain 95(1–2):15–21.

Hentall ID, Noga BR, Sagen J. (2001) Spinal allografts of adrenal medulla block nociceptive facilitation in the dorsal horn. J Neurophys 85(4):1788–1792.

68. Bone-Seeking Radiopharmaceuticals to Palliate Painful Bone Metastases

McEwan AJ. (2000) Use of radionuclides for the palliation of bone metastases. Semin Radiat Oncol 10(2): 103–114.

Index